Chapters in Text That Correspond to *Older Adults: Recommended B...*
and Curricular Guidelines for Geriatric Nursing Care...

American Association of Colleges of Nursing and The John A. Hartford Foundation Institute for Geriatric Nursing

P9-AGE-085

1. Recognize one's own and others' attitudes, values, and expectations about aging and their impact on care of older adults and their families: **Chapters 1, 21**

2. Adopt the concept of individualized care as the standard of practice with older adults: **Throughout all chapters**

3. Communicate effectively, respectfully, and compassionately with older adults and their families: **Throughout all chapters, especially Chapters 14, 20, 21, 23, 25, 26**

4. Recognize that sensation and perception in older adults are mediated by functional, physical, cognitive, psychological, and social changes common in old age: **Chapters 4, 7, 8, 14, 15, 18, 23, 24, 25, 27**

5. Incorporate into daily practice valid and reliable tools to assess the functional, physical, cognitive, psychological, social, and spiritual status of older adults: **Chapters 2, 4, 5, 6, 23, 25, 27 and throughout all chapters**

6. Assess older adults' living environment with special awareness of the functional, physical, cognitive, psychological, and social changes common in old age: **Chapters 3, 6, 7, 8, 10, 15, 16**

7. Analyze the effectiveness of community resources in assisting older adults and their families to retain personal goals, maximize function, maintain independence, and live in the least restrictive environment: **Chapters 14, 15, 16, 17, 18, 23, 24 and throughout all chapters**

8. Assess family knowledge of skills necessary to deliver care to older adults: **Chapters 6, 7, 8, 9, 11, 16, 20**

9. Adapt technical skills to meet the functional, physical, cognitive, psychological, social, and endurance capacities of older adults: **Chapters 7, 8, 10**

10. Individualize care and prevent morbidity and mortality associated with the use of physical and chemical restraints in older adults: **Chapters 15, 23**

11. Prevent or reduce common risk factors that contribute to functional decline, impaired quality of life, and excess disability in older adults: **Chapters 7, 8, 10, 11, 12, 14, 15, 23, 25**

12. Establish and follow standards of care to recognize and report elder mistreatment: **Chapter 18**

13. Apply evidence-based standards to screen, immunize, and promote healthy activities in older adults: **Chapters 3, 10 and throughout all chapters**

14. Recognize and manage geriatric syndromes common to older adults: **Chapters 7, 8, 9, 12, 13, 15, 23, 25**

15. Recognize the complex interaction of acute and chronic co-morbid conditions common to older adults: **Chapter 10 and throughout all chapters**

16. Use technology to enhance older adults' function, independence, and safety: **Chapters 15, 16, 22**

17. Facilitate communication as older adults transition across and between home, hospital, and nursing home, with a particular focus on the use of technology: **Chapters 16, 17, 20**

18. Assist older adults, families, and caregivers to understand and balance "everyday" autonomy and safety decisions: **Chapters 16, 17, 18, 20**

19. Apply ethical and legal principles to the complex issues that arise in care of older adults: **Chapters 17, 18, 26**

20. Appreciate the influence of attitudes, roles, language, culture, race, religion, gender, and lifestyle on how families and assistive personnel provide long-term care to older adults: **Chapters 1, 21, 22**

21. Evaluate differing international models of geriatric care: **Chapter 1**

22. Analyze the impact of an aging society on the health care system: **Chapters 1, 3, 17**

23. Evaluate the use of payer systems on access, availability, and affordability of health care for older adults: **Chapter 17**

24. Contrast the opportunities and constraints of supportive living arrangements on the function and independence of older adults and on their families: **Chapters 17, 20, 22**

25. Recognize the benefits of interdisciplinary team participation in care of older adults: **Chapters 1, 25, 26 and throughout all chapters**

26. Evaluate the utility of complementary and integrative health care practices on health promotion and symptoms management for older adults: **Chapters 3, 10, 11, 13, 26**

27. Facilitate older adults' active participation in all aspects of their own health care: **Chapter 3 and throughout all chapters**

28. Involve, educate, and when appropriate, supervise family, friends, and assistive personnel in implementing best practices for older adults: **All chapters**

29. Ensure quality of care commensurate with older adults' vulnerability and frequency and intensity of care needs: **Chapter 17 and throughout all chapters**

30. Promote the desirability of quality end-of-life care for older adults, including pain and symptom management, as essential, desirable, and integral components of nursing practice: **Chapters 11, 26**

NURSE CREDENTIALING PROGRAMS
HEALTH SCIENCES DIVISION

evolve

∴ *To access your Student Resources, visit:*

http://evolve.elsevier.com/Ebersole/TwdHlthAging/

Evolve® Student Resources for *Ebersole: Toward Healthy Aging: Human Needs and Nursing Response,* **Seventh Edition,** offer the following features:

Student Resources

- **Review/Critical Thinking Questions**
  This collection of questions is designed to review important content and test knowledge and understanding.

- **Animations**
  Animations visually enhance the material presented in the text.

- **Videos**
  Videos of assessment of the older adult provide real-life learning situations.

- **WebLinks**
  Links to hundreds of websites have been carefully chosen to supplement the content of each chapter of the text.

Toward Healthy Aging

Human Needs & Nursing Response

Toward Healthy Aging

Human Needs & Nursing Response

SEVENTH EDITION

Priscilla Ebersole, PhD, RN, FAAN
Professor Emerita
San Francisco State University
San Francisco, California

Patricia Hess, PhD, APRN, GNP, NAP
Professor Emerita
San Francisco State University
San Francisco, California

Theris A. Touhy, DNP, APRN, BC
Associate Professor
Christine E. Lynn College of Nursing
Florida Atlantic University
Boca Raton, Florida

Kathleen Jett, PhD, GNP, BC
Associate Professor
Christine E. Lynn College of Nursing
Florida Atlantic University
Boca Raton, Florida

Ann Schmidt Luggen, PhD, RN, GNP
Professor Emerita, Nursing
Northern Kentucky University
Highland Heights, Kentucky

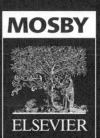
MOSBY
ELSEVIER

11830 Westline Industrial Drive
St. Louis, Missouri 63146

TOWARD HEALTHY AGING: HUMAN NEEDS AND NURSING RESPONSE ISBN: 978-0-323-04730-2
Copyright © 2008 by Mosby, Inc., an affiliate of Elsevier Inc.

All rights reserved. No part of this publication may be reproduced or transmitted in any form or by any means, electronic or mechanical, including photocopying, recording, or any information storage and retrieval system, without permission in writing from the publisher. Permissions may be sought directly from Elsevier's Rights Department: phone: (+1) 215 239 3804 (US) or (+44) 1865 843830 (UK); fax (+44) 1865 853333; e-mail: healthpermissions@elsevier.com. You may also complete your request online via the Elsevier website at http://www.elsevier.com/permissions.

Notice

Knowledge and best practice in this field are constantly changing. As new research and experience broaden our knowledge, changes in practice, treatment and drug therapy may become necessary or appropriate. Readers are advised to check the most current information provided (i) on procedures featured or (ii) by the manufacturer of each product to be administered, to verify the recommended dose or formula, the method and duration of administration, and contraindications. It is the responsibility of the practitioner, relying on their own experience and knowledge of the patient, to make diagnoses, to determine dosages and the best treatment for each individual patient, and to take all appropriate safety precautions. To the fullest extent of the law, neither the Publisher nor the Authors assume any liability for any injury and/or damage to persons or property arising out of or related to any use of the material contained in this book.

The Publisher

Previous editions copyrighted 1981, 1985, 1990, 1994, 1998, 2004

Library of Congress Control Number 2007931464

Acquisitions Editor: Catherine Jackson
Developmental Editor: Amanda Sunderman Politte
Publishing Services Manager: Deborah L. Vogel
Senior Project Manager: Jodi M. Willard
Design Direction: Julia Dummit
Text Designer: Julia Dummit

Cover art, "Flowers," was produced by Meryl Tankoos, a participant in the Adult Day Center of the Louis and Anne Green Memory and Wellness Center, Christine E. Lynn College of Nursing, Florida Atlantic University. The art program is called "Artful Memories" and is offered three times per week to interested participants. Classes are taught by a professional artist. Special thanks to Dr. Denise Sparks, Administrator of the Memory and Wellness Center, who helped make it possible for us to use this beautiful painting.

Printed in Canada

Last digit is the print number: 9 8 7 6 5 4 3 2 1

**Working together to grow
libraries in developing countries**

www.elsevier.com | www.bookaid.org | www.sabre.org

ELSEVIER   BOOK AID International   Sabre Foundation

About the Authors

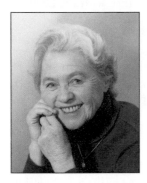

Priscilla Ebersole, PhD, RN, FAAN, has been involved in gerontological nursing for over 35 years. She has conducted national and international workshops and seminars on aging. Her expertise is in the fields of geropsychiatric nursing, middle age, and aging. She earned a baccalaureate, magna cum laude, at San Francisco State University; a master's and post-master's from the University of California at San Francisco; a doctorate at Columbia Pacific University; and a certificate in gerontological nursing from the University of Southern California. Dr. Ebersole has held appointments in the Applied Gerontology Certificate Program at San Francisco State University and at the Ethel Percy Andrus Gerontology Center at the University of Southern California, and she is a professor emerita in the School of Nursing, San Francisco State University. From 1981 to 1984 she was on leave from the School of Nursing at San Francisco State University to act as the field director of a gerontological nurse practitioner project funded by the W.K. Kellogg Foundation and administered by the Mountain States Health Corporation in Boise, Idaho. In 1988 Dr. Ebersole was a visiting professor at Case Western Reserve University and occupied the Florence Cellar–endowed gerontological nursing chair. In 1987 she was named Educator of the Year by the American College of Health Care Administrators. Dr. Ebersole was inducted into the Hall of Fame at San Francisco State University in 1997 and was awarded honorary membership in the National Association of Directors of Nursing Administration in Long-Term Care in 2000. In 2006 she was recognized by the National Gerontological Nurses Association and the National Conference of Gerontological Nurse Practitioners for her leadership roles and was named as an Honorary Alumna of the Frances Payne Bolton School of Nursing at Case Western Reserve University. She was the editor of the *Geriatric Nursing Journal* for 15 years and resigned the editorship in 2006 to become Editor Emerita. Dr. Ebersole and Dr. Patricia Hess co-authored five editions of *Toward Healthy Aging: Human Needs and Nursing Response* and a sixth edition with an additional author, Dr. Ann Luggen. Dr Ebersole's most recent text, *Geriatric Nursing: Growth of a Specialty*, was co-authored with Dr. Theris Touhy.

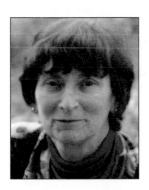

Patricia Hess, PhD, APRN, GNP, NAP, has earned certificates in gerontological nursing from the Ethel Percy Andrus Gerontology Center, the University of Southern California at Los Angeles, and Holy Names College. She received her BSN degree from the Francis Payne Bolton School of Nursing at Case Western Reserve University, a master's degree from the University of Colorado at Boulder, and a doctorate from Walden University. In 1986 she completed the geriatric nurse practitioner program at the University of California School of Nursing/School of Medicine at San Francisco. She is also a member of the National Academies of Practice. She has been involved in gerontologic nursing for over 40 years and has conducted workshops and seminars on aging. Her expertise is in the areas of health promotion and wellness, dying and death, and the education of students and staff regarding the specific needs of the aged in acute care settings. She is a professor emerita at San Francisco State University, and she held an appointment in the Applied Gerontology Certificate Program at San Francisco State University. Currently she is teaching Healthy Aging at satellite campuses of Samuel Merritt College.

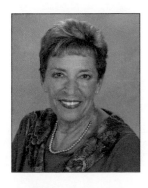

Theris A. Touhy, DNP, APRN, BC, has been a clinical specialist in gerontological nursing and a nurse practitioner for 30 years. Her expertise is in the care of older adults in nursing homes and of those with dementia. The majority of her practice as a clinical nurse specialist and nurse practitioner has been in the long-term care setting. She received her BSN degree from St. Xavier University in Chicago, a master's degree in care of the aged from Northern Illinois University, and a Doctor of Nursing Practice from Case Western Reserve University. Dr. Touhy is an associate professor in the Christine E. Lynn College of Nursing at Florida Atlantic University, where she has served as Assistant Dean of Undergraduate Programs. She teaches gerontological nursing and long-term, rehabilitation, and palliative care nursing in both the undergraduate and graduate programs. Her research is focused on spirituality in aging and at the end of life, caring for persons with dementia, and caring in nursing homes. Dr. Touhy was the recipient of the Geriatric Faculty Member Award from the John A. Hartford Foundation Institute for Geriatric Nursing in 2003, is a two-time recipient of the Distinguished Teacher of the Year in the Christine E. Lynn College of Nursing at Florida Atlantic University, and was awarded the Marie Haug Award for Excellence in Aging Research and the Cushing and Robb Award for Advanced Study in Nursing from Case Western Reserve University. She is co-author with Dr. Priscilla Ebersole, Dr. Patricia Hess, and Dr. Kathleen Jett of *Gerontological Nursing and Healthy Aging* and is co-author with Dr. Ebersole of *Geriatric Nursing: Growth of a Specialty.*

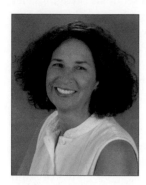

Kathleen Jett, PhD, GNP, BC, has been actively engaged in gerontological nursing for over 30 years. Her clinical experience is broad, from her roots in public health and long-term care, to clinical direction of a hospice, administrator of an assisted living facility, researcher and teacher, and advanced practice as both a clinical nurse specialist and nurse practitioner. The thread that ties all of her work together has been a belief that nurses can make a difference in the lives of older adults. Dr. Jett received her bachelor's, master's, and doctoral degrees from the University of Florida, where she also holds a graduate certificate in gerontology. A board-certified gerontological nurse practitioner, Dr. Jett was inducted into the National Academies of Practice in 2006. In 2000 she was selected as a Summer Scholar by the John A. Hartford Foundation Institute for Geriatric Nursing. She is currently an associate professor at the Christine E. Lynn College of Nursing at Florida Atlantic University. There she coordinates the graduate program in nursing education. Dr. Jett received an award of excellence in undergraduate teaching in 2005 and in 2006 was selected as the College's Distinguished Teacher of the Year. In addition to teaching and writing, Dr. Jett is actively engaged in a program of research aimed at reducing health disparities by improving the health literacy and health communication of elders and their health care providers.

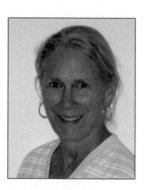

Ann Schmidt Luggen, PhD, RN, GNP-CS, CNAA, has been involved in gerontological nursing since she was a research assistant and teaching assistant with the Robert Wood Johnson Teaching–Nursing Home grant at the University of Cincinnati/Maple Knoll Village in the early 1980s. Her MSN is in medical-surgical and oncology nursing, and her doctorate is in gerontological oncology. She has been certified as a gerontology clinical nurse specialist and nurse practitioner and as an administrator at the advanced level, and she has done a postdoctorate in long-term care nursing administration at the University of Kentucky. She has also served as president of the Ohio Gerontological Nurse Practitioners and has been on the board of the National Gerontological Nursing Association for 10 years. She has served on the steering committee of the National Conference of Gerontological Nurse Practitioners. She was a core member of the new Greater Cincinnati Gerontological Nursing Association and the Cincinnati Oncology Nursing Association. She has presented at conferences nationally, regionally, and locally; has published numerous manuscripts; and has written and edited 10 books, including the first core curriculum for gerontological nursing. She has been the editor of a national geriatric nursing newsletter, writes a geriatric column for *Advances for Nurse Practitioners,* and has been an editor for *Geriatric Nursing* for more than 10 years. Dr. Luggen is professor emerita of the graduate program at Northern Kentucky University, having taught the nursing administration and the geriatric nurse practitioner programs.

For my children, nine grandchildren, two great-grandchildren, and the elders I have worked with, who have enriched my personal and professional life.

PRISCILLA EBERSOLE

To all the older adults who have contributed to my knowledge on aging by allowing me to be a part of their life. They have been examples of "aging in place" in illness or health. Through them I have seen adaptations that allowed them to live to their potential and have facilitated the healthy aging texts. To all my students who have embraced gerontological nursing as a specialty and are now disseminating what they have learned and care about to other health care providers and students. You are the future of gerontological nursing. Lastly, to the gerontological nurse practitioners who, though relatively small in number, strive to keep the older adult at his or her optimum wellness.

PATRICIA HESS

To my wonderful husband Bob, my children Danial, Andrew, and Peter, my daughter-in-law Amber and soon to be daughter-in-law Rose, and my friends-in-law Bill and Terry Capps, whose love and support provide the meaning in my life. To Colin Keating Touhy and Molly Capps Touhy, my beautiful grandchildren, who make growing older the most special time of my life. And to the wonderful and wise older people who have taught me how to care for elders and to their nurses and caregivers, who daily live out the words of this text.

THERIS A. TOUHY

To my husband Steve, who is a source of support through thick and thin. Without his willingness to keep me supplied with food, the long hours sitting in front of the computer and writing would not have been possible. To our four children and four wonderful grandchildren, who always remind me that the best part of life is the time we spend together and that the older we get, the more we have loved and the more adventures we have shared.

KATHLEEN JETT

I dedicate this edition to Priscilla Ebersole, who has been a friend, colleague, and mentor for many years and through joys and sorrows. Her retirement will leave a major gap in gerontological nursing.

ANN SCHMIDT LUGGEN

Contributors

Melissa Bernstein, PhD, RD, LD
Assistant Professor of Nutrition
Nutrition Department
Rosalind Franklin University
Chicago, Illinois

Gregory G. Gulick, DO, MPH, MA
Internal Medicine
St. Anthony's Primary Care
St. Petersburg, Florida;
Adjunct Professor,
Florida Atlantic University
Boca Raton, Florida

Ellis Quinn Youngkin, PhD, RNC, ARNP
Professor and Associate Dean
Christine E. Lynn College of Nursing;
Women's Health Care Nurse Practitioner
University Student Health Services
Florida Atlantic University
Boca Raton, Florida

Reviewers

Lois Kazmier Halstead, PhD, RN
Associate Dean, College of Nursing
Rush University
Chicago, Illinois

Kathleen Mitchell, DNS, MEd, MN, GNPC
Professor, School of Nursing
William Carey College
New Orleans, Louisiana

Judith L. Roy, RN, BSN, BC
Staff Development Coordinator
Maine Veteran's Home
Scarborough, Maine

Amy Silva-Smith, PhD, APRN, BC, ANP
Assistant Professor
Nurse Practitioner Program Coordinator
Beth-El College of Nursing and Health Sciences
University of Colorado—Colorado Springs
Colorado Springs, Colorado

Cheryl Ross Staats, MSN, RN, APRN, BC
Associate Clinical Professor, School of Nursing
The University of Texas Health Science Center
　at San Antonio
San Antonio, Texas

Joyce McCullers Varner, MSN, RN, GNP-BC, GCNS
Clinical Assistant Professor, College of Nursing
University of South Alabama
Mobile, Alabama

Preface

This seventh edition has been prepared by Theris A. Touhy, Kathleen Jett, and Ann Schmidt Luggen. We are delighted to have such capable professionals—all three gerontological nurse practitioners—who are willing to take on this intense and arduous task with such devotion and competence. Their commitment to providing the most current thinking in gerontological nursing and their philosophical devotion to healthy aging and wellness are essential to the integrity of this text.

This text is designed to provide nurses, faculty, and students with the most current information about best practices in gerontological nursing based on the most current research. Through their expertise, commitment, dedication, advocacy, and compassion, gerontological nurses who work with older adults in all settings will continue to be leaders in creating models that truly change the culture of existing systems of care. Nurses play an essential role in creating environments of care in which older adults can reach their full potential by thriving, not merely surviving, in the latter part of life. Our hope is that the nursing practice of those who read this book will be enriched, just as ours has been, by sharing the wisdom and beauty of older adults.

The first edition of *Toward Healthy Aging: Human Needs and Nursing Response* was published in 1981, and in the intervening 26 years the face of aging in the United States has changed dramatically. The baby boomers are now entering the ranks of the elders, medical expertise and technology is keeping elders alive longer, and there is increased interest in providing end-of-life care that will ensure a dignified and meaningful death. Many more nurse practitioners are practicing as primary care providers, guided by advanced knowledge and meticulous practice. This is the only comprehensive text that has endured through the many changes and has kept abreast of them. Gerontological nursing has come of age and is no longer the stepchild of nursing and medicine.

Priscilla Ebersole
Patricia Hess

In 1981, Dr. Priscilla Ebersole and Dr. Patricia Hess published the first edition of *Toward Healthy Aging: Human Needs and Nursing Response,* which has been used in nursing schools across the globe. Their foresight in developing a textbook that focuses on health, wholeness, beauty, and potential in aging made this book an enduring classic. In 1981 few nurses chose this specialty, few schools of nursing included content related to the care of elders, and the focus of care was on illness and problems. Today gerontological nursing is a strong and evolving specialty with a solid theoretical base and practice grounded in evidence-based research. Dr. Ebersole and Dr. Hess set the standards for the competencies required for gerontological nursing education and the promotion of health while aging. Many nurses, including us, have been shaped by their words, their wisdom, and their passion for care of elders. Now, 26 years later, it is our privilege to co-author the seventh edition of this text. We thank these two wonderful pioneers and mentors for the opportunity to build on such a solid foundation. We hope that we have kept the heart and spirit of their work, for that is truly what has inspired us and so many others to care for elders with competence and compassion.

We believe that *Toward Healthy Aging* is the most comprehensive gerontological nursing text available. The content ranges from biological, such as the etiology of common conditions and geropharmacology, to caring for persons with dementia, to understanding Medicare and aging and nursing in rural and frontier settings. Although Maslow's Hierarchy of Needs is the organizing framework, it includes additional theoretical frameworks for a range of situations.

Toward Healthy Aging is an appropriate text for both undergraduate and graduate students and is an excellent reference for nurses' libraries. This edition makes an ideal supplement to health assessment, medical-surgical, community, and psychiatric and mental health textbooks in programs that do not have a freestanding gerontological nursing course.

Within the covers the reader will find the latest information to be used in providing the highest level of care to adults as they age. The content is consistent with the AACN *Older Adults: Recommended Baccalaureate Competencies and Curricular Guidelines for Geriatric Nursing Care* developed by the AACN in collaboration with the John A. Hartford Foundation Institute for Geriatric Nursing at New York University. It goes further in emphasizing application of the goals set forth by *Healthy People 2010* and the need to provide evidence-based care. New chapters entitled *Health Assessment in Gerontological Nursing* (Chapter 6) and *Nutritional Needs* (Chapter 9) add to the text's value. In addition, this text includes specific strategies to promote healthy aging, case studies and opportunities for critical thinking, and comprehensive resources for further study.

We have been honored to work with Dr. Ebersole and Dr. Hess to provide a rich and useful edition of a classic text. We hope that the readers benefit from using it as much as we did in revising it!

Theris A. Touhy
Kathleen Jett
Ann Schmidt Luggen

Acknowledgments

This book would not have been possible without the support and guidance of the staff at Elsevier. Catherine Jackson, Acquisitions Editor, quietly and consistently voiced her support of the potential future success of the new edition and of the abilities of all of the co-authors. Amanda Politte, Developmental Editor, has been the person with the patience and persistence to pull the work from us and put it together in a way that will be useful to the readers. Her careful work with the artwork and artist is especially appreciated in bringing to you a fresh look. Jodi Willard, Senior Project Manager, skillfully made sure that we wrote in coherent sentences—not an easy thing to do. We also acknowledge our reviewers, contributors, and previous authors, for without their efforts, this edition would not have been possible. We also would like to thank our expert gerontological nursing colleagues, Sharon Stahl Wexler, PhD, RN, BC, and Catherine O'Neill D'Amico, PhD, RN, CNAA, for their preparation of the website materials for the book. And finally, we acknowledge the past and future readers who, we hope, will provide us with enough feedback to keep us honest in any future writing.

Priscilla Ebersole
Patricia Hess
Theris A. Touhy
Kathleen Jett
Ann Schmidt Luggen

Contents

CHAPTER 13
The Use of Herbs and Supplements in Late Life, 323

CHAPTER 14
Sensory Function, 338

CHAPTER 15
Mobility, 370

CHAPTER 1

Gerontological Nursing and an Aging Society

Theris A. Touhy

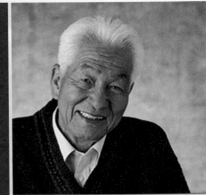
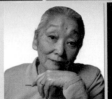
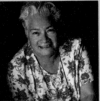

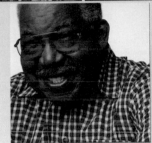

A YOUTH SPEAKS

Until my grandmother became ill and needed our help, I really didn't know her well. Now I can look at her in an entirely different light. She is frail and tough, fearful and courageous, demanding and delightful, bitter and humorous, needy and needed. I'm beginning to think that old age is the culmination of all the aspects of living a long life.

Jenine, 28 years old

A MIDDLE-AGER SPEAKS

Nursing care of the aged brings one in touch with the most basic and profound questions of human existence: the meanings of life and death; sources of strength and survival skills; beginnings, ending, and reasons for being. It is a commitment to discovery of the self—and of the self I am becoming as I age.

Stephanie, middle-aged faculty

AN ELDER SPEAKS

I'm 95 years old and have no family or friends that still survive. I wonder if anyone will be there for me when I leave the planet, which will be very soon I am sure. Mothers deliver, but who will deliver me into the hand of God?

Name withheld

LEARNING OBJECTIVES

On completion of this chapter, the reader will be able to:

1. Identify several viewpoints that influence the way aging is perceived.
2. Specify demographic changes related to the aging experience in the twenty-first century.
3. Develop the beginnings of a personal philosophy of aging.
4. Recognize the great diversity of older adults.
5. Understand the many factors that facilitate or hinder the aging process.

6. Compare various gerontological nursing roles and requirements.
7. Discuss nursing research studies on care of older adults and the role of gerontological nurses in research.
8. Discuss several formal geriatric organizations and their significance to nurses.
9. Identify several factors that have influenced the progress of gerontological nursing as a specialty practice.

THE STUDY OF AGING

In the past, both religious and secular movements have affected the way individuals viewed aging. Puritans thought the process of aging was a sacred pilgrimage to God, and as such, the righteous elders were revered. During the Victorian Age, it was believed that youth was the symbol of growth and expansion. Later, when the need to provide for an expanding population became more pressing, youthful energy, westward migration, and enormous material progress made elders seem

Special thanks to Priscilla Ebersole, the previous edition contributor, for her content contributions to this chapter.

out of touch and they were sometimes viewed with sentimental indulgence or irritation. The traditions of the elders seemed cumbersome and a hindrance to progress. In the scientific search for longevity, it was thought that mountain-climbing tribes high in the Andes and the Georgian Alps held the secret, lending a picture of reaching ever upward. Now space rockets silhouetted against the sky before launch represent symbols of generativity and emblems of our belief in the potential for an ever-expanding universe of possibilities throughout the life course. There seem to be infinite variations on the metaphors of aging all over the world. What we make of aging, it seems, depends on how we see it.

As we look to the future, our society will have more people older than 65 years than ever before in our history. This will change the face of aging as we know it now and present many challenges as well as many opportunities for our future. Attitudes toward older adults have shifted along with societal changes. A "reverse ageism" is apparent today, largely attributable to gerontology professionals of the "baby boom" confronting their own aging and desperately hoping they will be a part of the elite and vigorous older survivors: sexy, active, involved, and simply amazing. Some are. Many are simply gradually growing older and confronting the changes that can normally be expected. That is what this textbook is all about. How does one maximize the experience of aging and enrich the later years regardless of the physical and psychological changes that commonly occur? Nurses have a great responsibility to help shape a world in which older people can thrive and grow, not merely survive.

Words, statistics, and research data can only paint a picture of how aging looks. The most significant learning regarding the intricacies and challenges of aging and survival strategies comes from discussions with elders themselves. They are our role models, and their diversity makes it possible for us to develop greater understanding of life if we only listen to what they say and that which is unsaid. Many years ago, Irene Burnside (1975), one of the geriatric nursing pioneers, said it beautifully:

> Listen to the aged for they will tell you about living and dying.
>
> Listen to the aged for they will enlighten you about problem-solving, sexuality, grief, sensory deprivation, and survival.
>
> Listen to the aged for they will teach you how to be courageous, loving and generous.
>
> They are a distinguished faculty without formal classrooms, tenure, sabbaticals. They teach not from books but from long experience in living.

GERONTOLOGY

Gerontology is the scientific study of the effects of time on human development, specifically the study of older persons. It is at the opposite end of the spectrum from embryology and often includes several decades before death. Gerontology, by virtue of the Greek origin of the word *geron* (old man), should mean the study of old men, but many more women than men grow old. Healthy older men and women frequently elude the attention of gerontologists; thus study samples of elders, most likely taken from institutionalized subjects, have often been extrapolated to the healthier population. In fact, it is not yet certain what healthy old age can be; this will not be known until optimum social and biological conditions exist for growing older.

A large part of the study of aging comes from attending to older adults and the aging person in ourselves and how we perceive our own aging. These are fundamentally important to gerontology. Inquisitions into and curiosity about aging are as old as curiosity about life and death itself. Much that was thought to have been correct about aging has been shown through research to be half-truth, myth, or supposition. In developing a science and philosophy of aging, one essentially builds on personal experience; ultimately we all do this. How else can we measure the impact of dreams, fantasies, meditation, courage, love, grief, and the phenomena of living?

Gerontology began as an inquiry into the characteristics of long-lived people, and we are still intrigued by them. In 1000 BC, the average life span was 18 years and people who lived to old age were curiosities, stimulating reverence, speculation, and myth. Anecdotal evidence was used in the past to illustrate issues assumed to be universal. Only in the past 40 years have serious and carefully controlled research studies flourished. Theoreticians and researchers most commonly interested in the study of aging are sociologists, psychologists, and biologists. Their conceptual bases underlie their perspective regarding survival issues. Nursing draws from its own body of knowledge, as well as from all of these disciplines, to describe, monitor, protect, and evaluate the quality of life experienced by the old.

An individual ages biologically, psychologically, sociologically, and spiritually as a unitary being. A disciplinary rather than a humanistic perspective sometimes makes it appear that these are separate components of existence. There is such overlap that disciplinary lines are no longer appropriate in planning care. Multidisciplinary approaches and care programs are essential and are rapidly becoming the method of providing health care.

The Biomedicalization of Aging

The term *geriatrics* was coined by an American physician, Ignatz Nascher, around 1900 because he recognized that the medical care of older people involved special considerations, much as did the field of pediatrics. Nascher authored the first textbook on medical care of the elderly in the United States in 1914 (Nascher, 1914).

Aging has been seen as a biomedical problem that must be reversed, eradicated, or held at bay as long as possible. Therefore the impact of disease, morbidity, and impending death on the quality of life and the experience of aging has provided the impetus for much of the study by gerontologists. In this way, aging has inevitably been seen through the distorted lens of disease. Nevertheless, it is difficult to study such a complex and elusive condition as "healthy aging" without looking at the physical manifestations of function and lifestyle. Chronic disorders, not amenable to cure but requiring long-term adaptation and management, have not been attractive to medicine and nursing until recently. However, we are finally recognizing that aging and disease are separate entities although frequent companions. One of the dilemmas is a lack of clear understanding of normal aging processes. We may never know which changes occur over time because of assaults of the environment and which changes occur because the vital life centers are running out of resources. The trend toward the medicalization of the study of aging has influenced the general public as well. The biomedical view of the "problem" of aging is reinforced on all sides. However, the unquestioning public acceptance of medical authority has been considerably diminished as more and more individuals seek alternative health care methods, as well as diagnose and manage their own care through the Internet.

Who Will Care for an Aging Society?

The demand for gerontological nurses and other health professionals prepared to deliver care to growing numbers of older people across the globe is critical. In the United States, older adults account for 50% of all hospital days, 70% of home care visits, and 90% of long-term care residents (National Center for Health Statistics, 2004). Newly licensed nurses report 62.5% of their patients are older than 65 years (Berman et al., 2005). Although interest in gerontological nursing and the numbers of nurses prepared academically are increasing, the projected need for gerontological nurses in all settings is expected to reach 1.1 million by 2030 (Klein, 1997).

A growing concern is the lack of adequate staffing, particularly professional nurses, in nursing homes. Current federal standards require only one registered nurse (RN) in the nursing home for 8 hours per day—a figure quite shocking considering the ratio of RNs to patients in acute care, even with drastic shortages in that setting. More RN direct-care time per resident in nursing homes is associated with fewer pressure ulcers, fewer hospitalizations, fewer urinary tract infections (UTIs), less weight loss, fewer catheterizations, and less deterioration in the ability to perform activities of daily living (ADLs) (Horn et al., 2005). Despite increases in acuity level of nursing home patients and the positive relationship between registered nurse staffing and quality of nursing home care, care continues to be provided in U.S. nursing homes almost devoid of professional nurses. RN staffing levels declined 25% between 1999 and 2003, from 0.8 hours to 0.6 hours/resident day. A study by the Centers for Medicare & Medicaid Services (CMS) revealed that RN staffing levels below 0.75 hours/resident day can jeopardize the health and safety of residents, and yet approximately 97% of nursing homes do not meet these standards (Mezey and Harrington, 2005).

To improve quality of care in nursing homes, it is essential that staffing increases in nursing homes. Harrington (2005) suggests that a minimum percentage of Medicare payments be designated for nurse staffing as well as limits on administrative costs and profit margins. She further suggests that minimum state and federal nurse staffing levels be set at 4.1 total nursing hours and 0.75 RN hours/resident day.

An expert panel on nursing home care convened by the John A. Hartford Foundation Institute for Geriatric Nursing (Harrington et al., 2000) made comprehensive recommendations for improved RN staffing, increased gerontological nursing education requirements for all staff (including a bachelor of science in nursing [BSN] degree for directors of nursing), and increased staffing ratios for RNs, licensed practical nurses (LPNs), licensed vocational nurses (LVNs), and nursing assistants. Additional recommendations were that most nursing homes should have a full-time gerontological clinical nurse specialist (CNS) or gerontological nurse practitioner (GNP) on staff. Efforts to improve the nursing care of older adults through enhanced education are discussed on p. 8.

Geriatric medicine faces similar challenges. Older people make up 60% of all visits to cardiologists, 53% of visits to urologists, 48% of all patients in critical care, and 63% of patients with cancer (Berman et al., 2005). There are fewer than 7000 certified geriatricians (approximately 1 per 5000 Americans ages 65 years and older). This is far short of the estimated current need for 14,000 geriatricians or projections of a need for 36,000 geriatricians by 2030. Attracting students of all disciplines to geriatrics and improving the competency of current practitioners in care of older adults are essential to meet the needs and demands of a burgeoning aging population. "The consequences of inaction will be profound" (American Geriatrics Society, 2005, p. S246).

Organizations Devoted to Gerontological Research and Practice

The Gerontological Society of America (GSA) demonstrates the need for interdisciplinary collaboration in research and practice. The divisions of Biological Sciences, Clinical Medicine, Behavioral and Social Sciences, Social Research, and Policy and Practice include individuals from myriad backgrounds and many disciplines who affiliate with a section based on their particular function rather than their educational or professional credentials. Nurses can be found in all sections and occupy important positions as officers and committee chairs in the GSA. The nurses' special interest group, which, 30 years ago, met informally in a small hotel suite, now attracts 150 to 200 members and is the most rapidly growing membership contingent.

This mingling of the disciplines based on practice interests is also characteristic of the American Society on Aging (ASA). Other interdisciplinary organizations have joined forces to strengthen the field. The Association for Gerontology in Higher Education (AGHE) has partnered with GSA, and the National Council on Aging (NCOA) is affiliated with ASA. These organizations and others have encouraged the blending of ideas and functions, furthering our understanding of old age and of the integration necessary for optimum care. International gerontology associations such as the International Federation on Aging and the International Association of Gerontology and Geriatrics also have interdisciplinary membership and offer the opportunity to study aging internationally.

The American Medical Directors Association is a professional association of medical directors, physicians, and nurse practitioners practicing in the long-term care continuum, dedicated to excellence in patient care by providing education, advocacy, information, and professional development. The American Geriatrics Society is a professional organization of health care providers dedicated to improving the health and well-being of older adults. Both of these organizations have monthly journals and practice protocols for the care of older adults. These excellent evidence-based practice protocols are available on their websites.

Organizations specific to gerontological nursing include the National Gerontological Nursing Association (NGNA), the National Conference of Gerontological Nurse Practitioners (NCGNP), the National Association Directors of Nursing Administration in Long Term Care (NADONA/LTC) (also includes assisted living RNs and LPNs/LVNs as associate members), and the Canadian Gerontological Nursing Association (CGNA). The CGNA, founded in 1985, addresses the health needs of older Canadians and the nurses who care for them. The CGNA has developed Standards of Practice for Gerontological Nursing. In 2003 an alliance was formed with the NGNA to exchange information and share mutual goals and opportunities for the advancement of both groups (Mantle, 2005).

DEVELOPMENT OF GERONTOLOGICAL NURSING

Efforts to determine the appropriate term for nurses caring for older people have included *gerontic nurses, gerontological nurses,* and *geriatric nurses.* None of these terms is restrictive. We presently prefer the use of the term *gerontological nurse.*

Gerontological nursing has emerged as a circumscribed area of practice only within the past 5 decades. Before 1950, gerontological nursing was seen as the application of general principles of nursing to the older adult client with little recognition of this area of nursing as a specialty similar to obstetric, pediatric, or surgical nursing. Whereas most specialties in nursing developed from those identified in medicine, this was not the case with gerontological nursing since health care of the elderly was traditionally considered within the domain of nursing (Davis, 1985). In examining the history of gerontological nursing, one must marvel at the advocacy and perseverance of nurses who have remained deeply committed to care of older adults despite struggling against insurmountable odds over the years. We are proud to be the standard-bearers of excellence in care of older people (Box 1-1). For a comprehensive review of the history of the specialty, including Dr. Ebersole's interviews with the geriatric nursing pioneers, the reader is referred to *Geriatric Nursing: Growth of a Specialty* (Ebersole and Touhy, 2006).

The origins of gerontological nursing are rooted in England and began with Florence Nightingale as she accepted a position in the Institution for the Care of Sick Gentlewomen in Distressed Circumstances. Nightingale's concern for the frail and sick elderly was continued by Agnes Jones, a wealthy Nightingale-trained nurse, who in 1864 was sent to Liverpool Infirmary, a large Poor Law institution. The care in the institution had been poor, diet meager, and nurses often drunk. But Miss Jones, under the tutelage of Nightingale, improved the care dramatically, as well as reduced the costs.

In the United States, almshouses were the destination of the destitute older people and were insufferable places with "deplorable conditions, neglect, preventable suffering, contagion, and death from lack of proper medical and nursing care" (Crane, 1907, p. 873). As early as 1906, Lavinia Dock and other early leaders in nursing addressed the needs of the elderly chronically ill in almshouses in the American Journal of Nursing (AJN). Dock and her colleagues cited the immediate need for trained nurses and pupil education in almshouses, "so that these evils, all of which lie strictly in the sphere of housekeeping and nursing,—two spheres which have always been lauded as women's own—might not occur" (Dock, 1908, p. 520-523). In 1912 the American Nurses' Association (ANA) Board of Directors appointed an Almshouse Committee to continue to oversee nursing in these institutions. World War I distracted them from attention to these needs. But in 1925, the AJN advanced the idea of a specialty in the nursing care of the aged.

With the passage of the Social Security Act of 1935, federal monies were provided for old-age insurance and public assistance for needy older people not covered by insurance. To combat the fear of almshouse placement, Congress stipulated that the Social Security funds could not be used to pay for care in almshouses or other public institutions. This move is thought to have been the genesis of commercial nursing homes. During the next 10 years, many almshouses closed and the number of private boarding homes providing care to elders increased. Because retired and widowed nurses often converted their homes into such living quarters and gave care when their boarders became ill, they can be considered the first geriatric nurses and their homes the first nursing homes. Two nursing journals in the 1940s described centers of excellence for geriatric care: the Cuyahoga County Nursing Home in Ohio and the Hebrew Home for the Aged in New York. An article in the AJN by Sarah Gelbach (1943) recommended that nurses should have not only an aptitude for working with the elderly but also specific geriatric education. The first textbook on nursing care of the elderly was published by Newton and Anderson in 1950, and the first published nursing research on chronic disease and the elderly (Mack, 1952) appeared in the premier issue of Nursing Research in 1952 (Ebersole and Touhy, 2006).

In 1962 a focus group was formed to discuss geriatric nursing, and in 1966 a geriatric practice group was convened. However, it was not until 1966 that the ANA formed a Division of Geriatric Nursing. The first geriatric standards were published by the ANA in 1968, and soon after, geriatric nursing certification was offered. Geriatric nursing was

BOX 1-1   Professionalization of Gerontological Nursing

1906	First article published in American Journal of Nursing (AJN) on care of the elderly
1925	AJN considers geriatric nursing as a possible specialty in nursing
1950	Newton and Anderson publish first geriatric nursing textbook
	Geriatrics becomes a specialization in nursing
1962	American Nurses Association (ANA) forms a national geriatric nursing group
1966	ANA creates the Division of Geriatric Nursing
	First master's program for clinical nurse specialists in geriatric nursing developed by Virginia Stone at Duke University
1970	ANA establishes Standards of Practice for Geriatric Nursing committee, chaired by Dorothy Moses; included Lois Knowles and Mary Shaunnessey
1973	ANA defined Standards of Practice for Geriatric Nursing
1974	Certification in geriatric nursing practice offered through ANA; process implemented by Laurie Gunter and Virginia Stone
1975	Journal of Gerontological Nursing published by Slack; first editor, Edna Stilwell
1976	ANA renames Geriatric Division "Gerontological" to reflect a health promotion emphasis
	ANA publishes Standards for Gerontological Nursing Practice; committee chaired by Barbara Allen Davis
	ANA begins certifying geriatric nurse practitioners
	Nursing and the Aged edited by Burnside and published by McGraw-Hill
1977	First gerontological nursing track funded by Division of Nursing and established by Sr. Rose Therese Bahr at University of Kansas School of Nursing
1979	Education for Gerontic Nursing written by Gunter and Estes; suggested curricula for all levels of nursing education
	ANA Council of Long Term Care Nurses established; group first chaired by Ella Kick
1980	Geriatric Nursing first published by AJN; Cynthia Kelly, editor
1981	ANA Division of Gerontological Nursing issues statement regarding scope of practice
1983	Florence Cellar Endowed Gerontological Nursing Chair established at Case Western Reserve University, first in the nation; Doreen Norton, first scholar to occupy chair
	National Conference of Gerontological Nurse Practitioners established

1984	National Gerontological Nurses Association established Division of Gerontological Nursing Practice becomes Council on Gerontological Nursing (councils established for all practice specialties)
1986	ANA publishes survey of gerontological nurses in clinical practice
1987	ANA revises and issues Scope and Standards of Gerontological Nursing Practice
1989	ANA certifies gerontological clinical nurse specialists
1990	ANA establishes a Division of Long-Term Care within the Council of Gerontological Nursing
1992	ANA redefines long-term care to include life span approach
	John A. Hartford Foundation funds a major initiative to improve care of hospitalized older patients: Nurses Improving Care for Healthsystem Elders (NICHE)
1993	National Institute of Nursing Research established as separate entity
1994	ANA redefines Scope and Standards of Gerontological Nursing Practice
1996	John A. Hartford Foundation establishes the Institute for Geriatric Nursing at New York University under the direction of Mathy Mezey
2000	Recommended baccalaureate competencies and curricular guidelines for geriatric nursing care published by the American Association of Colleges of Nursing and the John A. Hartford Foundation Institute for Geriatric Nursing
2001	ANA, in collaboration with the National Gerontological Nursing Association, National Association Directors of Nursing Administration in Long Term Care, and the National Conference of Gerontological Nurse Practitioners, publishes revised Scope and Standards of Gerontological Nursing Practice and reaffirms the need for competent gerontological nursing
2003	Nurse Competence in Aging (funded by the Atlantic Philanthropies Inc.) initiative to improve the quality of health care to older adults by enhancing the geriatric competence of nurses who are members of specialty nursing associations (ANA, American Nurses Credentialing Center [ANCC], John A. Hartford Foundation Institute for Geriatric Nursing)
2004	Nurse Practitioner and Clinical Nurse Specialist Competencies for Older Adult Care published by the American Association of Colleges of Nursing and the Hartford Institute for Geriatric Nursing
	ANA Scope and Standards of Practice for all registered nurses referenced to include care of older adults

the first specialty to establish standards of practice within the ANA. In 1976 the Division of Geriatric Nursing changed its name to the Gerontological Nursing Division to reflect the broad role nurses play in the management of the elderly. In 1984 the Council of Gerontological Nursing was formed and certification for GNPs and CNSs became available. Nursing was the first of the professions to develop standards of gerontological care and the first to provide a certification mechanism to ensure specific professional expertise through credentialing (Ebersole et al., 2005).

The 2001 Scope and Standards of Gerontological Nursing Practice identifies levels of gerontological nursing practice (basic and advanced), standards of clinical gerontological nursing care, and gerontological nursing performance. In light of the increasing numbers of older adults who will be cared for by nurses, the 2004 ANA Scope and Standards of Practice for all registered nurses now also includes specific reference to care of older adults. Required knowledge and skills necessary for the practice of basic gerontological nursing are listed in Box 1-2.

Long-term care and custodial care have historically been neglected by medicine and nursing. Elders with complex chronic conditions and acutely painful problems were largely ignored by the professions and society at large. Visionaries such as Barbara Lee of the W.K. Kellogg Foundation; Robert Butler, first Director of the Institute on Aging; and Linda Aiken of the Robert Woods Johnson Foundation recognized the need and opportunities for improving the situation. Teaching nursing homes were developed, as were numerous other nursing home sites that made the commitment to staff the facility with an advanced practice gerontological nurse (APGN) on a full-time basis. Immediacy of care improved, transfers to hospitals decreased, and staff morale was enhanced as more knowledge was brought to bear on the problems and conditions of elder residents. This innovative model has been called the most significant experiment to improve nursing home care in the past decade (Strumpf, 1994).

For 40 years the ANA and others have been attempting to make gerontological nursing visible and integral to nursing education. In 1990 the John A. Hartford Foundation began investing in gerontological nursing and in the past decade has granted $35 million in various educational and clinical demonstrations of effective programmatic changes in the provision of care to older people (Mezey and Fulmer, 2002). The John A. Hartford Foundation commitment is the largest of any foundation in nursing and has stimulated curricular reform, the development of academic centers of excellence, and predoctoral and postdoctoral scholarships, fostering excellence in education, research, and practice in gerontological nursing.

There is a continued need to increase the numbers of faculty with preparation in gerontological nursing and to enhance the numbers of students and graduates choosing to work in the specialty. Ensuring gerontological nursing competency in all students graduating from a nursing program is an imperative for improvement of health care to older adults. The John A. Hartford initiatives have produced curriculum materials and competency guidelines that can be obtained by undergraduate nursing programs and institutions so that best practices can be defined and centers of excellence evaluated and publicized (http://www.aacn.nche.edu/education/gerocomp.htm).

The Nurses Improving Care for Healthsystem Elders (NICHE) program of the Hartford Institute for Geriatric Nursing has developed several models of nursing care practice to prevent iatrogenesis and improve outcomes for older patients in hospitals, including acute care of the elderly (ACE) units, placement of a geriatric resource nurse (GRN) on units that care for the elderly, and quality cost models of transitional care (Mezey et al., 2004a, 2004b). Used at more than 150 hospitals nationwide, NICHE provides hospitals with the tools to improve quality of care to older patients.

BOX 1-2   Knowledge and Skills for Basic Gerontological Nursing

- Recognize the right of competent older adults to make their own care decisions, and assist them in making informed choices.
- Establish a therapeutic relationship with the older adult to facilitate development of the plan of care, which may include family participation as needed.
- Use current gerontological standards to initiate, develop, and adapt the older adult's plan of care while involving the patient, family, and other providers as needed.
- Recognize age-related changes based on an understanding of physiological, emotional, cultural, social, psychological, economic, and spiritual functioning.
- Collect data to determine health status and functional abilities to plan, implement, and evaluate care.
- Participate and collaborate with members of the interdisciplinary team.
- Participate with older adults, their families if needed, and other health professionals in ethical decision making that is centered on the older adult, empathetic, and humane.
- Serve as an advocate for older adults and their families.
- Teach older adults and families about measures that promote, maintain, and restore health and functional performance; promote comfort; foster independence; and preserve dignity.
- Refer older adults to other professionals or community resources for assistance as necessary.
- Identify common chronic/acute physical and mental health processes and problems that affect older adults.
- Apply the existing body of knowledge in gerontology to nursing practice and intervention.
- Exercise accountability to older adults by protecting their rights and autonomy, recognizing and respecting their decisions about advance directives.
- Facilitate palliative care and comfort during the dying process to preserve dignity.
- Support the surviving spouse and family members, providing strength, comfort, and hope.
- Use the standards of gerontological nursing practice and collaborate with other health care professionals to improve the quality of care and quality of life of older adults.
- Engage in professional development through participation in continuing education, involvement in state and national professional organizations, and certification.

From American Nurses Association: *Scope and standards of gerontological nursing practice*, pp 8-9, Washington, DC, 2001, The Association.

Other encouraging signs include an award of $5 million to enhance the competence of nurses caring for older adults. The grant was funded by Atlantic Philanthropies and is being implemented through a strategic alliance between ANA and the Hartford Institute for Geriatric Nursing. Recognizing the critical need for a nursing workforce prepared to deliver quality health care to the nation's aging population, and in light of the fact that few of the nation's 2.2 million practicing nurses have received any preparation in gerontological nursing in their educational programs or on the job, the Nurse Competence in Aging Initiative is designed to improve the quality of health care to older adults by enhancing the gerontological competence—the attitudes, knowledge, and skills—of nurses who are members of specialty organizations. The initiative will provide grant and technical assistance to more than 50 specialty nursing associations with membership of more than 400,000 nurses, develop a web-based comprehensive gerontological nursing resource center (*www.geronurseonline.org*), and conduct a national gerontological nursing certification outreach (*www.hartfordign.org/nca*).

Gerontic Nurse Pioneers and Leaders[*]

The foundation of gerontic nursing (we use the term "gerontic" in this section in honor of Laurie Gunter, who first worked with ANA to certify geriatric nurses) as we know it today was built largely by a small cadre of nurse explorers between 30 and 50 years ago, many of whom are now gone. Gerontic nursing was defined and shaped by these few nurse pioneers who saw, early on, that older individuals had special needs and required the most subtle, holistic, and complex nursing care.

These gerontic nurse pioneers presented seminal thought and investigated new ideas related to the care of older people; refuted mythical tales and fantasies of aging; and found realities through investigation, clinical observation, practice, and documentation, setting in motion activities that markedly influenced the course of the aging experience. They saw new possibilities and a better future for older people.

When interviewed, most were quite matter-of-fact and had not thought of themselves as pioneers. "It was there to be done." "Someone needed to do it." "Well, I wouldn't say I was really a pioneer...have you spoken to...?" They saw something that others had not seen before, but because it was self-evident to them, it did not seem at all remarkable. One said, "You asked why I established the [gerontology academic] chair and I haven't yet given you a precise answer; I must give that some more thought" (Florence Cellar).

Some demonstrated a very personal connection to the elderly that involved a certain view of humanity from a more universal or spiritual perspective than is commonly held—a stark awareness of the interdependence of generations and individuals. With humor, grace, and dignity they tell what old age means to them.

Who were these individuals who paved the way to the future of gerontic care? There are many to whom we owe the origins of gerontic nursing as a specialty, many unnamed or presently unrecognized. To name only a few and some of their outstanding accomplishments:

Sister Rose Therese Bahr	Vitally involved in the development of the National Gerontological Nurses Association
Terri Brower	Generated gerontology curricula and the first relevant nursing research
Kathleen Buckwalter	Present editor of the Journal of Gerontological Nursing; for more than 30 years has consistently studied the care of elders with dementia and mentored numerous students interested in these disorders
Irene Burnside	Mentored numerous nurses interested in geriatric nursing
Florence Cellar	Donated funds to establish first gerontological nursing chair in the nation
Barbara Allen Davis	Generated gerontological interest and foci at ANA
Terry Fulmer	Co-director of the John A. Hartford Foundation Institute of Geriatric Nursing; has generated seminal research on elder abuse
Laurie Gunter	Established geriatric certification requirements at ANA
Mary Harper	Developed dynamic programs for elderly veterans; instrumental in guiding development of geropsychiatric programs
Cynthia Kelly	First editor of Geriatric Nursing Journal
Ella Kick	Developed humanistic care strategies in long-term care
Lois Knowles	Instrumental in developing first geriatric nursing standards
Barbara Lee	Sponsored development of geriatric nurse practitioner programs through Kellogg Foundation funding
Mathy Mezey	Director of the National Teaching Nursing Home Project and presently director of the nationally influential John A. Hartford Foundation Institute for Geriatric Nursing
Dorothy Moses	Developed first gerontology radio and television programs for lay public in San Diego
Mary Quinn	Has generated seminal research on elder abuse and undue influence
Sister Marilyn Schwab	Conceived, developed, and administered national model nursing home
Doris Schwartz	Coauthored the first textbook related to geriatric nursing care; developed interdisciplinary alliances
Eldonna Shields-Kyle	Created staff development curricula for nursing homes
Bernita Steffl	Political advocate for the elderly in Arizona; contributed to understanding of sexuality and aging

---

[*] Interview data collected by Priscilla Ebersole between 1990 and 2001.

Edna Stilwell	First editor of Journal of Gerontological Nursing
Virginia Stone	Developed first graduate program in gerontological nursing
Neville Strumpf and Lois Evans	Researched the dangers of restraints and led the way to the decreased use of restraints throughout the United States
Thelma Wells	Numerous research projects and publications relevant to understanding the older adult; particular expertise in study and care of urinary incontinence
Mary Opal Wolanin	Research, mentorship, and seminal work in understanding confusion and aging
May Wykle	Research in minority elder health; Florence Cellar Professor of Gerontological Nursing

Some characteristics apparent in this select group are independence and innovation, interpersonal investment, persistence, practicality, assertiveness, strong will, and ability to earn the respect of others both within and outside the nursing profession (Box 1-3). In addition, they expended incredible amounts of energy.

Mary Opal Wolanin particularly remembers the "pneumonia nurse" as one of the first in the genre of the geriatric nurse. "These nurses, by sheer nursing skill and devoted care, literally held the life of the pneumonia-stricken elder in their hands. This was in the days before penicillin...much less third- and fourth-generation antibiotics" (Wolanin, 1995). We are relearning respect for the virulence, morbidity, and mortality of many diseases we thought had all but disappeared but have now adapted to the best antibiotics available. We continue to need adventurous nurses who can find new and better ways to care for the elderly and the young and who can facilitate self-care in the most efficacious manner.

Gerontological Nursing Education

Most nurses will care for older people during the course of their careers. However, schools of nursing have only recently begun to include gerontological nursing content in their curricula and most still do not have freestanding courses in the specialty similar to courses in maternal/child or psychiatric nursing. Often the content has been difficult to promote because faculty may not have the expertise or enthusiasm, it is regarded as an extra requirement that overloads the already extensive informational requirements of the accrediting organizations, it is thought to be "integrated" throughout the program, and students tend to be most interested in critical care and maternity care. Some of this is because of age identification and some because the highly technical care is intriguing and challenging in a specific and concrete way that is not true of the subtle complexities of geriatric care. Yet, many educational institutions have incorporated dynamic courses in aging into their curricula. Box 1-4 presents a study comparing the nature of nursing work in long-term care (LTC) and the intensive care unit (ICU). Results of the study suggest that ICU nursing work is a biomedically intensive environment whereas LTC is a nursing intensive environment (Leppa, 2004).

A recent survey conducted by the John A. Hartford Foundation Institute for Geriatric Nursing, in collaboration with the American Association of Colleges of Nursing (AACN), compared gerontological content in baccalaureate programs with baseline data collected in 1997. Results

---

BOX 1-3   Wisdom from Gerontic Nurse Pioneers*

- We need to remind ourselves constantly that the purpose of gerontic nursing is to prevent untimely death and needless suffering, always with the focus of doing with as well as doing for, and in every instance to attempt to preserve personhood as long as life continues. (Doris Schwartz)
- Aging individuals are persons, not burdens or problems, and nurses can be educated to a more positive attitude about the older adult and can aid in implementation of professional behaviors to upgrade care of older citizens in America. (Sr. Rose Therese Bahr)
- There is always an interesting person there, sometimes locked in the cage of age. I think I have helped at least a few of my students with this approach, "You see me as I am now, but I see myself as I've always been and all the things I've been—not just an old lady." (Bernita Steffl)
- I am less fearful of medical afflictions that befall me in my old age than I am of the system and the professionals to whom my care may be entrusted. (Bernita Steffl)
- Among the first lessons that I learned from working with older patients was of patience and perseverance. I found

that if they were treated as normal human beings and one took the time to talk to them, and above all listen to what they had to say, they responded normally. (Dorothy Moses)
- I believe that one of the most valuable lessons I have learned from those who are older is that I must start with looking inside at my own thinking. I was very guilty of ageism. I believed every myth in the book, was sure that I would never live past my seventieth birthday, and made no plan for my seventies. Probably the most productive years of my career have been since that dreaded birthday, and I now realize that it is very difficult, if not impossible, to think of our own aging. (Mary Opal Wolanin)
- I am opposed to anyone going into the field of geriatric nursing until she has experienced the human condition at many points—vicariously through literature and our culture or by close observation. This field demands maturity since recognizing the diversity of aging people is very important in caring for the elderly during acute illness, chronic illness, and wellness. We need a broad knowledge base and a broader mind. (Mary Opal Wolanin)

*Interview data collected by Priscilla Ebersole between 1990 and 2001. For a more comprehensive discussion, see Ebersole P, Touhy T: *Geriatric nursing: growth of a specialty*, New York, 2006, Springer.

suggest that there has been a "fundamental shift in baccalaureate curriculum toward incorporation of a greater amount of gerontological content, integration of content in a greater number of nursing courses, and more diversity of clinical sites used for gerontological nursing experiences" (Berman et al., 2005, p. 268). Although these results are encouraging, there is a continued need to increase the numbers of faculty with preparation in gerontological nursing and to enhance the numbers of students choosing to work in the specialty.

Gerontological Nursing Roles

A gerontological nurse may be a generalist or a specialist. The generalist functions in a variety of settings—hospital, home, subacute and long-term care facilities, community—providing nursing care to individuals and their families. The gerontological nursing specialist has advanced preparation at the master's level and performs all the functions of the generalist but has developed clinical expertise, as well as an understanding of health and social policy and proficiency in planning, implementing, and evaluating health programs. Gerontological nursing roles encompass every imaginable venue and circumstance. Many nurses have created their own roles, some as care managers, in industrial health care, in neighborhood clinics, in national organizations, in retirement centers, in mobile clinics, and in entrepreneurial ventures. The more traditional institutionalized nursing roles in critical care, acute care, post–acute care, long-term care, and community centers are in dire need of individuals with gerontological nursing expertise. The opportunities are limitless because we are in a rapidly aging society.

One of the most important roles emerging in the past few decades is that of advanced practice gerontological nurses

---

BOX 1-4   Evidence-Based Practice: The Nature of LTC Nursing Work

PURPOSE

This pilot study explored the nature of nursing work in LTC nursing home environments and compared it to the nature of nursing work in ICU environments.

SAMPLE/SETTING

The LTC pilot study involved responses from 113 licensed staff from 35 nursing units in 9 LTC facilities in the metropolitan Seattle area. Nursing units included those with both heavy and light care patients, subacute care, Medicare units, and dementia units. The data about ICU nursing came from a pilot study conducted by Mitchell et al. (1989), which involved responses from 42 RNs in an ICU unit in the Seattle area

METHODS

Focus groups of 5-7 key informants (RNs and LPNs/LVNs) utilizing the Leatt Measure of Nursing Technology (1981). This instrument operationalizes and measures the nature of nursing work in terms of uncertainty (percentage of patients with more than one diagnosis and with complex nursing problems and how much nursing intuition or judgment is required in providing care); variability (percentage of patients with similar health problems on the unit and the variety of nursing techniques used); and instability (percentage of patients requiring frequent observation and care or specialized monitoring and potential emergency situations). Discussions were tape recorded, transcribed verbatim, and analyzed for common themes using constant comparative analysis. Data from the LTC nurses were then compared with data from a pilot study of 42 RNs in an ICU in the same geographical area.

FINDINGS

The nature of work in LTC and ICU environments is comparable in terms of work uncertainty, variability, and instability. Long-term care nursing scores for uncertainty and variability in nursing work were as high as ICU scores. Range of scores on the nursing work instability subscale was considerably lower than the ICU mean scores, with the subacute unit mean most closely approaching the ICU mean. The LTC respondents emphasized the complexity of the medical and psychosocial needs of their patients and families as one theme in the nature of their work. In LTC, nurses must attend to individual patient needs as well as the needs of the wider care community and how other patients, family members, and nursing staff are affected by care provided, especially in the dementia units. LTC nurses felt that the instability scale focused on mechanical technology and patient instability is not always reflected in the use of technical procedures and devices in this setting. Respondents discussed the fragility of their patients, the importance of knowing their patterns, and the need for astute observational skills to detect subtle changes that could indicate a change in physiology.

IMPLICATIONS

ICU and LTC require different nursing skills, judgment, and knowledge but the results of this study suggest that the work of nurses in LTC is as complex and demanding as ICU nursing work and there are many similarities in terms of uncertainty and nursing judgment, patient variability, and instability. LTC nursing work is performed on multiple levels (individual, family, patient groups, patient–nursing assistant groups) across the continuum of care (rehabilitation, subacute, custodial, and palliative) and presents a wide variety of opportunities for student learning and professional nursing practice. "The ICU work environment is a biomedically intensive environment and the LTC nursing environment is a nursing intensive environment...highly autonomous and centered on nursing care" (Leppa, 2004, p. 32). Further study is needed to explore the breadth of nursing work in LTC from the perspective of LTC nurses and patients. A better understanding of the complexities of this type of nursing work may help attract more students and nurses to this setting. LTC nursing work is challenging, highly autonomous, requires specialized knowledge and skills, and should be seen as different, not as "less than" because it does not involve as much medical technology.

Data from Leppa, CJ: The nature of LTC nursing work, *J Gerontolog Nurs* 30(3):26-33, 2004.
LTC, Long-term care; *ICU*, intensive care unit.

(APGNs) as major service providers. APGNs include GNPs and gerontological nursing clinical specialists. The educational and training programs arose from evident need, particularly in long-term care settings. These are nurses who have completed a master's program in gerontological nursing and have been certified by the ANA. Practice privileges vary from state to state, but the federal Medicaid and Medicare programs allow for individual provider numbers and direct reimbursement.

Advanced practice nurses have demonstrated their skill as well as cost-effectiveness across a variety of settings. The role of APGNs in nursing homes is well established, and the positive outcomes of their care include increased patient and family satisfaction, decreased costs, less-frequent hospitalizations and emergency room visits, and improved quality of care (Dowling-Castronova, 2000; Mezey et al., 2004a). The APGN is and will continue to be a major influence on quality of care in nursing homes and other settings.

Presently, 54 educational programs prepare APGNs and 3677 gerontological nurse practitioners and 677 gerontological clinical nurse specialists are certified (fewer than 6% of all advanced practice nurses). Approximately 9000 nurses are certified as gerontological nursing generalists (fewer than 1% of all RNs) (Mezey et al., 2004a). These numbers are far short of projected need for nurses competent in care of older people. There are 15,108 adult nurse practitioners and 34,933 certified family nurse practitioners (Moore, 2006), many of whom are caring for older people. Some have had intensive attention in their curricula to gerontological nursing care, but some have not and must learn on the job. Major problems are the lack of faculty with the necessary level of gerontological nursing expertise, sparse attention to gerontological nursing in basic nursing programs, and the routing of federal grants for education in medicine and nursing to family practice.

To increase competency in gerontological nursing, Mezey and Fulmer (2002) suggest that graduate programs should be "gerontologicalized" and all nurse practitioner graduates should have gerontological nursing competencies to meet the health care needs of a rapidly growing older adult population. The AACN published competencies for nurse practitioner (NP) and CNS programs preparing advanced practice nurses in specialties other than gerontological nursing who will work with older adults (*www.aacn.nche.edu/ Education/Hartford/OlderAdultCare.htm*).

Gerontological nurses are practitioners, educators, managers, researchers, consultants, politicians, inventors, entrepreneurs, and social advocates. Wherever gerontological nurses are found, their mission is to preserve function, enhance health, and enhance the quality of life and dying. Some anecdotes provide a look at poignant moments in the lives of gerontological nurses (Box 1-5).

AGING TODAY

A revolution is occurring in gerontological nursing as older adults are gaining full status and recognition in society. The "baby boomer" generation (the parents of the present young adults and most nursing students) are entering the ranks of the "young-old" (those 50 to 70 years old). The very old and the elite-old (those 90 years and older) are the fastest growing segment of the aging population as technologic advances have facilitated their survival.

Demographics of Aging

Demography, the statistical study of the size and distribution of population, is extremely significant in gerontology. The decennial census occurs every 10 years, and thus the 2000 census was especially important because it will dictate national concerns and policies regarding aging, as well as future directions.

Aging in the United States. The total population of the United States, according to latest figures in the U.S. Statistical Abstract (U.S. Census Bureau, 2007) is 281,296,639. Of these, 35.1 million persons are older than 65 years, making up 12.4% of the population. About 20.5 million of these are older women, and 14.4 million are older men. The number of older adults is expected to double within the next 25 years. By 2030, almost 1 in 5 Americans (72 million people) will be 65 years or older. The age-group 85 years and older is now the fastest growing segment of the U.S. population (U.S. Census Bureau, 2001).

In 2002 the life expectancy for infant girls in the United States was 79.7 years, whereas for boys it was 74.1 years. However, among African-Americans, life expectancy was 68.8 years for men and 75.6 years for women, evidence of important health disparity. In the United States, more than 36% of people older than 65 years live alone. However, for

---

BOX 1-5 Caring Moments in Gerontological Nursing

Quentin was 89 years old and blind and lived in a county nursing home. When his body began filling with fluid, Martha Debbie Dixon, RN, asked him what he would most like to do. His response, "One more time before I die, I want to feel the grass under my feet." Martha got Quentin dressed except for shoes and stockings and then took off her own shoes and stockings and both walked out into the warm summer evening. When she asked how he felt, his response was, "(the grass) Soft and moist with dew and oh, so good, I'm almost in heaven."

A woman who had been married 58 years was dying of lung cancer. Her husband was at her bedside most of the time trying to help with her care and keep her comfortable. When she became comatose and near death, he seemed lost. The nurse (*name withheld*) suggested he sit by her side and reminisce with her as dying persons often can hear even when they cannot respond. He spent 3 hours talking and reminiscing with her. After she died, he said, "You can't know what a great gift you gave us. I talked all about our life together. You helped us to die in love" (Hudacek, 2000, p. 77).

men older than 75 years, 69.3% live with a spouse, whereas only 31% of women older than 75 years live with a spouse (U.S. Census Bureau, 2001) (Figure 1-1). Florida (17.6%), Pennsylvania (15.6%), and West Virginia (15.3%) have the highest percentages of people 65 years and older. About 77% of persons older than 65 years lived in metropolitan areas (50% in suburbs, 27% in central cities), and 23% lived in non-metropolitan areas. In the comparatively mobile population of the United States, the experience of aging is greatly influenced by where one lives (Table 1-1) (Administration on Aging, 2001).

Gender Issues. Women, particularly culturally and ethnically diverse women, face great challenges as they age. White women are twice as likely as white men to be poor in old age, and single African-American and Latin women are four times more likely to live in poverty than white men as they grow older. More than 40% of older Latinas and black women who live alone are living in poverty. Across the world, the United States has one of the highest poverty rates for older women among industrialized countries. The problems of aging are largely problems of older women. Factors influencing the poverty status of older women include pay inequity, occupational segrega-

tion, caregiving responsibilities, longer life expectancy, rising health care costs, and women's work patterns, all of which reduce pension earnings, public assistance benefits, and personal savings (Hounsell and Riojas, 2006).

Diversity of Aging in the United States. Minority elders make up more than 16.1% of all older Americans. Between 1999 and 2030, the older minority population (older than 65 years) is projected to increase by 217%, compared with 81% for the older white population. The number of African-Americans elders will increase by 128%; the population of Asian-American elders will increase by 301%; Hispanic-American elders will grow 322%; and Native Americans and Alaska Native elders will increase by about 193%. By 2050, the percentage of the older population that is non-Hispanic white is expected to decline from 84% to 64%. Among all ethnic and racial groups, the Hispanic older population is projected to grow the fastest, from about 2 million in 2000 to more than 13 million by 2050 (Figure 1-2).

Although the health status of racial and ethnic groups has improved over the past century, disparities in major health indicators between white and non-white groups are growing (*www.aoa.gov*). Increasing the numbers of health care providers from different cultures as well as ensuring cultural

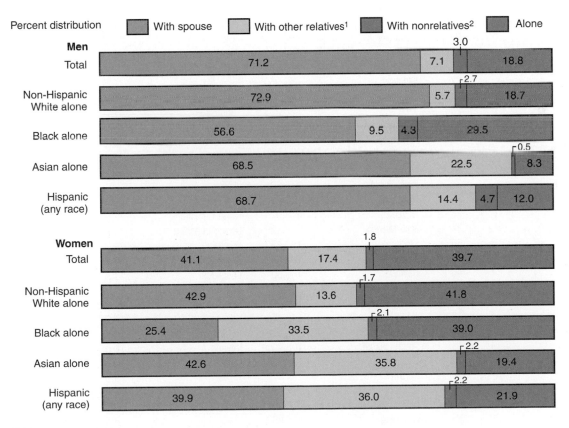

[1]No spouse present
[2]No spouse or other relative present
Note: The reference population for these data is the civilian noninstitutionalized population.

FIGURE 1-1 Living arrangements of population older than 65 years by gender, race, and ethnicity. (Redrawn from U.S. Census Bureau, 2003.)

TABLE 1-1

Population Ages 65 and Over Ranked by State: 2000

	Population Age 65 and Over		Percent of State's Population Age 65 and Over	
Rank	State	Number	State	Percent
1	California	3,595,658	Florida	17.6
2	Florida	2,807,597	Pennsylvania	15.6
3	New York	2,448,352	West Virginia	15.3
4	Texas	2,072,532	Iowa	14.9
5	Pennsylvania	1,919,165	North Dakota	14.7
6	Ohio	1,507,757	Rhode Island	14.5
7	Illinois	1,500,025	Maine	14.4
8	Michigan	1,219,018	South Dakota	14.3
9	New Jersey	1,113,136	Arkansas	14.0
10	North Carolina	969,048	Connecticut	13.8
11	Massachusetts	860,162	Nebraska	13.6
12	Virginia	792,333	Massachusetts	13.5
13	Georgia	785,275	Missouri	13.5
14	Missouri	755,379	Montana	13.4
15	Indiana	752,831	Ohio	13.3
16	Tennessee	703,311	Hawaii	13.3
17	Wisconsin	702,553	Kansas	13.3
18	Arizona	667,839	New Jersey	13.2
19	Washington	662,148	Oklahoma	13.2
20	Maryland	599,307	Wisconsin	13.1
21	Minnesota	594,266	Alabama	13.0
22	Alabama	579,798	Arizona	13.0
23	Louisiana	516,929	Delaware	13.0
24	Kentucky	504,793	New York	12.9
25	South Carolina	485,333	Oregon	12.8
26	Connecticut	470,183	Vermont	12.7
27	Oklahoma	455,950	Kentucky	12.5
28	Oregon	438,177	Indiana	12.4
29	Iowa	436,213	Tennessee	12.4
30	Colorado	416,073	Michigan	12.3
31	Arkansas	374,019	District of Columbia	12.2
32	Kansas	356,229	South Carolina	12.1
33	Mississippi	343,523	Minnesota	12.1
34	West Virginia	276,895	Illinois	12.1
35	Nebraska	232,195	Mississippi	12.1
36	Nevada	218,929	North Carolina	12.0
37	New Mexico	212,225	New Hampshire	12.0
38	Utah	190,222	Wyoming	11.7
39	Maine	183,402	New Mexico	11.7
40	Hawaii	160,601	Louisiana	11.6
41	Rhode Island	152,402	Maryland	11.3
42	New Hampshire	147,970	Idaho	11.3
43	Idaho	145,916	Washington	11.2
44	Montana	120,949	Virginia	11.2
45	South Dakota	108,131	Nevada	11.0
46	Delaware	101,726	California	10.6
47	North Dakota	94,478	Texas	9.9
48	Vermont	77,510	Colorado	9.7
49	District of Columbia	69,898	Georgia	9.6
50	Wyoming	57,693	Utah	8.5
51	Alaska	35,699	Alaska	5.7

From U.S. Census Bureau, 2001.

NOTE: The reference population for these data is the resident population.

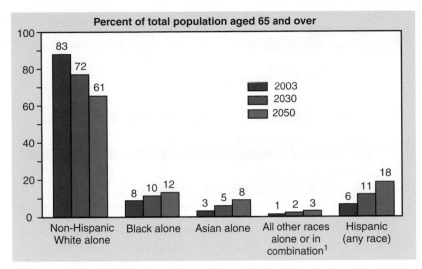

¹The race group "All other races alone or in combination" includes American Indian and Alaska Native alone, Native Hawaiian and Other Pacific Islander alone, and all people who reported two or more races.
Note: The reference population for these data is the resident population.

FIGURE 1-2 Diversity of the older population. (Redrawn from U.S. Census Bureau, 2004.)

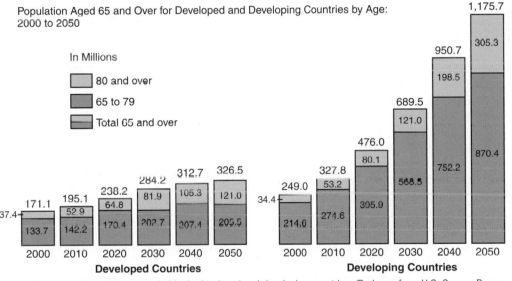

FIGURE 1-3 The population 65 years and older in developed and developing countries. (Redrawn from U.S. Census Bureau, 2004.)

competence of all providers is essential to meet the needs of a rapidly growing, ethnically diverse elderly population. One of the two major goals of *Healthy People 2010* is to eliminate health disparities. Chapter 21 discusses gender and cultural issues in aging in more detail.

Global Aging. The world population, now totaling more than 6 billion people, is getting older. Projections by the United Nations show that by 2050, more people will be older than 60 years than younger than 15 years. In fewer than 50 years, one person in five will be older than 60 years. Western Europe and Japan already have more older people than young people, and they will be joined by the rest of Asia in 2040 and the United States shortly after. Asia, Latin America, and Africa are already home to more than two thirds of the world's older people. The growing number of

older people in the world's population results from a combination of increased life expectancy and reduced fertility (Figure 1-3).

Japan (81.5 years) and Sweden (80.1 years) continue to have the longest life expectancy (United Nations Population Division, 2002). Of course, these statistics are influenced by the infant mortality rates, which are lowest in Sweden (3.4 deaths per 1000 live births) and Japan (3.3 deaths per 1000 live births). The infant mortality rate at birth in the United States is 6.8 per 1000 live births. The aged dependency, or support ratio, is almost 4 to 1 in developed countries and projected to be 2 to 1 by 2050 (AARP, 2001) (Figure 1-4).

Even in the poorest countries, life expectancy is increasing and the number of older people is increasing. In 2015, 67% of the world's older people will live in developing countries. Older people in developed and developing countries

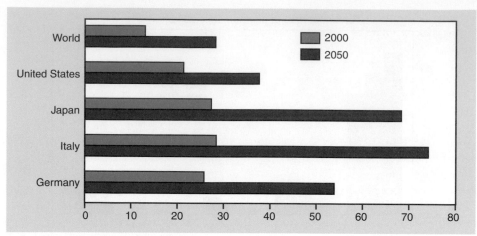

FIGURE 1-4 Aged dependency ratios, world total, and selected countries, 2000 and 2050. (These ratios include the number of persons age 65 years per every 100 persons ages 20 to 64 years.) (Redrawn from U.S. Census Bureau, International Data Base, 2001.)

face different challenges as they age. James Martin, in an address to the International Federation on Aging in 2006, calls this a century of extremes. In the United States, we are studying regenerative medicine and predicting that people could live to 120 years, whereas in Botswana, life expectancy is 27 years. Around the world, 100 million older people live on $1 or less per day. Poverty, hunger, and lack of access to basic life necessities are all too common in developing countries for people of all ages. Of older people in developing countries, 80% have no regular income, lack of food is a serious cause of ill health, and older widows are among the poorest and most vulnerable groups.

The human immunodeficiency virus (HIV)/acquired immunodeficiency syndrome (AIDS) epidemic has had devastating economic, social, physical, and psychological effects on older women and men, especially in sub-Saharan Africa. Almost 13 million children have lost one or both parents to HIV/AIDS, the vast majority in sub-Saharan Africa. As many as 9 of 10 orphans are cared for by their extended family, mainly the grandparents (*www.helpage.org*). As we study how to care for older people, it is important to remember that our view must be expanded to include older people across the globe who have very different needs. More details on international aging can be found in The International Plan of Action on Ageing Report available at *www.un.org/esa/socdev/ageing/ageipaa3.htm*.

Chronological Age

Chronology is becoming a less-significant factor to consider in aging. "Old" is a relative concept based on how one acts and feels physically, mentally, socially, and culturally. One can feel old when competing with younger folk or feel young when much healthier or younger looking than age contemporaries. In the United States, the chronological age of 65 years is the standard by which one is awarded the status of senior citizen, whether or not it is desired. In 1935, 65 years was chosen as the age at which a person could receive benefits and services under Social Security. As people live and work longer, the eligibility age for Social Security benefits is increasing. The

Do you consider yourself young, middle-aged, old, or very old?

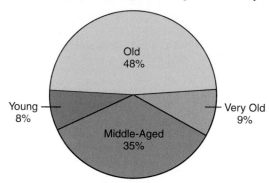

Nearly half of people 65 and older consider themselves to be middle-aged or young. There are no noticeable male-female or education group differences. Only 15% of people age 75+ consider themselves "very old."

FIGURE 1-5 Age self-identification. (Redrawn from National Council on the Aging, Inc., American perceptions of aging in the 21st century, telephone survey, Jan-Feb 2000. Available at *www.ncoa.org*.)

category of old is arbitrary and varies with time, place, cohort, and perception. "Old age," categorically, is likely to last for 25 additional years if one is healthy at age 65. Because of the great variations between a 65-year-old and an 85-year-old, old age has been further categorized into young-old (65 to 74 years); middle-old (75 to 84 years); and old-old (85 years and older) (Figure 1-5). From the gerontological nursing perspective, functional age, or the ability to perform ADLs, is a more essential measure of age than chronological age.

The Old. The parents of the baby boomers, the children of the Great Depression, make up the majority of the present old numerically. Some immunizations became available in their childhood, but many parents feared them and most children had all of the "childhood" diseases, such as measles, mumps, chickenpox, and whooping cough. Some had tuberculosis, poliomyelitis, and smallpox. Malnutrition was rampant among the poorer people. Dental care was neglected. In areas where the water was "soft," lacking minerals, teeth were soft and cavity prone. "Pigeon chest," a malformation of the rib cage caused by lack of vitamin D, was common. Goiter and myxedema were less common but were present regionally because of unrecognized iodine deficiencies. These problems were identified and almost eradicated before the next generation, the baby boomers, came along.

The survivors in this generation are called the "notch" babies; few in number at birth, even fewer survived childhood, adolescence, and World War II. War and patriotism molded their young adulthood. Most of these elders are fairly sturdy, but their adolescent and young adult lifestyles contributed to many problems that are now evident. The use and abuse of cigarettes and alcohol were considered sophisticated. A double standard prevailed in the expectations of men and women. Exercise was not valued by most because desirable work was steadily becoming less physically strenuous, and physical exertion was still associated with hard work. Remote memories of poverty and deprivation haunted many of them and propelled them into excesses when such were available and affordable. Few gave much thought to their own aging when in their middle years because most were preoccupied with providing for their children the things they had missed. Saving for children's college education was a high priority.

Nonagenarians and Centenarians. There is an expanding group of the very old, those now older than 90 years, who remain mobile and active. They are genetically hardy. These are an extraordinarily select group of individuals who have managed to survive the numerous dangers and diseases of childhood and, with the advancement of medical science, have overcome disorders that would have killed their parents. Some remember the influenza pandemic of 1918 in which numerous young and vital individuals died within a few hours of developing influenza (Cantor, 2002). Many of these present elders, because of the rigorous conditions of survival in their youth, are now living well into their 90s.

This generation raised their families during the depths of the Great Depression. Desperation was prevalent in the country at the time. Few were able to achieve a higher education, and many did not even complete grade school. The bulk of the working population were farmers, agricultural workers, factory workers, miners, and clerks. Unemployment was rampant. Individuals worked very hard for the essentials of existence and felt fortunate if they were employed. Henry Ford became famous for offering wages of $5 a day and producing assembly-line cars that made automobiles available to the common person. These individuals, who are the last to remember traveling by horse and wagon, have also flown across the nation in supersonic jet airplanes. Older people of today have been catapulted through socioscientific periods too numerous to mention. The shifts in human thought, technical capacities, and modes of life that have occurred within the single lifetime of the very old are stunning. These include the agrarian age, the industrial age, the atomic age, the space age, the microelectronic age, and the cyberspace age as we are all connected by the World Wide Web.

This generation has experienced more hardship and more lifestyle disruption and change than any of which we are aware. Federal aid, Social Security, the Works Progress Administration, and numerous other New Deal programs were instituted as survival measures during the depths of the Depression. Few of these individuals thought much about old age, and many say they are surprised to have lived so long. These elders rarely throw anything away because every scrap has potential value when one has known early deprivation. Many of them arrived in the United States in early childhood as steerage passengers, emigrating with their parents from Europe.

Centenarians, the "elite-old," are approached with some awe as our society seeks routes to longevity. About 1 in 10,000 people in developed countries lives to be a hundred or more (Christensen, 2001). A select few of these expert survivors have experienced the turning of 2 centuries. Many are bright and alert and have an unequaled personal history. The number of centenarians in the United States has doubled every decade since 1970. Currently, about 40,000 centenarians are in the United States. Centenarians are the fastest growing segment of our population; the second fastest is the age-group 85 years and older.

About 30% of centenarians have no children or siblings still living. Most centenarians are female (85%) and come from families in which longevity is common. Though there are fewer men, they are less likely than women to have significant mental or physical disabilities at that age (Christensen, 2001). Thirty percent of centenarians have no evidence of dementia (Silver et al., 2001). They are often sought for their opinions on the key to longevity. The supposition is that because they have lived so long they know the secrets to learning, growing, and thriving. Various centenarians have recommended such things as a daily highball, hard work, church attendance, healthy diets, or the continuation of sexual activity. Unfortunately, few agree and the myths abound. Lifestyle factors that do seem significant include diet, maintaining proper weight, exercise, avoidance of smoking, social connections, and how well a person handles stress (Christensen, 2001; Mentes, 2006).

Researchers in the United States, France, Italy, Denmark, and China are studying centenarians. Belle Boone Beard, who died in 1984, conducted several thousand interviews with centenarians during 40 years of study. Elsner and colleagues (1999) carry on her work and are concerned that little thought is being given to the ethical and policy considerations for this fastest growing segment of the population. Many questions and conflicting findings still exist regarding both the physiological and psychological adaptation of centenarians. Most centenarians are likely to be extremely frail and vulnerable both mentally and physically. Several websites offer a fascinating look at centenarians including pictures and video (*www7.nationalgeographic.com/ngm/0511/feature1/index.html* and *www.grg.org*).

Attitudes Toward Aging

Attitudes toward aging are inextricably tied to history and culture. Views of aging in any era or ethnic group are influenced by expected life span, economic conditions, social expectations, and the way these are dealt with in the media, arts, and literature of the time. A unique situation exists in our society. Rapid change and cataclysmic shifts in lifestyles, universal threats to survival, a shrinking world and an expanding universe, and previously undreamed of possibilities and opportunities have created remarkable differences in the life experience of each generation.

Ageist attitudes may be excessively positive or negative, depending on one's tendency to stereotype individuals based on their age. Older people, collectively, have often been seen in negative terms; however, a most striking change in attitudes toward aging has occurred in the past 20 years. Undoubtedly, this will continue to change as the baby boomers reach retirement age. The impact of media presentation is enormous, and we are gratified to see robust images of aging; fewer older people are portrayed as victims or those to be pitied, shunned, or ridiculed by virtue of achieving old age.

Attitudes of Elders. Attitudes of older people toward other elders are often far more rejecting than those of younger persons. Older persons with mental disabilities are particularly vulnerable because they represent the fears of their healthier contemporaries. In senior centers and retirement centers, the cliques of highly functioning elders are quite noticeable.

Attitudes of Children. Children are able to identify with older persons and feel comfortable with them in direct proportion to their frequency of contact. Those who see elders frequently are more aware of the reality of aging persons. Closeness with grandparents is highly correlated with attitudes young people hold toward older persons. Attitudes of school-age children and adolescents are generally positive regarding older people. These tendencies could be sustained and cultivated by giving more attention to aging in public school curricula. To decrease stereotypic notions, students in some schools are given opportunities to work with the elderly. Generally, persons who are younger and who have had extensive contact with the well elderly have the most positive regard for older people.

Attitudes of Health Care Students. Few students or professionals set out early on to be gerontology specialists. They enter the field most often by accident, by job opportunity, or through a revered mentor. Often, in nursing, it was an early serendipitous experience of a student caring for a physically debilitated or dependent elder who had amazing fortitude and courage that fostered an interest in the field. For many others it was intimate contact with grandparents, often in a caregiving capacity, that instilled the desire to care for elders. For those inspired, it is usually a combination of events. When nurses do become involved in caring for elders, their attitudes are usually very positive.

Research and Aging

In the nearly 4 decades since the institution of Medicare and Medicaid, growth has been colossal in gerontology as a scientific pursuit. Federal and foundation dollars in support of research and research training attracted many to the field of aging.

Some of the major problems in aging research are that the older people, although statistically ranging from 65 to 115 years old, are often grouped into a single category. We would no more think of categorically comparing the experience of a 3-year-old and a 13-year-old than we would compare apples and oranges. Studies of older people often include those 50 years old, eligible for certain memberships and discounts based on age deference, and the 104-year-old residing in a nursing home. These are considered as a group, though they have few if any similar characteristics. Some researchers extrapolate from studies of young adults or institutionalized elders, and conclusions are attributed to older people in general. A great deal of cross-sectional research and small samples are also suspect.

Research and gerontological knowledge are strongly influenced by federal bulletins that are distributed nationwide to indicate the type of research most likely to receive federal funding. These are published in requests for proposals (RFPs). In a very real way, the "alzheimerization" of aging has come about because, since the establishment of the National Institute on Aging (NIA) in 1971, the study of Alzheimer's disease has been awarded the largest share of research dollars for aging. Alzheimer's disease remains a primary area of research concentration, with a considerable focus on etiology, prevention, and medications that may halt or slow progress of the disease.

The investigators of the Baltimore Longitudinal Studies of the Aged have been collecting data and periodically publishing findings for almost 40 years. These studies were initially restricted to males, but more recently studies of females have been included as well. Several substantial longitudinal studies of older people are now presenting current evidence about elders from several cohorts.

The NIA, the National Institute of Nursing Research, the National Institute of Mental Health, and the Agency for Health Care Research and Quality continue to make significant research contributions to our understanding of older people. The meaning and experience of aging remain elusive, complex, and highly individualistic. Phenomenological studies have the potential to provide some of the richest information about the lived experience of aging. Also, in both quantitative and qualitative research, the study of ethnically diverse older people is most lacking.

Nursing Research

Gerontological nursing research and practice have evolved to the point where best practice standards are being published and distributed through several organizations. Nurses have generated significant research in the care of older adults. The 2002 issue of the *Annual Review of Nursing Research* (vol 20) is devoted entirely to gerontological nursing (Fitzpatrick, 2002). *Geriatric Nursing: Growth of a Specialty* (Ebersole and Touhy, 2006) also discusses the past, present, and future of nursing research. Numerous nursing research studies over the past 2 decades are cited, described, and analyzed. Issues most relevant to present concerns in care of older adults include end-of-life care, cultural diversity, tele-health management, pain management (especially in dementia), caregiver concerns, and health promotion.

Nursing research that has significantly affected the quality of life of older persons gains more prominence each decade. Some of the most important studies have investigated methods of caring for individuals with dementia (Buckwalter et al., 1999), reducing falls and the use of restraints (Strumpf and Evans, 2003; Strumpf et al., 1998), pain management (Ferrell, 1999), delirium (Foreman et al., 2001), and humane end-of-life care (Matzo and Sherman, 2003). Hinshaw (2000) notes that most research regarding health and illness of older adults has been in the following areas: ADLs and maintaining independence, managing cognitive impairment and depression, and providing supportive care environments for older people. She suggests that we need research that will identify those at risk of losing function, interventions for enhancing and maintaining memory, and interventions to enhance optimism and self-esteem. She sees a need for a stronger emphasis on intervention research and more interdisciplinary collaboration to ensure relevance of nursing research to practice. Gerontological nurse scholars and researchers May Wykle and Ruth Tappen identified areas in most need of gerontological nursing research (Ebersole and Touhy, 2006) (Box 1-6).

The Politics of Aging

The actual development of gerontology has probably been more influenced by political expediency than by any other factor, but politics and economics are so intermeshed that they can rarely be untangled. In the United States, the first real interest in aging emerged in the 1930s, when a population of older persons, who were largely impoverished, became demographically significant. Under the Roosevelt administration and the National Recovery Act (NRA) in the mid-1930s,

the United States began moving toward a socialistic political control that persists today, although it is often assailed by conservative policymakers. During the 1940s, the study of aging was set aside to devote attention to the more pressing problems of national defense and developments in weaponry. However, interest in aging rose rapidly after World War II.

Today, funding for social services is often tied to stringent governmental requirements. Although we hear about shifting the funding responsibility from federal agencies to state agencies, we have yet to see the full effects of this in action. One of the paradoxes that hinders the delivery of services to older people in the United States is that America is both a capitalistic and a socialistic society, with health care moving rapidly into a highly competitive marketing mode. Therefore life-sustaining services are now designed for profit, although we simultaneously federally subsidize them. See Box 1-7 for a summary of important political developments in the field of aging.

White House Conferences on Aging. The purpose of the White House Conferences on Aging (WHCoA) is to make recommendations to the President and Congress to help guide national aging policies. The first WHCoA, in 1961, paved the way for the establishment of the Older Americans Act, the Administration on Aging, and the Medicare program. After the second WHCoA, the National Institute on Aging was established in 1971 with Robert Butler as the first director. The commitment to sustain these programs sometimes seems tenuous, although politicians are well aware of the strength of elders' votes and therefore are likely to enact laws that will accrue votes. Older people, although a large part of the voting population, are highly individualistic and as yet have not formed a political power block except on issues such as erosion of Social Security or reduction of Medicare and Medicaid. The greatest congressional threats to these programs, as they vie for the defense dollars, will

---

BOX 1-6   Future Directions for Gerontological Nursing Research as Suggested by Wykle and Tappen

- Staffing patterns and the most appropriate mix to improve care outcomes in long-term care settings
- The influence of culture, diversity, ethnicity on aging
- Health disparities and health literacy
- Factors contributing to successful aging, health promotion, and wellness in the upcoming Baby Boomer generation
- Retirement decisions of the Baby Boomers, how they are made and how they are changing from our current knowledge level
- Dementia as a chronic illness and staying well with the disease
- Caregiving, particularly intergenerational
- Values and attitudes of the current generation toward aging and their expectations
- Interventions to assist with the increasing prevalence of drug and alcohol abuse and other mental health problems of the current and future generations of older adults

- Integration of current best practice protocols into settings across the continuum in cost-effective and care-efficient models
- Models of acute care designed to prevent negative outcomes in elders
- Strategies to increase preparation in gerontological nursing and increased recruitment of the brightest and best into gerontological nursing
- Models of interdisciplinary practice
- Health promotion and illness management interventions in the assisted living setting; role of professional nurses and advanced practice nurses in this setting; aging in place
- Development of models for end-of-life care in home and nursing home

From Ebersole P, Touhy T: *Geriatric nursing: growth of a specialty*, New York, 2006, Springer.

BOX 1-7 Political Events Influencing Aging

1935   Social Security Act signed by Franklin D. Roosevelt.

1937   National Institute of Health established; first of the special institutes to study diseases common to older people.

1948   Hospital Construction and Facilities Act (Hill-Burton) provided funds for construction of long-term care facilities.

1950   First National Conference on Aging held in Washington, D.C.

1951   Federal Committee on Aging and Geriatrics created to coordinate federal programs for the aging.

1952   First Federal-State Conference on Aging held in Washington.

1956   Special Staff on Aging established within U.S. Department of Health, Education, and Welfare. Federal Council on Aging replaced Intradepartmental Working Group on Aging.

1959   Senate subcommittee authorized to consider problems of the elderly and aging. Federal Council on Aging reconstituted at Cabinet level.

1960   First appropriation passed for Section 202, Housing Act of 1959, authorizing direct loans for housing for the elderly.

1961   First White House Conference on Aging held in Washington. Senate Special Committee on Aging established as advocate for older Americans.
First Annual Conference of State Executives held in Washington.

1962   Federal Council on Aging became President's Council on Aging.

1963   John F. Kennedy sent Congress the first presidential message on elderly citizens; designated May as Senior Citizens Month. Special Staff on Aging became Office of Aging in HEW's new Welfare Administration.

1965   President Johnson signed Older Americans Act, creating Administration on Aging (AOA). Amendments to the Social Security Act established Medicare program. Foster Grandparent Program initiated by Office of Economic Opportunity and Administration on Aging.

1967   Age Discrimination in Employment Act brightened job outlook for Americans 40 to 65 years old.

1970   Older Americans White House Forums held across the nation to identify problems and issues for upcoming White House Conference on Aging.

1971   Second White House Conference on Aging held in Washington.
Cabinet-level Domestic Council Committee on Aging created.
ACTION—the federal volunteer agency—established and given responsibility for senior volunteer programs previously administered by AOA.

1972   New act passed establishing Nutrition Program for the Elderly to be administered by AOA.

1973   Amendments to Older Americans Act called for state agencies on aging to establish area agencies on aging to plan for comprehensive, coordinated service delivery systems for older people at the local level.
Establishment of a National Clearinghouse on Aging and a Federal Council on the Aging with members appointed by the President.

Amendments included a separate Older Americans Community Employment Act with responsibility for administering given to Department of Labor.
Federal Aid Highway Act of 1973 provided funds for a demonstration program of public transportation in rural areas with an emphasis on the needs of the elderly and handicapped.

1974   Research on Aging Act established National Institute on Aging within National Institute of Health, Robert N. Butler appointed Director.
Amendments to Urban Mass Transportation Act of 1964 made funds available to nonprofit private organizations and corporations for transportation vehicles and equipment for the elderly and handicapped. National Mass Transportation Act mandated reduced fares for the elderly and handicapped on all public transportation systems assisted by the Act.

1975   House of Representatives Special Committee on Aging established.
Amendments to the Older Americans Act establish four new priority areas under Title IV:
   a. Transportations
   b. Home Services
   c. Legal Services
   d. Residential Repair and Renovation

1976   Title V of the Older Americans Act received an appropriation for the first time since inception of the Act in 1965. Five million dollars was appropriated "to pay part of the cost of acquisition, alteration, or renovation of community facilities that will serve as multipurpose Senior Centers."

1977   Title V re-funded at rate of $20 million annually.

1981   Third White House Conference on Aging held in Washington, D.C.
Mandatory retirement laws revised.

1982   T. Franklin Williams appointed director of National Institute of Aging.

1983   Diagnostic Related Groups (DRGs) instituted by the Health Care Financing Administration to control costs of Medicare.

1984   Sexual discrimination in pension benefit payments outlawed by U.S. Supreme Court.

1988   Medicare Catastrophic Coverage Act.

1989   Medicare Catastrophic Coverage Act repealed.

1991   Fourth White House Conference on Aging stalled. AOA funds cut drastically.

1992   Proposals from multiple sources for rescue of health care system.

1995   Fourth White House Conference on Aging (WHCoA). Focused on preservation of Medicare, Medicaid, Social Security, and the Older Americans Act (OAA).

1996   Majority of elders moved through Medicare changes to managed care systems.

1998   Congress considers privatizing Social Security.

2000   Numerous methods of reducing drug costs are proposed.

2004   Prescription drug plans instituted.

2005   Medicare payment for preventive benefits expanded.
Continued proposals for privatization of privatizing Social Security.
Fifth WHCoA.

demonstrate the strength of elders, their diverse opinions, and their collective power on certain issues.

The most recent WHCoA, held in 2005, focused on the aging of today and tomorrow, including the 78 million baby boomers who began to turn 60 in 2006. The top 10 resolutions voted by delegates are presented in Box 1-8.

Older Americans Act. The Older Americans Act (OAA), instituted after the 1961 WHCoA, established a vehicle for delivering community-based services through state Area Agencies on Aging (AAAs). AAAs have some flexibility in services provided, but they generally include senior centers, nutrition sites, in-home services for frail elderly, elder abuse prevention programs, long-term care ombudsmen, employment services, legal assistance, pre-retirement counseling, health promotion, and respite care. Federal appropriations and services have historically increased markedly each year as the numbers of older people have increased. Now seniors fear that these may not continue. The current political agenda is to transfer much of the responsibility for provision of services to the states, the cities, and the individual. This could mean more individual autonomy in the future. At present, the transferring of responsibility has greatly increased the burdens to families. Recently the Administration on Aging (AOA) has given considerably more attention to the needs of caregivers of older people (Greene, 2002).

The Business of Aging

Aging is not only a phase of life, a philosophy, or an experience—it is big business. Major marketing attention has been extended to the elderly as businesses grasp the market potential of the upcoming young-old. Even the revered American Association of Retired Persons (AARP) is designed primarily to provide services, education, and conveniences to the well-heeled, well-educated young-old. The AARP offers insurance for every purpose, travel and cruise packages, luxurious retirement facilities, and art objects, all marketed to the anticipated tastes and needs of vital and prosperous elders.

The revival of 1940s and 1950s memorabilia, music, and nostalgia all reflect market trends that stir memories of childhood in active young-elders. In addition to a large market of well elders, there is an enormous market for those needing assistive devices, supplies, and equipment for management of chronic disorders. Herbs and supplements claim an increasing share of the market, but the greatest of all is in the pharmacological market. Annual expenditures for prescription drugs exceed all other health care costs except hospitals and physicians. The advertising and business world is beginning to create niches for gerontologists as they realize the benefits of their special skills as applied to marketing. However, concerns are growing that elders are prime targets for anti-aging scams (U.S. Senate Special Committee on Aging, 2001).

GERONTOLOGICAL NURSING AND AGING: THE FUTURE

Baby boomers are looming on the horizon. A healthier old age seems to be within reach for the population in general and particularly for the segment dubbed "baby boomers." They are informed and educated, have been alerted to the importance of beginning to prepare early for a good old age, and expect a much higher quality of life as they age than did their elders. More and more of them find that they are caregivers to the older members of their family, sometimes as many as two generations, and have a very personal understanding of the needs of elders. These almost-elders are giving us new perspectives on the aging process. They and the numerous longitudinal studies of aging now in progress are changing the concepts of aging and the field of gerontology. Interest is increasing in anti-aging medicine and prolongevity (significant extension of the human life span and/or average life expectancy without lengthening suffering and infirmity) (Binstock, 2003). Yet much depends on world economics, and unrest exists among these individuals as they contemplate the possibility of insufficient resources in their final years.

There is no typical baby boomer. Although it has been fashionable to consider the baby boomers en masse, they are extremely diverse, differing by as much as 19 birth years, separated by race, culture, and socioeconomic status. To plan well for their retirement years, we must consider the following:

- Their diversity
- The uncertain political and economic future
- Potential major shifts in lifestyle expectations
- Radical differences in health care delivery systems
- Progress in technology and medical management of some disorders and an increase in iatrogenic disorders
- Shifts in values and ethics that will profoundly affect daily life

---

BOX 1-8   Top 10 Resolutions of the 2005 WHCoA

- Reauthorize the Older Americans Act within the first 6 months following the 2005 WHCoA
- Develop a coordinated, comprehensive long-term care strategy by supporting public and private sector initiatives that address financing, choice, quality, service delivery, and the paid and unpaid workforce
- Ensure that older Americans have transportation options to retain their mobility and independence
- Strengthen and improve the Medicaid program for seniors
- Strengthen and improve the Medicare program
- Support geriatric education and training for all health-care professionals, paraprofessionals, health profession students, and direct care workers
- Promote innovative models of non-institutional long-term care
- Improve recognition, assessment, and treatment of mental illness and depression among older Americans
- Attain adequate numbers of health care personnel in all professions who are skilled, culturally competent, and specialized in geriatrics
- Improve state and local based integrated delivery systems to meet 21st century needs of seniors

Data from News from the 2005 White House Conference on Aging (WHCoA). Available at *www.whcoa.gov.*

Articles about menopause proliferate, midlife crises abound, and anxiety about the future is rampant. Will there be income support, adequate retirement, available health care, disability benefits, and all the things the present generation of the old have relied on? The major concerns of baby boomers are health, finances, job security, sending children to college, and caring for parents. They have been called the "sandwich generation," because they try to meet the needs of "boomerang" children (those young adults who repeatedly return home because they cannot generate sufficient incomes to live independently) and elderly parents. Often they are also the primary caretakers of grandchildren. Shirley Chater (a nurse and a former director of Social Security) called them the "double whopper" generation. Gerontologists, marketing strategists, and the age industry are attempting to predict anticipated challenges.

Many uncertainties remain about the conditions, status, and benefits baby boomers will experience. Some of the major concerns are based in the shift of lifestyles away from the traditional family. Single parents, blended families, limited parenthood, unmarried parents, and gay and lesbian parents all represent lifestyles that may or may not produce children willing or available to assist parents as they age (see Chapter 20 for further discussion of caregiving roles and responsibilities).

Global challenges must be considered as well. Policies are needed that will adequately meet income, health, and long-term care needs for women as well as men throughout the world. The following are some of the issues and strategies that have been proposed for consideration by the international community (AOA International Division, 2002). First and foremost, especially in some of the less-developed countries, is that women and men should have equal access to resources, the right of inheritance, and ownership of land. Others include the following:

- Adapt economic security systems that protect young and old, and remove gender biases.
- Provide access to basic education and lifelong learning opportunities.
- Teach the continuity of life to children at very young ages.
- Promote healthy lifestyles and avoidance of risk behaviors.
- Ensure universal and affordable access to adequate health care.
- Support age-integrated environments using universal design principles.
- Provide training, counseling, financial assistance, and social service supports to adapt to the changing needs of families and their vulnerable members.

Many other suggestions can be retrieved from *www.ban-gate. aoa.dhhs.gov*. The message is that a much better distribution of resources and opportunities to all ages and cultures worldwide is essential if civilization is to endure.

Historically, nurses have always been in the front lines caring for older adults. They have provided hands-on care, supervision, administration, program development, teaching, and research and to a great extent are responsible for the rapid advance of gerontology as a profession. Gerontological nursing research has gained wide acceptance in the scientific community and has shown that better care is possible and should be expected. Nurses have been and continue to be the mainstay of care of older adults (Mezey and Fulmer, 2002; Wykle and McDonald, 1997).

The solid foundation built by the geriatric nursing pioneers and the current leaders in the specialty; the commitment of gerontological nurses to "tackle difficult but exceptionally meaningful issues that impact profoundly on the health and quality of life for older adults" (Mezey and Fulmer, 2002, p. M440); the opportunities for decision making, independent action, and innovation; and the significant contribution of gerontological nursing research to improved patient outcomes and health policy position the specialty for continued growth, recognition, contribution, and value to society. Dare we say that gerontological nursing will be the most needed specialty in nursing as the number of older people continues to increase and the need for our specialized knowledge becomes even more critical in every specialty and every health care setting (Ebersole and Touhy, 2006)? As Mezey and Fulmer (2002) have suggested, we need to ensure that, in the future, all older adults will be cared for by a nurse who has received special preparation in gerontological nursing.

KEY CONCEPTS

- Although the population as a whole is aging, the greatest categorical increase by group percentage is occurring among those 85 years old and older.
- Old age must be studied as a complex phenomenon with biopsychosocial and spiritual aspects affecting the manner in which an individual ages.
- Each cohort of older people is in some ways distinctly different from others, and individual older persons become more unique the longer they live. Thus one must be careful in attributing any specific characteristics to "old age."
- Normal old age cannot be easily measured as compared with young or middle adulthood.
- It is expected that as the majority of baby boomers become categorically old, in about the year 2010, many changes will occur in the experience of aging in the United States.
- The serious study of gerontology in the United States is comparatively new, reaching back only about 50 years.
- The number of centenarians is increasing rapidly, and the study of their lives holds fascination for many scientists and laypersons.
- Political actions and appropriations have had far-reaching influence on the individual experience of aging, chiefly through Medicare, Medicaid, and Social Security.
- With the advance of medical science, there has been a tendency to prolong the lives of the old and to consider their medical needs predominant.
- Nursing has led the field in gerontology because nurses were the first professionals in the nation to be certified as geriatric specialists.
- Certification assures the public of nurses' commitment to specialized education and qualification for the care of older people.

LONG-TERM CARE **ACUTE CARE** **COMMUNITY CARE**

Provide a milieu for living and holistic support in illness and dying

Support patient in achieving highest level of autonomy possible in situation

Make clients and families aware of options and resources
Involve clients in citizens' councils and political action groups
Support legislation affecting opportunities for older adults

Teach resident and families
Counsel resident and families
Learn about and use community resources, advise family and patient of same
Establish short-term and long-term goals: evaluate progress toward both periodically
Secure and maintain health, recreation, and social history

Provide appropriate information to patient and families about treatment plan, medications, and diagnosis in collaboration with physician

Teach clients and families
Cousult and collaborate with agencies and multiprofessional representatives
Educate clients to self-responsibility for health

Plan and coordinate care
Teach ancillary personnel
Communicate resident's needs in written and verbal form

Collaborate with multiprofessionals, patient, and family to develop a comprehensive care plan
Supervise ancillary personnel

Promote health through clinic and home contact
Provide appropriate resources
Identify health, social, or economic needs
Counsel clients and family members

Give treatments, medications, and rehabilitative exercises
Observe and evaluate patient response to treatment, medication, and care plan
Teach health care maintenance to staff and residents

Recognize implications of geriatric syndromes for patient care (e.g., falls, UI, delirium)
Protect patient from injury, iatrogenic disease, excess disability
Perform physical and psychological assessment and integrate in nursing care plan
Initiate action as outlined in evidence-based protocols regarding various conditions

Report case findings and make appropriate referral
Assess environmental safety
Assess response to illness and ability to follow treatment regimen
Provide information about medications and treatments

Keep physician aware of changes in residents' conditions
Institute life-saving measures in the absence of a physician
Perform physical assessment of residents
Ensure adequate medical, dental, and podiatric care for residents
Maintain hydration, nutrition, aeration, and comfort

Provide emergency treatment as needed for cardiopulmonary crisis, amelioration of shock, hemorrhage, convulsions, poisoning
Alert physician to changes in patient status and abnormal findings of tests
Maintain hydration, nutrition, aeration, and comfort

Provide health surveillance
Identify health, social, and economic need
Assist client and family to modify patterns detrimental to health
Evaluate deviations from normal and advise clients of appropriate action
Identify existing or impending illness
Encourage health promotion activities

Nursing function in caring for older adults in institutions and in the community.

Human Needs and Wellness Diagnoses

Self-Actualization and Transcendence
(Seeking, Expanding, Spirituality, Fulfillment)
Continues learning
Develops creative practice concepts
Seeks personal growth and enlightenment
Seeks spiritual growth and supports it in others
Seeks intellectual stimulation

Self-Esteem and Self-Efficacy
(Image, Identity, Control, Capability)
Is recognized for competence
Is professionally respected
Exerts leadership when needed
Seeks adequate resources and opportunities

Belonging and Attachment
(Love, Empathy, Affiliation)
Expresses genuine concern for clients
Affiliates with professionals and nonprofessionals
Supports colleagues appropriately
Demonstrates compassion

Safety and Security
(Caution, Planning, Protections, Sensory Acuity)
Protects self from contact with hazardous materials
Protects self from contracting infectious conditions
Protects self from injury by use of appropriate body mechanics
Follows established protocols and legal requirements

Biological and Physiological Integrity
(Air, Fluids, Comfort, Activity, Nutrition, Elimination, Skin Integrity)
Recognizes and honors own need for rest and relaxation
Develops habits that encourage healthy bodily functions

These are not all the possible wellness diagnoses that may be identified. The above are examples of nursing diagnoses that should be considered when planning care for the older adult.

- Requirements for accreditation of nursing programs should include solid evidence of special study in the care of older adults.
- The major U.S. organizations devoted exclusively to nurses caring for older people are the National Gerontological Nursing Association, the National Conference of Gerontological Nurse Practitioners, and the National Association Directors of Nursing Administration in Long Term Care.
- Clinical research in gerontological nursing is becoming more prevalent because nurses are better prepared and more confident in conducting research.
- The major changes in health care delivery have resulted in numerous revised, refined, and emergent roles for nurses in the field of gerontology.
- Advanced practice nurses have either nurse practitioner qualifications or clinical nurse specialist education. Advanced practice role opportunities for nurses are numerous and are seen as potentially saving money in health care delivery while facilitating more holistic health care.
- Gerontological nurses who desire to do so have found many opportunities for independent practice.
- Gerontological nursing at its best requires specialized education, maturity, commitment, and sensitivity.

STUDY QUESTIONS

What do you think are the triggering events that have increased your interest in aging persons?

Name five beliefs you have that are based on your experience with aging people. Discuss these and locate references within the text that either support or refute your belief.

Complete the Expectations Regarding Aging Survey, and discuss (Sarkisian CA et al: Development of the 12-item Expectations Regarding Aging [ERA-12] Survey, *Gerontologist* 45:240-248, 2005).

What are some of the sociocultural factors that have influenced our present views of older people?

How has the history of aging influenced our present concerns about aging?

How do you picture yourself at the age of 80? What do you hope for in your old age?

What do you think are the primary concerns for your parents or older relatives as they grow older? What are their views on growing older? What advice would they give to younger people about growing old?

Discuss your thoughts about the relevance of the nursing educational system to the actual care of older people.

Discuss your expectations of and obligations toward professional organizations that relate to nursing and gerontology.

Survey your community for available positions in nursing, and summarize the areas of need and those that are being neglected.

Interview a supervising nurse in each of the following settings: hospital, emergency department, home care, hospice, and nursing home. Ask the supervising nurses what they consider to be the greatest needs in the care of older adults within their settings. Ask what they consider to be the advantages of their setting in the care of older people.

Compare variations in institutional and community roles in gerontological nursing, and discuss some of the underlying differences.

Prioritize some of the immediate needs in the field of gerontological nursing and how these might best be addressed.

Discuss some of the pioneers in gerontic nursing and how their contributions and thoughts have affected your feelings about gerontic nursing.

Write a short essay (two or three pages) about the old person you have enjoyed or most respected in your lifetime.

Develop a collage depicting themes of aging.

Explore literature and identify attitudes toward aging conveyed in the literature.

Carefully examine the photograph of an unknown elder. Make up a story about him or her.

RESEARCH QUESTIONS

What aspects of gerontological nursing roles do nurses find most gratifying?

Why do so few students choose gerontological nursing as a field of practice? What factors might encourage more interest in the specialty?

Why do nursing home nurses stay, and why do they leave?

What is the actual time spent in baccalaureate nursing programs on clinical experiences caring for older people?

What is the actual time in the curriculum of baccalaureate nursing schools spent on content related only to the care of older people?

At what age or in which circumstances are individuals most likely to begin considering their own aging?

What are the most frequently held assumptions related to the experience of aging?

What effect has the changing intergenerational structure had on attitudes toward aging?

What are the concerns of younger people and baby boomers related to aging?

RESOURCES

American Association of Colleges of Nursing
www.aacn.nche.edu/

American Geriatric Society
www.americangeriatrics.org

American Medical Directors Association
www.amda.com

American Nurses Association
www.nursingworld.com

American Nurses Credentialing Center
www.nursingworld.org/ancc/

American Society on Aging
www.asaging.org

Canadian Gerontological Nursing Association
www.cgna.net

Creating Careers in Geriatric Advance Practice Nursing
www.aacn.nche.edu/Education/Hartford/creating.htm

Faculty Development in Geriatric Nursing—Mather Lifeways
www.matherlifeways.com/Re_facultydevelopment.asp

Gerontological Society of America
www.geron.org

Geronurse Online
www.geronurseonline.org

Hartford Institute for Geriatric Nursing
www.hartfordign.org

Help Age International
www.helpage.org/

International Association of Gerontology and Geriatrics
www.iagg.com.br/webforms/iaggMission.aspx

International Federation on Aging
www.ifa-fiv.org/en/accueil.aspx

International Plan of Action on Aging
www.who.int/gb/ebwha/pdf_files/EB115/B115_29-en.pdf

John A. Hartford Centers of Geriatric Nursing Excellence
University of California: San Francisco
www.Nurseweb.ucsf.edu/www./hcgne.htm
University of Arkansas for Medical Sciences
hartfordcenter.uams.edu
Oregon Health Science and Science University
www.ohsu.edu/hartfordcgne/
University of Pennsylvania
www.nursing.upenn.edu/centers/hcgne/
University of Iowa
www.nursing.uiowa.edu/Hartford/

National Association Directors of Nursing Administration in Long Term Care
www.nadona.org

National Conference of Gerontological Nurse Practitioners
www.ncgnp.org

National Gerontological Nursing Association
www.ngna.org

Nurse Competence in Aging
www.ana.org/anf/nca/htm

Springer Publishing Series on Geriatric Nursing
www.springerpub.com/store/SSGN/html

REFERENCES

Administration on Aging (AOA): *Geographic distribution—a profile of older Americans,* 2001. Available at *www.aoa.gov/aoa/stats/profile/2001/6.html.*

Administration on Aging (AOA), International Division, Department of Health and Human Services: *Strategies for a society for all ages,* Oct 2002. Available at *www.aoa.dhhs.gov/international/soc-allage-eng.html.*

American Association of Retired Persons (AARP): *Global aging: achieving its potential,* Washington, DC, 2001, The Association.

American Geriatrics Society Core Writing Group of the Task Force on the Future of Geriatric Medicine: Caring for older Americans: the future of geriatric medicine, *J Am Geriatr Soc* 53(suppl 6):245-256, 2005.

Berman A et al: Gerontological nursing content in baccalaureate programs: comparison of findings from 1997 and 2003, *J Prof Nurs* 21(5):268-275, 2005.

Binstock R: The War on "Anti-Aging Medicine," *Gerontologist* 43(1):4-14, 2003.

Buckwalter KC et al: Managing cognitive impairment in the elderly: conceptual, intervention and methodological issues, *Online J Knowl Synth Nurs* 6:10, Nov 1999.

Burnside IM: Listen to the aged, *Am J Nurs* 75(10): 1801, 1975.

Cantor N: *In the wake of the plague,* New York, 2002, Harper Collins.

Christensen D: Making sense of centenarians: genes and life style help people live through a century, *Science News Online* 159(10): 156, 2001. Available at *www.sciencenews.org.*

Crane C: Almshouse nursing: the human need, *Am J Nurs* 7:872-881, 1907.

Davis B: Nursing care of the aged: historical evolution, *Bull Am Assoc Hist Nurs* 47, 1985.

Dock L: The crusade for almshouse nursing, *Am J Nurs* 8(7): 520, 1908.

Dowling-Castronova A: Gerontological nursing—advanced practice. In Fitzpatrick J, Wallace M, editors, *Geriatric Nursing Research Digest,* New York, 2000, Springer.

Ebersole P et al: *Gerontological nursing and healthy aging,* ed 2, St. Louis, 2005, Mosby.

Ebersole P, Touhy T: *Geriatric nursing: growth of a specialty,* New York, 2006, Springer.

Elsner RJF et al: Ethical and policy considerations for centenarians—the oldest-old, *Image J Nurs Sch* 31(3):263, 1999.

Ferrell BR: The marriage: geriatric and oncology, *Geriatr Nurs* 20(5):238-240, 1999.

Fitzpatrick JJ, editor: *Annu Rev Nurs Res* 20, 2002 (entire issue devoted to geriatric nursing research).

Foreman M et al: Delirium in elderly patients: an overview of the state of the science, *J Gerontolog Nurs* 2(4):12-20, 2001.

Fulmer TT: Elder mistreatment, *Annu Rev Nurs Res* 20:369, 2002.

Gelbach S: Nursing care of the aged, *Am J Nurs* 43(12):1113, 1943.

Greene R, Administration on Aging (AOA): *American Society on Aging (ASA) CAREPro Project report,* ANA, Philadelphia, July 1, 2002.

Harrington C: Addressing the dramatic decline in RN staffing in nursing homes, *Am J Nurs,* 105(9), 25, 2005.

Harrington C et al: Experts recommend minimum staffing standards for nursing facilities in the United States, *Gerontologist* 40(1):5-16, 2000.

Hinshaw AS: Nursing knowledge for the 21st century: opportunities and challenges, *J Nurs Scholarsh* 32(2):117, 2000.

Horn S et al: RN staffing time and outcomes of long-stay nursing home residents, *Am J Nurs* 105(11):58-70, 2005.

Hounsell C, Riojas A: Older women face tarnished "golden years," *Aging Today* 7,9 March-April, 2006.

Hudacek S: *Making a difference: stories from the point of care,* Indianapolis, Ind, 2000, Center Nursing Press, Sigma Theta Tau International Society of Nursing.

Klein S, editor: *A national agenda for geriatric education,* New York, 1997, Springer.

Leppa CJ: The nature of LTC nursing work, *J Gerontolog Nurs* 30(3):36-43, 2004.

Mack M: Personal adjustment of chronically ill old people under home care, *Nurs Res* 9-30, 1952.

Mantle JH: Personal communication, March 2, 2005.

Matzo ML, Sherman DW: *Quality nursing care for the older adult at the end of their life,* St. Louis, 2003, Mosby.

Mentes J: On being 100 and healthy, *J Gerontolog Nurs* 32(4):6, 2006.

Mezey M, Fulmer T: The future history of gerontological nursing, *J Gerontol A Biol Sci Med Sci* 57(7):M438-441, 2002.

Mezey M, Harrington C: Addressing the dramatic decline in RN staffing in nursing homes, *Am J Nurs* 105(9):25, 2005.

Mezey M et al: A perfect NICHE for gerontology nurses, *Geriatr Nurs* 23(3):118, 2002 (entire issue devoted to models of geriatric nursing practice).

Mezey M et al: NPs in nursing homes: an issue of quality, *Am J Nurs* 104(9):71, 2004a.

Mezey M et al: Nurses improving care to healthsystem elders (NICHE): implementation of best practice models, *J Nurs Adm* 34(10):451-457, 2004b.

Mezey M et al: Nursing expertise in caring for older adults, *Am J Nurs* 104(9):72, 2004c.

Mitchell P et al: AACN demonstration project: profile of excellence in critical care nursing, *Heart Lung* 18:219-222, 1989.

Moore V: Senior Operations Specialist, American Nurses Credentialing Center. Personal communication, June 29, 2006.

Nascher I: *Geriatrics*, Philadelphia, 1914, P. Blakiston's Son & Co.

National Center for Health Statistics (2004).

Sarkisian CA et al: Development of the 12-item Expectations Regarding Aging (ERA-12) Survey, *Gerontologist* 45: 240-248, 2005.

Silver MH et al: Cognitive functional status of age-confirmed centenarians in a population-based study, *J Gerontol B Psychol Sci Soc Sci* 56(3):134-140, 2001.

Strumpf NE: Innovative gerontological practices as models for health care delivery, *Nurs Health Care* 15(10):522-527, 1994.

Strumpf NE: The dynamic partnership of Lois K. Evans and Neville E. Strumpf. In Ebersole PR: Geriatric nursing leaders. *Geriatr Nurs* 24(2): 110-112, 2003.

Strumpf NE et al: *Restraint-free care: individualized approached for frail elders*, New York, 1998, Springer.

United Nations Population Division: *World population highlights, Nov 2002*. Available at *www.un.org/esa/population/unpop.htm*.

U.S. Census Bureau: *Statistical abstract of the United States: 2002*, ed 122, Washington, DC, 2001, U.S. Government Printing Office.

U.S. Census Bureau: The 2007 Statistical Abstract: The National Data Book. Accessed February 17, 2007, from *www.census.gov/compendia/statab/population*.

U.S. Senate Special Committee on Aging: *Swindlers, hucksters and snake oil salesmen: hype and hope marketing anti-aging products to seniors*, serial no 107-114, Washington, DC, 2001, U.S. Government Printing Office.

Wolanin MO: Personal communication, San Antonio, Tex, Sept 1995.

Wykle M, McDonald P: The past, present and future of gerontological nursing. In Dimond J et al, editors: *A national agenda for geriatric education*, New York, 1997, Springer.

CHAPTER 2

Theories of Aging

Kathleen Jett

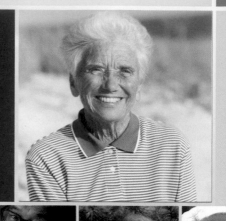
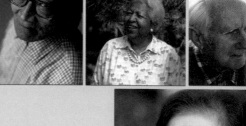
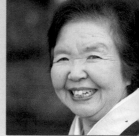

A STUDENT LEARNS

Due to the fact that some periods of life are set apart by certain events, it is generally assumed that a period labeled "Old Age" begins with a definite entrance at a certain year or following some outward event which manifests its beginning. However, unless there is a sudden onset of one of the chronic bodily disorders associated with age, we cannot detect an external symbol of entrance into old age.

Tatyana Urisman, age 30

AN ELDER SPEAKS

When I was a young girl Einstein was proposing the molecular theory of matter, and we still believed there were some truths that were beyond dispute. We had never heard of DNA or RNA and only knew of genes in the most rudimentary theoretical sense. Now truth is the greatest of all the theories of relativity, and I hear that scientists believe there is a gene that is controlling my life span. I really hope they find it before I die.

Bessie, age 72

LEARNING OBJECTIVES

On completion of this chapter, the reader will be able to:

1. Discuss the origins of the definitions of aging.
2. Differentiate stochastic from nonstochastic theories of biological aging.
3. Recommend strategies to promote healthy aging that are consistent with the state of the science of biological theories of aging.
4. Compare and contrast the major sociological theories of aging, and discuss.
5. Use at least one sociological theory of aging to support or refute commonly provided social services for older adults living in the community.
6. Create strategies to foster the highest level of wellness in aging based on the theories of Jung, Erikson, Peck, and Maslow.
7. Explain how personality may influence the lived experience of aging.

Theories are an attempt to explain phenomena, to give a sense of order, and to provide a framework from which we can view the world. People have been trying to explain the phenomena of aging since at least when history was first recorded (Birren and Schroots, 2001). For much of that time, scientists have been trying to use the information to try to reverse the process, to find the illusive "fountain of youth."

Although we have not yet come to a conclusion on why we age, we do know that aging is a process that begins at conception and continues until death (Ignatavicius and Workman, 2005). Aging in humans is influenced by changes in all aspects of personhood, be they biological, psychological, social, functional, or spiritual. Taken together, we come to know the person as he or she ages. A gerontological nurse can make an impact on health and wellness regardless of age.

The extant theories of aging are no longer thought to be in competition with each other. Instead, each offers a view of different and often overlapping aspects of the changes we

Special thanks to Patricia Hess, the previous edition contributor, for her content contributions to this chapter.

associate with aging. Only when considering them together can we begin to understand aging and begin to set our priorities in promoting health in late life.

This chapter provides the reader with an overview of the prominent theories of aging—those addressing biological, psychological, and sociological processes.

WHAT IS AGING?

In everyday language, aging is most often described in terms of chronology, or by the measurement of time since birth. In the United States one becomes "old" at 65 years or when one qualifies for retirement income. In other countries this number varies. Chronological aging is tied to social aging. Social age is measured by age-graded behaviors carrying an expected status and role within a particular culture or society. Transitions are often marked by ritual, for example, the retirement party, the receipt of the "gold watch." Type of dress, language, and role participation are reflections of social aging. Some groups define aging in functional terms that one becomes "old" when one is no longer able to perform one's usual activities (Jett, 2003).

Biological aging is viewed as an expression of the declining functional capacity of the most basic structures in the cells, which in turn affects the functioning of the organism, be it a yeast cell or a human being. Through the study of biorhythms, functional capacity has been found to change not only slowly over time but also in the course of the day and night (Erren et al., 2003). Circadian rhythms, or day/night shifts in capacity and function, are time and light dependent and regulate many hormonal and enzymatic processes. Some evidence exists that biorhythms are altered and become less consistently rhythmic during the aging process.

BIOLOGICAL THEORIES OF AGING

The biological theories of aging today have evolved from the early consideration of the changes over the life span of the organism. Two opposing meta-theoretical views formed the foundations for biological life span developmental theories. Although they differ significantly, both viewpoints agree that, in the end, the body as an organism becomes disorganized or chaotic and is no longer able to sustain itself and death ensues. The first view is that biological characteristics are both basic and complex. As a diminution of energy evolves over time, the organism becomes less capable of maintaining both the basic and complex characteristics; the basic characteristics are maintained at the expense of more complex characteristics. With the loss of the complex characteristics, the organism eventually becomes increasingly chaotic before death.

The contrasting view is that people, as living organisms, tend to differentiate with aging and replace basic characteristics with those of increasing complexity. Unable to maintain the complexity indefinitely, the differentiation yields to disorganization, again before death. Birren and Schroots (2001) suggested that the ultimate disorganization begins when the central nervous system control mechanisms lose their effectiveness in maintaining the dynamic equilibrium necessary to adapt to changes in the internal and external environment.

In recent years there has been considerable research on the biological theories of aging with an emphasis on the cell and the molecules and components within the cell. A great deal of bench research has been conducted in an attempt to unlock the "secrets of the cell."

Cellular Functioning

An understanding of the biological theories of aging requires a basic understanding of the functions of the cell. The architectural basis of an organism begins with the cell and cell division. Cell division, or doubling, continues as the organism grows. The organs and systems within the organism develop at different rates. Throughout the organism's life span, most but not all the cells are able to continue to divide and replicate themselves into newer, theoretically identical cells. As long as the cell can reproduce through division, it is alive. Two of the elements of the cell, deoxyribonucleic acid (DNA) and ribonucleic acid (RNA), serve as templates for reproduction, ensuring the same genetic components appear in the new cells.

Changes to the cell that decrease its ability to replicate are attributed to aging. Some of these changes occur independent of any external or pathological influences (Davidovic et al., 2003). The major biological questions are (1) what triggers the process of aging and (2) can it be stopped or modulated.

Biological theories of aging are divided into two major groups: stochastic and nonstochastic (Box 2-1). Stochastic theories propose that aging is a series of adverse cellular events that cause replicative errors. These errors occur randomly and accumulate over time. When the errors accumulate to a critical point, cell death occurs. Nonstochastic theories propose that the replicative errors associated with aging and death are intrinsic, predetermined, and timed—that is, programmed.

Stochastic (Error) Theories

The error theories propose that aging is the result of an accumulation of errors in the synthesis of cellular DNA and RNA, the basic building blocks of the cell (Short et al., 2005). With each replication, more errors occur until the cell is no longer able to function and dies (Sonneborn, 1979). When enough cells die, the organism dies. One of the variations of the error theory is that of the *Somatic Mutation Theory* recognizing the errors stimulated when the cells are exposed to x-ray radiation or chemical. Although the errors of mutation can be demonstrated, their association to the aging process is not clear (Finch and Ruvkun, 2001; Jacobs, 2003; Kirkwood and Proctor, 2002). Another version of this theory, known as the *Error-Catastrophe Theory of Aging*, has not been supported in research (Hipkiss, 2003). The three additional error theories discussed here are *Wear and Tear*, *Cross-Linkage*, and *Free Radicals*.

BOX 2-1 Biological Theories of Aging

STOCHASTIC THEORIES

The error theories propose that aging is a result of an accumulation of errors in the synthesis of cellular deoxyribonucleic acid (DNA) and ribonucleic acid (RNA), the basic building blocks of the cell (Short et al., 2005). With each replication, more errors occur until the cell can no longer function and dies.

Wear-and-Tear Theory

The wear-and-tear theory proposes that errors result when cells wear out over time because of continued use. Cells are aggravated by the harmful effects of internal and external stressors, which include injurious metabolic by-products. These may cause a progressive decline in cellular function and the death of an increasing number of cells.

Cross-Linkage Theory

This theory describes aging in terms of the accumulation of errors through a process of cross-linking, or stiffening of proteins in the body. Cross-linking is initiated by blood glucose as it attaches itself to a protein, causing a chain reaction of bonding or "cross-linking" between protein molecules. As they link, they become stiff and thick and less able to function.

Free Radical Theory

Free radicals are randomly produced natural by-products of cellular metabolism of oxygen and are always present to some extent. They are molecules that contain unpaired ions (electrical charge) and are highly reactive to molecules in the cell membrane. As the free ion charge latches onto other molecules, damage occurs, especially to the membranes of unsaturated lipids such as mitochondria and lysosomes. The body produces antioxidant substances to counter these effects, but it is believed that, with aging, more free radicals are produced and the ability of the body to counter the effects of them is decreased as well.

NONSTOCHASTIC THEORIES

The nonstochastic theories are those in which the changes of aging are attributed to a process that is programmed and thought to be predetermined.

Programmed Theory

The initial premise of the programmed aging theories, or as they were originally called, *biological* or *genetic clock theories*, begins with the assumption that the cell and organism have a genetically determined life span and life process (Hayflick, 1996).

Immunity Theory

In this case, the emphasis is on the senescence of the immune cells from the damage from the proliferation of free radicals (De la Fuente, 2002; Effros et al., 2003). Animal studies have demonstrated that the cells of the immune system become increasingly more diversified with age and predictably lose some of their self-regulatory ability (Miller, 1996; Strehler, 1960; Walford, 1983). Age-related changes in the immune system lead to decreased efficiency and is seen clinically as reduced immune functioning and may be associated with increased rates of infection and cancer. It is also thought to lead to an auto-aggressive phenomenon in which normal cells are misidentified as alien and are attacked by the body's own immune system. This phenomenon is used to explain the increase of autoimmune disorders as we age (Meiner and Lueckenotte, 2006).

Wear-and-Tear Theory. One of the earliest of the contemporary theories is based on wear and tear. The Wear-and-Tear Theory proposes that cell errors are the result of "wearing out" over time because of continued use. Cells are aggravated by the harmful effects of internal and external stressors, which include injurious metabolic by-products. These may cause a progressive decline in cellular function or the death of an increasing number of cells. Striated muscle, heart muscle, muscle fibers, nerve cells, and the brain are non-replaceable when destroyed by wear and tear or by mechanical or chemical injury.

This theory was first proposed in 1882 (Hayflick, 1988). Its proponents point to the evidence of microscopic damage to striated and smooth muscle fibers and nerve cells produced from "wear." However, strongly conflicting studies have found that the body can repair and increase function of the older, worn muscles through daily exercise.

Cross-Linkage Theory. Much effort is being directed at consideration of the cross-linkage theory of aging. This approach describes aging in terms of the accumulation of errors through a process of cross-linking, or stiffening of proteins in the body. Cross-linking is initiated by blood glucose through a process of glycosylation or glycation. The glucose attaches itself to a protein, which causes a chain reaction of bonding or "cross-linking" between protein molecules. As they link, they become stiff and thick. The new cross-linked proteins are called AGEs, or *advanced glycation end-products.*

Because collagens are the most plentiful proteins in the body, this is where the cross-linking can be seen most easily in the form of stiffened joints and roughened skin. Skin that was once smooth, silky, firm, and soft becomes drier, saggy, and less elastic with age. Collagen is also a key component of the lungs, arteries, and tendons, and similar changes can be seen there (see Chapter 4). Cross-linking may also cause cholesterol to attach to cell walls, leading to atherosclerosis, and the lens to cloud and stiffen, leading to cataracts.

Substances that may act as cross-linking agents include unsaturated fats and metal ions such as aluminum, zinc, and magnesium. Many medications taken by older adults (e.g., antacids, anticoagulants) contain aluminum and may exacerbate cross-linking, although a causative effect has not yet been clarified. We do know that the metals are also associated with damage from free radicals (see the Free Radical Theory section that follows) and are under investigation (Valko et al., 2005).

One area of promise is that related to diabetes in younger persons. Those with high levels of free blood glucose also have high levels of AGEs with resultant early "aging" of the organs. Finding ways to interrupt the linking may show us new and effective strategies to maximize health and function with diabetes and while aging (NIA, 2003).

Free Radical Theory. Proponents of the free radical theory claim that errors are the result of random damage from free radicals. Free radicals are natural by-products of the cellular metabolism of oxygen and are always present to some extent. In the immune system, free radicals are useful for destroying bacteria and other foreign substances. Free radicals are molecules that contain unpaired ions and therefore an extra electrical charge. They exist only momentarily but are highly reactive to molecules in the cell membrane. As the free ion charge latches onto other molecules, damage occurs, especially to the membranes of unsaturated lipids such as mitochondria and lysosomes. Some of the oxygen that would have been used for energy in the form of adenosine triphosphate (ATP) is no longer available. This process is called *lipid peroxidation.*

It is known that exposure of the organism to environmental pollutants and other stressors increases the production of free radicals and increases the rate of damage. The best known of the environmental pollutants include smog and ozone, pesticides, and radiation. Other environmental sources thought to cause increases in free radicals are gasoline, by-products in the plastic industry, and drying linseed oil paints (Hampton, 1991; Sharma, 1988).

In youth, naturally occurring vitamins, hormones, enzymes, and antioxidants are present to neutralize the free radicals as needed (Valko et al., 2005). However, when the accumulation of the damage caused by the action of the free radicals occurs faster than the cells can repair themselves, cell death occurs (Grune et al., 2001).

In simplistic terms, the free radical theory of aging, first proposed by Harman (1956), advocates that, over time, the production of free radicals increases and the body's ability to neutralize them decreases (De la Fuente, 2002). This theory continues to stimulate a great deal of cutting-edge research and thought by some as having the most promise for both the explanation of aging and the potential to reverse some of the signs of aging (Balaban et al, 2005, NIA, 2003). It is also referred to as oxidative stress theory.

Free Radicals and Antioxidants. Significant research is also underway to understand the effect of substances with antioxidant effects, that is, the ability to counter the effects of the free radicals. The effects of vitamins and dietary supplements have been particularly examined. These products were thought to either affect oxidation rates (and therefore the production of free radicals) or affect the accumulation of the free radicals (and therefore affect the potential damage to the cell).

Studies of vitamin E found that deficiencies (rare) increase excessive lipid oxidation. At normal cellular levels of vitamin E, an antioxidant effect is seen as a slower oxidation rate occurs, especially on low-density lipoproteins (AHRQ,

2003; Scheer, 1996; Valko et al., 2005). However, when taken to an organism level, research into the therapeutic effects of vitamin E, especially in heart disease, has been conflicting (AHRQ, 2003).

Vitamin C, the hormone melatonin (Valko et al., 2005), coenzyme Q10, niacin, and several naturally occurring enzymes (including mutase, catalase, and glutathione peroxidase) are thought to have antioxidant features as free radical scavengers (Hampton, 1991). More recently there is evidence of the scavenging antioxidant activity of BHT, BHA, and selenium (Valko et al., 2005). The scavengers are able to degrade, neutralize, or detoxify free radicals, thereby minimizing the ensuing damage. Again, when taken to the cellular level, the use of vitamin C supplementation may reduce free radicals but has not been supported for prevention in cardiovascular disease, and coenzyme Q10 has had mixed results (AHRQ, 2003). A number of other substances with antioxidant properties include tumeric, cloves, capsaicin, and red chilies, and this number is growing (Borek, 2006).

The current and evolving evidence relating to the action of free radicals and the substances with potential to counter some deleterious effects also appears to have the potential for being invaluable in the promotion of the healthiest aging possible. Vitamin therapy, healthy environments, and monitoring the food (especially antioxidants) one consumes may soon take on special meaning relating to both health today and longevity in the future.

Nonstochastic Theories

The nonstochastic theories are those in which the changes of aging are attributed to a process that is programmed and thought to be predetermined. Much of the contemporary work on programmed aging has evolved from the groundbreaking of Hayflick and Moorehead (1981).

Programmed Aging Theory. The initial premise of the programmed aging theories, or as they were originally called, *biological clock theories*, begins with the assumption that the cell and organism have a genetically determined life span and life process. The development, maturation, and cessation of activity such as menopause, thymic atrophy, graying of hair, and myriad other changes are considered normal programmed changes of aging rather than indicators of potential pathology.

In the original experiments with human diploid cell strains, Hayflick and Moorehead (1981) found that cells replicated themselves only a limited number of times before dying. The number of cell divisions is proportional to the life span of the species. Translated into human terms, it was predicted that the maximum possible life expectancy is 110 to 120 years old (Hayflick, 1996). It is interesting to note that the original Hayflick and Moorehead work (1981) found that living cells could be preserved by keeping them at subzero temperatures for long periods. However, when thawed years later, the cells continued to replicate from the point at which they had been interrupted. The total number of replications remained constant. Although the concept of finite cell replications is recognized, the translation into maximum human longevity has been challenged by the emergence of several extremely long-lived people (Box 2-2).

Gene Theory. The genetic influence on aging is irrefutable; however, how it is manifested remains elusive. Biologists are beginning to locate genes that govern cellular mortality, and they are attempting to identify genes that are responsible for the "on-off switch" (Darrach, 1992; Recer, 2000; Schlessinger, 2000). A gene responsible for premature aging (Werner's syndrome) has been identified (King, 1996), causing excitement in biogerontological circles.

The research focus now is on the acknowledged grouping of "old genes" or those that have or will have detrimental effects over time that may or may not follow a set path. These genes can be divided into those that regulate the cellular response to oxidative stress (see Free Radical Theory), those that regulate inflammatory responses (see Immunity Theory) and those that affect overall metabolism (see Caloric Restriction Theory). Although the leap has not yet been made between organisms such as nematodes and fruit flies to humans, the work is progressing (Nemoto and Finkel, 2004).

Immunity Theory. Closely tied to the free radical theory is the immunity theory of aging. In this case, the emphasis is on the senescence of the immune cells from the damage from the proliferation of free radicals (De la Fuente, 2002; Effros et al., 2003). The immune system in the human body is a complex network of cells, tissues, and organs that function separately and together to protect the body from substances from the outside, such as pathogens. Through this protective, self-regulatory action, the body attempts to maintain homeostasis and functioning. Self-regulatory immunity is controlled by B lymphocyte (humoral) and T lymphocyte (cellular) systems. In the simplest terms, the specialized lymphocytes protect the body against invasion by infection or other matter considered foreign, such as tissue or organ transplants. The results of animal studies have demonstrated that the cells of the immune system become progressively more diversified with age and somewhat predictably lose

some of their self-regulatory ability (Miller, 1996). The T lymphocytes show more signs of "aging" than do the B lymphocytes. The T cells are thought to be responsible for hastening the age-related changes caused by autoimmune reactions as the body battles itself.

Graft-versus-host reaction experiments with mice have demonstrated significantly higher rejection rates of tissue grafts in older mice than in younger mice. This has led to the postulation that greater cell aberration occurs with age and that cell self-regulation is greatly lacking (Makinodan, 1990). This might be one reason why wound healing slows as we age, despite proper diet, rest, and care.

Whereas *replicative senescence* is the term used to apply to the cell's faltering ability to reproduce, *immunosenescence* is the term used to describe the age-related change in the immune system leading to decreased efficiency and seen clinically as reduced immune functioning and increased rates of infection and cancer. Immunosenescence also leads to an auto-aggressive phenomenon in which normal cells are misidentified as alien and are attacked by the body's own immune system. This phenomenon is used to explain the increase of autoimmune disorders as we age (Meiner and Lueckenotte, 2006).

Autoimmune disorders and aging may be correlated, as evidenced by several shared characteristics. Both processes exhibit lymphoid depletion and hypoplasia, thymic atrophy, and increased plasma cells in lymphoid organs. The most relevant pathological change that can be evidenced in the immune system with age is thymic atrophy. T-cell–dependent immunity is probably related to decreased circulating thymic hormone levels (Figure 2-1). As early as 1969 (Quinti et al., 1981), thymic transplants, as well as the administration of young thymocytes or thymic extract to patients, were shown to be able to correct several age-dependent immunological impairments, such as antibody formation. Autoimmune and

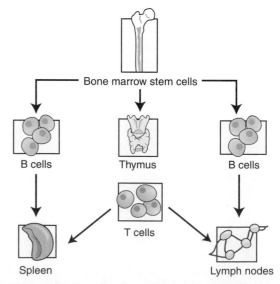

FIGURE 2-1 Cellular traffic of the immune system. (Modified from Finch C, Hayflick L, editors: *Handbook of the biology of aging,* New York, 1977, Van Nostrand Reinhold).

BOX 2-2   A Remarkably Long Life

On August 4, 1997, Mme Calment of Arles France died a rich woman at the age of 122 years and 4½ months, a super centenarian. In 1965, when she was 90 years old, her lawyer recognized the value of the apartment in which she lived and owned and made her, what turned out to be, the deal of a lifetime. In exchange for the deed to the apartment, he would pay her a monthly "pension" for life and she could live in the apartment the rest of her life. Over the next 32 years she was paid three times the apartment's value. She also outlived the lawyer, his son, her husband of 50 years, her daughter, and her only grandson. An active woman, she took up fencing at 85 and was still riding a bike at 100. She smoked until she was 117 and preferred a diet rich in olive oil (NIA, 2003; Nemoto and Finkel, 2004).

immunodeficient diseases in older adults illustrate the impact of the immunological theory on aging. Cell-mediated immunity decreases in older persons and may be responsible for decreased survival (Wayne et al., 1990).

An increasing number of health problems common to late life are being considered in terms of impaired immune functioning and autoimmunity. For example, individuals who require immunosuppressants are 80 times more vulnerable to cancer than those who do not receive such therapy (Makinodan, 1990). Alzheimer's disease, rheumatoid conditions, atherosclerosis, hypertension, and thromboembolism are among those being studied in relation to immunity. Some of the recent and potentially highly productive work has come from those studying human immunodeficiency virus (HIV) disease pathogenesis, finding replicative senescence of the CD8 T cells (Effros, 2003).

Emerging Biological Theories

Several areas appear to also hold promise in the ongoing search to understand biological aging (Box 2-3). In many ways, these newer approaches take the best of the past theories and extend them with emerging research findings. These include the theories of neuroendocrine (pacemaker) control, caloric restriction, and DNA-related possibilities.

Neuroendocrine Control or Pacemaker Theory. The neuroendocrine system regulates many essential activities related to the organisms' growth and development. The neuroendocrine (or pacemaker) theory focuses on the changes in these systems over time. For example, the female reproductive system is controlled by a combination of the endocrine and the nervous systems rather than the ovaries. From birth, it is expected that the reproductive system will slowly decline in functioning until menopause and, after that time, reproduction is not possible. It may be that common neurons in the high brain centers act as pacemakers that regulate the biological clock during development and aging and slow down and eventually "shut off" at the predetermined time (Guardiola-Lemaitre, 1997; Hayflick, 1996).

Aging is manifested in a slowing down or activity imbalance of the pacemaker neurons, affecting neural, muscular, and secretory function as evidenced in involution, reproduction, loss of fertility, decreased muscle strength, less ability to recover from stress, and impaired cardiovascular and respiratory activity. Specifically, the performance of an organism is linked to a variety of control mechanisms that regulate the interplay between different organs and tissues. Homeostatic adjustment declines, with consequent failure to adapt, followed by aging and death. Aging and death may be considered homeostatic failure. Understanding the aging of the reproductive cycle may help us better understand the process of biological aging because of the interconnectedness of the many neurotransmitters.

Much of the current research in this area is on the examination of the effect of hormones on neuroendocrine functioning over time, especially dehydroepiandrosterone (DHEA) and melatonin. DHEA is produced by the adrenal glands, and the amount secreted diminishes with time. Adding DHEA to the diets of experimental animals appears to have increased their longevity as will as bolstered their immune response (Legrain and Girard, 2003; Perrini et al., 2005). Melatonin, produced by the pineal gland, has been found to be a powerful regulator of biological rhythms and antioxidant. Its secretion is markedly reduced as one ages (Srinivasan et al., 2005). Other hormones under examination in relation to aging are growth factors, estrogen, and testosterone (NIA, 2003).

BOX 2-3　Emerging Biological Theories of Aging

NEUROENDOCRINE CONTROL OR PACEMAKER THEORY

The neuroendocrine system regulates many essential activities related to the organisms' growth and development. The neuroendocrine (or pacemaker) theory focuses on the changes in these systems over time. It may be that common neurons in the higher brain centers act as pacemakers that regulate the biological clock during development and aging and slow down and eventually "shut off" at the predetermined time. Much of the current research in this area is on the examination of hormones on neuroendocrine functioning over time, especially dehydroepiandrosterone (DHEA) and melatonin.

CALORIC RESTRICTION (METABOLIC) THEORY

Some animal studies since the 1930s have found that reductions in caloric intake by 30% have multiple positive effects, such as increasing the life span, slowing metabolism, lowering body temperature, and delaying the onset of most age-related diseases (NIA, 2003). In particular, caloric restriction has been found to reduce the level of lipid peroxidation and subsequent damage from oxidation. Speculation is that lower body temperature slows body biochemical reactions and lowers levels of pentosidine, a substance found to strongly correlate with onset of age-related diseases (Bokov et al., 2004).

GENETIC RESEARCH

As the human genome is being mapped, scientists continue to examine the role that both genetics and RNA has in both random and programmed aging and may eventually be able to explain senescence. Among the findings include that of the existence of telomeres, which serve as a type of capping of the ends of the chromosomes. With each cellular reproduction, the telomere is shortened, until a time when the telomere disappears and the cell can no longer reproduce and dies. Abnormal cells such as cancer cells produce an enzyme called *telomerase*, which actually lengthens the telomeres, enabling the cells to continue to reproduce. Learning to manipulate telomerase may have significant implications for both controlling cellular reproduction and aging.

Caloric Restriction (Metabolic) Theory. Another area of more recent interest is the effect of caloric restriction (Box 2-4). Animal studies since the 1930s have found that reductions in calories by 30% have multiple positive effects, such as increasing the life span, slowing metabolism, and delaying or reducing the onset of most age-related diseases (NIA, 2003). In particular, caloric restriction has been found to reduce the level of lipid peroxidation (see Free Radical Theory) and subsequent damage from oxidative stress (Bokov et al., 2004).

In a study on monkeys in 1987, researchers at the National Institute on Aging found that reducing their caloric intake by 30% led to lower body temperature. Speculation is that a lower body temperature slows body biochemical reactions and lowers levels of pentosidine, a substance that has been found to strongly correlate with onset of age-related diseases. Cutting calories may increase monkey life span by 30% to 50% (Ciabattari, 1996).

Research has also shown that dietary restriction hastens DNA repair. The theory of aging based on the accumulation of DNA damage in somatic cells is an old one, but it was unknown whether repair of DNA was gradually diminished in the aging process. These studies have shown that DNA repair processes are involved in aging, and not only does restricted caloric intake slow DNA error accumulation during aging but also it facilitates the repair process, resulting in longer-lived mice. The success of caloric restrictions on life extension of mice dates back to Cornero, who in 1507, because of illness at age 40, limited his food intake to 12 ounces a day and lived another 60 years.

More recently, the caloric restriction research has been challenged in that the effects have not been consistent in every experimental species; however, the area is still one of promise and has stimulated other hypotheses related to longevity (Masoro, 2006). Caloric restriction as a means of extending one's life span is being considered, along with high altitudes, decreased environmental temperature (Walford et al., 2002), and decreased core body temperature (Rosenfeld, 1985).

BOX 2-4   Research Highlights: Caloric Restriction

Walford (1986), a renowned and respected gerontologist and theorist in aging research, addresses this approach to life extension in The 120-Year Diet. Walford and seven other scientists lived in Biosphere 2, located in the Arizona desert, for 2 years and found themselves unexpectedly having to live on limited but nutrient-rich food and enforced caloric restrictions. The results were a positive effect on their hematologic, hormonal, and other biochemical parameters. Despite the drastic weight loss by all, both physical and mental activity remained at a high level. The situation was similar to the effect on caloric restrictions on experimental monkeys (Walford et al., 2002). A very important question is asked: Would people who are not living in a controlled environment tolerate or accept this drastic change in eating habits?

Genetic Research. As work on the human genome continues, new discoveries emerge. One of these with interesting implications for understanding aging from the perspective of the "biological clock" (see Programmed Aging Theory) is that related to the discovery of telomeres and the action of telomerase. It has been found that each chromosome is capped, so to speak, with structures known now as *telomeres*. With each cellular reproduction, the telomere is shortened until a time when the telomere disappears and the cell is no longer able to reproduce and dies (Figure 2-2). In striking contrast, abnormal cells, such as cancer cells, produce an enzyme called *telomerase*, which adds telomeres to the ends of the chromosome with each cell division (Keyes and Marble, 1998; NIA, 2003). Learning to manipulate telomerase may have significant implications for both controlling cellular reproduction and aging.

• • •

As more cell types are studied, the expression or repression of specific genes is appearing. It is hoped that more research will lead to the discovery of other pathways and key changes in gene expression used by other cells to establish senescence (Pereira-Smith and Bertram, 2000; Smith and Pereira-Smith, 1996). Biogerontological research has demonstrated that longevity is frequently considered to be related to enhanced metabolic capacity and the response to stress, as well as multiple mechanisms of aging (Jazwinski, 1996).

Although all these theories provide possible clues to aging, they also raise many questions and stimulate con-

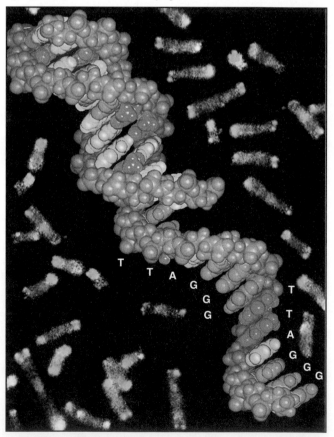

FIGURE 2-2 DNA Model. (From Jerry Shay and The University of Texas Southwestern Medical Center at Dallas; Office of News and Publications; 5323 Harry Hines Boulevard; Dallas, TX 75235.)

tinuing research. Many signs of normal aging may be the result of either random or programmed intrinsic cell death. Although strong evidence exists of genetic and therefore uncontrollable factors, significant environmental factors also may influence the speed at which we age. The frequency of mutations in mammalian aging is influenced by genetic mutation of autoimmune reactions, metabolic rate, genetic background, and environmental factors. In the past few years, the investigation of cellular senescence has expanded to additional cell types, such as endothelial cells and T lymphocytes. Whereas many cells show a limited life span, others appear to be able to replicate for undetermined periods.

Although a number of biological theories of aging have been proposed. None of them have been disproved, and each has a varying amount of evidence or support. A unifying theory does not yet exist that explains the mechanics and causes underlying the biological phenomenon of aging. Biological theories of aging can be addressed from a molecular, cellular, or systems level point of view. It is apparent that some theories emerge from others and that one or more theories could be superimposed on others. When taken together, each theory in its own right provides a clue to the aging process. However, many unanswered questions remain. Scientists in their continual search for truth persist in piecing together the puzzle of aging. New and exciting data concerning biological theories of aging have emerged recently through the application of more sophisticated methods of unlocking the secrets of the cell. We are beginning to confirm some of the previous suppositions and to develop a more thorough understanding of the genetic, molecular, and biochemical basis of cellular changes of aging.

▲ Promoting Healthy Aging: Implications for Gerontological Nursing

In time, the student will begin to develop an eclectic approach to theories of aging as he or she becomes familiar with the many facets of the aging process. Knowledge of the theories can be used in the very subjective consideration of successful and healthy aging.

In the promotion of healthy aging at any chronological age, the nurse can play an important role. Helping persons identify pollutants in their environments, from those associated with industrial emission to ultraviolet light to second-hand smoke, may profoundly affect health, even at a cellular level. The same can be said about smoking cessation and stress reduction. As more is learned about the effect of antioxidants and the substances in which they are found, the gerontological nurse can use the knowledge of biological theories of aging to encourage the healthiest diets and judicious use of neutraceutical and dietary supplements. With an understanding of potential changes in immunity, the conscientious nurse can take an active role in promoting specific preventive strategies such as the use of immunizations (especially influenza and pneumococcal) and the avoidance of exposure to others with infections (Box 2-5).

SOCIOLOGICAL THEORIES OF AGING

In sharp contrast to the biological theories of aging, sociological theories attempt to explain and predict the changes in roles and relationships in middle and late life with an emphasis on adjustment. The basic theories were developed in the 1960s and 1970s, studying primarily the most frail of elders residing in institutional settings. Most of these theories have persisted with little modification since that time and originally had a notable absence of the consideration of culture as an influencing factor. They must be viewed within the context of the historical period from which they emerged. Some of the theories continue to generate interest and thought, such as modernization and exchange theories, and others, such as disengagement theory, are no longer considered relevant. Other theories are evolving (Box 2-6). In contrast to the biological theories of aging, the sociological theories are not always based on empirical evidence because of methodological problems in measurement. They nonetheless have the significant potential for helping us understand the world around us and moving toward and into healthy aging.

Role Theory

One of the earliest explanations of how older adults adjust to aging was proposed by Cottrell in 1942 and offered as role theory. The theory has endured largely because of its significant face validity. From a contemporary perspective, role theory can be enhanced through a consideration of both social and cultural expectations of the person, family, and community.

Persons all over the world are engaging in roles that are consistent with their chronological age. As individuals evolve through the various stages in life, their roles evolve as well. The young adult often functions in the role of student, moving on to life partner and parent, and later grandparent. The timing of some of these roles is biologically driven

---

BOX 2-5   Areas of Potential Nursing Assessment and Education Consistent with the Biological Theories of Aging

- Engage in exercise and muscle training. (Wear And Tear)
- Avoid skin dryness and joint stiffening. (Cross-link)
- Avoid environmental pollutants and unnecessary radiation. (Free Radical)
- Watch for research related to the effect of unsaturated fats and heavy metals on cell health. (Cross-Link)
- Watch research on the use and presence of antioxidants. (Free Radical)
- Avoid stress. (Free Radical, Immunity)
- Avoid situations that decrease immune functioning in the body, e.g., chronic stress, malnutrition, excessive exercise. (Immunity).
- Watch for research related to the use of DHEA and melatonin. (Neuroendocrine)
- Maintain body weight no greater than ideal body weight. (Caloric Restriction)

BOX 2-6 Sociological Theories of Aging

ROLE THEORY

As individuals evolve through the various stages in life, their roles evolve as well. This theory proposes that the ability of an individual to adapt to changing roles over the life course is a predictor of adjustment to personal aging.

ACTIVITY THEORY

This theory sees activity as necessary to maintain life satisfaction and positive self-concept. The focus is on the individual's need to maintain a productive life for it to be a happy one. The productivity of middle life is thought to be best replaced with equally as engaging pursuits in late life (Maddox, 1963).

DISENGAGEMENT THEORY

Disengagement theory proposed that the withdrawal of elders from their roles earlier in life was necessary to allow the transfer of power to the younger generations. The transfer of power allowed for the maintenance of social equilibrium and an expression of mutually agreed upon roles. Disengagement was viewed as an adaptive and healthy behavior. Although this theory has been discounted by gerontologists and elders themselves, it continues to spark discussion and comparison.

CONTINUITY THEORY

According to continuity theory, individuals tend to develop and maintain a consistent pattern of behavior, substituting one role for a similar one as one matures. Late life (including roles, responsibilities, and activities) is a reflection of a continuation of life patterns (Havinghurst et al., 1968).

AGE-STRATIFICATION THEORY

Historical context is a key component of age-stratification theory. According to this theory, elders exist in cohorts or strata, or others who have shared similar historical periods in their lives, with age-graded systems of expectations and rewards. Age cohorts have been exposed to similar events, conditions, and global, environmental, and political circumstances (Riley et al., 1972). The definitions of the age-strata are usually social and cultural expressions of the definitions of aging as well as who and when one is placed in a stratum.

SOCIAL EXCHANGE THEORY

Social exchange theory is based on the consideration of the cost-benefit model of social participation (Dowd, 1980). According to this theory, social interactions are based on exchanges. The resources of one are exchanged for those of the other of equal value. Roles and skills can be offered to another in exchange for needed resources. The value of the exchanges may determine the social status of the participants. Older adults are often viewed as unequal partners in the exchange and may need to depend on metaphorical reserves of contributions to the pool of reciprocity.

MODERNIZATION THEORY

Modernization theory attempts to explain the social changes that have resulted in the devaluing of both the contributions of elders as well as the elders themselves. The status and therefore value of elders are lost when their labors are no longer considered useful, when kinship networks are dispersed, when the information they hold is not longer useful to the society in which they live, and when the culture in which they live no longer reveres them.

(e.g., parenthood), whereas other roles transcend time, such as volunteer and child. The theory proposes that the ability of an individual to adapt to changing roles over the life course is a predictor of adjustment to personal aging. Actual and potential conflicts in valuing of roles are explained in the Modernization Theory section later in this chapter.

Age Norms. An offshoot of role theory addresses the phenomena of "age norms." Age norms are socially and culturally constructed expectations of behavior at times in one's life and in pre-established roles. Norms are shared expectations that present "shoulds" or "oughts" for behaviors associated with specific roles. Age norms and age constraints are concepts that underscore the belief that persons of a given age fulfill roles and conduct their lives in a manner that is socially and culturally expected and acceptable.

Age norms have the potential to artificially open and close roles to individuals. They are based on the assumption that chronological age and relationships imply roles. For example, in the white mainstream American culture, the predominant expectation is that daughters or daughters-in-law will provide care to aging parents in need (NASUA, 2003). Although this opens up roles for the woman, it closes the role for the son or son-in-law. In other cultures, this role may not be so limited (Jett, 2002). Older adult men and

women are expected to "act their age" and refrain from such things as the loud, noisy, all-night parties and trendy clothing that are expected of many young adults.

Aging may lead to role discontinuity whereby a previous role becomes obsolete and no longer valued and may lead to problems with adjustment in late life. As some roles are completed, newer ones may not immediately appear or be embraced. Persons who have been preoccupied with the work role of middle age may experience significant loss on retirement or may simply replace the work role with intense volunteer activity. Persons who must either relinquish or assume a role involuntarily are at particular risk for problems with adjustment. They may lose the role of spouse with the death of a partner or lose the role of a parent with the death of a child. Others, of necessity, take on the role of parenting younger family members whose own parents are unable to fulfill their own roles. This new parenting role may be at great emotional, physical, and financial expense of the elders and now a topic of increasing interest (see Chapter 20).

Activity Theory

Activity theory also attempted to predict and explain how individuals adjusted to age-related changes by looking at one's level of activity and productivity. In 1953 Havinghurst and Albrecht first proposed that successful aging meant active aging. The focus is on the individual's need to maintain a productive life for it to be a happy one. The theorists saw activity as necessary to maintain life satisfaction and positive self-concept. The productivity of middle life is thought to be best replaced with equally as engaging pursuits in late life (Maddox, 1963). Activity meant that the person is able to "stay young." The theory was based on three assumptions: (1) it is better to be active than inactive; (2) it is better to be happy than unhappy; and (3) only the person herself or himself can judge life's success (Havinghurst, 1972).

This theory has continued to enjoy favor as it is still consistent with Western society's emphasis on work, wealth, and productivity. Failure to remain active and productive is viewed by many as signs of failure in late life or unsuccessful aging (Hooyman and Kiyak, 2005). However, activity theory fails to account for the wide variation in the influence of culture, health, economic status, and lifestyle on the levels of activity chosen or possible at any particular stage in life, especially late life.

Disengagement Theory

Disengagement theory was a direct challenge to activity theory and shifted the focus away from the individual to the individual aging within society. Disengagement theory viewed the withdrawal of elders from their roles and activities earlier in life necessary to allow the transfer of power to the younger generations. Disengagement theory suggests that "aging is an inevitable, mutual withdrawal or disengagement, resulting in decreased interaction between the aging person and others in the social system he [or she] belongs to" (Cumming and Henry, 1961, p. 2). The transfer was viewed as necessary for the maintenance of social equilibrium and an expression of mutually agreed upon roles. Disengagement was viewed as an adaptive and healthy behavior in contrast to the persistence of engagement that is seen as necessary for happiness in activity theory.

Disengagement theory has been largely discounted by gerontologist and elders themselves. It is now widely accepted that an elder's withdrawal is not necessarily a good thing for society. It has also been found that in some cultures persons achieve even greater prestige, power, and influence as they are recognized as elders (Sokolovsky, 1997).

Continuity Theory

Continuity theory was based on the early work of Havinghurst and colleagues and challenged both activity theory and disengagement theory. According to continuity theory, individuals tend to develop and maintain a consistent pattern of behavior, substituting one role for a similar one as one matures. Late life roles, responsibilities, and activities are a reflection of a continuation of life patterns (Havinghurst et al., 1968). Personality is seen not only to be enduring but also becoming more entrenched and pronounced as one ages. Three ideas important to this perspective, inferred from Neugarten and associates (1968), remain fundamental to beliefs about the older individual:

- In normal aging, personality remains consistent.
- Personality influences role activity and investment in role activity.

- Personality influences life satisfaction regardless of role activity.

Similar to role theory, continuity theory has survived because of its face validity; that is, on the surface it seems to make sense. It is difficult to test empirically.

Age-Stratification Theory

Age-stratification theory is a newer approach to understanding the role, reactions, and adaptations of older adults. Like continuity theory, it specifically challenges activity theory and disengagement theory. Age-stratification theory goes beyond the individual to the age structure of society (Marshall, 1996). Age structure can take a number of different forms, including the conceptualization of "young," "middle-aged" and "old" or Thomas' (2004) proposal of the state of "elderhood" following "childhood" and "adulthood."

Historical context is a key component of age-stratification theory. Elders exist in cohorts, or others who have shared similar historical periods in their lives, with age-graded systems of expectations and rewards. They have been exposed to similar events, conditions, and global, environmental, and political circumstances (Riley et al., 1972). For example, a cohort effect can be seen with men born between 1920 and 1930 who were very likely to have been active participants in World War II and the Korean War. In comparison, men born in the United States between 1940 and 1950 were likely to have been involved in the Vietnam Conflict, an entirely different experience. It is not surprising that these two groups of men have different perspectives and different health problems. Likewise, most white women born between 1920 and 1930 were raised with what are known as traditional values and roles and may have either never worked outside the home or been limited to lower-paying "women's work," such as housekeeping, teaching, and nursing. In contrast, women born between 1930 and 1940 had pressure to work outside the home and also had considerably more opportunities, partially as a result of the feminist revolution of the 1960s. Hooks (2000) reminds us that race must be considered when understanding cohort effects.

This theory may be particularly useful in understanding aging within a global context. The definitions of the age-strata are usually social and cultural expressions of aging as well as who and when one is placed in a stratum. The cohort effect can be used as a powerful tool for understanding the potential life experiences of persons from not only different cultures but also different parts of the world (see Chapter 21).

Social Exchange Theory

Again challenging both activity theory and disengagement theory, social exchange theory is based on the consideration of the cost-benefit model of social participation (Dowd, 1980). It explains that withdrawal or social isolation is the result of an imbalance in the exchanges between older persons and younger members of society and that the balance is what determines one's happiness and social support at any point in time.

According to this theory, social interactions are based on exchanges. The resources of one are exchanged for those of the other of equal value. For example, for the wage-earner, the resources of one's time and effort are exchanged for monetary compensation. Roles and skills can be offered to another in exchange for needed resources. The value of the exchanges may determine the social status of the participants.

Older adults are often viewed as unequal partners in the exchange and may need to depend on metaphorical reserves of contributions to the pool of reciprocity. This may be seen in the expectation of elderly African-Americans for care as "pay back" for their providing care to others earlier in their lives (Jett, 2002; 2006). Other elders care for young grandchildren so that their adult children can work. For this they may receive total support (e.g., room, board, income). Although this exchange may appear uneven, it can also be viewed from the more holistic perspective of a lifetime of exchanges and contributions.

Modernization Theory

Modernization theory attempts to explain the social changes that have resulted in the devaluing of both the contributions of elders and the elders themselves. Historically (before about 1900 in the United States), materials and political resources were controlled by the older members of the society (Achenbaum, 1978). The resources included not only their time, as shown in the examples just described, but also their knowledge, traditional skills, and experience. They held power through property ownership, including decision making related to food distribution. Older women often held important religious and cultural roles of instructing youth and controlling ceremony (Sokolovsky, 1997).

According to the modernization theory, the status and therefore value of elders are lost when their labors are no longer considered useful, kinship networks are dispersed, the information they hold is no longer useful to the society in which they live, and the culture in which they live no longer reveres them (Hendricks and Hendricks, 1986). It is proposed that these changes are the result of advancing technology, urbanization, and mass education (Cowgill, 1981).

Treatment of the elderly in modern Japan was long considered evidence of the inaccuracy of the theory. Historically, Japanese elders were given the highest status and held the greatest power. This did not seem to change with the industrialized advances after World War II. However, today Japan not only is a highly modern country from an industrial point but also is showing signs of "modernization" in social relations with it elders (Sokolvsky, 1997). Other researchers have also found support of the modernization theory, with changes observed in other societies such as India (Dandekar, 1996; Vincentnathan and Vincentnathan, 1994) and Taiwan (Silverman et al., 2000).

▲ Promoting Healthy Aging: Implications for Gerontological Nursing

The sociological theories of aging provide the gerontological nurse with much useful information and a background for facilitating healthy aging and adaptation (Box 2-7). Although they have been neither proved nor disproved,

---

BOX 2-7 Areas of Potential Nursing Assessment and Educations Consistent with the Sociological Theories of Aging

- Currently held roles, role satisfaction, and emerging roles (Role)
- Individual's and family's expectations of age norms and effect on self-esteem (Role)
- Current level of activity and satisfaction with such (Activity)
- Effect of changes in health on usual roles and activities (Role, Activity)
- Cultural beliefs and expectations related to roles, activity, and both engagement and disengagement related to these (Role, Activity, Disengagement)
- Usual life patterns and personality and attention to any change in these as an indication of a potential problem (Continuity)
- Knowledge of the historical context of the individual and potential influence on perception and responses (Age-Stratification)
- Complexity of social support and network (Social Exchange)
- Opportunities for contributions of knowledge to society (Modernization)
- Sense of self and self-worth (Modernization)

---

many of the ideas they contain have withstood the test of time. The theories have been adapted and applied to contemporary aging in many ways, from the concept of senior centers (activity theory) to nursing assessments of social support (social exchange theory). And, unfortunately, the disengagement theory is still applied any time one incorrectly accepts depression and isolation as a "normal" part of aging.

PSYCHOLOGICAL THEORIES OF AGING

Psychological theories presuppose that aging is one of many developmental processes experienced between birth and death. Life, then, is a dynamic process. Like the nonstochastic theories, most psychological theories use a life span developmental approach and describe the step-wise progression through predictable stages. Although these are widely accepted because of their face validity, like the sociological theories they are not well suited to testing or measurement (Box 2-8).

Jung's Theories of Personality

Psychologist Carl Jung (1971), a contemporary of Freud, proposed a theory of the development of personality throughout life, from childhood to old age. He was one of the first psychologists to define the last half of life as having a purpose of its own, quite apart from species survival. Late life is considered distinctly different from early life.

"We cannot live the afternoon of life according to the program of life's morning, for what was great in the morning

---

BOX 2-8 Psychological Theories of Aging

JUNG

According to Jung (1971), a personality is either extroverted (oriented toward the external world) or introverted (oriented to the subjective inner world of the individual). With chronological age, the person is able to move from extraversion to introversion, from a focus on outward achievement to one of acceptance of the self and awareness that both the accomplishments and challenges to a lifetime can be found within oneself.

ERIKSON

Erikson (1993) theorized a predetermined order of psychological development and specific tasks that one needed to master in a step-wise fashion. The task of middle age is proposed as generativity. Failure to accomplish this stage results in stagnation. The task of late life is that of ego integrity as opposed to ego despair. Ego integrity, drawing from a Freudian perspective, implies a sense of completeness and cohesion of the self. It is also described as the achievement of late life wisdom.

PECK

Peck (1968) advanced the work of Erikson, describing tasks that could lead to ego integrity. All three of his tasks addressed the individual coming to terms with the aging process through transcending and differentiating the self from a preoccupation with ego, body, and roles.

MASLOW

Maslow's hierarchy ranked the needs of the person from the most basic (related to the maintenance of biological integrity) to the most complex (associated with self-actualization). Like Erikson, Maslow proposed that the higher levels cannot be met without first meeting the lower-level needs. In other words, moving toward healthy aging is an evolving and developing process. As more basic-level needs are met, the satisfaction of higher-level needs is possible, with ever-deepening richness to life, regardless of one's age.

BOX 2-9 Research Highlights: Caring Throughout Life

In 1927 Dr. Herbert Stolz established the Institute of Child Welfare under the aegis of the Institute of Human Development and began a longitudinal study of the health and development of every third child born in Berkeley, California (an elite college town) for the ensuing 18 months. The original sample totaled 248 infants. The children are now septuagenarians. Their parents, now mostly nonagenarians, were interviewed by the Eriksons. Their preoccupation at this last stage of life was caring. For many, caring remained focused on children and grandchildren and seemed a vicarious way of continuing vital involvement in living. Others had grown beyond the central focus of the family, and their caring had more universal and altruistic components. For most of these very old, concern for their septuagenarian children dominated their thoughts. Reflecting on the successes of their children seemed to confirm their own parenting. As the dialectic around caring is cultivated, the elder is challenged "to accept from others that caring which is required and to do so in a way that is itself caring" (Erikson et al., 1986, p. 74).

---

will be little at evening, and what in the morning was true will at evening become a lie" (Jung, 1933, p. 108).

According to this theory, a personality is either extroverted and oriented toward the external world or introverted and oriented to the subjective inner world of the individual. Jung suggested that aging results in a movement from extraversion to introversion.

Beginning perhaps at midlife, individuals begin to question their own dreams, values, and priorities. The potential for resultant crisis of emotional upheaval is a step in the process of personality development. With chronological age and personality development, Jung proposed that the person is able to move from a focus on outward achievement to one of acceptance of the self and awareness that both the accomplishments and challenges to a lifetime can be found within oneself. The development of the psyche and the inner person is accompanied by a search for personal meaning and the spiritual self. This personality of late life can easily be compared to Erikson's ego integrity and Maslow's self-actualization, which are described in the following sections.

Developmental Theories of Erikson and Peck

Psychologist Eric Erikson is well known for articulating the developmental stages and tasks of life, from early childhood to later "elderhood." Most students have studied Erikson's 8-stage or task model. Erikson (1993) theorized a predetermined order of development and specific tasks that were associated with specific periods in one's life course. He proposed that one needed to successfully accomplish one task before complete mastery of the next was possible and originally articulated these in "either/or" language. He proposed that persons would return again and again to the task that had been poorly resolved in the past.

Erikson's task of middle age is generativity, or that which establishes oneself and contributes in meaningful ways for the future and future generations. Failure to accomplish this stage results in stagnation.

What has been called the "final task" of late life is that of ego integrity as opposed to despair. Ego integrity, drawing from a Freudian perspective, implies a sense of completeness and cohesion of the self. It is also described as the achievement of late life wisdom.

In later years, as octogenarians, Erikson and his wife Joan reconsidered his earlier work from the perspective of their own aging and a group of their cohorts (Erikson et al., 1986). They modified their "either/or" stance of the developmental tasks to the recognition of the balance of each of the tasks (Box 2-9). That is, within each person there is dialectic—the ego in a simultaneous state of integrity and despair; and the new goal of one achieving balance in the two. In 1986 they wrote, "The process of bringing into balance feelings of integrity and despair involves a review of and a coming to terms with the life one has lived thus far" (Erikson et al., 1986, p. 70).

Peck (1968) expanded on the original work of Erikson with the identification of discrete tasks of late life that, when taken together, achievement would result in ego integrity. Peck's tasks represent the process or movement toward Erikson's final stage.

- *Ego differentiation versus work role preoccupation:* The person no longer defines herself or himself by life work role but in individual personhood.
- *Body transcendence versus body preoccupation:* The body and changes are accepted as part of life rather than as a source of identity and focus.
- *Ego transcendence versus ego preoccupation:* The person sees oneself as part of a greater whole rather than an individual requiring special attention.

To achieve integrity using Peck's theoretical model, one must develop the ability to redefine self, to let go of occupational identity, to rise above body discomforts, and to establish meanings that go beyond the scope of self-centeredness.*

Maslow's Hierarchy of Human Needs

Another well-known theory with applications to aging is that of Maslow's Hierarchy of Needs (1954). This combines the bio-psycho-social needs of the individual. As far back as Hippocrates and Galen, the basic needs of all living people were recognized as the need for air, fluids, nutrition, hygiene, elimination, activity, and skin integrity. Along with these is the basic need for comfort or relief from suffering. The hierarchy ranks needs from the most basic, related to the maintenance of biological integrity, to the most complex, associated with self-actualization. Like Erikson, Maslow proposed that the higher levels cannot be met without first meeting the lower-level needs. In other words, moving toward healthy aging is an evolving and developing process. As basic-level needs are met, the satisfaction of higher-level needs is possible, with ever-deepening richness to life, regardless of one's age. Although it has been tested, this theory may be less culturally biased than others.

• • •

Many questions about late life development remain unanswered. Do biological differences exist between persons of different races and ethnicities, and how does this influence the aging of the human body? How does aging within a culture affect the individual, family, and community? How do people change in the later years? What is the reason for and purpose of aging? What is one meant to accomplish in the last half of the life span? What are the expected internal and external resources? What is the meaning of this last part of the life span? These are not new questions. Theories about them

---

*The reader is reminded that all existing theories were developed from a Eurocentric perspective and may have less usefulness when describing aging within other cultures, especially those that are collective rather than individualistic (see Chapter 21).

BOX 2-10	**Historical Figures and Their Beliefs About Aging**
Aristotle	Disengagement, interiority
Cicero and Montaigne	Self-discovery, pursuit of gentility and complexity
Plato	Development of wisdom
	Metamorphosis of the soul
Galen	Statesmanship and responsibility
Villanova	Moderation and humoral balance critical to vitality
Leonardo da Vinci	Coping with reality of physical decline
Cornaro	Restricted diet and moderation for long life
Sanctorius	Decay of body "spirits" leading to "universal hardness of fibres"
Fothergill	Effects of mind on body
	Positive attitudes recommended
Rush	Importance of heredity
Charcot	Latency periods of disease that only appear in old age

have been debated since the early Greeks; Plato, Aristotle, Cicero, and Montaigne sought the answers (Box 2-10). There are still many areas of adult development and aging that have been minimally explored and may be the essence of development in maturity and late life.

▲ Promoting Healthy Aging: Implications for Gerontological Nursing

Although different theories will resonate with different nurses, Maslow's theories of the hierarchy of human needs provide an organizing framework for this text. It can be used to better understand individuals and their concerns at any particular time and in any particular situation. And, finally, it can serve as a guide to set priorities in nursing interventions to promote healthy aging (Figure 2-3).

The gerontological nurse works to ensure that, first, the basic needs of the older adult are met and realizes that only then are higher levels of wellness possible. The person with dementia may begin to wander or become agitated because of the need to find a toilet, not knowing where to look. Until the toileting needs are met, the nurse's attempt to comfort or redirect is likely to be ineffective and frustrating. The person who lives alone but is unable to shop or cook will be distressed and perhaps irritable until arrangements can be made for home-delivered meals, either commercially or through a friend or family member.

As basic needs are met, a person will feel safe and secure. The person will likely sleep better and feel more comfortable interacting with others. While interacting with others, people

**Maslow's Hierarchy of Needs and Areas of Potential Nursing Assessment
and Education Consistent with the Theories of Aging**

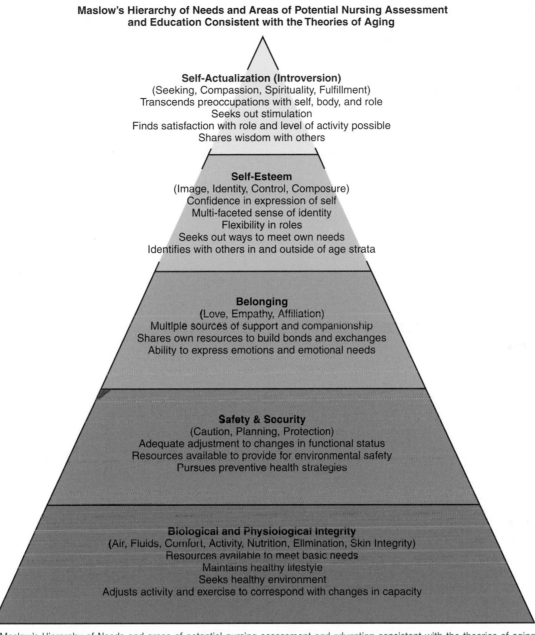

Self-Actualization (Introversion)
(Seeking, Compassion, Spirituality, Fulfillment)
Transcends preoccupations with self, body, and role
Seeks out stimulation
Finds satisfaction with role and level of activity possible
Shares wisdom with others

Self-Esteem
(Image, Identity, Control, Composure)
Confidence in expression of self
Multi-faceted sense of identity
Flexibility in roles
Seeks out ways to meet own needs
Identifies with others in and outside of age strata

Belonging
(Love, Empathy, Affiliation)
Multiple sources of support and companionship
Shares own resources to build bonds and exchanges
Ability to express emotions and emotional needs

Safety & Security
(Caution, Planning, Protection)
Adequate adjustment to changes in functional status
Resources available to provide for environmental safety
Pursues preventive health strategies

Biological and Physiological Integrity
(Air, Fluids, Comfort, Activity, Nutrition, Elimination, Skin Integrity)
Resources available to meet basic needs
Maintains healthy lifestyle
Seeks healthy environment
Adjusts activity and exercise to correspond with changes in capacity

FIGURE 2-3 Maslow's Hierarchy of Needs and areas of potential nursing assessment and education consistent with the theories of aging. (Modified from Ebersole P et al: *Gerontological nursing and healthy aging,* ed 2, St Louis, 2005, Mosby.)

often begin to meet their needs of belonging. Maslow sees people as social beings with a need to belong to something outside of themselves. These needs are met through memberships in churches, synagogues, mosques, and civic or social organizations and through ties to family and friends. After retirement, a member of a work organization may replace the belonging need with special interest groups. If it is not replaced, there is a risk for isolation and depression. When a person moves to live with a child in a distant city or into an assisted living facility or nursing home, meeting belonging needs can be especially challenging and the nurse may work with the elder to form new alliances and associations. The nurse works to create environments in which meaningful relationships and activities can remain a part of the elder's life.

A person whose basic needs are met, who feels safe and secure, and who has a sense of belonging will also have self-esteem and self-efficacy. In other words, people will accept and honor who they are and will feel that they have some personal power and self-confidence; they will know that they are important as people and that they inherently have value. Self-esteem is not something someone can give to anyone else. It is, however, something that others can negatively influence through ageist attitudes and behavior. For example, anytime the nurse assumes that a patient cannot do something based solely on the person's age, the nurse is being ageist and is actually belittling the individual. Unfortunately, this is commonly seen but can be challenged by the knowledgeable and sensitive gerontological nurse.

Finally, some people reach Maslow's highest level of wellness, that of self-actualization. Self-actualization is seen as people reaching out beyond themselves and finding meaning in their lives and a sense of fulfillment. It is a way to achieve the sense of integrity described by Erikson. It is a way of finding continuity in what otherwise can be seen as a disconnected or fragmented life. And according to Jung, it is a natural state of development.

This may not seem possible for all, but the nurse can foster this in unique and important ways. One of the authors (KJ) was asked to speak to a group in a nursing home about death and dying. To her surprise, the room was not filled with staff, as she had expected, but with the frailest of elders slumped in their wheelchairs. Instead of the usual lecture, she talked about legacies and asked the silent audience, "What do you want people to remember about you? What made your life worthwhile?" Without exception, each member of the audience had something to say, from "I had a

beautiful garden" to "I was a good mother" to "I helped design a bridge." Meaning can be found for life everywhere—you just have to ask.

KEY CONCEPTS

- Aging is a gradual process of change over the course of time. Each species may have an expected life span for humans, long thought to be 120 years; this belief has been recently challenged by long-lived individuals, the supercentenarians.
- It is unknown at this time what changes over time are the result specifically of aging, disease, lifestyle, or environmental impact.
- A number of biological theories contribute to our understanding the cellular process of aging; however, at this time none can stand alone as the explanation of the aging process and why it occurs.
- Most sociological theories of aging propose coping patterns of individuals approaching late life.

CASE STUDY: One Woman's Aging Experience

Jennie attained the remarkable age of 100 years the day before Christmas. There were numerous celebrations of her birthday by friends and family. She was delighted and surprised because little had been made of her birthday in previous years. She always explained it away by the fact it was so near Christmas. Aside from joint pains, difficulty in breathing at times (even though she had never smoked), frequent falls, and limited energy, she considered herself healthy, had rarely been ill enough to see a physician, and had only recently begun taking a medication for her heart. Jennie sometimes woke during the night with urinary urgency and then had difficulty falling asleep again. At those times she would sip a shot of brandy and read until she fell asleep. During the day she wore a protective pad because she tended to leak urine when she coughed or laughed. Jennie said, "This getting old is like the one-hoss shay*: everything falls apart." Jennie had a large network of friends and an attentive family, though she was well acquainted with grief and loss. Her husband of 75 years had died 3 years before, and she had left her lovely home and beloved dog when she moved into the retirement center at age 97. She was deeply spiritual but not religious in a ritualized sense. Her great-granddaughter was majoring in gerontology at the local university and often talked to Jennie about her life and remarkable adaptation in an attempt to find the key to her longevity.

Based on the case study, develop a nursing care plan using the following procedure†:

- List Jennie's comments that provide subjective data.
- List information that provides objective data.
- From these data, identify and state, using accepted format, two nursing diagnoses you determine are most significant to Jennie at this time. List two of Jennie's strengths that you have identified from the data.
- Determine and state outcome criteria for each diagnosis. These must reflect some alleviation of the problem identified

in the nursing diagnosis and must be stated in concrete and measurable terms.
- Plan and state one or more interventions for each diagnosed problem. Provide specific documentation of the source used to determine the appropriate intervention. Plan at least one intervention that incorporates Jennie's existing strengths.
- Evaluate the success of the intervention. Interventions must correlate directly with the stated outcome criteria to measure the outcome success.

Critical Thinking Questions

1. Discuss Jennie's physical changes as they relate to the biological theories of aging.
2. Jung talked about elders' movement toward introversion and meaning in late life. Does Jennie fit this pattern?
3. Consider the sociological theories of aging and discuss how each would or would not apply to Jennie.
4. Where on Maslow's Hierarchy of Needs would you place Jennie and why?
5. Imagine you are Jennie, and discuss with your great-granddaughter your thoughts about your own aging.
6. Discuss the meanings and the thoughts triggered by the student's and elder's viewpoints as expressed at the beginning of the chapter. How do these vary from your own experience?
7. Imagine yourself at 90 years old, and describe the lifestyle you will have and the factors that you believe account for your long life.
8. Organize a debate in which each individual attempts to convince others of the logic of one particular concept of aging.
9. List and discuss the psychological tasks of aging that you believe will be most difficult for you to accomplish.
10. Describe in a brief essay the characteristics of the oldest person you have known.

---

* A "one-hoss shay" was a cart drawn by a horse, popular around 1910.
† Students are advised to refer to their nursing diagnosis text and identify possible or potential problems.

- Psychological theories of aging are particularly culture- and cohort-bound and must be studied with that in mind. Jung and Erikson have made major contributions to our understanding of aging from the psychological perspective.
- It is becoming more generally accepted that personality characteristics, as well as biological characteristics, are to some degree inherent in the individual.

RESEARCH QUESTIONS

What physical changes can be attributed strictly to the aging of an organism?

What environmental factors have the potential to affect longevity?

What factors in relationships have the potential to contribute to survival?

What are the identifiable factors in extreme longevity?

What caloric distribution of carbohydrates, proteins, and fats contributes to longevity?

REFERENCES

Achenbaum WA: *Old age in a new land*, Baltimore, 1978, Johns Hopkins Press.

Agency for Healthcare Research and Quality (AHRQ): *Effect of supplemental antioxidants vitamin C, vitamin E, and coenzyme Q10 for the prevention and treatment of cardiovascular disease*, Summary Evidence Report/Technology assessment No 83, AHRQ Pub No 03-E042, Rockville, Md, 2003, The Agency. Available at *www.ahrq.gov*. Accessed March 7, 2006.

Balaban RS et al: Mitochondria, oxidants, and aging, *Cell* 120(4): 483, 2005.

Birren J, Schroots JJF: History of geropsychology. In Birren J, Schaie K, editors: *Handbook of the psychology of aging*, ed 5, San Diego, 2001, Academic Press.

Bokov A et al: The role of oxidative damage and stress in aging, *Mech Ageing Dev* 125(10-1):811, 2004.

Borek C: Aging and antioxidants: fruits and vegetables are powerful armor, *Adv Nurse Pract* 14(2):35-38, 2006.

Ciabattari J: *Parade's special intelligence report: another reason to diet*, *Parade Magazine*, p 8, Aug 4, 1996.

Cottrell L: The adjustment of the individual to his age and sex roles, *Am Soc Rev* 7:617, 1942.

Cowgill D: Aging and modernization: a revision of the theory. In Kart C, Manard B, editors: *Aging in America: readings in social gerontology*, Palo Alto, Calif, 1981, Mayfield.

Cumming E, Henry W: *Growing old*, New York, 1961, Basic Books.

Dandekar K: *The elderly in India*, Thousand Oaks, Calif, 1996, Sage.

Darrach B: The war on aging, *Life Magazine* 15(10):32-43, 1992.

Davidovic M et al: The privilege to be old, *Gerontology* 49(5):335, 2003.

De la Fuente M: Effects of antioxidants on immune system ageing, *Eur J Clin Nutr* 56(3):S5, 2002.

Dowd JJ: *Stratification among the aged*, Monterey, Calif, 1980, Brooks Cole.

Effros RB: Replicative senescence: the final stage of memory T cell differentiation? *Curr HIV Res* 1(2):153, 2003.

Effros RB et al: In vitro senescence of immune cells, *Exp Gerontol* 38(11-12):1243-1249, 2003.

Erikson EH: *Childhood and society*, New York, 1993, Norton.

Erikson EH et al: *Vital involvement in old age: the experience of old age in our time*, New York, 1986, Norton.

Erren TC et al: Light, timing of biological rhythms, and chronodisruption in man, *Naturwissenschaften* 90(11):485, 2003.

Finch CE, Ruvkun G: The genetics of aging, *Annu Rev Genomics Hum Genet* 2:435, 2001.

Grune T et al: Age-related changes in protein oxidation and proteolysis in mammalian cells, *J Gerontol A Biol Sci Med Sci* 56(11): B459-467, 2001.

Guardiola-Lamaitre B: Toxicology of melatonin, *J Biol Rhythms* 12(6):693, 1997.

Hampton J: *The biology of human aging*, Dubuque, Iowa, 1991, William C Brown.

Harman D: Aging: a theory based on free radical and radiation chemistry, *J Gerontol* 11:298, 1956.

Havinghurst RJ et al: Disengagement and patterns of aging. In Neugarten BL, editor: *Middle age and aging*, Chicago, 1968, University of Chicago Press.

Havinghurst RJ: *Developmental tasks and education*, New York, 1972, David McKay.

Havinghurst RJ, Albrecht R: *Older people*, New York, 1953, Longmans, Green.

Hayflick L: Why do we live so long? *Geriatrics* 43(10):77, 1988.

Hayflick L: *How and why we age*, New York, 1996, Ballantine Books.

Hayflick L, Moorehead PS: The serial cultivation of human diploid cell strains, *Exp Cell Res* 25:585, 1981.

Hendricks J, Hendricks CD: *Aging in mass society: myths and realities*, Boston, 1986, Little, Brown.

Hipkiss AR: Errors, mitochondrial dysfunction and ageing, *Biogerontology* 4(6):397, 2003.

Hooks, B: *Feminist theory: From margin to center*, Cambridge, MA, 2000, South End Press.

Hooyman NR, Kiyak HA: *Social gerontology: a multidisciplinary perspective*, ed 7, New York, 2005, Pearson.

Ignatavicius DD, Workman ML: *Medical-surgical nursing: critical thinking for collaborative care*, ed 5, St Louis, 2005, Saunders.

Jacobs HT: The mitochondrial theory of aging: dead or alive? *Aging Cell* 2(1):11, 2003.

Jazwinski SM: Longevity, genes, and aging, *Science* 273(5721):54, 1996.

Jett KF: Making the connection: seeking and receiving help by elderly African-Americans, *Qual Health Res* 12(3):373, 2002.

Jett KF: The meaning of aging and the celebration of years among rural African-American women, *Geriatr Nurs* 24(5):290, 2003.

Jett KF: Mind-loss in the African American community: a normal part of aging, *J Aging Stud* 20(1):1, 2006.

Jung CG: *Modern man in search of a soul*, San Diego, 1933, Harcourt, Brace & World.

Jung CG: The stages of life. In Campbell J, editor: *The portable Jung*, New York, 1971, Viking Press (translated by RFC Hull).

Keys SW, Marble M: In vivo data demonstrate critical role for telomeres, *Cancer Weekly Plus*, p 11, May 4, 1998.

King W: Scientists find gene link to aging: landmark discovery made in patients suffering from Werner's syndrome, *San Francisco Examiner*, p A-18, Apr 12, 1996.

Kirkwood TBL, Proctor CJ: Somatic mutations and ageing in silico, *Mech Ageing Dev* 124(1):85, 2002.

Legrain S, Girard L: Pharmacology and therapeutic effects of dehydroepiandrosterone in older subjects, *Drugs Aging* 20(13): 949, 2003.

Maddox G: Activity and morale: a longitudinal study of selected elderly subjects, *Soc Forces* 42:195, 1963.

Makinodan T: Gerontologic research. In Beck J, editor: *The 1990 year book of geriatrics and gerontology,* St Louis, 1990, Mosby.

Marshall VW: The state of theory in aging and the social sciences. In Binstock RH, George LK, editors: *Handbook of aging and the social sciences,* ed 4, San Diego, 1996, Academic Press.

Maslow A: *Motivation and personality,* New York, 1954, Harper & Row.

Masoro EJ: Caloric restriction and aging: controversial issues, *J Gerontol* 61A(1):14, 2006.

Meiner S, Lueckenotte A: *Gerontologic nursing,* ed 3, St Louis, 2006, Mosby.

Miller RA: The aging immune system: primer and prospectus, *Science* 273(5721):70, 1996.

National Association of State Units on Aging (NASUA): *The aging network implements the national family caregiver support program,* Washington DC, 2003, Administration on Aging.

National Institute of Aging (NIA): *Aging under the microscope: a biological quest,* NIH Pub No 02-2759, Bethesda, Md, 2003, Government Printing Office. Available at *www.nia.nih.gov.* Accessed March 19, 2006.

Nemoto S, Finkel T: Ageing and the mystery at Arles, *Science* 429:149-152, 2004.

Neugarten B et al: Personality and patterns of aging. In Neugarten B, editor: *Middle age and aging,* Chicago, 1968, University of Chicago Press.

Peck R: Psychological developments in the second half of life. In Neugarten B, editor: *Middle age and aging,* Chicago, 1968, University of Chicago Press.

Pereira-Smith OM, Bertram MJ: Replicative senescence, *Generations* 24(1), 2000.

Perrini S et al: Associated hormonal declines in aging: DHEAS, *J Endocrinol Invest* 28(3):85, 2005.

Quinti I et al: T-dependent immunity in aged humans: evaluation of T-cell subpopulations before and after short-term administration of thymic extract, *J Gerontol* 36:6, 1981.

Recer P: Showing your age? Quality-control genes at fault, study finds, *San Francisco Examiner,* p A-11, Mar 31, 2000.

Riley MW et al: *Aging and society: a sociology of age stratification,* vol 3, New York, 1972, Russell Sage Foundation.

Rosenfeld A: *Prolongevity,* New York, 1985, Alfred A Knopf.

Scheer JF: Jack of all nutrients: coenzyme Q19, *Better Nutrition* 58(8):48, 1996.

Schlessinger D: Alleles and aging: the effects of different forms of genes on aging and longevity, *Generations* 24(1):36, Fall/Winter 2000.

Sharma R: Theories of aging. In Timiras PS, editor: *Physiologic basis of geriatrics,* New York, 1988, Macmillan.

Short KR et al: Decline in skeletal muscle mitochondrial function with aging in humans, *Proc Natl Acad Sci USA* 102(15):5618, 2005.

Silverman P et al: Modeling life satisfaction among the aged: a comparison of Chinese and Americans, *J Cross Cult Gerontol* 15:289, 2000.

Smith JR, Pereira-Smith OM: Replicative senescence: implications for in vitro aging and tumor suppression, *Science* 273:63-7, 1996.

Sokolovsky F, editor: *The cultural context of aging: worldwide perspectives,* ed 2, Westpoint, CT: 1997.

Sonneborn T: The origin, evolution, nature and causes of aging. In Behnke J et al, editors: *The biology of aging,* New York, 1979, Plenum Press.

Srinivasan V et al: Melatonin, immune function and aging, *Immun Ageing* 29(2):17, 2005.

Strehler B, editor: *The biology of aging, symposium, no 6,* Washington, DC, 1960, American Institute of Biological Science.

Thomas WH: *What are old people for: how elders will save the world,* New York, 2004, VanderWky & Burnham.

Valko W et al: Metals, toxicity and oxidative stress, *Curr Med Chem* 12(10):1161, 2005.

Vincentnathan SB, Vincentnathan L: Equality and hierarchy in untouchable intergenerational relations and conflict resolutions, *J Cross Cult Gerontol* 9:1, 1994.

Walford RL: *Maximum life-span,* New York, 1983, Norton.

Walford RL: *The 120-year diet: how to double your vital years,* New York, 1986, Pocket Books.

Walford RL et al: Caloric restriction in Biosphere 2: alterations in physiologic, hematologic, hormonal, and biochemical parameters in humans restricted for a 2-year period, *J Gerontol A Biol Sci Med Sci* 57A(6):B211, 2002.

Wayne SJ et al: Cell-mediated immunity as a predictor of morbidity and mortality in subjects over 60, *J Gerontol* 45(2):M45, 1990.

CHAPTER 3

Health and Wellness

Theris A. Touhy

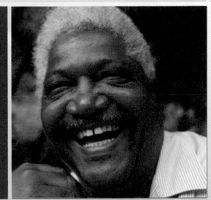

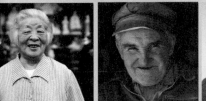

A STUDENT SPEAKS

I was so surprised when I went to the senior center and saw all those old folks doing tai chi! I feel a bit ashamed that I don't take better care of my body.

Maggie, age 24

AN ELDER SPEAKS

Just a change in perspective! I can choose to be well or ill under all conditions. I think, too often we feel like victims of circumstance. I refuse to be a victim. It is my choice and I have control.

Maria, age 86

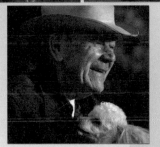

LEARNING OBJECTIVES
On completion of this chapter, the reader will be able to:

1. Discuss how health promotion and prevention activities can lead to a compression of morbidity for older people.
2. Define health and wellness.
3. Compare the difference between the health/wellness concept offered in the health and wellness and medical models.
4. Discuss the five dimensions of wellness.
5. Explain wellness in the context of chronic illness.
6. Identify gender differences that affect health/wellness and chronic illness.
7. Explain how and if the goals of wellness for elders can be accomplished.

HEALTH

As society moves into the twenty-first century, the long-existing but ignored concept of illness prevention and health promotion has emerged as individuals recognize that the present "health care" system does not meet their needs. Only recently have older people been considering health in a proactive manner. Older adults are now being strongly encouraged through media and health care systems to take personal responsibility for their own health through knowledge and behavioral change. Terms increasingly heard in the health arena now are *empowerment of the individual, prevention,* and *health promotion.*

Healthy People 2000/2010

The U.S. Department of Health and Human Services publications (USHHS) *Healthy People 2000* (1991) and *Healthy People 2010* (2000a) offer direction for the achievement of a better quality of life across the life span in the United States through measures that are directed at the reduction and prevention of health risks, unnecessary disease, disability, and death. The goals set forth by *Healthy People 2010* include (1) increasing quality and years of healthy life, and (2) eliminating health disparities. A summary of the *Healthy People 2000* objectives for adults 65 years of age and older appears in Box 3-1. The leading health indicators

Special thanks to Patricia Hess and Priscilla Ebersole, the previous edition contributors, for their content contributions to this chapter.

BOX 3-1   Summary Objectives for Adults Age 65 and Older *(Healthy People 2000)*

HEALTH STATUS

Reduce

- Suicide among white males
- Death by motor vehicle accidents (age 70+)
- Death from falls and fall-related injury, particularly age 85+
- Death from residential fires
- Hip fractures
- Number of persons who have difficulty performing two or more personal care activities so as to enhance independence
- Significant visual impairment
- Epidemic-related pneumonia and influenza deaths
- Pneumonia-related days of restricted activity

Increase

- Years of healthy life to at least 65 for blacks and Hispanics

RISK REDUCTION

Increase

- The percentage of individuals who regularly participate in light-to-moderate activity for at least 30 minutes a day
- Immunization levels for pneumococcal influenza among the chronically ill older population

- The percentage of older persons who receive, within appropriate intervals, screening and immunization services and at least one counseling service

SERVICES AND PROTECTION

Increase

- Percentage of recipients of home food service
- Percentage of older adults who have the opportunity to participate yearly in at least one organized health promotion program through senior centers, life care facilities, or community-based settings serving the older adult
- Percentage of states in the United States that have design standards for signs, signals, markings and lighting, and other roadway environmental improvements to enhance visual stimuli and protect the safety of older drivers and pedestrians
- The proportion of primary care providers who routinely review with their patients prescribed and over-the-counter medications each time a new medication is prescribed
- The usage of the oral care system
- The proportion who receive clinical breast examinations and mammograms
- The number of women age 70+ with uterine cervix who receive Pap tests

From U.S. Department of Health and Human Services, *Healthy People 2000,* Pub No (PHS) 91-50212, Washington, DC, 1991, U.S. Government Printing Office.

BOX 3-2   Healthy People 2010 Leading Health Indicators

- Physical activity
- Overweight and obesity
- Tobacco use
- Substance abuse
- Responsible sexual behavior
- Mental health
- Injury and violence
- Environmental quality
- Immunization
- Access to health care

From National Center for Health Statistics: *Data 2010: The* Healthy People 2010 *database,* Washington, DC, 2002, Centers for Disease Control and Prevention.

and focus areas of *Healthy People 2010* are shown in Boxes 3-2 and 3-3. Largely, the *Healthy People 2010* goals do not comprehensively address the health of individual elders but address the public health system in response to the 2002 Institute of Medicine study (Institute of Medicine, 2002; USHHS, 2000a) (Box 3-4).

The intent of these proposals is not only to lengthen life but also, more important, to improve quality of life and functional independence of older people. The ultimate goal for the elderly is to delay illness, prevent the ill from becoming disabled, and assist those who are disabled to function and prevent further disability. Health promotion activities and attention to healthy lifestyle habits such as those suggested by the *Healthy People* initiatives can postpone and reduce

morbidity for older people. The term *compressed morbidity*, discussed by Fries (1989), refers to the postponement of illness and disability caused by chronic illness and is a key public health goal (Morley and Flaherty, 2002). Table 3-1 presents a summary of progress toward *Healthy People 2000* and *2010* goals for older Americans.

Health and Wellness

In the medical arena, health is considered to be the absence of disease. Conformity to physical and mental capacity norms indicates one's health status. Therefore the more observable the evidence, the more definite the degree of health that can be declared or the diagnosis that can be affixed. Those biological and physiological capacities not considered essential for the performance of *well* activity are less likely to be considered significant.

The emergence of a strong holistic health movement has refocused on a clear definition and operational approach to health and wellness. The holistic approach has long been in existence but has received little attention. Dunn (1961) saw health in a holistic context and defined it as an integrated method of functioning that is oriented toward maximizing the potential of which the individual is capable within the environment in which he or she is functioning. Maslow recognized this as self-actualization. The holistic definition does not limit health to just its physical or mental or even social aspects but, rather, incorporates all of these facets in the total picture.

Sometimes *health*, per se, seems to be a limiting term that does not encompass the breadth that the terms *well-*

BOX 3-3   Healthy People 2010 Focus Areas

- Access to quality health services
- Arthritis, osteoporosis and chronic back conditions
- Cancer
- Chronic kidney disease
- Diabetes
- Disability and secondary conditions
- Educational and community-based programs
- Environmental health
- Family planning
- Food safety
- Health communication
- Heart disease and stroke
- HIV
- Immunization and infectious diseases
- Injury and violence prevention
- Maternal, infant and child health
- Medical product safety
- Mental health and mental disorders
- Nutrition and overweight
- Occupational safety and health
- Oral health
- Physical activity and fitness
- Public health infrastructure
- Respiratory diseases
- Sexually transmitted infections
- Substance abuse
- Tobacco use
- Vision and hearing

From U.S. Department of Health and Human Services: *Healthy People 2010,* Washington, DC, 2000, U.S. Government Printing Office. Available at *www.healthypeople.gov.*

BOX 3-4   Healthy People 2010 Objectives for the Public Health Infrastructure

- Increase access to information systems to apply data and information to public health practice.
- Increase public awareness of leading health indicators, health status indicators, and priority needs.
- Increase nationwide use of geographic information systems.
- Increase proportion of population-based *Healthy People 2010* objectives for which national data are available for all population groups identified for the objective.
- Increase availability of leading health indicators for select populations.
- Increase proportion of *Healthy People 2010* objectives that are tracked regularly at the national level.
- Increase proportion of *Healthy People 2010* objectives that are released within 1 year of data collection.
- Increase incorporation of specific competencies in essential public health systems and personnel systems.
- Increase integration of curricula specific to competency in public health services.
- Increase proportion of agencies that provide continuing education to develop competency in essential public health services for all their employees.

From U.S. Department of Health and Human Services: *Healthy People 2010,* Washington, DC, 2000, U.S. Government Printing Office.

ness and *well-being* suggest. Spector (1996) indicates that we find it difficult to define health without the use of some form of medical jargon, whereas "well is a state of being, an attitude...it is more than the absence of illness...it is an ongoing adaptational process" (Travis, 1977). Wellness involves one's whole being—physical, emotional, mental, and spiritual—all of which are vital components. For older people, health also includes the element of physical function. Spector (1985) and Markides and Mindel (1987) add the dimension of culture to the holistic health approach. Accordingly, what is considered wellness to the individual must include his or her cultural orientation. Culture cannot be relegated to a subposition under any other health component. It must stand equally so that health care providers can realize and more adequately respond to the significance of culture in the attainment of well-being. Culture affects a person's understanding of health as well as health behaviors (Box 3-5).

Perhaps Pender and colleagues (2002) have synthesized this most difficult concept from all the preceding definitions by defining health as "the actualization of inherent and acquired human potential through satisfactory relationships with others, goal-directed behavior and competent personal care while adjustments are made as needed to maintain stability and structural integrity." And yet, no specific definition of health can really convey the entirety of it (Pender et al., 2002; Spector, 1996).

The meaning that we attribute to health is continuing to change, and now the increasing focus is on prevention. Health is also being seen as a more expansive phenomenon with multiple dimensions: biopsychosocial, spiritual, environmental, and cultural (Pender et al., 2002). Change in any of these dimensions affects the health of an individual in a positive or negative manner. A change initiates (triggers) a behavioral change that can lead to empowerment. Empowerment may open many options for improving one's health. A positive approach to health emphasizes *strengths*, *resilience*, *resources*, and *capabilities*, rather than existing pathology.

Confusion often arises when the definitions of health, wellness, and well-being are used interchangeably by the general public and medical practitioners when discussing an individual's condition. The wellness model refers to health as one aspect in the achievement of wellness. The wellness approach suggests that every person has an optimum level of functioning for each position on the wellness continuum to achieve a good and satisfactory existence (well-being) (Figure 3-1). Even in chronic illness and dying, an optimum level of wellness and well-being is attainable for each individual.

Nurses have been among those caregivers who have attempted to provide care using the holistic philosophy, but they continue to struggle to make it integral to patient care. In an attempt to meld the broader health/wellness concepts and initiate a more positive approach to the capacities of older people, we offer this working definition for the care of the older individual: Wellness is the best achievable balance between

TABLE 3-1

National Report Card on Healthy Aging: How Healthy Are America's Seniors?

Indicator	Data for Persons Age 65 or Older[a] (Data Year)	*Healthy People 2000* Target	Grade (Pass/Fail)[b]	*Healthy People 2010* Target
HEALTH STATUS				
1. Physically unhealthy days (mean number of days in past month)	5.5 (2001)	c	c	c
2. Frequent mental distress (%)[d]	6.3 (2000-2001)	c	c	c
3. Oral health: Complete tooth loss (%)	22.4 (2002)	20	Fail	20
4. Disability (%)[e]	30.8 (2001)	c	c	c
HEALTH BEHAVIORS				
5. No leisure time physical activity in past month (%)	32.9 (2002)	22	Fail	20
6. Eating 5+ fruits and vegetables daily (%)	32.4 (2002)	50	Fail	N/A[f]
7. Obesity (%)[g]	19.5 (2002)	c	c	15
8. Current smoking (%)	10.1 (2002)	15	Pass	12
PREVENTIVE CARE AND SCREENING				
9. Flu vaccine in past year (%)	68.6 (2002)	60	Pass	90
10. Ever had pneumonia vaccine (%)	63.0 (2002)	60	Pass	90
11. Mammogram within past 2 years (%)	77.2 (2002)	60	Pass	70
12. Ever had sigmoidoscopy or colonoscopy (%)	58.3 (2002)	40	Pass	50
13. Up-to-date on select preventive services (%)[h]				
Men	34.4 (2002)	c	c	c
Women	33.4 (2002)	c	c	c
14. Cholesterol checked within past 5 years (%)	85.4 (2001)	75	Pass	80
INJURIES				
15. Hip fracture hospitalizations (per 100,000 persons)	525 (men) 1127 (women) 877 (total) (2002)	607 (total)	Fail	474 (men) 416 (women) NA (total)[i]

[a] Data for Indicators 1-14 were collected by CDC's Behavioral Risk Factor Surveillance System (BRFSS). Data for Indicator 15, hip fracture hospitalizations, come from CDC's National Center for Health Statistics, National Hospital Discharge Survey.

[b] Grade is based on the attainment of *Healthy People 2000* targets.

[c] Indicators 1, 2, 4, and 13 are more recently developed measures and, as such, do not have *Healthy People 2000* targets. Data related to Indicator 7, obesity, were combined with the overweight category in *Healthy People 2000,* and therefore obesity has no individual *Healthy People 2000* target.

[d] Frequent mental distress is defined as having had 14 or more mentally unhealthy days in the previous month. Data from the 2000 and 2001 BRFSS are combined here to get a sufficient sample size.

[e] Disability was defined on the basis of an affirmative response to either of the following two questions on the 2001 BRFSS: "Are you limited in any way in any activities because of physical, mental, or emotional problems?" or "Do you now have any health problem that requires you to use special equipment, such as a cane, wheelchair, a special bed, or a special telephone?"

[f] *Healthy People 2010* segments the nutrition target into multiple categories of fruits and vegetables.

[g] *Healthy People 2000* defined a target for overweight but not obesity. Because current standards separate these two conditions, obesity data are included in this report. The *Healthy People 2010* definition of obesity is a body mass index (BMI) of >30 kg/m^2.

[h] For men, three services are included: flu vaccine in past year, ever had a pneumonia vaccine, and ever had sigmoidoscopy or colonoscopy. For women, these same three services plus a mammogram within past 2 years are included.

[i] *Healthy People 2010* has separate hip fracture hospitalization targets for men and women and no target for the total number.

one's environment, internal and external, and one's emotional, spiritual, social, cultural, and physical processes. Figure 3-2 illustrates the interrelationship of the facets that compose health and successful aging. Each aspect is like a petal, anchored to the center and overlapping the other petals, each affecting the whole. Alterations in or loss of a petal can change the overall effect or appearance and its wholeness.

To achieve wellness or assist an individual to attain wellness potential, one needs to consider the dimensions of wellness: self-responsibility, nutritional awareness, physical fitness, stress management, and environmental sensitivity

(Pender et al., 2002, pp. 20-22). Each of these is discussed later in this chapter.

Measurements of a population's health status rely on life expectancy, morbidity, and death tables. These figures provide information on illness but do not reveal the extent to which the living are affected by these conditions. They do not indicate the health status, only the illness. For example, in morbidity tables people who are actually functioning at a high level of wellness are assigned to illness categories. Persons compiling these tables do not consider that the person with health disorders, malignancies, and other conditions may be

BOX 3-5   Evidence-Based Practice: Definitions of Health Among Diverse Groups of Elders

PURPOSE

To explore late-life definitions of health and similarities and differences in the meaning of health for elders from several different ethnic groups.

SAMPLE/SETTING

Two groups each of African American elders, Hispanic elders, Mandarin and Cantonese-speaking Chinese, and Eastern European. Age of participants was 59-87 and all resided in the Los Angeles area.

METHOD

Focus group methodology with analysis of transcripts.

FINDINGS

The meaning of health that emerged consisted of three domains of health: physical, psychological and spiritual, and social. The concept of physical health encompassed two major categories: somatic (basic body functioning and absence of physical illness) and functioning and activity. Most participants defined health as the ability to maintain one's activities. Psychological health included a positive attitude, happiness, not worrying, having an active mind, and creativity. The spiritual component of health included an approach to life rather than formal religious participation. Many mentioned having a sense of gratitude for life and the importance of a good heart. The social domain included maintaining social contacts, giving and receiving support from family and friends, and meaningful involvement in community and cultural activities.

African American, Eastern-European American and the Hispanic American participants identified the domain of physical health as primary. However, there were between-group distinctions, with African Americans focusing on the absence of illness or symptoms as primary in defining health; Eastern-Europeans focused on functional ability; and Hispanic Americans focused on not having to go to the doctor. For Chinese-Americans, the primary domain was psychological-spiritual.

IMPLICATIONS

The way elders of different ethnic and cultural groups view health is an important consideration in the planning of culturally competent health promotion programs. Values and beliefs about health differ across cultural and ethnic groups and programs must be modified to be appropriate for the cultural and ethnic values of health for specific populations. For example, the African American orientation to defining health as absence of symptoms presents challenges to health promotion activities targeted at risk factors. For the Chinese-Americans, psychological and spiritual domains were more important than physical health, an area not usually included in health promotion. Participant's definitions of health were based on a strengths model but health care activities still are primarily focused on a problem-based model with the focus on disease prevention.

Data from Damron-Rodriguez J et al: Definitions of health among diverse groups of elders: implications for health promotion, *Generations* 29(2).11-16, 2005.

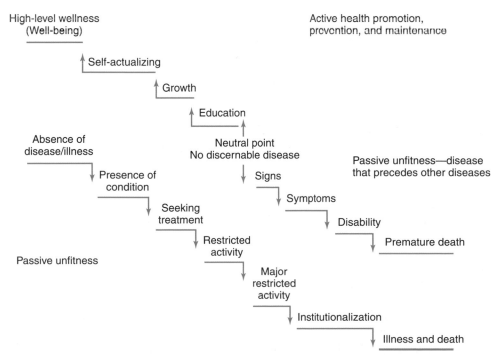

FIGURE 3-1 Comparisons of wellness/health and traditional medical continuum.

able to attain and function at a high level of wellness and be a contributing member of the community. Many older people with multiple chronic conditions continue to report that they have excellent or good health although racial and ethnic differences exist in self-reported health (Table 3-2). Chapter 21 discusses culture and aging in more depth. The wellness approach is perhaps the most equitable in the evaluation of the older individual's potential for maximum functioning.

Healthy Aging

The concept of healthy aging encompasses many of the elements of wellness just discussed. Important aspects of healthy aging are physical health, mental health, and an engagement with life (Rowe and Kahn, 1997). In a concept analysis of healthy aging (Hansen-Kyle, 2005, p. 52), the following definition emerged: "Healthy aging is the process of slowing down, physically and cognitively, while resiliently adapting and compensating in order to optimally function and participate in all areas of one's life (physical, cognitive, social, and spiritual)." The concept of healthy aging is a multidimensional process and is uniquely defined by each individual. The assumption that old age is a downhill course may be realistic from a physiological point of view. It is also recognized that the overall physical functioning of the body is determined mainly by the available energy and adaptive capacities.

The conviction by nurses and other caregivers that older people are individuals with declining health generates responses that include treating the older person as ill and feeble or potentially so. It is therefore expected by some that attempts to reverse conditions or situations, maintain a level of ability, or institute preventive health measures are useless for older people. Nothing could be further from the truth; all old people are improvable (Bortz, 1991). Historically, the principles of disease prevention and health promotion have not been aggressively applied to the problems of older adults. The focus has been on managing illnesses rather than on reducing risks, maintaining optimal function, and decreasing disability associated with illness.

Although the risk of disease and disability increases with advancing age, poor health is not an inevitable consequence of growing older. Much can be done to prevent or delay the onset of chronic illnesses and functional limitations in older adults as well as to minimize the impact of chronic illnesses when they do occur. The proportion of older people who are disabled has shown a downward trend in the past 10 years. Key strategies for improving the health of older people developed by the U.S. Centers for Disease Control and Prevention (CDC) are shown in Box 3-6. Adopting healthier behaviors such as regular physical activ-

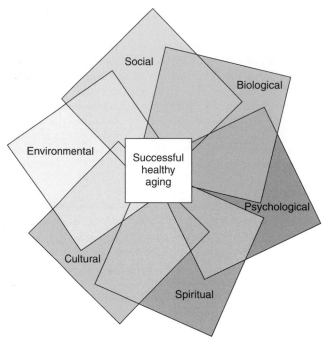

FIGURE 3-2   Healthy aging. (Developed by Patricia Hess.)

TABLE 3-2

Self-Reported Health Status of Older People by Race and Ethnicity

	HEALTH STATUS (2004)			
	Total	**White**	**African American**	**Hispanic**
N =	1.202	942	314	318
	%	%	%	%
Excellent/Good (Total)	**79**	**81**	**70**	**66**
Excellent	37	38	28	30
Good	42	43	42	36
Fair/Poor (Total)	**21**	**19**	**30**	**34**
Fair	16	14	24	28
Poor	5	5	6	6

From American Association of Retired Persons: *Images of aging in America 2004.* Available at *www.aarp.org/research/academic/images_of_aging.html.*

ity, healthy diet, a smoke-free lifestyle, and regular health screenings can dramatically reduce a person's risk for many chronic illnesses, including the leading causes of death and disability (Figures 3-3 and 3-4).

The most prevalent chronic conditions in individuals older than 75 years are much more common in women. One must consider the population predominance of women older than 75 years and the possibility that only the hardy men survive beyond 75 years. Racial and ethnic differences in health status continue with the leading causes of death and disability dramatically higher among racial and ethnically diverse populations in the United States. Elimination of health disparities is the focus of many national programs, including REACH 2010 (Racial and Ethnic Approaches to Community Health) sponsored by the CDC (*www.cdc.gov/programs/health07.htm*). Prevention and treatment of chronic illness is discussed more fully in Chapter 10 and culture and aging in Chapter 21.

BOX 3-6	**Key Strategies for Improving the Health of Older People**

1. Healthy lifestyle behaviors
2. Injury prevention
3. Delivery of culturally appropriate clinical preventive services
4. Immunization and preventive screenings
5. Self-management techniques for those with chronic illnesses

Modified from U.S. Department of Health and Human Services (USHHS), Centers for Disease Control and Prevention (CDC), *Healthy aging: preventing disease and improving quality of life among older Americans*, Washington, DC, 2006, U.S. Government Printing Office; Lang J et al: Healthy aging: priorities and programs of the Centers for Disease Control and Prevention, *Generations* 29(2):24-29, 2005.

HEALTH CONTINUUM

The medical interpretation of the health continuum is that if the individual is in good health or is well, disease or impairment is absent. Figure 3-1 indicates the progression along the traditional health continuum. When an individual develops a condition, it is expected that treatment will be sought to resolve the ailment. At this point, the individual begins the descent to dependency and despondency, either temporarily or for an extended period. The role of the individual is more passive than active. This dilemma is common in the older adult.

Health care continues to be based on acute cause and cure, the traditional medical model. In the early 1900s, this was an appropriate approach to health care: individuals contracted diseases that medical science could hope to cure (e.g., smallpox, diphtheria, syphilis, tuberculosis, polio, appendicitis). Today, however, chronic diseases and illnesses are the predominant conditions. Chronic disease or illness does not have a single cause, nor does it have a cure (Fries, 1992). Instead, it has a universal progression based on risk factors that may begin and remain unseen for decades before the condition surfaces in a pathological state. Examples include heart disease, diabetes mellitus, arthritis, and cancer. Another issue in the medical model is that if the older person's malady does not fit an already existing disease entity or diagnostic category, it is generally written off as a "sign of old age."

When one uses the wellness or holistic approach, which has been suggested as a more appropriate model for older people, one regards the health and wellness continuum from a more positive direction and the role of the individual is more active. The traditional or medical model of health questions whether everyone is capable of reaching or maintaining a high

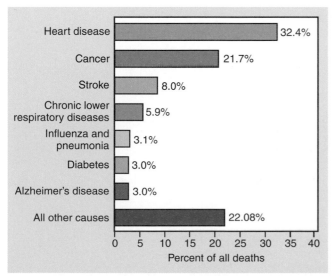

FIGURE 3-3 Causes of death among U.S. adults ages 65 years and older. (Redrawn from Centers for Disease Control and Prevention, National Center for Health Statistics. *National Vital Statistics Report, 2002.*)

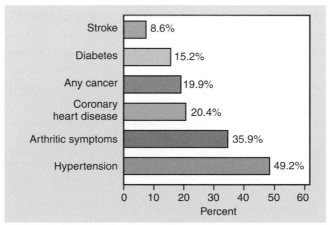

FIGURE 3-4 Prevalence of selected chronic conditions among adults ages 65 years and older, 2000-2001. A respondent was considered to have "arthritic symptoms" if he or she answered "yes" to the following questions: "During the past 12 months, have you had pain, aching, stiffness, or swelling in or around a joint?" and "Were these symptoms present on most days for at least 1 month?" (Redrawn from Centers for Disease Control and Prevention, National Center for Health Statistics. *National Health Interview Survey, 2000-2001.*)

level of wellness. The wellness model places wellness within the grasp of all persons, regardless of age or physical condition. The significance for the older person is a new and positive approach to what the nurse and other caregivers call "healthy." Wellness begins with the individual and stimulates the desire for growth and change. This means nurturing the physical self, expressing emotions more freely, improving personal decision making, becoming more creative with others, staying in touch with the environment despite physical incapacities, and improving health practices (Hey, 1996).

The wellness continuum picks up where the traditional medical model leaves off. Instead of a downward negative trajectory for the health of the older adult, focused on deterioration, the wellness model rises and moves in a positive direction (see Figure 3-1). The individual may reach plateaus in his or her ascension to higher-level wellness. The person may also regress because of an illness event, but the event can be a stimulus for growth potential and a return to moving up the wellness/health continuum (Figure 3-5). The division between the traditional and wellness continuums is a neutral point, where no discernible illness or weakness exists. Wellness is not given to a person; rather, it is a state of being and feeling that one strives to achieve through motivation and health practices. An individual must work hard to achieve wellness just as he or she must work hard to perform competently at a job.

Wellness and self-actualization develop through learning and growth. Education for wellness concerns the pursuit of the five dimensions of wellness: self-responsibility, nutritional awareness, physical fitness, stress management, and sensitivity to the environment. All these dimensions are crucial to one's wellness. Incorporation of these five dimensions into a lifestyle facilitates individual growth and attainment of Maslow's self-actualization and Erikson's eighth stage of growth and development, integrity. Growth and self-actualization are one's ultimate reward.

Wellness means more than preventive medicine. Preventive medicine is largely offensive in its approach to illness, employing vaccinations and screenings to avoid illness, whereas wellness is a collaborative effort between an individual and the primary care provider to maximize the quality of life. Wellness encourages health promotion and life enhancement, as well as addresses risk factors that can lead to disease and chronic illness if ignored.

DIMENSIONS OF WELLNESS
Self-Responsibility

Self-responsibility, or self-efficacy, implies control and places one's wellness in one's own hands. It says to the individual, "Your body is your house; how you maintain your body is your choice." It has a strong effect on one's health behavior. Many older people are not attuned to their body messages and have little or no knowledge about their health status, whereas others are attuned to negative rather than positive messages. Often the older person places the responsibility for keeping well in the hands of the nurse or others who give care. As a result of abdicating control over their own wellness, dependent behavioral expectations and roles evolve among the family, the caregiver, and the client.

Times are changing. The self-help movement for taking care of one's health needs has expanded enormously in the past few years. Governmental agencies have changed their focus to health promotion and disease prevention, necessitating client involvement in health outcomes. People are responding to these approaches and taking control of their lives. People are learning how to be in touch with their body signals and to take and seek action accordingly.

BOX 3-7   Steps for Health Behavior Change

PRECONTEMPLATION

Extended time period
Negative aspects of undesirable behavior stay in the periphery of the mind

CONTEMPLATION

Toy with ideas of change
Examine behavior problem
Consider balance between cost and benefit
May take a long time

PREPARATION

Intention to change unites with plan of action
Concrete steps to be taken within the next month

ACTION

Actual steps taken to modify behavior
Person feels empowered and in control of life
Frequently relies on support from others
Takes 1 day at a time

MAINTENANCE

Begins 6 months after action
Prevention of relapse
Lasts a lifetime

From Jitrarnontree N: *Evidence-based protocol. Exercise promotion: walking in elders,* Iowa City, Iowa, 2001, University of Iowa Gerontological Nursing Interventions Research Center, Research Dissemination Core; Prochaska JO et al: *Johns Hopkins medical health letter: health after 50,* Baltimore, 1996, Johns Hopkins Medical Institutions.

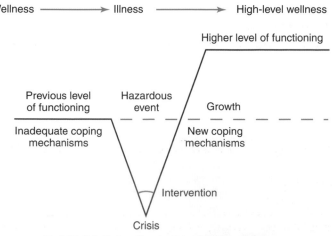

Wellness ⟶ Illness ⟶ High-level wellness

FIGURE 3-5 Growth potential: crisis as a challenge.

A significant time lag always occurs between change and acceptance of new ideas. Older people today are taking control of their lives and bodies; they are taking initiative and becoming empowered to educate themselves by actively seeking out those who can provide the particular information about their physical and mental needs, nutrition, and management of stress. Media blitzes and the Internet have made enormous differences in their ability to obtain desired information. Efforts that are most successful build group responsibility and social processes that are intrinsic to the self-health focus of the movement.

Change of health care behaviors is often difficult. The five steps of change are *precontemplation, contemplation, preparation, action*, and *maintenance* (Jitrarnontree, 2001; Prochaska, 1994). An individual may spend months in precontemplation and contemplation before he or she considers the benefits of action. Once the action occurs, maintenance begins about 6 months later. It is not uncommon and should not be considered a failure if an individual has to make several cycles through the stages before the desired effect is achieved. Behavioral researchers have shown that, in the example of smoking, 85% of smokers who eventually quit recycled back through precontemplation and contemplation stages. However, each relapse taught them something new to try in the next cycle. Box 3-7 outlines the steps in health behavior change.

The nurse can empower, enhance, and support the older person's movement toward self-responsibility by exploring with the person the underlying situations that may be creating a wellness imbalance and discussing alternatives available to him or her. There is general agreement about what examinations are important for persons 50 years of age and older, as well as a timetable for such examinations and tests. Table 3-3

TABLE 3-3

Suggested Examinations for Preventive Health Maintenance for Persons 50 Years of Age and Older

Examinations and Tests	Population Group	Frequency
Lipid disorders screening: TC and HDL-C	All persons	Every 1-3 years for men 35 and women 45 and older unless high risk
Pelvic examination and screening for cervical cancer	Women	Annually until age 70. After age 70, screening no longer necessary if 3 or more documented, consecutive, technically satisfactory/normal negative cervical cytology tests within past 10 years
Breast self-examination	Women	Monthly
Mammogram	Women	Ages 50-70 years: Every 1-2 years Age 70 years or older: Shared decision making
Osteoporosis screening	Women	Women 65 years or older regardless of risk factors
Digital rectal examination	All persons	Annually for women with pelvic examination; every 2 years for men
Sigmoidoscopy/colonoscopy	All persons	Initial screening at age 50 unless high risk Sigmoidoscopy every 5 years, or double-contrast barium enema every 5 years, or colonoscopy every 10 years
Stool for occult blood	All persons	Annually
Prostate examination	Men	Annually
Blood pressure	All persons	Every office visit and, at a minimum, every 2 years. More frequent monitoring is recommended if blood pressure is 120/80 or higher or risk factors are present
Diabetes mellitus screening	Age 65 years or older	Fasting plasma glucose every 3 years and at clinical discretion
Eye examination	All persons	Annually after age 50
Glaucoma test	All persons	Every 3 years after age 55; every year if family history
Depression screening	All persons	With annual examination
Screening for tobacco use	Pregnant women; All adults	With annual examination
Dental examination and cleaning	All persons	Yearly for those with teeth; cleaning every 6 months, every 2 years for denture wearers
Hearing test	All persons	Every 2-5 years
Immunizations		
Flu vaccine	All persons (well and with chronic conditions)	Annually for age 65 and older
Pneumonia vaccine	All persons (well and with chronic conditions)	Once after age 65 or older; booster may be needed after 5 years; ask physician
Tetanus booster	All persons	Every 10 years
Hepatitis B	Those at risk	Complete series

Compiled from AARP strategies for good health; *Healthy People 2000*, Washington, DC, 1991, U.S. Government Printing Office; Agency for Healthcare Research and Quality: *Guide to clinical preventive services 2005: recommendations of the U.S. Preventive Services Task Force* (www.pda.ahrq.gov).

lists the suggested preventive examinations that should be sought to maintain good health for those older than 50 years, according to the group involved and the frequency of testing. Medicare has recognized the value of prevention and Medicare Part B now includes coverage for a number of preventive services (Box 3-8). However, many older adults have not had all the recommended screenings covered by Medicare (USHHS, CDC, 2006). See Figure 3-6 for a preventive checklist for elders.

Nutritional Awareness

The nation as a whole is obese and remains undernourished because of an imbalanced diet. The nutrition of the elderly reflects this current dietary practice of food intake and use. During the period from 1999 to 2002, 69% of Americans ages 65 years and older were overweight or obese. The prevalence of obesity among adults 65 years of age and older increased from roughly 12% in 1990 to 19% in 2002. Weight problems among older adults increase the risk of disabilities related to cardiovascular disease, diabetes, and arthritis and are associated with increased functional limitations and decreased physical performance. Predictions are that if current increases in weight gain continue, by 2020 the prevalence of persons 50 to 69 years old who have difficulty bathing, dressing, or walking across a room will increase by 18% to 22% (Center for the Advancement of Health, 2006).

Undernutrition and malnutrition are also common problems among older adults in all settings. As people age, a number of physiological factors affect eating and appetite.

BOX 3-8 Medicare Coverage for Preventive Services

- One-time "Welcome to Medicare" physical exam
- Cardiovascular screening (cholesterol, lipid, triglyceride levels)
- Breast cancer screening mammograms (once every 12 months)
- Cervical and vaginal cancer screening (Pap test and pelvic exam once every 24 months unless high risk)
- Colorectal cancer screening (fecal occult blood every 12 months, flexible sigmoidoscopy every 48 months, screening colonoscopy once every 24 months if at high risk), barium enema (instead of colonoscopy or sigmoidoscopy) every 24 months for high risk or every 48 months if not at high risk)
- Prostate cancer screening (digital rectal exam every 12 months, PSA test once every 12 months)
- Influenza, pneumococcal, hepatitis B immunizations
- Bone mass measurements (once every 24 months for people at risk for osteoporosis or more often if medically indicated).
- Diabetes screening, supplies, and self-management training (fasting plasma glucose test, glucose monitors, test strips, lancets, diabetes self-management training)
- Glaucoma tests (once every 12 months for people at high risk for glaucoma)

From *Guide to Medicare's Preventive Services.* Available at *www.cms.gov.*

Psychological factors (depression, loneliness, isolation) can lead to reduced appetite and weight loss. Eating habits evolve from childhood, and specific dietary preferences and ethnic diets, although favored by an individual, may not provide the best nutrition.

Nutritional awareness involves learning about the foods that will make the body respond in a physically and emotionally healthy way. Heightened awareness is learning about "live" foods (fresh food, not canned or frozen) and nutrient-dense foods. Older people frequently depend on fast foods, prepared foods, and soft foods because of their convenience and the ease with which they can be carried and consumed. However, those foods are more expensive and contain many empty calories in addition to high amounts of salt, fats, and sugar. In the older adult, caloric needs decrease but the need for nutrients does not change. Selection of food should be directed toward the highest nutritional density.

The problem with nutritional awareness among older adults is the lack of nutritional education. Through reading, counseling, and classes, older people can learn to select and use "live" food in endless ways. Nutritional education might stimulate creative meal planning and bring to light both the economic benefits and the joy of new discoveries. Older people can be made more cognizant that good nutrition can prevent some of the chronic conditions that occur during old age. Problems such as constipation need not occur if the diet includes sufficient quantities of raw fruits and vegetables and whole wheat grains.

Caloric intake for most older individuals is uncertain; many do not eat the recommended 1200 to 1400 calories per day, whereas others eat well over this amount. In general, though, elders' appetites seem to diminish as they age. Older people may need to take a vitamin supplement. If older individuals are insecure about their nutrient intake from food, taking a daily supplement that supplies no more than 100% of the recommended amount of any nutrient will suffice. Beyond that, however, they risk distorting the body's nutrient requirements and suffering toxic effects from nutrient excess. Those who are not exposed to sunshine may need vitamin D supplementation.

We are what we eat, and if older people are to take control of their mind, body, and spirit to provide themselves with the highest level of wellness possible, it is essential that they become active in their nutritional intake. Older persons who are institutionalized and capable of making food selections should be allowed to do so, not only from the menu offered but also by perhaps forming a dietary selection group to plan menus with the dietitian or the institution's administration.

In summary, few older individuals eat an adequate diet. Nutrition is discussed in more depth in Chapter 9.

Physical Fitness

Few factors contribute as much to health in aging as being physically active. Despite a large body of evidence about the benefits of physical activity to maintain and improve function, especially in frail older adults, 33% of men and 50% of

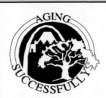

Saint Louis University Division of Geriatrics
Passport to Aging Successfully*

Please complete this questionnaire before seeing your physician and take it with you when you go.

SAINT LOUIS UNIVERSITY

NAME _____ AGE _____

BLOOD PRESSURE   lying down: _____ standing: _____

WEIGHT   now: _____ 6 months ago: _____ change: _____

HEIGHT   at age 20: _____   now: _____

CHOLESTEROL   LDL: _____   HDL: _____

VACCINATIONS   ☐Influenza (yearly)   ☐Pneumococcal   ☐Tetanus (every 10 years)

TSH   Date: _____   FASTING GLUCOSE   Date: _____

Do you SMOKE? _____

How much ALCOHOL do you drink? _____ per day

Do you use your SEATBELT? _____

Do you chew TOBACCO? _____

EXERCISE: How often do you

   do endurance exercises (walk briskly 20 to 30 minutes/day or climb 10 flights of stairs) _____/week

   do resistance exercises? _____ /week   do balance exercises? _____ /week

   do posture exercises? _____ /week   do flexibility exercises? _____ /week

Can you SEE ADEQUATELY in poor light? _____

Can you HEAR in a noisy environment? _____

Are you INCONTINENT? _____

Have you a LIVING WILL or durable POWER OF ATTORNEY FOR HEALTH? _____

Do you take ASPIRIN daily (only if you have had a heart attack or have diabetes)? _____

Do you have any concerns about your PERSONAL SAFETY? _____

When did you last have your STOOL TESTED for blood? _____

When were you last screened for OSTEOPOROSIS? _____

Are you having trouble REMEMBERING THINGS? _____

Do you have enough FOOD? _____

Are you SAD? _____

Do you have PAIN? _____

If so, which face best describes your pain?

😄	🙂	😐	🙁	😟	😣
0	1	2	3	4	5

MALES
Do you have trouble passing urine? _____

Have you discussed PSA testing with your doctor? _____

What is your ADAM score? _____

FEMALES
When was your last Pap smear? _____

When was your last mammogram? _____

Do you check your breasts monthly? _____

Are you satisfied with your sex life? _____

*This questionnaire is based on the health promotion and prevention guidelines developed by Gerimed® and Saint Louis University Division of Geriatric Medicine.

FIGURE 3-6 "Passport to Aging Successfully" for patients. This is available for patients at *www.thedoctorwillseeyounow.com*. (Reprinted with permission from *www.thedoctorwillseeyounow.com* and interMDnet Corporation, New York, NY.)

BOX 3-9 Healthy People 2010 Physical Activity and Fitness Goals and Objectives (Adults)

- Reduce the proportion of adults who engage in no leisure-time physical activity.
- Increase the proportion of adults who engage regularly, preferably daily, in moderate physical activity for at least 30 minutes per day.
- Increase the proportion of adults who engage in vigorous physical activity that promotes the development and maintenance of cardiorespiratory fitness 3 or more days per week for 20 or more minutes per occasion.
- Increase the proportion of adults who perform physical activities that enhance and maintain muscular strength and endurance.
- Increase the proportion of adults who perform physical activities that enhance and maintain flexibility.

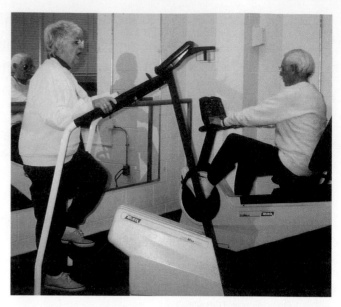

Today's older adult is interested in maintaining strength and endurance. (From Black JM, Hawks JH: *Medical-surgical nursing: clinical management for positive outcomes,* ed 7, St. Louis, 2005, Saunders.)

women older than 75 years engage in no physical activity (CDC, 2004). Only 4% of sedentary older adults have met the *Healthy People 2010* physical activity and strength training objectives (Struck and Ross, 2006) (Box 3-9). The prevalence of inactivity varies by race, gender, and ethnic group, with older women and black elders having higher rates of inactivity (Hughes et al., 2005a). The levels of physical activity among older adults have not improved over the past decade in the United States. Inactivity poses serious health hazards to young and old alike. It can lead to hypertension, coronary artery disease, obesity, tension, chronic fatigue, premature aging, depression, poor musculature, and inadequate flexibility (see Chapters 7, 8, and 15).

Many older people believe that they are too old to begin or participate in an active fitness program, but even with chronic conditions, a fitness program is possible. Even a small amount of time (at least 30 minutes of moderate activity several days a week) can improve health. The fundamental issue often overlooked is that each individual requires a program of activity that will work best for him or her. No matter how nutritionally aware, practiced in self-responsibility, or able to cope with stress, without physical fitness, one will not be fit or well.

Exercise: A Guide from the National Institute on Aging, provides specific information on exercise and fitness for older adults. The guide discusses the four types of exercises that are important in helping older people improve their health:

Endurance exercises include continuous movement involving large muscle groups that is sustained for a minimum of 10 minutes. These types of exercises increase breathing and heart rate and improve the health of the heart, lungs, and circulatory system. Examples of endurance exercises are swimming, bicycling, walking briskly, tennis, dancing, and gardening (mowing, raking). Initially, endurance exercises should be for a short duration and gradually increased.

Strength training (resistance) exercises build muscles and increase muscle strength by moving or lifting some type of resistance such as hand/ankle weights or resistance bands that require some physical effort. These exercises should be performed at least twice a week.

Balance exercises improve standing and gait and help prevent falls. Tai chi exercises have been shown to be of benefit for older people (Box 3-10).

Flexibility exercises keep the body limber and increase range of motion. These exercises should be performed at least 3 days a week (Resnick et al., 2006; Struck and Ross, 2006). Yoga is another form of exercise that can be practiced regardless of one's condition.

Fitness involves aerobic capacity, body structure, body composition, balance, muscle flexibility, and muscle strength. The most well-known type of fitness program is aerobic activity. The goal of aerobic activity is to fortify the body against stress. Aerobic activity such as jogging, swimming, and tennis is not out of reach for many older people. Doing the activity fast is not as important as is sustaining the endeavor long enough to accelerate the respiratory and cardiac rate sufficiently to reap benefits. Regular sustained aerobic exercise of the type and duration that will benefit the heart and blood vessels has been found to produce higher levels of high-density lipoproteins (HDLs) and lower blood triglyceride and cholesterol levels. Exercise also affords more efficient use of carbohydrates and a decreased resistance to insulin. Activity is discussed in greater depth in Chapters 7 and 15. Those older persons who have continued to be active and to exercise as a part of their everyday lifestyle continue to feel happier and healthier and look younger than those who were active but have now abandoned fitness.

A number of fitness activities are open to those who are capable of walking and being relatively active. Brisk walking for a sustained period of 10 to 15 minutes will tone the leg and arm muscles, provide improved oxygen exchange, and increase heart function. Some older people enjoy dancing,

BOX 3-10   Evidence-Based Practice: Influence of Intense Tai Chi Training on Physical Performance and Hemodynamic Outcomes in Transitionally Frail Older Adults

PURPOSE

This study explores the extent and time course over which tai chi (TC) impacts measures of physical performance and cardiovascular function in older adults who are becoming frail.

SAMPLE/SETTING

311 participants ranging in age from 70 to 97 (M 80.9) who were living in 20 independent congregate living facilities in the greater Atlanta area.

METHOD

A 48-week randomized trial was provided to 291 women and 20 men who were transitionally frail (older than 70 years old and had fallen at least once in the past year). Participants were randomized to either TC exercise or wellness education (control) interventions. Physical performance (gait speed, reach, chair-rises, 360 degree turn, picking up an object from the floor, and single limb support) and hemodynamic outcomes (heart rate and blood pressure) were obtained at baseline and after 4, 8, and 12 months.

RESULTS

The TC training had a positive impact on body mass index, systolic blood pressure, and heart rate as well as on chair rises. Fall occurrences were also reduced. Positive outcomes became apparent after 4 or 8 months of training and persisted through completion of the intervention.

IMPLICATIONS

TC exercise programs have positive benefits for frail older adults, including improved cardiovascular performance, decreased falls, and increased functional ability, and these benefits are demonstrated after at least 4 months of training.

Data from Wolf S et al: The influence of intense tai chi training on physical performance and hemodynamic outcomes in transitionally frail older adults, *J Gerontol A Biol Sci Med Sci* 61A(2):184-189, 2006.

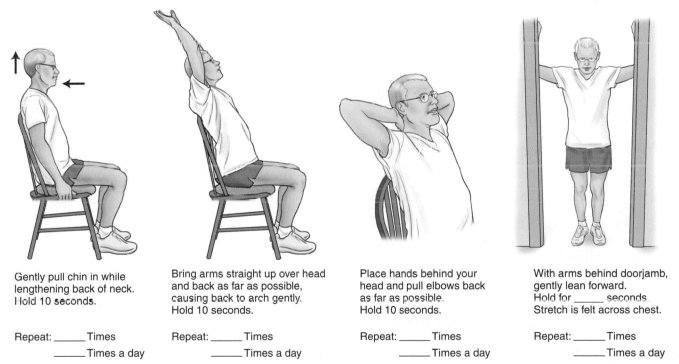

Gently pull chin in while lengthening back of neck. Hold 10 seconds.

Repeat: _____ Times
_____ Times a day

Bring arms straight up over head and back as far as possible, causing back to arch gently. Hold 10 seconds.

Repeat: _____ Times
_____ Times a day

Place hands behind your head and pull elbows back as far as possible. Hold 10 seconds.

Repeat: _____ Times
_____ Times a day

With arms behind doorjamb, gently lean forward. Hold for _____ seconds. Stretch is felt across chest.

Repeat: _____ Times
_____ Times a day

FIGURE 3-7 Examples of stretching exercises. (Adapted from Burke MM, Laramie JA: *Primary care of the older adult: a multidisciplinary approach,* St Louis, 2000, Mosby.)

which can be as strenuous as programmed exercise. For those older people who are limited in ability or confined to a chair, exercises can be done from a sitting position, which will accomplish many of the same benefits as if the individual were ambulatory.

Body balance is important to prevent falling. Muscle flexibility facilitates full range of motion for life's many activities that require stretching, bending, and reaching. (Figure 3-7 demonstrates stretching exercises to maintain and increase flexibility.) Muscle strength should be such that one can exert force and control over movement of the body. Easily accessible household objects, such as 1-pound bags of rice or beans, unopened ½-pound or 1-pound cans, or partially filled quart or ½-gallon water bottles, can be used for weight lifting in sustained, continuous repetitions to strengthen arm muscles. Also, various wrist and ankle weights can be purchased in sporting goods stores. Figure 3-8 illustrates a progression for strengthening the upper body with dumbbells.

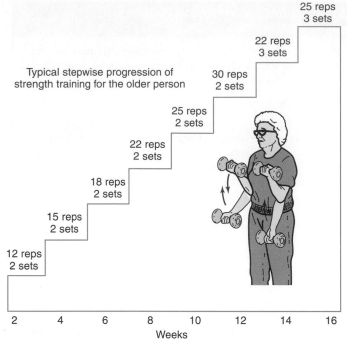

Typical stepwise progression of strength training for the older person

12 reps 2 sets
15 reps 2 sets
18 reps 2 sets
22 reps 2 sets
25 reps 2 sets
30 reps 2 sets
22 reps 3 sets
25 reps 3 sets

Weeks
2 4 6 8 10 12 14 16

FIGURE 3-8 An approach used in progressing an older person's dumbbell exercise program. The approach can be applied to other forms of strengthening programs. (From *Geriatrics* 47(8):34, 1992. Copyright 1992 by Advanstar Communications, Inc. Advanstar Communications, Inc. retains all rights to this article.)

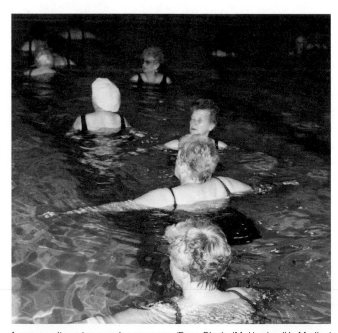

A community water exercise program. (From Black JM, Hawks JH: *Medical-surgical nursing: clinical management for positive outcomes,* ed 7, St. Louis, 2005, Saunders.)

Regardless of age or situation, the older person may find some activity that will be suitable to his or her condition. Table 3-4 compares sedentary and active approaches to daily living. Assisted living facilities and nursing homes should develop ongoing exercise programs for all residents. Studies have shown improvement in strength, walking speed, and

TABLE 3-4

Sedentary and Active Approaches to Daily Living

Sedentary	Active
Take the elevator or escalator.	Climb the stairs.
Call on the phone.	Walk down the hall, or walk next door.
Drive to lunch.	Walk to lunch.
Sit in a chair throughout a meeting.	Get up quietly and walk about the room.
Park right next to your destination.	Park some distance away from your destination.
Use the TV remote control.	Get up and walk to the TV when you want to change the channel.
Remain sedentary at your desk.	Take several minutes to do arm and leg exercises.
Visit with your colleagues in the "break room."	Take a walking break while you visit.

From Pender NJ et al: *Health promotion in nursing practice,* ed 4, Upper Saddle River, NJ, 2002, Prentice Hall.

functional abilities of frail nursing home residents with diagnoses ranging from arthritis to lung disease and dementia (Fiatarone et al., 1994; Hughes et al., 2005b). Following are examples of myriad ways in which elders keep fit:

- Em, an 84-year-old nursing home resident, jogged every morning in place for about 5 minutes and then briskly walked around the outside of the facility. Although she occasionally had lapses of memory, she was vital, erect, and interested in life around her.
- Nellie, 83 years old, began swimming to ease the discomfort of a short left arm, the residual effect of poliomyelitis, and for a frozen shoulder. She became an award-winning synchronized swimmer with 20 gold medals, 12 blue ribbons, and 13 trophies to her credit. Nellie continued to exercise this way despite the need to wear cataract goggles.
- At age 64, Dick became an avid wind surfer.
- In 1977, 91-year-old Madame Alexandra Baldina-Kasloff, prima ballerina in the early 1900s with the Bolshoi Theater, Moscow, was still participating in 90-minute workouts with her dance students.
- Hans Selye was known to swim for 30 minutes in the morning and ride his bicycle through the McGill University campus and then swim another 30 minutes in the evening and lift weights until his death in 1982 at age 75.
- Ada, age 82, still runs daily.
- Anabel, age 70, just completed her one-hundredth marathon.
- Woody, age 83, is a surfer.
- The Sun City Aqua Suns, synchronized swimmers, range in age from 68 to 88 years.
- Catherine, who died at age 106, walked to the bathroom three times each day; this was her activity. It was

BOX 3-11 Suggestions for Exercise Programs for Older Adults

- Provide appropriate screening before beginning an exercise program.
- Provide information on the benefits of exercise, emphasizing short-term benefits such as sleeping better.
- Clarify the misconceptions associated with exercise (fatigue, injury).
- Assess for declines in function, and discuss how exercise can minimize these declines.
- Assess barriers to exercise and how to overcome.
- Provide an "exercise prescription" that specifies what exercises and how often the person should exercise. Include daily and long-term goals.
- Goals should be specific, achievable, and match the older person's perceived needs and health and cognitive abilities, as well as their interests.
- Provide choices as to types of exercises, and design the program so that the person can do it at home or elsewhere when formal training ends.
- Provide self-monitoring methods to assist in visualizing progress.

- Group-based programs and exercising with a buddy may be more successful.
- Try to make the program fun and entertaining (walking with favorite music, socializing with friends).
- Discuss potential exercise side effects and any symptoms that should be reported.
- Share stories about your own personal exercise program and the benefits.
- Follow up frequently on progress, and provide reinforcement.
- Begin with low-intensity physical activity for sedentary older adults.
- Initiate low-intensity activities in short sessions (less than 10 minutes), and include warm-up and cool-down components with active stretching.
- Progression from low to moderate intensity is important to obtain maximum benefits, but activity level changes should be instituted gradually.
- Lifestyle activities (e.g., raking, gardening) can build endurance when performed for at least 10 minutes.

Data from Cress ME et al.: Best practices for physical activity programs and behavior counseling in older adult populations, *J Aging Phys Act* 13(1):61-74, 2005; Jitrarnontree N: *Evidence-based protocol. Exercise promotion: walking in elders.* Iowa City, Iowa, 2001, University of Iowa Gerontological Nursing Interventions Research Center, Research Dissemination Core; Schneider JK et al: Exercise training program for older adults: incentives and disincentives for participation, *J Gerontolog Nurs* 29(9):21-31, 2006; Struck B, Ross K: Health promotion in older adults: prescribing exercise for the frail and home bound, *Geriatrics* 61(5):22-27, 2006; Resnick B et al: Screening for and prescribing exercise for older adults, *Geriatrics Aging* 9(3):174-182, 2006.

difficult for her to do this, but without it she no longer would have walked or been able to sustain herself. The nurse who is knowledgeable in aging, age changes, health risk factors, and exercise science can develop and lead exercise programs for older adults. Goals for intensity, duration, and frequency of participation in physical activity should be established with the older adult with emphasis on changing sedentary behavior to active behavior at any level. Older people would benefit greatly from nurse-led programs designed specifically for the older adult that deal with their health conditions such as arthritis, diabetes, obesity, hypertension, and low self-esteem. Suggestions for initiating an exercise program with older people are summarized in Box 3-11.

Stress Management

Attitudes toward various life events determine one's perceptions of pleasure or displeasure. Uncontrollable events in daily life are responsible for many of the stresses experienced by the individual, but the individual also creates many stress situations. Selye (1974) defined *stress* as the body's response to any nonspecific demand placed on it, whether pleasant or not.

Any stressor (physical or psychological) will initiate stimulation and elevation of the enzymes in the adrenal glands to produce the major stress hormones: epinephrine, norepinephrine, and adrenal corticoids. These hormones are responsible for activating biochemical changes in the nervous, endocrine, and immune systems, which in turn affect all organ systems. Sustained stress can lead to such physical consequences as heart disease, hypertension, bowel irrita-

tion, and skin disorders. These conditions, when identified with stress as a major factor, are called *stress-related diseases*.

Most people recognize visible manifestations of stress such as increased body movement or language, irritability, sweaty or clammy hands, insomnia, and accelerated heart rate. The body responds to stress through the general adaptation syndrome (fight or flight). Fight or flight is an inborn response and part of the human character. It is frequently referred to as that "extra squeeze of adrenaline." At times it provides the individual with what seems to be superhuman power to escape from danger or the necessary stamina to complete essential detailed information by a deadline.

The general adaptation syndrome (Selye, 1956) comprises the alarm reaction, the stage of resistance, and the stage of exhaustion. Most stressors produce change only in the first two stages; more serious stressors lead to the exhaustion stage and thus death. However, exhaustion does not always terminate in death; when only part of the body is involved, the exhaustion stage may be reversible. For example, this frequently is the situation in exercise or local or regional infections. The hormonal activity initiated by the alarm reaction triggers the sympathetic nervous system to respond by elevating the blood pressure, pulse, and respirations and increasing metabolism and blood flow to the muscles. Biochemical changes begin, and the varied defense mechanisms of the body attempt to organize as a united front. At this point, while the body is mobilizing its forces, the individual's resistance is lowered. Once mobilization of defenses is completed, resistance rises to meet the threat. Adaptive capacity of the body is used to establish the individual at a new level of functioning or return the person to the prestress level—in other words, a return to a balanced state.

Adaptive energies are finite. When an individual is stressed over long periods, adaptive capacity is taxed and adaptive reserves are depleted. Minor happenings become major events, causing the body to remain mobilized in a ready state. When stressed again, one is forced to deal with or handle the stress at a lower threshold. Homeostasis remains tenuous and terminates eventually in illness or an irreversible state of exhaustion: death.

Older people are more frequently in a position of decreased ability to cope with daily hassles, cumulative life events, and other stressors because of their waning adaptive capacity. The deficits in adaptability are most evident in neuroendocrine interaction and in the separate responsiveness of the nervous and endocrine systems. Whether stress is physical or emotional, older people require more time to recover or return to prestress levels than when they were younger. In other words, the rate of recovery decreases with increasing age (Pender et al., 2002). Stress inventories are helpful in determining areas and degrees of stress, but it is wise to keep in mind that these tests have flaws. Stress inventories do not weigh individual differences; they relate to generalized stresses. What is stressful to one individual may not be perceived as such by another. It is also important to note that some individuals thrive on stress, whereas others require peace, quiet, and tranquility. Further discussion of stress can be found in Chapter 24.

Various means of stress reduction exist. Some individuals use one; others use a combination of methods. Most people believe relaxation is best achieved by being in tune with one's feelings. With an understanding of one's feelings and thoughts, the individual is more able to deal with these emotions and direct them positively to minimize the frequency of stress-involved responses. Exercise is one of the best antistress activities. Other methods include 10 to 20 minutes each day of deep relaxation, yoga, prayer, deep breathing, or fantasizing or daydreaming to remove oneself from stressful situations.

Meditation. Meditation is a form of relaxation and coping with stress. Meditation has many forms. In Eastern tradition, meditation involves working toward a psychological state termed *transcendental awareness* that restricts the focus or attention to an object of meditation, a physiological process, or an internal sensation. Mastery over attention develops an awareness that allows every stimulus to enter into consciousness devoid of our natural selection process; the ordinary cognitive process is stopped. To truly quiet the mind, practice and perseverance are necessary. Dramatic changes in lifestyle are not necessarily inherent in effective meditation. Two forms of meditation practiced in Western culture are Zen meditation and transcendental meditation. Both of these induce a state of relaxation.

Biofeedback. Biofeedback is a technique of getting feedback from the body's internal processes. By observing monitoring devices, persons can learn to influence heart rate,

circulation, and muscle tension. Biofeedback is a learned skill in stress control and explores the body-mind connection. It is particularly useful in conjunction with a wide variety of relaxation techniques. Machines show the individual the body-mind connection by providing visual or auditory signals to help the person develop awareness and then gain control of a specific autonomic function such as heart rate, blood pressure, muscle tension, or body temperature. Once learned, feelings that evoke the desired responses on the machine are applied by the person to everyday stresses without the aid of the machine. If the skill has been well learned and practiced, the results will be helpful to the person in stressful situations.

Autogenic Training. Autogenic training is a system of total body biofeedback or self-regulation without machinery; it is a combination of yoga and autosuggestion. Anyone without excessive hearing impairment or inability to concentrate can learn to regulate involuntary psychological and physiological processes through autogenics. Autogenics has been found to be effective in treatment of disorders of the gastrointestinal, circulatory, and endocrine systems, as well as anxiety, irritability, and fatigue. It can be used to increase resistance to stressors, reduce or eliminate sleep disorders, and modify pain.

Additional Methods of Stress Reduction

Progressive Relaxation. Relaxation decreases muscle activity and activity in the sympathetic and parasympathetic nervous systems. Relaxation results in decreases in oxygen consumption of the body, metabolic rate, respiratory rate, heart rate, premature ventricular contractions, both systolic and diastolic blood pressure, and muscle tension and an increase in alpha brain waves. Progressive relaxation, a method developed by Edmund Jacobson in 1938, can be achieved through tension-relaxation techniques of specific muscles or muscle groups or, without tension, through the countdown method, imagery, or recall of pleasant events or experiences.

Arranging One's Environment. Arranging one's environment to reduce the potential for stress is also possible. Designing a quiet environment, a place where one can take a momentary break to reenergize, is a way to reduce stress. For older people, the proximity of familiar belongings and environment can do much to reduce stress. Stress arises not only from worry, anger, expectations, and demands but also from loneliness, noise, and lighting. One should preplan to prevent stress from occurring or, if it does occur, to be ready for it. Application of what one has learned from a previous situation can help dissipate the intensity of stress. Occasionally getting lost in some creative pursuit is an excellent means of dealing with stress. For some, knitting is helpful, whereas others find that painting a pastoral scene or the side of the house works well. Just stroking a pet or watching fish swim in an aquarium can serve as a tranquilizer to stress. Others enjoy fishing, a game of golf, reading a book, or listening to music. Still others find writing poetry a means of releasing frustration and stress. Physical activity is an appropriate means of handling stress for some individuals

Developing Selfishness. It is important to clearly understand what the older person's goals are and to make sure that those goals are really expressive of self and are not goals that someone else wants fulfilled. Acceptance of someone else's goals can create much stress. Frequently, older people are caught in this situation, when an individual trying to help imposes expectations on the older person.

Perhaps one of the better ways of handling stress was expressed by Selye in an interview (Cherry, 1978) in which he recommends the practice of altruistic egotism; that is, look out for oneself first and give pleasure to self and others. *Eustress,* a term coined by Selye, is a balance of selfishness and altruism (altruistic egotism) that facilitates self-care and through which an individual has the desire and energy to care about others. Most individuals who exhibit stress-linked disease tend to be either too selfish or too self-sacrificing.

All methods and means to achieve stress management are open to all ages. Stress management requires education and change, which in itself can be stressful. In this technological society, stress reduction includes changing the environment, avoiding excessive change, time control, and time management. However, if stress management is taught in the context of eustress, that is, taking stress and making it work positively for you, the individual will gain in ability to control the stress in life.

Environmental Sensitivity. More attention is beginning to be focused on physical, social, and personal environmental spaces and their relationship to stress and health. The physical components of environmental sensitivity (air, water, and land mass) and the social components (government, economics, and culture) are avenues through which the individual's health and wellness can be enhanced or limited. In midlife,

one creates his or her own personal environment by career, job, friends, and lifestyle choices. However, the individual's influence on physical and social environment is more limited than in the personal sphere. One can consider where to live based on pollution, energy conservation measures, and food sources available, but if a work situation or a relocation is mandated, there is little one can do. Older people are often confronted with social and economic issues that force environmental changes against their wishes.

Poor water quality, air pollution, natural disasters, and extreme heat are examples of environmental pollutants that can be harmful to older people. The Environmental Protection Agency (EPA) has instituted an Aging Initiative to raise awareness of environmental hazards and to implement prevention strategies. Such efforts will benefit all citizens, and by protecting the environment, we protect our health. Older adults have been shown to have an increased susceptibility to air pollution and greater chance of requiring hospitalization for chronic obstructive pulmonary disease, asthma, and pneumonia during episodes of poor air quality. In 2002, 46% of the older adult population lived in countries with poor air quality, compared with 26% in 2000. Efforts to reduce air pollution such as clean-air regulations can decrease the negative consequences for all age-groups (Sykes, 2005). Excessive heat or cold can be hazardous for older people and cause many deaths. Chapter 16 discusses these conditions and hypothermia and hyperthermia.

Developing elder-friendly communities and increasing opportunities to "age in place" can enhance the health and well-being of older people. Many state and local city governments are assessing the community and designing interventions to enhance the ability of older people to remain in their homes and familiar environments. These interventions range from adequate transportation systems to home modifications and universal design standards for barrier-free housing (Wallace, 2005). Figure 3-9 presents elements of an elder-friendly community.

Addresses Basic Needs

- Provides appropriate and affordable housing
- Promotes safety at home and in the neighborhood
- Ensures no one goes hungry
- Provides useful information about available services

Promotes Social and Civic Engagement

- Fosters meaningful connections with family, neighbors, and friends
- Promotes active engagement in community life
- Provides opportunities for meaningful paid and voluntary work
- Makes aging issues a community-wide priority

Optimizes Physical and Mental Health and Well-Being

- Promotes healthy behaviors
- Supports community activities that enhance well-being
- Provides ready access to preventive health services
- Provides access to medical, social, and palliative services

An Elder-Friendly Community

Maximizes Independence for Frail and Disabled

- Mobilizes resources to facilitate "living at home"
- Provides accessible transportation
- Supports family and other caregivers

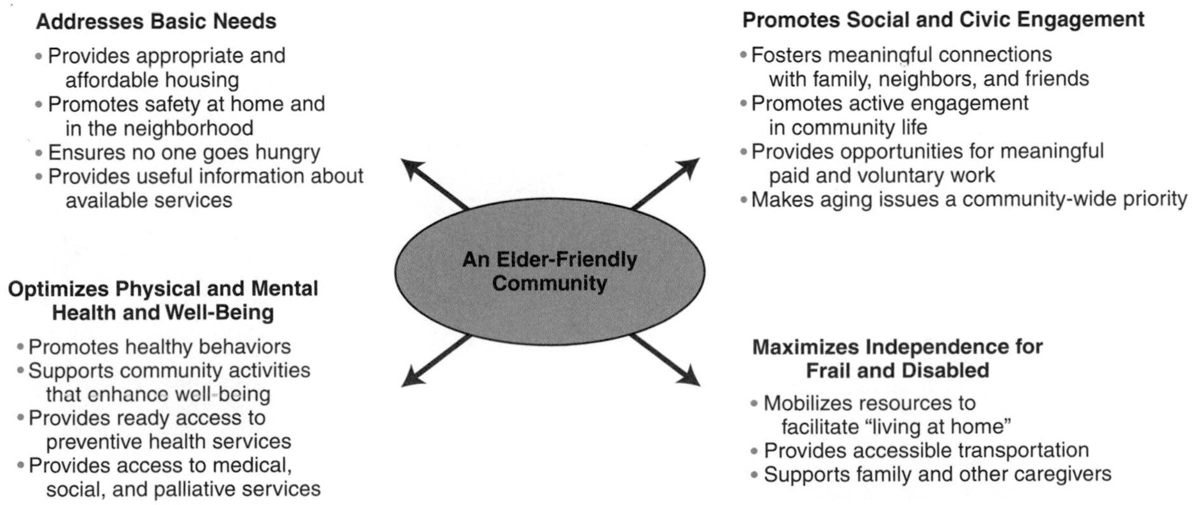

FIGURE 3-9 Essential elements of an elder-friendly community. (From AdvantAge Initiative, Center for Home Care Policy and Research, Visiting Nurse Service of New York [*www.vnsny.org/advantage/*]).

Personal space should be designed to include the opportunity for increasing self-development and experience, for receiving helpful feedback, and for establishing roles that are judged important. Personal environment should also facilitate time to be with friends, provide a supportive network, allow for enjoyment of beauty and nature, and provide abundant opportunities to give and receive affection and reinforce wellness behavior. The personal environment of many older persons living in the community and in institutions is devoid of the ingredients that make and reinforce a state of wellness. Again, instead of watching the older person languish or by chance discover means of improving his or her personal spaces, the caregiver's role should be to help the individual learn about opportunities and ways to design a better, happier, and healthier personal environment. Within confines, this is done in nursing care facilities that allow the older individual in residential care to bring a limited number of meaningful items and have easy access to the beauty of nature.

The sights and sounds confronting the older person and the opportunities to socialize, to make friends, and to feel wanted and perhaps loved should be important to the caregiver. Directly or indirectly, all of one's senses are affected by and affect the environment. Without this fifth dimension, wellness will not be of a high level. All dimensions are interrelated and influence one's state of health and wellness.

States (1986) uses the environmental components of the individual's room, the home, the neighborhood, and the planet at large as a basis of environmental sensitivity. Figure 3-10 provides a graphic view of the interrelation between environment and the four dichotomous elements: sick-well; dependent-independent; immobile-mobile; and malnourished–well-nourished.

▲ PROMOTING HEALTHY AGING: IMPLICATIONS FOR GERONTOLOGICAL NURSING

Environmental press (or demand) is a term used to describe the demands that social and physical environments make on the older person to adapt, respond, or change. Individuals usually function best when environmental press is slightly higher than the level at which they adapt. The environment should challenge them to try to function at their best level without overwhelming them. If environmental press is far below the person's adaptation level, sensory deprivation, dependence, learned helplessness, and functional decline can occur. It is important to assess the older person's health and functional ability to find an appropriate balance to promote adaptation and a better fit between the person and his or her physical and social environment to enhance quality of life (Hooyman and Kiyak, 2005).

Gerontological nurses use a holistic approach to enhance wellness in older people. The focus is on maximizing strengths, minimizing limitations, facilitating adaptation, and encouraging growth for all older people. Healthy aging does not mean the absence of disease; rather, it means achieving the highest level of personal wellness no matter the health condition. A wellness approach centers on assisting older people to meet as many of Maslow's defined needs as possible (Figure 3-11).

Nursing interventions for wellness may include the following:
* Identifying and stating strengths the individual demonstrates
* Discussing healthy lifestyle modifications
* Encouraging the reduction of personal and environmental risk factors

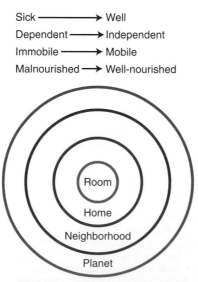

FIGURE 3-10 Environmental sensitivity. (Redrawn from States D: Personal conversation, San Francisco, 1986.)

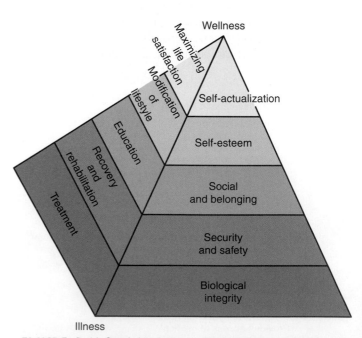

FIGURE 3-11 Correlation between illness-wellness continuum and Maslow's hierarchy of needs. (Developed by Patricia Hess.)

Human Needs and Wellness Diagnoses

Self-Actualization and Transcendence
(Seeking, Expanding, Spirituality, Fulfillment)
Maintains a healthy lifestyle
Takes preventive health measures
Seeks out stimulating interests
Manages stress effectively

Self-Esteem and Self-Efficacy
(Image, Identity, Control, Capability)
Exerts choices appropriately
Seeks out services when appropriate
Plans and follows a healthful regimen

Belonging and Attachment
(Love, Empathy, Affiliation)
Has an effective support network
Able to cope appropriately
Develops reciprocal relationships

Safety and Security
(Caution, Planning, Protections, Sensory Acuity)
Able to perform functional ADLs
Exercises to maintain balance and prevent falling
Makes effective changes in his or her environment
Follows recommended health screening for his or her age
Seeks health information

Biological and Physiological Integrity
(Air, Fluids, Comfort, Activity, Nutrition, Elimination, Skin Integrity)
Engages in aerobic exercise
Engages in stretching and toning body
Maintains adequate and appropriate nutritional intake
Practices health maintenance

These are not all the possible wellness diagnoses that may be identified. The above
are examples of nursing diagnoses that should be considered when planning care
for the older adult.

- Assisting the individual to devise methods of improving function, halting disabilities, and adapting lifestyle to reasonable expectations of self
- Providing access to resources when possible
- Referring appropriately and when needed

KEY CONCEPTS

- Wellness is a concept, not a condition. It is human adaptation at the most individually satisfying level in response to internal and external existing conditions.
- Wellness incorporates the holistic health movement, which assumes that health involves biopsychosocial and spiritual components of existence.
- Even in chronic illness and the dying process, an optimum level of wellness and well-being is attainable for each individual.
- *Health* is a term that is subsumed under *wellness* and indicates behaviors that are preventive of biopsychosocial problems.
- Pender (1987, 1996; Pender et al., 2002) states that health is "the actualization of inherent and acquired human potential through satisfactory relationships with others, goal-directed behavior, and competent personal care while adjustments are made as needed to maintain stability and structural integrity."
- Prevention is the key to postponing the onset of chronic illness. As life expectancy increases, the onset of chronic illnesses and related disabilities are compressed (postponed) to a shorter time closer to the end of life.
- *Healthy People 2000,* a document developed by the U.S. government, provides measurable goals by which to indicate our population's progress toward health.
- The goal of *Healthy People 2010* for the elderly is to prevent disability, delay illness, and modify its disabling effects as much and for as long as possible.
- Wellness includes behaviors fundamental to healthy adaptation, such as self-responsibility, physical fitness, stress management, nutritional awareness, and environmental sensitivity.
- The "medicalization" of our society has brought about the common belief that the absence of disease is health.
- The wellness model reinforces the belief that self-care and satisfactory adaptation are uniquely and individually defined.

CASE STUDY: Wellness in Late Life

Rhonda recently celebrated her ninetieth birthday with a large number of family and friends attending from far and near. She said, "That was the best day of my life! I was married three times but none of the weddings were as exciting as this. I have attained what I would never have thought possible when I was 50. Yes, life has been a struggle. One husband died in the Second World War, one was abusive and we were divorced, and the last husband, a wonderful man, developed Alzheimer's and I cared for him for 6 years. My children sometimes wonder how I have managed to keep such a positive outlook. I believe my purpose in living so long is to be an example of aging well."

Rhonda is frail and thin, and she has advanced osteoarthritis for which she routinely takes ibuprofen and calcium tablets. She does not tolerate dairy products, so she uses lactose-free products. She eats sparingly but likes almost all foods and is concerned about good nutrition. She daily rides the stationary bike in her apartment and last year walked a mile each day but has not regained her full function since a broken hip last June. While she was immobilized, she developed pressure wounds on her heels and coccyx but recently went to a wound center at a nearby hospital and is being treated effectively. She religiously follows the routine. As for religion, she says, "The closer I get to dying, the more I wonder what it is all about but I really just enjoy every day. Of course, I got depressed when I fell and broke my hip and I don't enjoy using the walker when I go out of the apartment but I feel blessed to have so many good people in my life."

Based on the case study, develop a nursing care plan using the following procedure*:

- List Rhonda's comments that provide subjective data.
- List information that provides objective data.

- From these data, identify and state, using accepted format, two nursing diagnoses you determine are most significant to Rhonda at this time. List two of Rhonda's strengths that you have identified from the data.
- Determine and state outcome criteria for each diagnosis. These must reflect some alleviation of the problem identified in the nursing diagnosis and must be stated in concrete and measurable terms.
- Plan and state one or more interventions for each diagnosed problem. Provide specific documentation of the source used to determine the appropriate intervention. Plan at least one intervention that incorporates Rhonda's existing strengths.
- Evaluate the success of the intervention. Interventions must correlate directly with the stated outcome criteria to measure the outcome success.

Critical Thinking Questions

1. What lifestyle changes might you suggest for Rhonda, and what would be your reason for doing so?
2. Where would you place Rhonda in the continuum of wellness? Explain your reasons for doing so.
3. Construct a definition of health that seems to you to incorporate the essential elements of a holistic perspective.
4. Discuss your thoughts about wellness as it relates to the medical concerns about old age.
5. Define wellness for yourself. What would you want to change in your life to achieve a sense of wellness?
6. Discuss the concept of wellness while dying and your thoughts about this issue.

---

* Students are advised to refer to their nursing diagnosis text and identify possible or potential problems.

RESEARCH QUESTIONS

Which physical conditions are most likely to impede the capacity for wellness?

Do most elders believe there is a state of wellness in spite of physical illness?

What are the factors that indicate one is in a state of "wellness"?

Is the physical deteriorative mode of defining old age related to the medical model or individual perceptions?

What are the variables that indicate a dying person is in a state of "wellness"?

How many people older than 50 years can explain wellness?

What do elders believe about the concept of "wellness"?

RESOURCES

American Association of Retired Persons, Reimagining America: How America can grow older and prosper, 2005
www.aarp.org

American Association of Retired Persons, Images of Aging in America 2004 (includes media presentation)
www.aarp.org/research/academic/images_of_aging.html

American Senior Fitness Association
www.seniorfitness.com

Armchair fitness video programs
www.srmchairfitness.com

Centers for Disease Control and Prevention
Health, United States, 2006
www.cdc.gov/nchs/data/hus/hus06.pdf

Centers for Disease Control and Prevention
The state of aging and health in America 2004
www.cdc.gov/aging

Davis et al.: Mirror, mirror on the wall: An update on the quality of American health care through the patient's lens, The Commonwealth Fund, April 2006
www.cmwf.org

Exercise: A guide from the National Institute on Aging
www.nia.nih.gov/HealthInformation/Publications/ExerciseGuide/

Exercise prescription for older adults with arthritis pain: Consensus practice recommendations
www.guideline.gov

Gentle chair yoga with Vera Paley (VHS or DVD with companion photo guide).
Louis and Anne Green Memory and Wellness Center, Florida Atlantic University
www.fau.edu/memorywellnesscenter

He W, Sengupta M, Velkoff V, DeBarros K: 65+ in the United States, 2005
www.census.gov

National Center for Chronic Disease Prevention and Health Promotion (Growing stronger, strength training for older adults, [downloadable book])
www.cdc.gov/nccdphp/dnpa/

NIH Senior Health (exercises for older adults)
www.seniorhealth.gov/exercise

Racial and ethnic approaches to community health (REACH 2010)
www.cdc.gov/programs/health07.htm

REFERENCES

Bortz WM: *We live too short and die too long*, New York, 1991, Bantam Books.

Center for the Advancement of Health: A *new vision of aging: helping older adults make healthier choices*, Washington DC, March 2006.

Centers for Disease Control and Prevention (CDC): *The burden of chronic diseases and their risk factors: national and state perspectives 2004*, Atlanta Ga: U.S. Department of Health and Human Services.

Cherry L: On the real benefits of eustress, *Psychol Today* 11(10):60, 1978.

Cress ME et al: Best practices for physical activity programs and behavior counseling in older adult populations, *J Aging Phys Act* 11(1):61-74, 2005.

Dunn HL: *High-level wellness*, Arlington, Va, 1961, RW Beatty.

Fiatarone M et al: Exercise training and nutritional supplementation for the physical frailty in very elderly people, *New Engl J Med* 330:1769-1775, 1994.

Fries JF: Health promotion and the compression of morbidity, *Lancet* 1:481-483, 1989.

Fries JF: *Where in health are we going? Healthy aging: challenges and choices for health professionals*, Conference, San Francisco, Oct 1-4, 1992.

Hansen-Kyle L: A concept analysis of healthy aging, *Nurs Forum* 40(2):45-57, 2005.

Hey RP: Healthy, wealthy, and wise, *AARP Bull* 7:6, July/Aug 1996.

Hooyman N, Kiyak H: *Social gerontology: a multidisciplinary perspective*, ed 7, Boston, 2005, Pearson.

Hughes S et al: Promoting physical activity among older people, *Generations* 29(2):54-59, 2005a.

Hughes S et al: Characteristics of physical activity programs for older adults: results of a multisite survey, *Gerontologist* 45(5):667-675, 2005b.

Institute of Medicine: *The future of the public's health in the 21st century*, Washington, DC, 2002, National Academy Press.

Jitramontree N: *Evidence-based protocol. Exercise promotion: walking in elders*, Iowa City, Iowa, 2001, University of Iowa Gerontological Nursing Interventions Research Center, Research Dissemination Core.

Lang J et al: Healthy aging: priorities and programs of the Centers for Disease Control and Prevention, *Generations* 29(2):24-29, 2005.

Markides KS, Mindel CH: *Aging and ethnicity*, vol 163, Newbury Park, Calif, 1987, Sage Library of Social Research.

Morley J, Flaherty J: It's never too late: health promotion and illness prevention in older persons, *J Gerontol A Biol Sci Med Sci* 57A(6):M338-M342, 2002.

National Center for Health Statistics: *Data 2010. The Healthy People 2010 database*, Washington, DC, 2002, Centers for Disease Control and Prevention.

National Center for Health Statistics: *Healthy people: tracking the nation's health*, 2002, Centers for Disease Control and Prevention. Available at *www.cdc.gov/nchs/about/otheract/hpdata2010/201indicators.htm*.

Pender N: *Health promotion in nursing practice*, Norwalk, Conn, 1987, Appleton-Century-Crofts.

Pender N: *Health promotion in nursing practice*, ed 3, Stamford, Conn, 1996, Appleton & Lange.

Pender NJ et al: *Health promotion in nursing practice*, ed 4, Upper Saddle River, NJ, 2002, Prentice Hall.

Prochaska JO: *Changing for good*, New York, 1994, Avon Books.

Resnick B et al: Screening for and prescribing exercise for older adults, *Geriatrics Aging* 9(3):174-182, 2006.

Rowe JW, Kahn RL: Successful aging, *Gerontologist* 37(4):433-440, 1997.

Selye H: *The stress of life*, New York, 1956, McGraw-Hill.

Selye H: *Stress and distress*, New York, 1974, Lippincott.

Spector RE: *Cultural diversity in health and illness*, Norwalk, Conn, 1985, Appleton-Century-Crofts.

Spector RE: *Cultural diversity in health and illness*, ed 4, Stamford, Conn, 1996, Appleton & Lange.

States D: Personal conversation, San Francisco, 1986.

Struck B, Ross K: Health promotion in older adults: prescribing exercise for the frail and home bound, *Geriatrics* 61(5):22-27, 2006.

Sykes K: A healthy environment for older adults: the aging initiative of the Environmental Protection Agency, *Generations* 29(2):65-69, 2005.

Travis J: *Wellness workbook: a guide to high level wellness*, Mill Valley, Calif, 1977, Wellness Resource Center.

U.S. Department of Health and Human Services (USHHS): *Healthy People 2000*, Pub No (PHS) 91-50212, 1-8, 22-27, 587-591, Washington, DC, 1991, U.S. Government Printing Office.

U.S. Department of Health and Human Services (USHHS): *Healthy People 2010*, ed 2, Washington, DC, 2000a, U.S. Government Printing Office.

U.S. Department of Health and Human Services (USHHS): *Tracking Healthy People 2010*, Washington, DC, 2000b, U.S. Government Printing Office.

U.S. Department of Health and Human Services (USHHS), Centers for Disease Control and Prevention (CDC), *Healthy aging: preventing disease and improving quality of life among older Americans*, Washington, DC, 2006, U.S. Government Printing Office.

Wallace S: The public health perspective on aging, *Generations* 29(2):5-10, 2005.

Wolf S et al: The influence of intense tai chi training on physical performance and hemodynamic outcomes in transitionally frail older adults, *J Gerontol A Biol Sci Med Sci* 61A(2):184-189, 2006.

CHAPTER 4

Physiological Changes with Aging

Kathleen Jett

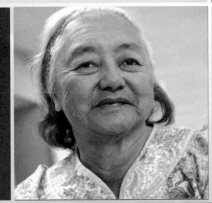

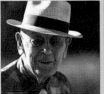

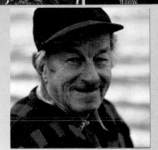

AN ELDER SPEAKS

Strange how these things creep up on you. I really was surprised and upset when I first realized it was not the headlights on my car that were dim but only my aging night vision. Then I remembered other bits of awareness that forced me to recognize that I, that 16-year-old inside me, was experiencing normal changes that go along with getting old.

Sally, age 60

LEARNING OBJECTIVES

On completion of this chapter, the reader will be able to:

1. Identify and discuss the normal age-related changes that occur in the following systems: integumentary, musculoskeletal, cardiovascular, respiratory, renal and urological, endocrine, gastrointestinal, nervous and special senses, reproductive, and immune.
2. Discuss the implications of the normal age-related changes in the human body on the promotion of healthy aging.
3. Begin to differentiate normal changes with aging from potentially pathological conditions.
4. Identify nursing interventions that promote healthy physiological aging.

Aging is a universal experience that some say begins at the moment of birth. The aging of the body is a normal part of the life of the person and is never pathological. However, the aging process is a wholly unique experience with each person and even each organ system aging at a different rate. Although questions about the process abound, all agree that the associated physiological changes are cumulative and affect the continuum of biological, psychological, social, and environmental processes (Figure 4-1). Three of the most important results of the physiological changes are the loss or decrease in compensatory reserve, the progressive loss in the efficiency of the body to repair damaged tissue, and decreased immune response.

Individual variations are significant at every age and in every part of the body and depend on a number of factors. The factors are either intrinsic (coming from within) or extrinsic (coming from without). Many of the normal changes with aging are intrinsic and less modifiable. Extrinsic changes are usually specific to one's way of life, such as smoking, lack of exercise, excessive exposure to sun, or traumatic injury.

Changes in body structure and function are lifelong alterations that begin to take on significance internally and externally in the fourth and fifth decades. External signs are the clues by which most people judge aging. Physical evidence of aging ranges from wrinkling and loss of elastin, to decreased muscle mass, decreased bone density, decreased vision, graying of the hair, and decreased hearing. However, these signs can be deceptive. Skin can become deeply wrinkled or hair can turn gray early in adult life. Today, individuals have at their disposal cosmetic surgery, hair coloring, makeup, and clothing choices that can make a person look younger than his or her chronological age.

Several of the age-related changes are similar to those seen in the presence of pathological conditions, and differentiating them from those which are expected is sometimes difficult. Many internal changes mimic disease manifestations

Special thanks to Patricia Hess, the previous edition contributor, for her content contributions to this chapter.

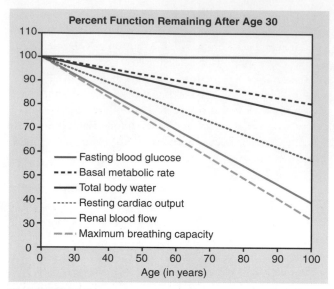

FIGURE 4-1 Changes in biological function with age. (Modified from Shock NW: In Carlston LA, editor: *Nutrition in old age, Tenth Symposium of the Swedish Nutrition Federation,* Uppsala, Sweden, 1972, Almquist & Wiksell.)

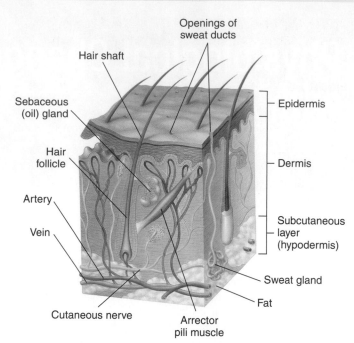

FIGURE 4-2 Structure of the skin. (From Thibodeau GA, Patton KT: *Anatomy & physiology,* ed 5, St Louis, 2003, Mosby.)

and might be interpreted as a pathological state in need of medical attention. On the other hand, normal changes can mask early signs of disease processes, for example, when the changes are incorrectly attributed to aging, such as urinary incontinence. This dichotomous situation makes it important for those who care for older adults to carefully explore the changes that do occur rather than immediately categorize them as either pathological or normal. The individual must be evaluated as a whole being for a correct interpretation of the changes that are occurring. Although normal age changes have usually been studied in concert with the most common pathological or disease conditions seen in late life, it is important for the gerontological nurse to be aware that they are not one and the same.

This chapter provides a detailed look at the changes in the human body that are considered a normal part of aging. The purpose of the chapter is to provide the nurse with the knowledge necessary to begin to differentiate normal changes from potential pathology. The nurse will then be better able to analyze his or her assessment findings so that changes that are suggestive of pathology can be evaluated further and changes that are clearly part of the aging process can be identified as such. With the identification, the gerontological nurse can facilitate healthy aging and adaptation to life's changes. Healthy aging can be defined as the ability to adapt to the normal changes and either the continuation or the adoption of a health-promoting and health-protecting lifestyle.

THE INTEGUMENT

The integument is the largest organ of the body (Figure 4-2). It provides clues to hereditary, dietary, physical, and emotional conditions and health. It serves as a means of communication and enables us to experience touch, warmth, cold,

and pain. It protects the internal organs, helps regulate body temperature, serves as an efficient vehicle for the excretion of salts, water, and organic wastes, and stores fat. It also helps protect the person from the damage of ultraviolet rays and produces vitamin D. Finally, the integument gives each person his or her unique and changing appearance. The integument is composed of the skin, hair, and nails. The skin is made up of three layers: the epidermis, the dermis, and the underlying subcutaneous layers between the skin and the muscles. The age-related changes in skin, hair, and nails are obvious to others and may be the first things noticed and attributed to "old age" See Box 4-1 for actions that promote healthy aging and potential implications for gerontological nursing.

Skin

Extrinsic causes of skin changes include environmental factors such as exposure to pollutants, chemicals, or solar radiation. Sun exposure increases the extent and speed of the normal changes in the aging skin. Characteristic thinning, dryness, roughness, wrinkles, and lightening are to be expected. These changes may affect the absorption of some topical medications. Increased incidence of skin cancers are usually the result of a lifetime of solar exposure (see Chapter 8), and the increased number of allergic rashes, irritations, and infections are thought to be associated with lessened immunity (see Chapter 2). Intrinsic changes occur gradually over time.

Epidermis. The epidermis is the outer layer of skin composed primarily of tough keratinocytes and squamous cells. Melanocytes produce melanin, which gives the skin color. The epidermis is in a constant state of renewal through regeneration, cornification, and shedding.

BOX 4-1 Promoting Healthy Skin While Aging

- Avoid excessive exposure to ultraviolet light.
- Keep moisturized.
- Avoid drying soaps.
- Always use sunscreens.
- Keep well hydrated.

The epithelium in the healthy young adult renews itself every 20 days, whereas epithelial renewal in an older adult may require 30 or more days because the keratinocytes become smaller and regeneration slows. This has significant implications for the slowed wound healing seen in the older adult (Gosain and DiPietro, 2004).

The number of melanocytes in the epidermis deceases about 10% to 20% per decade (Saxon and Eaton, 2002). Fewer melanocytes means a lightening of the overall skin tone, regardless of original skin color, and a decrease in the amount of protection from ultraviolet rays. However, in some areas of the skin, melanin synthesis is increased. Pigment spots (freckles and nevi) enlarge and can become more numerous with increased exposure to natural and artificial light. The new development of lentigines is common, and they are referred to as "age spots" or "liver spots." They are frequently found on the backs of the hands, wrists, and faces of light-skinned persons older than 50 years. Thick, brown, raised lesions with a "stuck on" appearance (seborrheic keratoses) are also common and of no clinical significance.

Dermis. The dermis is a supportive layer of connective tissues that provide stretch, recoil, and tensile strength. It lies just beneath the epidermis and is composed of elastin, collagen, and fat cells. It also supports blood vessels, nerves, hair follicles, and sebaceous (oil), eccrine (sweat), and apocrine glands. A thin basement membrane holds the dermis to the epidermis.

The dermis loses about 20% of its thickness with aging (Friedman, 2006a). The thinness of the dermis is what causes older skin to look more transparent and fragile. Dermal blood vessels are reduced, which accounts for resultant skin pallor and cooler skin temperature. Collagen synthesis decreases, causing the skin to "give" less under stress and tear more easily. Its absence also is a major factor in slowing the rate of wound healing. Elastin fibers thicken and fragment, leading to loss of stretch and resilience and the "sagging" appearance. The impact of the change in elastin has implications for a number of other systems as well.

Several of the structures found in the dermis have age-related reductions in functioning. Vascular hyperplasia causes more pronounced varicosities, benign cherry angiomas, and venous stars. At the same time, the decreased (about 60%) vascular supply to hair bulbs and eccrine, apocrine, and sebaceous glands decreases their size and function. The eccrine gland efficiency diminishes by about 15%, causing a decrease in spontaneous sweating in heat. Sebaceous glands secrete sebum, which protects the skin by preventing the evapora-

tion of water from the keratin or horny layer of the epidermis; sebum possesses bactericidal properties. With aging, the glands enlarge yet secrete 23% less sebum each decade, beginning after puberty (Chiu, 2000; Gilchrest, 2000). Nerve density decreases. Sensory and end-organ activity is gradually diminished beginning at age 10 years, and by 90 years of age one third of sensory function is altered. Light touch, vibratory, and corneal sensitivity and two-point discrimination are decreased (Chiu, 2000; Gilchrest, 2000). The effect of normal aging on the sensation of pain is unclear.

Hypodermis. Beneath the dermis and above the muscles lies the subcutaneous tissue of the hypodermis. It contains connective tissues, blood vessels, and nerves, but the major component is subcutaneous fat or adipose tissue. The primary purposes of the adipose tissue are to store calories and provide thermal regulation. It also provides shape and form to the body and acts as a shock absorber against trauma (The Merck Manual of Geriatrics, 2006).

Lean muscle is replaced by fat, yet subcutaneous fat is reduced and with it some degree of thermal regulation, especially related to hypothermia. It is not uncommon to hear older adults complain that they are cold or are seen wearing a sweater or sitting with a lap blanket. Windy, dry, cold weather can accelerate loss of body heat by evaporation, and subsequent hypothermia may lead to death by decreasing core body temperature (Cunningham and Brookbank, 1988).

Hyperthermia is also potentially problematic because of the reduced efficiency of the eccrine (sweat) glands. The glands become fibrotic, and surrounding connective tissue becomes avascular. These changes cause a decline in the efficiency of the body's cooling mechanism. The older the adult, the less likely the person is able to perspire freely. This results in an increased risk for heat exhaustion and heat stroke in warm environments.

Subcutaneous fat also seems to "shift" locations with aging. The diminution of the subcutaneous fat layer around the orbit of the eye creates a sunken appearance of the eyes. Landmarks become more prominent, and muscle contours are easily identified. Skinfold thickness, a measure of subcutaneous fat content, is markedly reduced in the forearm with age. Women older than 45 years begin to see the skinfolds on the back of their hands rapidly diminish, even if weight gain is substantial. At the same time, the amount of adipose tissue increases in the abdomen and in women, the thighs, even without a change in actual body weight.

Hair

Hair becomes gray as melanin production in the hair bulb decreases. Regardless of gender, 50% of the population older than 50 years have gray or partly gray hair. At times, the hair color may turn shades of yellow or yellow-green.

Vertex and frontal and temporal hair loss in some men is prominent beginning in the late teens or early 20s, and by 60 years of age, 80% of men are substantially bald. The amount of hair in the ears, nose, and eyebrows of older men increases (Luggen, 2005). Women may experience the same pattern of hair loss as men, but it is less pronounced. However, about 20 million women in the United States are affected by hair loss, and for 75% of them this becomes noticeable by age 85 years (Luggen, 2005). As a result of the altered balance of estrogen and androgens in women after menopause, excessive unwanted terminal hair can occur in the face and chin area. Axillary and pubic hair diminishes in quantity and thickness and, in some instances, disappears. Race, gender, sex-linked genes, and hormonal balance influence the maximum amount of hair that one has and the changes that will occur throughout life. Persons of Asian descent are less hairy than whites, and Native Americans may have little or no body hair (Rossman, 1986). In both men and women, hair becomes sparser; hair on the head thins, and leg hair may be completely lacking, especially in women who are not taking estrogen replacement. This latter finding is often misinterpreted as a sign of peripheral vascular disease.

Diffuse alopecia occurs in both genders with aging. It can also occur because of iron deficiency, hypothyroidism, autoimmunity, systemic diseases, medications, anabolic steroids, chronic renal failure, hypoproteinemia, or inflammatory skin diseases. Granulomatous disorders such as sarcoidosis and inflammatory disorders such as discoid lupus or lichen planus can cause hair loss because of scarring.

Nails

Nails of the fingers and toes thicken and change shape, color, and growth rate, in part as a result of decreased circulation. Nails become more brittle, flat, or concave (rather than convex) with longitudinal striations, and in persons with darkly pigmented skin, pigmented bands may appear in the nails. Nails may yellow or appear grayish with poorly defined or absent lunulae. Toenails grow at a 15% slower rate than fingernails (Cornell, 1986). Brittle nails with splitting ends or layers occur commonly in middle-aged women and elders of both genders. With age, the cuticle becomes less thick and wide. Vigorous manipulation of the cuticle may lead to further retardation of the already slowed nail growth. Although not a normal part of aging, onychogryphosis (nail plate thickens and distorts) and the fungal infection onycholysis are common. Vertical ridges (onychorrhexis) may appear as a result of poor nutrition, micro-trauma, and disease (AGS, 2006).

THE MUSCULOSKELETAL SYSTEM

A functioning musculoskeletal system is necessary for the body's movement in space, for gross responses to environmental forces, and for the maintenance of posture. This complex system comprises bones, joints, tendons, ligaments, and muscles. Although none of the age-related changes to the musculoskeletal system are life-threatening, any of them could affect one's ability to function and therefore one's quality of life. Some of the changes are visible to others through the person's appearance in stature and posture and have potential to affect the individual's self-esteem as well.

> **BOX 4-2** Promoting Healthy Bones and Muscles
>
> - Ensure regular intake of vitamin D and calcium.
> - Engage in regular weight-bearing exercise, e.g., tai chi.
> - Engage in regular flexibility and balance exercises, e.g., yoga.
> - For women: consider preventive pharmacotherapeutics.

Suggested nursing interventions to promote healthy aging of bones and muscles can be found in Box 4-2.

Structure and Posture

Changes in stature and posture are two of the obvious outward signs of aging and are caused by multiple developmental factors involving skeletal, muscular, subcutaneous, and fat tissue. These changes may begin to be seen as early as the fifth decade (Manolagas, 2000). Vertebral disks become thin as a result of dehydration, causing a shortening of the trunk. When combined with a slight curving of the cervical vertebra, height is lost. The long bones, which are not affected, take on the appearance of disproportionate size. A stooped, slightly forward-bent posture is common. The stooped posture is often accompanied by slightly flexed hips and knees and somewhat flexed arms, bent at the elbows. To maintain eye contact, it may be necessary to tilt the head backward, which makes it appear that the person is jutting forward. Posture and structural changes occur primarily because of calcium loss from bone and as a result of atrophic processes of cartilage and muscle (Figure 4-3).

Accompanying the changes in posture, shoulder width decreases because of shrinkage of the deltoid muscles and acromion processes. Chest width and pelvis width increase, and abdominal length decreases while its girth increases. An overall picture of a disproportionate individual may be seen, as if the person needs to be "stretched out a bit."

Bones

Bones comprise both organic tissue and inorganic products, especially minerals. Bone is not static; instead, it is active, constantly changing tissue. Bone integrity is maintained by a balance in the ongoing and cyclic resorption and renewal of bone minerals, especially calcium. The density of the bone mass can continue to increase until the person is in his or her 30s and then declines (Crowther, 2006). With age, disequilibrium in bone maintenance develops when the resorption is more rapid than the deposition of new minerals. Aging bone is composed of about one-third minerals and two-thirds connective tissue, the reverse of childhood bone development. Because of the reduction in estrogen at menopause, loss of bone mass is four times more common in older women than in men. As the reduction is a normal part of aging, so is the decreased bone mass (also referred to as *bone mineral density* or *BMD*). Susceptible women who are not taking hormone replacement after menopause may lose up to 50% of their cortical bone mass by the time they are 70 years old (Crowther, 2006). The loss of bone density in

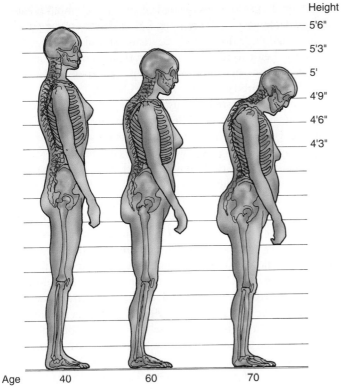

Height

— 5'6"

— 5'3"

— 5'

— 4'9"

— 4'6"

— 4'3"

Age   40   60   70

FIGURE 4-3 Normal spine at age 40 years and osteoporotic changes at ages 60 and 70 years. These changes can cause a loss of as much as 6 to 9 inches in height. Note the exaggerated thoracic and lumbar curves at age 70 years. (From Ignatavicius DD et al: *Medical-surgical nursing: a nursing process approach*, ed 5, Philadelphia, 2006, Saunders.)

women is most rapid in the first 5 to 10 years after menopause (Brucker and Youngkin, 2002). Excessive loss of BMD results in the pathological condition known as *osteoporosis* (see Chapter 15).

Reduced BMD is responsible for changes in physical appearance and in a significant increase in the risk for accidental injury. Osteoporosis of the cervical spine results in a C-shaped or kyphotic neck. Resorption of the bone in the mandible leads to poorly fitting dentures and painful sensations when chewing or biting. But by far the most important issue related to osteoporosis is the increased risk for fall-related fractures (Box 4-3). Such injuries increase with age, as does the associated morbidity and mortality (see Chapter 15).

Joints, Tendons, and Ligaments

The junction between two or more bones is called a *joint*. The joints make movement possible. Tendons and ligaments are bands of connective tissue that bind the bones to each other and allow the joints to articulate. Cartilage is a very fibrous tissue that lines the joints and supports specific body parts, such as the ears and nose.

Age-related changes in articular cartilage result from biochemical changes: increases in transglutaminase and possibly calcium pyrophosphates. As the cartilage in the joints dries, it becomes thinner, which results in less movement or pain as bones rub on bones. Knee cartilage decreases in

BOX 4-3   Research Note: Tai Chi Decreases Fear of Falling

A group of 291 women and 20 men between the ages of 70 and 97 years were provided with either a wellness education program or an intense tai chi exercise program. All participants were considered frail at the time of the study. At 8 months and at 12 months, the group who were receiving the tai chi exercise program were significantly less fearful of falling when compared with the wellness program alone group.

Data from Sattin RW et al: Reduction in fear of falling through intense tai chi exercise training in older, transitionally frail adults, *J Am Geriatr Soc* 53(7):1168-1178, 2005.

thickness a quarter of a millimeter per year, most likely because of wear and tear (Manolagas, 2000). Worn-down cartilage around joints produced by continuous flexing over the years coupled with stray pieces of cartilage and diminished lubricating fluid in the joints can lead to slower and painful movement at times. With progressive loss of articular cartilage, the common pathological condition of arthritis may develop (see Chapter 15).

Cartilage in the intervertebral disks shrinks and contributes to the loss of height. The cartilage in the nose and ears continues to grow throughout life, leading to the change in facial appearance in late life.

Ligaments, tendons, and joints show the result of cellular cross-linkage over time (see Chapter 2). They become dryer and stiffer, resulting in hardened, more rigid, less flexible movement and predisposing these structures to tears. They can also weaken with disuse and deconditioning. Tendons may shorten and move out of their usual positions in the presence of rheumatoid arthritis (RA), a painful and debilitating condition. Although RA is usually first diagnosed in persons in their 30s and 40s, when present in late life coping with it becomes more problematic when superimposed on the normal changes with aging (see Chapter 15).

Muscles

The three types of muscles are skeletal, smooth, and cardiac. Skeletal muscle is essential for movement, posture, and heat production, and much of it is under voluntary control. The smooth muscle is under the control of the autonomic nervous system and is found throughout the body, primarily in the lining of the organs and blood vessels. Cardiac muscle is a special muscle found only in the heart.

Age-related changes to muscles are known as *sarcopenia* and seen almost exclusively in the skeletal muscle. Muscle tissue mass decreases (atrophies) while adipose tissue increases. Muscle mass can continue to build until the person is in his or her 50s. However, between 30% and 40% of skeletal muscle mass of a 30-year-old may be lost by the time the person is in his or her 90s (Crowther, 2006). Half of the loss may be caused by physical inactivity, a change in the central and peripheral nervous system that decreases the motor units to muscle cells, and reduced skeletal protein synthesis.

The loss of maximum isometric contractile force is associated with loss of muscle mass, which decreases 20% in the sixth decade and up to 50% by the eighth decade (Manolagas, 2000). Strength and stamina decrease from 65% to 85% of the maximum strength an individual had at 25 years of age.

THE CARDIOVASCULAR SYSTEM

The cardiovascular system comprises the blood (see Chapter 5), the blood vessels, the lymphatics, and the heart. The cardiovascular system is responsible for the transport of oxygen and nutrient-rich blood to the organs and the transport of metabolic waste products to the excretory organs. The most relevant age-related changes in this system are myocardial and blood vessel stiffening, decreased beta-adrenoreceptor responsiveness, and impaired autonomic reflex control of the heart rate (McCance, 2006). In health, the age-related changes in the system are minimal and have little or no effect on its ability to function except when the need for blood flow is increased or in illness (Table 4-1). However, the prevalence of cardiovascular disease, particularly heart disease, is so high that it is sometimes mistaken for normal in late life. Indeed, heart disease is the number-one cause of death worldwide, even though much of it is preventable.

Heart

Radiological silhouette of the four-chambered healthy human heart shows a slight but clinically insignificant increase in size (Lakatta, 2000). Generally, the atrium increases about 20% in size between 18 and 93 years of age (Lakatta, 1993). Studies suggest that the left ventricle wall thickens up to 50% between ages 25 and 80 years as a result of the increase in myocyte size but that this is an adaptation that enhances filling capacity (Taffet and Lakatta, 2003). A fourth heart sound (S4) is not uncommon in a healthy elder.

Electrocardiogram changes with aging under normal circumstances are minimal. PR, QRS, and QT intervals lengthen slightly. Catecholamines and other enzymes that influence the effect of the force and speed of heart contractions diminish in amount, producing a longer interval be-

tween contractions, a weakened cardiac force, and a greater energy demand on heart muscle. Lower contractile strength, reduced cardiac output, and enzymatic stimulation together cause the heart to respond to the work demand with less efficient performance and greater energy expenditure than would be required at a younger age (Oskvig, 1999).

Because the heart is a muscle, it requires a rich and dependable blood supply. The coronary arteries serve that purpose. However, one of every two persons age 60 years and older may have some narrowing of the coronary arteries, but only about 50% of those have clinical signs of coronary artery dysfunction (Taffet and Lakatta, 2003). By age 60 years, the maximum coronary artery blood flow provides the cardiovascular system with 35% less blood than in earlier years. Contraction of the older heart is prolonged, most likely because of the slower release of calcium into the myoplasm during systole. Reduced efficiency and contractile strength of the heart muscle are reflected in decreased maximum heart rate, stroke volume, cardiac output, ejection fraction, and oxygen uptake (Oskvig, 1999). The decline in work response of the left ventricle at rest is a reflection of decreased stroke volume and cardiac output and a delay in heart muscle irritability and contractile recovery. This decline is also referred to as *reduced cardiac reserve* or *presbycardia*.

Despite these limitations, the healthy older heart is able to sustain adequate function for everyday life. Diminished cardiac output and reserve become significant only when the person is physically or mentally stressed by illness or emotion. Sudden demands for extra oxygen and energy may result in inadequate cardiac response, attributed to the presbycardia just noted. It takes longer for the heart to accelerate to both meet the sudden demand and return to a resting state. For the gerontological nurse, this means that the increased heart rate one might expect to see when the person is in pain, anxious, febrile, or hemorrhaging may not be evident. Instead, the nurse must depend on other signs of distress in the older patient. Similarly, the older heart may not be able to adequately compensate for other physical condi-

TABLE 4-1
Cardiovascular Function in Elderly Persons

Determinant	Resting Cardiac Performance	Exercise Cardiac Performance
Cardiac output	Unchanged or slightly decreased in women only	Declines because of a decrease in heart rate and stroke volume
Heart rate	Slightly decreased	Increases less than in younger people, possibly because of decreased cardiovascular response to catecholamines; overall slight decrease
Stroke volume	Slightly increased	Slight increase
Ejection fraction	Unchanged	Increases more from rest to exercise in younger people than in older people
Afterload	Increased	Uncertain
End-diastolic volume	Unchanged	Smaller for women
End-systolic volume	Unchanged	Lesser increase
Contraction	Increased because of prolonged relaxation	Decreases with vigorous exercise*
Cardiac dilation	No change	Increases at end-diastole and end-systole
VO$_2$ max	Not applicable	Declines because of a decline in skeletal muscle mass

Data from Gerstenblith G, Lakatta EG: Aging and the cardiovascular system. In Willerson JT, Cohn JN, editors: *Cardiovascular medicine,* New York, 1995, Churchill Livingstone.
*As measured by end-systolic volume/systolic blood pressure (ESV/SBP), an index of contractility.

tions that impose added cardiac demand such as infection, anemia, pneumonia, cardiac arrhythmias, surgery, diarrhea, hypoglycemia, malnutrition, avitaminosis, circulatory overload, and drug-induced and noncardiac illnesses such as renal disease and prostatic obstruction. In these circumstances, the gerontological nurse must be diligently alert to signs of rapid decompensation of both the previously well elder and one who is already medically fragile.

Valves. Four valves control the flow of blood in, out, and within the heart. When the competence of the valve is compromised, a small amount of blood may "leak" backward during the heart's contraction or relaxation. The sound of the backflow is described as a *murmur* and is rated or graded on a six-point scale, from "one" as insignificant to "six" as life threatening, and named according to its associated valve and timing (during systole or diastole). Some older adults have aortic and mitral murmurs that were chronicled from childhood. Generally those murmurs are not as prominent as murmurs that occur in late life.

In normal aging, the valves may be thicker and stiffer as a result of lipid deposits, collagen degeneration, and fibrosis, making slight incompetence and mild systolic murmurs an expected finding. Late-life valvular changes may be exacerbated by earlier rheumatic infections and arteriosclerosis. Aortic and mitral valves are most commonly affected and result in slight to moderate regurgitation of blood. At least 50% of elders have a systolic murmur that is a grade one or two. Murmurs that are diastolic are always indicative of a serious problem in cardiac hemodynamics and are always considered pathological (Lakatta, 2000).

Conductivity. As a completely unique muscle, the heart alone has the capacity to produce its own stimulation for movement, that is, contraction alternated with relaxation. The origin of the stimulation is in specialized pacemaker cells found in the sinoatrial (SA) node, the atrioventricular (AV) node, and the bundle of His. The beating movement produces "heart sounds," heard as S1 and S2 in the healthy heart.

During the third and fourth decades of life, and accelerating in the sixth decade, SA node cells decrease in number as myocardial fat, collagen, and elastin fibers increase. The number of SA cells at age 75 years is only 10% of that which existed at age 20 years (Taffet and Lakatta, 2003). Similarly, the AV node and the bundle of His lose a number of conductive cells into the fourth decade and the left bundle between the fifth and seventh decade (Miller, 1990).

Despite these changes in the conductivity, the aging heart is able to adapt. This means that the resting rate remains unchanged with age but the maximum heart rate is achieved with decreased activity. Sinus rates of fewer than 60 beats per minute are common in the elderly and do not necessarily indicate SA node disease. Significant interference with the blood flow to the SA node, either by occlusion or by narrowed arteriosclerotic vessels, can produce arrhythmias in late life as it would at any age. Slight arrhythmias, such as skipped or occasional extra beats, become more common in

with aging and may be a normal consequence of aging (Saxon and Eaton, 2002). Key instructions for older adults in promoting a healthy heart can be found in Box 4-4.

Blood Vessels

The major blood vessels involved in circulation are the veins and arteries. The heart propels the oxygen-rich blood from the heart through the highly elastic and flexible arteries. They are expected to expand and contract depending on the body's need for oxygen. The movement of the muscles around the veins and the valves within them carry blood back to the heart and lungs for reoxygenation. Several of the same age-related changes seen in the skin and muscles affect the intima of the blood vessels, especially the arteries.

The most significant change is related to elasticity. Elasticity affects blood vessel integrity, particularly the arteries. Elasticity is diminished because of changes in collagen, elastin, and possible cross-linking (see Chapter 2). In addition, vessel walls thicken as a result of reorganization of the cellular and extracellular matrix (Taffet and Lakatta, 2003). Elastic fibers fray, split, straighten, and fragment. Calcium that leaves the bone is deposited in the vessels. This chemical and anatomical alteration decreases the lumen size of the vessels and causes uneven blood flow to various organs. There is little flow change to the coronary arteries or the brain, but perfusion to other tissues and organs is reduced. The reductions in the perfusion of the liver and kidneys can be significant and affect medication metabolism (Oskvig, 1999). When the changes go beyond those expected with aging, it is usually attributed to atherosclerosis or arteriosclerosis.

Systolic blood pressure increases with aging as a result of a number of factors. Arterial wall stiffening consistently increases and baroreceptor activity decreases, which is thought to be associated with increased catecholamine levels. Dietary intake of sodium also is significant (Lakatta, 2000; McCance, 2006). In studies of rural Chinese elders who have diets of less than 1 gram per day of sodium, no increases in blood pressure were found (Taffet and Lakatta, 2003).

Less dramatic changes are found in the veins, although they do become somewhat stretched and the valves are less efficient. Pooling of blood increases the venous pressure, diminishing the effectiveness of peripheral valves. This means that edema develops more quickly, especially in the lower extremities, and that the older adult is more at risk for deep vein thrombosis because of the potential increased

---

BOX 4-4 Promoting a Healthy Heart

- Engage in regular exercise.
- Eat a low-fat, low-cholesterol, balanced diet.
- Maintain tight control of diabetes.
- Do not smoke, and avoid exposure to smoke.
- Avoid environmental pollutants.
- Practice stress management.
- Minimize sodium intake.
- Maintain ideal body weight.

sluggishness of the venous circulation. The normal changes with aging, when combined with long-standing but unknown weakness of the vessels, may become visible in marked varicosities and explain the increased rate of stroke and aneurysms in older adults.

THE RESPIRATORY SYSTEM

The respiratory system is the vehicle for ventilation and gas exchange, particularly the transfer of oxygen into and the release of carbon dioxide from the blood. It includes the nose, pharynx, larynx, trachea, bronchi, bronchioles, alveolar ducts, and alveoli. The respiratory structures also depend on the musculoskeletal and nervous systems for full function. The respiratory system matures by age 20 years and begins to decline in healthy individuals after 25 years of age (Table 4-2). Although subtle changes occur in the lungs, thoracic cage, respiratory muscles, and respiratory centers in the central nervous system, the changes are small and, for the most part, insignificant. The specific age-related changes include loss of elastic recoil, stiffening of the chest wall, inefficiency in gas exchange, and increased resistance to air flow (Figure 4-4). Respiratory problems are common but almost always attributed to exposure to environmental toxins (e.g., pollution, cigarette smoke) rather than the aging process (Sheahan and Musialowski, 2001).

Like the cardiovascular system, the biggest change is in the efficiency, in this case, of gas exchange. Under usual conditions, this has little or no effect on the performance of customary life activities. However, when an individual is confronted with a sudden demand for increased oxygen, a respiratory deficit may be evident.

Like one of the changes in older skin, infection is an increased risk because of a diminished immune response; however, in the lungs this risk is compounded by two additional age-related changes. The cilia, which normally act as brushes to repel foreign substances or propel mucus out of the trachea, are less responsive and less effective. Tockman (2000) and Anderson (2000) suggest that the importance of age to mucociliary transport is not fully established but may be clinically significant in the recurrence of respiratory infections. Neurologically, a diminished cough reflex is a normal age-related change. When other clearing mechanisms are intact, the cough reflex is not essential for respiratory clearance.

TABLE 4-2
Age-Related Changes in the Respiratory System

Respiratory Function	Pathophysiological Changes	Clinical Presentation
Mechanics of breathing	Increased chest wall compliance Loss of elastic recoil Decreased respiratory muscle mass and strength	Decreased vital capacity Increased reserve volume Decreased expiratory flow rates
Oxygenation	Increased ventilation/perfusion mismatch Decreased cardiac output Decreased mixed venous oxygen Increased physiological dead space Decreased alveolar surface area available for gas exchange Reduced CO_2 diffusion capacity	Decreased PaO_2 Increased A-a oxygen gradient
Control of ventilation	Decreased responsiveness of central and peripheral chemoreceptors to hypoxemia and hypercapnia	Decreased V_T Increased respiratory rate Increased minute ventilation
Lung defense mechanisms	Decreased number of cilia Decreased effectiveness of the mucociliary clearance Decreased cough reflex Decreased humoral and cellular immunity Decreased IgA production	Decreased ability to clear secretions Increased susceptibility to infection Increased risk of aspiration
Sleep and breathing	Decreased ventilatory drive Decreased upper airway muscle tone Decreased arousal	Increased frequency of apnea, hypopnea, and arterial oxygen desaturation during sleep Increased risk of aspiration Snoring Obstructive sleep apnea
Exercise capacity	Muscle deconditioning Decreased muscle mass Decreased efficiency of respiratory muscles Decreased reserves	Decreased maximum oxygen consumption Breathlessness at low exercise levels
Breathing pattern	Decreased responsiveness to hypoxemia and hypercapnia Change in respiratory mechanics	Increased respiratory rate Decreased V_T Increased minute ventilation

From Meiner S, Lueckenotte AG: *Gerontologic nursing*, ed 3, St Louis, 2006, Mosby; modified from Pierson DJ, Kacmarek RM, editors: *Foundations of respiratory care*, New York, 1992, Churchill Livingstone.

When impairment such as dysphagia or decreased esophageal motility is present, these normal changes significantly increase the risk for aspiration and its sequela (Anderson, 2000; Tockman, 2000).

Airways

Nose. With age and especially in men, the nose elongates downward as support of the upper and lower lateral cartilage weakens. The subsequent droop of the end of the nose can restrict airflow at the nasal valve junction. Narrowing of this valve in the presence of minor septal deviations that were no problem in one's younger years can cause breathing problems in one's later years (Sheahan and Musialowski, 2001).

Trachea and Larynx. Stiffening of the larynx and tracheal cartilage occurs as a result of calcification. Voice pitch increases for men and decreases for women, but substantially more so for elders who are in poor health. Breathlessness in speech is the result of less air passing through and the incomplete closure of the glottis. More limited mobility of the jaw may also contribute to this.

Chest Wall and Lung

Ossification or rigidity of the costal cartilage and the downward slant of the ribs create a less compliant, more rigid rib cage, which limits chest expansion. Intercostal and accessory muscles and the diaphragm become more compliant, or "floppier," as a consequence of muscle weakness. The potential for greater lung expansion exists but cannot be realized because of the structural limitations that develop in the thoracic walls. Some elastic recoil is lost as well (see earlier comments regarding changes in elastin in the skin). This reduced efficiency of air expulsion found in the older population resembles emphysema but is considered normal and is referred to as "senile emphysema" (Anderson, 2000; Tockman, 2000). The extent of change is the critical factor in differentiating normal from pathological conditions.

If skeletal defects such as kyphoscoliosis or arthritic costovertebral joints are present, this situation is exacerbated by further reducing the size of the chest cavity area in which the lungs can expand. These changes have the potential to increase dead space, decrease vital capacity, and decrease expiratory flow (Anderson, 2000; Tockman, 2000).

The elastin and collagen changes result in a decrease of the outward movement and the inward pull, with the result of slightly smaller total lung capacity, increased residual capacity and residual volume, and early airway closure. As a result of these chest wall changes, by the age of 70 years, respiratory muscle strength and endurance may decrease by up to 20% (McCance, 2006).

After age 30 years, the alveoli progressively enlarge and thus structurally resemble the air sac changes associated with emphysema. The elastin fibers in the alveolar walls are bound to the respiratory and terminal bronchioles, which help maintain the small airway patency at low lung volumes. The loss of the elastin attachment causes an increase in compliance, collapse of the small airways, and uneven alveolar ventilation, trapping air and increasing dead space (Anderson, 2000; Tockman, 2000). The alveolar dilation with the loss of alveolar attachments and the increase in the number of collapsed small airways, a physiological change, is called *senile lung* or *alveolar duct ectasia* (Campbell and Lefrak, 1978; Tockman, 1995) and is seen in some individuals older than 60 years. This creates an increase in lung resonance with percussion.

Total lung capacity is not significantly altered but, rather, is redistributed. Residual capacity increases with the diminished inspiratory and expiratory muscle strength of the thorax. Incomplete lung expansion does not provide for inflation of the lung bases and leads to basilar lung collapse and hyperinflation of the lung apices. The auscultation of slight atelectasis is common. Greater diaphragmatic motion is needed because of the restriction of the costal structures and the general overall change in muscle strength of the body. The lack of basilar inflation, ineffective cough response, and a less efficient immune system, as noted, pose potential problems, especially for persons who are sedentary, bedridden, or limited in activity.

Oxygen Exchange

The effectiveness of gas exchange is measured in blood gas analysis and reported in pH, PCO_2, and PO_2. Whereas the pH and PCO_2 do not change with aging, the PO_2 declines because of the changes already discussed. The maximum PO_2 possible at sea level can be estimated by multiplying the person's age by 0.3 and subtracting the product from 100. For

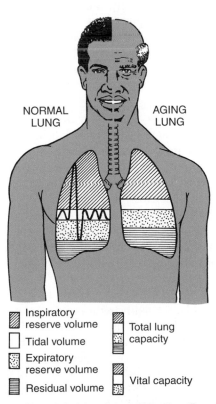

NORMAL LUNG   AGING LUNG

Inspiratory reserve volume

Tidal volume

Expiratory reserve volume

Residual volume

Total lung capacity

Vital capacity

FIGURE 4-4 Changes in lung volumes with aging. (From McCance KL, Huether SE, editors: *Pathophysiology: the biological basis for disease in adults and children*, ed 5, St Louis, 2006, Mosby.)

BOX 4-5   Promoting Healthy Lungs

- Obtain pneumonia immunization.
- Obtain annual influenza immunization.
- Avoid exposure to smoke and pollutants.
- Do not smoke.
- Avoid persons with respiratory illnesses.
- Seek prompt treatment of respiratory infections.
- Wash hands frequently.
- Eat meals in relaxed atmosphere.
- Practice thorough oral hygiene.

example, the maximum PO_2 of a 60-year-old is 82 as calculated ($100 - [60 \times 0.30]$) compared with 73 in a 90-year-old ($100 - [90 \times 0.03]$) (McCance, 2006).

Chemoreceptor function is altered or blunted at the peripheral and central chemoreceptor sites or in the integrating central nervous system pathways. This means that compensatory response to either hypercapnia or hypoxia is decreased. In healthy men between 64 and 73 years, response to hypoxia is 51% less and to hypercapnia is 41% less than in younger adults. This response is independent of mechanical lung changes and is attributed to the neuromuscular drive to breathe. Maximum inspiration and expiration pressures, which have declined as a result of chest wall inflexibility, reduce functional respiratory reserve and increase risk for respiratory failure. Compensatory responses are significantly hindered in situations of stress.

Reliable pulmonary function values that depict normal respiratory function specific to the older adult are difficult to obtain. The absence of reliable pulmonary function values on which to evaluate the respiratory status of the older adult requires that the nurse use other methods to assess the person's respiratory ability and needs, such as attention to respiratory rate and evidence of shortness of breath or cyanosis. Key instructions for older adults in promoting healthy lungs can be found in Box 4-5.

THE RENAL AND UROLOGICAL SYSTEMS

The renal and urological systems are composed of two kidneys, two ureters, a bladder, and a urethra. The renal system is responsible for regulating water and salts and maintaining the acid-base balance in the blood. The kidneys, the primary organs in the renal system, are highly vascular. They produce the hormone *erythropoietin*, which stimulates the bone marrow to produce red blood cells, and the enzyme *rennin*, which helps regulate blood pressure. The urological system is responsible for storing and excreting toxins and other fluids released by the kidneys.

The kidneys are the primary organs responsible for regulation of the chemical composition of the body and blood and fluid volume. In middle adulthood, each kidney has about 1 million nephrons, the basic working units of the kidney (Saxon and Eaton, 2002). Within each nephron is a tightly coiled collection of capillaries and a renal tubule,

called a *glomerulus*. With each beat of the heart, blood passes through the glomerulus for filtering; a small amount of the resulting filtrate is excreted as urine, and the remainder is returned back to the blood for further use by the body. The rate at which fluid filters from the blood through the glomerulus is the glomerular filtration rate (GFR). Urine flows through the tubules and eventually to the bladder for storage awaiting voluntary excretion through urination. Creatinine is a substance that is not reabsorbed and therefore is a good measure of the GFR and a proxy measure of kidney function. Two types of age-related changes occur to the urinary system—anatomical and functional.

Kidneys

Like other organs, in health the renal system continues to function adequately. Indeed, the age-related loss of nephrons, kidney mass, and ability to concentrate urine ordinarily leads to little change in the body's ability to regulate its body fluids and the ability to maintain adequate fluid homeostasis under usual circumstances.

The size and function of the kidneys begin to decrease in the fourth decade and are significantly decreased by the middle of the sixth decade; the kidney is 20% to 30% smaller by the end of the eighth decade (Saxon and Eaton, 2002). The kidney contour remains relatively smooth. Kidney mass and weight decrease mainly in the cortical portion where the reduction in number of glomeruli corresponds to the weight loss of the organ. By the eighth decade, age-related glomerular sclerosis is evident, which is in proportion to that found elsewhere in the body. The cause of sclerosis of the glomeruli is unknown. Microscopically, the renal tubules develop diverticula in the distal portion of the nephron. In general, these changes pose little threat to well-being unless nephron function is abruptly reduced by an acquired renal disease or a sudden salt or water load or deficit (Wiggins, 2003).

Renal Vessels

Renal blood flow decreases 50% by the time one is 80 years of age or about 10% per decade of adult life. This is caused by the changes in the renovascular bed (Horowitz, 2000). Preglomerular arterioles become obliterated, resulting in loss of blood flow. As with the glomerulus, the large renal vessels show evidence of sclerosis with age but it does not narrow the vessel lumen. Smaller vessels do not show this change. Only 15% of elders who are normotensive have sclerotic changes in the renal arterioles, so the implications for healthy aging are present.

Ureters, Bladder, and Urethra

The ureters, bladder, and urethra are muscular structures with the same changes found elsewhere. Some tone and elasticity are lost. This is most notable in the bladder, where it is accompanied by loss of bladder holding capacity. The capacity declines from about 500 to 600 mL of urine in the younger adult to about 250 mL in the older adult (Saxon and Eaton, 2002). Weakened contractions during emptying can lead to residual urine in the bladder. Changes to the extent to cause urinary incontinence, or the involuntary loss of urine, increase in frequency but should never be considered a normal part of aging (see Chapter 9).

Glomerular Filtration Rate

The changes in renal function are seen in the reductions in the GFR. GFR begins to decline at about 40 years of age and continues after that. The GRF may be reduced by about 50% by the time the person is 75 years old (Huether, 2006a). The presence of creatinine in the blood is directly related to muscle mass and is a product of muscle metabolism. The GFR is measured by the creatinine clearance, or the rate at which creatinine is filtered from the blood, and also changes with age. Urine creatinine, secondary to loss of muscle mass, alters the expected relationship of serum creatinine to the creatinine clearance. A linear decline begins at about age 40 years with a rate of 0.8 mL/min/1.73 m^2/year (Lindeman, 2000). However, up to one third of older adults do not exhibit a decline in GFR, suggesting that factors other than age-related changes may be responsible for altered renal function (Lindeman, 2000). Plasma creatinine clearance is constant throughout life. The decline in urine creatinine clearance is an important indicator for appropriate drug therapy in older adults (see Chapter 10). The GFR is a calculated number (see Chapter 12).

Regardless of the filtration rate, the ability to concentrate urine decreases. This means that the older adult cannot tolerate either dehydration or fluid overload as well as a younger adult. Hyperkalemia is more common as a result of this reduced efficiency. Sudden large changes in pH or fluid load can quickly lead to either hypervolemia or hypovolemia. Hypovolemia can quickly lead to renal insufficiency. These changes in function are especially important to the gerontological nurse when caring for the person who is exposed to changes in the environment, from renal-toxic medications to high temperatures, or for the person who has functional limitations affecting his or her ability to obtain adequate fluids.

THE ENDOCRINE SYSTEM

The endocrine system, working in tandem with the neurological system, provides the mechanism for the regulation and integration of body activities. The endocrine system effects control through the production and secretions of hormones by glands throughout the body. Hormones are responsible for and control reproduction, growth and development, maintenance of homeostasis, response to stressors, nutrient balance, cell metabolism, and energy balance. Two principles must be kept in mind when considering hormonal control and effects: (1) a particular hormone may have an effect on many body systems and functions, and (2) one body function may require the coordinated action of many hormones. The primary glands of the endocrine system are the pituitary, thyroid, parathyroid, adrenal, pineal, and thymus. The pancreas, the ovaries, and the testes are not glands, but they contain endocrine tissue.

The current view of endocrine changes in older adults is one of increased molecular disorderliness (Table 4-3). In contrast to the other systems, there are no consistent or predictable changes that affect function, with few exceptions (Hill, 2006).

Thyroid Gland

Slight changes occur in the structure and function of the thyroid gland, which may explain the increased incidence of hypothyroidism in older adults (Huether, 2006b). Some atrophy, fibrosis, and inflammation occur. Although other evidence of change is inconclusive at this time, diminished secretion of TSH and T4 and decreased plasma triiodothyronine (T3) appear to be age related. Serum T3 decreases with age (Cotter and Strumpf, 2002), perhaps as a result of decreased secretion of thyroid-stimulating hormone (TSH) by the pituitary gland. When thyroid replacement is needed, the older adult usually requires lower doses than younger adults.

Parathyroid Gland

Age-related changes in parathyroid hormone (PTH) secretion have been proposed as the explanation for alterations in calcium homeostasis, but the research has been inconclusive. It is known that persons consume less calcium as they age and that malabsorption may occur as well. When combined with the slight reduction in PTH, the hypocalcemia of hyperparathyroidism may occur. On the other hand, mild, persistent hypercalcemia is observed in healthy older adults as well.

TABLE 4-3
Aging Changes in the Endocrine System

Hyporesponsiveness	Hyposecretion	Degradation Changes	Hypersecretion
Increased connective tissue, pigment and structure changes in target tissue	Plasma insulin-like growth factor	Thyroid hormones	Norepinephrine
Decreased receptor-ligand binding	T3	Cortisol	Parathyroid hormone
Insulin resistance	Aldosterone	Aldosterone	Atrial natriuretic peptide
	Active renin	Inactive to active renin conversion	Glucagon
	Calcitonin	Norepinephrine clearance	
	Arginine vasopressin		
	Growth hormone		

From Meiner S, Lueckenotte AG: *Gerontologic nursing*, ed 3, St Louis, 2006, Mosby.

Adrenal Glands

Like the other glands, the adrenal gland becomes more fibrous. Although this does not affect the maintenance of glucocorticoid levels, it does decrease the metabolic clearance rate of glucocorticoids. The leaner one is, the less cortisol is used by the body. As the lean-to-fat ratio changes with aging, so might the use of cortisol. The higher cortisol levels may lead to a decrease in cortisol secretion. Although it is not yet known, these changes may affect the circadian patterns of adrenocorticotropic hormone (ACTH) and cortisol secretion (Huether, 2006b).

Endocrine Pancreas

The endocrine pancreas secretes insulin, glucagon, somatostatin, and pancreatic polypeptides. The secretion of these substances does not appear to decrease to any level of clinical significance in late life. However, for reasons unknown, the tissues of the body often develop decreasing sensitivity to insulin. When combined with increased needs for insulin in obesity, the result is often the development of diabetes type two. Older adults have the highest rate of diabetes type two than any other group, with significant variation by ethnicity and region (see Chapter 10).

Diseases associated with this system can occur with any age; however, the complex interrelationships between this system and others makes attributions to the aging process nearly impossible.

THE DIGESTIVE SYSTEM

The digestive system includes the gastrointestinal tract (GI tract) and the accessory organs that aid in the system's purpose of digestion. Like the endocrine system, few true age-related changes affect function. However, a number of common health problems can have a great effect on the digestive system. Changes in other systems can also affect GI structure and function. Age-related changes can be seen as early as the 50s (Huether, 2006c). The GI tract includes the mouth, pharynx, esophagus, stomach, small intestine, and large intestine.

Mouth and Teeth

A well-lubricated mouth and adequate dentition are important in the initiation of digestive activity. The breakdown of food begins as it enters the mouth and is broken apart by the teeth (mastication) and is prepared for digestion by the action of saliva.

Age-related changes affect both the teeth and mouth. With the wear and tear of years of use, the teeth eventually lose enamel and dentin and then they become more vulnerable to caries (cavities). The roots become more brittle and break more easily. For reasons unknown, the gums are also more susceptible to periodontal disease. As a result of these changes, teeth may be lost. Taste buds decline in number, and salivary secretion lessens. A very dry mouth (xerostomia) is common. Even in health, when combined, these changes all have the potential to decrease the pleasure and comfort of eating, which could lead to anorexia and subsequent weight loss. A number of medications taken for common health problems can quickly exacerbate potential problems, especially xerostomia. When the gerontological nurse administers medications to an older adult or conducts medication education, he or she should warn persons about this potential (see Chapter 12).

Esophagus

In youth, food passes quickly through the esophagus to the stomach because of the strong and coordinated contractions of associated muscle and peristalsis. In aging, the contractions increase in frequency but are more disordered and therefore propulsion is less effective. This, combined with the overall decrease in effective peristaltic action of the esophagus, causes a condition known as *presbyesophagus*. The sluggish emptying of the esophagus also forces the lower end to dilate, sustaining greater stress in this area and possibly causing digestive discomfort. Pathological processes that are seen in increasing frequency in older adults include gastroesophageal reflux disease (GERD) and hiatal hernias.

Stomach

Aging is also associated with decreased gastric motility and volume and reductions in the secretion of bicarbonate and gastric mucus (Huether, 2006c). The reductions are caused by age-related gastric atrophy and result in hypochlorhydria (insufficient hydrochloric acid). Decreased production of intrinsic factor can lead to pernicious anemia if the stomach is not able to utilize ingested B_{12} vitamins. The protective alkaline viscous mucus of the stomach is lost because of the increase in stomach pH. This makes the stomach more susceptible to peptic ulcer disease, particularly with the use of nonsteroidal antiinflammatory drugs. Loss of smooth muscle in the stomach delays emptying time, which may lead to anorexia or weight loss as a result of distention, meal-induced fullness, and the feeling of satiety (Price and Wilson, 2002).

Small Intestine

The small intestine is a 5- to 6-meter–long muscular tube in which nutrients are absorbed from the food contents into the bloodstream. The functional units are the villi, small inpouchings in the intestinal folds. They also secrete some of the digestive enzymes necessary for digestion and absorption.

The age-related changes include those related to smooth muscles noted earlier and those related to the villi, the anatomical structures essential for absorption. The villi become broader and shorter and less functional. Nutrient absorption is affected; proteins, fats, minerals (including calcium), vitamins (especially B_{12}), and carbohydrates (especially lactose) are absorbed more slowly and in lesser amounts (Huether, 2006c).

Large Intestine

The large intestine, about 1.5 meters long, transports food residue, unabsorbed gastric secretions, shed epithelial cells, and bacteria from the small intestine to the rectum for expulsion in defecation. Transport is caused by segmental movements of muscles called *peristalsis*. Although peristalsis is slowed somewhat with aging, it should not be to the extent to cause problems with defecation even though there is blunted response to rectal filling. In other words, constipation, often thought of as a normal part of aging, is not. Instead, constipation is more often the result of side effects of medications and life habits, immobility, inadequate fluid intake, and lack of attention to the gastrocolic reflex. The role of the gerontological nurse and elimination needs are presented in Chapter 7.

Accessory Organs of Digestion

The accessory organs include the liver, gall bladder, and pancreas. Each contributes in unique ways in the digestive process.

Liver and Gallbladder. The liver is second only to skin in organ size. It is a highly vascular organ dependent on blood from both the arterial and venous systems. Among other things, the liver produces bile and bile salts, key ingredients for intestinal emulsion and absorption of fats. The bile is stored in the gall bladder until it is needed during the digestive process. The liver is able to store blood for use as needed and is the primary site of the metabolism for most toxic substances (e.g., medications, alcohol) that enter the bloodstream.

The liver continues to function throughout life even with a decrease in volume and weight (mass). The weight decreases by 25% between ages 20 and 70 years in both men and women. The decrease in mass brings with it a concomitant decrease in liver blood flow. Increased lipofuscin (brown pigment) in the hepatocytes turns the liver brown. This pigment is the remnant of a lifelong buildup of unexcreted metabolic residue of lipids and proteins, but it is not clinically significant (Horowitz, 2000). Protein synthesis and the rate of degradation result in the accumulation of abnormal protein with a corresponding inability to break down protein. Liver regeneration is slowed but not greatly impaired. Liver function tests remain unaltered with age; changes are indicative of a pathological process (see Chapter 5). Alertness for changes in hepatic health is especially important relative to the metabolism of medications and other toxins.

There does not seem to be a specific change in the gallbladder; however, the incidence of gallstones increases (Huether, 2006c). This is possibly caused by the increased lipogenic composition of bile from biliary cholesterol. The decrease in bile salt synthesis increases the incidence of cholelithiasis and cholecystitis (Hall, 2003). In addition, the decrease in bile acid synthesis causes a reduction in hydroxylation of cholesterol. This, in conjunction with a decrease in hepatic extraction of low-density lipoprotein (LDL) cholesterol from the blood, increases the level of serum cholesterol in the older adult.

Exocrine Pancreas. The exocrine pancreas secretes enzymes and alkaline fluids that are essential for digestion. The pancreas functions in both the endocrine and the digestive

---

BOX 4-6 **Promoting Healthy Digestion**

- Practice good oral hygiene.
- Wear properly fitting dentures.
- Seek prompt treatment of dental caries and periodontal disease.
- Eat meals in relaxed atmosphere.
- Maintain adequate intake of fluids.
- Provide time for response to gastrocolic reflex.
- Respond promptly to urge to defecate.
- Eat a balanced diet.
- Avoid prolonged periods of immobility.
- Avoid tobacco products.

---

systems. Although the pancreas becomes more fibrotic, has increased fatty acid deposits, and atrophies slightly, these changes should not affect function. However, the overall reduction in the volume of pancreatic secretions may explain the increase in intolerance to fatty foods as one ages. Key instructions for the promotion of healthy digestion are provided in Box 4-6.

THE NERVOUS SYSTEM

The nervous system is the most complex of all and functions both alone and in tandem with all the other systems. The nervous system is divided into the central nervous system (CNS) and the peripheral nervous system (PNS). In combination with the endocrine system, it is responsible for the maintenance of homeostasis. The nervous system effects and is affected rapidly through the impulses of the neurons, the basic nerve cells. The neurons generate electrical and chemical impulses by selectively changing their cell membranes and communicating these changes to other neurons by the release of chemicals known as *neurotransmitters*.

Although many neurophysiological changes occur with aging, they do not occur in all older persons and do not affect all the same way. For example, the presence of neurofibrillary tangles is a classic sign of dementia and found in the brains of all persons with Alzheimer's disease, but they are found also in the brains of persons without dementia. Although it is very difficult to show a true cause and effect of age-related changes in the nervous system, some changes appear to be consistent (Table 4-4). Cognitive changes are discussed in Chapter 23.

The Central Nervous System

Most of the changes seen in the aging nervous system are found in the CNS. The CNS is divided into three functional components: the higher level brain (cerebral cortex), the lower level brain (basal ganglia, thalamus, hypothalamus, cerebellum, and brainstem), and the spinal cord. The brain is divided into three areas (the cerebrum, the cerebellum, and the brainstem) and into two hemispheres (right and left). Each hemisphere is divided into four lobes (frontal, temporal, parietal, and occipital). Each CNS neuron has a body (soma), fingerlike projections (dendrites), and a single

TABLE 4-4

Significant Changes in the Aging Nervous System

Neurological Components	Changes
CENTRAL NERVOUS SYSTEM	
Neurons	Shrinkage in neuron size and gradual decrease in neuron numbers
	Structural changes in dendrites
	Deposit of lipofuscin granules, neuritic plaque, and neurofibrillary bodies within the cytoplasm and neuron
	Loss of myelin and decreased conduction in some nerves, especially peripheral nerves (PN)
Neurotransmitters	Changes in the precursors necessary for neurotransmitter synthesis
	Changes in receptor sites
	Alteration in the enzymes that synthesize and degrade neurotransmitters
	Significant decreases in neurotransmitters, including acetylcholine (Ach), glutamate, serotonin, dopamine, and gamma-aminobutyric acid
PERIPHERAL NERVOUS SYSTEM	
Motor	Muscular atrophy—decrease in muscle bulk
	Decrease in electrical conduction
Sensory	Decrease in electrical conduction
	Atrophy of taste buds
	Alteration in olfactory nerve fibers
	Alteration in the nerve cells of the vestibular system of the inner ear, cerebellum, and proprioception
Reflexes	Altered electrical conduction of the nerve caused by myelin loss
	Altered reflex responses (ankle, superficial reflexes)
Reticular formation	Physiological changes in the reticular activating system (RAS) results in decreased stages 3 and 4 of the sleep cycle
AUTONOMIC NERVOUS SYSTEM	
Basal ganglia	Slowing of autonomic nervous system response as a result of structural changes in the basal ganglia

From Meiner S, Lueckenotte AG: *Gerontologic nursing*, ed 3, St Louis, 2006, Mosby.

axion. The neurons in the lobes and in the brainstem undergo age-related changes (Figure 4-5).

With aging, the number of neurons found in the CNS decreases with the correlating decrease in brain weight and size. This change in size is seen primarily in the frontal lobe and appears as "atrophy" on computed tomography (CT) scans or magnetic resonance imaging (MRI). By itself, this is considered a clinically insignificant finding. There is also decreased adherence of the dura mater to the skull, fibrosis, thickening of the meninges, narrowing of the gyri, widening of the sulcus, and increase in the subarachnoid space (Sugarman, 2006).

Cellular changes include loosening of the dendrite structure in the neuron, the deposition of amyloid and lipofuscin, and the presence of neurofibrillary tangles, senile plaques, and Lewy bodies (Sugarman, 2006). Lipofuscin is a yellow-brown pigment seen in older cells, but its effect is not yet fully known. It may be associated with the disruption of protein synthesis. "Neurofibrillary tangles" describes the physical appearance of the neuron that is the result of changes in neural fiber proteins. Their exact effect is not yet known. Senile plaques represent areas of nerve degeneration that can be found in the interstitial spaces of the cerebral cortex of the older brain. But again, the precise implication of this change is unknown.

Sleep disturbances may also be a normal part of aging resulting from changes in the reticular formation (RF). The RF is a set of neurons that extend from the spinal cord, through the brainstem, and into the cerebral cortex. With aging, a loss of deep sleep (stages 3 and 4) may be seen. Elders spend more time in bed to get the same amount of "sleep" as the time in light sleep increases in proportion to deep sleep (Friedman, 2006b). However, excessive daytime somnolence is not expected and should lead to a thorough assessment of causative factors aside from aging, especially side effects of medication and depression.

A subtle change in cognitive and motor functioning occurs in the very old. Mild memory impairments and difficulties with balance may be seen as normal age-related changes in neurodegeneration and neurochemistry (see Chapter 23). Changes in neurotransmitters occur with the decreasing levels of choline acetylase, serotonin, and catecholamines. Other enzymes such as monoamine oxidase (MAO) increase. Redundancy of brain cells may forestall the effects of these changes, but the exact number of cells required for certain functions is not known.

The Peripheral Nervous System

The PNS is composed of cranial nerves projecting from the brain and spinal nerves in either afferent or efferent pathways. The PNS includes the somatic nervous system and the autonomic nervous system (ANS). The latter is divided between the parasympathetic and the sympathetic nerves. The somatic nerves include the cranial nerves and others that carry information to and from the brain. The ANS activates

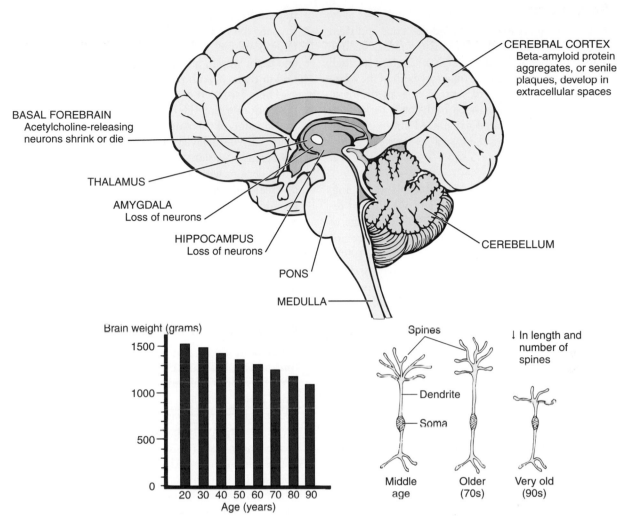

FIGURE 4-5 Changes in the brain with aging. (From Meiner SE, Lueckenotte AG. *Gerontologic nursing*, ed 3, St Louis, 2006, Mosby. *Bottom left and right*, modified from Sekoe DJ: Aging brain, aging mind, *Sci Am* 267:133-142, 1992. Copyright 1992 by Scientific American, Inc. All rights reserved. *Top*, Courtesy Carole Donner, Tucson, Ariz.)

smooth muscle, glands, and the cardiac muscle; it is entirely motor. The ANS works in association with other systems (e.g., endocrine) to maintain homeostatic equilibrium and is controlled to some extent by higher brain centers.

The best overall descriptors of the age-related changes to the PNS are a slowness of functioning and prolonged recovery phases after activation, especially of the ANS. The age-related changes are discussed in detail as they relate to proprioception, senses, and sense organs. For a discussion of common consequences of sensory changes, see Chapter 14.

Proprioception. Proprioception, the awareness of one's position in space, is a combined product of neurological and muscular feedback. Kinesthetic perception enables a person to automatically respond to changes in environmental conditions. In a younger person, this response is not only automatic but also almost instantaneous and, in many cases, protects the person from accidental injury. For example, a 20-year-old is walking on a smooth surface when suddenly an irregularity in the surface is encountered. The person is likely to trip. However, instead of falling, the body quickly adjusts the center of gravity and continues on—perhaps not even noticing what has happened. This ability decreases as the person ages; kinesthetic perception becomes less reliable, and falls, with or without injury, are much more likely to occur. Both the awareness of the threat to one's position and the speed of response to the change are age-related changes in the neurological system. Conditions such as arthritis, stroke, some cardiac disorders, or damage to the structures of the inner ear may affect peripheral and central mechanisms of mobility. Further discussion of sensory alterations appears in the following section and in Chapter 14.

SENSORY CHANGES

A number of changes occur as a result of the intrinsic aging process of the sensory organs and their association with the nervous system. Other changes are extrinsic and linked to the environment. One cannot totally escape diminution of smell, sight, sound, and touch.

Smell Perception

Sensitivity to odors increases through adolescence and then declines after age 60 years, with an increasing rate of decline after 80 years (Huether and DeFriez, 2006). Changes in smell are attributed to loss of cells in the olfactory bulb of the brain and a decrease in the number of sensory cells in the nasal lining. This change has implications both for appetite (decreases in) and for safety related to reduced ability to smell toxic substances in the environment such as smoke or gas.

Taste Perception

A very gradual decline in taste perception occurs with aging. The number of fungiform papillae (location of taste bud receptors) on the tongue decreases up to 50% by the age of 50 years (Jackson and Owsley, 2003). Loss of taste buds begins in the sixth decade and gradually progresses (Wilson, 1995). Taste buds atrophy, lose efficiency in relaying flavor, and decline in number. Sweet taste decreases because of a decrease in amylase in the saliva (Huether and DeFriez, 2006).

In crude taste, the number of nerve endings, papillae, and taste buds decreases. This is, however, more pronounced when estrogen or protein deficiencies exist (Wilson, 1995). Changes are accelerated in the presence of dental problems, medications, or smoking.

As a result, higher concentrations of flavor are required, especially for sodium, although all of the primary taste qualities are affected: sweet, salty, bitter, and sour (Horowitz, 2000). However, taste changes alone in the healthy person are modest and not considered to be significant. The most important potential effect is on appetite when in combination with any loss of smell as just noted or with special diets, such as low-sodium diets.

Tactile Perception

Tactile sensitivity (somatesthesia) decreases with age because of skin changes and is associated with reduced functioning of some of the sensory neurons. This is particularly striking in the fingertips, palms of the hands, and lower extremities (Meisami, 1995). However the extent of neuropathy seen in older adults (e.g., with diabetes) makes it difficult to pinpoint tactile changes as a normal part of aging. Normal and pathology-induced changes in somatesthesia are closely tied to those of pain perception.

There has been conflicting evidence on changes in pain perception in the older adult. However, some agree that the transmission of the pain impulse from the site of pain to the brain may be delayed. The delay creates some potentially dangerous situations, especially for the frail or dependent elder. Persons with limited activity, such as those confined to a wheelchair or to bed, may not feel the pressure on bony prominences or the body messages to change position, resulting in pressure ulcers. Transmission of hot and cold impulses may be delayed long enough for the individual to sustain significant tissue damage to some part of the body, such as with burns. However, the gerontological nurse cannot presume that an older adult, even one with limited cognition, has a reduced pain perception.

Eye and Vision Changes

Changes in eye structure begin early, are progressive in nature, and are both functional and structural (Table 4-5). The structures most affected are the cornea, anterior chamber, lens, ciliary muscles, and retina (Huether and DeFriez, 2006). All the age-related changes affect visual acuity and accommodation. These changes, particularly presbyopia (decreased near vision as a result of aging), begin to become noticeable in the fourth decade for many people. They are not usually great problems but are mainly an inconvenience. Although presbyopia is first seen between 45 and 55 years of age, 80% of those older than 65 years have fair to adequate far vision past 90 years of age. Nearly 95% of adults older than 65 years wear glasses for close vision (Burke and Laramie, 2000), and 18% also use a magnifying glass for reading and close work. Extraocular changes have both cosmetic and comfort effects. Key aspects of promoting eye health can be found in Box 4-7.

TABLE 4-5

Changes in the Eye Caused by Aging

Structure	Change	Consequence
Cornea	Thicker and less curved	Increase in astigmatism
	Formation of a gray ring at the edge of limbus (arcus senilis)	Not detrimental to vision
Anterior chamber	Decrease in size and volume caused by thickening of lens	Occasionally exerts pressure on Schlemm canal and may lead to increased intraocular pressure and glaucoma
Lens	Increase in opacity	Decrease in refraction with increased light scattering and decreased color vision (green and blue); can lead to cataracts
Ciliary muscles	Reduction in pupil diameter, atrophy of radial dilation muscles	Persistent constriction (senile miosis): decrease in critical flicker frequency*
Retina	Reduction in number of rods at periphery, loss of rods and associated nerve cells	Increase in the minimum amount of light necessary to see an object

From McCance KL, Huether SE: *Pathophysiology: the biologic basis for disease in adults and children*, ed 5, 2006, St Louis, Mosby.
*The rate at which consecutive visual stimuli can be perceived as separate.

BOX 4-7   Promoting Healthy Eyes

- Protect eyes from ultraviolet light.
- Avoid eye strain; use a bright light when needed.
- See health care provider promptly for changes in vision.
- Have yearly dilated eye examination.

Extraocular. Like the skin elsewhere, the eyelids lose elasticity and drooping (senile ptosis) may result from this and from skin atrophy. In most cases, this is a concern only for appearances. In extreme cases, it can interfere with vision if the lids sag far enough over the lower lid margin. Spasms of the orbicular muscle may cause the lower lid to turn inward. If it stays this way, it is called *entropion*. With the curling of the lid, the lower lashes also turn inward, causing irritation and scratching of the cornea. Surgery may be needed to prevent permanent injury. Decreases in the orbicular muscle strength may result in *ectropion*, or an out-turning of the lower lid. Without the integrity of the trough of the lower lid, tears run down the cheek instead of bathing the cornea. This and an inability to close the lid completely lead to excessively dry eyes and the need for artificial tears. The person also may need to tape the eyes shut during sleep.

A reduction of goblet cells in the conjunctiva is another cause for drying of the eyes in the older adult. Goblet cells produce mucin, which slows the evaporation of tear film, and are essential for eye lubrication and movement (Tumosa, 2000).

Ocular. The cornea is the avascular transparent outer surface of the eye globe that refracts (bends) light rays entering the eye through the pupil. With aging, the cornea becomes flatter, less smooth, and thicker, with the changes noticeable by its lackluster appearance or loss of sparkling transparency. The result is the increased incidence of astigmatism. For the person who was myopic (near-sighted) earlier in life, this change may actually improve vision.

The anterior chamber is the space between the cornea and the lens. The edges of the chamber include the canals that control the volume and movement of aqueous fluid within the space. With aging, the chamber decreases slightly in size and volume capacity because of thickening of the lens. Resorption of the intraocular fluid becomes less efficient with age and may lead to eventual breakdown in the absorption process. If the change is greater, it can lead to increased intraocular pressure and the development of glaucoma (Huether and DeFriez, 2006).

Within the anterior chamber is the iris. The iris is a ring of muscles inside the anterior chamber surrounding the opening into the eye (the pupil) that gives the eye color and regulates the amount of light that reaches the retina. The iris becomes paler in color as a result of pigment loss and increases in the density of collagen fibers. A normal age-related change in the iris is related to other neurological changes—that is, slowed response to sensory stimuli, in this case, to light and dark. Slowness to dilate in dark environments creates moments when elders cannot see where they are going. Because of the slow ability of the pupils to accommodate to changes in light, glare can be a major problem. Glare is a problem created not only by sunlight outdoors but also by the reflection of light on any shiny object, such as headlights or polished linoleum floors (Meisami et al., 2002). Persistent pupillary constriction is known as *senile miosis*.

At the edges of the cornea and the iris is a small ring known as the *limbus*. In some older adults, a gray-white ring or partial ring, known as *arcus senilis*, forms 1 to 2 mm inside the limbus. It does not affect vision and is composed of deposits of calcium and cholesterol salts.

The lens, a small, flexible, biconvex, crystal-like structure just behind the iris, is most responsible for visual acuity as it adjusts the light entering the pupil and focuses it on the retina. Age-related changes in the lens are probably universal. The constant compression of lens fibers with age, the yellowing effect, and the inefficiency of the aqueous humor, which provides the lens with nutrition, all have a role in altered lens transparency. Lens cells continue to grow but at a slower rate than previously. The lens can no longer focus (refract) close objects effectively and assessed as decreased accommodation. Changes to the suspensory ligaments, ciliary muscles, and parasympathetic nerves contribute to the decreased accommodation as well. Finally, light scattering increases and color perception decreases.

Lens opacity (cataracts) begins to develop around the fifth decade of life. The origins are not fully understood, although ultraviolet rays of the sun contribute, with cross-linkage of collagen creating a more rigid and thickened lens structure (see Chapter 14).

Intraocular. Intraocular changes occur as well, although these are not usually assessed by the registered nurse but are by the advanced practice nurse. The vitreous humor, which gives the eye globe its shape and support, loses some of its water and fibrous skeletal support with age. Opacities other than cataracts can be seen by the person as lines, webs, spots, or clusters of dots moving rapidly across the visual field with each movement of the eye. These opacities (floaters) are bits of coalesced vitreous that have broken off from the peripheral or central part of the retina. Mostly they are harmless but annoying until they dissipate or one gets used to them. However, if the person sees a shower of these and a flash of light, immediate medical attention is required because it might indicate serious retinal problems (Meisami et al., 2002; Tumosa, 2000).

The retina, which lines the inside of the eye, has less distinct margins and is duller in appearance than in younger adults. Fidelity of color is less accurate with blues, violets, and greens of the spectrum; light colors such as reds, oranges, and yellows are more easily seen. Color clarity diminishes by 25% in the sixth decade and by 59% in the eighth decade. Some of this difficulty is linked to the yellowing of the lens and impaired transmission of light to the retina, and the fovea may not be as bright. Drusen (yellow-white) spots may appear in the area of the macula (Tumosa, 2000). As long as these changes are not accompanied by distortion of objects or a decrease in vision, they are not clinically significant. Finally, the number of rods and associated nerves at the periphery of the retina is reduced, resulting in peripheral vision that is not as discrete or is absent (Tumosa, 2000). Arteries in back of the eye may show atherosclerosis and slight narrowing. Veins may show indentations (nicking) at the arteriovenous crossings if the person has a long history of hypertension.

Auditory Changes

Like the eye, age-related changes affect both the structure and function of the ear (Table 4-6). Some hearing loss affects about one third of all adults between ages 65 and 74 years and about one half of those ages 75 to 79 years. This high-frequency, sensorineural loss is known as *presbycusis*. More than 10 million elders have hearing loss (Williams, 2000). The ear includes outer, middle, and inner sections. Key aspects of promoting healthy ears can be found in Box 4-8.

Outer Ear. When observing the external ear, the prominent feature is the auricle, or pinna. With aging, it loses flexibility and becomes longer and wider as a result of diminished elasticity. The ear lobe (lobule) sags, elongates, and develops wrinkles. Together these changes make the ear appear larger. The periphery of the auricle develops coarse, wiry, stiff hair in men. The tragus also becomes larger in men.

The auditory canal behind the tragus narrows, causing inward collapsing. Stiffer and coarser hair lines the ear canal. Cerumen glands atrophy, causing thicker and dryer cerumen, which is more difficult to remove and a substantial cause for hearing loss (see Chapter 14).

Middle Ear. The tympanic membrane (eardrum), which separates the external ear from the middle ear, vibrates in response to sound. With aging, it becomes dull, less flexible, somewhat retracted, and gray in appearance. This vibrating membrane in turn stimulates the bones (ossicles) of the middle ear. The ossicle joints between the malleus and stapes often calcify, causing joint fixation or reduced vibration of these bones and therefore reduced sound transmission contributing to presbycusis.

Inner Ear. The ossicles end at the open window, the entrance to the inner ear. For functional hearing, each of the organs contained within must be functioning. With normal aging, they do continue to function; however, their sensitivity decreases. Vestibular sensitivity decreases as a result of degeneration of the organ of Corti in the cochlea and otic nerve loss. Changes in the efficiency of the cochlea and hair cells of the organ of Corti are responsible for the impaired transmission of sound waves along the nerve pathways of the brain and are considered to be the most common cause of presbycusis. Sounds can still be heard but not always clearly (see Chapter 14).

Atrophy of the organ of Corti begins in middle age and causes sensory hearing loss. Loss of cochlear neurons that occurs in late life, even with the preservation of the organ of Corti, is a neural hearing loss and is considered to be related to genetic factors. Familial tendencies in middle life associated with electrophysiological function of the organ of Corti are the basis of metabolic hearing loss (Gulya, 1995). Altered motion of the cochlear ducts may occur in middle age and is considered to be cochlear conductive hearing loss. The role of basilar membrane stiffening as a possible cause of this type of hearing loss is speculated. All these types of loss are presbycusis. Many elders have a combination of causes for their hearing deficit. Unilaterally or bilaterally, impairment of the aging otic nerve can cause a condition known as *tinnitus*, a buzzing, clicking, roaring, ringing, or other sound in the ear. Tinnitus becomes most acute at night or in quiet surroundings.

TABLE 4-6
Changes in Hearing Caused by Aging

Changes in Structure	Changes in Function
Cochlear hair cell degeneration	Inability to hear high-frequency sounds (presbycusis, sensorineural loss); interferes with understanding speech; hearing may be lost in both ears at different times
Loss of auditory neurons in spiral ganglia of organ of Corti	Inability to hear high-frequency sounds (presbycusis, sensorineural loss); interferes with understanding speech; hearing may be lost in both ears at different times
Degeneration of basilar (cochlear) conductive membrane of cochlea	Inability to hear at all frequencies, but more pronounced at higher frequencies (cochlear conductive loss)
Decreased vascularity of cochlea	Equal loss of hearing at all frequencies (strial loss); inability to disseminate localization of sound
Loss of cortical auditory neurons	Equal loss of hearing at all frequencies (strial loss); inability to disseminate localization of sound

From McCance KL, Huether SE: *Pathophysiology: the biologic basis for disease in adults and children,* ed 5, 2006, St Louis, Mosby.

BOX 4-8 Promoting Healthy Ears

- Avoid exposure to excessively loud noises.
- Avoid injury with cotton-tipped applicators and other cleaning materials.
- Use assistance devices as appropriate, e.g., hearing aids.
- See health care provider promptly for sudden changes in hearing.

THE REPRODUCTIVE SYSTEM

The reproductive systems in men and women serve the same physiological purpose—human procreation. Several organs in the system also can be a source of physical pleasure and a means of physical intimacy between persons. Age-related changes are under both nervous and hormonal control. Although both aging men and aging women undergo changes, the changes affect women significantly more than men. Women lose the ability to procreate after the cessation of ovulation and menses (menopause), whereas men remain capable their entire lives. A discussion of sexuality in late life can be found in Chapter 19.

The Female Reproductive System

Menopause is a universal experience for women, usually by the time they are in their early 50s. It follows a period known as *perimenopause*. Perimenopause is the transition period 5 to 10 years before the cessation of menses, when 90% of women note variability in the frequency and quality of menstrual flow. Follicular loss accelerates after about 37 to 38 years of age (Deneris and Huether, 2006). Both symptoms and timing depend on a number of factors including genetics, health, lifestyle, and concurrent medications. During this time, reproductive hormone levels fluctuate significantly, especially estradiol and estrone. As the level of these two decreases, the body responds with increases in follicle-stimulating hormone (FSH) and luteinizing hormone (LH) in an attempt to compensate.

As menopause signals the end of the reproductive phase in a woman's life, several other age-related changes occur, particularly in breast tissue and urogenital structures. As ovarian function decreases, the breast tissue involutes. During the premenopausal period (approximately between 35 and 50 years of age), mammary tissue decreases moderately. After menopause, the glandular tissue in the breasts decreases even further and is replaced with fat and connective tissue. Older breasts are smaller and less firm.

At the same time, a number of changes in the urogenital structures occur. Outwardly, the labia majora and minora become less prominent and pubic hair thins. The ovaries, cervix, and uterus slowly atrophy. The vagina shortens, narrows, and loses some of its elasticity, typical of aging muscle and skin. Vaginal walls also lose their ability to lubricate quickly, especially if the woman is not sexually active. The vaginal epithelium changes considerably; the pH rises from 4.0 to 6.0 before menopause to 6.5 to 8.0 afterward (Deneris and Huether, 2006). The vaginal changes result in the potential for dyspareunia (painful intercourse), trauma during intercourse, and more susceptibility to infection. Menopause is also often accompanied by lowered libido in women; however the mechanism of this is not known.

The Male Reproductive System

Although men have the ability to produce sperm from puberty on, they also experience changes in functioning of the reproductive and urogenital organs in late life. The changes are usually more subtle and noticed only as they accumulate, beginning when men are in their 50s. In normal, healthy aging, the testes atrophy, lose weight, and soften. The seminiferous tubules thicken, and obstruction caused by sclerosis and fibrosis could occur, which will decrease spermatogenic capacity. Although sperm count does not decrease, fertility may be reduced because of the higher number of sperm lacking motility or because of structural abnormalities. Erectile changes are also seen: more stimulation is needed to achieve a full erection, ejaculation is slower and less forceful, and refractory periods are longer (Deneris and Huether, 2006). As with women, alterations in hormone balances may play a part in the age-related changes in men. Testosterone level is reduced in all men but not enough to be considered a true deficiency in most. A secondary factor may be a decrease in the sensitivity of the target tissues to hormones.

By the age of 80 years, the prevalence of prostatic enlargement is up to 80% (Kamel and Dornbrand, 2004). The condition known as *benign prostatic hypertrophy (BPH)* is so common that some are beginning to call it a normal part of aging. The only time it is considered a problem is when the enlargement is such that it causes compression of the urethra. As a result, the man may experience urinary retention leading to repeated urinary tract infections and/or overflow incontinence. Intervention is pursued only when the symptoms of BPH interfere with the man's quality of life (Kamel and Dornbrand, 2004).

THE IMMUNE SYSTEM

The immune system functions to protect the host from invasions from foreign substances and organisms. To do so, it must be able to differentiate the self from the non-self (Kishiyama, 2006). The immune system includes many of the systems already discussed, including white blood cells, bone marrow, thymus, lymph nodes, and spleen.

A number of age-related changes have been described as having implications for the increased risk for infection in the older adult. For example, the skin is thinner and therefore less resistant to bacterial invasion. The reduced number of cilia in the lungs lead to the increased risk for pneumonia. The friability of the urethra increases the risk for urinary track infections, especially in women. But perhaps the most important of all is the reduced immunity at the cellular level. Cellular immunity has been the subject of intense scrutiny and is discussed in Chapter 2.

Late life brings a decrease in T-cell function resulting from a decrease in innate immunity, adaptive immunity, and self-tolerance. The response to foreign antigens decreases, but immunoglobulins increase, creating an autoimmune response not associated with autoimmune diseases, which usually occur before middle age (Michel, 2000; Proust, 2000). Being alert for signs and symptoms of autoimmune changes is probably as important as prevention and protection from infection for the older adult (Box 4-9).

OTHER CHANGES WITH AGING

Body Composition

Alteration in body weight occurs as lean body mass declines and body water is lost: 54% to 60% in men; 46% to 52% in women (Kee and Paulanka, 2000) (Figure 4-6). Fat tissue increases until 60 years of age; therefore body density is higher in youth because of the density of muscle versus the lightness of fat. From 25 to 75 years of age, fat content of the body increases by 16%. Cellular solids and bone mass decline; extracellular water, however, remains relatively constant. The water loss has significant implications for the dramatically increased risk for dehydration.

Temperature Regulation

An age-related change that is also especially important to the gerontological nurse is that related to temperature regulation. Early studies by Stengel (1983) found oral temperature norms in well elders significantly lower in women older than 80 years than in younger women. Older men consistently had an even lower temperature than women of comparable age. The old-old may have a temperature of 96.8° F with an average range of 95° to 97° F. By tympanic membrane thermometer, the temperature may be 96° F (Hogstel, 1994). These findings emphasize the need to carefully evaluate the basal temperature of older adults and recognize that even low-grade fevers (98.6° F) in the elderly may signify serious illness. *Because of this and because of a delayed immune response, a lack of fever (greater than 98.6° F) cannot be used to rule out an infection.*

The older adult is also at risk for hypothermia and hyperthermia because of reduced responsiveness to environmental changes of temperature. The changes that affect this include decreased shivering, slowed metabolic rate, decreased vasomotor response, diminished or absent sweating, and decreased perception of heat and cold (Huether and DeFriez, 2006). The nurse must be alert for potential problems for the frail or functionally impaired elder who may depend on others for care.

BOX 4-9	Healthy People 2010 Immunization Rates

Objective 1-9c: Reduce hospitalizations for preventable pneumonia or influenza—persons 65 years and older
Baseline: 10.6 persons per 10,000 (1996)
2010 Target: 8.0 persons per 10,000

Objective 14-5: Reduce invasive pneumococcal infections
Baseline and 2010 Target:

OBJECTIVE		RATE PER 100,000	
		1997 Baseline	2010 Target
	New invasive pneumococcal infections		
14-5b	Adults 65 years and older	62	42
	Invasive penicillin-resistant pneumococcal infections		
14-5d	Adults 65 years and older	9	7

From U.S. Department of Health and Human Services: *Healthy People 2010: national health promotion and disease prevention objectives,* Washington, DC, 2000, The Department.

Proportion of Body Weight Represented by Water

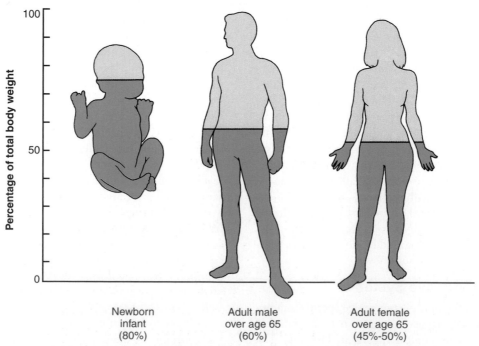

FIGURE 4-6 Changes in body water distribution. (From Thibodeau GA, Patton KT: *Structure and function of the body,* ed 12, St Louis, 2004, Mosby.)

It can be concluded that complex functions of the body decline more than simple body processes; that coordinated activity, which relies on interacting systems such as nerves, muscles, and glands, has a greater decremental loss than single-system activity; and that a uniform and predictable loss of cell function occurs in all vital organs. Yet most older adults are able to function effectively within the physical dictates of their body and continue to live to a healthy old age, capable of wisdom, judgment, and satisfaction.

Many of the age changes that occur have been discussed here and will be elaborated further in subsequent chapters.

KEY CONCEPTS

- Age-related changes that are observable and measurable occur over time and are focused chiefly on physiological and biological changes.
- The rate of aging of body systems and functions varies enormously.
- Individuals normally and gradually lose bone mass, structural integrity of organs, and specificity of bodily processes in the course of aging.
- Physical appearance inevitably changes with a downward shift of skin and tissue integrity brought about by the pressure of gravity over time.

Human Needs and Wellness Diagnoses

Self-Actualization and Transcendence
(Seeking, Expanding, Spirituality, Fulfillment)
Is able to cope with adverse physical conditions
Expresses self appropriately
Overcomes physical adversity with spirituality

Self-Esteem and Self-Efficacy
(Image, Identity, Control, Capability)
Has a strong self-esteem
Has multiple hobbies
Solves problems effectively
Is well groomed

Belonging and Attachment
(Love, Empathy, Affiliation)
Expresses an adequate sense of belonging
Participates in group activities
Appropriately expresses affection toward others

Safety and Security
(Caution, Planning, Protections, Sensory Acuity)
Adapts to changes in sensory acuity
Problem solves satisfactorily
Has adequate mobility
Travels alone

Biological and Physiological Integrity
(Air, Fluids, Comfort, Activity, Nutrition, Elimination, Skin Integrity)
Has adequate cardiac output
Has intact skin
Maintains adequate nutrition
Maintains adequate fluid intake
Has sufficient range of motion

These are not all the possible wellness diagnoses that may be identified. The above are examples of nursing diagnoses that should be considered when planning care for the older adult.

CASE STUDY: Changes with Aging

Mrs. Rodriguez is a 60-year-old Latina woman who lives with her daughter and her family. Her granddaughter Elana has just started nursing school and has become more aware of her grandmother's health. She has noticed the following conditions, which she is afraid are signs of health problems.

Mrs. Rodriguez is complaining about her knees; they are feeling stiffer, especially in the morning. She is having difficulty reading her crossword puzzles and states that the letters are just too small. She hasn't noticed it, but those around her find that she understands them better when they look at her while they are speaking. She is also complaining that she gets out of breath easily, especially when she is climbing the steps to her second-floor room—something she has done without difficulty for years.

Based on the case study, develop a nursing care plan using the following procedure*:

- List Mrs. Rodriguez's comments that provide subjective data.
- List information that provides objective data.
- From these data, identify and state, using accepted format, two nursing diagnoses you determine are most significant to Mrs. Rodriguez at this time. List two of Mrs. Rodriguez's strengths that you have identified from the data.
- Determine and state outcome criteria for each diagnosis. These must reflect some alleviation of the problem identified in the nursing diagnosis and must be stated in concrete and measurable terms.

- Plan and state one or more interventions for each diagnosed problem. Provide specific documentation of the source used to determine the appropriate intervention. Plan at least one intervention that incorporates Mrs. Rodriguez's existing strengths.
- Evaluate the success of the intervention. Interventions must correlate directly with the stated outcome criteria to measure the outcome success.

Critical Thinking Questions

1. As a student, you have already taken a course on the normal changes with aging. What advice do you have for Elana?
2. Which of the age-related changes has the potential to have the most effect on one's quality of life?
3. Which of the age-related changes has the most implications for the risk for infection in an older adult?
4. For each system, suggest additional strategies to promote healthy aging in the presence of normal age-related changes to the system.
5. An older patient says to the nurse, "I think the older I get, the more falling apart I am. I seem to be good for nothing!" What response from the nurse will recognize normal changes with aging but foster self-esteem at the same time?

* Students are advised to refer to their nursing diagnosis text and identify possible or potential problems.

- Lubrication of joints, elasticity, enzymatic processes, and cellular fluids diminish during aging.
- In healthy aging, changes to the heart and lungs do not affect everyday activity. However, these changes can become significant if the body is stressed.
- Hormonal and endocrine changes are significant in the aging process.
- Nervous system acuity and sensory acuity are diminished in aging, and these losses are often compensated for with the use of accoutrements or aids.

RESEARCH QUESTIONS

Where do individuals seek knowledge of the aging process?
Is chronological age more significant than physiological age in determining functional efficacy?
When does one become aware of changes in function that are related to aging? Which change is likely to appear first? How much influence does environment have on reduced hearing capacity?
How do age-related changes differ in males and females?

REFERENCES

American Geriatric Society (AGS): *Geriatric review syllabus*, ed 6, New York, 2006, The Society.

Anderson W: Aging and the lung. In Beers MH, Berkow R, editors: *The Merck manual of geriatrics*, ed 3, Whitehouse Station, NJ, 2000, Merck Research Laboratories.

Brucker MC, Youngkin EQ: What's a woman to do? Exploring HRT questions raised by the woman's health initiative, *AWHONN Lifelines* 65: 408-417, 2002.

Burke MA, Laramie JA: *Primary care of the older adult: a multidisciplinary approach*, ed 2, St Louis, 2000, Mosby.

Campbell EJ, Lefrak SS: How aging affects the structure and function of the respiratory system, *Geriatrics* 33:68, 1978.

Chiu N: Aging and the skin. In Beers MH, Berkow R, editors: *The Merck manual of geriatrics*, ed 3, Whitehouse Station, NJ, 2000, Merck Research Laboratories.

Cornell RC: Aging and the skin: what is normal aging, *Geriatr Med Today* 5(pt 20):24, 1986.

Cotter V, Strumpf NE: *Advanced practice nursing with older adults*, New York, 2002, McGraw-Hill.

Crowther CL: Structure and function of the musculoskeletal system. In McCance KL, Huether SE, editors: *Pathophysiology: the biological basis for disease in adults and children*, ed 5, St Louis, 2006, Mosby.

Cunningham WR, Brookbank JW: *Gerontology: the psychology, biology, and sociology of aging*, New York, 1988, Harper & Row.

Deneris A, Huether SE: Structure and function of the reproductive systems. In McCance KL, Huether SE, editors: *Pathophysiology: the biological basis for disease in adults and children*, ed 5, St Louis, 2006, Mosby.

Friedman S: Integumentary function. In Meiner SE, Lueckenotte AG: *Gerontologic nursing*, ed 3, St. Louis, 2006a, Mosby.

Friedman S: Pain, temperature regulation, sleep, and sensory function. In McCance KL, Huether SE, editors: *Pathophysiology: the biological basis for disease in adults and children*, ed 5, St Louis, 2006b, Mosby.

Gilchrest B: Aging and the skin. In Beers MH, Berkow R, editors: *The Merck manual of geriatrics*, ed 3, Whitehouse Station, NJ, 2000, Merck Research Laboratories.

Gosain A, DiPietro LA: Aging and wound healing, *World J Surg* 28(3):321-326, 2004.

Gulya AJ: Ear disorders. In Abrams WB et al, editors: *The Merck manual of geriatrics*, ed 2, Whitehouse Station, NJ, 1995, Merck Research Laboratories.

Hall K: Effect of aging on gastrointestinal function. In Hazzard WR et al, editors: *Principles of geriatric medicine and gerontology*, New York, 2003, McGraw Hill.

Hill C: Endocrine function. In Meiner SE, Lueckenotte AG: *Gerontologic nursing*, ed 3, St. Louis, 2006, Mosby.

Hogstel MO: Vital signs are really vital in the old-old, *Geriatr Nurs* 15(5):253, 1994.

Horowitz M: Aging and the gastrointestinal tract. In Beers MH, Berkow R, editors: *The Merck manual of geriatrics*, ed 3, Whitehouse Station, NJ, 2000, Merck Research Laboratories.

Huether SE: Structure and function of the renal and urologic systems. In McCance KL, Huether SE, editors: *Pathophysiology: the biological basis for disease in adults and children*, ed 5, St Louis, 2006a, Mosby.

Huether SE: Mechanisms of hormonal regulation. In McCance KL, Huether SE, editors: *Pathophysiology: the biological basis for disease in adults and children*, ed 5, St Louis, 2006b, Mosby.

Huether SE: Structure and function of the digestive system. In McCance KL, Huether SE, editors: *Pathophysiology: the biological basis for disease in adults and children*, ed 5, St Louis, 2006c, Mosby.

Huether SE, DeFriez CB: Pain, temperature regulation, sleep, and sensory function. In McCance KL, Huether SE, editors: *Pathophysiology: the biological basis for disease in adults and children*, ed 5, St Louis, 2006, Mosby.

Jackson GR, Owsley C: Visual dysfunction, neurodegenerative diseases, and aging, *Neurol Clin* 21(3):709-728, 2003.

Kamel H, Dornbrand L: Health issues of the aging male. In Landefeld CS et al: *Current geriatric diagnosis and treatment*, New York, 2004, McGraw-Hill.

Kee JL, Paulanka BJ: Fluids and their influence on the body. In Kee JL, Paulanka BJ: *Handbook of fluids, electrolytes and acid-base imbalances*, Albany, NY, 2000, Delmar.

Kishiyama JL: Disorders of the immune system. In McPhee SJ, Ganong WF, editors: *Pathophysiology of disease: an introduction to clinical medicine*, ed 5, Lange, 2006, McGraw-Hill.

Lakatta E: Cardiovascular regulatory mechanisms in advanced age, *Physiol Rev* 73(2):413, 1993.

Lakatta EG: Aging in the cardiovascular system. In Beers MH, Berkow R, editors: *The Merck manual of geriatrics*, ed 3, Whitehouse Station, NJ, 2000, Merck Research Laboratories.

Lindemann RD: Aging and the kidney. In Beers MH, Berkow R, editors: *The Merck manual of geriatrics*, ed 3, Whitehouse Station, NJ, 2000, Merck Research Laboratories.

Luggen AS: Rapqunzel no more: hair loss in older women, *Adv Nurse Pract* 13(10):28-33, 2005.

Manolagas S: Aging musculoskeletal system. In Beers MH, Berkow R, editors: *The Merck manual of geriatrics*, ed 3, Whitehouse Station, NJ, 2000, Merck Research Laboratories.

McCance KL: Structure and function of the cardiovascular systems. In McCance KL, Huether SE, editors: *Pathophysiology: the biological basis for disease in adults and children*, ed 5, St Louis, 2006, Mosby.

Meisami E: Aging of the sensory system. In Timiras PS, editor: *Physiological basis of aging and geriatrics*, ed 2, Boca Raton, Fla, 1995, CRC Press.

Meisami E et al: Sensory systems: normal aging, disorders, and treatments of vision and hearing in humans. In Timiras PS, editor: *Physiological basis of aging and geriatrics*, ed 3, Boca Raton, Fla, 2002, CRC Press.

Michel J: Aging and the immune system. In Beers MH, Berkow R, editors: *The Merck manual of geriatrics*, ed 3, Whitehouse Station, NJ, 2000, Merck Research Laboratories.

Miller RA: Aging and the immune response. In Schneider EL, Rowe JW, editors: *Handbook of biology of aging*, ed 3, San Diego, 1990, Academic Press.

Oskvig RM: Special problems in the elderly, *Chest* 115(suppl 2):158-164, 1999.

Price S, Wilson L: *Pathophysiology: clinical concepts of disease processes*, ed 6, St Louis, 2002, Mosby.

Proust J: Aging and the immune system. In Beers MH, Berkow R, editors: *The Merck manual of geriatrics*, ed 3, Whitehouse Station, NJ, 2000, Merck Research Laboratories.

Rossman I, editor: *Clinical geriatrics*, ed 3, Philadelphia, 1986, Lippincott.

Saxon SV, Eaton MJ: *Physical change and aging: a guide for the helping professionals*, ed 4, New York, 2002, Springer.

Sheahan SL, Musialowski R: Clinical implications of respiratory system changes in aging, *J Gerontolog Nurs* 27(5):26, 2001.

Stengel GB: Oral temperature in the elderly, *Gerontologist* 23:306, 1983 (special issue).

Sugarman RA: Structure and function of the neurologic system. In McCance KL, Huether SE, editors: *Pathophysiology: the biological basis for disease in adults and children*, ed 5, St Louis, 2006, Mosby.

Taffet GE, Lakatta EG: Aging of the cardiovascular system, In Hazzard WR et al, editors: *Principles of geriatric medicine and gerontology*, New York, 2003, McGraw Hill

The Merck Manual of Geriatrics (online): Age-related changes in skin structure and function, 2006 (website): www.merck.com/mrkshared/mmg/sec15/ch122/ch122b.jsp. Accessed July 1, 2006.

Tockman MS: The effects of aging on the lungs: lung cancer. In Abrams WB et al, editors: *The Merck manual of geriatrics*, ed 2, Whitehouse Station, NJ, 1995, Merck Research Laboratories.

Tockman MS: Aging and the lung. In Beers MH, Berkow R, editors: *The Merck manual of geriatrics*, ed 3, Whitehouse Station, NJ, 2000, Merck Research Laboratories.

Tumosa N: Aging and the eye. In Beers MH, Berkow R, editors: *The Merck manual of geriatrics*, ed 3, Whitehouse Station, NJ, 2000, Merck Research Laboratories.

Wiggins J: Changes in renal function, In Hazzard WR et al, editors: *Principles of geriatric medicine and gerontology*, New York, 2003, McGraw Hill.

Williams TF: History and physical examination. In Beers MH, Berkow R, editors: *The Merck manual of geriatrics*, ed 3, Whitehouse Station, NJ, 2000, Merck Research Laboratories.

Wilson WR: Nose and throat disorders. In Abrams WB et al, editors: *The Merck manual of geriatrics*, ed 2, Whitehouse Station, NJ, 1995, Merck Research Laboratories.

CHAPTER 5

Laboratory Values and Diagnostics

Kathleen Jett

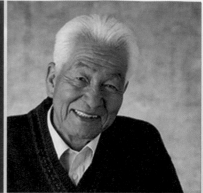

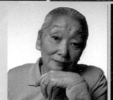 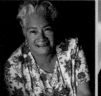

A STUDENT SPEAKS

I always thought that as people got older, their blood sugars went up a little and that was OK. Now I realize that an elevation in fasting glucose means a problem regardless of one's age.

Susan, age 20

AN ELDER SPEAKS

Every time I turn around somebody wants my blood. They say that they need to "watch me closely" but I am not sure what that has to do with my blood. What if they take too much and it causes me to get sick?

Sung Ye, age 92

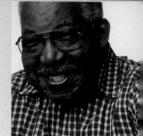

LEARNING OBJECTIVES

On completion of this chapter, the reader will be able to:

1. Identify the laboratory values that increase or decrease with normal aging.
2. Understand the implications and deviations of key abnormal laboratory values in the older adult.
3. Define cautions the nurse should take when interpreting laboratory values in the older adult.
4. Discuss strategies that can be used to maximize the quality of the laboratory testing.
5. Discuss the key laboratory tests used to monitor common health problems.

The nurse's knowledge related to laboratory values and diagnostics tests takes on special meaning when working with older adults. The older a person is, the more difficult is the interpretation of findings and the more important are the nurse's skills. These skills include basic interpretation and those required to obtain or supervise specimen collection, from the specific techniques, such as venipuncture and urine collection, to the timing of the procedure and awareness of influences on the results. For nurses working in long-term care settings, some knowledge of interpretation is especially important to ensure that the persons with abnormalities in their laboratory results are treated promptly and appropriately. Advanced practice nurses are responsible for diagnostic and prescriptive responses to these results.

In this chapter the reader will be provided information about (1) common laboratory and diagnostic tests seen in gerontological nursing, (2) variations in findings that may be a normal change with aging and those that are indications of possible pathology, (3) factors influencing variations in laboratory and diagnostic results, and (4) the gerontological nurse's responsibility in promoting health and preventing adverse events.

Laboratory findings are often reported in relationship to a range of normalized values or reference ranges and referred to as "normal limits" within specific parameters. Although it would be convenient to have adjusted ranges for older adults, this has not been possible because of the large variation within this group of persons and the increasing number

Special thanks to Ann Schmidt Luggen, the previous edition contributor, for her content contributions to this chapter.

of factors that influence the results. Instead, we must take the knowledge of normal changes and consider the person in terms of his or her unique health status and needs. Although small variations in laboratory findings can occur in persons of any age, several of them are more likely to be seen in the older adult; the older the adult, the more likely the change.

HEMATOLOGICAL TESTING

Hematological testing refers to that which is associated with the blood and lymph and their component parts. Blood is composed of red blood cells, white blood cells, and cell fragments called *platelets*. Together the cells float in a fluid matrix called *plasma*. Although several age-related hematological changes are occurring mainly from changes in the bone marrow, few of these are clinically significant (Beers and Berkow, 2000). However, a number of common conditions may impair the hematological system, such as inadequate nutrition, sensory deficits, and impaired physical mobility.

Several laboratory tests are used to measure and diagnose hematological health. The hemogram includes counts of the platelets, white blood cells, and red blood cells, as well as the calculation of a hematocrit and indices. A complete blood count (CBC) is a hemogram plus a differential count (see discussion that follows). One of the basic laboratory measures that reflect hematopoietic functioning is iron studies. The erythrocyte sedimentation rate uses red blood cells in the measurement of systemic inflammation.

Red Blood Count

Red blood cells (RBCs), or erythrocytes, are biconcave, disk-shaped cells whose primary function is to transport molecules of hemoglobin, which in turn transports and exchanges oxygen and carbon dioxide throughout the body. Because the erythrocytes have no nucleus of their own, they cannot reproduce. With the red blood cell's average life span of 120 days, the body is in constant need of replenishment. Red blood cells are produced primarily by the bone marrow, the tissue found inside the spaces of the long bones. No evidence exists that the number of red blood cells produced decreases in healthy aging (Beers and Berkow, 2000). However, for unknown reasons, the amount of bone marrow in the body diminishes from birth through age 30 years; then it stabilizes. At about age 70 years, it diminishes again (Beers and Berkow, 2000). As a result, the speed in which new blood cells can be produced in late life (called *decreased marrow reserve*) is reduced. This becomes a potential problem only for the older adult with an acute illness or bleeding.

The number of red blood cells is measured by a count of the absolute number found in a cubic millimeter (mm^3) of whole blood and reported in the RBC count. Other indices of RBCs are mean corpuscular volume (MCV), mean corpuscular hemoglobin (MCH), and mean corpuscular hemoglobin concentration (MCHC). Hemopoietic functioning is measured in the hemoglobin and hematocrit.

Hemoglobin and Hematocrit. Hemoglobin is the main component of the red blood cell. It is a conjugated protein whose main function is to transport oxygen from the lungs to the tissues and carbon dioxide from the tissues to the lungs. It contains iron atoms and the red pigment *porphyrin*. It is the iron atom that combines easily with both oxygen and carbon dioxide to permit the work of the RBC. Each saturated gram (g) of hemoglobin carries 1.39 mL of oxygen, and therefore the hemoglobin concentration, not the red blood count, is a measurement of anemia in a person and in warm-blooded animals.

The term *hematocrit* means "to separate blood." It is the relative percentage of packed RBCs to plasma in blood in which the two have been separated (often referred to as "spun down"). The hematocrit is measured as part of a CBC and is also a marker of levels of anemia. It is not a good measure of overall blood volume. Although they measure different aspects of the RBC, the hematocrit and hemoglobin are comparative numbers, with the hemoglobin approximately one third of the hematocrit (Nicoll et al., 2004). For example, a person with a hemoglobin of 12 g/dL will have a hematocrit of approximately 36%. A hemoglobin equal to or less than 5 g/dL or over 20 g/dL is considered a "critical value" in which the person is in extreme jeopardy and requires urgent intervention (Pagana and Pagana, 2006).

In healthy young adults, hemoglobin levels are slightly higher in men than in women. Most studies suggest that these relative levels remain unchanged in healthy late life (Berghe et al., 2004). Others have found a slight decline in those older than 90 years (Sarkozi, 2002). However, the older adult is at significant risk for reductions in hemoglobin in the presence of chronic illness or malnutrition (Pagana and Pagana, 2003). Significant reductions in iron levels are diagnosed as an anemia. For persons who are medically fragile and have multiple and prolonged chronic diseases, the presence of anemia of chronic disease is common. Elevations in hematocrit and hemoglobin may be the result of a pathological process but are more often an early sign of hypovolemia from malnutrition, dehydration, or severe diarrhea (Beers and Berkow, 2000). The volume depletion must be corrected before an accurate interpretation can be done.

White Blood Cells

White blood cells (WBCs), or leukocytes, are divided primarily into two types—granulocytes (neutrophils, basophils, and eosinophils) and agranulocytes (monocytes and lymphocytes). They defend the body against foreign substances through the process of phagocytosis, in which the cells encapsulate and destroy the invader. They also transport and distribute naturally occurring antibodies. They are found mainly in the interstitial fluid until they are needed and then travel to the site of invasion or infection. The number of WBCs is regulated largely by the endocrine system and by the need for a particular type of cell (Box 5-1). Each cell has a life span of 13 to 20 days, after which it is destroyed in the lymphatic system and excreted in feces (Pagana and Pagana, 2006). They are produced by the bone marrow and thymus and are stored in the

BOX 5-1	Functions of the Types of White Blood Cells
CELL TYPE	**CELL FUNCTION**
Neutrophils	Stimulated by pyogenic infections, to fight bacteria
Eosinophils	Stimulated by allergic responses, to fight antigens and parasites
Basophils	Stimulated by the presence of allergens, transport histamine
Lymphocytes	Stimulated by the presences of viral infections
Monocytes	Stimulated by severe infections including viral, parasitic, and rickettsial

Data from McPhee S, Ganong W: *Pathophysiology of disease: an introduction to clinical medicine*, pp 115-143, New York, 2006, McGraw-Hill; and Meiner SE, Lueckenotte AG: *Gerontologic nursing*, ed 3, St Louis, 2006, Mosby.

lymph nodes, spleen, and tonsils. Like RBCs, WBCs are measured in cells per cubic millimeter (mm³) of whole blood and are reported in the WBC count and CBC. The average adult has 5000 to 10,000 WBCs/mm³. WBC count of less than 2500 or more than 30,000 mm³ is considered critical (Pagana and Pagana, 2006). When used diagnostically, the WBC count is examined and reported as a differential, or by the relative percentage of each of the five types of cells. The differential alone is of limited use and always must be considered with the complete WBC count. If some of the counts in the differential are elevated, it must be determined if this is an absolute increase or just an increase in the number relative to the changes in the WBC count.

In the healthy older adult, the total leukocyte count is unchanged from earlier life. In younger adults, the presence of infection or inflammation is commonly manifested with an elevated temperature, lymph node enlargement, and increase in total WBC count, which resolve as the condition is treated. However, in the older adult, these signs may be absent or not seen until the person is quite ill or septic. Rather than an increase in the total lymphocytes, only the number of neutrophils (bands) may be increased, called *bandemia* or a *left shift*. And the shift may be very subtle (Desai and Isa-Pratt, 2002). This lack of or delayed response means a diminished ability to respond to the intrusion of foreign substances. Scientists have studied this phenomenon as they examine the immunity theory of aging (see Chapter 2). This change has significant implications for the gerontological nurse. Waiting for the "usual signs" of infection in an older adult may result in his or her death. Instead, the nurse must be alert for more subtle signs of illness such as new onset or increased confusion, falling, or incontinence and report these changes earlier rather than later.

Exacerbating an already potentially dangerous situation is the frequency in which older adults experience a decrease in leukocytes caused by commonly prescribed medications and common medical conditions. Drugs that cause decreases include antibiotics, anticonvulsants, antihistamines, antimetabolites, cytotoxic agents, analgesics, phenothiazines, sulfonamides, and diuretics (Pagana and Pagana, 2006). On the other hand, increases in leukocytes may be a side effect of several drugs including allopurinol, aspirin, heparin, steroids, and triamterene (Pagana and Pagana, 2006).

Neutrophils. The largest percentage of WBCs are neutrophils (55% to 70%), which are produced daily in the bone marrow (Pagana and Pagana, 2006). Neutrophils play an important part in the localization of infections by phagocytizing bacteria. They are called *polymorphonuclear leukocytes (PMNs)*, or "polys." Neutrophilia, or increased neutrophils, may be an indicator of infections, connective tissue diseases such as rheumatoid arthritis, malignancies, medications such as corticosteroids, trauma, and metabolic conditions such as gout, uremia, thyrotoxicosis, and lactic acidosis (Desai and Isa-Pratt, 2002). All are common conditions in late life.

Lymphocytes. Lymphocytes are divided into two types: T cells and B cells. The differential does not separate out T cells and B cells but, rather, counts them together. In some disease situations such as HIV/AIDS, it is important to separate them, but rarely. T cells are produced by the thymus and are active in cell-mediated immunity; B cells are produced in the bone marrow and are involved in the production of antibodies, or humoral immunity. In adulthood, 80% of lymphocytes are T cells, with a slight decrease in T cells and increase in B cells with aging. Monoclonal gammopathy, common in older adults, is a T-cell lymphocyte dysfunction (Beers and Berkow, 2000).

Monocytes. Monocytes are the largest of the leukocytes. When converted to tissue macrophages, they are able to quickly fight viral, bacterial, parasitic, and rickettsial infections through phagocytosis. Monocytes are immature macrophages. In contrast to the mature cells, they may be present for months or even years before they migrate to an inflammatory site to phagocytose microorganisms, dead RBCs, and foreign debris.

Eosinophils and Basophils. Eosinophils are involved in allergic reactions. They ingest antigen-antibody complexes induced by IgE-mediated reactions to attack allergens and parasites. High eosinophil counts are found in people with type I allergies such as hay fever and asthma. Eosinophils are involved in the mucosal immune response, which is known to diminish in late life (Beers and Berkow, 2000). Increased eosinophils in the peripheral blood smear may also be caused by infections such as tuberculosis or pulmonary fungal infections, rheumatoid arthritis, ulcerative colitis, regional enteritis, seasonal allergic rhinitis, atopic dermatitis, solid tumor cancers, and various lymphomas and leukemias (Desai and Isa-Pratt, 2002). Basophils transport histamine, a factor in immune and antiinflammatory responses. They are not involved in bacterial or viral infections.

Platelets

Platelets are small, irregular particles known as *thrombocytes*, an essential ingredient in clotting. They are formed in the bone marrow, the lungs, and the spleen and are released when a blood vessel is injured. As they arrive at the site of injury, they become "sticky," forming a plug of the site to stop the bleeding and help trigger what is known as the *clotting cascade* (Thibodeau and Patton, 2003). Some decrease in platelet "stickiness" may occur with age, although this is poorly understood (Beers and Berkow, 2000). Often the abnormal platelet count is found serendipitously with the CBC (Desai and Isa-Pratt, 2002). Causes include vitamin B_{12} and folate deficiencies (diminished production); leukemias, lymphomas, and solid tumor cancers; medications (estrogen and thiazides); radiation; alcohol; infection; immune disorders, such as systemic lupus and polyarteritis nodosa; and hepatitis (Beers and Berkow, 2000). At platelet levels below 50,000/mm^3, the gerontological nurse must carefully observe for both overt and covert signs of bleeding, including spontaneous bleeding. If the platelet count falls below 20,000/mm^3, spontaneous bleeding can occur, and if less than 40,000/mm^3, prolonged bleeding after procedures (e.g., venipuncture, rectal exam) can occur (Pagana and Pagana, 2006).

COMMON DIAGNOSTICS RELATED TO HEMATOLOGICAL TESTING

Erythrocyte Sedimentation Rate

The erythrocyte is the largest cell in whole blood. It is measured by the rate at which a erythrocyte falls to the bottom of a test tube in 1 hour. This is known as the *erythrocyte sedimentation rate (ESR),* also referred to as the "sed rate." The calculated measurement of the rate of settling of erythrocytes is a proxy measure for the presence or absence of inflammation or necrosis in the body and is related to changes in the plasma proteins. The ESR is reported in millimeters per hour (mm/hr). The ESR may be slightly elevated in normal, healthy older adults (10 to 20 mm/hr) (Kane et al., 2004). In many cases, the cause of an elevated ESR is unknown and the person is asymptomatic. In other cases, the increase is caused by the presence of chronic inflammatory processes such as rheumatic disease or cancer. The ESR is highly nonspecific and cannot be used for the diagnosis of any one disorder; however, it is used most often for monitoring inflammatory conditions such as polymyalgia rheumatica, temporal arteritis, or rheumatoid arthritis (Moore, 2006). If a person of any age has an unexplained rise in ESR, further testing is indicated.

Iron Studies

When the number of red blood cells or the hemoglobin and hematocrit are found to be decreased, the person may have an anemia. Although not a normal change with aging, anemia is a common pathological finding in older adults, especially in those with long-standing chronic disease or renal insufficiency. Sometimes the person is symptomatic or the anemia is the result of a major bleeding episode, but often it is an incidental finding of a hemogram. The gerontological nurse should be able to recognize the potential for the anemia and to monitor its treatment. The advanced practice gerontological nurse must be able to diagnose and treat the anemia as appropriate.

Although a number of types of anemia exist, they all result in a reduced capacity for the transport of oxygen and carbon dioxide. Progressive anemia that is untreated or not responsive to treatment will result in the person's death. Recall that the major component of the hemoglobin of the RBC is iron. Diagnostic testing for anemia begins with what are referred to as "iron studies." Iron studies include iron, ferritin, total iron-binding capacity (TIBC), and transferrin measures. Any of these alone is an inadequate measure because of the complexity of their interrelationships. In the presence of reduced hemoglobin, additional tests measuring folic acid and vitamin B_{12} may also be indicated.

Iron. Iron enters the body through the intestines during the digestion of iron-containing foods such as dark-green, leafy vegetables and red meats. Transferrin is the plasma protein that is responsible for transporting the iron into bone marrow to be used later in the production of hemoglobin. The serum concentration of iron is determined by a combination of its absorption and storage, as well as the breakdown and synthesis of hemoglobin. The iron in the hemoglobin is necessary not only for the transportation of oxygen and carbon dioxide but also for controlling protein synthesis in the mitochondria, essential for generating energy in the cells (Freedman and Sutin, 2002). Serum iron (Fe^{++}) is reported in micrograms per deciliter (mcg/dL). The TIBC measures the combination of the amount of iron and the amount of transferrin available in the blood serum.

To maintain health, it is very important to have adequate stores of iron. With adequate iron stores, the body is able to respond quickly to stress and the demand for increased oxygen and energy and to replenish iron lost through bleeding. Ferritin is a complex molecule made up of ferric hydroxide and a protein and can be measured as a reflection of the body iron stores. Taken together with serum iron transferrin and blood indices (MCV, MCH, MCHC), the type of anemia one has may be determined and appropriate treatment initiated.

Iron deficiency anemia is the most common form of anemia in older adults (Moore, 2006). In most instances, changes in serum iron reflect blood loss from the gastrointestinal or genitourinary tract. In promoting healthy aging, the gerontological nurse must be alert for nutritional deficits and signs of blood loss in older persons in all types of settings. Anemia of chronic disease is very common in the long-term care setting. One of the first signs of anemia may be fatigue, which may be confused with a side effect of a medication or falsely attributed to normal aging.

B Vitamins

The two B vitamins that are especially important to hematological health are folic acid and B_{12}. Folic acid, one of the eight B vitamins that make up the B-complex group, is necessary for the normal functioning of both RBCs and WBCs related to deoxyribonucleic acid (DNA) synthesis (Nicoll et al., 2004). Folic acid is formed by bacteria in the intestines. It is stored in the liver. It is also contained in eggs, milk, leafy vegetables, yeast, liver, and fruit. Decreases in folic acid may indicate protein-energy malnutrition, several types of anemia, and liver and renal disease. It is more common among persons with chronic alcohol abuse. Although folic acid levels do not decrease in healthy aging, the nurse must be alert for signs of actual or potential nutritional disturbances. Folic acid (nanograms per milliliter [ng/mL]) is usually measured in conjunction with that of B_{12} levels.

Vitamin B_{12} (cobalamin) is a coenzyme of folic acid; together they are important for the maturation of the normal erythrocyte and DNA synthesis. Vitamin B_{12} is obtained only from the ingestion of animal protein and requires intrinsic factor in the stomach for absorption. The B_{12} anemia that results from lack of intrinsic factor is known as *pernicious anemia*. Vitamin B_{12} deficiency is a pathological finding that is found with increasing frequency in late life, with a prevalence of 10% to 15%, most likely the result of malabsorption from gastric atrophy or hypochlorhydria (Johnson and Sullivan, 2004). Tests of B_{12} and folate are now part of the standard workup for dementia (Sink and Yaffee, 2004). If untreated, vitamin B_{12} deficiency may ultimately be fatal. Other clinical manifestations include glossitis, increased lactate dehydrogenase (LDH) levels, paresthesias of feet and hands, and vibratory and proprioception disturbances. Ataxias will also occur without treatment. Cerebral manifestations include memory impairment, change in taste and smell, irritability, and somnolence.

BLOOD CHEMISTRY STUDIES

Blood chemistry studies include an assortment of laboratory tests that are used to identify and measure circulating elements and particles in the plasma and blood: glucose, proteins, amino acids, nutritive materials, excretion products, hormones, enzymes, vitamins, and minerals. Some of these are used for screening and others for monitoring specific health problems or treatments. Some tests are individually selected, but many are done in "panels" or grouped in clusters with a variety of names, including "Chem-7" or "BMP" (basic metabolic panel) or "SMA-16" or "CMP" (complete metabolic panel), among others. The nurse must become familiar with the names and test components used by the laboratory that provides services to her or his individual patient. In this chapter we address only the most common tests of blood chemistry used in caring for older adults (Table 5-1).

Hormones

In the older man and postmenopausal woman, the hormones that receive the most attention are those related to the thyroid gland: triiodothyronine (T_3), thyroxine (T_4), and thyroid-stimulating hormone (TSH). Although changes in thyroid function are not a normal part of aging, the incidence of disturbances, especially hypothyroidism, is seen with increasing frequency (Beers and Berkow, 2000). Screening for thyroid disease is a component of the primary health care of older adults, especially women and persons with depression, anxiety, dementia, or cardiac arrhythmias. A fully functioning thyroid gland (or its replacement) is necessary to maintain life. The laboratory tests that measure thyroid function include the T_4, T_3, free T_4 and free T_3, and TSH. TSH is produced by the pituitary to stimulate the thyroid to produce T_3 and T_4.

Although all the above are commonly included in a thyroid panel, a serum free T_4 and TSH are all that are required for most initial diagnoses. If the person has a goiter, a thyroid scan with technetium may be necessary (Gambert and Miller, 2004). In most cases, treatment (especially thyroid replacement) can be monitored easily with the TSH alone.

Hypothyroidism is the most common disturbance seen in older adults, affecting between 0.9% and 17.5%, with prevalence increasing with age (Gambert and Miller, 2004). The most common causes are autoimmune thyroiditis, prior radioiodine treatment, and subtotal thyroidectomy. Hypothyroidism can also be iatrogenic, from provider-prescribed thyroid replacement that is not adequately monitored. In diagnosis, the clinical picture is combined with laboratory findings, especially a markedly elevated TSH and reduced total and free T_4 (Table 5-2).

Hypothyroidism is seen alone and in a combination of other autoimmune and cardiac conditions. The accuracy of the laboratory findings are easily affected by concurrent environmental conditions and drug intake (Table 5-3). In subclinical hypothyroidism, diagnosis may be made on the basis of clinical assessment alone. Although the T_3 is of very limited value, it is usually included in a "thyroid panel." There is an age-associated decrease in the ability of the body to convert T_4 to T_3 (so that it can be used). The subsequent lack of T_3 will cause the pituitary to increase the production of TSH, producing hypothyroidism.

Hyperthyroidism, or thyrotoxicosis, is significantly less common. Its prevalence in community-living elders is thought to be 1% to 3% and is more common in women (Gambert and Miller, 2004). It is usually caused by multinodular and uninodular toxic goiter rather than the Graves' disease that is seen in younger adults. Hyperthyroidism can also be caused by iodine-containing substances, such as the cardiac drug *amiodarone* (Beers and Berkow, 2000). Finally, like hypothyroidism, hyperthyroidism can be iatrogenic, or from inadequately monitoring thyroid replacement. Special caution must be used for chronic use of doses over 0.15 mg/day of L-thyroxin. Hyperthyroidism is diagnosed with a low or normal serum T_4 and a low TSH (see Table 5-2). The nurse is in a key position to monitor the thyroid function of the patient by ensuring timely and appropriate laboratory testing of TSH.

Electrolytes

Gerontological nurses are frequently called on to promptly interpret electrolyte reports and respond to these in some way. An adjustment of a medication dosage, an increase or decrease in the patient's fluid intake, or a new medication may be needed, or transferring the patient from one location to another (e.g., nursing home to hospital, general unit to intensive care unit) may need to be considered. A minor electrolyte imbalance may have little effect in a younger adult but may have significantly deleterious results in an

TABLE 5-1

Hematology: Implications for Aging

Test Name	Adult Normals	Older Adult Normals	Significance of Deviations
Red Blood Cells	4.2-6.1 million/mm^3	Unchanged with aging	*Low:* hemorrhage, anemia, chronic illness, renal failure, pernicious anemia *High:* high altitude, polycythemia, dehydration
Hemoglobin	12-18 g/dL	Values may be slightly decreased	*Low:* anemia, cancer, nutritional deficiency, kidney disease *High:* polycythemia, CHF, COPD, high altitudes, dehydration
Hematocrit	37%-52%	Values may be slightly decreased	*Low:* anemia, cirrhosis, hemorrhage, malnutrition, rheumatoid arthritis *High:* polycythemia, severe dehydration, severe diarrhea, COPD
White Blood Cells (total)	5000-10,000/mm^3	Unchanged with aging	*Low:* drug toxicity, infections, autoimmune disease, dietary deficiency *High:* infection, trauma, stress, inflammation
Neutrophils	55%-70%	Unchanged with aging	*Low:* dietary deficiency, overwhelming bacterial infection, viral infections, drug therapy *High:* physical and emotional stress, trauma, inflammatory disorders
Eosinophils	1%-4%	Unchanged with aging	*Low:* increased adrenal steroid production *High:* parasitic infections, allergic reactions, autoimmune disorders
Basophils	0.5%-1%	Unchanged with aging	*Low:* acute allergic reactions, stress reactions *High:* myeloproliferative disease
Monocytes	2%-8%	Unchanged with aging	*Low:* drug therapy: predispose *High:* chronic inflammatory disorders, tuberculosis, chronic ulcerative colitis
Lymphocytes	20%-40%	Unchanged with aging	*Low:* leukemia, sepsis, SLE, chemotherapy, radiation *High:* chronic bacterial infection, viral infections, radiation, infectious hepatitis
Folic Acid	5-25 ng/mL	Unchanged with aging	*Low:* malnutrition, folic acid anemia, hemolytic anemia, alcoholism, liver disease, chronic renal disease *High:* pernicious anemia
Vitamin B$_{12}$	160-950 pg/ml	Unchanged with aging	*Low:* pernicious anemia, inflammatory bowel disease, atrophic gastritis, folic acid deficiency *High:* leukemia, polycythemia, severe liver dysfunction
Total Iron-Binding Capacity (TIBC)	250-460 mcg/dL	Unchanged with aging	*Low:* hypoproteinemia, cirrhosis, hemolytic anemia, pernicious anemia *High:* polycythemia, iron deficiency anemia
Iron (Fe)	60-180 mcg/dL	Unchanged with aging	*Low:* insufficient dietary iron, chronic blood loss, inadequate absorption of iron *High:* hemochromacytosis, hemolytic anemia, hepatitis, iron poisoning
Uric Acid	4.0-8.5 mg/dL	May be slightly increased	*Low:* lead poisoning *High:* gout, increased ingestion of purines, chronic renal disease, hypothyroidism
Prothrombin Time (PT)	11.0-12.5 seconds	Unchanged with aging	*High:* liver disease, vitamin K deficiency, warfarin (Coumadin) ingestion
Partial Thromboplastin Time (PTT)	60-70 seconds	Unchanged with aging	*Low:* early stages of disseminated intravascular coagulation, metastatic cancer *High:* clotting factor deficiency, cirrhosis, vitamin K deficiency, heparin administration
Platelets	150,000-400,000/mm^3	Unchanged with aging	*Low:* hemorrhage, thrombocytopenia, SLE, pernicious anemia, chemotherapy, infection *High:* malignancy, polycythemia, RA, iron deficiency anemia

From Meiner S, Lueckenotte AG: *Gerontologic nursing,* ed 3, St Louis, 2006, Mosby; adapted from Pagana KD, Pagana TJ: *Diagnostic and laboratory test reference,* ed 6, St Louis, 2003, Mosby; Pagana KD, Pagana TJ: *Manual of diagnostic and laboratory tests,* ed 2, St Louis, 2004, Mosby.
CHF, Congestive heart failure; *COPD,* chronic obstructive pulmonary disease; *SLE,* systemic lupus erythematosus; *RA,* rheumatoid arthritis.

TABLE 5-2

Interpreting Thyroid Testing Results

TSH	Free T$_4$	Cause	Response
Increased (>10 mU/L)	Low	Clinical hypothyroidism Inadequate replacement therapy	Usually requires treatment
	Normal	Subclinical hypothyroidism	Treatment depends on presence of signs and symptoms
	High	Hypothalamic/pituitary disorder	Referral to an endocrinologist for further testing
Decreased (<0.1 mU/L)	Low	Euthyroid sick syndrome Hypothalamic/pituitary disorder	Referral to an endocrinologist for further testing
	Normal	Subclinical thyrotoxicosis T$_3$ thyrotoxicosis (if T$_3$ is elevated)	Referral to an endocrinologist for monitoring
	High	Clinical thyrotoxicosis Excessive replacement therapy	Referral to an endocrinologist for further testing and treatment Adjust dosage and retest

Adapted from Margolis S, Reed R: Thyroid disease. In Hamm R et al: *Primary care geriatrics: a case-based approach,* ed 4, pp 517-524, St Louis, 2002, Mosby; data from Bauer D, McPhee J: Thyroid disease. In McPhee S, Ganong W: *Pathophysiology of disease: an introduction to clinical medicine,* pp 567-588, New York, 2006, McGraw-Hill.

TABLE 5-3

Factors Affecting Laboratory Testing of Thyroid Functioning

Test	Increased Result	Depressed Result
TSH	Potassium iodide and lithium	Severe illness, aspirin, dopamine, heparin, and steroids
T$_3$	Estrogen and methadone	Anabolic steroids, androgens, phenytoin, propranolol, reserpine, and salicylates
T$_4$	Estrogen, methadone, and clofibrate	Anabolic steroids, androgens, lithium, phenytoin, and propranolol

Modified from Pagana KD, Pagana TJ: *Manual of diagnostic and laboratory tests,* ed 2, St Louis, 2004, Mosby.

TABLE 5-4

Signs and Symptoms of Disturbances in Sodium Levels

	Hyponatremia	Hypernatremia
Signs	Plasma Na$^+$ <130 mmol/L (approximately) Drop in BP (in hypovolemia) Tachycardia (in hypovolemia)	Plasma Na$^+$ >150 mmol/L (approximately) Poor skin turgor Dry mucous membranes
Symptoms	Mental status changes	Mental status changes

Data from Beck L: Renal system, fluid and electrolytes. In Landefeld S et al: *Current geriatric diagnosis and treatment,* pp 247-356, New York, 2004, Mc-Graw-Hill.

older adult, especially one who is medically fragile. Dehydration is the most common form of electrolyte disturbance in the elderly, especially for those residing in long-term care facilities (Mentes, 2006). Excess water loss can be the result of any number of things including medications, immobility, confusion, infections, or diarrhea.

Electrolytes are inorganic substances that include acids, bases, and salts. In solution, they break up and form negatively (anions) or positively (cations) charged particles known as *ions.* Their blood levels are reported as solitary measurements or as a part of panels, such as the Chem-7 or the SMA-12 or 16 noted earlier. The most common electrolytes of concern in gerontological care include sodium, potassium, calcium, and glucose.

Sodium and Chloride. The test for sodium is a proxy index of body water. It measures the amount of sodium in circulating blood. The regulation of sodium is necessary for the maintenance of blood pressure, the transmission of nerve impulses, and the regulation of body fluids in and out of the cells (Moore, 2006) (Table 5-4). The movement of the fluids affects blood volume and is tied to thirst (Grodner et al., 2004). Sodium balance is further influenced by renal filtration and blood flow, cardiac output, and glomerular filtration rate (GFR). The laboratory sodium levels indicate the balance between ingested sodium and that which is excreted by the kidneys. Changes in sodium (Na$^+$) are always accompanied by changes in chloride (Cl$^-$) because they are predominantly found in combinations as sodium chloride.

Like other balances in the human body, in ordinary activity, aging changes are not apparent in function or health. However, because of the age-associated loss of nephrons and decreased GFR in normal aging, it is much more difficult for the body to respond to crises in sodium depletion or overload. Aging is associated with impaired water conservation and sodium balance, especially in times of stress (Beers and Berkow, 2000). Hyponatremia (low sodium) occurs with excessive water retention; hypernatremia (elevated sodium) occurs with excessive water loss.

Hyponatremia is diagnosed when one's plasma sodium concentration drops below about 136 mmol/L and is accompanied by chloride levels of less than 90 mmol/L and usually a decreased osmolality (<270 mOsm/kg) (Beck, 2004). It is a common disorder seen in the older population with a prevalence from 7% in community-living elders to as high as 15% to 20% in those in hospitals and long-term care settings. The most common cause of hyponatremia in older adults is caused by the kidney's inability to excrete free water. Other causes include hyperglycemia, gastrointestinal (GI) fluid loss via vomiting, excessive sweating, pancreatitis, bowel obstruction, thiazide diuretic therapy, syndrome of inappropriate antidiuretic hormone (SIADH), hypothyroidism, congestive heart failure, cirrhosis, and acute and chronic renal failure (Desai and Isa-Pratt, 2002). Hyponatremia is one of the most common causes of delirium in older adults. Mental status changes and other central nervous system (CNS) effects can be seen with levels equal to or less than 125 to 130 mEq/L (Beck, 2004). Hypovolemic hyponatremia is always accompanied by a significant drop in postural blood pressure and tachycardia as the body attempts to compensate. In the most severe cases, hyponatremia can result in a high rate of morbidity and mortality.

Hypernatremia is an elevation of plasma sodium (>145 mEq/L) in which loss of water is excessive without concurrent loss of sodium. This is a common problem in ill older adults in hospital and long-term care facilities (Desai and Isa-Pratt, 2002). The prevalence in this group is up to 30% with a mortality rate of 42% (Beck, 2004). Low body weight is a risk factor. The mortality rate for this is 40% in hospitalized elders, especially if it occurs quickly and is severe (>160 mEq/L). When sodium levels are more than 155 mEq/L, mental status changes should be expected. Signs of water loss such as diminished skin turgor, dry mucous membranes, and orthostatic hypotension may or may not be evident in the older adult. Severely high Na^+ may cause hemiparesis, stupor or coma, and seizures. Hypernatremia is accompanied by elevated plasma chloride (>110 mEq/L) and increase osmolality (>300 mOsm/kg) (Beck, 2004).

Potassium. Potassium (K^+) is an electrolyte found in both intracellular and extracellular fluid. Differing from sodium, it is found primarily within the cells themselves. Potassium is essential in maintaining cell osmolality, muscle functioning, and transmitting nerve impulses. It is also a key component in the maintenance of acid-base balance. Serum potassium levels decrease as lean body mass decreases, because most potassium (75%) is stored in lean body mass (Beers and Berkow, 2000). Both hypokalemia (reduced potassium levels) and hyperkalemia (elevated potassium levels) are seen in the laboratory findings of older adults and are often the result of drug therapy or inadequate monitoring for drug side effects. Chronic hyperkalemia may be seen in persons suffering from acute renal failure. The signs and symptoms of a disturbance in potassium levels may not be evident until it is severe (Box 5-2).

Hypokalemia is associated with cardiac arrhythmias and may cause glucose intolerance and renal tubular dysfunction. Mild hypokalemia is asymptomatic. Severe hypokalemia (K^+ <2.5 mEq/L) produces muscle weakness, cramping, confusion, fatigue, paralytic ileus, atrial and ventricular ectopy and tachycardia, fibrillation, and sudden death (Beers and Berkow, 2000). The electrocardiogram (ECG) will demonstrate a characteristic response to hypokalemia. Chronic hypokalemia may lead to significant renal tubular dysfunc-

---

BOX 5-2 Signs and Symptoms of Disturbances in Potassium Levels

HYPOKALEMIA	HYPERKALEMIA
Generalized muscle weakness	Impaired muscle activity
Fatigue	Weakness
Muscle cramps	Muscle pain/cramps
Constipation	Increased GI motility
Ileus	Bradycardia
Flaccid paralysis	Cardiac arrest
Hyporeflexia	ECG changes:
Hypercapnia	P wave flattened
Tetany	T wave large, peaked
ECG changes:	QRS broad
QT interval prolonged	Biphasic QRS-T
T wave flattened or	complex
depressed	
ST segment depressed	

For additional information, see Fukagawa M et al: Fluid and electrolyte disorders. In Tierney L et al, editors: *Current medical diagnosis and treatment*, pp 865-895, New York, 2006, McGraw-Hill.

---

tion. The most common causes are over-diuresis and GI losses through vomiting and diarrhea. Other causes or risk factors include low K^+ intake, pernicious anemia therapy, leukemias and lymphomas, parenteral nutrition, increased catecholamine release such as with a myocardial infarction, head trauma, delirium tremens, and hypothermia (Desai and Isa-Pratt, 2002).

Hyperkalemia (K^+ >5 mEq/L) is most commonly exhibited by a shift of K^+ from the intracellular to the extracellular compartment, which increases the plasma concentration. Body stores may be normal or low (Beers and Berkow, 2000). It may also be caused by decreased renal excretion of K^+ (Desai and Isa-Pratt, 2002). Common causes of hyperkalemia in the elderly patient include the concurrent use of potassium-sparing diuretics and prescribed potassium supplements, excessive K^+ intake in the presence of acute or chronic renal failure, hyperglycemia, nonsteroidal antiinflammatory drugs (NSAIDs), angiotensin-converting enzyme (ACE) inhibitors, and beta-blocking drugs. High K^+ may be asymptomatic until cardiac toxicity occurs (Beers and Berkow, 2000). Characteristic ECG changes indicate the problem. It causes ventricular arrhythmias, vague weakness, paresthesias, flaccid paralysis, ventricular fibrillation, and asystole.

Calcium and Phosphorus. Calcium (Ca^{++}) is essential for blood clotting, nerve conduction, muscle functioning, and enzymatic activity. Only about 1% of the body's calcium is found in the blood; the remainder is stored in the bones and teeth. The serum calcium level is maintained by release or resorption of bone calcium, depending on the body's needs. Because the serum levels do not change with aging but calcium metabolism does, the result is decreased bone stores. When a significant amount of the stores is lost, osteoporosis (porous bones) is diagnosed. Only a small percentage of ingested calcium is bio-available and must be accompanied by an adequate amount of vitamin D.

About half of the circulating (serum) calcium is bound to proteins, especially albumin. A person with a low albumin level will present with an artificially low serum calcium. This is especially common in medically fragile persons, such as those residing in skilled nursing facilities. The measurement of serum calcium must be adjusted to determine the actual serum calcium using a standard formula (add 0.8 mg/dL to the total calcium concentration for each 1 g/dL decrease in albumin below its normal concentration of 4 g/dL).

When the person has true hypocalcemia, causes include hypoparathyroidism, vitamin D deficiency, acute pancreatitis, or malignancy. Medications that can cause hypocalcemia include loop diuretics, calcitonin, bisphosphonates, phenobarbital, fluoride, and radiographic contrast dyes (Pagana and Pagana, 2006).

True hypercalcemia may be caused by hyperparathyroidism, lithium therapy, malignancy, vitamin A or D intoxication, hyperthyroidism, granulomatous diseases, immobilization, and drugs such as thiazides and theophylline (Pagana and Pagana, 2006). Transient hypercalcemia can result from dehydration. Mild hypercalcemia is asymptomatic and easily detected. Related abnormalities include hypertension, muscular weakness, irritability, GI disturbances, renal colic, bone cysts, polyuria, and diminished bone mass (Beers and Berkow, 2000).

Calcium levels are inversely related to phosphorus levels—the excess serum levels of one cause the kidneys to excrete the other. Phosphorus is a mineral found mostly in the bones and in combination with calcium with the rest found within the cells. It is required for the generation of bony tissue and functions in the metabolism of glucose and lipids. Phosphorus levels are slightly decreased and worsened with long-term use of antacids.

Glucose. Glucose is the most common sugar used by the body for energy. For optimal functioning, the levels of fasting glucose in the body must be maintained between about 70 and 110 mg/dL. Although the required levels do not change with aging, the signs and symptoms of the persons with elevations or reductions may change. For many older adults, even slight hypoglycemia can result in confused and depressed CNS activity. At the same time, many are able to tolerate hyperglycemia well and the typical signs of polydipsia and polyuria may be absent. The diagnostic criteria for altered glucose metabolism are based on either fasting or random blood glucoses in a variety of circumstances (Box 5-3). The glycosylated hemoglobin (A1c) should not be used for diagnostic purposes but is used for monitoring treatment (Halter, 2003). The reliability and validity of the results of laboratory testing highly depends on the timing of the sampling and current medications, especially steroids.

Although the criteria for diagnosis do not change, age-related changes are recognized in glucose metabolism and in the prevalence of diabetes. As many as 50% of all persons with diabetes are older than 60 years, and approximately 25% of the persons older than 60 years have diabetes (Halter, 2003). Fasting glucose levels are in the higher normal range, and the ability to return to normal levels after a glucose chal-

---

BOX 5-3   Diagnostic Criteria Used in the Diagnosis of Diabetes

A diagnosis of diabetes mellitus (DM) is made using standard criteria.

ONE random plasma glucose ≥200 mg/dL when exhibiting symptoms
OR
TWO of any one or a combination of positive tests on different days
- Fasting plasma glucose (FPG) ≥126 mg/dL (NOTE: these are not blood glucoses that you get with an Accu-Chek)
- Oral glucose tolerance test (OGTT) ≥200 mg/dL 2 hours after glucose
- Random plasma glucose ≥200 mg/dL without symptoms

From National Institute of Diabetes and Digestive and Kidneys Disorders: *Diagnosis of diabetes.* 2005. Available at *www.niddk.nih.gov.* Accessed May 31, 2006.

---

lenge or after eating is more dramatically changed. These changes appear to be most related to a decrease in the insulin sensitivity of the tissues. It is not known if this change is the result of the tendency for less physical activity or the normal changes in body adiposity (see Chapter 4).

Urine glucose testing, once commonly done, does not correlate well with serum glucose (Desai and Isa-Pratt, 2002). In some patients, glucose spills into the urine even when plasma glucose is normal. There is great individual variability. It is no longer advised to use urine glucose levels to manage diabetes but, rather, plasma glucose levels.

The nurse is often responsible for ensuring the quality of the collection of laboratory specimens. In relation to glucose testing, it is important that interpretation of findings is within the context of time since meals or snacks as well as medications used and administered and concurrent medical problems.

Alkaline Phosphatase

An important enzyme test for aiding in the identification of liver and bone disease is the serum alkaline phosphatase (ALP). ALP increases slightly with age in both men and women but is more notable in women (Mauk, 2005). Increases may be related to extrahepatic sources such as renal insufficiency, bone disorders, malabsorption, statin use, improper specimen handling, intestinal mucosa disturbances, heavy alcohol consumption, systemic infection, pancreatitis, and neoplasms. Low ALP levels occur with hypothyroidism, pernicious anemia, hypophosphatemia, and medications such as estrogens, theophylline, clofibrate, and alendronate. Food ingestion can cause an artificial increase in ALP; therefore the specimen must be drawn when the person has been fasting.

Uric Acid

Uric acid is a naturally occurring end product of purine metabolism. It is usually measured in serum chemistry studies but is also found in the urine. Two thirds of the amount normally produced is excreted in the kidneys and the rest in the stool. Elevations in uric acid levels are found when there is either an overproduction or an underexcretion. The measurement of uric acid levels are indicated in the evaluation of renal failure or leukemia, or, most often, in the diagnosis or treatment of gout. A number of conditions and situations can result in increased uric acid levels, including binge alcohol drinking; medications, especially thiazide diuretics; surgery; or acute medical illness. The levels also increase slightly with age and vary between men and women (Blumenthal, 2004; Nicoll et al., 2004).

Although elevated uric acid levels are associated with gouty arthritis, the diagnosis is made more on the clinical presentation than the laboratory findings. Chronic hyperuricemia means that the person is at risk for gout but it does not confirm gout. An individual may have symptoms at levels just over the normal range and may have no symptoms at a significant elevation (Blumenthal, 2004). Most people who have elevated uric acid levels never have symptoms, and 30% of those who have an acute attack have normal uric acid levels (Desai and Isa-Pratt, 2002).

Prostate-Specific Antigen

Prostate cancer is the second leading cause of cancer death among men in the United States, and the risk increases with age. The risk of developing prostate cancer is 2.01% for men older than 50 years but jumps to 6.46% for men older than 60 years. The majority (75%) of prostate cancer is seen in men older than 75 years and is more common in African-American men than any other ethnic group (USPTF, 2002).

The primary screening tools for prostate cancer are the digital rectal examination (DRE) and prostate-specific antigen (PSA). The DRE may stimulate the release of the antigen; therefore the PSA must always come before the DRE. A cutoff point of 4.0 ng/mL is the standard; however, it has only a 63% to 83% sensitivity for prostate cancer so it can miss a significant number of persons with disease and also has a number of "false positives"—elevations in men without cancer (USPTF, 2002). A number of causes of increased levels of PSA exist in addition to prostate cancer, including infection, physical activity, rectal stimulation during DRE or sexual activity, benign prostatic hyperplasia, and ejaculation within 1 day of the laboratory test. When the PSA and DRE results are combined, the overall value of the screens increases.

LABORATORY TESTING FOR CARDIAC HEALTH

Heart disease remains the number-one cause of death for all persons (Ebersole et al., 2005). As a result, the gerontological nurse must be knowledgeable about the most common laboratory testing related to cardiac function. These include measures following acute cardiac events for tests associated with cardiac health risk determination.

Acute Cardiac Events

Older adults who appear to have acute and unexpected changes that may be related to an ischemic event need immediate transportation to an emergency department for evaluation. Once there, initial testing for an acute cardiac event or acute myocardial infarction (AMI) will include an ECG and cardiac enzymes or tissue markers.

Creatine Kinase. The cardiac enzyme *creatine kinase (CK)* is present in various parts of the body and in several forms of isoenzymes. The isoenzyme CK-MB is associated with cardiac tissue, and laboratory values are used in the diagnosis of AMI, myocardial muscle injury, unstable angina, shock, malignant hyperthermia, myopathies, and myocarditis (Pagana and Pagana, 2006). The CK-MB rises 3 to 6 hours after an AMI occurs. It peaks at 12 to 24 hours (unless the infarction extends) and returns to normal after 12 to 48 hours; therefore it is not a useful measure after that period of time. Drugs commonly used by the elderly that can cause false elevations include anticoagulants, aspirin, clofibrate, dexamethasone, furosemide, captopril, colchicine, alcohol, lovastatin, lidocaine, propranolol, and morphine. For the best diagnosis, the CK-MB is used as a comparative measure with troponin.

Troponin. Troponin I and troponin T are the best cardiac markers available and have become the gold standard for diagnosis of an AMI when compared with the CK-MB. They are very specific for cardiac tissue necrosis beginning 2 to 8 hours after an acute event, and elevations may persist up to 3 weeks (Rich, 2004). Normal levels of troponin I are up to 0.60 ng/mL (Moore, 2006).

Testing and Monitoring Cardiovascular Risk and Health

Increasing attention has been given to three biochemical markers that are believed to have value in the detection of heart disease or in the assessment for risk of cardiovascular disease. These are C-reactive protein (hs-CRP), homocystine, and brain natriuretic peptide (BNP). Tests for lipids continue to be important for both determining health risk and monitoring treatment.

C-Reactive Protein. C-reactive protein (CRP) is one of the serum analytes that is released in the acute phase of inflammation. Inflammation is present not only after cardiac events but also after injury, surgery, and infections. Inflammation is also being considered as an early sign of vascular changes and indications of increased risk for coronary artery disease (Ryan and Wilson, 2006). It is thought that CRP levels will rise earlier in the inflammatory process and may one day replace the ESR discussed earlier; however, at this time the routine use of this test as a screen is very controversial.

Homocystine. Homocystine is a naturally occurring amino acid that is produced in the metabolism of animal and plant proteins. A standardized normal level has not yet been determined, but most studies define hyperhomocysteinemia at approximately 15 micromoles/L (Chamberlain, 2005). Elevated homocystine levels have been associated with an increased risk for cardiovascular disease and stroke. They are higher in persons who smoke, who have high cholesterol, and who have systolic hypertension and may be genetically influenced as well (Zubrod and Holman, 2004).

Brain Natriuretic Peptide. Brain natriuretic peptide (BNP) is a neurohormone secreted by the ventricles in response to excessive stretching and pressure that is found in cardiomegalia (Prahash and Lynch, 2004). It has been found to be elevated in persons with heart failure or left ventricular dysfunction. BNP is being used with increased frequency as a marker of the extent of heart disease.

Lipids. Dyslipidemia indicates a health risk regardless of one's age and is a major predictor of coronary heart disease. Laboratory testing for lipids is usually done as a "lipid panel" and includes both cholesterol and triglyceride. It is done both as a health screen and for monitoring the response to treatment, usually with lipid-lowering medications and/or diet. For the most accurate results, the person should have fasted 12 to 15 hours before the test.

Cholesterol. Cholesterol is a sterol compound necessary in the body to stabilize the cell membranes. Cholesterol is metabolized in the liver where it is combined with low-density lipoprotein (LDL), high-density lipoprotein (HDL), and very-low-density lipoproteins (VLDLs) for transportation in the bloodstream. Men's cholesterol levels slowly increase from puberty until about age 60 years. They then appear to stabilize and rise again after age 80 years. The cholesterol levels of women continue to rise slightly after age 60 years. The increases in aging are seen primarily in LDL, with the HDL remaining more stable (Gambert and Miller, 2004). A "total cholesterol" is the measurement of overall cholesterol in the blood and is of little diagnostic value. The lipid panel provides the total cholesterol as well as the LDL-C and the HDL-C breakdown (Table 5-5). The LDL can also be calculated, but this may result in an underestimate when compared with the direct LDL (Moore, 2006).

Drugs that increase cholesterol include adrenocorticotropic hormone, anabolic steroids, beta-adrenergic blocking agents, corticosteroids, phenytoin, sulfonamides, thiazides, and vitamin D. Drugs that decrease serum cholesterol levels include allopurinol, androgens, bile salt binding agents, captopril, chlorpropamide, clofibrate, colchicine, erythromycin, isoniazid, lovastatin, monoamine oxidase (MAO) inhibi-

tors, neomycin (taken orally), niacin, and nitrates. Low serum cholesterol is indicative of severe liver disease or malnutrition (Pagana and Pagana, 2006). A total cholesterol level below 160 mg/dL in a frail elder is a risk factor for increased mortality (Johnson, 2002).

Triglycerides. Triglycerides are the primary lipids found in the blood and bound to a protein. They are produced in the liver and circulated in the blood. Excess blood levels are deposited into fatty tissue. Triglycerides peak at midlife. Abnormal triglyceride levels may indicate obesity, alcohol abuse, or estrogen use. Severely elevated triglyceride levels (>2000 mg/dL) is a strong risk factor for pancreatitis (Gambert and Miller, 2004).

TESTING FOR BODY PROTEINS

Total Protein

Body proteins are measured by amount of albumin and globulin in the serum, the majority being the latter. Serum albumin is a measure of nutritional status. Globulins are important in the functioning of antibodies and in the maintenance of osmotic pressure.

Serum Albumin

Serum albumin and globulin are used most often as measures of nutritional status but also are an indicator of liver function (Pagana and Pagana, 2006). Although they are commonly ordered, they are neither sensitive nor specific for nutritional health and a slight decrease is a normal change of aging. Corticosteroids, insulin, phenazopyridine, and progesterone increase protein levels. Dehydration will show a deceptive increase in albumin levels. Albumin levels decrease with overhydration, liver and renal disease, malabsorption, and changes in position from an upright to a supine position during the blood draw (Johnson and Sullivan, 2004). The half-life of albumin is about 3 weeks, so changes are not quickly apparent except in sudden and acutely severe conditions. Pre-albumin (transthyretin) has a half-life of only 2 to 3 days and is therefore a more sensitive marker for change. A low pre-albumin level can confirm poor nutritional status and serve as a monitor for active treatment. However, albumin levels are most useful as an indicator of the severity of illness and the risk of mortality.

TABLE 5-5

Interpreting Lipid Panels

Total Cholesterol		LDL Cholesterol		HDL Cholesterol		Triglycerides	
<200	Desirable	<100	Optimal	<40	Low	<150	Normal
200-239	Borderline high	100-128	Near optimal	>60	High	150-199	Borderline high
≥240	High	130-159	Borderline high			200-499	High
		160-189	High			>500	Very high
		≥190	Very High				

Data from Grundy S et al: Implications of recent clinical trials for the National Cholesterol Education Program Adult Treatment Panel III guidelines, *Circulation* 110:227-239, 2004.

LABORATORY TESTS OF RENAL HEALTH

Renal functioning decreases substantially with age (see Chapter 4), but in most cases the body is able to compensate adequately and with only slight increases in laboratory findings. Dietary intake of protein, metabolism, and previous physical activity contribute to the increase in these values along with reduction in lean body mass. Any more marked alternations in laboratory findings are not expected as a "normal part of aging." However, because of the frequency of health problems and medications that further affect renal health, measuring and monitoring renal functioning is particularly important to the older adult and the gerontological nurse. The most common measures to show early variation in illness or problems with medication use affecting the kidneys are the blood urea nitrogen (BUN) and creatinine.

Blood Urea Nitrogen

Urea is the end product of protein metabolism. The serum chemistry test for BUN is a measurement of the nitrogen portion of urea and is used as a gross measurement for renal functioning. The changes over time in the BUN may be more important than any one laboratory result, especially in considering renal insufficiency or renal failure (Beck, 2004). Protein intake affects BUN, and many drugs increase the levels. Some are allopurinol, aminoglycosides, cephalosporins, furosemide, methotrexate, aspirin, bacitracin, gentamicin, carbamazepine, probenecid, corticosteroids, propranolol, thiazides, and tetracyclines (Pagana and Pagana, 2006).

Creatinine

Creatinine is a by-product of the breakdown of muscle creatinine phosphate that is normally produced in energy metabolism. As long as muscle mass remains the same, the serum creatinine is constant. Therefore reduced muscle mass of normal aging will result in a decreased creatinine level. Impaired excretion (renal) will result in an increase. Although the measurement of creatinine is a more accurate reflection of renal health than the BUN, it also can overestimate renal function in the elderly. For the most accurate measure of both renal status and changes related to treatment, it is necessary to calculate the creatinine clearance.

The Cockcroft-Gault equation was developed to estimate creatinine clearance (CrCl) using the serum creatinine value and the person's age. This is frequently used by clinicians in estimating doses when prescribing drugs for elders with probable diminished renal function (Desai and Isa-Pratt, 2002). It replaces obtaining a 24-hour urine collection for creatinine clearance, which is difficult to do, especially in frail elders. The formula for men is as follows:

$$\frac{(140 - \text{Age}) \times \text{Weight in kg}}{(72 \times \text{Serum creatinine})}$$

In women, because of their smaller muscle mass, the value is multiplied by 0.85 or 85%.

It is especially important to calculate and monitor creatinine clearance in the administration of potentially nephrotoxic medications like allopurinol. Other medications for which CrCl is especially important are aminoglycosides, ACE inhibitors, and NSAIDs (Beck, 2004).

MONITORING FOR THERAPEUTIC BLOOD LEVELS

Several medications commonly prescribed require close monitoring of blood levels. Each has a narrow therapeutic window; in other words, at levels too low, their effect may be negligible and at levels too high, they may become toxic and result in adverse drug events. Although this applies to several antibiotics in use (e.g., vancomycin), this discussion is restricted to medications that may be considered "routine" in the lives of older adults.

Coagulation Time: Prothrombin Time/ Partial Thromboplastin Time/ International Normalized Ratio

Prothrombin is produced by the liver and is a key component in the clotting of blood. For the body to produce prothrombin, it must have adequate intake and absorption of vitamin K. In clotting, prothrombin is converted to thrombin as the first part of the coagulation cascade. The prothrombin time (PT) is the most sensitive to deficiencies in vitamin-K–dependent clotting factors II, VII, IX, and X. It is not sensitive to fibrinogen deficiencies and heparin (Nicoll et al., 2004).

The PT is among those tests that the gerontological nurse will see most often and one of the most important ones relating to the immediate needs of the patient. The nurse is responsible for securing testable samples and initially interpreting them. The nurse practitioner is responsible for ensuring the correct use of the test and for initiating or adjusting medications and treatments related to the test results. In the past, measurement and monitoring coagulation status depended on the interpretation of the PT. However these results were so unstable from patient to patient and laboratory to laboratory, the interpretations were fraught with errors. Today the international normalized ratio (INR) is a calculated rating with significantly greater reliability.

Anticoagulation therapy has become the mainstay of the treatment of atrial fibrillation and stroke prevention (e.g., after surgery). Any person who is taking the drug *warfarin* (Coumadin) must have periodic measure of the PT/INR. Too high an INR may result in severe and life-threatening bleeding. A PT of 30 seconds or more is considered a panic level, one that requires immediate intervention (Nicoll et al., 2004). An increased PT is seen in inadequate anticoagulation medication doses, liver disease, vitamin K deficiencies, bile duct obstruction, and salicylate intoxications. It also may be increased with the concomitant use of such drugs as allopurinol, cholestyramine, clofibrate, and sulfonamides (Pagana and Pagana, 2006). Too low an INR removes the preventive action of the therapy and suggests a hypercoagulation state. For persons who are receiving the anticoagulant *heparin*, the partial prothrombin time (PTT) is used to monitor coagulation status and drug dosage.

Cardiac Rate Control: Digoxin Level

Digoxin (Lanoxin) is a drug that is commonly used to control ventricular response to chronic atrial fibrillation. It is initiated slowly and carefully to prevent too rapid a reduction in heart rate. Once the patient's dose is stabilized, the nurse monitors the effect of the medication by measuring the heart rate before drug administration and by observing for signs of adverse effects (see Chapter 10). Monitoring may also include periodic blood levels. The normal therapeutic range is 0.9 to 2.0 ng/mL with toxicity occurring at levels above 3.0 ng/mL. However, because of the normal changes with aging that affect pharmacokinetics, a sub-therapeutic dose may be quite effective for some persons and toxicity may be evident at levels below 3.0 ng/mL. The nurse can use the blood level only as a general guide, and it must be combined with the clinical presentation (including heart rate) of the person.

Antiseizure: Phenytoin (Dilantin) Levels

Phenytoin is a commonly prescribed medication used for the prevention and control of seizures. Like warfarin and digoxin, it has a narrow therapeutic window; the blood levels should remain between 10 and 20 mcg/mL at all times. Breakthrough seizure activity may occur with levels below 10 mcg/mL and toxicity at levels above 20 mcg/mL. However, like digoxin, both control of seizure and toxicity can be found at low levels. Again, the patient must be carefully and individually treated. In preparing laboratory specimens and reports, it is essential to consider the results within the context of timing of previous dosages and possible food or other drug interactions.

Thyroid Hormone Levels

See Hormones on pp. 92 and 94.

URINE STUDIES

Urine is produced by the kidneys, and the ureters carry waste products for excretion from the bladder. The most common test that will involve the nurse is the urinalysis. The nurse is often involved with collecting and testing urine as a part of specific urine studies. The nurse may help the patient collect the specimen and send it to the laboratory but also may perform point-of-care testing and initial analysis. The most important aspects of urine studies are in collection technique and procedures related to storage.

Urinalysis

The urinalysis or analysis of the urine is done both macroscopically by the nurse at the bedside and microscopically in the laboratory. In healthy aging, the findings should not differ from findings at a younger age, but abnormalities are frequently found because of the high rate of diabetes and urinary tract infections experienced by older adults.

The urinalysis begins with obtaining what is called a "clean-catch specimen." This is one in which the contamination by skin flora is minimized through preparation of the genital area (Table 5-6). For persons with complete urinary incontinence, it may be necessary to obtain a catheterized specimen. If the patient has an indwelling catheter, the specimen is obtained by aspirating from the specimen port using a 25-gauge needle. The specimen should be tested or sent to the laboratory immediately. It may be refrigerated for up to 2 hours if absolutely necessary. But any specimen that has not been properly stored or tested promptly should be disposed of and a new one obtained. The cleaner and fresher the specimen, the more accurate is the analysis.

The point-of-service (bedside) analysis by the nurse begins with an observation of the specimen for color, odor, and clarity. Colorless urine may be the result of large fluid intake or recent caffeine intake. Dark urine often is the result of poor fluid intake or the presence of microscopic blood or bacteria. Clarity is hindered by the presence of phosphate crystals after a high-protein meal or the presence of a large number of bacteria. A strong or foul odor is suggestive of either a state of dehydration (concentrated urine) or bacteriuria.

The bedside analysis usually concludes with what is called a "urine dip," in which a pre-treated strip is dipped into the urine and the colors that appear are compared with a standardized chart. Although the bedside analysis is used often, because of the high rate of false negatives and false positives, it should be used only as a screening tool and combined with the clinical assessment of the person. The remainder of the obtained sample is often sent to the laboratory for the microscopic analysis. Both the laboratory and the bedside analyses will measure the urine specific gravity, pH, and presence of urine protein, glucose, ketones, blood, bilirubin, nitrates, and leukocytes (see Table 5-1). The results are recorded and reported to the person's health care provider as indicated.

Specific gravity measures the density of urine relative to the density of water. Urine is 95% water. This test is helpful in determining the adequacy of the renal concentrative mechanism; it measure hydration (Desai and Isa-Pratt, 2002). Specific gravity in the adult is normally between 1.005 and 1.030. These values decrease with aging. This decline has been related to the 33% to 50% decline in the number of nephrons, which impairs the ability of the kidney to concentrate urine.

The pH indicates acid-base balance of the urine. An alkaline pH is usually caused by bacteria (which may indicate a urinary tract infection), a diet high in citrus fruits and vegetables, or intake of sodium bicarbonates. Acidic urine occurs with starvation, dehydration, and diets high in meats and cranberries.

Urine protein can be a sensitive indicator of kidney function. It is normally not present in urine except perhaps in trace amounts in concentrated urine. In dilute urine, it is pathological and should always be considered with the specific gravity of the urine. Ketones, blood, and glucose should

TABLE 5-6

Technique for Obtaining Clean-Catch Midstream Voided Specimen

A clean-catch midstream specimen is the best clinically effective method of securing a voided specimen for urinalysis. It is not a simple procedure and requires patient education and active assistance of the female patient.

EQUIPMENT

Antiseptic towelettes
Disposable gloves if assistance of patient is required
Sterile specimen container

PROCEDURE

Nursing Action	Rationale/Amplification
Male Patient	
1. Instruct the patient to expose glans and cleanse area around the meatus.	1. The urethral orifice is colonized by bacteria. Urine readily becomes contaminated during voiding.
2. Allow the initial urinary flow to escape.	2. The first portion of urine washes out the urethra and contains debris.
3. Collect the midstream urine specimen in a sterile container.	3. The midstream sample reflects the status of the bladder.
4. Avoid collecting the last few drops of urine.	4. Prostatic secretions may be introduced into urine at the end of the urinary stream.
5. Either test or send specimen to laboratory immediately.	5. If a culture is needed, it should be performed as soon as possible to avoid multiplication of urinary bacteria and lysis of cells.
Female Patient	
1. Ask the patient to separate her labia to expose the urethral orifice. If no one is available to assist the patient, she may sit backward on the toilet seat facing the water tank or sit on (straddle) the wide part of the bedpan.	1. Keeping the labia separated prevents labial or vaginal contamination of the urine specimen. By straddling the toilet seat/bedpan, the patient's labia are spread apart for cleansing.
2. Cleanse the area around the urinary meatus with towelettes: a. Wipe the perineum from the front to the back. b. Dispose of the towelette and repeat.	2. The urethral orifice is colonized by bacteria. Urine is readily contaminated during voiding.
3. While the patient keeps the labia separated, instruct her to void forcibly.	3. This helps wash away urethral contaminants.
4. Allow initial urinary flow to drain into bedpan (toilet) and then catch the midstream specimen in a sterile container; make sure that the container does not come in contact with the genitalia.	4. The first portion of urine washes out the urethra. Have patient remove the container from the stream while she is still voiding.
5. Test or send the specimen to the laboratory immediately.	5. Too long an interval between collection and analysis causes contaminants to multiply in the urine and cells to lyse.

all remain negative at any age. Ascorbic acid and aspirin can cause false-negative results for glucose. Ketones may be positive in high-protein diets, "crash" diets, or starvation. Blood is never normal in urine.

Nitrates and/or leucocytes are often found in the presence of infection. A urinalysis suggestive of the presence of bacteria indicates the need for further testing, most often a culture of the urine, and a subsequent testing of sensitivity of the bacteria to antibiotics. This is often ordered as a "U/A [or urine analysis] C & S as indicated."

IMPLICATIONS FOR THE NURSE IN THE LONG-TERM CARE SETTING

Laboratory tests and regular screening tests are commonly employed when caring for a nursing home resident. Laboratory tests are often viewed positively because they are a fast and accurate way to assess some key parts of the older person's physical status. Protocols for establishing routine laboratory testing procedures for long-term care vary widely from

one institution to the next. Gerontological nurses advocate good resident care by requesting laboratory tests and developing protocols to comply with recommended minimum standards for screening and monitoring laboratory tests for elderly residents in long-term care institutions.

In summary, collecting and monitoring laboratory values are important nursing responsibilities. This can be particularly important for the gerontological nurse because some laboratory values change slightly with aging and the older person may be more sensitive to changes in homeostasis (see Chapter 4). The variance of values at both ends of the laboratory range could be misinterpreted as abnormal or questionable when they are within normal range for that gender and age-group. The "normal ranges" in the population older than 65 years are often different from those of the younger population, and these differences should be and are slowly being established so that we have standards to indicate real pathological age-related differences

Laboratory values are helpful tools in understanding clinical signs and symptoms, although clinical decisions based on laboratory values alone are not enough for treatment of the whole person. Abnormal laboratory results trigger comprehensive patient assessments, obtaining information about clinical signs and symptoms, patient history, and psychosocial and physical examination. The nurse synthesizes this information along with the interpretation of laboratory values to establish the most appropriate care in collaboration with the person's nurse practitioner or physician.

KEY CONCEPTS

- In most laboratory measures, there is little difference in the results between a younger adult and an older adult.
- Because of more limited reserves, the older adult is often more sensitive to slight variations in biological parameters.
- The laboratory criteria used in the diagnosis of diabetes and thyroid disease do not differ according to age.
- The nurse is often responsible for the initial interpretation of laboratory results. The nurse cannot depend entirely on laboratory values when considering the possibility of medication toxicity.
- The nurse may be responsible for the accurate and appropriate collection of laboratory specimens.

- Medications and chronic disorders complicate the measurement of laboratory values in elders because most elders are taking several medications at any given time that may interact to alter the reliability of laboratory measurements.

RESEARCH QUESTIONS

In what way does food and alcohol intake affect the accuracy of laboratory test results?

Summarize laboratory values that are considered "critical" and require some type of immediate response.

REFERENCES

Beck LH: Renal systems, fluid and electrolytes. In Landefeld CS et al: *Current geriatric diagnosis and treatment*, New York, 2004, McGraw-Hill.

Beers MH, Berkow R: *The Merck manual of geriatrics*, ed 3, Whitehouse Station, NJ, 2000, Merck Research Laboratories.

Berghe C et al: Prevalence and outcomes of anemia in geriatrics: a systematic review of the literature, *Am J Med* 116(7):3, 2004.

Blumenthal DE: Geriatric rheumatology. In Landefeld CS et al: *Current geriatric diagnosis and treatment*, New York, 2004, McGraw-Hill.

CASE STUDY: Evaluating Laboratory Results

An 84-year-old white male, Mr. Jones, is being admitted to the nursing home where you work. He has a history of heart disease, hypertension, diabetes, constipation, and anemia of chronic disease. You find that he denies any fever, chest pain, numbness or tingling, leg swelling, or palpitations. His diabetes has been under fairly good control while at home, but he has difficulty telling you how much insulin he has been taking. His skin is slightly warm to the touch. He is lethargic, but you notice that he also has some muscle twitching. He has an order to have blood tests done today, including a CBC and a complete metabolic panel. You request it and get the following results later in the evening. Medications are lisinopril 20 mg/day, Lasix 40 mg/day, potassium 5 mEq/day, insulin 30/70 12 units every morning, laxative as needed, multivitamin daily.

	Result	Normal Range
Sodium	135 mEq/L	136-148 mEq/L
Potassium	5.8 mEq/L	3.5-5.3 mEq/L
Chloride	110 mEq/L	97-108 mEq/L
Glucose	60 mg/dL	70-110 mg/dL
BUN	36 mg/dL	10-20 mg/dL
Creatinine	3.7 mg/dL	0.6-1.2 mg/dL
Albumin	2.4 g/dL	3.5-5.8 g/dL
WBCs	$31.2 \times 10^3/mm^3$	$3.8\text{-}10.8 \times 10^3/mm^3$
RBC	$4.0 \times 10^6\ \mu L$	$4.4\text{-}5.8 \times 10^6\ \mu L$
HGB	10.2 g/dL	13.8-17.2 g/dL
HCT	30.6%	41.0%-50.8%

Based on the case study, develop a nursing care plan using the following procedure*:
- List Mr. Jones' comments that provide subjective data.
- List information that provides objective data.

- From these data, identify and state, using accepted format, two nursing diagnoses you determine are most significant to Mr. Jones at this time. List two of Mr. Jones' strengths that you have identified from the data.
- Determine and state outcome criteria for each diagnosis. These must reflect some alleviation of the problem identified in the nursing diagnosis and must be stated in concrete and measurable terms.
- Plan and state one or more interventions for each diagnosed problem. Provide specific documentation of the source used to determine the appropriate intervention. Plan at least one intervention that incorporates Mr. Jones' existing strengths.
- Evaluate the success of the intervention. Interventions must correlate directly with the stated outcome criteria to measure the outcome success.

Critical Thinking Questions

1. Which of the laboratory findings are not within normal limits?
2. Are there any deviations in the results that are consistent with normal aging? If so, which ones and why?
3. Are there any deviations in laboratory results that would be expected in persons with prolonged chronic illness like Mr. Jones? If so, what are they and why are they expected?
4. Which of the above deviations from normal are potentially the most dangerous for Mr. Jones at this time? If so, why?
5. Could any of the abnormal blood tests be related to his medications?
6. Are there any results that need prompt referral to Mr. Jones' primary care provider? If so, which one(s)?

* Students are advised to refer to their nursing diagnosis text and identify possible or potential problems.

Chamberlain KL: Homocystine and cardiovascular disease: a review of current recommendation for screening and treatment, *J Am Acad Nurs Pract* 17(3):90-95, 2005.

Desai SP, Isa-Pratt S: *Clinician's guide to laboratory medicine*, ed 2, Cleveland, 2002, Lexi-Comp.

Ebersole P et al: *Gerontological nursing and healthy aging*, ed 2, St Louis, 2005, Mosby.

Freedman ML, Sutin DG: Blood disorders and their management. In Tallis RC et al, editors: *Brocklehurst's textbook of geriatric medicine and gerontology*, ed 6, Edinburgh, 2002, Churchill Livingstone.

Gambert SR, Miller M: Endocrine disorders. In Landefeld CS et al: *Current geriatric diagnosis and treatment*, New York, 2004, McGraw-Hill.

Grodner M et al: *Foundations and clinical applications of nutrition: a nursing approach*, St Louis, 2004, Mosby.

Halter JB: Diabetes mellitus. In Hazzard WR et al, editors: *Principles of geriatric medicine and gerontology*, New York, 2003, McGraw-Hill.

Johnson LE: Nutrition. In Ham RS et al, editors: *Primary care geriatrics*, ed 4, St Louis, 2002, Mosby.

Johnson LE, Sullivan DH: Nutrition and failure to thrive. In Landefeld CS et al: *Current geriatric diagnosis and treatment*, New York, 2004, McGraw-Hill.

Kane RL, Ouslander JG, Abrass IB: *Essentials of clinical geriatrics*, ed 5, New York, 2004, McGraw-Hill.

Mauk KL: *Gerontological nursing: competencies for care*, Boston, 2005, Jones & Bartlett.

Mentes J: A typology of caps and oral rehydration: problems exhibited by frail nursing home residents, *J Gerontolog Nurs* 32(1):13-19, 2006.

Moore SA: Laboratory and diagnostic tests. In Meiner SE, Lueckenotte AG: *Gerontologic nursing*, ed 3, St Louis, 2006, Mosby.

Nicoll D et al: *Pocket guide to diagnostic tests*, ed 4, New York, 2004, McGraw-Hill.

Pagana KD, Pagana TJ: *Mosby's diagnostic and lab test reference*, ed 6, St Louis, 2003, Mosby.

Pagana KD, Pagana TJ: *Manual of diagnostic and laboratory tests*, ed 3, 2006, St Louis, Mosby.

Prahash A, Lynch T: B-type natriuretic peptide: a diagnostic, prognostic, and therapeutic tool in health failure, *Am J Crit Care* 13(1):46, 2004.

Rich MW: Cardiac disease. In Landefeld CS et al: *Current geriatric diagnosis and treatment*, New York, 2004, McGraw-Hill.

Ryan M, Wilson AM: C-reactive protein in cardiovascular disease, *Long-Term Care Interface* 7(5):40-46, 2006.

Sarkozi L: Biochemical tests. In Tallis RC et al, editors: *Brocklehurst's textbook of geriatric medicine and gerontology*, ed 6, Edinburgh, 2002, Churchill Livingstone.

Sink KM, Yaffee K: Cognitive impairment and dementia. In Landefeld CS et al: *Current geriatric diagnosis and treatment*, New York, 2004, McGraw-Hill.

Thibodeau GA, Patton KT: *Structure and function of the body*, ed 12, St Louis, 2003, Mosby.

USPTF (US Preventive Task Force): Screening for prostate cancer: recommendations and rationale, Rockville, Md, 2002, AHRQ. Available at *www.ahrq.gov/clinic/3rduspstf/prostatescr/prostaterr/htm*. Accessed June 29, 2006.

Zubrod G, Holman JR: Novel biochemical markers of cardiovascular risk: a primary care primer, *Consultant* 44(10):1509-1513, 2004.

CHAPTER 6

Health Assessment in Gerontological Nursing

Kathleen Jett

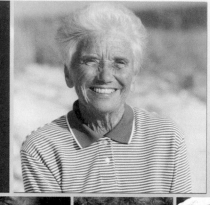

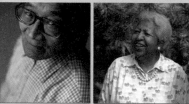
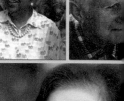

AN ELDER SPEAKS

Whenever I go to one of my doctors I feel like they are rushing through and never really give me a good examination. Then I had an appointment with a nurse practitioner who specialized in us older folks. I couldn't believe the difference. I not only felt listened to but I also felt like I got the best exam I have had in a long time. I am sure it will help me get better!

Henry at age 76

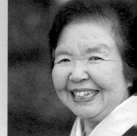

LEARNING OBJECTIVES

On completion of this chapter, the reader will be able to:

1. Explain what is necessary to consider when obtaining assessment data from an elder of another cultural background.
2. List the essential components of the comprehensive health assessment of an older adult.
3. Discuss the advantages and disadvantages of the use of standardized tools in the gerontological assessment.

4. Describe the purpose of the inclusion of functional assessment when caring for an older adult.

In the promotion of healthy aging, gerontological nurses conduct skilled and detailed assessments of and with the persons who entrust themselves to their care. The process of assessment of older adults is strikingly different from that of younger adults in that it is more comprehensive even when problem-oriented. If a complete and comprehensive assessment is needed, this is usually performed by a number of members of the health care team, led by the nurse. A comprehensive assessment requires not only physical data but also an integration of the biological, psychosocial, and functional aspects of the person. Inquiries into physiological and anatomical function, growth and development, family relationships, group involvement, and religious and occupational pursuits are included. Questions regarding genetic background, although important, have less significance for the elderly because genetic consequences usually appear earlier in life.

Assessment of the older adult requires special abilities of the nurse: to listen patiently, to allow for pauses, to ask questions that are not often asked, to observe minute details, to obtain data from all available sources, and to recognize normal changes associated with late life that might be considered abnormal in one who is younger (see Chapter 4). In gerontological nursing, assessment takes more time than does assessment of younger adults because of the increased medical and social complexities of older adults. The quality and speed of the assessment is an art born of experience. Novice nurses should neither be expected nor expect themselves to do this proficiently but should expect to see both their skills and the amount of information obtained increase over time. According to Benner (1984), assessment is a task for the expert. However, an expert is not always available. By using assessment tools, reasonably reliable data may be obtained by nurses at all skill levels.

The assessment provides information critical to the development of a plan of action that can enhance personal health status, decrease the potential for or the severity of chronic conditions, and assist the individual to gain control over health through self-care. The nurse can consider the results of assessment as a snapshot of an individual's health status at the time it is completed. Periodic assessment of physical, functional, social, and mental status in health and illness allows for a comparison with a baseline and for that which nursing care can be planned or adjusted. Health assessment is a complex process that requires entire textbooks to address in detail. In this chapter we provide an overview of parts of the assessment and discussion of tools that are particularly unique or helpful in caring for the older adult.

THE HEALTH HISTORY

The initiation of the health history marks the beginning of the nurse-client relationship and the assessment process. The health history is collected either verbally in a face-to-face interview or through the clarification of a written history completed by the patient or patient's proxy beforehand. The latter method is usually much faster than the former. If the elder has limited English proficiency, a knowledgeable interpreter is needed and the interview will generally take about double the amount of time (see Box 21-2).

Any health history form or interview should include a patient profile, a past medical history, a review of symptoms and systems, a medication history (prescribed and over-the-counter remedies including herbals and dietary supplements), a family history (especially parents and siblings), and a social history. The social history of the older adult should include the current living arrangements, economic resources to deal with current health issues, amount of family and friend support if needed, and the types of community resources available if needed. It should also include the identification of those who are involved in health care decision making. Finally, if functional status is measured by self-report or by proxy, this is also routinely collected at the time of the health history.

To meet the needs of our increasingly diverse population of elders, the use of questions related to the explanatory model (Kleinman, 1980) is recommended to complement the standard health history (Box 6-1). The responses will better enable the nurse to understand the elder and plan culturally appropriate and effective interventions. See also Chapter 21.

When a more comprehensive assessment is needed, additional components are included, with data often collected using well-established tools. Additional areas are psychological parameters such as cognitive and emotional well-being; caregiver stress or burden; the individual's self-perception of health; and patterns of health and health care, education, family structure, plans for retirement, and living environment. For those living at home, a home safety assessment can be very helpful. Areas or problems not frequently addressed by the care provider or mentioned by the elder but should be addressed are sexual dysfunction, depression, incontinence, alcoholism, hearing loss, and memory loss or confusion (Ham, 2002).

PHYSICAL ASSESSMENT

The health history is usually followed by the physical assessment or examination. Although the manual techniques of the examination do not differ significantly from those used with younger persons, knowledge of the normal changes with aging (see Chapters 4 and 5) is essential for the appropriate analysis of the data obtained. When assessing persons from ethnically distinct groups, is it also necessary to be aware of cultural rules of etiquette and taboos that influence the examination (Box 6-2).

However, because of the complex interrelationship among the parts of the complete assessment process, the use of a model or tool when performing the physical assessment may be very helpful. The website of the John A. Hartford Institute for Geriatric Nursing (*www.hartfordign.org*) provides a compilation of key tools used in assessment in their "Try This" series.

BOX 6-1 The Explanatory Model for Culturally Sensitive Assessment

1. How would you describe the problem that has brought you here? (What do you call your problem; does it have a name?)
   a. Who is involved in your decision making about health concerns?
2. How long have you had this problem?
   a. When do you think it started?
   b. What do you think started it?
   c. Do you know anyone else with it?
   d. Tell me what happened to that person when dealing with this problem.
3. What do you think is wrong with you?
   a. How severe is it?
   b. How long do you think it will last?

4. Why do you think this happened to you?
   a. Why has it happened to the involved part?
   b. What do you fear most about your sickness?
5. What are the chief problems your sickness has caused you?
6. What do you think will help clear up this problem? (What treatment should you receive; what are the most important results you hope to receive?)
   a. If specific tests, medications are listed, ask what they are and do.
7. Apart from me, who else do you think can make you feel better?
   a. Are there therapies that make you feel better that I do not know? (May be in another discipline?)

Modified from Kleinman A: *Patient and healers in the context of culture: an exploration of the borderland between anthropology, medicine, and psychiatry,* Berkeley, 1980, University of California Press; Pfeifferling JH: A cultural prescription for mediocentrism. In Eisenberg L, Kleinman A, editors: *The relevance of social science for medicine,* Boston, 1981, Reidel.

BOX 6-2 Key Points to Consider in Observing Cultural Rules and Etiquette

- Social organization and expectations (e.g., roles of family members and friends)
- Communication style, especially in the health care setting
- Use of personal space and eye contact
- General health orientation related to time (past, present, future)
- Appropriate wording of greetings
- Appropriate use of names
- Appropriateness of touch, especially between genders

FANCAPES is an assessment model and tool that can be used with frail elders but is less useful for the active and healthy elder. It uses a survival-needs framework with an emphasis on function. The acronym FANCAPES represents Fluids, Aeration, Nutrition, Communication, Activity, Pain, Elimination, and Socialization and social skills. The information provided is helpful in the appraisal of the older person's ability to meet his or her needs and the extent to which assistance is necessary. FANCAPES can be used in all settings, may be used in part or total (depending on the need), and is easily adaptable to the functional pattern grouping if nursing diagnoses are used in planning care.

FANCAPES

Fluids. Evaluation of fluids requires an assessment of the client's state of hydration and those physiological, situational, and mental factors that contribute to the maintenance of adequate hydration. Attention is directed to the ability of the person to obtain adequate fluids independently, to express thirst, to swallow effectively, and to evaluate medications that affect intake and output (see Chapters 7 and 12).

Aeration. Aeration refers to the adequacy of oxygen exchange. Observations include respiratory rate and depth at rest and during activity; talking, walking, and situations requiring added exertion; and the presence or absence of edema in the extremities or abdomen. At a minimum, breath sounds should be auscultated and medications reviewed to evaluate their effects on aeration. A determination of oxygen saturation level should be done any time that respiratory compromise is suspected.

Nutrition. Nutrition assessment includes mechanical and psychological factors in addition to the type and amount of food consumed. It is also necessary to ascertain the person's ability to bite, chew, and swallow. Persons who are edentulous may have dentures that fit improperly or are not worn. Alterations in diet because of culture, medical restrictions, available economic resources, and living conditions should be considered. Visual and neurological impairment, which might interfere with the person's ability to prepare a meal or feed himself or herself, should be noted (see Chapter 14). Functional or economic status may interfere with obtaining groceries or foods for special diets (see Chapter 17).

Communication. Communication includes sending and receiving verbal and nonverbal information in the external world. Assessment of communicative ability includes the determination of sight and sound acuity; voice quality; and adequate function of the tongue, teeth, pharynx, and larynx. Appraisals of the person's ability to read, write, and understand the spoken language of the nurse should be ascertained. This is an important issue, since an undetected limitation of these skills can lead to erroneous conclusions or to the patient's inability to follow directions.

Activity. Although the ability to ambulate is a major component in activity assessment, activity includes more than movement or exercise. The nurse assesses the person's ability to eat, toilet, dress, and groom; to prepare meals; to dial the telephone; and to move about with or without assistive devices. Coordination and balance, finger dexterity, grip strength, and other abilities necessary in daily life should also be assessed.

Pain. Pain, both physical and mental, is important to consider. The presence and absence of pressure and discomfort are key aspects of pain assessment. Information about recent losses or visible symptoms of anxiety may help identify persons in pain. The manner by which a client customarily attains relief from pain or discomfort will provide further information (see Chapter 11).

Elimination. Bladder and bowel elimination are assessed and include evidence of urinary dribbling or incontinence, use of assistive devices or altered body structures resulting from surgical intervention, and medications that affect voiding and intestinal peristalsis. The nurse and patient will need to find words that they both understand when talking about bowel and bladder functioning. The words used in health care, such as "stooling" or "voiding," should be avoided unless it is known that they are understood (see Chapter 7 for discussion of incontinence).

Socialization and Social Skills. Examination of socialization and social skills assesses the individual's ability to negotiate in society, to give and receive love and friendship, and to feel self-worth. Assessment focuses on the individual's ability to deal with loss and to interact with other people in give-and-take situations.

Functional Assessment

Whereas the emphasis of FANCAPES is on physical functioning and helps organize the physical part of the appraisal, a full functional assessment is broader. A formal functional assessment can be defined as the evaluation of a person's ability to carry out basic tasks for self-care and tasks needed to support independent living. A thorough functional assessment will help the gerontological nurse work toward healthy aging by accomplishing the following:

- Identifying the specific areas in which help is needed or not needed
- Identifying changes in abilities from one period of time to another

- Determining the need for specific service(s)
- Providing information that may be useful in assessing the safety of a particular living situation

The major tools used in functional assessment are those that assess the individual's ability to perform the tasks needed for self-care (i.e., those needed to maintain one's health) and, separately, those tasks needed for independent living (i.e., those needed to maintain one's home). Self-care activities are known as *activities of daily living (ADLs)* and are international as well as cross-cultural in nature. ADLs usually are listed on tools as eating, toileting, ambulation, bathing, dressing, and grooming. Three of these tasks (grooming, dressing, bathing) require higher cognitive function than the others.

The instrumental activities of daily living (IADLs) are tasks needed for independent living, such as cleaning, yard work, shopping, and money management. The successful performance of IADLs requires a higher level of cognitive and physical functioning than the ADLs. For persons with dementia, the progressive loss of the ability to perform IADLs begins with those that require the highest cognitive functions, such as handling finances and shopping.

Numerous tools are available that describe, screen, assess, monitor, and predict functional ability. Generally, the assessment does not break down a task into its component parts, such as picking up a spoon or cup or swallowing water, when assessment of eating is done; instead, eating is seen as a total task. Most of the tools result in a score of some kind—a rating of the person's ability to do the task alone, to need assistance, or to not be able to perform the task at all. The ratings are done by self-report, proxy, or observer. The tools are beneficial in their ability to serve the purposes just noted. However, most are not sensitive to small changes and can be used only as part of a holistic assessment.

Activities of Daily Living

Katz Index. The Katz Index (Katz et al., 1963) developed in 1963 serves as a basic framework for most of the measures of ADLs since that time. There are several versions of the Katz Index; one is based on a 3-point scale and allows one to score client performance abilities as independent, assistive, dependent, or unable to perform. Another version of the tool assigns 1 point to each ADL that can be completed independently and a zero (0) if it cannot. Scores will range from a maximum of 6 (totally independent) to 0 (totally dependent). A score of 4 indicates moderate impairment, whereas 2 or less indicates severe impairment (Figure 6-1).

	Independence (1 point) NO supervision, direction, or personal assistance	Dependence (0 points) WITH supervision, direction, personal assistance, or total care
BATHING Points:_____	(1 point) Bathes self completely or needs help in bathing only a single part of the body such as the back, genital area, or disabled extremity.	(0 points) Needs help with bathing more than one part of the body, getting in or out of the tub or shower. Requires total bathing.
DRESSING Points:_____	(1 point) Gets clothes from closets and drawers and puts on clothes and outer garments complete with fasteners. May have help tying shoes.	(0 points) Needs help with dressing self or needs to be completely dressed.
TOILETING Points:_____	(1 point) Goes to toilet, gets on and off the toilet, arranges clothes, cleans genital area without help.	(0 points) Needs help transferring to the toilet, cleaning self, or uses bedpan or commode
TRANSFERRING Points:_____	(1 point) Moves in and out of bed or chair unassisted. Mechanical transferring aids are acceptable.	(0 points) Needs help in moving from bed to chair or requires a complete transfer.
CONTINENCE Points:_____	(1 point) Exercises complete self-control over urination and defecation.	(0 points) Is partially or totally incontinent of bowel or bladder.
FEEDING Points:_____	(1 point) Gets food from plate into mouth without help. Preparation of food may be done by another person.	(0 points) Needs partial or total help with feeding or requires parenteral feeding.

| TOTAL POINTS: _____ | 6 = High (patient independent) | 0 = Low (patient very dependent) |

FIGURE 6-1 Katz Index of Independence in Activities of Daily Living. (From Katz S et al: Progress in development of the index of ADL, *Gerontologist* 10(1):20-30, 1970.)

BOX 6-3   Instrumental Activities of Daily Living

1. Telephone:
   I: Able to look up numbers, dial, receive and make calls without help
   A: Able to answer phone or dial operator in an emergency but needs special phone or help in getting number or dialing
   D: Unable to use telephone
2. Traveling:
   I: Able to drive own car or travel alone on bus or taxi
   A: Able to travel but not alone
   D: Unable to travel
3. Shopping:
   I: Able to take care of all shopping with transportation provided
   A: Able to shop but not alone
   D: Unable to shop
4. Preparing meals:
   I: Able to plan and cook full meals
   A: Able to prepare light foods but unable to cook full meals alone
   D: Unable to prepare any meals

5. Housework:
   I: Able to do heavy housework (e.g., scrub floors)
   A: Able to do light housework but needs help with heavy tasks
   D: Unable to do any housework
6. Medication:
   I: Able to take medications in the right dose at the right time
   A: Able to take medications but needs reminding or someone to prepare them
   D: Unable to take medications
7. Money:
   I: Able to manage buying needs, write checks, pay bills
   A: Able to manage daily buying needs but needs help managing checkbook, paying bills
   D: Unable to manage money

From *Multidimensional Functional Assessment Questionnaire*, ed 2, by Duke University Center for the Study of Aging and Human Development with permission of Duke University, 1978.
I, Independent; *A*, assistance; *D*, dependent.

This scoring puts equal weight on all activities, and the determination of a cutoff score is completely arbitrary. Despite these limitations, the tool is useful because it creates a common language about functioning for all caregivers involved in planning overall care and discharge.

Barthel Index. The Barthel Index (Mahoney and Barthel, 1965) is probably the tool most commonly used in rehabilitation settings to measure the amount of physical assistance required when a person can no longer carry out ADLs independently. It has proved to be especially useful as a method of documenting improvement of a patient's ability. The Barthel Index ranks the functional status as either independent or dependent and then allows for further classification of independent into intact or limited; and dependent into needing a helper or unable to do the activity at all. Instruction is needed in the use and scoring of this tool before using it.

Functional Independence Measure. The Functional Independence Measure (FIM) is widely used and the most comprehensive functional assessment tool for rehabilitation settings. It includes measure of ADL, mobility, cognition, and social functioning. It was developed through the work of a number of experts and has been thoroughly tested. Ordinarily the tool is completed by the joint efforts of the interdisciplinary team and used for both planning and evaluation of progress. Considerable training is required to accurately use the FIM (Granger and Hamilton, 1993); however, its use is encouraged.

Instrumental Activities of Daily Living

The original scoring tool for IADLs was developed by Lawton and Brody (1969). Both the original tool and the subsequent iterations again use the self-report, proxy, and observed formats with the three levels of functioning (independent, assisted, and unable to perform). The pros and cons of using these are the same as the measures of ADLs. Box 6-3 gives an example of a self-rated instrument for IADLs.

The ADLs and IADLs can also be measured based on performance or demonstration of such. These tools overcome the problems associated with self-report and proxy report and yield more objective measurement of functional status. They take longer to conduct; the cutoff scores are subjective and arbitrary. The three performance tests related to mobility are simple and quick: the ability to stand with feet together in a side-by-side manner and in a tandem and semi-tandem position, a timed walk of 8 feet, and a timed rise from a chair and return to a seated position five times (Box 6-4).

Function and Cognition

When assessing both functional status and cognitive abilities, slightly different tools are indicated. The Blessed Dementia Score (Blessed et al., 1968) is based on a 22-item tool that can be scored from 0 to 30. The higher the score, the greater the degree of dementia. This tool incorporates aspects of ADLs, IADLs, memory, recalling events, and finding one's way outdoors. The Clinical Dementia Rating Scale (Morris, 1993) and the Global Deterioration Scale (Reisberg et al., 1982) also assess both functional and cognitive abili-

BOX 6-4 Functional Performance Tests

STANDING BALANCE

Instructions: Semi-tandem stand.* The nurse:
a. First demonstrates the task. (The heel of one foot is placed to the side of the first toe of the other foot.)
b. Supports one arm of the older adult while he or she positions the feet as demonstrated above. The elder can choose which foot to place forward.
c. Asks if the person is ready; then releases the support and begins timing.
d. Stops timing when the older adult moves the feet or grasps the nurse for support or when 10 seconds have elapsed.

*Start with the semi-tandem stand. If it cannot be done for 10 seconds, then the **side-by-side** test should be done. If the semi-tandem can be accomplished for the requisite 10 seconds, follow the same instructions as above, except the **full tandem** requires placing the heel of one foot directly in front of the toes of the other foot.

SCORING	FULL TANDEM	SEMI-TANDEM	SIDE-BY-SIDE
0	_____	<10 seconds or unable	<10 seconds or unable
1	_____	<10 seconds or unable	10 seconds
2	<3 seconds or unable	10 seconds	_____
3	3 to 9 seconds	10 seconds	_____
4	10 seconds	10 seconds	_____

Standing Balance Score: _____

WALKING SPEED

Instructions: The nurse:
a. Sets up an 8-foot walking course with an additional 2 feet at both ends free of any obstacles.
b. Places an 8-foot rigid carpenter's ruler to the side of the course.
c. Instructs the older adult to "walk to the other end of the course at your normal speed, just like walking down the street to go to the store." Assistive devices should be used if needed.
d. Times two walks. **The fastest of the two is used as the score.**

Scoring
0 Unable
1 >5.6 seconds
2 4.1 to 5.6 seconds
3 3.2 to 4 seconds
4 <3.2 seconds
Walking Speed Score: _____

CHAIR STANDS

Instructions: The nurse:
a. Places a straight-backed chair next to a wall.
b. Asks the older adult to fold the arms across the chest and stand up from the chair one time. If successful:
c. Asks the older adult to stand and sit five times as quickly as possible.
d. Times from the initial sitting position to the final standing position at the end of the fifth stand.
Scores are for the five rise-and-sits only. If the older adult performs fewer than five repetitions, the score is 0.

Scoring
0 Unable
1 >16.6 seconds
2 13.7 to 16.5 seconds
3 11.2 to 13.6 seconds
4 <11.2 seconds
Chair Stands Score: _____

Total of all performance tests (0-12) _____

Modified from Guralnik JM et al: A short physical performance battery assessing lower extremity function: association with self-reported disability and prediction of mortality and nursing home admission, *J Gerontol Med Sci* 49(2):M85-M94, 1994; Bennett JA: Activities of daily living: old-fashioned or still useful? *J Gerontolog Nurs* 25(5):22-29, 1999.

ties and also are used to stage dementia. Determining the functional and cognitive stage of the dementia can allow the nurse to provide considerable anticipatory teaching to both the family and other caregivers.

MENTAL STATUS ASSESSMENT

Older adults are at great risk for impaired mental capacity. In late life, cognitive ability is easily threatened by any disturbance in health or homeostasis, and the incidence of dementing illnesses such as Alzheimer's disease increases in proportion to age. Altered or impaired mental status may be the first sign of anything from a heart attack to a urinary tract infection. Gerontological nursing requires skills in basic assessment of mental status, especially cognitive abilities and mood, and sensitivity to subtle changes in cognition, which may indicate a reversible health problem.

Cognitive Measures

Mini-Mental State Examination. The tool most often seen is probably the Mini-Mental State Examination (MMSE) by Folstein et al. (1975). The MMSE is a 30-item instrument that is used to screen for cognitive deficiencies and is one of the tools used in the determination of a diagnosis of dementia or delirium. It tests orientation, short-term memory and attention, calculation ability, language, and construction (Figure 6-2). To ensure that the results of this test are valid and reliable, it must be administered exactly as it is written. It cannot be given to persons who cannot see or write or who are not proficient in English. A score of 30 suggests no impairment, and a score of 26 or less suggests a potential dementia; however, adjustments are needed for educational level (Osterweil et al., 2000). It has not yet been standardized cross-culturally. In the long-term care setting, the MMSE is administered by either the nurse or the social

---

MMSE Sample Items

Orientation to Time
"What is the date?"

Registration
"Listen carefully. I am going to say three words. You say them back after I stop. Ready? Here they are...
APPLE (pause), PENNY (pause), TABLE (pause). Now repeat those words back to me." [Repeat up to 5 times, but score only the first trial.]

Naming
"What is this?" [Point to a pencil or pen.]

Reading
"Please read this and do what it says." [Show the examinee the words on the stimulus form.] CLOSE YOUR EYES

FIGURE 6-2 Mini-Mental State Examination. (If using this tool, it is recommended that the original instructions found in this article are reviewed, especially for persons with visual or manual limitations. Score must be adjusted for low education levels. Not standardized for non–English-speaking persons.) Reproduced by special permission of the Publisher, Psychological Assessment Resources, Inc., 16204 North Florida Avenue, Lutz, Florida, 33549, from the Mini Mental State Examination, by Marshal Folstein and Susan Folstein, Copyright 1975, 1998, 2001 by Mini Mental LLC, Inc. Published 2001 by Psychological Assessment Resources, Inc. Further reproduction is prohibited without the permission of PAR, Inc. The MMSE can be purchased from PAR, Inc. by calling (800) 331-8378.

worker as part of the collection of period data for the Minimum Data Set (MDS) (see Appendix 6-A).

Short Portable Mental Status Questionnaire. A second tool that tests cognitive ability is the Short Portable Mental Status Questionnaire (SPMSQ) (Pfeiffer, 1975). The tool covers 10 questions that assess the person's orientation, remote memory, concentration, and calculation ability (Box 6-5). The SPMSQ can be used with individuals who have a short attention span and cannot sit long enough for the MMSE to be administered. Its value as an assessment tool is its ease of administration and the fact that it requires no equipment. It can be administered reliably with little preparation, and the established norms account for educational level. It is difficult to accurately use the normal cutoff points (three wrong answers) for patients with delirium because of its variable presentation. It has not been standardized for use cross-culturally with non–English-speaking groups.

Clock Drawing Test. The Clock Drawing Test, which has been used since 1992 (Mendez et al., 1992; Tuokko et al., 1992), is a screening tool that differentiates cognitively intact persons from those with cognitive impairment. To complete the Clock Drawing Test, the individual

must be able to adequately hold a pen or pencil because it does require some manual dexterity. It would not be appropriate to use with individuals who are blind or who have severe arthritis, Parkinson's disease, or stroke that affects their dominant hand. It is unknown if it can be used with a person without writing skills. A person is presented with either a blank piece of paper or a paper with a circle drawn on it. He or she is then asked to draw the face of a clock that says it is 3:45. Scoring is based on both the position of the numbers and the position of the hands (Box 6-6). This tool does not establish criteria for dementia, but if performance on the clock drawing is impaired, it suggests the need for further assessment.

Mood Measures

The tools just mentioned are used in the assessment of cognitive ability. Additional measurements may be needed of affective state or mood, especially the presence or absence of depression, a common and too often unrecognized problem in late life. Persons with untreated or under-treated depression are more functionally impaired and will have prolonged hospitalizations and nursing home stays, lowered quality of life, and perhaps shortened length of life (see Chapter 25). Persons with depression may appear as if they have dementia, and many persons with dementia are also depressed. The interconnection between the two calls for skill and sensitivity of the nurse to ensure that elders receive the most appropriate and effective care possible.

Beck Depression Inventory. The Beck Depression Inventory (BDI) (Beck, 1987) is one of the most widely used self-administered tools in the identification of depression. The 21 items are divided between affective symptoms (e.g., I feel sad) and physical symptoms (e.g., I am having trouble sleeping). The BDI is used for screening, measuring severity of depression, and monitoring changes over time, such as response to treatment.

Zung Depression Scale. The Zung Self-Rating Depression Scale (Zung, 1965) has 20 items and is also commonly used with older adults. The items are similar to those in the BDI and are rated on frequency of occurrence from 1 to 4, or "a little of the time" to "most of the time." Elders may score inaccurately higher (indicating more depression) because of the number of physical complaints that are associated with normal aging or frequently used medications rather than because of true depression.

Geriatric Depression Scale. The Geriatric Depression Scale (GDS), developed by Yesavage et al. (1983), is a 30-item tool designed for gerontological patients and based almost entirely on psychological discriminators. A short version is also available (Box 6-7). The GDS has been extremely successful in determining depression because it deemphasizes physical complaints, libido, and appetite. Although not without problems, it is viewed as a more accurate measure of depression in the elderly than other tools. It cannot be used in persons with dementia or cognitive impairment (Osterweil et al., 2000).

ASSESSMENT OF SOCIAL SUPPORT

A comprehensive assessment of an older adult and his or her family would be incomplete without an evaluation of social networks and support. Assessment of social support considers an individual's surrounding network of intimates, friends, and family. Tools to adequately measure social networks have been in development for a number of years. However, the many nuances and configurations of social support networks make standardized measurements difficult. One tool that has shown some usefulness is the Family APGAR. Although it was designed for younger families, it has potential for use with elders and their families.

Family APGAR

The Family APGAR (Smilkstein, 1978) explores five specific family functions: Adaptation, Partnership, Growth, Affection, and Resolution (Figure 6-3). A score of less than 3 points of a possible 10 points indicates a highly dysfunctional family (at least as perceived by the person). A 4- to 6-point score suggests moderate family dysfunction. Although these results alone should not be considered definitive for family dysfunction. The APGAR tool is useful in the following situations:

- Interviewing a new patient
- Interviewing a person who will be caring for a chronically ill family member
- After adverse events (e.g., death, diagnosis of cancer)
- When the patient history suggests family dysfunction

If an elder has more intimate social relationships with friends than with the spouse or family or is without family or spouse, the Friend APGAR should be used. The questions

---

BOX 6-5 Short Portable Mental Status Questionnaire (SPMSQ)

1. What is the date today (month/day/year)?
2. What is the day of the week?
3. What is the name of this place?
4. What is your telephone number?
5. How old are you?
6. When were you born (month/day/year)?
7. Who is the current president of the United States?
8. Who was the president just before him?
9. What is your mother's maiden name?
10. Subtract 3 from 20 and keep subtracting each new number you get, all the way down.

Scoring
0-2 errors = intact
3-4 errors = mild intellectual impairment
5-7 errors = moderate intellectual impairment

From Pfeiffer E: A short portable mental status questionnaire for the assessment of organic brain deficit in elderly patients, *J Am Geriatr Soc* 23(10):433-441, 1975.

BOX 6-6 Clock Drawing Test

INSTRUCTIONS

On a blank piece of paper:
    Ask the elder to draw a circle.
    Ask the elder to place the numbers inside the circle.
    Ask the elder to place the hands at 3:45.

SCORING

Draws closed circle	Score 1 point
Places numbers in correct position	Score 1 point
Includes all 12 correct numbers	Score 1 point
Places hands in correct position	Score 1 point

INTERPRETATIONS

Errors such as grossly distorted contour or extraneous markings are rarely produced by cognitively intact persons.
Clinical judgment must be applied, but a low score indicates the need for further evaluation.

Data from Mendez MF et al: Development of scoring criteria for the clock drawing task in Alzheimer's disease, *J Am Geriatr Soc* 40(11):1095-1099, 1992; Tuokko H et al: The Clock Test: a sensitive measure to differentiate normal elderly from those with Alzheimer disease, *J Am Geriatr Soc* 40(6):579-584, 1992.

BOX 6-7   Geriatric Depression Scale, Short Form

Patient _____ Examiner _____ Date _____

Directions to patient: Please choose the best answer for how you have felt over the past week.

Directions to examiner: Present questions VERBALLY. Circle answer given by patient. Do not show to patient.

1. Are you basically satisfied with your life?	yes	**no (1)**
2. Have you dropped many of your activities and interests?	**yes (1)**	no
3. Do you feel that your life is empty?	**yes (1)**	no
4. Do you often get bored?	**yes (1)**	no
5. Are you in good spirits most of the time?	yes	**no (1)**
6. Are you afraid that something bad is going to happen to you?	**yes (1)**	no
7. Do you feel happy most of the time?	yes	**no (1)**
8. Do you often feel helpless?	**yes (1)**	no
9. Do you prefer to stay at home rather than go out and do things?	**yes (1)**	no
10. Do you feel you have more problems with memory than most?	**yes (1)**	no
11. Do you think it is wonderful to be alive now?	yes	**no (1)**
12. Do you feel pretty worthless the way you are now?	**yes (1)**	no
13. Do you feel full of energy?	yes	**no (1)**
14. Do you feel that your situation is hopeless?	**yes (1)**	no
15. Do you think that most people are better off than you are?	**yes (1)**	no

Total: Please sum all boldfaced answers (worth one point) for a total score. _____

Score: 0-4 No depression; 5-10 Mild depression; ≥11 Severe depression.

From Patient Plus: Geriatric Depression Score. (2006). EMIS and Patient Information Publications. Accessed, March 7, 2006, from www.patient.co.uk/showdoc/40002438. Format modified slightly from original. From Yesavage JA et al: Development and validation of a geriatric depression screening scale: A preliminary report, *J Psychiatr Res* 17(1):37-49, 1982-1983.

---

are the same as in the Family APGAR but with the word *Friend* substituted for *Family*.

An additional value of this instrument is the ability to assess the caregiver's perception of emotional and social support with a new diagnosis of Alzheimer's disease of a relative. Also, a number of tools are specifically designed to measure the burden of the caregiver role.

SPIRITUAL ASSESSMENT

Spiritual well-being, whether it is associated with a formal religious practice or nonreligious intangible elements, has been recognized as important in the lives of many, including older adults. Spiritual needs are broader and more personal than religion. They transcend the physical and psychosocial elements of the person and are probably an important aspect of self-actualization as defined by Maslow. Nurses tend not to deal with spiritual needs of patients because they are thought to be too personal. However, if nurses are to care for the whole person, spiritual needs must be part of the assessment process. Although a concise tool has yet to be developed, the aspects that would be included in both assessment and subsequent interventions are listed in Box 6-8. (See Chapter 27.)

ENVIRONMENTAL SAFETY ASSESSMENT

Environmental safety is an issue for persons at all ages. For persons with limitations in cognition, mobility, vision, or hearing or are at risk for a fall-related injury, safety is espe-

cially important. Nurses in every setting are responsible for promoting the safety of the persons under their care.

The most common assessments related to safety are administered by home health nurses and occupational therapists. In general, they consist of lists of potential dangers and the status of the danger (present or absent) and provide suggestions or an opportunity for planning to reduce the potential dangers. Often nurses think of safety related to the risk for falling, but fire hazards, poisoning, and problems with temperature (hypothermia or hyperthermia) exist as well. Unfortunately, many older persons who have lived in their homes for many years are also in potential danger because of increased crime and victimization. Figure 6-4 provides an example of a tool that could be used in a home safety assessment. See also Chapter 15 for a more detailed discussion of mobility and environmental safety.

INTEGRATED ASSESSMENTS

In some cases an integrated approach is used rather than a collection of separate tools. The most well known is the classic Older American's Resources and Service (OARS) developed by Dr. Eric Pfeiffer (1979) and colleagues at Duke University. The Patient Appraisal and Care Evaluation (PACE) tool was designed particularly for use in long-term care settings but has been used in the home as well (USDHHS, 1978). The Comprehensive Assessment and Referral Evaluation tool (CARE) was designed for assessment of functional status and mental health (Gurland

The following questions have been designed to help us better understand you and your friends. Friends are nonrelatives from your school or community with whom you have a sharing relationship.

The following questions have been designed to help us better understand you and your family. You should feel free to ask questions about any item in the questionnaire.

"Family" is the individual(s) with whom you usually live. If you live alone, consider family as those with whom you now have the strongest emotional ties. Comment space should be used if you wish to give additional information or if you wish to discuss the way the question applies to your family. Please try to answer all questions.

For each question, check only one box

	Almost always	Some of the time	Hardly ever
I am satisfied that I can turn to my friends for help when something is troubling me.	☐	☐	☐

Comments:

I am satisfied with the way my friends talk over things with me and share problems with me.	☐	☐	☐

Comments:

I am satisfied that my friends accept and support my wishes to take on new activities or directions.	☐	☐	☐

Comments:

I am satisfied with the way my friends express affection, and respond to my emotions, such as anger, sorrow, or love.	☐	☐	☐

Comments:

I am satisfied with the way my friends and I share time together.	☐	☐	☐

For each question, check only one box

	Almost always	Some of the time	Hardly ever
I am satisfied that I can turn to my family for help when something is troubling me.	☐	☐	☐

Comments:

I am satisfied with the way my family talks over things with me and shares problems with me.	☐	☐	☐

Comments:

I am satisfied that my family accepts and supports my wishes to take on new activities or directions.	☐	☐	☐

Comments:

I am satisfied with the way my family expresses affection and responds to my emotions, such as anger, sorrow, or love.	☐	☐	☐

Comments:

I am satisfied with the way my family and I share time together.	☐	☐	☐

Who lives in your home?* List by relationship (e.g., spouse, significant other,† child, or friend).

Please check the column below that best describes how you now get along with each member of the family listed.

Relationship	Age	Sex	Well	Fairly	Poorly
_____	___	___	☐	☐	☐
_____	___	___	☐	☐	☐
_____	___	___	☐	☐	☐
_____	___	___	☐	☐	☐

If you don't live with your own family, please list below the individuals to whom you turn for help most frequently. List by relationship (e.g., family member, friend, associate at work, or neighbor).

Relationship	Age	Sex	Well	Fairly	Poorly
_____	___	___	☐	☐	☐
_____	___	___	☐	☐	☐
_____	___	___	☐	☐	☐
_____	___	___	☐	☐	☐

*If you have established your own family, consider home to be the place where you live with your spouse, children, or significant other; otherwise, consider home as your place of origin (e.g., the place where your parents or those who raised you live).

†"Significant other" is the partner you live with in a physically and emotionally nurturing relationship but to whom you are not married.

FIGURE 6-3 The Family APGAR. (Reprinted with permission from Smilkstein G et al: Validity and reliability of the family APGAR as a test of family function, *J Fam Pract* 15(2):303-311, 1982.)

BOX 6-8   Assessing Spiritual Distress

BRIEF HISTORY

Losses
Challenges to belief, value system
Separation from religious and cultural ties
Death
Personal and family disasters

SYMPTOMS (DEFINING CHARACTERISTICS) SUCH AS THE FOLLOWING

Unmet needs
Threats to self
Change in environment, health status, self-concept, etc.
Questioning meaning of own existence
Depression
Feeling of hopelessness, abandonment, fear

ASSESSMENT OF THE CAUSE OF SPIRITUAL DISTRESS

Depletion anxiety
Helplessness, hopelessness
Perceived powerlessness
Medication reaction
Hormonal imbalances

---

et al., 1977). These and other tools were considered in the development of the MDS, the major assessment tool currently used in skilled nursing facilities. In the home care setting, the Outcomes and Assessment Information Set (OASIS), a computerized assessment tool, is universally used at this time. All these tools are quite comprehensive and therefore quite lengthy. Once completed, they serve as a resource for a detailed plan of care. The Fulmer SPICES Tool serves as a guide for a much shorter but still comprehensive assessment.

Older American's Resources and Service (OARS)

The OARS assessment tool is designed so that each component can be used individually. This enables it to be added to or integrated into self-designed tools. It was designed to evaluate ability, disability, and the capacity level at which the person is able to function. Five dimensions are considered for assessment: social resources, economic resources, physical health, mental health, and ADLs. Each component uses a quantitative rating scale: 1—excellent; 2—good; 3—mildly impaired; 4—moderately impaired; 5—severely impaired; and 6—completely impaired. At the conclusion of the assessment, a cumulative impairment score (CIS) is established, which can range from the most fit (6) to total disability (30). This aids in establishing the degree of need. Information considered in each domain includes the material in the following sections.

Social Resources. The social resources dimension of the OARS evaluates the social skills and the ability to negotiate and make friends (the number of times friends are seen, the number of telephone conversations). In the assessment interview, is the person able to ask for things from friends, family, and strangers? Is a caregiver (or caregivers) available if needed? Who are they, and how long are they available? Does the elder belong to any social network or group, such as a special interest or church group?

Economic Resources. Data about monthly income and sources (Social Security, Supplemental Security Income, pensions, income generated from capital) are needed to determine the adequacy of income compared with the cost of living and food, shelter, clothing, medications, and small luxury items. This information can provide insight into the elder's relative standard of living and point out areas of need that might be alleviated by use of additional resources.

Mental Health. Consideration is given to intellectual function, the presence or absence of psychiatric symptoms, and the amount of enjoyment and interaction the person gets from life.

Physical Health. This includes the diagnosis of major and common diseases of older persons, the type of prescribed and over-the-counter medications the person is taking, and the person's perception of his or her health status. Excellent physical health includes participation in regular vigorous activity, such as walking, dancing, or biking, at least twice each week. Seriously impaired physical health is determined by the presence of one or more illnesses or disabilities that are severely painful or life threatening or require extensive care.

Activities of Daily Living. The ADLs included in the OARS are walking, getting into and out of bed, bathing, combing hair, shaving, dressing, eating, and getting to the bathroom on time by oneself. The IADLs measured include tasks such as dialing the telephone, driving a car, hanging up clothes, obtaining groceries, and taking medications and having correct knowledge of their dosages.

Fulmer SPICES

The Fulmer SPICES, an overall assessment tool of older adults (Wallace and Fulmer, 2007), has proved reliable and valid in use with older adults whether they are healthy or frail and whether they are in acute, skilled nursing, or long-term care facilities or at home. The acronym *SPICES* refers to six common syndromes of the elderly that require nursing interventions: Sleep disorders, Problems with eating or feeding, Incontinence, Confusion, Evidence of falls, and Skin breakdown. Nurses are encouraged to make a 3 × 5 card with this acronym on it and carry it with them to use as a reference when caring for older adults (Figure 6-5). It is a

	Okay (y/n)	Plan to improve	
Basic Structure Intact roof Solid floors and stairs Functioning toilet (or outhouse) Source of fresh water Wheelchair ramp			X | Client | Clinician
Temperature Control Fan/air-conditioner Proper use of heating pads Proper hot water heater temperature Adequate heat/insulation			Clinician's signature _____
Nutrition Kitchen condition/food storage Evidence of alcohol use Pests			
Fire Prevention and Response Use of kerosene heaters Use of open gas burners on stove for heat Smoking in bed Use of oxygen Dangerous electrical wiring Smoke alarms Exit plans in case of fire			
Self-Injury/Violence Prevention Locks Method of calling for help Proximity of neighbors Surrounding criminal activity Emergency phone numbers by telephone Loaded guns/knives Household toxins Water/bathtub Power tools			
Medication Management Duplicate medicines, outdated drugs, pill box Correct labeling Storage safety, accessibility, refrigeration Caregiver familiarity Wandering control (for confused patients) Doortap latches, special locks Fenced yards with hidden latches Identifcation bracelets Electronic wandering alarms			Date _____

FIGURE 6-4 Guidelines for home safety assessment. (Modified from Yoshikawa TT et al: *Practical ambulatory geriatrics*, ed 2, St Louis, 1998, Mosby.)

system for alerting the nurse of the most common problems that occur in the health and well-being of older adults, particularly those who have one or more medical conditions.

▲ PROMOTING HEALTHY AGING: IMPLICATIONS FOR GERONTOLOGICAL NURSING

Whether the nurse is working with a standardized instrument or creating a new one, the goal of assessment is always to assist the patient in improving his or her quality of life. The nurse is expected to collect data that are the most accurate and to do so in the most efficient yet caring manner

possible. The use of tools serves as a way to organize the collected data necessary for assessment and to be able to compare the data from time to time. Each tool has strengths and weaknesses as does each completed assessment. A number of factors complicate assessment of the older adult. These include the difficulty of differentiating the effects of aging from those originating from disease, the coexistence of multiple diseases, the underreporting of symptoms by older adults, atypical presentation or nonspecific presentation of illness, and the increase in iatrogenic illnesses.

Over-diagnosis or under-diagnosis occurs when the normal age changes are not considered; these include both physical changes and biochemical changes (see Chapter 4).

Patient Name:_____ Date_____

Spices	Evidence
Sleep disorders	
Problems with eating or feeding	
Incontinence	
Confusion	
Evidence of falls	
Skin breakdown	

FIGURE 6-5 SPICES. (Adapted from *Fulmer SPICES: an overall assessment tool of older adults.* Developed by Meredith Wallace and Terry Fulmer, Hartford Institute for Geriatric Nursing, New York University, New York, 2007.)

Under-diagnosis is far more common in the care of the elderly. Many symptoms or complaints are ascribed to normal aging rather than to a disease entity that may be developing. Difficulty in assessing the older adult with multiple chronic conditions is also a challenge. Symptoms of one condition can exacerbate or mask symptoms of another. The gerontological nurse is challenged to provide the highest level of excellence in the assessment of the elderly without burdening the person in the process.

KEY CONCEPTS

- Assessment of the physical, cognitive, psychosocial, and environmental status is essential to meeting the specific needs of the older adult and implementing appropriate interventions.
- Whether the data for an assessment tool are collected by self-report, by report-by-proxy, or through nurse observation will affect the quality and quantity of the data.
- Knowledge of how to use a particular gerontological assessment tool is needed to accurately administer it.
- Co-morbidity of many older adults complicates obtaining and interpreting assessment data.

RESEARCH QUESTIONS

What is the importance of measuring ADLs and IADLs in older adults?

For each ADL, develop a plan of interventions that you would institute to compensate for ADL deficits and that would still foster an elder's independence as much as is realistic.

What makes an assessment tool effective?

What tool or tools would be most appropriate for assessing an elder in the community, in the hospital, in long-term care, or in day care? Give your rationale for the choices.

CASE STUDY: A Complex Assessment

An 84-year-old white male, Mr. Desir, is originally from Haiti but is now living in the United States with his daughter. He speaks only Haitian Creole but is accompanied by his son-in-law, who is fluent in both languages. Mr. Desir fell at home and was found to have an irregular heartbeat and is being admitted to the hospital for evaluation. You have been assigned to do his admission assessment. He has a history of arthritis heart disease, hypertension, diabetes, and anemia of chronic disease. You find that he denies any fever, chest pain, numbness or tingling, leg swelling, or palpitations. His son-in-law tells you that he has been getting confused lately and may be a little depressed. Mrs. Desir is still in Haiti. She can take care of herself but had been having difficulty taking care of her husband. After processing the orders for tests and medications, you proceed with the assessment.

Based on the case study, develop a nursing care plan using the following procedure*:

- List Mr. Desir's comments that provide subjective data.
- List information that provides objective data.
- From these data, identify and state, using accepted format, two nursing diagnoses you determine are most significant to Mr. Desir at this time. List two of Mr. Desir's strengths that you have identified from the data.
- Determine and state outcome criteria for each diagnosis. These must reflect some alleviation of the problem identified in the nursing diagnosis and must be stated in concrete and measurable terms.

- Plan and state one or more interventions for each diagnosed problem. Provide specific documentation of the source used to determine the appropriate intervention. Plan at least one intervention that incorporates Mr. Desir's existing strengths.
- Evaluate the success of the intervention. Interventions must correlate directly with the stated outcome criteria to measure the outcome success.

Critical Thinking Questions

1. You know that you usually have only 20 to 30 minutes to do the complete assessment. In this situation, you know you will need more time and inform your supervisor. What will be your justification for the need for more time?
2. If you cannot do a complete head-to-toe examination and detailed history, list the parts you will do in order of priority.
3. Considering the patient's medical history and chief complaint, what deviations from normal are you expecting to find during your assessment?
4. Develop a list of actual and potential problems that will need to be addressed during Mr. Desir's hospital stay.
5. What strategies can you use to overcome the potential language barrier when family is not present?
6. Explore potential reference resources that will help you provide culturally competent care for this patient.

---

* Students are advised to refer to their nursing diagnosis text and identify possible or potential problems.

CASE STUDY: A Comprehensive Assessment

Eighty-year-old Mrs. Hernandez is newly admitted your acute care hospital unit. She is there for observation and testing after a witnessed syncopal episode. She lives with her 90-year-old husband, who has mild dementia, and her 60-year-old daughter. Her daughter admits to you that neither of her parents has been doing well and that the doctors "just haven't been able to figure it out." You know that Mrs. Hernandez will be receiving both neurological and cardiac testing. However, as a gerontological nurse you also know that she and her family may benefit most from a comprehensive evaluation. The decision of which assessments to do is within the scope of practice for nurses at your facility.

Based on the case study, develop a nursing care plan using the following procedure*:
- List Mrs. Hernandez's comments that provide subjective data.
- List information that provides objective data.
- From these data, identify and state, using accepted format, two nursing diagnoses you determine are most significant to Mrs. Hernandez at this time. List two of Mrs. Hernandez's strengths that you have identified from the data.
- Determine and state outcome criteria for each diagnosis. These must reflect some alleviation of the problem identi-

fied in the nursing diagnosis and must be stated in concrete and measurable terms.
- Plan and state one or more interventions for each diagnosed problem. Provide specific documentation of the source used to determine the appropriate intervention. Plan at least one intervention that incorporates Mrs. Hernandez's existing strengths.
- Evaluate the success of the intervention. Interventions must correlate directly with the stated outcome criteria to measure the outcome success.

Critical Thinking Questions

1. In caring for Mrs. Hernandez, which aspects of a more detailed evaluation will you conduct and in what order of priority?
2. What is your reason for selecting the type of assessment you will do, and what is the reason for your ranking?
3. Of the assessment tools that are available to you, which will be the most reasonable to perform within the limitations of an acute care setting?
4. How would any of your answers to the above change in a skilled nursing facility? Assisted living facility? In the home setting?

* Students are advised to refer to their nursing diagnosis text and identify possible or potential problems.

REFERENCES

Beck AT: *Beck depression inventory: manual*, San Antonio, 1987, Psychological Corporation.

Benner P: *From novice to expert*, Menlo Park, Calif, 1984, Addison-Wesley.

Blessed G et al: The association between qualitative measures of dementia and of senile change in the cerebral grey matter of elderly subjects, *Br J Psychiatry* 114(512):797-811, 1968.

Folstein MF et al: Mini-mental state: a practical method for grading the cognitive state of patients for the clinician, *J Psychiatr Res* 12(3):189-198, 1975.

Granger CV, Hamilton BB: The Uniform Data System for Medical Rehabilitation report of first admissions for 1991, *Am J Phys Med Rehabil* 72(1):33-38, 1993.

Gurland B et al: The comprehensive assessment and referral evaluation (CARE), *Int J Aging Hum Dev* 8(1):9-42, 1977-1978.

Ham RJ: Assessment. In Ham RJ et al, editors: *Primary care geriatrics: a case-based approach*, ed 4, St Louis, 2002, Mosby.

Katz S et al: Studies of illness in the aged: the index of ADL: a standardized measure of biological and psychosocial function, *JAMA* 185:914-919, 1963.

Kleinman A: *Patient and healers in the context of culture: an exploration of the borderland between anthropology, medicine, and psychiatry*, Berkeley, 1980, University of California Press.

Lawton MP, Brody EM: Assessment of older people: self-maintaining and instrumental activities of daily living, *Gerontologist* 9(3):179-186, 1969.

Mahoney FI, Barthel DW: Functional evaluation: the Barthel Index, *Md State Med J* 14:61-65, 1965.

Mendez MF et al: Development of scoring criteria for the Clock Drawing Task in Alzheimer's disease, *J Am Geriatr Soc* 40(11):1095-1099, 1992.

Morris JC: The clinical dementia rating (CDR): current version and scoring rules, *Neurology* 43(11):2412-2414, 1993.

Osterweil D et al: *Comprehensive geriatric assessment*, New York, 2000, McGraw-Hill.

Pfeiffer E: A short portable mental status questionnaire for the assessment of organic brain deficit in elderly patients, *J Am Geriatr Soc* 23(10):433-441, 1975.

Pfeiffer E: *Physical and mental assessment—OARS*. Workshop Intensive, Western Gerontological Society, San Francisco, April 28, 1979.

Reisberg B et al: The global deterioration scale for assessment of primary progressive dementia, *Am J Psychiatry* 139(9):1136-1139, 1982.

Smilkstein G: The Family APGAR: a proposal for a family function test and its use by physicians, *J Fam Pract* 6(6):1231-1239, 1978.

Tuokko H et al: The clock test: a sensitive measure to differentiate normal elderly from those with Alzheimer disease, *J Am Geriatr Soc* 40(6):579-584, 1992.

U.S. Department of Health and Human Services (USDHHS): *Working document on patient care management*, Washington, DC, 1978, U.S. Government Printing Office.

Wallace M, Fulmer T: Fulmer SPICES: An overall assessment tool for older adults (revised). Try This Series. (2007). Accessed March 6, 2007, from *www. hartfordign.org*.

Yesavage JA et al: Development and validation of a geriatric depression screening scale: a preliminary report, *J Psychiatr Res* 17(1):37-49, 1982-1983.

Zung WW: A self-rating depression scale, *Arch Gen Psychiatry* 12:63-70, 1965.

Minimum Data Set (MDS) Version 2.0 (Condensed) for Nursing Home Resident Assessment and Care Screening

Identification Information	Name, gender, birthday, Social Security and Medicare numbers, provider number, reasons for assessment
Background Information	Assessment reference date, date of entry, marital status, payment sources, responsible person, advance directives
Demographic Information	Date of entry, situation before admission, occupation, education, language, mental health history, and conditions related to MR/DD status
Customary Routine	Usual cycle of daily events, eating patterns, functional ability in activities of daily living, social involvement
Cognitive Patterns	Consciousness, memory, recall ability, decision-making skills, delirium, disordered thinking, changes in cognitive status
Communication/Hearing Patterns	Hearing, communication devices/techniques, modes of expression, speech clarity, ability to understand, changes in communication or hearing
Vision Patterns	Vision, specific limitations/difficulties, visual appliances
Mood and Behavior Patterns	Indicators of depression, anxiety, sad mood, mood persistence, mood changes, behavioral symptoms, changes in behavioral symptoms
Psychosocial Well-Being	Sense of initiative/involvement, unsettled relationships, past roles
Physical Functioning and Structural Problems	Activities of daily living (ADLs) self-performance: bed mobility, transfer, walking/locomotion, dressing, eating, toileting, personal hygiene, bathing, range of motion, modes of transfers, modes of locomotion, functional and rehabilitation potential, changes in ADL function
Continence in Last 14 Days	Self-control categories, bowel continence, bladder continence, bowel elimination pattern, appliances and programs, changes in urinary continence
Disease Diagnoses	Diseases, infections, other diagnoses
Health Conditions	Problem conditions, pain symptoms, pain site, accidents, stability of conditions
Oral/Nutritional Status	Oral problems, height and weight, weight changes, nutritional problems, nutritional approaches, parenteral or enteral intake
Oral/Dental Status	Oral status and disease prevention, tooth decay, disintegration; buccal cavity examination; dentures, bridges, missing teeth
Skin Condition	Ulcers, type of ulcers, history of unresolved ulcers, other skin problems or lesions, skin treatments, foot problems and care
Activity Pursuit Patterns	Time awake, time involved in activities, preferred activity settings, general activity preferences, prefers change in daily routines
Medications	Number of medications, new medications, injections, days received the following medications (antipsychotic, antianxiety, antidepressant, hypnotic, diuretic)
Special Treatments and Procedures	Treatments, procedures, and programs; intervention programs for mood, behavior, cognitive loss, nursing rehabilitation/restorative care, devices and restraints, hospital stays, emergency department visits, physician visits, physician orders, abnormal laboratory values
Discharge Potential and Overall Status	Discharge potential, overall change in care needs
Resident Participation in Assessment	Resident, family members, significant other

Resident's Name: _____   Medical Record No.: _____

1. Check if RAP is triggered.
2. For each triggered RAP, use the RAP guidelines to identify areas needing further assessment. Document relevant assessment information regarding the resident's status.
   - Describe:
     —Nature of the condition (may include presence or lack of objective data and subjective complaints).
     —Complications and risk factors that affect your decision to proceed to care planning.
     —Factors that must be considered in developing individualized care plan interventions.
     —Need for referrals/further evaluation by appropriate health professionals.
   - Documentation should support your decision making regarding whether to proceed with a care plan for a triggered RAP and the type(s) of care plan interventions that are appropriate for a particular resident.
   - Documentation may appear anywhere in the clinical record (e.g., progress notes, consults, flowsheets).
3. Indicate under the *Location of RAP Assessment Documentation* column where information related to the RAP assessment can be found.
4. For each triggered RAP, indicate whether a new care plan, care plan revision, or continuation of current care plan is necessary to address the problem(s) identified in your assessment. The Care Planning Decision column must be completed within 7 days of completing the RAI (MDS and RAPs).

A. RAP Problem Area	(a) Check if Triggered	Location and Date of RAP Assessment Documentation	(b) Care Planning Decision -- check if addressed in care plan
1. DELIRIUM	☐		☐
2. COGNITIVE LOSS	☐		☐
3. VISUAL FUNCTION	☐		☐
4. COMMUNICATION	☐		☐
5. ADL FUNCTIONAL/ REHABILITATION POTENTIAL	☐		☐
6. URINARY INCONTINENCE AND INDWELLING CATHETER	☐		☐
7. PSYCHOSOCIAL WELL-BEING	☐		☐
8. MOOD STATE	☐		☐
9. BEHAVIORAL SYMPTOMS	☐		☐
10. ACTIVITIES	☐		☐
11. FALLS	☐		☐
12. NUTRITIONAL STATUS	☐		☐
13. FEEDING TUBES	☐		☐
14. DEHYDRATION/FLUID MAINTENANCE	☐		☐
15. ORAL/DENTAL CARE	☐		☐
16. PRESSURE ULCERS	☐		☐
17. PSYCHOTROPIC DRUG USE	☐		☐
18. PHYSICAL RESTRAINTS	☐		☐

B. _____
1. Signature of RN Coordinator for RAP Assessment Process

2. ☐☐ _ ☐☐ _ ☐☐☐☐
   Month   Day   Year

_____
3. Signature of Person Completing Care Planning Decision

4. ☐☐ _ ☐☐ _ ☐☐☐☐
   Month   Day   Year

TRIGGER LEGEND

1 —Delirium	7 —Psychosocial Well-Being	13 —Feeding Tubes
2 —Cognitive Loss/Dementia	8 —Mood State	14 —Dehydration/Fluid Maintenance
3 —Visual Function	9 —Behavioral Symptoms	15 —Dental Care
4 —Communication	10A —Activities (Revise)	16 —Pressure Ulcers
5A —ADL-Rehabilitation	10B —Activities (Review)	17 —Psychotropic Drug Use
5B —ADL-Maintenance	11 —Falls	18 —Physical Restraints
6 —Urinary Incontinence and Indwelling Catheter	12 —Nutritional Status	

Modified from Minimum Data Set (MDS)—Version 2.0 for Nursing Home Resident Assessment and Care Screening, Form 1728HH, Des Moines, IA, 1995, Briggs Corporation.

CHAPTER 7

Managing Basic Physiological Needs

Ann Schmidt Luggen and Theris A. Touhy

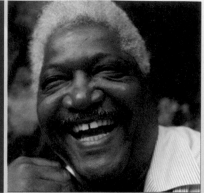

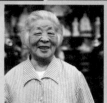

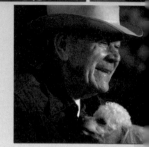

AN ELDER SPEAKS

I am an artist. I exercised sporadically, mostly walking. I wanted only to sleep and read after losing my significant other. I use a walker as I am battling congestive heart failure. I moved to a retirement community and started to exercise. In balance class twice a week, I walk laps on my own without using the bars, my walker, or a cane. I twist on a spinner without holding on as if spinning on a lazy Susan. In exercise class three times a week I march without support in a cardiovascular warm-up, I stretch from my neck to my toes, and I lift dumbbells for 20 to 40 repetitions. This is more exercise than I did in my whole life. I feel wonderful! I used to get angina, now it happens very rarely. I feel more confident. I think exercising is a lot of fun, especially when we crack up laughing about ourselves. In my free time, I am preparing all new works for an art exhibit.

Ruth, 87 years old (NIH, 2005)

AN ELDER SPEAKS

The years have changed the sleep patterns. Bedtime rituals take longer. Nature wakens me two or three times a night for trips to the bathroom. Sleep returns at once unless my mind turns on and it gets launched on a needless project. The earlier remedies are called on to slow down the activities, or the next day is a disaster. My 90-year-old aunt, who slept very little and lightly and lay awake many nights, said she went to the bathroom several times just for something to do instead of just lying there.

Ricarda, 90 years old

LEARNING OBJECTIVES

On completion of this chapter, the reader will be able to:

1. Identify age-related changes that affect basic biological support needs: elimination, rest and sleep, and activity.
2. List the types of outcomes that occur because of age-related changes in the basic biological support needs.
3. Describe the nursing assessment relevant to basic biological support needs.
4. Explain nursing interventions useful in the promotion of the individual's basic biological support needs.
5. Discuss individualizing nursing care plans for each of the basic biological support needs.

Life support or survival requirements for the older adult do not differ from those for younger human beings. Fluctuations in homeostatic balance of these needs, however, make each of these needs more precarious. Assessing and monitoring survival functions are basic to ensuring the person's opportunity to reach his or her highest level of health and wellness.

This chapter addresses these crucial needs in the context of the biological needs of Maslow's Hierarchy. Unless the biological needs are fulfilled adequately, the individual cannot be expected to maintain or reach the higher levels of coping and health. Attention has been devoted to elimination, rest, and activity because these are areas of function in which the nurse can make a significant difference in health and wellness. The nurse's role in the maintenance of neurological, renal, and cardiopulmonary function in older persons is indirect. Nurses cannot directly change the existing physiological or pathological conditions of heart, lungs, nervous system, or kidneys, but they can promote and maintain rest, exercise, and nutrition, which affect the function of these systems.

In assessing the life support needs of the elderly, two important questions should be considered: What is troubling the person, and what threatens his or her health or life? Keeping these two questions in mind will assist the gerontological nurse in providing the most appropriate and realistic approaches to the survival needs of older adults.

ELIMINATION

The body must remove waste products of metabolism to sustain healthy function, but bladder and bowel activity are fraught with social implications. Bladder and bowel function in late life, although normally only slightly altered by physiological changes of age, can develop problems severe enough to interfere with the ability to continue independent living and can seriously threaten the body's capacity to function and to survive. The effects of uncontrolled bladder and bowel action are a threat to the person's independence and well-being.

Elimination is a private matter, not publicized socially. However, the media advertise laxatives to maintain evacuation of fecal matter. Bowel preoccupation costs millions of dollars in laxative expenditures, mainly to the older person. As children, correct behavior in dealing with our own body waste is taught early. Deviations from this are socially unacceptable and can lead to chastisement, ostracism, and social withdrawal.

Bowel Function

The main functions of the colon and rectum are storing and passing feces. The passage of feces, or stool, is regulated by colonic contractions and peristaltic waves. Water is reabsorbed during this process, which decreases the volume of the stool. A person must sense fullness and identify that contents are in the rectum to coordinate function of the internal and external anus (Tabloski, 2006).

Attention to bowel function occurs when there is a deviation from what is perceived as normal elimination. It is a common stereotype that the elderly frequently complain to physicians and other health care personnel about problems, particularly constipation. Whatever the complaint, one needs to know exactly what the individual means when he or she says there is a problem. Bowel function problems that the nurse may encounter in care of older clients are constipation, fecal impaction, irritable bowel syndrome, and fecal or bowel incontinence.

Constipation. Constipation has different meanings to different people. Some individuals consider constipation infrequent bowel action; others perceive it as difficulty in passing feces. In one study, half of the elders who complained of constipation moved their bowels at least once a day (Edwards, 2002). To the health professional, constipation occurs when there are fewer than three bowel movements a week, hard stools, and difficulty with evacuation (McCance, 2006). It is the most common gastrointestinal (GI) complaint to the health care provider, with about 60% of community-based elders reporting laxative use (Beers and Berkow, 2006). About 74% of older adults in long-term care use laxatives daily.

Normal elimination should be an easy passage of feces, without undue straining or a feeling of incomplete evacuation or defecation. The urge to defecate occurs when the distended walls of the sigmoid and rectum, which are filled with feces, stimulate pressure receptors to relax the sphincters for the expulsion of stool through the anus. Evacuation of feces is accomplished by relaxation of the sphincters and contraction of the diaphragm and abdominal muscles, which raises intra-abdominal pressure.

Constipation appears to be a problem of the elder because of age-related physiological changes (Beers and Berkow, 2006). Rectal sensation is impaired, requiring larger volumes to elicit the sensation to defecate. Also, resting anal sphincter pressure is reduced and maximum sphincter pressure is diminished, predisposing to fecal incontinence. It is perhaps more correct to consider the extensive use of laxatives by older adults in the United States as a cultural habit. During earlier times, weekly doses of rhubarb, cascara, castor oil, and other types of laxatives were consumed and believed by many to promote health. This belief that cleaning out the colon was paramount to maintaining good health still persists in some groups.

Constipation is a symptom. It is a reflection of poor habits, postponed passage of stool, and many chronic illnesses—both physical and psychological. See Chapter 9 for nutritional causes of constipation. Numerous precipitating factors or conditions can cause or worsen constipation (Beers and Berkow, 2006). Box 7-1 lists these factors. Diet plays a significant role in problems with intestinal motility and constipation.

▲ Promoting Healthy Aging: Implications for Gerontological Nursing

Assessment. The precipitants and causes of constipation must be included in the evaluation of the patient. A review of these factors will also determine if a patient is at risk for altered bowel function. Ask specifically about the

BOX 7-1 Precipitating Factors for Constipation

PHYSIOLOGICAL

Dehydration
Insufficient fiber intake
Poor dietary habits

FUNCTIONAL

Decreased physical activity
Inadequate toileting
Irregular defecation habits
Irritable bowel disease
Weakness

MECHANICAL

Abscess or ulcer
Fissures
Hemorrhoids
Megacolon
Pelvic floor dysfunction
Postsurgical obstruction
Prostate enlargement
Rectal prolapse
Rectocele
Spinal cord injury

Strictures
Tumors

OTHER

Lack of abdominal muscle tone
Obesity
Recent environmental changes
Poor dentition

PSYCHOLOGICAL

Avoidance of urge to defecate
Confusion
Depression
Emotional stress

SYSTEMIC

Diabetic neuropathy
Hypercalcemia
Hyperparathyroidism
Hypothyroidism
Hypokalemia
Porphyria
Uremia

Parkinson's disease
Cerebrovascular disease
Defective electrolyte transfer

PHARMACOLOGICAL

ACE-inhibitors
Antacids: calcium carbonate,
    aluminum hydroxide
Antiarrhythmics
Anticholinergics
Anticonvulsants
Antidepressants
Anti-Parkinson's medications
Calcium channel blockers
Calcium supplements
Diuretics
Iron supplements
Laxative overuse
Nonsteroidal antiinflammatories
Opiates
Phenothiazines
Sedatives
Sympathomimetics

Adapted from Allison OC et al: Chronic constipation: assessment and management in the elderly, *J Am Acad Nurse Pract* 6(7):311, 1994; Tabloski PA: *Gerontological nursing,* Upper Saddle River, NJ, 2006, Pearson/Prentice Hall.

Rome Criteria for chronic constipation, which includes two of the following for 12 weeks out of 12 months (not necessarily consecutive weeks): straining, lumpy or hard stools, sensation of incomplete evacuation, sensation of anorectal blockage or obstruction, and two or fewer bowel movements per week (McCance, 2006). It is recognized that elderly people at high risk for constipation and subsequent impaction are those who are immobilized and debilitated or who have significant dementia. It is also important to know that confusion, increased agitation, incontinence, or unexplainable falls may be the only clinical symptoms of constipation in the older adult with dementia.

A physical examination is needed to rule out systemic causes of constipation. A neurological examination is important because constipation is a common problem of many neurological illnesses (Edwards, 2002). The assessment will also focus on the GI system and signs of dehydration. The abdomen is examined for bowel sounds, pain, localized masses (retained stool), distention, and evidence of prior surgery (Edwards, 2002).

A rectal examination is important to reveal painful anal disorders such as hemorrhoids or fissures that will impede the evacuation of stool and to evaluate sphincter tone, rectal prolapse, stool presence in the vault, strictures, masses, anal reflex, and enlarged prostate (Edwards, 2002). Bright red blood on rectal examination may indicate bleeding from internal or external hemorrhoids but possibly a more serious underlying condition (Tabloski, 2006).

Further diagnostic testing may be indicated; a barium enema, proctosigmoidoscopy, colonoscopy, abdominal x-ray film, or computed tomography (CT) scan of the abdomen may be done if the elder is able. Biochemical tests should include a complete blood count (CBC), fasting glucose, chemistry panel, and thyroid studies. These will rule out a number of causes of constipation such as diabetes, electrolyte imbalances, and hypothyroidism.

Other tests are available for chronic constipation. Colonic transit and anorectal function can be evaluated (Beers and Berkow, 2006). These tests include radiopaque markers, defecating proctography, and anorectal manometry.

Interventions. The first intervention is to examine the medications the patient is taking and eliminate those that are constipating or change to medications that do not cause constipation. Edwards (2002) states that it is better to start a bowel regimen with an empty colon, which may require the removal of impaction manually or the use of enemas. Any regimen should be started slowly and with the patient's preferences included to improve compliance. This will also avoid bloating and cramping gas pains that occur with a faster implementation time.

Non-pharmacological interventions for constipation that have been implemented and evaluated can be grouped into four areas: (1) fluid/fiber, (2) exercise, (3) environmental manipulation, and (4) a combination of these. Adequate hydration is the cornerstone of constipation therapy (Beers and Berkow, 2006). The use of bran fiber, fruit and vegetable fiber, and nuts is recommended. Bran fiber results in a functioning colon with higher fecal bulking action. However, it should be noted that starting an elder on this high-fiber diet should be done slowly; give one tablespoon each day (AM) and increase slowly over time. See Chapter 9 for more methods of nutritional management. The use of natural fibers will minimize or obviate the need for supplemental fibers such as psyllium and methylcellulose. Decreasing the fat in the diet is useful because fat slows the transit time of digestion. If megacolon or colonic dilation from bowel obstruction is suspected, fiber supplements are not advised; most of these patients are on a fiber-restricted diet.

Position. The squatting or sitting position facilitates bowel function if the patient is able. A similar position may be obtained by leaning forward and applying firm pressure to the lower abdomen or placing the feet on a stool. Massaging the abdomen may help stimulate the bowel.

Regularity. Establishing a routine for toileting promotes or normalizes bowel function (bowel retraining). The gastrocolic reflex occurs after breakfast or supper or after the main meal of the day and may be enhanced by a warm drink. Given privacy and ample time (a minimum of 10 minutes), many will have a daily bowel movement. It is helpful to have something to do while sitting on the toilet so that the elder is not preoccupied with bowel movements. Any urge to defecate should be followed by a response toward the bathroom.

Exercise. Exercise is important as an intervention to stimulate colon motility and bowel evacuation. Daily walking for 20 to 30 minutes is helpful, especially after a meal. Pelvic tilt exercises and range-of-motion (passive or active) exercises are beneficial for those who are less mobile or even bed-bound.

Laxatives. When changes in diet and lifestyle are not effective, laxatives are considered. One consideration is senna tea. Senna is an effective laxative stimulant that is safe for elderly patients and is nontoxic; because it is a stimulant, it may cause cramping. Senna is effective in small doses and has a local action that increases colon peristalsis. Another laxative often prescribed is cascara. They can both be taken orally or rectally. They can cause abdominal cramping and fluid and electrolyte disturbances, especially if impaction is present (Beers and Berkow, 2006). These stimulant laxatives should be used short term because they can cause dependency. Bulk laxatives such as Metamucil, Citrucel, and FiberCon increase the stool bulk and urge to defecate if taken with adequate fluids (Tabloski, 2006). Lactulose and sorbitol are osmotic agents that increase fluid in the colon and soften stools (Tabloski, 2006). They work slowly but are effective in frail elderly. Emollient laxatives or lubricants include mineral oil; however, mineral oil should not be used in the debilitated elder because of the risk of oil aspiration and vitamin depletion if used too often. Saline laxatives work by drawing water into the small bowel and stimulating peristalsis; the bowel empties within hours. These agents include Milk of Magnesia and Fleet Phospho-Soda. They should not be used in those elders with poor renal function if the agents contain magnesium, phosphate, or sulfate salts (Edwards, 2002). See Box 7-2 for an effective natural laxative recipe.

BOX 7-2 Natural Laxative Recipe That Really Works: Power Pudding

Standard recipe:
- 1 cup wheat bran
- 1 cup applesauce
- 1 cup prune juice

Mix and store in refrigerator. Start with administration of 1 tbsp/day. Increase *slowly* until desired effect is achieved and no disagreeable symptoms occur.

Enemas. Enemas can be used but not on a regular basis. Soapsuds and phosphate enemas irritate the rectal mucosa and should not be used (Edwards, 2002). Enemas of any type should be reserved for situations in which other methods produce no response or when it is known that there is an impaction. Normal saline or tap water enema at a temperature of about 105° F is the best choice. Perforation is a possibility, and the enema should be administered with care. The amount of water should be 500 to 1000 mL (Beers and Berkow, 2006). Oil retention enemas are used for refractory constipation (Reuben et al., 2006).

A program to prevent as well as treat constipation that incorporates a high-fiber diet, liberal fluid intake, daily exercise, and environmental modifications that promote a regular pattern of bowel elimination needs to be developed for each client. The interventions for clients in any setting are based on a thorough assessment. When prescribing opiates, a prevention program should always be put in place because these drugs delay gastric emptying and decrease peristalsis.

Fecal Impaction. This situation is a major complication of constipation. It is common in incapacitated and institutionalized elderly people. Symptoms of fecal impaction include malaise, urinary retention, incontinence of bladder or bowel, confusion, fissures, hemorrhoids, and intestinal obstruction. The causes are similar to those of constipation. Unrecognized, unattended, or neglected constipation eventually leads to fecal impaction and incontinence or paradoxical diarrhea, which results from a ball-valve effect that allows liquid stool to seep around the obstructing fecal mass during normal colon contractions. Removal of a fecal impaction is at times worse than the misery of the condition. Continued obstruction by the fecal mass may eventually impair sensation, leading to the need for larger stool volume to stimulate the urge to defecate, which contributes to megacolon (Edwards, 2002). Valsalva maneuvers done during straining at stool defecation can cause transient ischemic attacks and syncope, especially in frail elderly.

Management of fecal impactions requires the digital removal of the hard, compacted stool from the rectum with use of lubrication containing lidocaine jelly. Generally this is preceded by multiple enemas or an oil-retention enema to soften the feces in preparation for manual removal. Use of suppositories is not effective, because their action is blocked by the amount and the size of the stool in the rectum as compared with the capacity of the sphincter to dilate. Suppositories do not facilitate the removal of stool in the sigmoid, which may continue to ooze once the rectum is emptied.

Several sessions or days may be required to totally cleanse the sigmoid colon and rectum of impacted feces. Once this is achieved, attention should be directed to planning a regimen of prevention that includes adequate fluid intake, increased dietary fiber, administration of stool softeners if needed, and many of the other suggestions presented for prevention of constipation.

Fecal or Bowel Incontinence.

Fecal incontinence is defined as the inability to control the passage of stool or gas via the anus or involuntary loss of stool from the rectum at inappropriate times (Staab and Hodges, 1996). The prevalence of fecal incontinence is approximately 3% to 4% of community-dwelling elders, and approximately 16% to 60% of the institutionalized older people have some fecal incontinence (Richter, 1995). Often fecal incontinence is associated with urinary incontinence. Fecal incontinence, like urinary incontinence, has devastating social ramifications for the individuals and families who experience it. Contributing factors are similar to those for urinary incontinence. The factors affecting fecal incontinence include dementia, intestinal transit time, rectal factors (sensory), pelvic floor and sphincter tone, pelvic musculature, medications, muscular flaccidity, and the inability to get to the toilet when the urge to eliminate is present. Other factors distinct to bowel evacuation problems are long-term dependence on laxatives, lack of sufficient bulk in the diet, insufficient fluid intake, lack of exercise, hemorrhoids, and depression. Many instances of fecal incontinence result from fecal impaction, or the origin may be neurological. Serious illness accompanied by delirium and excessive doses of iron, antibiotic, and digitalis preparations may precipitate incontinence. Sedatives, too, can account for incontinence through depression of cerebral awareness and control over sphincter response.

▲ Promoting Healthy Aging: Implications for Gerontological Nursing

Assessment. Assessment should include a complete client history and a bowel record. The following questions should be included in a bowel incontinence assessment:

- What is the availability of the toilet or commode, and what is the time required to get to it?
- What medications, if any, is the older person taking that influence peristaltic action, lucidity, or fluid balance?
- How much bulk is provided in the food? (Pureed food does not help.)
- What manual dexterity is required to remove clothing once the older person is in the bathroom?
- Is there any neurological or circulatory impairment of the cerebral cortex?

Interventions. Fecal incontinence is a symptom. It requires that the patient be accepted as a person, that the incontinence problem not be advertised or ridiculed, and that the

person not be made to feel ashamed or guilty. A great deterrent to successful intervention in incontinence is inconsistency in implementing the planned strategy and unrealistic expectations of rapid, full recovery. Time and patience are essential ingredients of success. Nursing interventions should include several days' surveillance of the patient's bowel function. A chart similar to that used to monitor urinary incontinence can be constructed (see Figure 7-1 on p. 130).

Nursing intervention should work to manage and/or restore bowel continence. Therapies similar to those used in treating urinary incontinence are effective with fecal incontinence, such as environmental manipulation, diet alterations, bowel training, sensory reeducation, sphincter training exercises, biofeedback, electrical stimulation, medication, and/or surgery to correct underlying defects. Instituting a diet adequate in dietary fiber (6-10 g daily) will add bulk, weight, and form to the stool and improve colon evacuation of the sigmoid and rectum rather than produce a continuous or intermittent oozing of fecal material. This may assist in attaining more controlled and complete bowel movements.

When the incontinence has a cerebral or neurological cause, it is often necessary to identify triggers that initiate incontinence. For example, eating a meal stimulates defecation 30 minutes after completing the meal, or defecation occurs after the morning cup of coffee. If the fecal incontinence is only once or twice each day, it can be controlled by being prepared. Placing the individual on the toilet, commode, or bedpan at a given time after the trigger event facilitates defecation in the appropriate place at the appropriate time.

When fecal incontinence is continual, it may be necessary to develop a plan that controls the specific time of day when the individual has a bowel movement or movements. Generally, this is accomplished by establishing constipation for several days and evacuating the bowel (e.g., every fourth day) by enema or suppository. Diet plays a role in this also. Creating the proper diet will affect intestinal motility and help evacuation. Bowel training of this type allows for predictability of colon evacuation and more freedom and less embarrassment for the older person (Box 7-3). If protective garments are necessary, they will allow the patient more opportunity to participate actively in events and to be more mobile in the institutional community.

The effectiveness of interventions in fecal incontinence will be self-evident but will take time. As in treatment of urinary incontinence, goals must be realistic. It cannot be stated too often or too strongly that the nurse must always provide immaculate skin care to persons with incontinence because self-esteem and skin integrity depend on it.

Bladder Function

Normal bladder function requires an intact brain and spinal cord, a competent bladder, and active sphincters that will sustain maximum urethral pressure against rising bladder pressure. A full bladder increases pressure and signals the spinal cord and the brainstem center the desire to micturate. Social training then dictates whether micturition should be attended to or should be postponed until there is an appropriate

---

BOX 7-3 Bowel Training Program

1. Obtain bowel history, and establish a schedule for the bowel training program that is normal and comfortable for the patient and conforms to his or her lifestyle.
2. Ensure adequate fiber and fluid intake (normalize stool consistency).
   a. Fiber.
      (1) Add high-fiber foods to diet (dried fruit, dried beans, vegetables, and wheat products).
      (2) Suggest adding 1 to 3 tbsp bran or Metamucil to diet one or two times each day. (Titrate dosage based on response.)
   b. Fluid.
      (1) Two to three L daily (unless contraindicated).
      (2) Four oz of prune, fig, or pear juice (or a warm fluid) may be given daily as a stimulus (e.g., 30-60 min before the established time for defecation).
3. Encourage exercise program.
   a. Pelvic tilt, modified sit-ups for abdominal strength.
   b. Walking for general muscle tone and cardiovascular system.
   c. More vigorous program if appropriate.
4. Establish a regular time for the bowel movement.
   a. Established time depends on patient's schedule.
   b. Best times are 20 to 40 min after regularly scheduled meals, when gastrocolic reflex is active.

   c. Attempts at evacuation should be made daily within 15 min of the established time and whenever the patient senses rectal distention.
   d. Instruct patient in normal posture for defecation. (The patient normally sits on the toilet or bedside commode; for the patient who is unable to get out of bed, the left side-lying position is best.)
   e. Instruct the patient to contract the abdominal muscles and "bear down."
   f. Have the patient lean forward to increase the intra-abdominal pressure by use of compression against the thighs.
   g. Stimulate anorectal reflex and rectal emptying if necessary.
      (1) Insert a rectal suppository or mini-enema into the rectum 15 to 30 min before the scheduled bowel movement, placing the suppository against the bowel wall, or (2) insert a gloved, lubricated finger into the anal canal and gently dilate the anal sphincter.

From Basch A, Jensen L: Management of fecal incontinence. In Doughty DB: *Urinary and fecal incontinence: nursing management,* St Louis, 1991, Mosby.

---

opportunity to seek out toilet facilities. However, when the bladder contents reach 500 mL or more, the pressure is such that it becomes more difficult to control the urge to void. As volume increases, emptying the bladder becomes an uncontrollable act. The bladder of an older person retains its tonus, but the volume it can hold decreases. If cerebrovascular disease or dementia is present, the changes are exaggerated and bladder control diminishes. Nocturnal frequency is common in two thirds of women and men older than 65 years who do not take medication and in more than 80% of those elders with three chronic diseases (Wasson and Bruskewitz, 1990).

Many healthy older people are annoyed by frequency and some degree of urgency. The warning period between the desire to void and actual micturition is shortened or lost. Age-related changes, illness, cognitive impairments, difficulty in walking or handling a bedpan or urinal, and problems manipulating clothing may be responsible for some incontinence. Drugs that increase urinary output and sedatives, tranquilizers, and hypnotics, which produce drowsiness, confusion, or limited mobility, promote incontinence by dulling the transmission of the desire to micturate.

Urinary Incontinence. Incontinence, or the loss of ability to control the elimination of urine on an occasional or consistent basis, is one of the most prevalent symptoms encountered in care of older adults. Weiss (2005) commented that urinary incontinence (UI) is more prevalent than diabetes, Alzheimer's disease, and many other chronic conditions that have

prompted more attention and treatment. Incontinence causes considerable embarrassment and astronomical costs both socially and economically. The economic costs are $11.2 billion annually in the community and nearly $5.3 billion in long-term care settings (Fourcroy, 2001). UI costs exceed those of coronary artery bypass surgery and renal dialysis combined (Weiss, 2005). Estimates of costs and numbers of individuals enduring incontinence vary widely because many people isolate themselves and keep silent about the problem. About half of patients with UI have never discussed the concern with their primary care provider (Weiss, 2005).

UI affects 12% or more of the older adult population. Estimates are that approximately 10% to 30% of community-living elders, 30% to 35% of elders who are hospitalized, and 50% of elders living in nursing homes experience UI (Ham et al., 2002). Women are at least twice as likely as men to experience UI (Mason et al., 2003). Continence must be routinely addressed in the initial assessment of every older person, yet many older people do not bring up their concerns about incontinence and many health professionals do not ask. UI may become apparent when people are institutionalized, or episodes of UI may present only during a hospitalization, lifestyle change, or physiological disruption.

A recent survey of 1400 Americans revealed that despite the prevalence of UI, 64% of those experiencing symptoms were not doing anything to manage their condition. On average, adults waited 6 years after first experiencing symptoms before talking to a health care professional.

The common belief that incontinence is inevitable with age leads to inadequate assessment and treatment, and in fact, 38% of those surveyed believed loss of bladder control was just a part of natural aging (accessed 8/5/04 from *www. nafc.org/NAFCNewsRelease.asp*). Individuals may not seek treatment because of embarrassment in talking about the problem or because they do not know that successful treatments are available (Palmer and Newman, 2006). Older people want more education about bladder control, and nurses can take the lead in implementing approaches to continence promotion and public health education about UI (Palmer and Newman, 2006). Incontinence is not a result of advancing age, nor is it a disease. It is a symptom of existing environmental, psychological, drug, or physical disturbances and can become a catastrophic event when it interferes with mobility, sociability, and the ability to remain in one's home. Box 7-4 enumerates risk factors associated with urinary incontinence.

Consequences of Urinary Incontinence. Incontinence ushers in dependence, shame, guilt, and fear. Older people who are aware of a problem of continence are mortified by their state. Psychological consequences of UI include depressive symptoms as a result of anxiety and embarrassment about appearance and odor of urine. This can lead to restricted social activities, isolation, and avoidance of sexual activity. Physical consequences of UI include skin problems (rashes, breakdown, infection), pressure ulcers, urinary tract infections (UTIs), and falls. UI is one of the four independent risk factors for institutionalization. Other factors are cognitive impairment, dependence in ambulation, and being unmarried (Ham et al., 2002; Holroyd-Leduc and Straus, 2004).

Evidence-Based Practice. The Agency for Health Care Policy and Research (AHCPR) (now Agency for Healthcare Research and Quality [AHRQ]) increased awareness and knowledge about incontinence and has continued to disseminate factual information through the publication of the Clinical Practice Guideline, *Urinary Incontinence in Adults*, in 1992 and the updated version in 1996 (*www.guidelines.gov*). These were the first guidelines published by the Agency in response to the prevalence of UI and lack of evidence-based treatment. This information attempts to improve reporting, diagnosis, and treatment of the ambulatory and non-ambulatory individual and to educate health professionals and consumers about urinary incontinence (Fantl et al., 1996). The AMDA (1996) clinical practice guidelines on UI in long-term care are another valuable resource for nurses working in nursing homes (*www.amda.com*), and the "Nursing Standard-of-Practice Protocol: Urinary Incontinence in Older Adults Admitted to Acute Care" (Bradway and Hernly, 1998) is useful for nurses in acute care. The Center for Medicare and Medicaid Services (CMS) has published new interpretive guidelines for incontinence in long-term care settings (Schnelle and Ouslander, 2006). Wyman (2003) noted that despite a substantial amount of evidence-based practice protocols, a national clinical prac-

---

BOX 7-4   Risk Factors for Urinary Incontinence

- Immobility of chronic degenerative diseases
- Diminished cognitive status, dementia
- Delirium
- Medications (anticholinergic properties, sedatives, diuretics)
- Smoking
- Fecal impaction
- Low fluid intake
- Environmental barriers
- High-impact physical exercise
- Diabetes
- Stroke
- Estrogen deficiency
- Pelvic muscle weakness
- High caffeine intake
- Hysterectomy in older women
- Childhood enuresis
- Pregnancy
- Morbid obesity
- Environmental barriers

Modified from Fantl JA et al: Managing acute and chronic urinary incontinence. In *Clinical practice guideline: quick reference guide for clinicians*, no 2, 1996 update, AHCPR Pub No 97-0686, Rockville, Md, 1996, U.S. Department of Health and Human Services, Public Health Service, Agency for Health Care Policy and Research.

---

tice guideline, identification of competencies for both generalist and specialist practice, and a growing public awareness, UI continues to be underdetected, underdiagnosed, and undertreated across all practice settings. Some who have been diagnosed with UI do not receive treatment, particularly those with cognitive impairments. "Continence remains undervalued, and UI remains underassessed. Even though UI is a basic nursing care issue, nurses are not claiming it as one" (Mason et al., 2003, p 3). Educational competencies for beginning nursing practice in continence care are presented in Box 7-5.

Types of Urinary Incontinence. The types of UI categorized by symptoms are stress, urge, overflow, iatrogenic, mixed, and functional (Dash et al., 2004) (Table 7-1). Transient urinary incontinence, the result of functional and iatrogenic causes, can be remembered by the mnemonic *DRIP* (Box 7-6).

Stress incontinence occurs more often in elderly women and occurs when intraabdominal pressure exceeds urethral resistance. Muscles around the urethra become weak so even a small amount of urine may spontaneously pass. It occurs frequently in obese individuals, especially apple-shaped (rather than pear-shaped) individuals (Fourcroy, 2001). It is more common in white women than in African-American women, but research on UI in minorities is limited. Involuntary urine loss may occur when an individual sneezes, coughs, bends over, or lifts a heavy object. The amount of urine leakage usually is small, and the volume is low when postvoid residual urine is obtained or visualized by ultrasound.

BOX 7-5   Educational Competencies for Continence Care: Basic Preparation for Beginning Professional Practice

A professional nurse will be able to independently:

1. Obtain a focused health history to include the following:
   a. The presence of risk factors for urinary incontinence (UI) and medical conditions that may be contributing to UI and identifying patients at risk for the development of UI
   b. Confirming the presence and effect of UI subjectively
   c. A detailed exploration of the symptoms of UI and associated factors
   d. Medication review including prescription and nonprescription drugs to identify those patients whose medications may negatively affect urine control
   e. Bowel pattern to include frequency, consistency, and usage of any assistive products (e.g., dietary measures, prescription and nonprescription medications including suppositories and enemas)
   f. Functional, environmental, social, and cognitive factors that may contribute to or result in UI

2. Obtain an intake and output record that includes the following:
   a. Voiding records from patients that include time and onset of incontinent episodes, voiding pattern, 24-hour recording with diurnal and nocturnal frequency, amount voided, amount leaked, activity when leakage
   b. Intake record with 24-hour pattern of fluid intake that includes amount, frequency, and type of oral intake

3. Obtain diagnostic measures to detect evidence of urinary tract infection and other disorders contributing to incontinence that may include the following:
   a. Urinalysis or the use of a chemically treated dipstick to detect hematuria, pyuria, bacteriuria, glycosuria, or proteinuria
   b. Obtaining a clean-catch or catheterized urine specimen for culture and sensitivity if indicated
   c. Obtaining a catheterized urine specimen to detect amount of urine in bladder or postvoid residual (PVR) volume or bladder ultrasound

4. Conduct a physical examination that includes the following:
   a. Focused abdominal examination to estimate suprapubic fullness, to rule out palpable hard stool, and to evaluate bowel sounds
   b. Examination of the genitals, including skin integrity of perineum, appearance of urethral meatus, and presence of prolapse
   c. Rectal examination including evaluation of sphincter tone, perineal sensation, and presence or absence of fecal impaction
   d. Confirming the presence of UI objectively and evaluation of the force and character of urine stream during voiding with observation of actual toileting of client
   e. A functional assessment, including mobility, self-care ability, mental status examination, and communication patterns

5. Assess environment

6. Initiate nursing interventions that include the following:
   a. Strategies that promote bladder health (fluid hydration, caffeine reduction, bowel programs, dietary strategies, weight reduction, smoking and alcohol reduction)
   b. Educating and counseling patients and families (e.g., anatomy and physiology of genitourinary system, factors affecting continence, etiological factors related to UI treatment options available to patients who may benefit from scheduled voiding regimens without further testing)
   c. Identifying patients who require further evaluation before therapeutic intervention; collaborating with physicians or advanced practice nurses regarding diagnosis, intervention plan, expected outcomes, and ongoing evaluation
   d. Implementing scheduled toileting programs for functional incontinence and evaluating effectiveness
   e. Supervising nursing staff in the implementation of prompted voiding and scheduled toileting programs and evaluating effectiveness
   f. Evaluating patients with indwelling catheters for voiding trial and initiation of bladder training
   g. Teaching pelvic muscle exercises to patients at risk for developing stress incontinence
   h. Implementing bladder training programs for early symptoms of stress or urgency
   i. Implementing scheduled toileting programs for patients at risk for developing functional incontinence before UI develops
   j. Identifying patients who would benefit from assistive devices to maintain continence
   k. Recommending appropriate containment devices and topical therapy for prevention and management of skin breakdown

From Jirovec MM et al: Addressing urinary incontinence with educational continence-care competencies, *Image J Nurs Sch* 30(4):375-378, 1998.

Urge incontinence, or overactive bladder, is more common in younger women and is caused by central nervous system lesions such as stroke, demyelinating diseases, and local irritating factors such as bladder tumors or UTIs. Individuals sense the urge to void but cannot inhibit urination long enough to reach a toilet. The volume of urine lost is moderate, and episodes occur every few hours. Postvoid residual urine reveals a low volume.

Overflow incontinence is a result of neurological abnormalities of the spinal cord that affect the contractility of the detrusor muscle of the bladder. Any factor disrupting detrusor stability, such as drugs, tumors, strictures, and prostatic hypertrophy, will cause the bladder to become overdistended, leading to frequent or constant loss of urine. Postvoid residual urine volumes may be high.

Functional incontinence refers to a situation in which the lower urinary tract is intact but the individual is limited by environmental factors, musculoskeletal disability, or severe cognitive impairment. Urine is lost because the individual is unaware of the need to void or is unable to reach a toilet because of arthritis, Parkinson's disease, or, for hospitalized patients, their condition or raised side rails or restraints.

TABLE 7-1
Types of Incontinence and Associated Causal Factors

Type	Causal Factors
Stress	Obesity
	Estrogen deficiency
	Pelvic floor muscle weakness
	Radiation or prostate surgery
	Urethral sphincter weakness
	Drugs
Urge	Stroke
	Dementia
	Parkinsonism
	Urinary tract infection
	Detrusor overactivity or instability
	Drugs
Overflow	Fecal impaction
	Enlarged prostate
	Diabetic neuropathy
	Severe pelvic prolapse
	Drugs
Functional	Mobility limitations
	Cognitive impairment
	Depression
	Bipolar/schizophrenic disorders
	External factors:
	Restraints
	Caregiver inattention
	Drugs
	Environmental barriers
Iatrogenic	Extracellular fluid compartment:
	Congestive heart failure
	Chronic venous insufficiency
	Metabolic states:
	Glycosuria
	Calcemia
	Drugs

Adapted from Fantl JA et al: Managing acute and chronic urinary incontinence. In *Clinical practice guideline: quick reference guide for clinicians*, no 2, 1996 update, AHCPR Pub No 97-0686, Rockville, Md, 1996, U.S. Department of Health and Human Services, Public Health Service, Agency for Health Care Policy and Research; Miller CA: *Nursing care of older adults*, ed 2, Philadelphia, 1995, Lippincott; Palmer MH: *Urinary incontinence*, Gaithersberg, Md, 1996, Aspen; Resnick NM: Urinary incontinence. In Abrams WB et al, editors: *Merck manual of geriatrics*, ed 2, Whitehouse Station, NJ, 1995, Merck Research Laboratories; Staab AS, Hodges LC: *Essentials of gerontological nursing*, Philadelphia, 1996, Lippincott.

Iatrogenic incontinence is associated with medication side effects. This can be managed by decreasing the dosage of medication to maintain the primary drug effect but eliminate the secondary effects. It may be necessary to change a drug to another class of medication that is not associated with incontinence. Other iatrogenic causes of incontinence include expanded extracellular fluid compartmentalization with the development of nocturia and polyuria, such as occurs in heart failure, in chronic venous insufficiency, and in metabolic states such as polyuria with increased glycosuria or increased calcemia.

BOX 7-6   Causes of Acute or Transient Incontinence

D Delirium, depression, dehydration, dementia
R Restricted mobility, retention
I Infection, inflammation, impaction (fecal)
P Polyuria, pharmaceuticals

Modified from Kane RL et al: *Essentials of clinical geriatrics*, ed 3, New York, 1994, McGraw-Hill; Durrant J, Snape J: Urinary incontinence in nursing homes for older people, *Age Aging* 32:12-18, 2003; Bravo C: Urinary and fecal incontinence in dementia, *Rev Clin Gerontol* 14:129-136, 2004.

In *mixed incontinence*, more than one urinary incontinence problem exists in the same individual. These conditions can be caused by anatomical, physiological, or pathological factors (internal factors) or by outside factors, such as mobility, dexterity, motivation, and environment. Most older adults with UI have the mixed type, and treatment should be directed toward the most problematic symptoms.

▲ *Promoting Healthy Aging: Implications for Gerontological Nursing*

Assessment. Nurses are often the ones to identify urinary incontinence, but neither nurses nor physicians have been particularly aggressive in management. Assessment is multidimensional. It includes a health history, physical examination, and urinalysis. More extensive examinations are considered after the initial findings are assessed. A thorough health history should focus on the medical, neurological, and genitourinary history; medication review of both prescribed and over-the-counter drugs; a detailed exploration of the symptoms of the urinary incontinence; and associated symptoms and other factors. Nurses, in general, should be able to gather data that will help the physician or the advanced practice nurse in accurate diagnosis and treatment. Box 7-7 presents the assessment of urinary elimination.

One of the best ways to validate and describe incontinence problems is with a voiding diary (Figure 7-1). This is applicable to both community-dwelling and institutionalized elders. Accurate notations should be made of significant burning, itching, or pressure. The character of the urine (color, odor, sediment or clear) and difficulty starting or stopping the urinary stream should be recorded. Activities of daily living (ADLs) such as ability to reach a toilet and use it and finger dexterity for clothing manipulation should be documented. Older adults in the community can usually do this without much difficulty. Bladder diaries for those in long-term care are usually maintained by the staff. Bladder diaries enable not only identification of problems but also evaluation of the effectiveness of nursing interventions and treatment.

Use of problematic medications, such as sedatives, hypnotics, anticholinergics, and antidepressants, should be assessed. Diuretics, narcotics, calcium channel blockers, alpha-adrenergic agonists, minor tranquilizers, antispasmodics, and major tranquilizers are among the drugs contributing to UI. Caffeine and alcohol use should also be assessed. In summary, assessment of urinary incontinence can identify inconti-

BOX 7-7 Elements of an Incontinence Assessment

HISTORY

1. Onset
   a. Recent onset within past 6 months
   b. Onset within past 3 years
   c. Persistent problem for >3 years
2. Frequency
   a. Once each day or less
   b. At least once and up to twice each day
   c. Three times each day or more
   d. Nighttime only
3. Severity
   a. Small amounts of urine lost
   b. Moderate amounts of urine lost
   c. Large amounts of urine lost
4. Risk factors
   a. Smoking
   b. Caffeine intake
   c. Alcohol
   d. Inadequate fluid intake
   e. Chronic constipation
   f. Obesity
5. Psychological impact
   a. Concerned about UI
   b. Not concerned with UI because it is well managed
   c. Unaware of/denies UI
   d. Cost of managing UI burdensome
   e. Major change in lifestyle
   f. Social/family relationships adversely affected
6. Medical history
   a. Stroke
   b. Parkinson's disease
   c. Dementia
   d. CHF
   e. Diabetes
   f. Multiple or difficult vaginal deliveries
   g. Pelvic surgery
   h. Pernicious anemia
   i. Multiple sclerosis
   j. Kidney disease, stones, recurrent infection
   k. Back injury or surgery
7. Current management
   a. Pads/incontinence underwear
   b. Toileting regimen
   c. Catheters or devices
   d. Medication
   e. Skin care
8. Incontinence symptom profile
   a. Stress UI
      (1) Leakage with cough, sneeze, physical activity
      (2) UI in small amounts (drops, spurts)
      (3) No nocturia or UI at night
      (4) UI without sensation of urine loss
   b. Urge UI
      (1) Strong, uncontrolled urge before UI
      (2) Moderate/large volume of urine loss (gush)
      (3) Frequency of urination
      (4) Nocturia more than twice nightly
      (5) Enuresis
   c. Overflow UI
      (1) Difficulty starting urine stream
      (2) Weak or intermittent stream (dribbles) with change in position
      (3) Postvoid dribbling
      (4) Feeling of fullness after voiding
      (5) Voiding in small amounts frequently or dribbling
   d. Functional UI
      (1) Mobility or manual dexterity impairments
      (2) Sedative, hypnotic, central nervous system depressant, diuretic, anticholinergic, alpha-adrenergic antagonist
      (3) Depression, delirium, dementia
      (4) Pain

PHYSICAL EXAMINATION

1. Abdominal examination
   a. Normal
   b. Palpable bladder
   c. Abdominal masses
   d. Distended bowel
2. Genitals
   a. Normal
   b. Reddened, irritated tissue
   c. Discharge
   d. Infection
   e. Odor
   f. Lesions
3. Pelvic examination
   a. Vaginal inspection
      (1) Normal
      (2) Tissue pale, thin, dry
      (3) Pelvic organ descent with Valsalva maneuver
      (4) Lesions
   b. Pelvic muscle assessment
      (1) Palpable, voluntary contraction, rating 0 to 5
      (2) Unable to elicit voluntary contraction
4. Rectal examination
   a. Snug anal sphincter tone and good sensation
   b. Lax or absent anal sphincter tone
   c. Fecal impaction

FUNCTIONAL ASSESSMENT

1. Mobility
   a. Can use toilet with assistance
   b. Needs assistance or verbal prompting to toilet
   c. Unable to use toilet
2. Manual dexterity
   a. Independent
   b. Needs assistance
   c. Unable to use toilet
3. Cognitive function
   a. Intact
   b. Impaired Mini-Mental State Examination score (<24 abnormal)

ENVIRONMENTAL ASSESSMENT

1. Consider distance to bathroom
2. Assess bathroom for lighting, glare, grab bars, physical barriers
3. Determine caregiver willingness and ability to provide assistance
4. Assess need for toilet substitutes and adaptations (raised toilet seat, grab bars)
5. Consider adaptable clothing and devices to facilitate disrobing for toileting
6. Ensure proper assistive devices (wheelchair, walker, cane)

BLADDER DIARY

1. Record and review a bladder diary for 3 to 5 days including the following:
   a. Timing of voiding
   b. Volume voided
   c. Circumstances associated with UI episodes

IDENTIFY POSSIBLE DIAGNOSES OR CLINICAL IMPRESSION

1. Rule out other serious medical problems, assess and treat constipation and fecal impaction, check urine with dipstick

From Dash ME et al: Urinary incontinence: the Social Health Maintenance Organization's approach, *Geriatr Nurs* 25(2):81-89, 2004; Fantl JA et al: Managing acute and chronic urinary incontinence. In *Clinical practice guideline: quick reference guide for clinicians*, no 2, 1996 update, AHCPR Pub No 97-0686, Rockville, Md, 1996, U.S. Department of Health and Human Services, Public Health Service, Agency for Health Care Policy and Research; Yu LC et al: Profile of urinary incontinent elderly in long-term care institutions, *J Am Geriatr Soc* 38(4):433-439, 1990.
UI, Urinary incontinence; *CHF*, congestive heart failure.

"URO-Log" (Voiding Diary)
To be completed before your doctor's appointments.

Name _____   Date _____

Time of day	Type and amount of fluid intake	Type and amount of food eaten	Amount voided (in ounces)	Amount of leakage (small, medium, large)	Activity engaged in when leakage occurred	Was urge present?

FIGURE 7-1 Example of voiding diary. (From HIP, Union, SC.)

BOX 7-8   Therapeutic Modalities in the Treatment of Urinary Incontinence

SUPPORT MEASURES

Appropriate attitude
Accessible toilet substitutes (bedpan, urinal, commode)
Avoidance of iatrogenic complications (urinary tract infections, excessive sedation, inaccessible toilets, drugs adversely affecting the bladder or urethral function)
Protective undergarments
Absorbent bed pads
Behavioral techniques (bladder training, toilet scheduling, prompted voiding, conditioning, biofeedback, pelvic floor muscle exercises [PMEs])
Good skin care

DRUGS

Bladder relaxants
Bladder outlet stimulants

SURGERY

Suspension of bladder neck
Prostatectomy
Prosthetic sphincter implants
Urethral sling
Bladder augmentation

MECHANICAL DEVICES

Catheters
External (condom or "Texas" catheter)
Intermittent
Suprapubic
Indwelling

---

nence as either acute/transient (the result of temporary conditions that are amenable to medication, surgery, or psychological intervention) or established (the result of neurological involvement or damage to the urinary system). Transient incontinence is curable; established incontinence is treatable or controllable but not generally curable.

Interventions. When the problem is sufficiently understood, various therapeutic modalities and concomitant nursing interventions can be initiated. Selection of a modality and interventions will depend on the type of incontinence and its underlying cause and whether the outcome is to cure or to minimize the extent of the incontinence. Nursing interventions include appropriate assessment and develop-

ment and implementation of restorative therapeutic modalities (Box 7-8).

Attitude. Most health care personnel think of UI as "part of the job," with interventions more often directed toward prevention of skin breakdown and keeping people clean and dry than appropriate assessment and management (Taunton et al., 2005). Caregivers are often unaware of the many causes of incontinence and passively accept a client's urinary incontinence and believe that it is an inevitable part of aging, which may add to the elder's feelings of low self-worth, dependence, and social isolation. A recent study exploring women's experiences with UI while living in long-term care settings reported that the women experienced a loss of control and dignity, were embarrassed to talk about this problem, and were given very little assistance in maintaining continence (MacDonald and Butler, 2007). UI should be seen as a treatable concern. The nurse who cares for the incontinent person either in the community or in other types of facilities needs knowledge about UI and its treatment, sensitivity, insight, patience, and understanding. The fact that incontinence can be curable and that the nurse and other health care providers will work with the elder to resolve the incontinence is an important idea to foster in the elder who is not cognitively impaired. For those with cognitive impairment who can be routinely taken to the toilet, staying dry and maintaining normal patterns are important to self-esteem and dignity.

Toilet Accessibility. Accessibility to the toilet is an intervention that often is not considered in providing assistance for the person with UI. Environmental circumstances can contribute to incontinence. If the distance the older person must either walk or travel by wheelchair to reach the toilet is longer than the time between the onset of the desire to micturate and actual micturition, UI is certain to occur. Toilet substitutes for the infirm and ill have been around for hundreds of years. Four types are used: commodes for the bedside; over-toilet chairs for transport; bedpans for beds or commodes; and urinals for both men and women that can be used in bed, in a chair, or in a standing position. The criterion for use of a commode is that the toilet is too far for the elder's mobility or it requires too much energy for the elderly person to get to the toilet. A commode can also substitute for an inadequate number of available toilets. Urinals are generally used by men; however, bottle-shaped urinals have been designed for women and are used on occasion. They can be obtained from a surgical supply store or various mail-order catalogs (see Resources).

Protective Undergarments and Padding. A variety of protective undergarments or adult briefs are available for the older adults with incontinence. These products may be useful in addition to toileting programs and often relieve anxiety about "wetting" oneself. Disposable types come in several sizes determined by hip and waist measurements, or one size may fit all. Many of these undergarments look like regular underwear and contribute more to dignity than the standard "diaper." Referring to protective undergarments as diapers is demeaning and infantilizing to older people and should be avoided. The lining of these disposable pants may contain fiberfill or an absorbent polymer or gel substance. Polymer and gel substances are more absorbent and tend to keep a protective layer between the skin and wet material. Washable garments with inserts also do a reasonable job of containing urine. However, they tend to be made of plastic or rubber and therefore are hot and cause skin discomfort. If pants are going to leak, they will do so at the groin. It is important to fit them firmly but comfortably around the legs.

A variation of the standard draw sheet is a protective washable pad used along with a plastic sheet. The Australian Kylie pad is a sophisticated version of the draw sheet that is successful in keeping both the bed and the incontinent person dry. It is composed of two layers, with a water-repellent layer next to the individual. Urine is absorbed by the liner. Disposable protective pads are available, but it is important to know the amount and type of fill in the pads. A polymer gel is more economical. It is unwise to purchase pads because they are inexpensive if it means using several more per day than if more expensive and more absorbent pads were bought.

Lifestyle Modifications. Several lifestyle factors are associated with either the development or exacerbation of UI. These include dietary factors (increased fluid, avoidance of caffeine), weight reduction, smoking cessation, bowel management, and physical activity.

Behavioral Techniques. Behavioral techniques such as timed voiding, prompted voiding, bladder training, biofeedback, and pelvic floor muscle rehabilitation are recommended as first-line treatment of UI. These techniques are usually effective in urge and stress incontinence. In some instances the goal is not to regain a normal voiding pattern but to decrease the number of wetting episodes, to decrease laundry costs and use of absorbent protection, and to improve the person's quality of life and social activity. The methods are free of side effects and do not limit future options. However, they do require time, effort, practice, motivation, and education for both the patient and the caregiver. Cognitive status, UI and voiding patterns, mobility, and the need for psychological reinforcement to ensure adherence to the regimen determine the choice of program (Lekan-Rutledge and Colling, 2003). Scheduled voiding regimens may be combined with other interventions such as fluid modification, caffeine reduction, pelvic floor muscle exercises (PFMEs), or drug therapy (Wyman, 2003).

Timed voiding consists of a fixed toilet schedule at 2-hour intervals. This technique may be more useful in stress UI (Wyman, 2003). Bladder training uses an interplay of methods and teaches the individual to void at regular intervals and attempts to lengthen intervals between voidings. Bladder training has been effective in reducing the frequency of urge and stress incontinence in older women and may be even more effective when combined with PFMEs and reduction of caffeine (Wyman, 2003).

Prompted voiding is a scheduled toileting regimen that can be used with cognitively impaired residents who accept toileting. Prompted voiding may improve continence in 25% to 40% of incontinent residents in long-term care facilities. Many factors influence the success of prompted voiding and other toileting regimens in long-term care, including mobility of the residents, staffing ratios, motivation and education of staff, the need for ongoing reinforcement, and a shift in the expectations from incontinence to continence (Lekan-Rutledge, 2000; Schnelle et al., 1998).

Implementation of a UI assessment, prevention, and treatment program in long-term care is time consuming and staff intensive. Consistent implementation of systematic toileting programs, prompted voiding, or other programs to improve UI care requires consistent leadership, support of direct care staff, a multidisciplinary approach, and ongoing feedback and evaluation. Taunton et al. (2005) suggest that "consultation with an advanced practice nurse experienced in restorative continence management would be useful in developing initiatives to increase staff knowledge, modifying inhibiting attitudes, and standardizing the currently used informal interventions" (p. 43). The Centers for Medicare & Medicaid Services (CMS) guidelines for assessment of UI and treatment programs have become a major focus of nursing home inspections and quality improvement efforts. UI is in desperate need of further research, and gerontological nurses can take an active role in design and testing of models of care. Several models of UI management in long-term care that nurses can use in designing programs have been reported in the literature (Dixon, 2002; Lekan-Rutledge, 2000; Remsburg et al., 1999). See Box 7-9 for suggestions for caregivers who are toileting patients with dementia and Box 7-10 for interventions for noninstitutionalized elders.

Pelvic floor muscle rehabilitation includes PFMEs, vaginal weight training, biofeedback-assisted PFMEs, and electrical and magnetic stimulation. PFMEs are most effective for stress UI but also may be of benefit in urge and mixed UI in older women. Pelvic floor exercises (also called *Kegel exercises*) strengthen the periurethral and pelvic floor muscles. The contractions exert a closing force on the urethra. Correct identification of the pelvic floor muscles and adherence to the exercise regimen are key to success. To help identify the correct muscle groups, it may be helpful to tell the person to try to tighten the anal sphincter (as if to control the passage of flatus or feces) and then tighten the urethral/vaginal muscles (as if to stop the flow of urine). Wyman (2003) recommends 36 to 50 pelvic floor muscle contractions divided into two or three exercise sets performed daily or three times per week for 12 to 16 weeks. In several randomized controlled trials, Kegal exercises have shown more effectiveness than medication for urge UI (Weiss, 2005).

Vaginal weight training was introduced in Europe as an alternative for women who have difficulty identifying the pelvic floor muscles. Graded-weight vaginal balls or cones are worn during two 15-minute periods each day or are used in addition to PFMEs. When the weighted cone is placed in the vagina, the pelvic floor muscle contractions keep it from slipping out. Although this technique involves less time and is more easily taught than PFMEs, difficulty inserting the cones and discomfort have been noted as deterrents to use (Wyman, 2003).

Biofeedback uses both visual and auditory instruments to give the individual immediate feedback on how well he or she is controlling the sphincter, the detrusor muscle, and/or the abdominal muscles. Those who are successful learn to contract the sphincter and/or relax the detrusor and abdominal muscles automatically. Further research is indicated as to the effectiveness of this treatment, but women who have weak muscles or difficulty isolating muscles appear to benefit (Wyman, 2003). Table 7-2 provides a summary of behavioral modalities, the type of incontinence, outcomes, and appropriate populations for these approaches.

BOX 7-9   Hints for Caregivers Toileting Residents with Dementia

- Have the word "bathroom" or "toilet" on the door.
- Have a picture of a toilet on the door.
- Leave door to bathroom open to visualize toilet.
- Decrease clutter in and around the toilet.
- Increase environmental safety (i.e., use good lighting, hand rails, elevated toilet).
- Use simple verbal or behavioral cues.
- Hold out your hand and say pleasantly, "Come with me."
- Sing with the resident or use another pleasant distraction if resistant to toileting.
- Avoid complicated commands or questions (i.e., "Mr. Jones, is it time for you to go to the bathroom?").
- Avoid grabbing the resident's wrist and pulling.
- If the resident is nonresponsive, leave alone and return later.
- Stay with a routine.
- Use a familiar caregiver and only one person working with the resident.
- Have residents wear clothing with elastic waistbands or other easy-to-remove clothing.
- Stay pleasant and avoid confrontation or hurrying.
- Use timing with fluids and toileting.
- Avoid bladder irritants.
- Provide skin care cleanser, moisturizer, and protection.
- Keep containment garments simple and similar to regular underpants.

Adapted from Smith DB: A continence care approach for long-term care facilities, *Geriatr Nurs* 19(2):81-86, 1998.

BOX 7-10   Helpful Interventions for Noninstitutionalized Elders to Control or Eliminate Incontinence

- Empty bladder completely before and after meals and at bedtime.
- Urinate whenever the urge arises; never ignore it.
- A schedule of urinating every 2 hours during the day and every 4 hours at night is often helpful in retraining the bladder. An alarm clock may be necessary.
- Drink 1½ to 2 quarts of fluid per day before 8 PM. This helps the kidneys function properly. Limit fluids after supper to ½ to 1 cup (except in very hot weather).
- Drink cranberry juice or take vitamin C to help acidify the urine and lower the chances of bladder infection.
- Eliminate or reduce the use of coffee, tea, brown cola, and alcohol because they have a diuretic effect.
- Take prescription diuretics in the morning on rising.
- Limit the use of sleeping pills, sedatives, and alcohol because they decrease sensation to urinate and can increase incontinence, especially at night.
- If overweight, lose weight.
- Exercises to strengthen pelvic muscles that help support the bladder are often helpful for women.
- Make sure the toilet is nearby with a clear path and good lighting, especially at night. Grab bars or a raised toilet seat may be needed.
- Dress protectively with cotton underwear and protective pants or incontinent pads if necessary.

TABLE 7-2

Behavioral Intervention Options for Incontinence

Type of Incontinence	Intended Population	Behavioral Intervention	Purpose of Intervention	Expected Outcome
Urge, stress, mixed	Cognitively intact; able to discern urge sensation; able to understand or learn how to inhibit urge; able to toilet with or without assistance	Bladder training	Restore normal pattern of voiding and normal bladder function Inhibit involuntary detrusor contractions	↓ Number of wet episodes ↓ Amount of urine lost ↓ Number of voidings ↑ Bladder capacity ↑ Quality of life
Urge, functional	Cognitively impaired; functionally disabled; incomplete bladder emptying; caregiver dependent	Scheduled toileting	Timed with individual's voiding habits Decrease wet episodes; no attempt to regain normal voiding pattern	↓ Number of wet episodes ↓ Laundry costs and/or use of absorbent devices ↑ Quality of life ↑ Social activity
Functional, urge, mixed	Same as above	Habit training Mobility and access to toilet	Develop a pattern for voiding	↓ Frequency of incontinent episodes ↑ Comfort ↑ Quality of life
Urge, functional	Functionally able to use toilet or toileting device; able to feel urge sensation; able to request toileting assistance; caregiver is available	Prompted voiding	Heighten individual awareness of need to void	↑ Interaction between caregiver and individual ↓ Wet episodes
Stress, urge, mixed	Able to identify and contract pelvic muscles; able and willing to follow instructions and committed to actively participate	Pelvic floor training	Strengthen pubococcygeus muscle for efficient urethral closure during sudden increases in intravesical pressure	↑ Strength and size of pubococcygeus ↑ Duration of muscle contraction with increased urethral pressure ↓ Urine loss ↑ Ability to stop urine flow once initiated Self-report of ↓ urine loss ↑ Self-esteem; enhance quality of life ↓ Reliance on pads, panty liners, or absorbent products
Stress, urge, mixed	Cognitively intact Compliant with instructions Able to stand Has sufficient muscle strength to contract muscle and retain the lightest vaginal weight No pelvic organ prolapse	Vaginal weight training	Same as above	Same as above
Stress, mixed	Able to understand analog or digital signals using auditory or visual display Motivated, able to learn voluntary control through observation of biofeedback A health care provider who can appropriately assess the incontinence problem and provide behavior interventions	Biofeedback	Same as above	Same as above
Stress, urge, mixed	Able to discern stimulation	Electrical stimulation	Reeducation of pelvic muscle; inhibit bladder instability and improve striated sphincter and levator ani contractility and efficiency	↑ Resistance of the pelvic floor; block uninhibited bladder contractions

Adapted and compiled from Anderson MA, Braun JV: *Caring for the elderly client,* Philadelphia, 1995, FA Davis; Fantl JA et al: Managing acute and chronic urinary incontinence. In *Clinical practice guideline: quick reference guide for clinicians,* no 2, 1996 update, AHCPR Pub No 97-0686, Rockville, Md, 1996, U.S. Department of Health and Human Services, Public Health Service, Agency for Health Care Policy and Research.; Palmer MH: *Urinary incontinence,* Gaithersburg, Md, 1996, Aspen; Staab AS, Hodges LC: *Essentials of gerontological nursing,* Philadelphia, 1996, Lippincott.

Skin Care. Skin care maintains the first line of defense against infection. Skin that is in contact with urine should be washed gently with mild soap and warm water and then dried thoroughly. Application of a skin lubricant or an ointment, such as A & D or skin barrier cream, provides a thin protective layer to skin repeatedly exposed to urine. It is tempting to neglect an individual who is dependent and wears protective undergarments, but it is important that the person be checked every few hours for wetness to maintain skin intactness. To minimize the episodes of incontinence, it is prudent to establish the incontinence pattern and place the individual on a toilet or commode before voiding.

Medications. Pharmacological treatment is most often indicated for urge UI and overactive bladder (OAB). OAB symptoms include urgency, frequency, and nocturia with or without urge UI. Drugs for urge UI and OAB include anticholinergic (antimuscarinic) agents. The bladder is a smooth muscle that contains muscarinic receptors that are responsible for contractions. Commonly prescribed medications include oxybutynin (Ditropan) and tolterodine (Detrol). These medications are not first-line treatment, and behavioral therapies as just discussed are more effective and should be implemented first (Weiss, 2005). Undesirable side effects of anticholinergic medications, such as dry mouth, dry eyes, constipation, confusion, or the precipitation of glaucoma, are problematic, particularly in older people. Tolterodine and the newer forms of oxybutynin (long-acting and topical formulation) have been shown to have fewer side effects (Newman, 2003).

Surgery. Surgical intervention is appropriate for some conditions of incontinence. Surgical suspension of the bladder neck in women has proved effective in 80% to 95% of persons electing to have this surgical corrective procedure. Outflow obstruction incontinence secondary to prostatic hypertrophy is generally corrected by prostatectomy. Sphincter dysfunction resulting from nerve damage after surgical trauma or radical perineal procedures is 70% to 90% repairable through sphincter implantation. Complications for this type of surgery are greater than 20% and may require an additional surgery. A urethral sling of fascia increases urethral elevation and compression. Continence is restored in approximately 60% to 80% of clients who have this surgery (Newman and Palmer, 2003). Periurethral bulking has been added to the number of surgical procedures that address urinary incontinence. Collagen or polytetrafluoroethylene (PTFE) is injected into the periurethral area to increase pressure on the urethra. This adds bulk to the internal sphincter and closes the gap that allowed leakage to occur.

Nonsurgical Devices. Stress UI can be treated with intravaginal support devices, pessaries, and urethral plugs. An extracorporeal magnetic innervation chair (ExMI), approved by The U.S. Food and Drug Administration (FDA), may also be of benefit in stress UI. The ExMI strengthens pelvic floor muscles through application of a low-intensity magnetic field (Weiss, 2005). Another option is the pessary, which has been around for many years and has been used primarily to prevent uterine prolapse. The pessary is a device that is fitted into the vagina and that exerts pressure to elevate the urethrovesical junction or the pelvic floor. The patient is taught to insert and remove the pessary much like inserting and removing a diaphragm used for contraception. The pessary is removed weekly or monthly for cleaning with soap and water and then reinserted. Adverse effects include vaginal infection, low back pain, and vaginal mucosal erosion. Another concern is forgetting to remove the pessary (Newman and Palmer, 2003).

Catheters. Indwelling catheters may be appropriate for short-term use in hospitalized patients, but clinical guidelines indicate that indwelling catheter use is appropriate only when urethral obstruction or urinary retention is present, with the following conditions (Fantl et al., 1996; Newman and Palmer, 2003):

- Persistent overflow UI, symptomatic infections, or kidney disease
- Surgical or pharmacological interventions inappropriate or unsuccessful
- Contraindications to intermittent catheterization for retention
- When changes of bedding, clothing, and absorbent products may be painful or disruptive for a patient with an irreversible medical condition, such as metastatic terminal disease, coma, or end-stage congestive heart failure
- For patients with stage 3 or 4 pressure ulcers that are not healing because of continual urine leakage
- For patients who live alone without a caregiver or with a caregiver who is unable to routinely change the person's clothing and bed linens

Regulatory standards in nursing homes follow these same guidelines, and the use of indwelling catheters must be justified based on medical conditions and failure of other efforts to maintain continence. Long-term catheter use increases the risk of recurrent urinary tract infections leading to urosepsis, urethral damage in men secondary to urethral erosion, urethritis or fistula formation, and bladder stones or cancer (Newman and Palmer, 2003). UTIs are the most common infections in residents in long-term care. Asymptomatic bacteriuria is considered a benign condition in older people and should not be treated with antibiotics. Screening urine cultures should also not be performed in patients who are asymptomatic (Midthun et al., 2004). Symptomatic UTIs need antibiotic treatment, but it is important to observe the range of symptoms elderly patients may present. Fever, dysuria, and flank pain may not be present. Changes in mental status, decreased appetite, abdominal pain, new onset of incontinence, or even respiratory distress may signal a possible UTI in older people. Catheter care should consist of washing the meatal area with soap and water daily.

Intermittent catheterization (the periodic insertion of a sterile or clean catheter several times per day to empty the bladder) is frequently used in patients with spinal cord injuries and may be of benefit in other conditions. Complications occur less frequently in patients managed by clean intermittent catheterization than in those with indwelling catheters. The procedure may be problematic for many elders with limited dexterity.

External catheters (condom catheters) are sometimes used in male patients who are incontinent and cannot be toileted. Long-term use of external catheters can lead to fungal skin infections, penile skin maceration, edema, fissures, contact burns from urea, phimosis, UTIs, and septicemia (Newman and Palmer, 2003). The catheter should be removed and replaced daily and the penis cleaned, dried, and aired to prevent irritation, maceration, and the development of pressure areas and skin breakdown. If the catheter is not applied and monitored correctly, strangulation of the penile shaft could occur.

Evaluation. The success of interventions in urinary incontinence is measured against phased accomplishment such as the following:

1. The individual voids when placed or sits on the toilet.
2. The individual drinks at least 2000 mL of fluid daily.
3. The individual remains continent 25% of the time.
4. The individual has fewer accidents in each successive phase.
5. The individual is continent all the time.

"Caring for persons with elimination problems has been integral to basic nursing care since Florence Nightingale's time" (Wells, 1994, p. 110). Gerontological nurses have a pivotal role in continence care. It is important that nurses and other health care providers understand the causes of UI, risk factors, and evidence-based protocols for interventions. Competency in continence care needs to be included in the preparation for beginning nursing practice. Health promotion education, comprehensive assessments of UI, education of informal and formal caregivers, and use of evidence-based interventions should be part of individualized care for all older people experiencing UI symptoms. Gerontological nurses also need to be knowledgeable about appropriate products and devices as management options.

Failure to address continence promotion has enormous consequences for both the individual and society in terms of economics and burden of care. Gerontological nurses have an ethical responsibility to take action. Further research is needed, and research priorities include the following (Mason et al., 2003, p. 53):

- The prevalence and nature of UI in men, young women, and members of minority groups
- The effectiveness of various behavioral techniques, devices, and products and pharmacotherapy
- The effectiveness of primary prevention strategies
- Alternative models for educating and involving staff in primary and long-term care settings for improved management of incontinence

Resources listed at the end of this chapter will be valuable to the gerontological nurse as he or she prepares for practice. Gerontological nurses may wish to pursue advanced training and certification through specialty organizations such as The Society of Urologic Nurses and Associates (*www.suna.org*) and the Wound, Ostomy, and Continence Nurses Society (*www.wocncb.org*).

Meeting elimination needs is basic to the maintenance of biological and physiological integrity, but its importance reaches far higher on the hierarchy. Inadequate attention to this basic need can cause excess disability, cause insecurity, affect safety, cause social isolation and curtailment of meaningful activities and relationships, and interfere with the ability of the older person to achieve a meaningful and fulfilling life. Without an adequate knowledge base of continence care, meeting basic elimination needs with basic nursing care will remain mopping up accidents and putting on diapers.

REST AND SLEEP

The human organism needs rest and sleep to conserve energy, prevent fatigue, provide organ respite, and relieve tension. Sleep is an extension of rest, and both are physiological and mental necessities for survival. Rest depends on the degree of physical and mental relaxation. It is often assumed that lying in bed constitutes rest, but worries and other related stressors cause muscles throughout the body to continue to contract with tension even though physical activity has ceased. Attainment of rest depends on this interrelationship of psyche and soma. Body functions possess refractory times and rest periods in the continuous cycle of activity (biorhythms). Drastically or continually altered sleep and rest cycles disrupt homeostatic balance and create physical or mental aberrations. Sleep is a basic need. Rest occurs with sleep in sustained, unbroken periods. Sleep is restorative and recuperative and is necessary for the preservation of life.

Biorhythm and Sleep

Our lives are a series of rhythms that influence and regulate physiological function, chemical concentrations, performance, behavioral responses, moods, and the ability to adapt. Nearly one third of our lives are spent in sleep and rest. The pattern of sleep is a mirror of our health (Eliopoulos, 2001). The most obvious rhythm is the day/night cycle known as the *diurnal* or *circadian rhythm*. The most important and obvious biorhythm is the circadian sleep/wake rhythm. Abnormalities of this cycle, termed *circadian dysrhythmia*, are common among older adults (Beers and Berkow, 2000). They take a longer time to resolve than they do in younger adults.

Sleep itself is an active multiphase process. The hypothalamus is the sleep center of the body, and hypocretins are neuropeptides secreted here and promote wakefulness and rapid-eye-movement (REM) sleep (McCance, 2006). Sleep is promoted by prostaglandin D2, L-tryptophan, and growth factors.

Normal sleep has two phases that have been documented by electroencephalogram (EEG) (McCance, 2006). These are REM sleep and non-REM (NREM) sleep or slow-wave sleep. These two cycle in 90- to 110-minute intervals. Sleep changes occur in aging. Total sleep time is reduced, and elders take a longer time to fall asleep. Many theories exist as to the reason for these changes—lifestyle changes, physical challenges, lack of daily routine, circadian rhythm desynchronization, and use of sedatives. Older adults with good general health, positive

BOX 7-11 Sleep Structure

FOUR STAGES OF NON–RAPID-EYE-MOVEMENT (NREM) SLEEP

Stage 1
Lightest level
Easy to awaken
5% of sleep in young

Stage 2
Decreases with age
Low-voltage activity on electroencephalogram (EEG)
May cease in old age

Stage 3
Decreases with age
High-voltage activity on EEG
May cease in old age

Stage 4
Decreases with age
High-voltage activity on EEG
15% of sleep in elders

RAPID EYE MOVEMENT (REM) SLEEP

Alternates with NREM sleep throughout the night
Rapid eye movements are the key feature
Breathing increases in rate and depth
Muscle tone relaxed
85% of dreaming occurs

Adapted from Beers MH, Berkow R: *The Merck manual of geriatrics,* ed 3, Whitehouse Station, NJ, 2000, Merck Research Laboratories.

moods, and engagement in more active lifestyles and meaningful activities report better sleep and fewer sleep complaints. Poor sleep is an indicator of health status and requires investigation (National Sleep Foundation, 2007). Both cortisol and growth hormone are diminished in older individuals and probably affect sleep patterns. Sleep disorders usually occur earlier in men than in women, by about 10 years (McCance, 2006). Older adults are less able to tolerate sleep deprivation compared with younger adults. See Box 7-11 for structure of sleep.

Institutions that provide care for frail elders usually adhere to specific time schedules, which may not correspond to the person's biorhythm and may place the individual out of synchronization with his or her body functions. Attention to biorhythms can help establish the normal sleep/wake pattern of the person and identify the best times to introduce activities, periods of rest, and therapeutic measures.

Chronobiological Disorders. Similar to jet lag and swing-shift work, elders experience chronobiological disorders with aging. Similarly, winter/seasonal affective disorder is a chronobiological disorder. For most sighted people, dim-light melatonin onset begins at night, approximately 14 hours after awakening in the morning (Lewy, 2005). Circadian rhythms can be shifted by giving a person low-dose (<0.5 mg) melato-

nin, which convinces the body that it is sleep time. Melatonin is the chemical signal for darkness.

Bright-light therapy has been found to be effective, especially in elders who fall asleep early. It is helpful for readjusting sleeping schedules (Rosto, 2001). This author suggests exposure to bright outdoor light or the use of an indoor light box later in the afternoon to reset the circadian rhythm. The use of newer hypnotics such as zolpidem tartrate (Ambien) or zaleplon (Sonata) appear to cause little residual sleepiness and may be helpful in reestablishing a regular sleep pattern (Hill-O'Neill and Shaughnessy, 2002). These and other drugs should be used only short-term, intermittently 2 to 4 times/week and for no more than 3 to 4 weeks, and the person should be monitored closely for untoward reactions to the medications (Reuben et al., 2006). The medication should be gradually stopped, and the elder may expect some rebound sleep difficulty, although less so with the newer hypnotics.

Sleep Disorders

Insomnia. *Insomnia* is defined as difficulty falling asleep or staying asleep. Insomnia can be classified by duration. Transient insomnia occurs in times of acute stress that may be caused by bereavement, hospitalization, or even retirement. Short-term insomnia occurs with prolonged stress, new medications, or stopping a medication, or it may occur because of a psychological disorder. Chronic insomnia lasts longer than 3 weeks and is what usually occurs with aging, but it may occur with chronic stress such as nursing home placement, losses, continued bereavement, a forced retirement, medications, or a psychiatric disorder (Beers and Berkow, 2000). Insomnia is more common in women and can be a serious problem to the older person and family. Its effects include mood changes, memory deficits, diminished concentration, poor judgment, impaired performance, and changes in the immune system (Fielo, 2001).

Two classifications for insomnia are the Diagnostic and Statistical Manual of Mental Disorders (DSM-IV-TR) and the International Classification of Diseases (ICD). Most primary health providers use the ICD classification; psychiatrists use the DSM criteria. Depression is a common cause of insomnia in older adults. The prevalence of insomnia is difficult to document, but the use of hypnotics is more common in older adults than in younger people. A number of drugs may cause sleep disturbances (Box 7-12). In addition to medications, depression, and daytime naps, other causes of insomnia include worry and anxiety, hospitalization, new environments, pain, heat or cold, dementia, Parkinson's disease, allergies, changes in routine, alcohol use or abuse, inadequate exercise, periodic limb movement of sleep (PLMS; also called *nocturnal myoclonus*), and restless leg syndrome (RLS) (Phillips, 2005; Reuben et al., 2006; Schoenfelder and Culp, 2001). In addition, melatonin, which is naturally secreted during evening hours and promotes sleep, is diminished in older adults.

Sleep Apnea. Sleep apnea is a disorder characterized by repetitive cessation (>10 seconds) of respiration during sleep (Reuben et al., 2006). It may be further characterized by

BOX 7-12   Drugs That Cause Sleep Disturbances

- Caffeine (prolongs sleep latency and interferes with sleep maintenance)
- Bronchodilators and sympathomimetics (stimulate central nervous system [CNS])
- Diuretics (if used late in the day, produce nocturia, waking the person)
- Decongestants, ephedrine, β-agonists, and methylxanthines (if used at night, prolong sleep initiation)
- Antihypertensives, α-agonists, and central-acting (CNS effects alter sleep physiology) (clonidine, methyldopa, reserpine)
- β-Blockers (cause nightmares; CNS effects cause changes in sleep physiology)
- Carbidopa and levodopa (cause nightmares)
- Benzodiazepines (cause rebound insomnia with discontinuation; tolerance with prolonged use)
- Other: alcohol, cortisone, nicotine, phenytoin, progesterone, quinidine, sedatives

BOX 7-13   Sleep Apnea Risk Factors

- Increasing age
- Enlarged neck circumference
- Male gender
- Anatomical abnormalities of the upper airway
- Family history
- Obesity
- Snoring
- Alcohol or sedative use
- Smoking
- Cardiac disorders
- Hypertension
- Nocturia
- Cognitive dysfunction
- Upper airway resistance/obstruction

Data from McCance KL, Huether SE. *Pathophysiology*, ed 5, St Louis, 2006, Mosby; McCullough P: *How well do you sleep?* Presentation at the Kentucky Council of Nurse Practitioners and Midwives, Lexington, Ky, April 2001; Phillips B: Sleep apnea, periodic limb movement, restless legs syndrome, and cardiovascular complications. In Sleep disorders in the geriatric population: implications for health, *Clin Geriatrics Suppl* Dec 2005, American Geriatric Society; Reuben D et al: *Geriatrics at your fingertips 2006-2007*, ed 8, New York, 2006, American Geriatric Society.

hypopnea—a transient reduction in airflow with diminished oxygen saturation for greater than 10 seconds during sleep. Daytime sleepiness is excessive, and/or cardiopulmonary function is altered. Obstructive sleep apnea accounts for about 90% of sleep apnea cases, affecting about 25% of those older than 65 years (Phillips, 2005), and occurs twice as often in men as in women (McCullough, 2001). Box 7-13 lists sleep apnea risk factors. When breathing is inadequate, a "fire alarm" goes off and the person is aroused from slumber, normal ventilation then occurs, and the person tries to go back to sleep. Sleep is then very fragmented and not restorative or refreshing. After months or years of living with this problem, severe psychological and physiological consequences may occur, including right-sided heart failure, hypertension, cardiac arrhythmias, and death (Drazen, 2002). Other consequences may include an increased number of automobile accidents, more work-related accidents, poor performance, depression, and decreased quality of life (McCullough, 2001).

Assessment includes information from the sleeping partner and consideration of a sleep study because assessment during sleep is important. The sleeping partner's sleep is often disturbed, and the partner may move to another room to sleep. Therapy will depend on the severity of the sleep apnea. Some of the clinical features of sleep apnea include gasping and choking on awakening; uncertainty of reason for awakenings; restless sleep; non-restorative sleep; poor memory and intellectual functioning; irritability and personality change; and morning headache or confusion (McCullough, 2001). The family will reveal that the person has daytime sleepiness, which is often unrecognized by the patient. If questioned about automobile accidents, the assessor will find that some accidents or some near-misses have occurred. The patient will sleep in inappropriate settings such as in social situations or at work.

Physical assessment often reveals that the individual is obese. The neck is often short and thick. The uvula is large, and the soft palate hangs low. Tonsils may be enlarged; adenoids are enlarged. The individual may have micrognathia or retrognathia, that is, small chin or receded chin. Look for upper airway tumors or cysts (McCullough, 2001).

Specific treatment of sleep apnea has the goals of reducing morbidity and mortality and increasing quality of life. There should be risk counseling about impaired judgment from sleeplessness and possibility of accidents if driving. The patient should be encouraged to lose weight, avoid alcohol and sedatives, stop smoking, avoid supine sleep positions by using pillows or sleeping in a chair, and avoid situations in which there would be sleep deprivation (McCullough, 2001). Medical interventions include nasal mask continuous positive airway pressure (CPAP), which presents the difficulty of compliance. Oxygen may be used because it can reduce arrhythmias; humidifiers, oral appliances, decongestants, nasal steroids, antihistamines, selective serotonin reuptake inhibitor (SSRI) antidepressants, and tricyclic antidepressants may also be used. Surgery to reconstruct the upper airway can be considered. This involves tonsillectomy, uvula surgery, and a number of other procedures; however, this is not very satisfactory in those older than 50 years. A newly available dental device is put over the teeth or dentures and is effective, although less effective than CPAP. It may be considered in those intolerant of CPAP (Phillips, 2005). In severe cases, tracheostomy is used to bypass the upper airway. It is interesting to note that because sleep apnea causes arrhythmias in older adults, pacemakers have been inserted. A significant finding with the pacemaker is that patients have fewer and less severe episodes of apnea if the pacemaker is set to achieve atrial overdrive (15 beats per minute faster than usual night heart rate without the pacer) (Drazen, 2002).

Nocturnal Myoclonus. The incidence of PLMS (nocturnal myoclonus) increases with age and may occur in up to 45% of community-based elders (Beers and Berkow, 2006). It may occur in up to 80% of those with RLS (McCullough, 2001). The etiology is unknown, although it has been suggested that the cause may be an age-related decrease in dopamine receptors because carbidopa-levodopa can be used to manage the myoclonus. PLMS occurs only during sleep. Often the patient is unaware of the occurrence; however, it is very disruptive to the sleep partner.

A diagnosis is difficult to make, but diagnostic criteria include insomnia or excessive sleepiness; repetitive highly stereotyped limb muscle movements such as extension of the big toes with partial flexion of ankle, knee, and sometimes hips; polysomnographic monitoring displays of repetitive episodes of muscle contractions and associated awakenings or arousals; and no evidence of a medical, mental, or other sleep disorder that might account for the symptoms (Reuben et al., 2006). The upper extremities also may move. Dopamine agonists such as bromocriptine, pergolide, pramipexole, or ropinirole are preferred. Carbidopa-levodopa is a good choice treatment—given 1 to 2 hours before bedtime. Second-line therapy is carbamazepine and gabapentin—drugs often used to manage seizure disorders.

Restless Leg Syndrome. RLS is characterized by the need to move the limbs and may have associated paresthesias or dysesthesias (Reuben et al., 2006). Motor restlessness is present and is exhibited by pacing the floor, stretching, flexing, body rocking, marching in place, tossing and turning in bed, and rubbing the legs. A vague discomfort is present, often in the calf of the leg. Symptoms are exacerbated by rest. It is often worse at night, and is relieved by activity. This can occur at any age but most severely affects those in middle to old age. It is often progressive but may have remissions. The cause is unknown but about 30% of cases report family history of RLS, and it can occur as a side effect of some pharmaceuticals (SSRIs, tricyclics, lithium, dopamine antagonists, caffeine). Other causes are iron deficiency, spinal and peripheral nerve lesions, and uremia.

Assessment focuses on the neurological examination, which is usually normal. A peripheral neuropathy or radiculopathy may be present. In secondary RLS, patients usually have one of the following: polyneuropathies, lumbosacral radiculopathy, amyotrophic lateral sclerosis (ALS), Parkinson's disease, multiple sclerosis, or poliomyelitis. It has also occurred after gastrectomy and with anemia (especially iron or folate deficiency), diabetes, cancers, chronic obstructive pulmonary disease (COPD), rheumatoid arthritis, hypothyroidism, renal failure, and amyloidosis (McCullough, 2001).

Diagnosis and management can be long and cumbersome. A number of laboratory tests can be performed to rule out certain conditions, such as anemia and diabetic neuropathy. If a neuroleptic drug is implicated, changing medications may stop the symptoms entirely. The person should avoid alcohol, caffeine, and nicotine. Sometimes warm or cool baths or whirlpool baths may help. Walking, stretching, and rubbing the legs usually help. Treatment of choice is gabapentin at bedtime only (Remmel et al., 2002). Bromocriptine may relieve chronic symptoms. In severe, refractory RLS, opioids or benzodiazepines may be necessary.

Sleep Disorders of Dementia. Patients with Alzheimer's disease (AD) have increased sleep fragmentation, longer time to sleep onset, diminished sleep efficiency, less total sleep time, and diminished slow-wave sleep (Ancoli-Israel, 2005). This becomes more pronounced with disease progression. Patients with AD and vascular dementia may also have a higher incidence of sleep apnea than elders without dementia. Suggestions for management include reviewing medications for those causing sleep disruption, providing only short daytime naps, relieving daytime boredom, and providing adequate daylight or light exposure.

In 1990, the National Institutes of Health (NIH) convened a conference to review the treatment for sleep disorders of older adults. Recently, NIH convened a task force to review sleep/wake disorders in elders with AD (Omnicare, 2006). The FDA developed guidelines/criteria for sleep disturbances in dementia stating that sleep problems associated with dementia are valid targets for pharmacological treatment. Few clinical trials have studied sleep problems in patients with dementia, but in one trial, triazolam was found ineffective, and in another, zolpidem demonstrated some improvement in sleep.

Sleep and Drugs. Drug tolerance, physical dependence, daytime delirium, drowsiness, and depression of mental alertness occur with chronic use of bedtime hypnotic agents. Some sedatives and tranquilizers are responsible for loss of equilibrium, falls, and fractures. Hypnotic drugs can induce night terrors, hallucinations, and such paradoxical effects as agitation instead of relaxation, hangover, depression, and changes in memory, balance, and gait. If hypnotic drugs are necessary, those that are the least disruptive to the sleep cycle should be employed, particularly the non-benzodiazepine hypnotics. The CMS has published guidelines for the use of sedatives/hypnotics in older adults with insomnia (Omnicare, 2006). Guidelines suggest not using these drugs for more than 10 consecutive days. If reducing the dose is unsuccessful, the 10-day limit may be exceeded. CMS suggests using lower doses than recommended and then increasing gradually until the functional status is improved. All these drugs should be used with caution in elders in a nursing facility. Good non-pharmacological options are back rubs, warm beverage, and listening to soothing audiotapes. If the resident does not fall asleep within an hour of the alternative therapy, then give the hypnotic. In one study, the use of the optional non-pharmacological treatment resulted in a 23% reduction in the use of hypnotics (Omnicare, 2006).

Other Factors Affecting Sleep. Gastric acid secretion, or gastroesophageal reflux disease, best known as *GERD*, is a common cause of sleeplessness. The diagnosis was rarely made 10 to 15 years ago but is very common in older adults. We have better methods of diagnosis and heightened professional awareness.

More than 20% more acid is produced during REM sleep (Remmel et al., 2002). Because the esophageal sphincter at the gastric inlet is more relaxed in elders, acid refluxes into the esophagus, which does not have the same protective lining as the stomach. Over time, the lining of the esophagus becomes scarred and protective secretions emerge, which causes secretions at the back of the throat, resulting in frequent coughing during sleep. The primary treatment is elevating the head of the bed (not just the mattress) 7 to 8 inches so that gravity keeps the secretions in the lower part of the esophagus. Other treatments for chronic GERD include avoidance of coffee and especially alcohol, which relaxes the sphincter even more. Useful medications with few side effects include Zantac, Prilosec, and Prevacid. Zantac and Prilosec are now available over the counter and are not covered under Medicare D prescription assistance plans.

▲ Promoting Healthy Aging: Implications for Gerontological Nursing

Assessment. Nurses are in an excellent position to assess sleep, to improve the quality of a person's sleep, and to study sleep or assist in sleep research by being available at customary sleep times. Sleep history interviews are important and should be obtained from all older clients and their family members. The nurse should learn how well the person sleeps at home, how many times the person is awakened at night, what time the person retires, and what rituals occur at bedtime. Rituals include bedtime snacks, watching television, listening to music, or reading, which, unless carried out, interfere with the individual's ability to fall asleep. Other assessment data should include the amount and type of daily exercise, favorite position when in bed, room environment, temperature, ventilation, illumination, activities engaged in several hours before bedtime, time from dinner and sleep, and sleep medications, as well as other medications taken routinely. Information about involvement in hobbies, life satisfaction, and perception of health status is also important to establish possible depression. The history should be cross-checked with the bedmate, family members, or caregiver. Some of the numerous medical conditions, the related reasons for sleep alterations in the elderly person, and possible interventions are listed in Table 7-3.

Subjective and objective measures of sleep assessment available to nurses include visual analog scales, subjective rating scales (e.g., 0-10 or 0-100), questionnaires that determine if one's sleep is disturbed, interviews, and daily sleep charts. The Pittsburgh Sleep Quality Index (PSQI) (Busse et al., 1989) can be used to measure the quality and patterns of sleep in older people (available at *www.hartfordign.org*, Try This Series). Objective measures include polysomnography

conducted in sleep laboratories, including EEGs and electromyograms (EMGs), and direct observation (Schoenfelder and Culp, 2001).

A nursing standard-of-practice protocol for sleep disturbances in elderly patients was developed as part of the Nurses Improving Care of the Hospitalized Elderly (NICHE) project supported by a grant from the John A. Hartford Foundation. Assessment standards are presented in Table 7-4. The assessment is to elicit information relative to indicators or defining characteristics of sleep disturbance. The sleep diary or log is noted as an important part of assessment. This information will provide an accurate account of the person's sleep problem and identify the sleep disturbance. Usually a family member or the caregiver, if the person is unable, records specific behaviors on a flowsheet. Two to four weeks is required to obtain a clear picture of the sleep problem. Important items to record are the following:

1. The number of times a person calls for assistance to the bathroom, pain medication, or subjective symptoms of inability to sleep, such as anxiety
2. If the person is out of bed
3. Whether the person appears to be asleep or awake on rounds or when checked
4. Episodes of confusion or disorientation
5. If sleep medication was given and if repeated
6. Time the person awakens in the morning (approximation)
7. Where the person falls asleep in the evening
8. Daytime nap

Interventions. Interventions begin after a thorough sleep history has been recorded. Management of disturbed sleep is directed at identifiable causes. Transient sleep disorders or short-term sleep problems do not require treatment with medications. For chronic sleep problems, use the lowest dose of the mildest drug first—for example, a hypnotic such as zolpidem (Ambien) or zaleplon (Sonata); trazodone (Desyrel) may be used if there is depression, because this antidepressant has good sleep profile. Although pharmacological treatment is clearly beneficial, the benefits may not persist over time, and side effects can be problematic (Griffith, 2002).

Non-pharmacological interventions are of benefit either alone or in combination with drug therapy as demonstrated from one research study (Griffith, 2002) looking at three treatment methods, one being placebo. The drug treatment in this study was beneficial for about 3 months, but subjects were less well maintained in the subsequent 21 months without the drug than those subjects with behavioral treatments. This is not surprising, because behavioral changes have a longer-lasting effect. It is interesting to note that the combined treatment of behavioral therapy plus drug therapy was less effective than behavioral therapy alone. The behavior treatment consisted of the following: associate bed with sleep or sex; do not go to bed unless sleepy; if unable to sleep in 15 minutes, go to another room and repeat as necessary; arise at the same time every morning; naps permitted until

TABLE 7-3

Causes, Reasons, and Potential Interventions for Sleep Alterations in the Older Adult

Causes	Reasons	Potential Interventions
Arthritis	Pain builds; joints stiffen during periods of activity; pain relief medicine may wear off	Provide comfortable pillows; offer pain medication before pain becomes too intense
Angina pectoris	Pain likely to occur during rapid-eye-movement (REM) sleep	Keep nitroglycerine at bedside
Chronic obstructive pulmonary disease (COPD)	Abnormal increases in alveolar tension; decrease in oxygen saturation; prone position causes dyspnea and stasis of mucus	Patient education regarding self-care; toilet before bedtime; use bronchial dilators; prevent fatigue; rest during day; no diuretics in late afternoon; caution to avoid cola, coffee, tea, chocolate; use sedatives and over-the-counter (OTC) medication with caution
Heart failure	Nocturnal dyspnea Nocturia	Appropriate cardiotonic regimen; extra pillows; do not take diuretics late in day or in the evening
Diabetes	Inadequate regulation of blood sugar may lead to glycosuria and nocturia; overly tight control of blood sugar Hypoglycemic attacks (can mimic anxiety attacks)	Control by diet, insulin, or oral medication Adjust diabetic regimen Teach regular, adequate caloric intake; bedtime snack
Disturbed sensory perception	Poor environmental lighting; visual difficulties; nocturnal hallucinations; alterations in REM/non-REM (NREM) cycle	Modify environment; check hearing aid; put glasses nearby; reduce noise at home or in hospital; reassure frequently
Alzheimer's disease (AD)	AD patients' sleep shows reduction in stages III and IV sleep early in disease; late in AD these stages disappear; daytime sleepiness increases as disease progresses	Assist staff and family with wandering behavior and sundowning syndrome; be sure person has comfortable chair in which to rest; strict scheduling of nighttime bed hours, day naps, and activity periods and needs; attention to sleep hygiene, relaxation, massage at bedtime; stop all drug treatment to see if normal sleep rhythm returns
Depression	Disturbed sleep pattern: problem falling asleep, early morning awakening, decreased total sleep time; barbiturate use can cause fragmented sleep and nightmares	Assess sleep; check for recent discontinued drugs; frequent reassurance; have same caregiver relate to client; antidepressants if depression diagnosed
Congestive heart failure	Fluid buildup produces symptoms	Restrict fluids at bedtime; prop up on pillows
Gastroesophageal reflux disease (GERD)	Gastric juices and stomach acid increases during REM sleep	Provide nightly preventive medicine
Alcoholism	Abnormal electroencephalogram (EEG) pattern results; as effects wear off, sleeper may awaken with withdrawal symptoms and a hangover	No alcoholic beverages; explain that reformed alcoholics may experience insomnia for a year or so after withdrawal of alcohol
Parkinsonism	Total wake time increases, decreased REM during the night	L-Dopa at bedtime may help decrease rigidity that occurs
Surgical procedures	Premature arousal related to blood drawn at 5 AM or 6 AM; anxiety and worry about outcome; pain	Analyze rituals and routines in place. Can they be changed? Keep pain-free; monitor vital signs frequently; promote rest
Cardiac	Discomfort caused by environment (noise, temperature, lights); postoperative psychosis (usually follows 24-day lucid interval)	Modify environment Establish therapeutic rapport early; instruct patient preoperatively; orient frequently when postoperative; elicit family support
Situational insomnia	On admission to institution; after visit by relative; after move to new residence; after recent loss or death	Establish one-to-one relationship; provide short-term use of hypnotic

Data from de Brun S. *Occup Health Nurs* 29:36, 1981; Hemenway J: Sleep and the cardiac patient, *Heart Lung* 9(3):453, 1980; Pacini C, Fitzpatrick J: Sleep patterns of hospitalized and nonhospitalized aged individuals, *J Gerontolog Nurs* 8(6):327, 1982; Raskind M, Eisdorfer C. *Drug Ther* 7(8):44, 1977; Wagner D. *Alzheimer's Disease and Related Disorders Newsletter* 5(1), 1985.

3 PM; education about sleep requirements; and corrections about mistaken concepts on how to promote sleep. The researcher states that the optimal management regimen may be to begin with a hypnotic, followed by behavioral therapy after discontinuing the hypnotic. This study was based on "stimulus control" or "sleep restriction therapy." Guidelines for stimulus control are listed in Box 7-14. A meta-analysis of treatment protocols revealed that 70% to 80% of patients will improve with behavioral therapy (Kirkwood, 2001). The patient who

is self-directed may benefit from these behavioral routines or other rules of sleep hygiene (Box 7-15). Other behavioral techniques include progressive muscle relaxation, meditation, hypnosis, and biofeedback. Often, referral to a specialist for education of these techniques is needed.

Bright-light therapy, as discussed on p. 136, helps reset the patient's biological clock. It is also used to treat depression. Bright-light therapy is given 30 minutes to 2 hours each day. Duration depends on the brightness of the light

TABLE 7-4

Nursing Protocol: Sleep Disturbance in Elderly Patients

Assessment	Health Promotion and Maintenance Intervention	Evaluation
Sleep-Wake Patterns Inquire about usual times for retiring and rising, time for falling asleep, frequency and duration of nighttime awakenings; frequency and duration of daytime naps; daytime physical and social activity	**Maintain Normal Sleep Pattern** Maintain usual bedtime/wake time Avoid staying in bed beyond waking hours Encourage to get up at regular time even if did not sleep well Schedule nighttime activities to provide uninterrupted periods of sleep of at least 2-3 hr	**Objective Evidence** Time required to fall asleep; should fall asleep within 30-45 min Time for awakening, at usual reported time Behavior, alertness, attention, ability to concentrate, reaction time
Have person provide a subjective evaluation of the quality of sleep Have person complete sleep log for 2 wk	Balance daytime activity and rest Encourage keeping daytime naps to a minimum Promote social interaction Encourage exercise before evening	Observe duration of sleep: patient should remain asleep for at least 4-hr intervals
Bedtime Routines/Rituals Inquire about activities performed by the individual before bedtime (e.g., personal hygiene, prayer, reading, watching TV, listening to music, snacks)	**Support Bedtime Routines/Rituals** Offer a bedtime snack or beverage Enable bedtime reading or listening to music Assist with aspects of personal hygiene at bedtime (e.g., bath) Encourage prayer or meditation Assist to establish a relaxing bedtime routine	**Subjective Evidence** Verbalizations about the quality and quantity of sleep (e.g., statements of difficulty falling asleep or frequent awakenings; having slept well; feeling well-rested/refreshed; an increased sense of well-being)
Medications Obtain information relative to all prescribed and self-selected over-the-counter medications used by person, especially sleep aids, diuretics, laxatives Determine types of medications and length of time used by person	**Avoid/Minimize Drugs That Negatively Influence Sleep** Pharmacological treatment of sleep disturbances is treatment of last resort Discontinue or adjust the dose or dosing schedule of any/all offending medications Consider drug-drug potentiation Administer medications to promote sleep (i.e., give diuretics at least 4 hr before bedtime)	
Diet Effects Obtain information about the consumption of caffeinated and alcoholic beverages	**Minimize/Avoid Foods That Negatively Influence Sleep** Discourage use of beverages containing stimulants (e.g., coffee, tea, sodas) in afternoon and evening Encourage use of food naturally containing L-tryptophan Provide snacks according to patient preference Generally discourage use of alcoholic beverages Decrease fluid intake 2-4 hr before bedtime Encourage to have lighter meal in evening	
Environmental Factors Evaluate noise, light, temperature, ventilation, bedding Inquire about distance of bathroom from bedroom Inquire about use of nightlights	**Create Optimal Environment for Sleep** Keep noise to an absolute minimum Set room temperature according to preference Provide blankets as requested Use nightlight as desired Provide soft music or white noise to mask noise Encourage bed and bedroom for sleep and not other activities Use light exposure during day and evening to maintain wakefulness	
Physiological Factors Evaluate breathing pattern with sleep, with attention to pauses Observe for periodic movement or jerking during sleep Inquire about sleeping position Note diagnoses of sleep disorders Note diagnoses of specific health problems that adversely affect sleep (e.g., CHF, COPD)	**Promote Physiological Stability** Elevate head of bed as required Provide extra pillows per preference Administer bronchodilators, if prescribed, before bedtime Use medical therapeutics (e.g., continuous positive airway pressure machine) as prescribed	

Modified from Foreman MD, Wykle M: Nursing standard-of-practice protocol: sleep disturbances in elderly patients, *Geriatr Nurs* 16(5):238, 1995.

Continued

TABLE 7-4

Nursing Protocol: Sleep Disturbance in Elderly Patients—cont'd

Assessment	Health Promotion and Maintenance Intervention	Evaluation
Illness Factors Inquire about pain, affective disturbances (e.g., depression, anxiety, worry, fatigue, and discomfort)	**Promote Comfort** Provide analgesia as needed 30 min before bedtime (Note that some over-the-counter analgesics may have caffeine) Massage back or feet to help relax Warm and cool compresses to painful areas as indicated Use relaxation methods—deep breathing, progressive relaxation, mental imagery Encourage to urinate before going to bed Keep path to bathroom clear/provide bedside commode	

BOX 7-14   Stimulus Control for Insomnia

- Go to sleep only with the intention of sleep and when sleepy.
- Use the bed only for sleep and sexual activity.
- If you cannot fall asleep, get up and go to another room. Stay up as long as needed to feel sleepy. Return to bed when sleepy. If unable to sleep again after 10 minutes, repeat and get up as long as needed.
- Set the alarm clock and get up at the same time every morning, regardless of how long you slept.
- Do not nap during the day.

Adapted from Kirkwood C: *Treatment of insomnia*, New York, 2001, Power-Pak, CE Publishers (website): *www.powerpak.com*.

BOX 7-15   Sleep Hygiene Rules

1. Have a regular bedtime and wakeup time, even on weekends.
2. Avoid naps. If you must nap, sleep no longer than 30 minutes in early afternoon.
3. Exercise at least 3 hours before bedtime.
4. Wind down during the evening; have a bedtime routine, such as brush teeth, set alarm clock, and read.
5. Limit caffeine (tea, cola, coffee, chocolate), nicotine, and diuretics, especially late in the day.
6. Do not use alcohol to sleep. It maintains a light sleep, not a restful deep sleep.
7. If you have reflux, eat the evening meal at least 3 to 4 hours before bedtime; have a light snack if needed before bedtime.
8. Give attention to the bed environment (comfortable bed, pillows between the knees, quiet, darkness, warm temperature).
9. Do not watch the clock, which increases anxiety and pressure to sleep; if anxious, take a warm bath.

Adapted from Beers MH, Berkow R: *The Merck manual of geriatrics*, ed 3, Whitehouse Station, NJ, 2000, Merck Research Laboratories; Sleep Clinic of San Francisco: *Rules for good sleep hygiene*, press release, Aug 30, 2001.

(Beers and Berkow, 2006). Outdoor light or a commercially made light box can be used. Room light and window light are inadequate.

Drugs should be a last resort and are not intended for long-term treatment. Rebound insomnia and episodes of confusion and nightmares are common when sleep medications are withdrawn. The key to selection of a hypnotic is to consider the half-life and the adverse effects of the agent. Long-acting benzodiazepines should not be used in elderly patients. They are twice as likely to fracture a hip compared with elders using short-acting or intermediate-acting benzodiazepines.

Evaluation. The nursing standard-of-practice protocol presented in Table 7-4 includes an evaluation component. Observation of the person when awake and asleep is necessary. Physiological changes observable for each stage of sleep reviewed previously can be evaluated to give clues to the phases of sleep cycle experienced. It is essential to obtain subjective evidence of the quality and quantity of sleep.

ACTIVITY

Activity is a direct use of energy in voluntary and involuntary physical and behavioral ways that alter the microenvironment and macroenvironment of the individual. The focus of this section is on physical activity. *Healthy People 2010* recommends that health professionals counsel physically inactive adults to increase their physical activity (U.S. Department of Health and Human Services, 2002). Chapter 3 discusses *Healthy People 2010* goals for physical activity and fitness for older adults. The Centers for Disease Control and Prevention (CDC) gives us current facts about exercise health behaviors of older adults (Schoenborn et al., 2006).

Age/Exercise

Nearly one half of adults ages 55 years and older engage in at least some light, moderate, or vigorous leisure-time physical activity. This may occur regularly or irregularly.

- About one half of adults ages 55 to 64 years exercise.
- About one fourth of adults age 85 years and older exercise.
- Adults ages 55 to 64 years and those 65 to 74 years old engaged in similar regular leisure-time activity (28.1% and 26.9%).
- Adults older than 75 years rarely engage in regular exercises/activities.

Ethnicity/Culture/Exercise

- Non-Hispanic white adults and non-Hispanic Asian adults were more likely than non-Hispanic black adults or Hispanic adults to engage in at least some leisure-time physical activity.
- Among adults ages 55 to 64 years, about 6 in 10 non-Hispanic white adults (60.8%) and non-Hispanic Asian adults (58%) engaged in some leisure-time physical activity compared with about 4 in 10 non-Hispanic black adults (43.5%) and Hispanic adults (41.9%).

Finance/Exercise

- Adults who were *not* poor were more likely than those who were poor to engage in some type of leisure activity.
- Adults with private health insurance coverage were twice as likely as those with public coverage to engage in some level of leisure-time activity.

Marital Status/Exercise

- Married adults were more likely than formerly married adults or adults who had never been married to engage in leisure-time activity. Among adults ages 55 to 64 years, 6 in 10 (60.2%) engaged in leisure-time physical activities compared with 5 in 10 formerly married adults (50.9%) and never-married adults 52.5%).

Strengthening

- All older age-groups participate rarely in activities designed to strengthen muscle.
- In adults ages 55 to 64 years, 17.2% do strengthening exercises.
- In adults age 85 and older, 7.2% do strengthening exercises.

Other Exercise Facts

From the National Institute on Aging (2002):

- Exercise helps older people feel better and enjoy life more, even if they think they are too old or too out of shape.
- The combination of lack of physical activity and poor diet is the second highest underlying cause of death in the United States (smoking is the leading cause).
- Regular exercise improves existing diseases and disabilities in older people. It improves mood and relieves depression.
- Staying physically active on a regular, permanent basis helps prevent certain diseases, such as cancers, heart disease, and diabetes, and disabilities as we grow older.

Public perceptions of the elderly and how they spend their time continue to reflect the belief that retirement ushers in the pursuit of sedentary, private, isolated activity and the assumption of a passive role in society. Physical activity is often the barometer by which an individual's health and wellness are judged. The inability to exercise, perform physical work, and complete activities of daily living is one of the first indicators of decline. Research in gerontological exercise physiology is relatively young, but results indicate that maintenance of a physically active lifestyle arrests, delays, or significantly improves age changes associated with cardiovascular, respiratory, and musculoskeletal function.

Physical inactivity is a risk factor for many conditions experienced by the elderly, including obesity, diabetes, and cardiovascular, respiratory, and musculoskeletal diseases. Regular exercise reduces mortality rates even for smokers

---

BOX 7-16   Key Points of Physical Fitness

Health Promotion: physical activity is one of the most important and effective therapeutic interventions in older adults. Physical activity is normal; inactivity is abnormal.

Health Benefits: benefits accrue independently of other risk factors and are proportional to the amount of physical activity that occurs. Those at greatest risk of an adverse event are those with the most to gain.

Health Guidelines: guidelines often found in the government or geriatric association literature often identify a role for physical activity in the management of chronic health problems such as osteoarthritis, osteoporosis, hypertension and cardiac disease, diabetes mellitus, and chronic lung diseases.

Healthy Walking: engaging in a brisk walk for at least 10 minutes at a time, and for 30 minutes each day, and 5 days each week will bring muscular and aerobic benefit. There is conclusive evidence that regular aerobic activity has great physical benefit.

5-A Framework: promoting physical activity is guided by this framework: assess, advise, agree, assist, and arrange. It's never too late.

Compiled from American Geriatric Society: *Geriatric review syllabus: a core curriculum in geriatric medicine,* ed 6, New York, 2006, The Society; Kennie D et al: Health promotion and physical activity. In Tallis RC, Fillit HM, editors: *Brocklehurst's textbook of geriatric medicine and gerontology,* ed 6, Spain, 2003, Churchill Livingstone.

---

and obese elders (Beers and Berkow, 2000). Indirect benefits of regular exercise include increased social interaction, increased sense of well-being, and improved quality of sleep.

The National Institute on Aging has a guide in Spanish to make health information about exercise available to Hispanic elders (National Institute on Aging, 2002). The guide has been extensively tested in Hispanic senior centers, ensuring cultural appropriateness. "It's never too late to start" is an accompanying "fotonovela" with a case study of an older woman who convinces her friends to join her exercise group.

Benefits. Direct benefits of exercise include preservation of muscle strength, increased aerobic capacity, greater bone density, and greater mobility and independence (Beers and Berkow, 2000). Regular exercise is known to increase insulin sensitivity and glucose tolerance and therefore is part of the management plan of anyone with diabetes. Exercise, if done on a regular basis, reduces systolic and diastolic blood pressures and can lessen the need for drug therapy. Exercise increases high-density lipoproteins (HDLs, or the so-called "good" lipoproteins) and lowers triglycerides. It is of benefit in mood disorders such as depression, so common in older adults. Karani and colleagues (2001) describe a study of 32 elderly people in a 10-week exercise program who improved in social functioning and depressive symptoms during the program. Other physical benefits include improved cardiac muscle tone, decreased percentage of body fat, improved ability to breathe deeply and effectively, reduced tension, better quality sleep, favorable bowel control, and appetite control. Box 7-16 presents key points of physical fitness.

Regular exercise can help prevent falls and injury by improving strength, balance, neuromuscular coordination, joint function, and endurance (Beers and Berkow, 2000). To avoid falls during active exercise, balance training should be part of the exercise program. Benefits in both physical and psychosocial aspects of function have been found for community-living and institutionalized elderly. All elders, whether frail or healthy, can benefit from various forms of exercise programs (Figures 7-2, 7-3, and 7-4).

Risks. Those who are frail or are sarcopenic should not engage in strenuous activity, nor should their joints be forced past the point of resistance or discomfort. If the frail have regularly participated in activity that the nurse deems too stressful to their musculoskeletal systems, it is important to keep in mind that an activity done for many years is not as difficult as if it were just introduced. When the activity is new, serious consideration should be given to levels of physical stress produced. Musculoskeletal injuries such as torn ligaments and muscles are common problems (Beers and Berkow, 2000). Risk of fractures increases rapidly with advancing age. The risk of sudden death is temporarily heightened during exercise, especially when the exercise is vigorous and the one exercising is poorly conditioned.

Many people are fearful of falling because of altered balance or the inability to reach or bend. Some fear that if they get down on the floor they will not be able to get up again. Sometimes all that is necessary to alleviate this fear is to ensure that the person has his or her glasses or other appliances that provide security, stability, and mobility. Activity should not be thought of as something to keep the person busy but should be purposeful to enhance his or her physical and mental well-being. Physical activity has therapeutic benefit beyond any potential risks (Kennie et al., 2003). (See Chapters 3 and 15.)

▲ Promoting Healthy Aging: Implications for Gerontological Nursing

Assessment. Healthy older adults who plan only to increase an activity, such as walking, or begin other light- or moderate-intensity activities may need no special evaluation or advice. They may simply review their plans with their nurse or other health professional (Kennie et al., 2003). An assessment should be initiated before allowing a less healthy older adult to participate in an exercise program, especially if a number of co-morbid conditions are present. Very frail and vulnerable elders need assessment by a professional exercise specialist and need to be followed to ensure benefit without compromising safety.

The assessment includes a medical history; knowledge of the individual's present physical activity level; any physical limitations; current medications; and emotional, psychological, and social needs. In addition to the medical history, a physical examination with emphasis on cardiovascular,

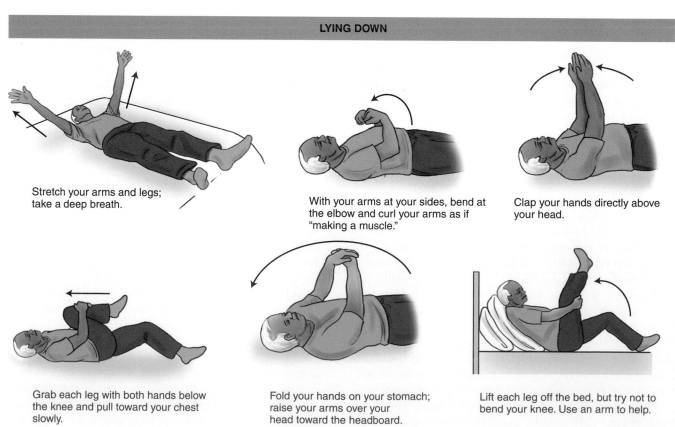

LYING DOWN

Stretch your arms and legs; take a deep breath.

With your arms at your sides, bend at the elbow and curl your arms as if "making a muscle."

Clap your hands directly above your head.

Grab each leg with both hands below the knee and pull toward your chest slowly.

Fold your hands on your stomach; raise your arms over your head toward the headboard.

Lift each leg off the bed, but try not to bend your knee. Use an arm to help.

FIGURE 7-2 Exercises: lying down, sitting, standing up, and walking places. (Redrawn from Johnson-Paulson JE, Kosher R: *Geriatr Nurs* 6[6]: 322-325, 1985.)

SITTING

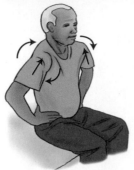

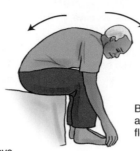

Bend forward and let your arms dangle; try to touch the floor with your hands.

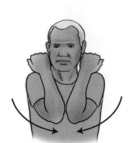

Shrug your shoulders forward, then move them in a circle, raising them high enough to reach your ears.

Touch your elbows together in front of you.

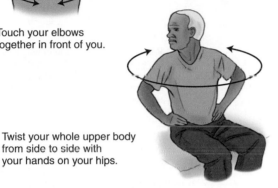

Twist your whole upper body from side to side with your hands on your hips.

While still sitting, move each of your knees up and down as if you are walking; each time your right foot hits the ground, count it as one. Lift your knee high.

STANDING UP

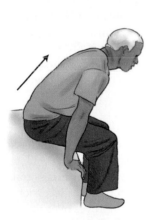

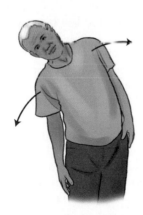

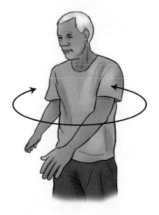

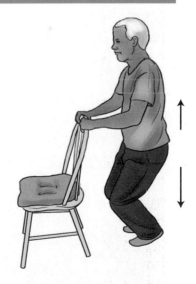

Using your arms, push off from the bed and stand up; if you get dizzy, sit down and try again.

With hands at your side, bend at the waist as far as you can to the right side, then to the left.

Keep your feet planted on the ground and twist your upper body at the waist from side to side with your arms swinging; when you twist to the right, count it as one.

While holding onto the edge of the bed or back of a chair, bend your knees slightly.

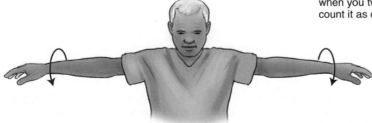

Hold your arms out and turn them in big circles.

FIGURE 7-2, CONT'D

Continued

WALKING PLACES

Walking is good exercise. It helps in toning muscles and in maintaining flexibility of joints and also is good exercise for the heart and circulatory system. Walking briskly for 20 minutes a day, 3 times a week can be as effective as jogging in conditioning the heart, but it does take a longer time to achieve the same effect as jogging. For those who cannot walk rapidly for long periods, walking to the point of muscular fatigue also helps maintain good muscle tone.

There are signs your body may give you to indicate you are overdoing exercise. Stop, rest, and if necessary call your physician if you experience any of these symptoms:

• SEVERE SHORTNESS OF BREATH
• CHEST PAIN
• SEVERE JOINT PAIN
• DIZZINESS OR FAINT FEELING
• HEART FLUTTERING

In all walking exercises, go only as fast as you are able to walk and still carry on a conversation. If you cannot, slow down.

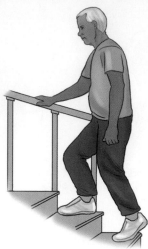

Walking upstairs requires effort. Place one foot flat on a step, push off with the other, and shift your weight. Use a railing for balance if necessary.

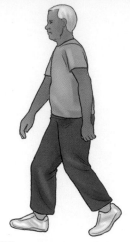

INSIDE

It is important to maintain walking ability. Determine how far you can walk and each day walk to 3/4 of that distance, building endurance. Wear supportive shoes and use whatever aids are necessary.

OUTSIDE

Wear soft-soled shoes with good support, i.e., jogging shoes. When walking, push off *from* your toes and land on your heels. Swing arms loosely at your sides. Begin with 10-minute walks and build to 20 to 30 minutes.

FIGURE 7-2, CONT'D

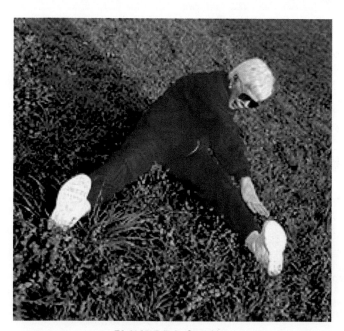

FIGURE 7-3 Stretching.

pulmonary, musculoskeletal, and neurological systems should be done.

The examination should focus on those aspects that may have an impact on functional status and that may give clues to potential risk. Attention should be focused on joint range of motion, flexibility, and strength. Previous injuries and the presence of active inflammation must be assessed. Conditions that must be stabilized before starting an exercise program include unstable angina, thrombophlebitis, cardiomyopathy, uncontrolled arrhythmias, uncompensated heart failure, high blood pressure (Beers and Berkow, 2000), and GERD.

Fitness Testing. Fitness testing may be warranted in some elders with chronic illnesses or disability and who are able to endure testing. Performance on a 7-minute walk test can help determine the intensity level to start fitness training (Beers and Berkow, 2000). It also provides feedback to the person as his or her performance improves over time.

The American College of Sports Medicine recommends exercise tolerance testing (ETT) for the elderly person before recommending a moderately intense or vigorous exercise program. This test provides information regarding metabolic equivalents and target heart rate of the older person. ETT for frail elderly people is not recommended. A frail elder's functional impairments may hinder the ability to perform an adequate test. The strength required for ETT may exceed the aerobic capacity of a frail elder. ETT is not essential for the elder who desires to start a simple walking program or perform a moderate level of exercise as a means to improve mobility and performance of activities of daily living.

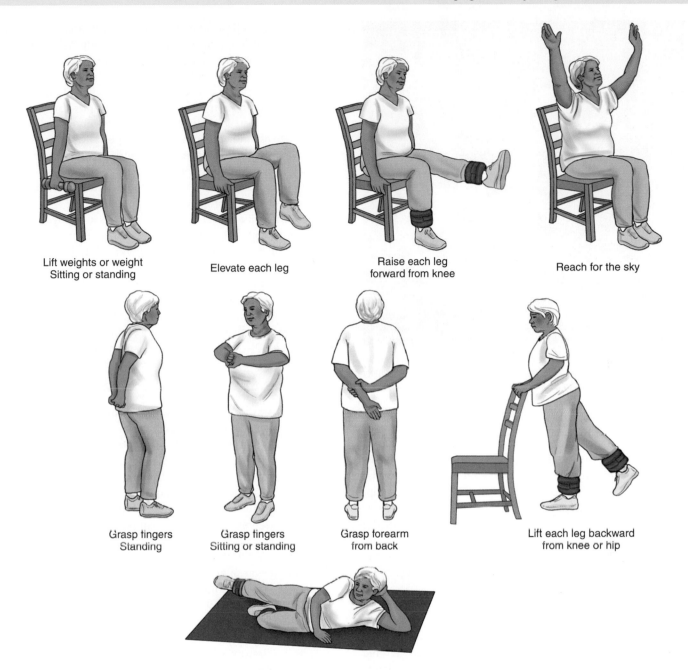

Lift weights or weight
Sitting or standing

Elevate each leg

Raise each leg
forward from knee

Reach for the sky

Grasp fingers
Standing

Grasp fingers
Sitting or standing

Grasp forearm
from back

Lift each leg backward
from knee or hip

Abduct each leg upward

FIGURE 7-4 Examples of strength-training exercises. (Modified from Centers for Disease Control and Prevention. *Growing Stronger. Strength Training for Older Adults: Exercises: Stage 1.* Available from www.cdc.gov/nccdphp/dnpa/physical/growing_stronger/exercises/index.htm. Accessed June 30, 2006.)

Exercise Supervision. Some patients should be supervised during exercise testing and the exercise program. This may be done in a rehabilitation center. These patients include those with acquired valvular heart disease, those with a recent myocardial infarction, congenital heart disease, angina, ventricular arrhythmias, severe coronary artery disease of three vessels or the main vessel, two previous myocardial infarctions, an ejection fraction of less than 30%, heart disease symptoms at rest or in very-low-intensity activity, and those who have a drop in systolic blood pressure with exercise (Beers and Berkow, 2000).

The risk of cardiac events in sedentary older women is greater than in younger individuals. Elderly women exercise less than elderly men and are at higher risk for deconditioning. However, a review of randomized, controlled exercise trials confirms a low rate of myocardial infarction and cardiovascular complications (George and Goldberg, 2001). A concern is the usual increase in blood pressure during resistance exercise. Large changes in blood pressure during exercise can be avoided if older women are educated about avoiding the Valsalva maneuver and maintaining normal breathing patterns.

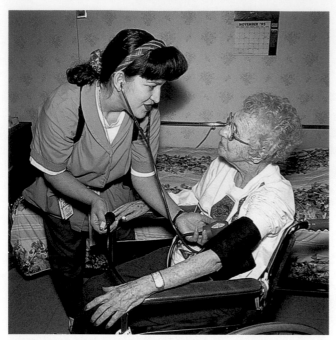

Assessment of the older person's medical and functional states should be performed before beginning an exercise program. (From Lewis SM, Heitkemper MM, Dirksen SR: *Medical-surgical nursing: assessment and management of clinical problems,* ed 7, St Louis, 2007, Mosby.)

Laboratory. Laboratory analysis should include a hematocrit ratio and a hemoglobin level (see Chapter 5). A low hematocrit ratio and hemoglobin level will increase the workload on the heart to maintain an adequate oxygen supply. In addition, analysis of electrolyte and fluid balance is necessary to evaluate conductivity and contractility of the cardiac muscle and its ability to function adequately. Lipid levels may be obtained to evaluate positive change, and thyroid studies may be obtained if this is a possible reason for inactivity.

Interventions

Exercise Prescription. Types of exercise may be prescribed that will be therapeutic for different patients: aerobic activity, resistance training, flexibility training, and balance training. The patients' levels of fitness and medical problems will be considered before prescribing. Those who are markedly deconditioned will need to start very slowly. For example, a patient with severe COPD can begin treadmill exercises at a slow rate (Beers and Berkow, 2000). Patients with difficulty standing can perform seated exercise programs using cuff weights or no weights for flexibility training. Elders with arthritis benefit from water exercises. The prescription is most effective if the nurse finds activities that the patient most enjoys.

The CDC recommends that all adults participate in at least 30 minutes of exercise over a 24-hour period and do it 5 days each week (2004). Three 10-minute activities meet the goal and may work best for elders who cannot do 30 minutes at one time. The ability to talk while exercising suggests how well or how long one can exercise; if one can talk easily while exercising, the exercise intensity level is low or moderate for that person. If talking is difficult, the intensity may be too high.

The elder may be able to integrate activity into daily life rather than doing a specific exercise. Examples are walking to the store instead of driving, golfing, swimming, hiking, raking leaves, and gardening. When especially low-intensity exercise is needed, the person can work for 2 to 3 minutes, rest for 2 to 3 minutes, and continue the pattern for 15 to 20 minutes. Patients who are deconditioned will improve markedly with this program.

Low-intensity aerobic exercise includes walking, cycling on level terrain, light stretching (flexibility) exercises, swimming on a float, and light housework. With low-intensity work, talking and singing are possible; there is no muscle pain, and the elder does not perspire (Beers and Berkow, 2000).

Moderate-intensity exercise includes walking fast, cycling fast, golfing with a cart or walking, light calisthenics, treading water, and heavy housework or yard work (Beers and Berkow, 2000). Talking is possible with moderate activity but singing is not. Perspiration occurs when activity is sustained. Muscles do not hurt or feel strained.

High-intensity exercises for the very fit include walking or jogging at 5 miles per hour (mph), cycling at 11 to 12 mph, swimming 0.5 mile in 30 minutes, playing tennis, and hiking. Talking will be difficult with high-intensity activities. Perspiration will occur, and with time, the muscles will feel weak or rubbery (Beers and Berkow, 2000). It is recommended that a rating of perceived exertion be used rather than self-monitoring the pulse rate during exercise, which is usually inaccurate and less revealing than the signs and symptoms just listed with each exercise level.

Walking is the most common exercise of older adults in the United States; about 50% walk for exercise (Beers and Berkow, 2000). The mortality rate is reduced 50% in those elders who walk at least 2 miles per day. Walking reduces the risk of new heart disease and falls and helps heal those with chronic heart disease.

The respiratory system indicates intolerance to activity when dyspnea is evident or when the respiratory rate increases during the activity. The cheeks, lips, and nail beds become red (flushed), pallid, or cyanotic with intolerance, and exercise should cease immediately. Fatigue, tiredness, and the need to sit down are additional signs of inability to tolerate the activity. Obviously, tightness and heaviness in the chest and tightness in the legs are indicative of activity that has gone too far. If nothing occurs within the expected tolerance level but the nurse notices that the person is slowing down, shows signs of decreased dexterity or coordination, and needs frequent rests, the person is not able to tolerate that level of activity.

A sustained brisk walk is one of the most popular and accessible forms of activity for the elderly. Those who have done little walking are encouraged to start slowly by first walking to the corner of the block and eventually being able to develop the capacity for distance walking of several miles. Those limited to institutional facilities should also be encouraged to increase the amount of walking. At first it may be only from the bed to the bathroom, then over time a walk down the hall, and eventually around the total facility. If the person can go outside, walking around the block might be a long-term goal. This exercise should be done on a regular basis, if not daily.

Exercise Programs. Participation in exercise programs is influenced by a number of factors. Among a group of mall walkers, those told to exercise by their physician perceived significantly greater susceptibility and severity of health problems if they did not walk than those not told by their physician to walk. Motivating the elderly person to change his or her behavior is not always easy, but usually, if the exercise or activity is one that the elder chooses, compliance will be greater.

The following variables reflect critical characteristics of exercise programs that improve long-term compliance:

1. Low to moderate intensity, duration, and frequency of exercise
2. Group participation and social pleasure
3. Emphasis on variety and pleasure, including use of games as exercise
4. Setting personal goals or developing contracts
5. Evaluation of response to training and clear demonstration of improvement
6. Involvement of friends, family, or spouse
7. Use of music
8. Positive feedback at each session
9. Enthusiastic leadership and role models

Enjoyment and individualization of the program to meet individual goals and needs are key factors in improving long-term participation. Another consideration for many older adults is the expense associated with the exercise program. Many elderly people have limited financial reserves for recreational purposes. These kinds of programs are free at some neighborhood senior centers.

It is also important that the individuals who conduct aerobic exercise programs and classes consider differences between the abilities of young and old. Classes are generally taught by young and fit persons who may become so involved in what they are doing that they are unaware that the elderly person may not be able to do the number of repetitions they consider necessary for strengthening muscles. These programs can damage the muscles, tendons, ligaments, and joints of the older adult. Training older fit women or men to lead aerobic exercise programs is helpful; participants can identify and bond with the leaders, which increases compliance. A variety of exercise programs exist for the elderly person. These programs need to be evaluated on an individual basis to determine if they are appropriate. The instructor's qualifications should be determined (AARP, 2006). The instructor must have the ability to deal with health conditions that will be present among class partici-

pants. If taking an aquatics class or swimming, find out if the pool is clean and if a lifeguard is on duty. Is the pool well lit, and are walking areas slippery? Sample programs for endurance, muscle strengthening, balance training, and flexibility are seen in Figures 7-2 and 7-4.

Senior Games. Senior centers throughout the United States have instituted physical fitness programs, which include Ping-Pong, bocce, golf, horseshoes, and many other activities enjoyed by many older adults. These activities incorporate rhythmic action and stretching and provide improvement in or maintenance of cardiopulmonary function, muscle tone, and mental stimulation.

All 50 states in the United States promote "Senior Games" in collaboration with public service and private corporations. These are Olympic-style competitions for men and women 55 years of age and older—even for those aged "100+". The 2007 games were held in Louisville, Kentucky, for a 2-week period and included such sports as archery, badminton, basketball, bowling, cycling, golf, horseshoes, race walking, racquetball, road racing, shuffleboard, softball, swimming, table tennis, tennis, track and field sports (e.g., javelin throw), a triathlon, and volleyball. The National Senior Games Association is a not-for-profit member of the U.S. Olympics Committee (National Senior Games Association, 2006).

Dancing. For those accustomed to it, ballroom, folk, or square dancing should be encouraged. This form of activity done properly can have as much aerobic benefit as workouts to music videotapes. Dancing is kind to the joints and can burn as many calories as swimming, biking, or walking. However, it should not be done as the only form of activity because it does not develop upper body strength in most situations. To enhance cardiovascular and respiratory fitness, one would have to engage in 20 to 30 minutes of sustained dancing. Dancing provides another means of obtaining pleasant, sociable, vigorous exercise, which tones the body and benefits cardiopulmonary and mental health.

Swimming. Swimming, one of America's most popular sports, or water exercise facilitates muscle tone and improves circulation, muscle strength, endurance, flexibility, and weight control; it can also be relaxing and a mood elevator. The benefits of aquatic activity or exercise therapy are that arm and leg movements against water are less painful and do not seem to require as much effort because of the buoyancy of the water. Some elders maintain a swimming program begun earlier in life; others enjoy this as a relaxing new way to become active and socialize. Those who do not know how to swim or who do not swim well might benefit from water exercise classes such as "water walking" held in the shallow end of the pool. The YWCA, many community health centers, and the American Red Cross offer classes in these types of activities. The Arthritis Foundation co-sponsors with the YMCA many aquatic exercise programs across the United

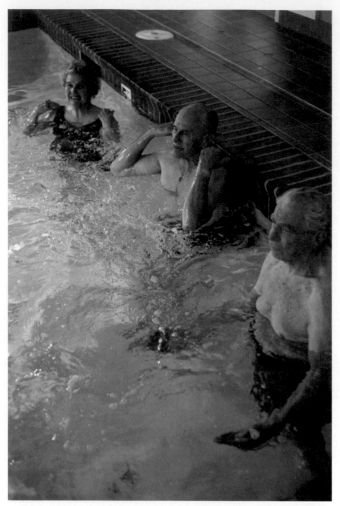

Aquatic exercise programs are beneficial for elders with mobility problems; improves circulation, muscle strength, and endurance; and provides socialization and relaxation. (Copyright © Getty Images.)

States. Not all are at the YMCA; some are at other neighborhood pools. One of the authors (AL) entered her zip code and found nearly 50 programs in her local area. Elders with mobility problems move at ease in water; many programs offer basic and advanced aquatic exercises.

Different Forms of Exercises. Tai chi can improve the quality of life for all people and especially for elders with arthritis, other musculoskeletal disorders, and balance problems. It includes agile steps and exercises that improve mobility, breathing, and relaxation. Some forms use 12 movements—6 basic and 6 advanced—and continue to challenge the participant by reversing the direction of the movements (Arthritis Foundation, 2006). It is said to increase energy, whereas other exercises dissipate energy. Many who practice it believe that it refreshes, calms, increases flexibility, and helps with arthritis pain (see Chapter 3).

The older adult can participate socially in a community class or at a health care center or even purchase or obtain from the library a video to practice at home. Tapes and videos

are available on tai chi for seniors (Tai Chi, 2006). In China and Japan, workers take tai chi breaks; students take tai chi in physical education classes, and seniors practice balance and calmness in small groups (see Chapter 3).

Yoga is another form of exercise that can be practiced regardless of one's condition. It is a method of concentration and meditation and can foster mental alacrity, independence, and good health in the late life through simple exercise, relaxation, meditation, and nutritional education.

Isotonic exercises train the cardiovascular and skeletal muscles. Isometrics work mainly with the cardiovascular system. Persons who are confined to a bed or chair or who are ambulatory can do these rhythmical tasks or calisthenics.

Exercise should be aerobic in nature and easily attained and not produce an oxygen debt. Numerous programs have been developed in which simplicity and flexibility of the program make it easily adaptable to a variety of settings. Guidelines include the following:

- Teach to avoid sudden twisting movements, rapid movements, and rapid transitions from one movement to the next.
- Avoid sustained isometric contractions of longer than 10 seconds.
- Assess ability to tolerate low-level activity without signs and symptoms of muscle fatigue, shortness of breath, angina, arrhythmias, abnormal blood pressure, or intermittent claudication.
- Stop exercising if arrhythmias, angina, or excessive breathlessness occurs.
- Avoid exercise during acute viral infections.
- Increase activity slowly by intensity, duration, and frequency.
- Monitor exercise intensity by perceived exertion and exercise heart rate.
- Perform a gradual, extended exercise warm-up (at least 15 minutes) to maximize flexibility and decrease muscle injury.
- Perform cool down for 5 to 10 minutes after exercising.
- Modify exercise program up or down based on individual responses.

Special Needs of Older Adults

It is also important to address the special needs of elderly people when initiating an exercise program. The elderly are less able to adapt to the environment during exercise. They should dress in layers to adjust to different environmental temperatures. Well-fitting footwear and stockings are essential to prevent injury if foot sensation is impaired such as that which occurs in diabetes mellitus and other neuropathic disorders. If perception is impaired, such as in diabetes, blisters and friction injuries may occur without the elderly person knowing it. Maintaining hydration is essential. Consumption of fluid before exercising and regularly while exercising is recommended. Environments with poor air quality should be avoided for exercise, including areas near roadways.

Often when beginning a physical exercise program, muscles will be sore. Warm, not hot, baths or soaks are excellent. Another way to minimize muscle soreness is a 5- to 10-minute cool down period of slow walking or stretching to keep the primary muscle groups active, to decrease venous pooling, and to increase venous return to the heart.

Nurses should capitalize more than they do on function—activities of daily living, such as providing the person with bath brushes to wash their own backs in the shower or bathtub and encouraging the person to dry body parts or rub the back dry with a towel. Reaching for objects while cleaning house can be included in an activity program, as can washing dishes in warm water to provide finger exercises. Warm water helps relieve stiffness and enables the fingers to move more easily without discomfort. Various exercises for bed, chair, and standing are presented in Figures 7-2 and 7-4. This does not cover the numerous maneuvers that exist but, rather, gives a sampling of possible movements.

Housekeeping activities can be utilized for strength and flexibility. Community-dwelling elders can be taught simple approaches in utilizing household chores for activity. The elderly in long-term care who are able and enjoy helping others could be encouraged to push wheelchairs, clean tables, and run errands.

Other activities that can be done while watching television or whenever there are a few spare minutes during the day are rolling a pencil between the hand and a hard surface, squeezing a rubber ball, lifting each leg 20 times, exaggerating the chewing motion of the jaw, holding the stomach in, tightening the buttocks, flexing the fingers, and rotating the head and the ankles. Figures 7-2 and 7-4 model these and other more formal exercises easy for the older person to do each day.

Activity, in general, should be paced and occur regularly every day. Activities that will help eliminate stiffness should be planned for the morning, when stiffness is most prevalent. Relaxation exercises should be considered before bedtime to help induce sleep. With any activity in which elders are involved, sufficient intermittent rest periods should be provided. An example of a small-group exercise program is presented in Box 7-17.

In summary, this chapter has looked at the life support needs individually. It is apparent that each area influences the function of others. Persons would not continue to survive if these needs could not be met independently or without the assistance of others. The quality and the overall perception of life can be augmented when the nurse monitors these specific functions and provides assistance to the elder needing support.

BOX 7-17   **Movements for Geriatric Patients**

The progression should be from smaller, more personal movements to larger ones that may involve communication with the rest of the group. Movements should begin slowly and later develop speed. The amount of balance required should be minimal at first and more later, when the patients feel more secure and uninhibited. A sample class might be as follows:

1. Scratch the small of your back against the chair. Now try your upper back, too.
2. Begin by pretending to wash your face, then your arms and shoulders and neck.
3. Stretch up as high as you can; now sink down as low as you can. Now try to reach as far forward as possible; now out to each side.
4. Can you nod your head up and down as if to say *"Yes?"* Now try *"No."* Now an even stronger *"No!"*
5. Let's try marching in place to the music. You may use one or both feet.
6. Let's try making circles with different parts of our body. Start with one shoulder. Try both shoulders. Try one hand, now the other hand. Can you reverse directions?
7. How about kicking one leg at a time up in the air as the music gets louder?

8. Let's have one half of the group kick while the other half stomps. Now let's reverse.
9. Can you now reach out as if you're trying to shake hands with the person across the circle from you?
10. Now try actually shaking hands with the person next to you. How about the person on the other side?
11. Now, let's all take a huge deep breath and stretch as tall and as long as possible. Now let the air out slowly and let your head, back, and arms deflate slowly as a balloon. Try it again; take in even more air. Now deflate even more slowly.

The above is a simple example of what can be done with a small group of 6 to 10 patients. It is advisable, if possible, to have an extra person present to help encourage patients and monitor safety.

The goals that may be achieved are many and varied. They include increased range of motion and strength, increased balance and coordination, and increased cardiovascular function if the class takes place for at least 20 minutes on a regular basis. Nonphysical goals may be greater social interaction, communication with others who are limited in function or disabled in the same or different ways, and greater self-awareness.

From Fond D. *Coordinator* 2:30, Mar 1983.

Human Needs and Wellness Diagnoses

Self-Actualization and Transcendence
(Seeking, Expanding, Spirituality, Fulfillment)
Recognizes that physiology does not limit spirit
Finds fulfillment in activities
suitable to limitations

Self-Esteem and Self-Efficacy
(Image, Identity, Control, Capability)
Maintains independence in ADLs and IADLs
to level of ability and competence
Makes appropriate lifestyle choices

Belonging and Attachment
(Love, Empathy, Affiliation)
Recognizes importance of companionship
Maintains close relationships
with some confidantes
Recognizes significance of relationships
to physical health and morale

Safety and Security
(Caution, Planning, Protections, Sensory Acuity)
Uses assistive devices as needed
Uses visual and hearing aids appropriately
Modifies living quarters to avoid accidents
Monitors medications for appropriate usage

Biological and Physiological Integrity
(Air, Fluids, Comfort, Activity, Nutrition, Elimination, Skin Integrity)
Aware of and responsive to subtle body signals
Adapts to changing physiological need
Exercises daily to extent of comfort, ability, and tolerance
Cares for skin to avoid bruises and lesions

These are not all the possible wellness diagnoses that may be identified. The above
are examples of nursing diagnoses that should be considered when planning care
for the older adult.

KEY CONCEPTS

- Interruptions in the basic requirements for nutrition, fluids, elimination, activity, and rest may trigger exacerbations of subclinical and chronic disorders.
- When basic needs are out of balance, it is common for the very old to exhibit mental status changes.
- Medications may interfere with adequate food intake and elimination.
- UI is a symptom of an underlying problem and needs thorough assessment. Many therapeutic modalities are available for treatment of UI.

- Deep, stage-4 sleep is not attained in late life. Older persons tend to be easily aroused. The nursing focus is to help them understand the changes and their sleep pattern and that their individual needs to obtain sufficient rest will vary.
- Sleep apnea is an interruption in breathing during sleep that has been linked to excess pharyngeal tissue, cardiac problems, cerebral infarction, and hypertension. It may be demonstrated by long periods without inspiring and loud snoring on expiration. The long periods of anoxia may have effects, over time, on cerebration.
- Physical activity (and the ease with which it is performed) is often the barometer by which an individual's health and wellness are judged.

CASE STUDY: Elimination

Stella, at 78 years old, had never had problems with her bowel movements. They had been regular—each morning about an hour after breakfast. In fact, she hardly thought about them because they had been so regular. While hospitalized for podiatric surgery last year, she never regained her usual pattern of bowel function. She was greatly distressed by this because it had been a symbol to her of her good health. Admittedly, she did not move about as much now or as well and had begun using a cane. And she had heard that pain medications sometimes made one constipated, so she tried to use them very sparingly despite the pain. She tried to reestablish her pattern of having a bowel movement every morning after breakfast but with little success. She now began to worry about constipation and to use laxatives. She thought, "This constipation really upsets me. I just don't feel like myself if I don't have a bowel movement every day."

Based on the case study, develop a nursing care plan using the following procedure*:

- List Stella's comments that provide subjective data.
- List information that provides objective data.
- From these data, identify and state, using accepted format, two nursing diagnoses you determine are most significant to Stella at this time. List two of Stella's strengths that you have identified from the data.
- Determine and state outcome criteria for each diagnosis. These must reflect some alleviation of the problem iden-

tified in the nursing diagnosis and must be stated in concrete and measurable terms.
- Plan and state one or more interventions for each diagnosed problem. Provide specific documentation of the source used to determine the appropriate intervention. Plan at least one intervention that incorporates Stella's existing strengths.
- Evaluate the success of the intervention. Interventions must correlate directly with the stated outcome criteria to measure the outcome success.

Critical Thinking Questions

1. What information will you need to obtain from Stella to help her determine the causes of her constipation?
2. What advice will you give Stella regarding the use of laxatives?
3. What dietary changes will you suggest to her, and how will you do this to motivate compliance?
4. What information regarding the relationship of medications to constipation will be useful to Stella?
5. When you are constipated, how do you feel?
6. Do you know any elders who focus a lot of their conversation on elimination? How do you handle that? How should you handle that?

* Students are advised to refer to their nursing diagnosis text and identify possible or potential problems.

CASE STUDY: Rest and Sleep

Gerald, 80 years old, had a sleeping disorder and was tired most of the day and lonely at night. His wife of 45 years had recently moved into her sewing room on the couch at night because she could no longer cope with his loud snoring. He sometimes even seemed to stop breathing, which kept her awake watching his abdomen rise and fall, or not. Sometimes he would awaken suddenly, gasping for air. However, he had tolerated it because he thought nothing could be done for it. Because it had become a threat to his marriage, he became motivated to investigate possible solutions. Gerald said to his nurse clinician, "This isn't anything, but it upsets my wife." Though he did not admit it, he was also worried because he was beginning to feel rather weak and listless during the day. When he had consulted the clinic nurse, Gerald was diagnosed with obstructive sleep apnea. He found that some very practical means of dealing with this problem of sleep apnea were available, and if these were not effective she had reassured him that additional medical interventions could be helpful.

Based on the case study, develop a nursing care plan using the following procedure*:

- List Gerald's comments that provide subjective data.
- List information that provides objective data.
- From these data, identify and state, using accepted format, two nursing diagnoses you determine are most sig-

nificant to Gerald at this time. List two of Gerald's strengths that you have identified from the data.
- Determine and state outcome criteria for each diagnosis. These must reflect some alleviation of the problem identified in the nursing diagnosis and must be stated in concrete and measurable terms.
- Plan and state one or more interventions for each diagnosed problem. Provide specific documentation of the source used to determine the appropriate intervention. Plan at least one intervention that incorporates Gerald's existing strengths.
- Evaluate the success of the intervention. Interventions must correlate directly with the stated outcome criteria to measure the outcome success.

Critical Thinking Questions

1. What lifestyle factors may be increasing Gerald's episodes of sleep apnea?
2. In what circumstances is sleep apnea particularly dangerous to health?
3. Compose a list of 10 questions you would ask Gerald to obtain a clear picture of factors contributing to his sleep apnea. Discuss the rationale behind each.
4. List some of the common methods for dealing with this problem that Gerald's nurse may have given to him.

* Students are advised to refer to their nursing diagnosis text and identify possible or potential problems.

CASE STUDY: Exercise and Activity

Tom, 75 years old, had lost his wife Ella a year ago and had been feeling down and tired much of each day. He had retired at age 70 from his job as a housing contractor and had spent much of his time with Ella. They had been married for 50 years. He now sometimes seemed to sit in front of the television most of the day without actually remembering what it was that he had seen. Many of the couple's friends had moved away or to retirement settings, and other than his daughter who lived about 45 minutes drive from his house, he rarely saw anyone any more. He had lived like this for nearly a year, and it had become his daily pattern of life. Tom took the initiative after a suggestion from his daughter to go to the local senior citizen center. He went and had lunch there nearly every day. At one point he was asked if he would allow a nursing student to spend time with him during her semester in a gerontology course. He agreed. In the course of her assessment, she (and he) found that his activity level was nearly completely sedentary. She gave Tom information about the ramifications of such a sedentary life. She pointed out that the center had an exercise class every day between 10 AM and 12 noon. Because he came every day (except Saturday and Sunday) for lunch, it seemed a good thing to do. Gerald said to his nursing student, "This isn't anything I am really interested in doing, but I will give it a try." Though he did not admit it, he was also worried because he usually felt weak and listless during the day after his lunch. When he did attend the first class, he found that there were basic exercises and more advanced ones for elders who had participated regularly for 6 months. He found after a few weeks that he was enjoying the social aspect of the exercise if not the exercise itself. After nearly a year of fairly regular participation, Tom began playing golf with some of the men from the center. Once he attended a dance.

Based on the case study, develop a nursing care plan for the nursing student using the following procedure*:
- List Tom's comments that provide subjective data.
- List information that provides objective data.
- From these data identify and state, using accepted format, two nursing diagnoses you determine are most significant to Tom at this time. List two of Tom's strengths that you have identified from these data.
- Determine and state outcome criteria for each diagnosis. These must reflect some alleviation of the problem identified in the nursing diagnosis and must be stated in concrete and measurable terms.
- Plan and state one or more interventions for each diagnosed problem. Provide specific documentation of the source used to determine the appropriate intervention. Plan at least one intervention that incorporates Tom's existing strengths.
- Evaluate the success of the intervention. Interventions must correlate directly with the stated outcome criteria to measure the outcome success.

Critical Thinking Questions

1. What lifestyle factors that Tom had developed after his wife Ella's death became dangerous to his health?
2. Compose a list of 10 questions you would ask Tom to obtain a clear picture of factors contributing to his activity level. Discuss the rationale behind each.
3. List some of the common methods for motivating Tom that his nursing student may have used.
4. Describe the level of activity that Tom should begin with and what symptoms he might expect as he increases his activity.

* Students are advised to refer to their nursing diagnosis text and identify possible or potential problems.

RESEARCH QUESTIONS

Elimination

What are the specific concerns elders harbor related to constipation?

Is concern with constipation a sociocultural artifact?

Do childhood training experiences affect one's eliminatory functions in late life?

What are the remedies for constipation most often deemed effective as perceived by elders?

Does fecal impaction affect urinary incontinence?

Rest and Sleep

How do sleep patterns correlate with various disease states?

How do sleep patterns change with each decade after age 50 years?

What is the average time of the total sleep cycle as experienced by a healthy individual older than 70 years?

How much does exercise contribute to a good night's sleep?

What is the effect of nonpharmacological interventions on sleep?

Activity

How does activity level affect various disease states? How do activity patterns change with each decade after age 50 years? How are they different in men and women?

What is the average time of activity Tom should plan to give each day as a man 70 years of age?

How does exercise contribute to one's sense of well-being?

RESOURCES*

Association of Women's Health, Obstetric and Neonatal Nurses (Continence Clinical Practice Guidelines and UI Information)
2000 I. Street, Suite 740
Washington, DC 20036
(202) 261-2400
www.awhonn.org

Home Delivery Incontinent Supplies Co., Inc
1315 Dielman Industrial Court
Olivette, MO 63132
(800) 269-4663
www.hdis.com

International Continence Society
www.continenceworldwide.org

*See the Resources section on p. 63 for additional resources on exercise and aging.

National Association for Continence
(Lay and Professional Education, UI Products)
PO Box 1019
Charleston, SC 29402
www.nafc.org

National Center on Sleep Disorders Research
www.nhibi.nih.gov/sleep

National Sleep Foundation
www.sleepfoundation.org

Society of Urologic Nurses and Associates
East Holly Ave, Box 56
Pittman, NJ 08071
(888) 827-7862
www.suna.org

Wound, Ostomy and Continence Nurses Society
4700 Lake Avenue
Glenview, IL 60025
(888) 224-WOCN
www.wocn.org

REFERENCES

American Association of Retired Persons (AARP): *Making a splash with water workouts* (website): *www.aarp.org/health/fitness/work_out/a2003-07-21-waterworkout.html*. Accessed June 30, 2006.

American Medical Directors Association (AMDA): *Clinical practice guideline: urinary incontinence* (website): *www.amda.com*, Columbia, Md, 1996, The Association.

Ancoli-Israel S: Sleep disturbances among patients with dementia. In Sleep disorders in the geriatric population: implications for health, *Clin Geriatrics Suppl* Dec 2005, American Geriatric Society.

Arthritis Foundation: *Aquatic program* (website): *www.arthritis.org/events/getinvolved/ProgramsServices/aquaticprogram.asp*. Accessed June 30, 2006.

Arthritis Foundation: Tai Chi from the Arthritis Foundation® (website): *www.arthritis.org/events/getinvolved/ProgramsServices/taichi.asp*. Accessed June 30, 2006.

Beers MH, Berkow R: *The Merck manual of geriatrics*, ed 3, Whitehouse Station, NJ, 2000-2006, Merck Research Laboratories.

Bradway C, Hernly S: Nursing standard-of-practice protocol: urinary incontinence in older adults admitted to acute care, *Geriatr Nurs* 19(2):98-102, 1998.

Busse D et al: The Pittsburgh Sleep Quality Index: a new instrument for psychiatric practice and research, *J Psychiatr Res* 28(2):193-213, 1989.

Centers for Disease Control and Prevention (CDC) and Merck Institute of Aging & Health: *The state of aging and health in America 2004* (websites): *www.cdc.gov/aging; www.miahonline.org; www.merck.com/mrkshared/mmg/home.jsp.*

Dash M et al: Urinary incontinence: the Social Health Maintenance Organization's approach, *Geriatr Nurs* 25:81-89, 2004.

Dixon D: The Wellspring model: implications for LTC, *Caring for the Ages* 3(3):18-21, 2002.

Drazen JM: Perspective, sleep apnea syndrome, *N Engl J Med* 346(6):390, 2002.

Edwards WF: Gastrointestinal problems. In Cotter VT, Strumpf NE, editors: *Advanced practice nursing with older adults*, New York, 2002, McGraw-Hill.

Eliopoulos C: *Gerontological nursing*, ed 5, Philadelphia, 2001, Lippincott.

Fantl JA et al: Managing acute and chronic urinary incontinence. In *Clinical practice guideline: quick reference guide for clinicians*, No 2, 1996 update, AHCPR Pub No 97-0686, Rockville, Md, 1996, U.S. Department of Health and Human Services, Public Health Service, Agency for Health Care Policy and Research.

Fielo S: The mystery of sleep: how nurses can help the elderly, *Nurs Spectr* Oct:30, 2001.

Fourcroy JL: Overactive bladder, *Adv Nurse Pract* 9(3):59-62, 2001.

George B, Goldberg N: The benefits of exercise in geriatric women, *Am J Geriatr Cardiol* 10(5):260, 2001.

Griffith R: *Treating insomnia in the elderly*, 2002 (website): *www.healthandage.com*.

Ham R et al: *Primary care geriatrics*, ed 4, St Louis, 2002, Mosby.

Hill-O'Neill KA, Shaughnessy M: Dizziness and stroke. In Cotter VT, Strumpf N, editors: *Advanced practice nursing with older adults*, New York, 2002, McGraw-Hill.

Holroyd-Leduc JM, Straus SE: Management of urinary incontinence in women: clinical applications, *JAMA* 291(8):997-999, 2004.

Karani T et al: Exercise in the healthy older adult, *Am J Geriatr Cardiol* 10(5):269, 2001.

Kennie D et al: Health promotion and physical activity. In Tallis RC, Fillit HM, editors: *Brocklehurst's textbook of geriatric medicine and gerontology*, ed 6, Spain, 2003, Churchill Livingstone.

Kirkwood C: *Treatment of insomnia*, New York, 2001, Power-Pak, CE Publishers (website): *www.powerpak*.com.

Lekan-Rutledge D: Diffusion of innovation: a model for implementation of prompted voiding in long-term care settings, *J Gerontol Nurs* 26(4):25-33, 2000.

Lekan-Rutledge D, Colling J: Urinary incontinence in the frail elderly: Even when it's too late to prevent a problem, you can slow its progress, *Am J Nurs* (suppl): 36-46, 2003.

Lewy AJ: Circadian rhythm disruptions in the older adult. In Sleep disorders in the geriatric population: implications for health, *Clin Geriatrics Suppl* Dec 2005. American Geriatric Society.

MacDonald DG, Butler L: Silent no more: Elderly women's stories of living with urinary incontinence in long-term care, *J Gerontol Nurs* 33(1):14-20, 2007.

Mason DJ et al: Changing UI practice, *Am J Nurs* 3(suppl):2-3, 2003.

McCance KL, Huether SE. *Pathophysiology*, ed 5, St Louis, 2006, Mosby.

McCullough P: *How well do you sleep?* Presentation at the Kentucky Council of Nurse Practitioners and Midwives, Lexington, Ky, April 2001.

Midthurn S et al: Urinary tract infections, *J Gerontolog Nurs* 30(6):4-9, 2004.

National Institute on Aging: *It's never too late to start* (exercise pamphlet, Spanish) (website): *www.nia.nih.gov/news/pr/2002*.

National Institute of Health Senior Health, *An exercise story* (website): *nihseniorhealth.gov/stories/ct_ruth.html/aug/2005*. Accessed on June 30, 2006.

National Senior Games Association (website): *www.seniorgames.org*. Accessed June 30, 2006.

National Sleep Foundation: Aging gracefully and sleeping well, 2007 (website). *www.sleepfoundation.org*. Accessed January 30, 2007.

Newman D: Stress urinary incontinence in woman, *Am J Nurs* 103(8):47-56, 2003.

Newman DK, Palmer MH, editors: The state of the science on urinary incontinence, *Am J Nurs* 3(suppl):1-58, 2003.

Omnicare: *Geriatric guidelines 2006*, Covington Ky, 2006, Omnicare.

Palmer M, Newman D: Bladder control: educational needs of older adults, *J Gerontolog Nurs* 32(1):28-32, 2006.

Phillips B: Sleep apnea, periodic limb movement, restless legs syndrome, and cardiovascular complications, *Clin Geriatrics Suppl* Dec 2005, American Geriatric Society.

Remmel K et al: *Handbook of symptom-oriented neurology*, ed 3, St Louis, 2002, Mosby.

Remsburg RE et al: Two models of restorative nursing care in the nursing home: designated versus integrated restorative nursing assistants, *Geriatr Nurs* 20(6):322-326, 1999.

Reuben D et al: *Geriatrics at your fingertips 2006-2007*, ed 8, New York, 2006, American Geriatric Society.

Richter JE: Functional disorders of the gastrointestinal tract. In Abrams WB et al, editors: *Merck manual of geriatrics*, ed 2, Whitehouse Station, NJ, 1995, Merck Research Laboratories.

Rosto L: Sleep and the elderly, *Advance for Providers of Post-Acute Care* 4(6):27, 2001.

Schnelle JF, Ouslander J: CMS guidelines and improving continence care in nursing homes: The role of the medical director, *J Am Med Dir Assoc* 7(2), 2006.

Schnelle JF et al: Developing rehabilitative behavioral intervention for long-term care: technology transfer, acceptance, and maintenance issues, *J Am Geriatr Soc* 46(6):771-777, 1998.

Schoenborn C et al, Centers for Disease Control and Prevention, U.S. Department of Health and Human Services, National Center for Health Statistics: *Health characteristics of adults 55 years of age and over: United States, 2000-2003*. Advance data from Vital and Health Statistics No 370, April 11, 2006.

Schoenfelder DP, Culp KR: Sleep pattern disturbance. In Maas ML et al, editors: *Nursing care of older adults: diagnoses, outcomes, and interventions*, St Louis, 2001, Mosby.

Staab A, Hodges LC: *Essentials of geriatric nursing*, Philadelphia, 1996, Lippincott.

Tabloski PA: *Gerontological nursing*, Upper Saddle River, NJ, 2006, Pearson/Prentice Hall.

Tai Chi for Health Institute, *Tai Chi for seniors* (website): *www.taichiforseniorsvideo.com/*. Accessed June 30, 2006.

Taunton R et al: Continent or incontinent: that is the question, *J Gerontolog Nurs* 31(9):37-44, 2005.

U.S. Department of Health and Human Services: *Healthy People 2010*, Hyattsville, Md, 2002, Public Health Service.

Wasson JH, Bruskewitz RC: Disorders of the lower genitourinary tract: bladder, prostate, testes. In Abrams WB et al, editors: *The Merck manual of geriatrics*, Rahway NJ, 1990, Merck Sharpe & Dohme, Research Laboratories.

Weiss B: Selecting medications for the treatment of urinary incontinence, *Am Fam Physician* 71(2):315, 2005.

Wells TJ: Nursing research on urinary incontinence, *Urol Nurs* 14(3):109-112, 1994.

Wyman J: Treatment of urinary incontinence in men and older women, *Am J Nurs* 3(suppl):38-45, 2003.

CHAPTER 8

Biological Maintenance Needs

Ann Schmidt Luggen and Kathleen Jett

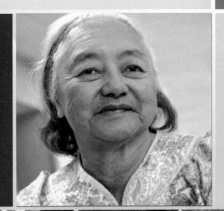
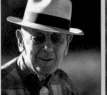
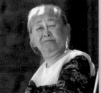

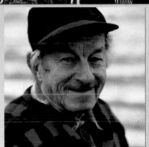

AN ELDER SPEAKS

My legs are so large and so heavy. I am hardly walking anymore.

AnnaLouise, 86 years old

LEARNING OBJECTIVES

On completion of this chapter, the reader will be able to:

1. Describe health promotion components of maintenance needs.
2. Identify common dental, foot, and skin problems of the elderly.
3. Use standard assessment tools to assess buccal cavity, feet, and skin.
4. Identify preventive, maintenance, and restorative measures for dental, foot, and skin health.
5. Establish selected nursing diagnoses on the basis of assessment for dental, foot, and skin health and care.
6. Make a plan of care for prevention and maintenance of dental, foot, and skin health.
7. Identify nursing interventions that promote healthy aging in the presence of alterations in oral or skin functioning.

Biological maintenance needs are not only essential to life but also have direct and indirect effects on one's psychosocial well-being. However, for some unexplainable reason, some patients are well cared for from neck to ankles, instead of from head to toe. Under normal circumstances, teeth and feet receive cursory or minimal attention in the overall care of the client. When care in an institutional setting is rushed because of a "busy day" or a "heavy assignment," the care of the teeth and feet is most frequently omitted. Skin care fares better. Much attention is directed to preventing and alleviating pressure, but other important integumentary influences such as friction, shearing force, moisture, and nutrition are not addressed as carefully.

In this chapter we discuss the basic needs necessary to maintain health and the nursing interventions to promote basic health while aging as related to the mouth, feet, and skin.

ORAL HEALTH

Oral health, especially dental health, is a basic need that is increasingly neglected with advanced age, debilitation, and limited mobility. One reason for this neglect may be the general assumption that most older people are edentulous. Some elders themselves may believe that losing their teeth is a natural consequence of growing old. For many years it was. Recall George Washington and his wooden false teeth. In the 1960s, more than 70% of elders older than 75 years were edentulous (American Geriatric Society [AGS], 2006). The problem with this attitude is that it has fostered neglect of an essential body part: the mouth. However, by the 1990s, fewer than 40% of those older than 75 years were edentulous, and that number is decreasing.

Orodental health can affect well-being in a variety of ways. The mouth is an important means for communication between people through speech, but much of socialization and pleasure is derived from food and drink. In terms of function, the teeth are necessary for chewing, or mastication (AGS, 2006). Orodental health is integral to general health. Gum or dental problems can put the person at risk for systemic disease. Poor oral function, poor hygiene, and chronic oral problems can raise concerns with self-presentation and fear of embarrassment that affect socialization and self-esteem. Aesthetically, the teeth support the lips and cheeks and maintain the usual distance between nose and mouth. Loss of teeth causes a dramatic change in one's appearance.

Aging teeth become worn, become darker in color, and tend to develop longitudinal cracks (Box 8-1). The dentin, or layer beneath the enamel, becomes brittle and thickens so that pulp space diminishes (AGS, 2006). It becomes less sensitive. The dentin becomes less susceptible to the effects of bacterial metabolites because permeability is lessened as a result of sclerosis of dentinal tubules. When teeth are lost, the alveolar bone beneath shrinks (see also Chapter 4).

Today the percentage of elders without natural teeth is more than 30%, primarily as a result of periodontitis, which occurs in about 95% of those older than 65 years. Nearly 50% of Americans ages 85 years and older have no natural teeth (AGS, 2006). More than one third of them have moderate to severe periodontal disease (CDC, 2004; National Institutes of Health, 2004). Prevalence of this disease is decreasing as knowledge increases and more people use fluorides, improve nutrition, engage in new oral hygiene practices, and take advantage of improved dental health care. However, the gerontological nurse in a caregiving role should realize that whether the teeth are natural or full or partial dentures, they need care.

In the existing health care system, dental care is a low priority, reflected by the absence or inadequacy of third-party reimbursement for the type of dental care needed by older adults. The number-one cause of tooth loss is the inability or the unwillingness of older adults to access and/or pay for restorative dental treatment when faced with a den-

tal disease or disorder, usually caries (AGS, 2006). Decades ago, dental care was extremely painful, and fear of the dentist still exists (Momeyer and Luggen, 2005). More than 100 million Americans still do not have access to fluoridated water to protect their teeth. Yet the per capita cost of water fluoridation over one's lifetime is less than the cost of one dental filling (Carmona, 2006). Dental insurance generally terminates when individuals reach 65 years of age or when the premium payments are too expensive, and the older adult population is less likely to go to the dentist compared with any other age-group (Centers for Disease Control and Prevention [CDC], 2001). Americans paid out of pocket for nearly one half of all dental care expenses in 2000; those older than 65 years paid more than three fourths of their dental expenses (Longley, 2004). Average out-of-pocket dental expenses are higher for the retired than the working population because national programs such as Medicare and Medicaid do not provide adequate reimbursement for tooth and dental repair. Although some states include certain dental services under Medicaid, those elderly people in nursing homes who are eligible for dental treatment often do not receive it. Elders are finding that even with insurance, their past employers and health maintenance organizations (HMOs) are paying less of the premiums and the policy holder is paying more. In one report, only 10.5% of elders did not pay any out-of-pocket expenses for dental care (Longley, 2004).

A report from the Centers for Disease Control and Prevention (CDC) indicates that both male and female elders have fewer dentist visits than any other age-group (HealthandAge, 2004). Black elders have the fewest dentist visits of any ethnic or racial group. Men do not care for their teeth as well as women do. Nearly 29% of women brush after every meal; 20.5% of men do (HealthandAge, 2004). Poor elders have about one-half the number of dentist visits as other poor age-groups. Gerontological nurses could promote healthy aging by referring them to a specific dentist who will develop an ongoing relationship with the older patient. Oral health problems are painful, costly, and preventable. Figure 8-1 shows the incidence of tooth decay over the life span.

BOX 8-1   Age Changes of the Buccal Cavity

- Decrease in the cellular compartment
- Loss of submucosal elastin in oral mucosa
- Loss of connective tissue (collagen)
- Increase in thickness of collagen fibers
- Decrease in function of minor salivary glands caused by fatty replacement of acini
- Decrease in number and quality of blood vessels and nerves
- Attrition on occlusive contact surfaces
- Enamel less permeable and teeth more brittle
- Tooth color change, yellowing
- Excessive dentin formation
- Diminished space for pulp
- Decrease in rate of cementin deposition
- Decrease in size of root canals
- Decrease in size and volume of tooth pulp
- Increase in pulp stones and dystrophic mineralization

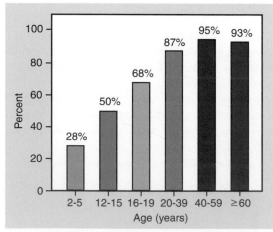

FIGURE 8-1 Dental decay over the life span.

Primary and secondary prevention strategies are effective in older adults with potential or actual dental problems (AGS, 2006; Rubenstein and Nahas, 1998). This approach will ensure good health in the successive levels of Maslow's Hierarchy of Needs (see Chapter 10).

Lack of teeth alters articulation of speech, jaw alignment, and general appearance. Persons without teeth rarely smile; they feel embarrassed and cover their mouths or withdraw from social contacts. The type and consistency of food chosen to eat become limited and monotonous. Frequently, those who are edentulous eat food that is inadequate and deficient in nutritive value. The appearance of the food is unappetizing. Further, oral pain is common and prevents eating normally. At least 7% of elders report having tooth pain twice during the past 6 months (CDC, 2001). Older adults in racial/ethnic minorities with low levels of education are more likely to report dental pain, which usually signifies advanced dental problems. Difficulty eating can be caused by lack of teeth, dental pain, ill-fitting dentures, infections, or temporomandibular joint (TMJ) problems, which can be caused by misalignment of teeth. Trouble with chewing is also related to educational level: 23% of those with 0 to 8 years of education have trouble chewing, whereas 10% of those with at least 13 years of education have problems (CDC, 2001; Vargas et al., 2001).

Common Oral Health Problems in Late Life

The primary risk factor for dental caries in older adults is poor oral hygiene (AGS, 2006). This commonly occurs because of loss of manual dexterity, loss of visual acuity, and loss of flexibility in the arms and shoulders. Eating inappropriate foods such as cakes, cookies, and gummy, sticky candies and drinking sweet drinks are other risk factors for caries at any age. Susceptibility to caries may be related to insufficient fluoride applied preventively during formative and young adult years. Heredity plays a role in susceptibility, as well as does nutrition (Mayo Clinic, 2005).

Dental caries is a major reason for tooth loss (see Figure 8-1). Caries, or decay, is demineralization and cavitation from bacteria and occurs throughout the life span (AGS, 2006). Older adults have more caries at the root surface because of periodontal diseases that expose the root surface. Advanced caries can result in necrosis of the remaining pulp, which then leads to painful abscesses. Even if the abscess does not cause a great deal of pain, treatment is essential because these infections can spread to every organ system.

Root Caries. Root caries can occur on any tooth surface. Most root caries are found on the proximal and buccal surfaces of the teeth, appearing initially as small, round, shallow, pigmented defects at the root surface. As these caries advance, they usually spread laterally and may undermine the tooth crown. With the new preventive measures available for tooth decay, the incidence has diminished. However, for the most economically or socially disadvantaged, the decline has not occurred. The percentage of older African-Americans and the

percentage of persons with very low incomes with untreated caries have increased since 1974; poor whites went from 33% in 1974 to 39% in 1994, and African-Americans went from 42% in 1974 to 47% in 1994 (Vargas et al., 2001).

Gingivitis and Periodontitis. Gingivitis and periodontitis are also major causes of tooth loss and are caused by accumulation of bacterial plaque on the teeth (Box 8-2). The bacteria invade periodontal tissues, causing an inflammatory response and destruction of connective tissues that support the tooth (Figure 8-2). Resulting problems cause loss of tooth anchorage and eventually the loss of teeth from bacterial sources. A number of drugs and medications aggravate periodontal disease. Phenytoin, calcium channel blockers, and cyclosporine cause gingival hyperplasia that bleeds easily. Antihypertensives, anticholinergics, and antipsychotics reduce saliva, which contains antimicrobials. If allowed to continue, the tooth loses stability and deep pockets around the tooth appear. Although the disease progresses and remits, it eventually leads to tooth loss if not stopped.

BOX 8-2   Contributing Factors in Periodontal Problems in Late Life

ANATOMICAL

Tooth malalignment
Thinning gingival mucosa

BACTERIAL

Plaque accumulation
Invasion of organisms at or below gum line
Food impaction

DRUGS AND METALLIC POISONS

Allergic responses
Phenytoin
Cytotoxins
Heavy metals (lead, arsenic, mercury)

EMOTIONAL AND PSYCHOMOTOR

Bruxism (grinding of teeth)
Cerebrovascular accident
Mental impairment

INTRINSIC (SYSTEMIC)

Endocrine
Metabolic
Altered immune system

MECHANICAL

Calculus
Retention of impacted food
Moveable and spreading teeth
Ragged-edged fillings and crown overhangs
Poorly designed or poorly fitting dentures

Data compiled from Ofstehage JC, Magilvy K: Oral health and aging, *Geriatr Nurs* 7:238, 1986; Papas AS et al: *Geriatric dentistry: aging and oral health*, St Louis, 1991, Mosby; Zach L et al: *Clinical geriatrics*, ed 3, Philadelphia, 1986, Lippincott.

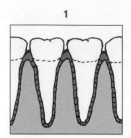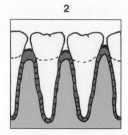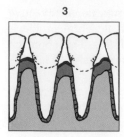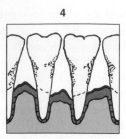

FIGURE 8-2 Progression of periodontal disease. *1,* Normal, healthy gingivae (gums). Healthy gums and bone anchor teeth firmly in place. *2,* Gingivitis. Plaque and its by-products irritate the gums, making them tender, inflamed, and likely to bleed. *3,* Periodontitis. If not removed, plaque hardens into calculus (tartar). As plaque and calculus continue to build up, the gums begin to recede (pull away) from the teeth and pockets form between the teeth and gums. *4,* Advanced periodontitis. The gums recede farther, destroying more bone and the periodontal ligament. Teeth—even healthy teeth—may become loose and need to be extracted. (Courtesy Karen L. Merrill, Wellesley, Mass.)

Gingivitis. Gum recession occurs with periodontal disease and after long periods of ignoring gingivitis. Periodontal changes should be minimal in the healthy aging, with adequate self-care or care from caregivers and health professionals. When care is inadequate, inflammation, swelling, pain, bleeding, unpleasant taste in the mouth, and discomfort from odors may occur; this is gingivitis. Tartar, or calculus, forms over plaque; if tartar is not removed regularly, gingivitis and then periodontal disease with gum recession will occur. Periodontal disease does not appear to be a specific disease of the elderly but the result of chronic gingivitis from young age through middle-aged adulthood. The prevalence of periodontal disease is about 6% in adults ages 25 through 34 years and 41% in those ages 65 years and older (Vargas et al., 2001).

Periodontitis. The signs of periodontal disease are the same regardless of one's age (Box 8-3). Tooth loss related to periodontal disease is similar in men and women. Elders in poverty are twice as likely to be edentulous as those above the poverty line (Vargas et al., 2001). About 52% of nursing home residents are edentulous. Further, 92% of elders with tooth loss have both upper and lower dentures. In this group, 24% of black elders and 19% of Hispanic elders do not use their dentures. In long-term care, 80% of those who lost all their teeth had both dentures but nearly 20% did not wear them (Vargas et al., 2001) and very frequently the dentures were misplaced or lost entirely.

Periodontitis can be a significant infection. It has been linked to diabetes complications, heart disease, and respiratory diseases, as well as tooth loss (CDC, 2000). Diabetes, when uncontrolled, heightens the risk for infection, as does estrogen deficiency and smoking. Oral infections warrant more attention and care than we have given. According to the CDC, although water fluoridation has drastically improved the incidence of tooth decay, has a minimal cost, and is a method of primary prevention, more than 100 million Americans have no access to it.

A direct relationship between cardiovascular disease and periodontal disease was published by the National Institutes of Health (NIH) in 2005. Older adults with certain bacterial growth causing periodontal disease also had thick carotid arteries—a strong predictor of stroke and heart attack (Luggen, 2005a). This study continues. The most common bacteria causing infection in the mouth are as varied as the articles discussing the topic. Some are *Streptococcus* organisms, *Actinobacillus actinomycetemcomitans*, *Porphyromonas gingivalis*, *Tannerella forsythia*, and *Treponema denticola*, as well as *Staphylococcus aureus* (45%), the latter causing most abscesses. Most of these are implicated in heart disease/arterial wall disease. Others include gram-negative bacteria such as enteric gram-negative bacilli (42%) and *Pseudomonas aeruginosa* (13%). It is thought that these pathogens that colonize dental plaque provide a reservoir for pneumonia in hospitalized elders (El-Solh et al., 2004). Of interest, more than 600 types of bacteria inhabit the mouth (Luggen, 2005a).

Xerostomia. Xerostomia (dry mouth) is a condition that results from salivary hypofunction. It contributes to periodontal disease (Momeyer and Luggen, 2005). Saliva neutralizes plaque, provides lubrication for the oral surfaces maintaining speech function and mastication, maintains the patency of taste pores, and protects from infection (AGS, 2006; Momeyer and Luggen, 2005; Reese, 2001). Xerostomia complaints are common in older adults. Many of the causes of dry mouth are related to medications, local diseases such as gland tumors, and systemic diseases. The medica-

---

BOX 8-3   Signs of Periodontal Disease*

- Gums bleeding when teeth are brushed (even a little bleeding is not normal; if you have a "pink" toothbrush, see your dentist)
- Red, swollen, or tender gums
- Detachment of the gums from the teeth
- Pus that appears from the gum line when the gums are pressed
- Teeth that have become loose or change position
- Any change in the way your teeth fit together when you bite
- Any change in the fit of partial dentures
- Chronic bad breath or bad taste

*Not limited to elders.

tions that are causative include anticholinergic agents (all of which cause dry mouth to a degree), antihistamines, the tricyclic antidepressants, antipsychotics, opiates, calcium channel blockers, phenytoin, hydrochlorothiazide, cyclosporine, and antiarrhythmics (AGS, 2006; Momeyer and Luggen, 2005).

Dry mouth makes eating, swallowing, tasting, and speaking difficult. Some of the causes of hyposalivation are radiation therapy to the head and neck, chemotherapy, and at least 400 common medications. Other causes include dehydration, tumors, duct obstruction, sarcoidosis, diabetes, Alzheimer's disease, acquired immunodeficiency syndrome (AIDS), and Sjögren's syndrome (a connective tissue disorder that includes decreased lacrimal and salivary gland function). The primary form of Sjögren's syndrome affects salivary and lacrimal glands; the secondary form includes a connective tissue disease, usually rheumatoid arthritis, scleroderma, or thyroiditis (Beers and Berkow, 2000).

Treatment includes discontinuing the offending drug; drinking more water; and avoiding sugary snacks, tobacco, alcohol, and beverages with caffeine, all of which increase mouth dryness. With some remaining secretion, stimulation occurs with sugarless candies, mints, and chewing gum. Pilocarpine, a cholinergic drug, can be prescribed but is to be avoided in those with Parkinson's disease, peptic ulcer, asthma, heart failure, urinary tract infection, and glaucoma.

Ageusia. Many older adults do not enjoy taste as they once did (ageusia). The number of taste receptors, however, remains consistent. Taste buds can be damaged by hot drinks, smoking, infections, antibiotics, exposure to metals and chemicals, periodontal problems, and inflammatory conditions in the mouth (Robb-Nicholson, 2003). The problem may be in other parts of the sensory system—olfactory (anosmia), thermal, tactile, or textural sensors (Reese, 2001). Olfactory changes are the most common cause of loss of taste. Hypothyroidism and liver disease can alter smell perception, as can rare disorders such as aneurysms and tumors in the brain (Robb-Nicholson, 2003).

Drugs, diseases, and tobacco use reduce or alter taste sensation. Examples of other causes are abrasive teeth, gastrointestinal (GI) disorders, allergies, salivary dysfunction, and diabetes. Loss of taste can occur as we age for a variety of reasons; often it is transient and/or treatable.

Loss of taste can be problematic because it may lead to a loss of interest in foods. This may lead to poor nutrition or eating foods with stronger tastes, such as salt. Salt should be avoided in some situations such as heart failure.

Stomatopyrosis. Stomatopyrosis (or burning mouth syndrome, scalded mouth syndrome, burning tongue syndrome, burning lips syndrome, glossodynia, and stomatodynia) is sometimes seen primarily in postmenopausal women (Beers and Berkow, 2000). It does occur in nearly 4% of U.S. middle-age and older adults—women 7 times more often than men (Mayo Clinic, 2004a). It is called *glossopyrosis* when it occurs on the tongue, but it can occur in any area of

the mouth. Often the tip of the tongue is affected (Knight, 2006). The person often complains of "taste phantoms," that is, taste sensations that occur in the absence of taste stimuli. Often the taste is bitter or metallic (Mayo Clinic, 2004a). Usually it occurs with no precipitant. However, it can occur with candidal infection or xerosis (50%) and is painful. Other investigators have found that ill-fitting dentures are causative. Some believe that ingredients in the dentures are the cause—methyl methacrylate monomer and other products—and have produced positive skin reactions on testing. Pain complaints indicate that it is worse late in the day and early evening. Proposed causes include poor oral hygiene with infrequent cleaning of dentures (Knight, 2006). It occurs in about 20% of elders who wear dentures. The burning pain increases and remits during the course of a day; nothing seems to alleviate the pain. Even changing the dentures has not alleviated the problem. If lesions are present, the diagnosis is incorrect and is probably candidiasis, which often causes a burning sensation. Prevention is the best management. Consultation with a dietitian may clarify the need for vitamin supplements. Proposed causes include deficiencies of vitamins B_1, B_2, B_6, and B_{12}; and deficiency of folic acid. However, vitamin replacement has not corrected the problem. Iron deficiency anemia has also been suggested as causative. Other possible causes are local trauma, especially excessive irritation from excessive teeth brushing and brushing the tongue, overuse of mouthwashes, and consuming too many acidic drinks (Mayo Clinic, 2004a).

Psychological problems have also been implicated in burning mouth syndrome. Depression, anxiety, and fear of cancer have been associated with the disorder (Mayo Clinic, 2004a). More recently, researchers have suggested that the cause is neuropathy—damaged nerves or dysfunctional nerves. Allergies to certain foods, food flavorings, food additives, fragrances, dyes, or other substances have also been described. Gastroesophageal reflux disease (GERD) has been implicated with the bitter stomach acids that reflux into the esophagus and often to the throat. A common medication for hypertension, the angiotensin-converting enzyme (ACE) inhibitors have been implicated in burning mouth syndrome. Diabetes and hypothyroidism have been postulated. Oral tissues may react to high blood sugars.

Screening and diagnosis include a thorough medical and nutritional history. Testing may include a complete blood cell count (CBC), allergy testing, oral swab culture or even biopsy, and blood for vitamin deficiencies. A consultation with a specialist may be in order—dermatologist, dentist, psychiatrist, or an ear-nose-throat (ENT) specialist (otorhinolaryngologist).

Treatment will depend on finding the cause. Some successful therapies include treating dry mouth (xerostomia) or Sjögren's syndrome, using nystatin for thrush or candida, managing the depression and/or anxiety, correcting nutritional deficiencies, correcting the ill-fitting dentures, treating neuropathy with gabapentin, avoiding foods to which one is allergic, avoiding medications that cause onset or worsening, detecting and treating bruxism (grinding teeth at night or clenching teeth during the day), managing the hypothyroidism, and keeping good control of diabetes. This is a treatable condition. It may take time and many professional visits. Short-term remedies may include avoiding cinnamon and mints, cigarette smoke, and alcohol-based mouthwashes, as well as leaving dentures out during the night (Mayo Clinic, 2004a). The person could try brushing the teeth with baking soda and chewing ice chips or sugar-free chewing gum.

Candidiasis. Candidiasis is a common infection in elderly persons. It presents as diffuse erythema with cracks at the corners of the mouth, erythema in denture areas, and white patches on the buccal mucosa. It results in taste dysfunction, pruritus, burning, and pain (AGS, 2006). Candidiasis resembles leukoplakia in that they both cause white patches in the oral cavity and, in some types of candidiasis, the white patches cannot be scraped away. The mouth is often painful, especially when the infection is beneath the dentures. Diagnosis is easily made by a smear and Gram stain. This infection is very common in older adults. The cause is usually an immunocompromising situation such as diabetes mellitus; antibiotics often given for an infection; salivary hypofunction; corticosteroids or inhaled steroids for asthma; or antineoplastics (AGS, 2006; Beers and Berkow, 2000). Treatment is a topical or systemic antifungal agent such as nystatin or clotrimazole. The dentures should be soaked in benzoic acid, chlorhexidine, or sodium hypochlorite and rinsed thoroughly and worn infrequently during treatment.

Leukoplakia. Leukoplakia is a thick lesion of squamous cells in the mucous membranes of the mouth that manifests as a slightly raised, slightly circumscribed white patch that cannot be scraped away. It is malignant or premalignant less than 10% of the time. Some "plakias" may be mixed red and white. When it is red, it is termed *erythroplakia* (AGS, 2006). Erythroplakia lesions are malignant or premalignant, and 93% of case biopsies reveal atypical cells. It is generally found on the lips, tongue, gums, or buccal mucosa. It is caused by exposure to tobacco tars including snuff, chewing tobacco, cigarettes, cigars, and pipes (Crowley, 2004). Leukoplakia should be followed closely; if it does not disappear in 2 weeks, the elder should consult a specialist: a dentist, oral surgeon, or ENT physician. A dentist or an oral surgeon should evaluate erythroplakia, and a biopsy should be taken immediately (AGS, 2006). A clinician may obtain a scraping (exfoliative cytology) for review by the laboratory. Early identification markedly improves the outcome.

Oral Cancers. Oral cancers occur more frequently in late life. About 30,900 new cases are found each year. Twice as many occur in men as in women. For all stages combined, the 5-year survival rate is 59% and 10-year survival rate is 48%. This has not changed significantly in the past 20 years—we can make a difference in terms of finding these lesions early through good oral examinations. See Box 8-4 for signs and symptoms the nurse clinician may elicit from a good assessment.

> **BOX 8-4**   **Oral and Throat Cancer Signs and Symptoms**
>
> - Persistent mouth pain
> - A sore in the mouth that does not heal or increases in size
> - White or red lumps or patches in the mouth
> - Cheek thickening
> - Difficulty moving the tongue, chewing, or swallowing
> - Swelling or pain in the jaw or difficulty moving the jaw
> - A persistent feeling that something is caught in the throat, soreness in the throat
> - Persistent mouth bleeding
> - Chronic irritation from jagged teeth or poorly fitting dentures
> - Pain around the teeth; loosening of the teeth
> - Numbness or loss of feeling of the tongue or elsewhere in the mouth
> - Voice changes
> - Lump or swelling in the neck
> - Severe pain in one ear—with a normal eardrum
>
> All these signs and symptoms should be referred to a specialist.

Oral cancers occur more commonly in black men than in whites (ACS, 2006a). Of interest, the new cases diagnosed have been dropping by 5% each year for the past 2 years. Incidence of oral cancer is different in other countries of the world (ACS, 2006a). It is much more common in Hungary and France than in the United States and much less common in Mexico and Japan. These differences are thought to be environmental.

Risk factors for oral cancer are tobacco use, alcohol use, and exposure to ultraviolet light, especially for cancer of the lips (ACS, 2006b). Pipe, cigar, and cigarette smoking are all implicated. Chewing tobacco is associated with an uncommon type of squamous cell carcinoma.

Other risk factors are age, irritation, poor nutrition, mouthwash with high alcohol content, and human papillomavirus (HPV) infection as a possible factor in 20% of oropharyngeal cancers; immune system suppression from immunosuppressant drugs; and gender. Eating a wholesome diet is preferable to adding vitamin supplements (ACS, 2006b). The ACS cancer prevention diet includes 5 servings of fruits and vegetables every day and whole grain foods from plant sources—cereals, grains, rice, pasta, and beans. Red meats should be eaten rarely, especially high-fat meats or processed meats.

Those who have the following are more likely to develop oral cancers: leukoplakia for longer than 3 weeks, erythroplakia (flat, red mucosal patches) of similar duration, ulcerations, dysplasias, and infection. Removing these lesions surgically does not prevent oral cancers from occurring as was previously thought (ACS, 2006b). Having an oral cancer predisposes one to a second primary cancer by up to 33%.

Chemoprevention has been studied in recent years. Isotretinoin (related to vitamin A) reduces the risk of a second cancer of the mouth and neck occurring (ACS, 2006b). However, it has no effect on preventing recurrence of the same cancer. Isotretinoin has serious side effects—eye problems, increase in blood cholesterol, and rashes—so it is not recommended for the general population. It is an option for those at high risk. Much research has shown that vitamin A supplements are not recommended. This vitamin does not reduce cancer risk (ACS, 2006b). Indeed, too much vitamin A can increase the risk for lung or prostate cancers. More studies are being conducted utilizing other retinoids, some aspirin-like medications, and immune system proteins that may help fight viral infections (interferons).

When a lesion in the oral cavity or neck is found, the patient is sent to a specialist, usually for a biopsy first. To grade a malignancy, more testing is usually necessary: dental x-rays; computerized tomography (CT), which allows one to see organs in 2-dimension "slices"; and magnetic resonance imaging (MRI) scan, which generates a picture without x-ray but, instead, through a powerful magnetic field with radio waves (Mayo Clinic, 2004b). The images can be viewed from any direction and any plane and help determine the extent of the original mass and any lymph node or organ involvement. Ultrasound is another diagnostic tool. It uses no radiation but, instead, combines high-frequency sound waves and computer processing. It provides information about the shape, texture, and consistency of tumors or cysts.

Therapy options are based on diagnosis and staging. Usually, patients will have surgery, radiation therapy, and chemotherapy either alone or in combination, depending on the stage. When discussing options, it is important that the patient consider all choices and how they affect overall health (ACS, 2006c). Some treatments may be curative but affect functions such as speech, chewing and swallowing, and disfigurement. Obtaining a second opinion is always a good decision. If detected early, these cancers can almost always be treated successfully (Mayo Clinic, 2004b).

▲ Promoting Healthy Aging: Implications for Gerontological Nursing

Assessment. Assessment of the oral cavity should be a regular part of nursing assessment (Box 8-5). It is much better preventive care to periodically inspect the person's mouth than to wait until a problem occurs. All persons, especially adults older than 50 years with or without dentures should have their gums, tongue, teeth (natural or dentures), and mucous membranes inspected on a regular basis. Federal regulations mandate an annual examination for those residing in skilled nursing facilities. Visits to the dentist should occur more often if oral disease is present. The American Cancer Society recommends an annual oral examination for everyone. Although the oral examination is best performed by a dentist, nurses can also provide basic screening examinations to persons without access to dental care (Figure 8-3).

BOX 8-5   Important Points of Oral Assessment

Salivation
Tongue:
- Texture
- Moisture
- Coloring

Palates
Gingival tissues (gums)
Teeth
Dentures/bridgework
Soft tooth debris
Lips:
- Texture
- Moisture
- Coloring

Voice
Swallowing ability

Modified from Danielson KH: Oral care and older adults, *J Gerontol Nurs* 14(11):6, 1988.

With dentures removed, gums are inspected for color and palpated for lesions and swelling. Ill-fitting dentures are responsible for ulcerations, which resemble cancerous lesions. Generalized inflammation, or sore mouth, is demonstrated by a reddened mucosa and a granular-looking outline of the denture bases along the gingival borders. Papillary hyperplasia is a warty papular type of condition of the palate created by the suction of the upper denture. Skinfolds at the mouth corners can overlap, causing lesions that resemble those seen in vitamin deficiencies such as riboflavin or an infectious process such as candidiasis. It is important not to overlook this possibility.

Teeth, if present, should be checked for jagged edges, fractures, lost fillings, caries, the number of teeth, and occlusion adequate for mastication. Dentures, if partial or full, should be removed and inspected for excessive wear, breakage, and rough spots. It is also necessary to learn when dentures were last checked by a dentist for relining, rebasing, and replacement, which is necessary whenever denture fit is too loose or causing pressure sores on the gums. This is especially important when the person has had a weight gain or loss of 10 or more pounds. Dentures may be hard to accept because they will never feel exactly like one's own teeth and because the mouth is always changing.

The tongue is inspected for color, swelling, and lesions and observed and palpated on all surfaces for tenderness and lesions. Check the movements of the tongue—up, down, straight out. The older patients of one of the authors (AL) enjoy it when asked to stick their tongues out at her! Observe for tremor. The mucous membranes, in general, should be observed for color, moistness, smoothness, and the appearance of lesions. Assessment should also consider and utilize the strengths of the older adult when developing nursing diagnoses and interventions for oral care. These strengths may include maintenance of dignity, increased socialization, the desire to be well

KAYSER-JONES BRIEF ORAL HEALTH STATUS EXAMINATION				

Resident's Name _____

Examiner's Name _____

Date _____

TOTAL SCORE _____

CATEGORY	MEASUREMENT	0	1	2
LYMPH NODES	Observe and feel nodes	No enlargement	Enlarged, not tender	Enlarged and tender*
LIPS	Observe, feel tissue, and ask resident, family or staff (e.g., primary caregiver)	Smooth, pink, moist	Dry, chapped, or red at corners*	White or red patch, bleeding or ulcer for 2 weeks*
TONGUE	Observe, feel tissue, and ask resident, family, or staff (e.g., primary caregiver)	Normal roughness, pink and moist	Coated, smooth, patchy, severely fissured or some redness	Red, smooth, white or red patch; ulcer for 2 weeks*
TISSUE INSIDE CHEEK, FLOOR, AND ROOF OF MOUTH	Observe, feel tissue, and ask resident, family, or staff (e.g., primary caregiver)	Pink and moist	Dry, shiny, rough, red, or swollen*	White or red patch, bleeding, hardness; ulcer for 2 weeks*
GUMS BETWEEN TEETH AND/OR UNDER ARTIFICIAL TEETH	Gently press gums with tip of tongue blade	Pink, small indentations; firm, smooth, and pink under artificial teeth	Redness at border around 1-6 teeth; one red area or sore spot under artificial teeth*	Swollen or bleeding gums, redness at border around 7 or more teeth, loose teeth; generalized redness or sores under artificial teeth*
SALIVA (EFFECT ON TISSUE)	Touch tongue blade to center of tongue and floor of mouth	Tissues moist, saliva free flowing and watery	Tissues dry and sticky	Tissues parched and red, no saliva*
CONDITION OF NATURAL TEETH	Observe and count number of decayed or broken teeth	No decayed or broken teeth/roots	1-3 decayed or broken teeth/roots*	4 or more decayed or broken teeth/roots; fewer than 4 teeth in either jaw*
CONDITION OF ARTIFICIAL TEETH	Observe and ask patient, family, or staff (e.g., primary caregiver)	Unbroken teeth, worn most of the time	1 broken/missing tooth, or worn for eating or cosmetics only	More than 1 broken or missing tooth, or either denture missing or never worn*
PAIRS OF TEETH IN CHEWING POSITION (NATURAL OR ARTIFICIAL)	Observe and count pairs of teeth in chewing position	12 or more pairs of teeth in chewing position	8-11 pairs of teeth in chewing position	0-7 pairs of teeth in chewing position*
ORAL CLEANLINESS	Observe appearance of teeth or dentures	Clean, no food particles/tartar in the mouth or on artificial teeth	Food particles/tartar in one or two places in the mouth or on artificial teeth	Food particles/tartar in most places in the mouth or on artificial teeth

Upper dentures labeled: Yes_____ No _____ None _____ Lower dentures labeled: Yes_____ No _____ None _____ Italic*—refer to dentist immediately

Is your mouth comfortable? Yes_____ No _____ If no, explain: _____

Additional comments:_____

FIGURE 8-3 Kayser-Jones Brief Oral Health Status Examination. (With permission of Jeanie Kayser-Jones, RN, PhD, School of Nursing, University of California, San Francisco.)

groomed and well dressed, and taking an active role in maintenance of one's own health.

Interventions

Care of the Teeth. Too often, older adults are seen by the dentist when it is too late to salvage the teeth. It is therefore imperative to conscientiously include appropriate dental care to maintain and preserve the existing teeth. Dental care begins at home and should be reinforced by the caregiver when the person requires assistance in meeting this activity of daily living. Prescribed oral hygiene for the individual with some or all teeth is to brush, floss, and use a fluoride dentifrice and mouth rinse daily. It is best if individuals can brush their teeth after each meal. Elders with cognitive problems or problems with dexterity require modified toothbrushes or regular assistance and dental prophylaxis more often than every 6 months (Beers and Berkow, 2000), especially if caries are present.

Teeth whitening products have hit the marketplace. As teeth yellow with aging, these agents have become a curiosity and then a purchase for many persons of any age, but especially at mid-life and beyond. These agents make teeth whiter, either by lightening teeth or by removing stain and discoloration (Mayo Clinic, 2006a). The two types are whitening toothpaste and peroxide-based whiteners or bleaching agents, which come as gels and strips. All toothpastes contain abrasives that remove stains; the new whitening toothpastes have gentle chemical or polishing agents that provide additional surface stain removal. They contain no bleaching agents. The bleaching agents are peroxide-based and bleach teeth; they actually change the yellowing tooth color. They remove deep and surface stains. They are weaker than the ones that are used in the dentist office. Whitening is not permanent and must be repeated periodically to maintain the whiteness. Coffee, tea, and red wine drinkers would need to use it more often than those who are not.

Mechanical Plaque Removal. A soft, round-bristled toothbrush minimizes the chance of traumatizing the gums yet stimulates the gums to retain firmness and adequate circulation. Dental experts recommend inclining the soft toothbrush at a 45-degree angle to the gum line and using a gentle scrubbing motion of short back-and-forth strokes over one or two teeth at a time. All surfaces—inner, outer, and chewing—should be brushed accordingly. For persons with more limited movement of their hands, it may be easier for the elder to use a child's toothbrush rather than an adult brush. A brush of this size and type is generally made of soft

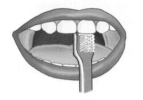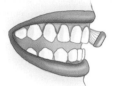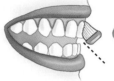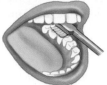

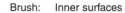
Brush: Inner surfaces   Outer surfaces   At a 45° angle   Biting surfaces

FIGURE 8-4 Correct toothbrushing.

bristles and is a third smaller than the adult brush. It is easier to brush individual teeth and into the back angles of the mouth. Another alternative is to use soft brushes with the newer electronic toothbrushes. Most have large handles for easier grasp, require little or no arm or wrist movement, provide a consistent motion, often have swivel activity and reach back areas well, and are relatively lightweight. Disclosure tablets or drops will stain the plaque that collects at the gum line and tooth appositions red or deep pink. It can help the person see the areas of plaque accumulation that otherwise are not visible on inspection. Brushing teeth routinely for approximately 2 minutes each time should adequately remove debris and stimulate the gums (Figure 8-4).

Interproximal Plaque Removal. Dental flossing is an integral part of the cleaning process; once a day is sufficient if done properly. The person should use about a 46-cm length of lightly waxed floss; a seesaw motion places the floss between the tooth surfaces; removal of plaque requires up-and-down movement under the gum line and side surfaces of teeth. Many people floss just between the teeth but forget to include under the gum line and the single surface of the last molar. Use of a commercial floss handle may provide the leverage and ease necessary for the person to continue flossing. If the floss handle is too delicate to grasp, the section on adaptive aids that follows suggests modifications. Persons with sensitive or ulcerated gums might find a Water Pik device appropriate. The forced water device cleans teeth and provides a gentle massage to the gums. However, because it can also force bacteria into the tissue, its use should be in consultation with the person's dentist.

Rinses. A variety of rinses are available for cosmetic or therapeutic purposes. Cosmetic rinses function primarily to refresh the mouth, but major disadvantages exist. First, depending on the brand, cosmetic rinses contain 6% to 29% alcohol by volume, which can be an oral tissue irritant and can exacerbate or create xerostomia. Second, undiagnosed alcoholism is a growing problem among the elderly, so caution is advised in the use of alcohol-containing rinses. A third disadvantage of cosmetic rinses is that the effect of the mouth-flushing rinse is transient and may mask underlying causes of oral disease.

Therapeutic rinses contain an agent that is beneficial to the surface of the teeth and the oral environment. Some therapeutic rinses require a prescription such as Peridex (chlorhexidine), which contains alcohol but is also a broad-spectrum antimicrobial agent that helps control plaque; it has an unpleasant taste and not all persons will persist in using it. The commercial product Listerine, which is in this same category, is an over-the-counter product that carries the American Dental Association approval, but it should not be used by persons on Antabuse or who have severe oral mucositis because it contains a high quantity by volume of alcohol (26.9%). Fluoride rinses such as the over-the-counter ACT and Fluorigard prevent caries development by incorporating fluoride into developing enamel, by enhancing or increasing remineralization of enamel, and by antibacterial action. Remineralizing rinses are used to replace calcium and phosphate lost from enamel or cementum during the caries process. One study of the association of vitamin D and periodontal disease (PD) in middle-aged and older adults found that vitamin D may be associated with PD independent of bone mineral density (Dietrich et al., 2004). Because low bone mineral density is prevalent in older adults (women and some men), taking doses of vitamin D seems to be a good thing.

Nurses sometimes use hydrogen peroxide or sodium bicarbonate with their patients in need of oral rinses (Coleman, 2002). No good evidence exists that these are particularly useful. In fact, evidence does exist that peroxide damages the oral mucosa. Bicarbonate is also unpleasant to taste, changes the mouth pH, and may cause mucosal burns if not diluted properly. Rinsing the mouth with plain water is also not sufficient because bacterial plaque will continue to form.

Adaptive Aids for Oral Care. The handle of a toothbrush or floss holder can easily be customized for elders with a grasp weakened by arthritis, stroke, or other conditions. Enlisting the elder's assistance and creativity in designing the home care device is important because he or she is the best judge of what works well. Box 8-6 and Figure 8-5 provide possible adaptations.

Assisting Dependent Elders. It is essential to provide oral care daily regardless of whether the individual is severely disabled, physically handicapped, comatose, or mentally incapable of carrying out his or her own oral hygiene. Debilitated elders are at a greater risk of developing oral disease. They take more medications; they produce less saliva; they lack resistance to bacterial toxins that cause periodontal disease; and they may eat softer foods, which tend to remain in their mouths longer. When the person is unable to carry out his or her own dental/oral regimen, it is the responsibility of the caregiver to do so, be it the nurse, nurses' aid, or family member.

Daily oral home care should be a part of general hygiene care. Having the proper equipment and using the appropriate techniques can greatly simplify the task and ensure better results. To make oral hygiene complete, the tongue should be brushed. With age, mouth organisms form a white coating on the tongue, and this coating must be brushed off. This can be done most easily at the time of brushing teeth. It is preferable to brush the tongue or wipe it with gauze when brushing the teeth after each meal. Cleaning the tongue may be difficult for some people because it elicits the gag reflex if brushed too far back on the tongue. A curved-bristle toothbrush for those who need assistance allows greater access to harder-to-reach dental surfaces. These are available commercially. They remove more plaque than straight-bristle brushes. The benefit to the caregiver is reduction in time and degree of difficulty in giving oral care. Use of disclosure liquid or chewing tablets helps the caregiver identify whether proper brushing and flossing were actually accomplished.

The type of dentifrice is not as important as the mechanical action employed in the teeth-cleaning process, although the dentifrice should contain fluoride. With the effects of fluoride in reducing gum line and root caries and preventing bacterial invasion of teeth, the use of a commercial fluoride toothpaste is beneficial.

Caregivers should be shown and provided with written instructions to reinforce the verbal instructions and demonstration. Box 8-7 provides directions for caregivers regardless of the setting.

Brushing after each meal is preferred. However, in the institutional setting, it may not be possible to brush a person's teeth three or four times each day, but if the teeth are thoroughly brushed for 2 minutes and flossed at least once in 24 hours, the integrity of the mouth can be maintained at a minimum level. It is common to see nurses using foam swabs with or without lemon glycerin. These swabs are ineffective for cleaning teeth and controlling plaque and should not be used other than to moisten the mouth for those who are nothing-by-mouth (NPO) status (Coleman, 2002).

Care of the Dentures. Those who are edentulous may wear complete dentures. Dentures help maintain adequate nutrition and psychologically aid to preserve appearance, social contacts, and relationships that a person has cultivated. Many elders believe that once they have dentures, oral care is no longer needed. Older adults with dentures should be taught the proper home care of their dentures and oral tissue. This prevents odor, stain, and plaque buildup and removes debris under dentures that causes

---

BOX 8-6 Toothbrush and Floss Holder Adaptations

Wrap handle with:
- Washcloth
- Aluminum foil
- Thin foam sheets

Insert handle into:
- Sponge ball
- Sponge hair roller
- Plastic bicycle handle grip

Secure to handle:
- Velcro or elastic strap to slip over hand
- Curved handle of nail brush with bristles removed; slip over fingers

---

BOX 8-7 Dental Care: Instructions for Caregivers

1. If the patient is in bed, elevate his or her head by raising the bed or propping it with pillows, and have the patient turn his or her head to face you. Place a clean towel across the chest and under the chin, and place a basin under his or her chin.
2. If the patient is sitting in a stationary chair or wheelchair, stand behind the patient and stabilize his or her head by placing one hand under the patient's chin and resting his or her head against your body. Place a towel across his or her chest and over the shoulders. (It may be helpful to secure it with a safety pin.) The basin can be kept handy in the patient's lap or on a table placed in front of or at the side of the patient. A wheelchair may be positioned in front of the sink.
3. If the patient's lips are dry or cracked, apply a light coating of petroleum jelly.
4. Brush and floss the patient's teeth as you have been instructed (sulcular brushing, if possible). It may be helpful to retract the patient's lips and cheek with a tongue blade or fingers in order to see the area that is being cleaned. Use a mouth prop as needed if the patient cannot hold his or her mouth open. If manual flossing is too difficult, use a floss holder or an interproximal brush to clean the proximal surfaces between the teeth. Use a dentifrice containing fluoride.
5. Provide the conscious patient with fluoride rinses or other rinses as indicated by the dentist or hygienist.

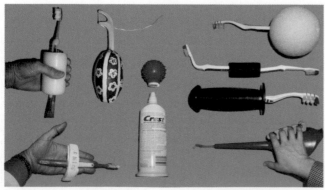

FIGURE 8-5 Adaptive aids for brushing. (From Darby M, Walsh M: *Dental hygiene: Theory and practice,* ed 2, St Louis, 2004, Saunders.)

From Papas AS et al: *Geriatric dentistry, aging and oral health,* St Louis, 1991, Mosby.

pressure and shrinkage of the underlying support structures. Dentures and other dental appliances such as bridges should be cleaned after each meal and anytime they are removed (Box 8-8).

Dentures must be worn constantly during the waking hours. They should be removed at bedtime to allow relief of the compression on the gums, cleaned, placed in an appropriate storage container, and replaced in the mouth on awakening. If the elder prefers to sleep with dentures in place, he or she should be encouraged to remove them for at least 4 hours during the day and relinquish them for daily cleaning. See Box 8-9 for tips on proper care of dentures. For cleaning, all surfaces of the dentures should be brushed with a denture brush or a medium-firm toothbrush. If removable bridges or other wires (or prong-type attachments) are present, these should be thoroughly cleaned to remove any debris and food. When cleaning dentures, fill the sink over which the washing will be done one-third or one-half full of water; hold the dentures close to the water so that if the dentures do slip, the water will break the fall and no damage will result.

Some immersion (soaking) cleaners assist in cleaning dentures (see Box 8-9). These products should be nonabrasive to the denture material, require little handling of the dentures, and reach all parts of the dentures. If used daily in conjunction with brushing, this should be sufficient to keep dentures clean. The elder or caregiver should always brush and rinse the dentures before and after the immersion soak. The gums, tongue, and palate should be cleansed by using a soft-bristled brush or by wiping the soft tissue with a gauze-wrapped finger. It does little for tissue integrity to clean the dentures and leave a residual film of debris on the gums. Gums, too, should be cleansed with a gloved finger wrapped in gauze or with a soft toothbrush to remove the film and residual food particles caught under dentures. This is an opportune time to massage the gums to increase circulation and inspect them for irritations.

Dentures are very personal and expensive possessions. In communal living situations of nursing homes, hospitals, and other care centers, dentures have often been misplaced, mixed up with others, or lost in the sheets and laundry. Dentists, laboratory technicians, and dental hygienists are now marking dentures. Some states require that all newly made dentures are marked with the client's identification. If dentures have not been marked, the caregiver can write the name, initial, or appropriate identification number on the dentures either on the buccal flange or on the palate using a non-toxic product. This is a temporary measure that must be repeated after a short time. This is not ideal, but it is better than not having dentures marked at all.

Broken or damaged dentures are a common problem after long or clumsy use. This generally happens when dentures are accidentally dropped during cleaning because of poor neuromuscular coordination or because they are slippery to handle. Do-it-yourself fix-it kits are not advisable.

BOX 8-8   Instructions for Denture Cleaning

1. Rinse your denture or dentures after each meal to remove soft debris.
2. Once a day, preferably before retiring, brush your denture according to the method described below. Then place it in a denture-cleaning solution and allow it to soak overnight or for at least a few hours. (Acrylic denture material must be kept wet at all times to prevent cracking or warping.)
3. Remove your denture from the cleaning solution and brush it thoroughly.
    a. Although an ordinary soft toothbrush is adequate, a specially designed denture brush may clean more effectively. (CAUTION: Acrylic denture material is softer than natural teeth and may be damaged by being brushed with very firm bristles.)
    b. Brush your denture over a sink lined with a washcloth and half-filled with water. This will prevent breakage if the denture is dropped.
    c. Hold the denture securely in one hand but do not squeeze. Hold the brush in the other hand. It is not essential to use a denture paste, particularly if dentures are soaked before being brushed to soften debris. Never use a commercial tooth powder because it is abrasive and may damage the denture materials. Plain water, mild soap, or sodium bicarbonate may be used.
    d. When cleaning a removable partial denture, great care must be taken to remove plaque from the curved metal clasps that hook around the teeth. This can be done with a regular toothbrush or with a specially designed clasp brush.
4. After brushing, rinse your denture thoroughly and insert it into your mouth.

From Papas AS et al: *Geriatric dentistry, aging and oral health,* St Louis, 1991, Mosby.

BOX 8-9   Take Care of Your Dentures

1. When your denture is out of your mouth, it should be stored in a water-filled container. This will prevent the denture material from drying out.
2. Place the container in a secure location where it will not be knocked onto the floor or disturbed by pets or children.
3. Never place your denture in hot water—use only cool or lukewarm water.
4. Never soak dentures with metal parts in bleach.
5. Never try to adjust or repair your denture. Let an expert do it.
6. Never use abrasive powders or a hard toothbrush to clean your denture.
7. Never soak your denture in a product that contains alcohol, such as mouthwash, or clean it with regular toothpaste.
8. ALWAYS rinse your denture thoroughly under running water before inserting it into the mouth.

From Papas AS et al: *Geriatric dentistry, aging and oral health,* St Louis, 1991, Mosby.

Broken dentures should be correctly repaired by a dental laboratory. Relining of dentures is usually a temporary measure; rebasing dentures is more successful. A new impression is made of the remaining dental ridge. The teeth are removed from the original pink denture and used in the new better-fitting denture base that has been adjusted to the changes in the dental ridges. This is less costly than a new denture because the original teeth are used. Prosthetic failure generally results from tissue changes in the mouth. These alterations can develop from the prostheses themselves, from the physical and emotional status of the wearer, and often from significant weight fluctuations.

Dentures should be checked once a year. The average time a denture base will be able to support the denture is 10 to 20 years. Many elders lose as much as 50% of supporting bone in as few as 5 to 10 years. Rapid bone loss occurs with ill-fitting dentures (loose dentures). Denture adhesive helps only temporarily.

Dental Implants. Not everyone can wear dentures, and the causes for elders' inability to wear dentures are diverse. During recent years, several new approaches to dealing with missing teeth have been devised, such as dental implants. Current research indicates that providing a stable prosthetic may be the single most important determinant in fulfilling client aesthetic expectations. Osseointegrated dental implants have become reliable and safely provide long-term prosthetic stability for edentulous clients of all ages. Dental implants are not an appropriate treatment for all persons. The basic objective of dental implantation is to provide an attachment mechanism for teeth or dentures. Dental implants can anchor lower or upper dentures, usually with a metal screw surgically placed into the jaw bones. They provide a method to replace partial or full dentures with fixed bridgework, provide a method of replacing a single tooth, improve chewing function and restore the feeling of natural tooth function, and improve the quality of life by removing the frustration associated with using dentures or removable bridgework.

The procedure is done in several steps, which cover approximately 3 to 5 months from start to completion. Elderly candidates for dental implantations must be fit enough to undergo minor oral surgery and have a jaw and mineral density that can accommodate the implant system. A major problem for implants is the lack of jaw bone that occurs in 10% of prospective patients. In addition, the candidate for implants can have no history of drug abuse (potential for misuse of pain management drugs) and must possess realistic expectations of the outcome. Cost of implants varies widely from area to area, but implants are very costly and are not covered by insurance. Figure 8-6 demonstrates several types of implant supports.

It cannot be emphasized too strongly how vital dental care is to the well-being in late life. For too long, health care providers have been too naive, unconcerned, or remiss in the maintenance of this important need, which influences so many other equally and more important physiological, psychological, and social needs. It is heartening to find that

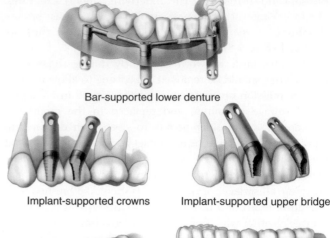

Bar-supported lower denture

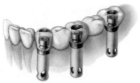

Implant-supported crowns

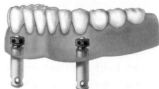

Implant-supported upper bridge

Implant-supported lower bridge   Ball-supported lower denture

FIGURE 8-6 Type of dental implant supports. (Courtesy Sulzer Calcitek, Inc., Carlsbad, Calif.)

dental schools include dental care of geriatric patients in their curricula and students receive practice by going into the community with mobile dental vans to senior centers and to visit homebound and institutionalized elders. More and more dentists are also making themselves available to persons residing in long-term care facilities.

HEALTHY FEET

The feet undergo a great deal of use, trauma, misuse, and neglect as a part of everyday living. Most older adults accept foot problems as an inescapable accompaniment of aging. Nurses and people in general have a fairly strong negative reaction to having contact with the feet. It is aesthetically unpleasant to many. Yet promoting healthy feet and good care of the feet can alleviate disability, pain, and the propensity for falling. It is for these reasons that the importance of feet to the well-being of the elderly is emphasized more extensively in this chapter than in most texts.

Feet influence the physical, psychological, and social well-being of the individual. Feet carry one's body weight, hold the body erect in an upright and stationary position, coordinate and maintain balance in walking, and must be rigid yet loose and adaptable enough to conform to the surfaces underfoot (all the while holding the legs and body in an upright position). Little attention is given to these valuable appendages until the feet interfere with ambulation and the ability to maintain independence.

Feet have been symbolically significant from biblical times, when respect and concern were shown by washing the feet, particularly of religious leaders and those held in esteem. The expressions "swept off our feet" (indicating sudden attraction or love), "cold feet" (when we are reluctant to do something), and "he has both feet on the ground" (indicating someone with a good deal of common sense) are examples of the metaphors we use to symbolize the meaningfulness we attribute to feet. We contend that the symbolic significance of the feet is present today, and attending to the feet is a gesture of response to the total individual.

Feet have a significant effect on one's productivity, amiability, and mobility. The effect is comparable to the influence that the automobile has had in our society. Like the automobile, if something is wrong, it is difficult to get around and the routine of the day is upset. Feet, like the automobile, are taken for granted and accorded little attention as long as they work. Unlike the automobile, though, the feet do not have easily replaceable parts. Neglect of the feet throughout one's earlier years can result in painful conditions later. Uncomfortable and painful feet may force the elderly person to become sedentary and deprived of social contacts. Foot discomfort can cause irritability, fatigue, and chronic complaints. Socrates is thought to have said, "To him whose feet hurt, everything hurts."

The person's feet are subjected to functional and physical neglect and traumatic stresses over the years. The residual effect from these varied stresses, compounded by a decreased ability to clearly see one's feet (because of visual impairment) or to bend and perform self-care to one's feet can result in conditions that need not exist or at least could be controlled.

Mobility may mean the difference between an independent, active community life, self-respect, motivation, and responsibility for one's health versus institutionalization (see Chapter 15). Even in an institution, foot problems may mean the difference between confinement to bed or wheelchair and the ability to ambulate in the protective setting.

Common Foot Problems in Late Life

The human foot has 26 bones, 33 joints, and more than 100 tendons, muscles, and ligaments (U.S. Food and Drug Administration [USFDA], 2006). It is a very complex structure, and much can go wrong. Some foot irregularities and problems are genetically inherited; however, many problems occur because of wear and tear and misuse of feet and the shoes we wear to protect them. Shoe styles affect the foot and can even affect the hip or leg.

When the older foot, subjected to long periods of stress, can no longer adapt to the stresses, inflammatory changes in bone and soft tissue occur and may manifest in mechanical disorders. See Box 8-10 for age-related foot changes.

With increasing age, many elders are less and less able to walk because of any of the conditions just mentioned. Lives can become more isolated, and dependency occurs. As walking slows or stops, osteopenia and sarcopenia occur, muscle mass is lost, and tissue atrophies. These affect the structure and function of the foot (AGS, 2006). See Box 8-11 for other key points. The number and severity of the problems increase with age. Major abnormalities occur gradually with

---

BOX 8-10   Age-Related Foot Changes

- Skin becomes drier, less elastic, and cooler.
- Subcutaneous tissue on dorsum and sides of foot thins.
- Plantar fat pad shrinks and degenerates.
- Toenails become brittle, thicken, and are less resistant to fungal infections.
- Degenerative joint disease decreases range of motion.

BOX 8-11   Key Points About Diseases/Disorders of the Older Foot

- Foot problems are common and have significant functional consequences for older persons.
- Proper shoes and orthotics can alleviate many foot problems.
- Peripheral skin problems may require topical medications, orthotics, proper footwear, and even débridement by a specialist.
- Systemic illnesses are associated with serious foot problems, and podiatric care is necessary.

Data from American Geriatric Society (AGS): *Geriatric review syllabus*, ed 6, New York, 2006, The Society.

---

discomfort, not described by the elder as pain. Without proper care and treatment, these conditions become disabling and a threat to the person's independence. Care of the foot often involves a team approach, including the person, the nurse, the podiatrist, and the person's primary health care provider.

Manifestations of degenerative processes in older persons include plantar fasciitis, atrophy of the plantar fat pad, and hammertoe formation (AGS, 2006). In the presence of these conditions, mobility and ambulation become limited and may worsen. Orthopedic foot disorders are caused by repetitive trauma, inflammation, osteoarthritis, rheumatoid arthritis, osteoporosis, and gout. These manifest as tendonitis, joint swelling, bursitis, neuritis, neuromas, stress fractures, residual deformities, and anterior imbalance. When foot pain is severe and lasting, stress fracture should be suspected if other explanations are not obvious.

The health of the foot can reflect systemic disease conditions or give clues to physical illness before their actual appearance. Sudden or gradual changes in nail or skin condition of the feet or appearance of recurring infections may be the precursors of more serious health problems. Rheumatological disorders such as the different forms of arthritis usually affect the other joints but can also affect the feet (see Chapter 15). Gout occurs most often in the joint of the great toe but is a systemic disease (see Chapter 15). Both diabetes and peripheral vascular disease commonly cause problems in the lower extremities and can quickly become life-threatening (see Chapter 10). Other, more localized common problems affecting feet are addressed in the following sections (Figure 8-7).

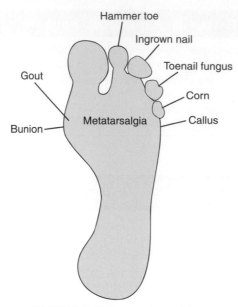

FIGURE 8-7 Common foot problems.

Corns. Corns (heloma), hyperkeratotic skin lesions, are conical-shaped layers of compacted skin usually on the dorsal surface of the proximal interphalangeal joint of smaller toes. They occur as a result of shearing, friction, and pressure on the skin rubbing against bony, protuberant areas of the toes when shoes are worn. Once the small, hard, white-to-yellow corn is established, continued pressure elicits pain. Unless the cause of the corn is removed, it will continue to enlarge and cause increasing pain. Soft corns (heloma molle) form in the same manner but occur between opposing surfaces of the toes. Both corns and calluses interfere with the ability to walk comfortably and wear shoes. If not managed, corns can become a primary irritant. This can produce localized avascularity that can precipitate ulceration (AGS, 2006).

Many elders manage these problems by following what they or their parents have done for years to correct their foot discomfort. Over-the-counter preparations for corns, in particular, damage normal tissue, as well as remove the corn; they do not treat the cause. Chemical burns and ulcerations from these products can result in the loss of toes or a leg for the person with diabetes, with neurological impairment, or with poor circulatory function to the lower extremities. Some people use razor blades and scissors to remove corns and calluses; this is a dangerous solution and is never recommended. Moleskin or lamb's wool can be used, with a hole cut in the center for the corn. This can be placed around the corn, protecting it from pressure without restricting circulation to healthy tissue. Soft corns between the toes can be eased by loosely wrapping small amounts of lamb's wool around the involved toe.

Calluses. Calluses (tyloma) are also layers of compacted skin that usually occur on the soles and heels of the feet because of chronic irritation and friction from shoes. Calluses can be eased with moleskin or lamb's wool applied to

those areas that receive undue friction. Moleskin adheres for several days or longer but should be removed when it becomes wet or excessively soiled. Removing moleskin should be done slowly to prevent tearing of skin. An emollient cream with a urea base, used routinely, will also be helpful in reducing keratosis and increasing hydration.

Bunions. Bunions (hallux valgus) are deviations or varus splaying of the first metatarsal (the joint of the great toe) with a valgus and rotational deformity of the phalanges of the great toe causing it to protrude medially (AGS, 2006). The first toe then drifts laterally (Hochburg et al., 2004). Bunions are long-standing residual effects from occupational activity and the influence of traumatic shoe styles. They are most common in women. Women's shoes, which draw the toes together, and the improper weight transmission and restrictive hosiery all contribute to the problem. Bunions are also thought to have a hereditary predisposition. Walking can be markedly compromised. Bunions may be treated with corticosteroid injections or antiinflammatory pain medications. A custom-made shoe should be considered. Shoes that provide forefront space (e.g., running shoes) work well. Surgery is available.

Hammertoe. Hammertoe is dorsiflexion of the metatarsophalangeal joint with plantar contraction of the proximal interphalangeal joint (AGS, 2006). It occurs most often in smaller toes but can occur in the hallux, or joint of the great toe. This condition limits the ability to walk. Variants of hammertoe are mallet toes and claw toes and cock-up toes, occurring when the contracture has no contact between the toe and the plane of support. The problem is related to atrophy of interossei muscles of the foot with contractures of the long extensor tendons. The deformity may be classified as flexible, semi-rigid, or rigid, based on the amount of flexibility when reducing the deformity. The toes may become rotated with osteoarthritis or dislocated and subluxed with rheumatoid arthritis. With these deformities, corns are likely to develop.

Metatarsalgia. Metatarsalgia is pain in the anterior metatarsal area. It may be caused from atrophy of the fat pad on the plantar surface of the foot, pressure from hammertoe deformities, degenerative changes, obesity, and imbalance (AGS, 2006; Beers and Berkow, 2000). Other causes include a narrow, high-arched foot, which focuses stress on the ball of the foot; legs that are unequal in length, thus adding stress to the metatarsal joints of the shorter leg; and flat feet. Relief is obtained with redistribution of the pressure away from the metatarsal head with the use of orthotics. Pain medications are helpful for symptomatic relief. Orthotics can be a reasonably priced alternative (rather than custom-made shoes) for the elder with foot problems.

Morton's Neuroma. Morton's neuroma is a painful, disabling deformity caused by entrapment of nerves of the foot. The affected nerves lie between the metatarsal heads, and the diagnosis is made by applying direct pressure on the plantar surface of the foot. Massage provides symptomatic relief of pain. Corticosteroid injections also provide temporary relief. For permanent correction, surgery must be done.

Plantar Fasciitis.   Pain on the sole of the foot is common and usually caused by a condition known as *plantar fasciitis* (AGS, 2006). When the pain is in the heel, it may be caused by stretching, straining, or tearing of the plantar fascial attachment on the calcaneus. A spur may develop from chronic stress on the attached area. Spurs are calcium growths on the foot bones. It is not uncommon to see a "pump bump," or Haglund's deformity (Beers and Berkow, 2000), on the posterior aspect of the heel; Haglund's deformity is a calcaneus exostosis. It may lead to bursitis because it creates pressure on the heel. Treatment is similar to that for other foot problems, with corticosteroid injections, anti-inflammatories, short-term opiates, avoiding walking barefoot, stretching exercises, or splinting (USFDA, 2006). In addition, physical therapy may be useful. Slippers should be worn when pain is acute.

Fungal Infections.   Fungal infections are very common in the foot, and the incidence increases with age (Habif, 2005). Nail fungus, onychomycosis, is characterized by degeneration of the nail plate with color changes to yellow or brown, brittleness, and hypertrophy of the nail (Figure 8-8). However, not all these changes are caused by fungus; 50% of thickened, dark nails may be attributed to other causes. Gross thickening of the nail plate may occur with tight-fitted shoes or other chronic trauma (Habif, 2005). Fungal infections are often caused by a tinea species with superficial invasion by *Trichophyton mentagrophytes* or *T. rubrum*. *Candida* species onychomycosis occurs nearly exclusively in chronic mucocutaneous candidiasis—a rare disease. Laboratory testing for dermatophytes makes the diagnosis definitive.

Diminished blood supply to the feet in elderly people often decreases the treatment options. Some of the pharmaco-

logical interventions may be contraindicated in the presence of liver compromise (see Chapter 12). For persons with circulatory compromise or diabetes, nail health should be monitored by a dermatologist or a podiatrist on a regular basis. Podiatrists often come to nursing home facilities monthly to care for persons with these common problems.

Hands should be washed each time the feet of a patient with a fungus infection are handled. Feet, especially between the toes, should be dry and exposed to sun and air. Topical application of antifungal drugs is of little value (Habif, 2005), although many older adults obtain these drugs over the counter. Systemic therapy is 50% to 80% effective, although the relapse rate is 15% to 20% in 1 year.

▲ Promoting Healthy Aging: Implications for Gerontological Nursing

The gerontological nurse is a proactive advocate for promoting the best foot health possible. Foot care is a prime factor in determining mobility and quality of life in retaining independence. Elders with painful foot problems and resultant activity limitations are usually forced to remain within the boundaries of their homes. Nursing care of the aging foot should be directed toward maintaining comfort and function, removing possible mechanical irritants, decreasing the likelihood of infection, and helping enhance and preserve maximum function. These goals are consistent with podiatric goals. The nurse has the important function of assessing the feet for clues to well-being and functional ability—not just bathing and applying lotion to the feet. Nurses can identify potential and actual problems and refer or seek podiatric assistance for the patient's foot problems.

Assessment.   Nursing care of the feet should include a thorough assessment. Figure 8-9 illustrates some of the important aspects to look for and evaluate, and it includes simple explanations of specific items to ensure uniform evaluation regardless of who performs the assessment. A foot assessment includes careful inspection of gait, postural deformities, physical limitations, and position of the foot with the heel strike. Inspect feet for irritation, abrasions, and other lesions; check for hazards to the maintenance of adequate circulation to the lower extremities and the existing circulatory status; and observe the individual's general mobility. A variety of tools are available, which speaks to the need for individualization to the client population with whom one is working and to the expertise of the individual who is doing the assessment and giving the care (Figure 8-10).

Assessment is the key to maintenance of the person's highest level of function and mobility (Box 8-12). Regular assessment of the feet is especially important for persons with diabetes, cardiac conditions, peripheral vascular disease, thyroid conditions, and renal conditions. Those individuals with residual foot and leg impairment from strokes may develop foot ulcers from pressure exerted by their shoes or braces and from pressure and persistent friction and irritation caused by altered walking patterns.

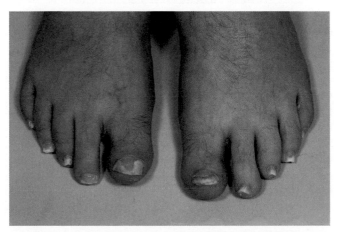

FIGURE 8-8 Onycholysis, yellowing, crumbling, and thickening of the toenails. (From Bolognia J et al: *Dermatology,* St Louis, 2003, Mosby.)

NURSING ASSESSMENT OF THE
GERIATRIC LOWER EXTREMITY

Patient Number _____
Date _____
R.N. Number _____

INSTRUCTIONS: FOR EACH ITEM, CIRCLE THE RESPONSE IN THE APPROPRIATE COLUMN, UNLESS DIRECTED OTHERWISE. CLARIFICATION OF ITEMS APPEAR IN THE FAR RIGHT COLUMN.

1. Mobility (check one)
   Walks without assistance _____ Walks with help of equipment _____
   Does not walk—uses wheelchair _____ Bedfast _____

2. Ask the client, "Does the condition of your feet or legs limit your activity in any way?"	YES	NO
If YES, describe. _____		
3. ASK THE CLIENT TO WALK APPROXIMATELY 10 FEET.		
Is there any gait disturbance?	YES	NO

REMOVE THE CLIENT'S SHOES AND STOCKINGS

	ACCEP-TABLE	UN-ACCEP-TABLE
4. Cleanliness of feet.		
5. Are the stockings a good fit?	YES	NO
6. Does the client usually wear well-fitting, leather (synthetic) shoes that cover the feet completely?	YES	NO
7. Does the client wear garters? (circular)	YES	NO 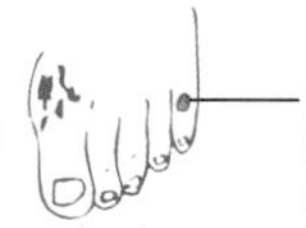

Dermatological assessment

8. Skin lesions		
a. Fissure between the toes?	YES	NO
b. Fissure on heel(s)?	YES	NO
c. Excoriation on legs or feet?	YES	NO
d. Corn(s)? (Figure 1)	YES	NO
e. Callus(es)?	YES	NO
f. Plantar wart?	YES	NO
g. Other, describe _____	YES	NO
9. Itching on legs or feet?	YES	NO
10. Rash on legs or feet?	YES	NO
11. INSPECT PRESSURE AREAS ON THE FEET FOR LOCALIZED AREAS OF REDNESS. ARE ANY PRESENT?	YES	NO
IF YES, WHICH FOOT?	RIGHT	LEFT
12. INSPECT LEGS, FEET, AND TOES FOR LOCALIZED SWELLING, WARMTH, TENDERNESS, REDNESS.		
Is any present?	YES	NO
If YES, specify location.	Rt. leg	Lt. leg
	Rt. foot	Lt. foot
13. Toenails		
a. Ingrown?	YES	NO
b. Overgrown (long)?	YES	NO
c. Thickened?	YES	NO
d. Yellow discoloration?	YES	NO
e. Black discoloration?	YES	NO

Figure 1 — Red, thickness

Corn: painful, circular area of thickened skin, appearing on skin that is normally thin.

Callus: Thickened skin, occurring on skin that is normally thick (i.e., soles).

Ingrown toenail: a "tender overhanging nail fold" (Bates, 1974)

FIGURE 8-9 Nursing assessment of the geriatric lower extremities. (From King PA: Foot assessment of the elderly, *J Gerontol Nurs* 4[6]:47-52, 1978.)

Interventions

Care of Toenails. The inability to provide self-care of the toenails is influenced by poor vision, hand tremors, the inability to bend, obesity, or increased nail thickness. Nails that are neglected or do not receive treatment may become unusually long and curved. This type of nail is known as *ram's horn* because of its appearance. Hard, thickened nails indicate inadequate nutrition to the nail matrix from trauma or poor circulation. Once the nail becomes thickened, it will remain so. These conditions should be brought to the attention of the podiatrist. Any attempt by the nurse or other caregiver to cut these nails may result in further damage to the matrix or precipitate an infection. This problem can be crippling if neglected.

Normal nails that become too long or begin to interfere with stockings, hose, or shoes should be cut straight across and even with the top of the toe (Figure 8-11). Nails that are hard can easily split, causing trauma to the matrix, pain, and possibly infection. Feet should be soaked in warm water for a very short time to soften the nails before they are clipped. Ideally, toenails should be trimmed after the bath or shower, but if this is not appropriate, soaking

Circulatory status (Questions 14-18 relate to FEET ONLY)

14. Do the feet have any red, reddish blue, or bluish discoloration?	YES	NO
15. Is there any brownish discoloration around the ankles?	YES	NO
16. Is the dorsalis pedis present? (Figure 2)	YES	NO
If NO, which foot?	RIGHT	LEFT
17. Is the posterior tibial pulse present? (Figure 3) If NO, which foot?	YES	NO
	RIGHT	LEFT
18. Is the skin dry?	YES	NO

The following relate to BOTH FEET AND LEGS

19. Is edema present?	YES	NO

CHECK THE TEMPERATURE OF THE LEGS AND THE FEET WITH THE BACKS OF YOUR FINGERS, COMPARING ONE EXTREMITY WITH THE OTHER.

20. Are the feet the same temperature?	YES	NO
21. Are the legs the same temperature?	YES	NO
22. Does the client have any pain in the legs or feet? If YES, DESCRIBE	YES	NO

INSPECT THE LEGS, SIDES OF ANKLES, SOLES, TOES FOR ULCERATION.

23. Is any ulceration present?	YES	NO
If YES, specify location.	Rt. leg	Lt. leg
	Rt. foot	Lt. foot

Structural deformities

24. Hallux valgus (bunion)? (Figure 4)	YES	NO
25. Hammer toes? (Figure 5)	YES	NO
26. Overlapping digits?	YES	NO

ASK THE CLIENT TO STAND

27. Are the legs the same relative size?	YES	NO
28. Are the legs the same relative length?	YES	NO
29. Are varicosities present?	YES	NO

Use three fingers on the dorsum of the foot usually just lateral to the extensor tendon of the great toe.

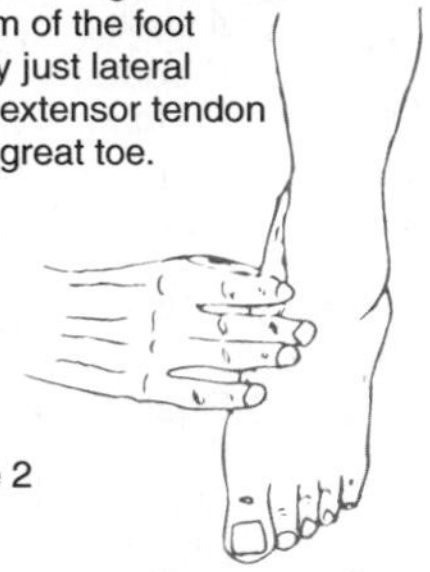

Figure 2

Curve your fingers behind and slightly below the medial malleolus of the ankle.

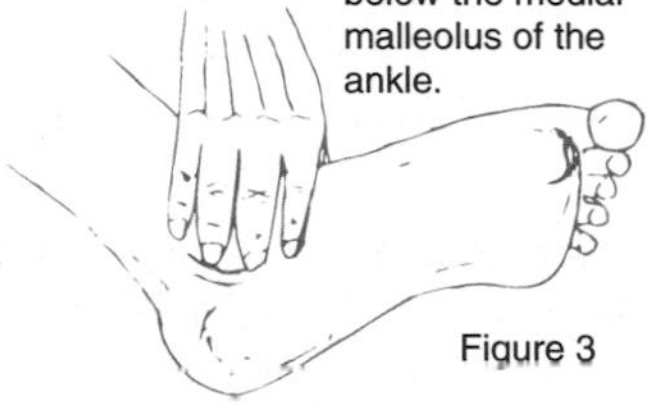

Figure 3

Figures 2 and 3. Questions 16 & 17. (The instructions and illustrations for palpating the pulses are from A Guide to Physical Examination, 1974, by Barbara Bates, M.D., used by permission of J.B. Lippincott.)

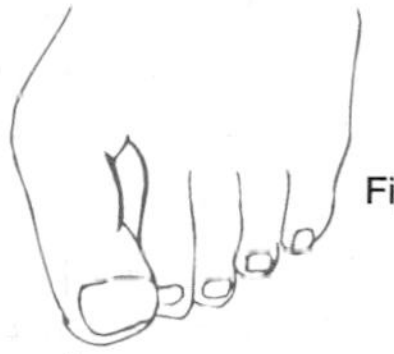

Figure 4

Hallux valgus (Outward deviation of great toe)

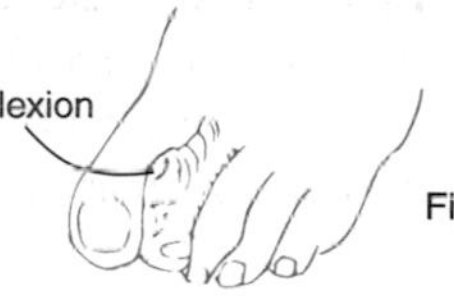

Flexion

Figure 5

Hammer Toe (Flexion contracture) (From N.J. Giannestras, Foot Disorders, p. 65, 1973.)

FIGURE 8-9, CONT'D

5 to 10 minutes will facilitate the procedure. Box 8-13 provides suggestions for a variety of foot soaks for specific aspects of foot care. Foot soaks are not recommended for elders with diabetes.

Shoes. Shoes should cover, protect, and provide stability for the foot, maximize toe space, and minimize the chance of falls. In essence, shoes should be functional. Shoes that provide enough forefoot space laterally and dorsally, such as running shoes, generally have a wide toe box and fit well. Depth inlay shoes made by the Alden Shoe Company (Middleborough, MA 02346) have been cited as providing significant relief. Extra depth in shoes for women is offered by Miller Shoes, now owned by Drew Shoe Company (252 Quarry Road, Lancaster, OH 43130).

Slip-on shoes are helpful for those who are unable to bend or lace shoes. Velcro closures are also useful to those who have limited finger dexterity. Low-heeled shoes with a wide toe box and a ridged sole minimize falls, place less stress on the legs and back, and are ideal for comfort.

Fitting shoes appropriately is useful in preventing foot ailments (National Institute on Aging, 2000). Our foot size

```
                              ASSESSMENT
Medical history
_____  Arthritis
_____  Diabetes
_____  Peripheral vascular disease
_____  Smoking
_____  Vision problems
_____  Falls in past year
Does client do a daily foot inspection?_____ yes_____ no, comments:
Footwear
                 Does client ever go barefoot?_____ yes_____ no, comments:
_____  Canvas or leather shoes
_____  Shoes fitted properly
_____  Socks
_____  Restrictive leg wear
_____  More than one pair of shoes
                 Appearance of footwear: _____
_____
_____
                 Type of footwear most often worn: _____
_____
Ambulation_____ with_____ without assistance.
Type of device used if assisted: _____
Color and temperature of extremity: _____
Presence of pedal pulses:        Right_____              Left_____
Structure
Presence of:                                     Location/remarks
_____ Bunions          _____ Spurs          _____
_____ Corns            _____ Ulcerations    _____
_____ Callus           _____ Cracks         _____
_____ Edema            _____ Dry skin        _____
_____ Hammertoes       _____ Blisters       _____
Description of toenails:_____
_____

Skills performed: Foot soak
                  Nail trim
Follow-up date:
```

FIGURE 8-10 Foot assessment tool. (From Ruscin C et al: Foot care protocol for the older client: a guide for working with clients to improve care of the feet, *Geriatr Nurs* 14[4]:210-212, 1993.)

changes as we grow older, and foot size increases as the day progresses. Usually, one foot is larger than the other. Shoes should be fitted to the largest foot. Select a shoe that is shaped like your foot. There should be about one-half inch of space (a "thumb's width") from the longest toe to the end of the inside of the shoe while standing. Shoes may "stretch" and become more comfortable. Make sure the shoe does not slip and ride up and down on the heel during walking. Take new shoes home and walk on the carpet to make sure they "work" right, and return them if they do not.

Dependent Edema. Circulation is less efficient in the lower extremities, especially the feet. Edema of the ankles and feet is evident after prolonged periods of sitting and standing. It is helpful if the elder does not wear constricting circular garters, socks with snug bands, or support hose, which constrict the feet. Sitting with the feet elevated on a footstool or hassock helps reduce edema and facilitates better venous circulation. Foot exercises are a means of reducing edema by encouraging more efficient venous return. Exercises can be done at any time. It may be helpful to develop the habit of doing foot exercises after rising and before going to bed. Other times would be during television commercials.

The exercises are simple, and in addition to helping reduce edema, they facilitate foot flexibility. Toe bends, or curling and relaxing the toes, should be done at least 5 times on each foot. These can be done one foot at a time or both feet together followed by rotating the feet at the ankles clockwise and then counterclockwise 5 to 10 times, and finally, bringing the knees to the chest 5 to 10 times. These exercises can be done consecutively or with short rest periods in between, depending on the stamina of the individual.

Foot Massage. Foot massage is another useful means of reducing edema, stimulating circulation, and improving pedal flexibility. Not only does massage aid in accomplishing these things, but also it relaxes the feet and stimulates relaxation of the rest of the body. However, not all elderly are candidates for foot massage, and the nurse needs to be particularly careful not to cause an alteration in the skin's integrity. Foot massage requires lubrication; the lotion or oil applied after the bath or shower can be used if the massage is done at that time. To give a foot massage, position yourself so that the client's feet are easily accessible; sit at the foot of the bed if the client is reclining, or sit opposite the client if he or she is seated, with the foot to be massaged cradled

---

BOX 8-12   Essential Data of Foot Assessment

OBSERVATION OF MOBILITY

Gait
Ambulation
Foot hygiene
Footwear

PAST MEDICAL HISTORY

Systemic diseases
Musculoskeletal problems
Vascular disease, ulcerations, or peripheral vascular disease
Vision problems
Falls
Trauma
Smoking history
Pain

BILATERAL ASSESSMENT

Color
Circulation
Pulses
Structures (hammer toe, bunion, overlapping digits)
Temperature
Dermatological aspects:
    Skin lesions (fissures, corns, calluses, warts, excoriation)
    Edema
    Itching
    Rash
    Toenails:
        Long, thick
        Discoloration

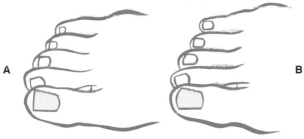

FIGURE 8-11 Cutting toenails. **A,** Correct method. **B,** Incorrect method.

BOX 8-13   Foot Soaks

CLEANSING

Add several drops of mild liquid soap or detergent to warm water.

CALLUS SOFTENING

Add ½ cup vinegar or ¼ cup baking soda to 1 qt of warm water.

DRY SKIN

Use warm water only.

WOUND OR MILD INFECTION

Add 2 tbsp of Epsom salts or 1 tsp of table salt to 1 qt of warm water.

Modified from Kaiser Permanente patient information sheet.

---

between your knees or resting on something comfortable for support.

Steady the foot to be massaged with one hand, and with the knuckles of the other hand make small, firm circles over the entire sole of the foot, including the heel (Figure 8-12, A and B). Light touch tends to tickle, whereas firmness does not; however, the feet of older adults may be more sensitive to pressure than those of the young, so the nurse must modulate the firmness of the massage accordingly. There is an overpowering urge when about to touch someone's feet to say, "I hope you aren't ticklish"—stifle that urge! The power of suggestion is tremendous. Use firm, smooth movements, and you should have satisfying results. You may also find that the person seems to converse spontaneously. Continue to massage the foot; support the foot with the fingers of both hands while the thumbs repeat the small circles over the entire sole of the foot. As you move your thumbs from the toes, you may find that the fingertips are less awkward when you massage around the ankle and the heel (Figure 8-12, C and D). When your fingers reach the heel, take one hand and gently lift the foot under the ankle, and with the other hand use the fingertips and thumb to firmly make circles on the heel. More pressure will be required here because of the thicker horny layer of skin (see Figure 8-12, D).

On the top of the foot, starting at the ankle, look at the long tendons that run from the base of the ankle to each toe.

Support the heel of the foot with one hand, and with the tip of the thumb on your other hand, firmly but gently run your thumb between each tendon groove and off between the toes (Figure 8-12, E). (This can be uncomfortable, so adjust your pressure.) Next grasp the foot between both hands; fingers should be touching on the sole of the foot, heels of the hands touching on the top of the foot (Figure 8-12, F). Press the heels of your hands firmly downward on the foot, and push up on the sole of the foot with your fingers (like breaking a cracker in half). At the same time, slide your hands toward the edges of the foot. Repeat this motion three times. With one hand, steady the foot, and with the thumb and forefinger of the other hand, grasp the base of the big toe. Gently stretch and rotate it from side to side, using a corkscrew motion, until your fingers slide off the tip of the toe. Do this to each toe in sequence (Figure 8-12, G). To finish the massage, place the foot between your hands; hold the foot gently for several seconds (Figure 8-12, H); replace it next to the other foot; gently pick up the other foot and

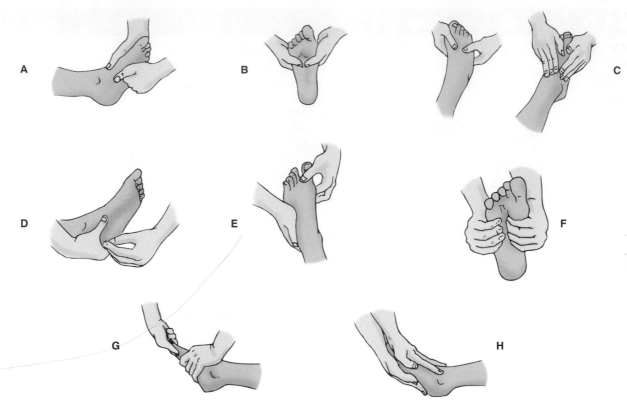

FIGURE 8-12 Foot massage. **A,** With knuckles, make small circles over sole of foot. **B** and **C,** With thumbs and fingers, make circles over entire foot. **D,** With tips of fingers, make circles on heel. **E,** Gently run thumb between tendon grooves from ankle to toes. **F,** As if breaking a cracker, move foot back and forth. **G,** Gently stretch and rotate each toe. **H,** End by placing foot between hands.

repeat the massage sequence. The nurse will find that foot massage can be easily modified to incorporate range-of-motion (ROM) exercises for the toes and ankles. In addition to foot massage, lukewarm oil (baby oil or mineral oil) applied to the feet followed by wrapping in warm moist towels and elevation for 10 to 15 minutes not only facilitates a few minutes of relaxation but also aids in improving integrity of the skin of the feet. Feet are then washed in sudsy warm water and dried thoroughly, or excess oil can simply be removed with a soft towel.

Diabetic foot care is similar to that suggested for good foot care but is critical. A summary of good foot care and diabetic foot care, identifying the similarities and differences, is presented in Table 8-1. If an individual follows the recommendations for diabetic foot care, feet can usually be maintained in comfort.

HEALTHY SKIN AND HAIR

Hair is our crowning glory. Though hair loss is common as we age, it is difficult to accept for both men and women, but especially for women. About 20 million women in the United States are affected by hair loss (Luggen, 2005b). Women experience hair loss later than men do, but often some hair loss is detected by age 50 and nearly 75% of women older than 65 years have noticeable hair loss. As part

of the integument, hair has biological, psychological, and cosmetic value for both men and women.

The skin has esthetic and cosmetic appeal. Artists have portrayed its delicate, flawless qualities, and poets have extolled its virtues through descriptive phrases. Today, art, poetry, and conversation still include similar depictions.

As the largest, most visible organ of the body, the skin serves as a "window" on the person (Kagan et al., 2002). The effects of time and exposure are visible (Merck, 2006a). Wrinkled skin, thinning epidermis, reduced barrier function, delayed healing, loss of elasticity, loss of immunological responses, increased number of inflammatory responses, loss of sensory perception, loss of sweating, and loss of thermoregulation with increased vulnerability to heat and cold occur with aging (see Chapter 4 and Box 8-14).

Vitamin D production is reduced—a 75% decrease between early and late adulthood in the precursor of vitamin D. Other reasons for insufficient vitamin D include lack of sun exposure in many elderly people, especially those who are institutionalized. Paradoxically, we know that avoidance of sun exposure is a cornerstone to prevention of skin cancer. It is suggested that small amounts of sun exposure, exposing hands, face, and arms for 15 minutes per day, three times per week, may be sufficient to ensure adequate levels of vitamin D (Fuller and Casparian, 2001). Poor intake of dairy products is another reason for insufficient vitamin D. The recommended

TABLE 8-1

Essentials of Good Foot Care: Standard and Diabetic

Standard Foot Care	Applicable to Both	Diabetic Foot Care
	Inspect feet daily for cuts, blisters, reddened areas, and scratches. Use a magnifying glass or mirror to inspect the feet, or have someone else do it for you if you cannot reach or see well.	
Wash feet daily (if unable to do by self, ask someone else).		Wash feet daily but DO NOT soak feet daily (causes excessive dryness).
	Blot dry rather than rub dry to avoid injury to sensitive skin. Pay particular attention to between toes.	
	Use emollients, cocoa butter, lanolin lotion, mineral oil, or vegetable oil to soften dry skin to help retain moisture and prevent cracking. DO NOT put between toes; it may contribute to fungal infections.	
		Dust lightly with unscented powder between toes (can prevent excessive perspiration).
	Soak toenails 10-15 minutes in warm water only on day you trim your toe nails.	
	Cut toenails straight across using a toenail clipper.	
	Never cut down the corners.	
Seek help if unable to trim toenails alone.		Have a podiatrist cut toenails if they are too thick to cut yourself or if you are unable to cut your toenails alone.
		DO NOT cut corns or calluses. Have a podiatrist treat them.
		DO NOT apply harsh chemical corn- and wart-removing products to the toes and feet. These can remove tissue as well as the corn or wart.
		DO NOT apply heating pads, chemical or battery operated, to feet.
	Wear clean socks, hose, stockings daily.	
	Cotton socks absorb perspiration for feet that sweat.	
	Keep feet warm with thick, fleecy insoles inside slippers to protect from cold, or wear cotton socks with comfortable slippers.	
		DO NOT walk barefooted at any time.
		Sandals for the beach protect the feet from hot sand, sharp objects, etc. At home, wear shoes or slippers.
	Wear comfortable, well-fitting shoes with broad toe space and low heels.	
Avoid shoes that do not feel comfortable or need to be "broken in."		Good quality athletic shoes, although expensive, outlast regular shoes and are less expensive in the long run.
		Shake out shoes before putting them on to remove foreign objects that might cause injury.
		Carefully break in new shoes. Begin by wearing shoes an hour a day, and gradually increase the time worn.
	DO NOT pop blisters. Infections can occur.	
If blister breaks, wash area, apply antiseptic, keep covered during the day, uncovered at night.		See physician immediately.

Modified from Dellasega C, Yonushonis MEH: Diabetes mellitus in the elderly. In Stanley M, Beare PG: *Gerontological nursing,* Philadelphia, 1995, Davis; Helfand AE, issue editor: *The aging foot: focus on geriatric care and rehabilitation,* 2(10):1, 1989; Jarvik L, Small G: *Parent care,* New York, 1988, Crown. *Continued*

TABLE 8-1

Essentials of Good Foot Care: Standard and Diabetic—cont'd

Standard Foot Care	Applicable to Both	Diabetic Foot Care
	Avoid wearing tight-fitting hose, tight stockings, or garters; DO NOT sit with crossed legs. All of these constrict blood flow to the lower extremities.	
	Review the condition of your orthotics regularly. Mark a date with a laundry marker as a reminder for the podiatrist to reevaluate the effectiveness of the device.	
	Stop smoking. Smoking constricts blood vessels, reducing blood flow to the lower extremities.	
	Report foot injuries promptly to the physician.	
		Call physician for any problems such as tenderness, redness, warmth, drainage, ingrown toenail, athlete's foot, pain in the feet or calves.

Modified from Dellasega C, Yonushonis MEH: Diabetes mellitus in the elderly. In Stanley M, Beare PG: *Gerontological nursing,* Philadelphia, 1995, Davis; Helfand AE, issue editor: *The aging foot: focus on geriatric care and rehabilitation,* 2(10):1, 1989; Jarvik L, Small G: *Parent care,* New York, 1988, Crown.

BOX 8-14   Structural and Functional Changes of the Aging Skin*

Compared with a healthy younger person, age-related changes are as follows:
- Epidermis (outer layer) thins gradually.
- Loss of integrity between epidermis and dermis increases susceptibility to trauma and shearing forces.
- Dermis becomes thin and less flexible.
- Dermis has fewer fibroblasts, resulting in decreased production of elastin (reduced skin elasticity) and collagen (decreased skin strength, increased wrinkling).
- Damaged skin is replaced slowly.
- Fewer Langerhans cells (immune surveillance cells) are present.

- Loss of melanocyte function, less tanning of skin, and less protection from sun occur, increasing likelihood of cancers.
- Pigmentation areas of melanin clumps form telangiectases on the face.

Photoaging effects seen in elderly people include the following:
- Elastin increases so that epidermis thickens and atrophies.
- Wrinkles develop.
- Loss of Langerhans cells increases.
- Loss of collagen increases.
- Predisposition to skin cancers increases.

*See Chapter 4.

---

amount of vitamin D has recently been increased for adults older than 50 years, and some researchers are urging even higher doses for the entire population, to prevent fractures (Fuller and Casparian, 2001).

Healthy skin, despite exposure to heat, cold, water trauma, friction, and pressure, maintains a homeostatic environment. Healthy skin is durable, pliable, and strong enough to protect the body by absorbing, reflecting, cushioning, and restricting various substances and forces that might enter and alter its function. It is sensitive enough to relay messages to the brain.

Common Skin Problems in Late Life

Many skin problems are seen in late life, both in the healthy older adult and in those compromised by illness or mobility limitations. Consensus in the literature is that the common skin problems of aging are xerosis (dry skin), pruritus, seborrheic keratosis, rosacea, stasis dermatitis, herpes zoster, and pressure ulcers. Photoaging not only affects the appearance but also can lead to the development of actinic keratosis and skin cancers. See Chapter 4 for a discussion of the normal changes with aging.

Xerosis. Xerosis (dry skin) is perhaps the most common problem associated with normal aging, although it is poorly understood. It may be linked to a dramatic age-associated decrease in epidermal filaggrin—a protein required for binding keratin filaments into macrofibrils. This leads to separation of dermal and epidermal surfaces, which compromises nutrient transfer between the two layers of skin (Merck, 2006b). Xerosis is also probably a reflection of alteration in lipid composition of the stratum corneum and other changes in the epidermis. The use of statins (HMG-CoA reductase inhibitors), commonly used in management of lipid disorders, may produce acquired severe xerosis and ichthyosis. Xerosis is frequently accompanied by pruritus, itching of the dry skin (see discussion that follows).

BOX 8-15   Causes of Pruritus in the Elderly Person

DERMATITIS

Atopic eczema
Dermatitis herpetiformis
Contact dermatitis
Seborrheic dermatitis
Nodular prurigo
Lichen simplex chronicus (neurodermatitis)
Xerosis (dry skin)
Microvascular (stasis dermatitis, erythema)
Exfoliative skin disorders

PAPULAR SCALING DISORDERS

Psoriasis
Lichen planus

DRUG REACTIONS

Drug withdrawal (delirium tremens)
Antidepressants
Opiates
Aspirin
Estrogens
Biological monoclonal antibodies
Vitamin B complex
Erythromycin estolate
Anabolic steroids
Cocaine
Progesterone
Testosterone
Antimalarials, e.g., quinidine
Tolbutamide

METABOLIC RESPONSES

Liver and biliary obstructive disorders
Renal failure (uremia)
Diabetes mellitus
Hypothyroidism
Thyrotoxicosis

NEOPLASTIC DISORDERS

Hodgkin's lymphoma
Other lymphomas
Prostate cancers
Brain tumors
Leukemias
Stomach cancer
Pancreatic cancer
Lung cancer
Colon cancers

HEMATOPOIETIC RESPONSES

Iron deficiency anemia
Polycythemia vera

PSYCHOGENIC ETIOLOGIES

Involutional psychoses
Hallucinatory aberrations (dementias)

INFECTIONS AND INFESTATIONS

Bacterial (impetigo, chlamydia)
Viral (herpes zoster)
Yeast infections (candidiasis, monilial intertrigo)
Parasitic (scabies, pediculosis)

Xerosis is a problem for 59% to 85% of elderly people (Hardy, 2001). It occurs primarily in the extremities, especially the legs, but can affect the face and trunk as well. Older skin becomes less efficient at holding moisture. The thinner epidermis allows more moisture to escape from the skin. Inadequate fluid intake has a systemic effect; it pulls moisture from the skin to assist in overall hydration of the body.

Exposure to environmental elements such as artificial heat in cold areas (called a "winter itch"), decreased humidity, use of harsh soaps, frequent hot baths, nutritional deficiencies, and smoking contribute to skin dryness and dehydration of the stratum corneum. Hospital care promotes dry skin through routine bathing, use of drying soap, prolonged bed rest, and the action of bed linen on the patient's skin. Repeated wetting and drying of the skin layer causes subsequent tissue drying.

Chapping, drying, and major skin changes occur more slowly and later in those individuals who routinely use emollient skin care products that afford good skin protection. Some skin care items contain moisturizers and sun-screening agents as well. Based on the number of commercial skin preparations on the market today, it is obvious that dry skin and protection from ultraviolet (UV) rays are recognized problems.

Pruritus. Pruritus (itching), an unpleasant cutaneous sensation, is a common result of xerosis and is a symptom, not a diagnosis or a disease; it is an additional threat to skin intactness. It is normal only when it is physiologically appropriate to remove a noxious stimulus from the skin, for example, parasitosis (Sood and Taylor, 2002). It is aggravated by heat, sudden temperature changes, gentle touch, pressure, vibration, electrical stimuli, sweating, contact with articles of clothing, fatigue, exercise, and emotional upheavals. However, pruritus is also a potential sign of systemic disorders such as hypothyroidism and hyperthyroidism, Hodgkin's disease, and other conditions, including lymphomas, chronic renal failure, obstructive biliary or hepatic disease, iron deficiency anemia, leukemias, parasitosis, human immunodeficiency virus (HIV) infection, and drugs (e.g., opioids, captopril, trimethoprim-sulfamethoxazole, salicylates, quinidine, antimalarials, chlorpropamide, phenothiazines—all drugs that cause cholestasis) (National Cancer Institute [NCI], 2006; Sood and Taylor, 2002). Intense nocturnal itching is a primary sign of scabies, which occurs with some frequency in nursing home facilities or sites of communal living. The gerontological nurse should always listen carefully to the patient's ideas of why the pruritus is occurring and what relieves it or does not relieve it. Box 8-15 lists the various causes of pruritus in the elderly person.

An itch is generally viewed as a primary sensory modality with similarities to pain (Bernhard, 2006). The sensation of the itch resides in free nerve endings in the epidermis and dermis, and the sensation is traced to conducting, histamine-responsive unmyelinated C-fibers, the same as some of the pain sensations (NCI, 2006). Itch is perceived in the somatosensory cortex with projections to the motor center causing the urge to scratch.

The urge to scratch is an ineffective response to the urge to remove the irritant itch from the skin. When one scratches, a counterstimulus is introduced, which is stronger than the original itch stimulus. The nerve messages become confused or eliminate the itching sensation by the intensity of the scratch stimulus.

Seborrheic Keratosis. Seborrheic keratosis is a benign growth that appears mainly on the trunk, face, neck, and scalp as single or multiple lesions. One or more benign lesions are present on nearly all adults older than 65 years. An individual may have dozens of these benign lesions. The keratosis is a waxy, raised, verrucous lesion, flesh-colored or pigmented in varying sizes (Figure 8-13). They have the appearance of being "stuck on the skin." Sebaceous keratotic lesions can at times be picked off with a fingernail, but the lesion soon returns. Generally, seborrheic keratoses are removed by a dermatologist for cosmetic reasons, by curettage and light cautery or by freezing with liquid nitrogen for 15 to 20 seconds. A variant is seen in darkly pigmented persons that occurs mostly on the face with numerous small, dark, possibly pedunculated papules (Beers and Berkow, 2000).

Rosacea. Rosacea is an inflammatory skin condition that begins most often at midlife between the ages of 30 and 50 years. It is characterized by vascular erythema, telangiectasia, and flushing, possibly with inflamed papules and pustules in symmetrical or asymmetrical areas of the face (Beers and Berkow, 2000; National Skin Centre [NSC], 2006). It may occur on the nose, cheeks, forehead, and chin, and

occasionally ocular lesions and/or dry eyes may be present. Occasional or chronic edema may occur. It occurs most often in women, but the severity is greater in men (NSC, 2006). It occurs more often in fair-skinned individuals.

In men mainly, rhinophyma can occur (Habif, 2005). It is caused by a deep inflammation of the nose and leads to an irreversible thickening of the skin. Long-term antibiotics are often required for this phenomenon. A drying topical therapy with sulfacetamide and sulfur has been found to be effective. The etiology is not known. It is thought to be related to endocrine abnormalities, focal infection, diet, vascular disorder, *Demodex folliculorum,* and psychological factors such as stress (NSC, 2006). It may be aggravated by sun exposure, alcohol, hot drinks, spicy foods, temperature extremes, and stress.

Persons with rosacea may have skin that is sensitive to cosmetics, although high-quality moisturizers are recommended as are oil-free cosmetic products. Sunscreens of sun protection factor (SPF) higher than 30 are recommended. Soaps should be mild, and alcohol or witch hazel products should be avoided. Cetaphil (a gentle cleansing lotion) or other similar products should be used. Eye involvement is common, including mild conjunctivitis with soreness, grittiness, burning, and tearing. More severe eye signs may be seen, such as blepharitis, chalazion, telangiectasis of the eyelids, conjunctival hyperemia, corneal vascularization and infiltrate, and corneal vascularization and thinning (Habif, 2005).

Treatments include avoiding precipitants such as red wine and hot food and drink, using sunscreens, and treating pustules with topical antibiotics. Topical metronidazole gel or sulfacetamide with sulfur are the most effective treatments, although others are used (Habif, 2005). An ophthalmologist or dermatologist should be consulted if the eye is involved.

Stasis Dermatitis. Stasis dermatitis is a chronic inflammatory eczematous dermatitis of the legs associated with chronic venous insufficiency and edema, dilated and varicose veins, and hyperpigmentation (Habif, 2005). It occurs in adults older than 70 years, and the prevalence is thought to be more than 20% (Flugman, 2005). It is a common chronic problem and frequently relapses. Those with this problem are at risk for cellulitis.

In venous insufficiency, the venous hypertension that occurs is caused by increased venous hydrostatic pressure that is transmitted to the dermal microcirculation (Flugman, 2005). This leads to increased permeability of dermal capillaries. Macromolecules such as fibrinogen leak out so that a fibrin cuff forms in more severe disease. These cuffs are not found in any other ulcers—only in venous hypertension. Stasis dermatitis may be exacerbated by edema, scratching, or contact dermatitis.

Venous stasis dermatitis is a risk factor for venous ulcers (see Chapter 10) and deep vein thrombosis (DVT). There is often a family or personal history of varicose veins or venous insufficiency (Habif, 2005). There may be a history of DVT, trauma, ulceration, or surgery.

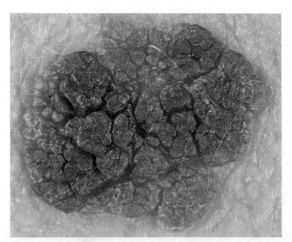

FIGURE 8-13 Seborrheic keratosis in an older adult. (From Habif TP: *Clinical dermatology: a color guide to diagnosis and therapy,* ed 4, St Louis, 2004, Mosby.)

Edema not drained by lymphatic or venous systems causes persistent swelling, redness (hemosiderin deposition), a woody induration, and pruritic eruptions. Chronic edema impairs healing, and even very small wounds may become large, chronic ulcerations and difficult to heal. Often the very swollen leg will weep fluids.

Other clinical findings or information in the history of stasis dermatitis include an insidious onset of pruritus affecting the extremities; increased swelling of the medial ankle at the end of the day; a reddish brown skin discoloration (an early sign of stasis dermatitis); and dependent leg edema. Dermatitis and pruritus can be chronic. The pruritus is a difficult symptom because scratching may cause infection; cellulitis and impetigo can be significant problems. Congestive heart failure worsens the peripheral edema (Flugman, 2005). Chronically congested legs may have local lymphatic disturbances and recurrent erysipelas, which causes elephantiasis (stasis papillomatosis) (Habif, 2005).

Herpes Zoster. Herpes zoster (HZ), or shingles, is frequently seen in older adults. The peak incidence occurs between ages 50 and 70 years. The lifetime risk of all people is 10% to 20% (Habif, 2005). Immunosuppressed elders are at greatest risk; however, HZ can occur in healthy people as well. The onset of this viral disease may be preceded by a prodrome of chills, fever, GI disturbance, malaise, and pain or paresthesias along the affected dermatome. Soon clusters of papulovesicles develop in the dermatomal distribution. A new preventive subcutaneous antiviral has been developed and is on the market. Most HZ occurs in the thoracic area (⅔ of cases); 10% to 20% are trigeminal, 10% to 20% are cervical, 5% to 10% are lumbar, and fewer than 5% are sacral (Habif, 2005).

HZ may be very painful and pruritic. As many as 20% of elderly patients may have postherpetic neuralgia (PHN) lasting weeks or months after resolution of the acute infection. HZ is infectious until dry crusts appear (Beers and Berkow, 2000).

Before diagnosis, the elder may complain of headache, photophobia, and malaise. Occasionally, local lymphadenopathy is present but no fever (Habif, 2005). Occasionally, the skin where the eruption *will* occur is painful or tender and is a predictive sign. Often the area is pruritic or burning. The ensuing papular eruption may follow one dermatome or two or more. The more dermatomes involved, the more serious the situation, especially if it involves the head. In most cases, the severity of the infection increases with age.

Early treatment of the infection with oral antiviral drugs (famciclovir or this antiviral family of drugs) substantially reduces the incidence of PHN, which is common with increasing age (40% in those older than 60 years) and increases in severity more than incidence with increasing age. Occasionally the antiviral therapy is given empirically to those who are immunocompromised or have trigeminal zoster. Topical drugs are not used.

Analgesics are usually needed—gabapentin, or newer variations of the drug (for neuropathic pain) and possibly opioids, depending on the level of the patient's pain. Post-HZ scarring and discoloration are common in elderly patients. A lidocaine patch has been used successfully on dry, non-open areas and has a Food and Drug Administration (FDA) indication for this use. Steroids have not been found to be effective in management. Oral antidepressants may be helpful especially when the pain is lasting.

Burow's solution (aluminum acetate 5%) diluted 1:20 or more helps remove crusts and soothes the skin. The crusts will drop off in 2 to 3 weeks. Gauze dressings can be applied after soaking in the solution, but they must be changed regularly, every 2 to 3 hours. Cool tap water can be used for wet dressings for 20 minutes at a time several times each day (Habif, 2005). This discourages bacterial overgrowth. The best early management is starting the antiviral agent as soon as possible for shortening the course of HZ.

Complications are common. The pain of PHN is the major cause of morbidity in HZ—74% of elders ages 70 years and older (Habif, 2005). The incidence and duration of pain increase with aging. Most adults younger than 30 years have no pain at all. Other complications include peripheral nerve palsies, encephalitis, myelitis, a contralateral hemiparesis syndrome, and when disseminated over the body, death. HZ recurs in about 6% of patients. Complications of HZ depend on the dermatome(s) involved. Eye involvement requires immediate consultation with an ophthalmologist. Encephalitis may occur, as well as motor neuropathies, such as Guillain-Barré syndrome, and urinary retention. With severe HZ or HZ affecting more than one dermatome, intravenous therapy of antivirals should be given. PHN is difficult to treat. The pain can be described as lancinating and intermittent, constant deep aching or burning, or dysesthetic pain that is provoked by trivial stimuli (Beers and Berkow, 2000). Diagnosis is made by a biopsy of a vesicle or a Tzanck smear; however, the diagnosis should be made clinically because the laboratory study takes weeks to complete. HZ is distinguished from herpes simplex by fluid culture or direct fluorescent antibody analysis if diagnosis is a problem. HZ also always occurs along a dermatome, whereas herpes simplex can occur anywhere and can vary in location.

Photoaging

In most elderly Americans, the obvious changes in the appearance of the skin are the result of chronic exposure to UV radiation from sun exposure (Merck, 2006b). Pale skin and the loss of melanocytes (10% to 20%) increase the vulnerability to UV radiation. This photoaging manifests as solar elastosis or exaggerated fine and coarse wrinkling of skin, sallowness, and telangiectases. Actinic purpura (solar, or senile purpura) that occur on the forearms of elders are thought to represent excessive numbers of red blood cells (RBCs) in photo-damaged connective tissue. The RBCs extravasate from fragile blood vessels and clear slowly. Stellate pseudoscars on the arms also are indicative of photoaging. Cigarette smoking increases the wrinkling and photoaging and risk for skin cancers. Photoaging causes diminished immunological and inflammatory responsiveness in the skin. Rough, red dysplastic areas of actinic keratoses are associated with severe skin damage and heightened risk for skin cancers.

Most sunscreens have many chemicals that absorb, reflect, or scatter light. Most absorb UVB rays. Most block UVA rays. Zinc oxide and titanium dioxide block both UVA and UVB rays. These and other sunscreens also block UV-induced vitamin D formation in the skin (Merck, 2006b). Therefore it is essential that older adults safeguard against osteopenia and osteoporosis by drinking vitamin D–fortified milk or orange juice or take vitamin D supplements, at least 800 international units (IU) per day (see Chapter 15).

Skin Cancers

Photoaging significantly increases the risk of both premalignant and malignant lesions in the older adult. Nearly 1 million cases of skin cancer are diagnosed each year (National Institutes of Health [NIH], 2000). More than 95% of these are basal cell carcinoma (BCC). They are highly treatable and rarely metastasize. However, local invasion can cause disfigurement and functional impairment if not detected and treated early. Other skin cancers seen are squamous cell carcinoma (SCC) and melanomas. Risk factors for nonmelanomatous skin cancers are listed in Box 8-16.

Actinic Keratosis. Actinic keratosis is a precancerous lesion, occasionally becoming a squamous cell carcinoma (Mayo Clinic, 2006b). It is the result of years of overexposure to the sun or UV light, which induces mutations. Risk factors are older age, fair complexion, blue eyes, and history of freckles in childhood. It is found on sun-exposed areas such as bald head, hands, face, ears, nose, upper trunk, and arms. Actinic keratosis is characterized by rough, scaly, sandpaper-like patches, pink to reddish-brown on an erythematous base (Mayo Clinic, 2006b) (Figure 8-14). Lesions may be single or multiple; they may be painless or mildly tender. Early recognition, treatment, and removal of this lesion are important to prevent serious problems later. Persons with actinic keratoses should use a protective sunscreen with a minimum SPF of 30. They should be seen by a dermatologist every 6 to 12 months for evaluation. These lesions are easily treated if discovered and diagnosed early.

Basal Cell Carcinoma. BCC appears after the fifth decade, affecting 800,000 Americans every year (Skin Cancer

Foundation [SCF], 2006). It used to occur mainly in older age-groups but is occurring more and more in younger middle-aged adults. It is more prevalent in light-skinned persons. It occurs in the basal (bottom layer) of the epidermis. It may be precipitated by extensive chronic sun exposure, chronic irritation, and chronic ulceration of the skin. Though it grows slowly, it can, if neglected, cause considerable disfigurement. Early detection and treatment are advisable, even though metastasis is rare. Suspicious lesions should always be referred to the dermatologist.

This neoplasm has the classic appearance of a pearly papule with prominent telangiectases (blood vessels), which leads to a centrally ulcerated area (Figure 8-15). However, its appearance actually varies greatly and is often overlooked or confused with a squamous cell lesion, often requiring a biopsy for confirmation of a diagnosis.

Other appearances of a BCC include the following:
- An open sore that bleeds, oozes, or crusts and remains for 3 or more weeks (SCF, 2006).
- A reddish patch or irritation, often on the chest, shoulders, arms, or legs. Sometimes this patch crusts, itches, or hurts.

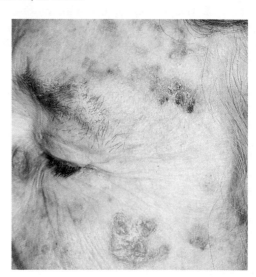

FIGURE 8-14 Actinic keratosis in an older adult in an area of sun exposure. (From Habif TP: *Clinical dermatology: a color guide to diagnosis and therapy,* ed 3, St Louis, 1996, Mosby.)

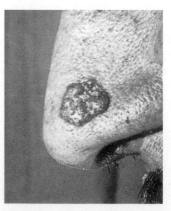

FIGURE 8-15 Basal cell carcinoma, the most commonly occurring skin cancer. (Courtesy Gary Monheit, MD, University of Alabama at Birmingham School of Medicine.)

BOX 8-16	**Risk Factors for Nonmelanomatous Skin Cancers**

- History of nonmelanomatous skin cancer
- Older age
- Light eyes
- Light skin
- Light hair
- Poor ability to tan
- Substantive cumulative lifetime sun exposure

Adapted from National Institutes of Health: *Screening for skin cancer including counseling to prevent skin cancer,* 2000 (website): *http://text.nlm.nih.gov/temppfiles/is/tempBRPg43432.html.*

- A shiny nodule or bump, pearly or translucent, pink or red or white in a lighter pigmented person and tan, black, or brown in darker-skinned elders and might be confused with a mole (nevus).
- A pink growth with a slightly rolled, elevated border and crusty interior is usually a BCC.
- A scarlike area, white, yellow, or waxy in color with poorly defined borders, may be a more aggressive form.

Squamous Cell Carcinoma.

Squamous cell carcinoma (SCC) is the second most common skin cancer and affects predominantly older adults. It accounts for 20% of all skin cancers (University of Maryland [UM], 2004). It is an invasive, primary cutaneous malignancy arising from the keratinocytes of the skin or mucosa (Habif, 2005). It usually is found on the head, neck, or hands of elderly people (Figure 8-16). It may evolve from actinic keratoses or de novo. Lifetime risk for development of a SCC is 4% to 14% (Habif, 2005). More than 100,000 new cases are diagnosed each year and result in 2500 deaths.

Sun exposure is the major cause, and it is more prevalent in pale or fair-skinned men and women who live in sunny locations. It is seen more on the leg in older women compared with men (Habif, 2005). Other risks for the development of this type of skin cancer include exposure to sources of UV light (frequently in tanning beds by the future generation of older adults), hydrocarbons, tobacco, chronic infections such as osteomyelitis, chronic inflammatory conditions, exposure to arsenic, burns, and human papillomavirus (HPV) (Habif, 2005).

SCC arising from actinic keratosis appears as a hypertrophic actinic keratosis (Habif, 2005). It has a persistent, red, poorly-defined base and an adherent yellow-white scale. Diagnosis is made by skin biopsy. SCC arising de novo appears with well-defined margins and is smooth, dull, red, firm, and dome-shaped with a crusted center in sun-exposed areas. The ear is an important place to look for SCCs. If the crust is removed, the smell may be foul because it is necrotic tissue. Invasion occurs locally and systemically in about 2% to 6% of cases and metastasizes in 2 to 3 years to regional lymph nodes (Habif, 2005).

SCCs on the lip, the ear pinna, and the genitals are most likely to metastasize. Other risk factors for metastasis are

tumors larger than 2.0 cm, invasion deeper than 0.4 cm, or both; decreased differentiation of tumor cells (fewer different types of cells); recurrent lesions; mucin-producing variant SCC; immunocompromised elders (older adults become more immunocompromised with natural aging); and tumor arising in a scar or a chronic wound (Habif, 2005). They are treated with wide excision, radiotherapy, and cryotherapy. New SCC lesions are apt to occur because of the skin damage already accrued.

Melanoma.

This frightening skin cancer is increasing in incidence—more rapidly than any other cancer over the past 10 years (SCF, 2006). Each year, 51,000 new cases are reported to the American Cancer Society in the United States (SCF, 2006) and result in 7000 deaths each year. The incidence has risen dramatically—in 1981 an American's lifetime risk was 1 in 250; today the risk is 1 in 87. In older adults, the superficial spreading melanoma is most common, accounting for about 60% of all melanomas (Beers and Berkow, 2000). It increases through the eighth decade. Nodular melanoma accounts for 15% of all melanomas and also occurs mostly in late life. Lentigo melanoma accounts for 5% to 10% of melanomas and occurs mainly in elderly patients. Mean age at diagnosis is 67 years.

Melanoma is very treatable if caught early; however, it metastasizes quickly. It originates often in a mole (nevus) or other growths on normal-appearing skin (UM, 2004). Any nevus that changes should be evaluated by a dermatologist or skin cancer specialist.

There are four basic types of melanoma, and they look different and occur on different areas of skin in the elder; three occur in situ and one is invasive from the start (SCF, 2006). They differ significantly from one another in appearance, behavior, and prognosis.

Superficial spreading melanoma (SSM) is the most common type (70%-80%) (Habif, 2005; SCF, 2006). It spreads over the skin for a long period before invading the skin. A nurse following a patient for a long period will note this change as will caregivers and the elder himself or herself if observant. It begins as a flat or slightly raised discolored patch with irregular borders and somewhat geometric form. It may be tan, brown, black, red, blue, or white. It may be a change in an older mole (usually), or it may arise de novo (occasionally). It occurs mainly on the trunk in men, legs in women, and upper back in both men and women. These occur in younger older adults.

Lentigo maligna (LM) accounts for about 5% to 10% of all melanomas (Habif, 2005). Like SSM, it remains close to the surface for some time, appearing as a flat (macule) or mildly elevated, mottled tan, brown, or dark-brown coloration (Figure 8-17). This type of in-situ (intraepidermal) melanoma is the one that occurs most often in elderly people with fair skin color (SCF, 2006). It is seen on chronically sun-damaged skin on the face, ears, arms, and upper trunk. It is the most common form seen in Hawaii.

LM progresses to invasive LM melanoma (LMM) in 5% of patients (Habif, 2005). It occurs equally in men and women, most often elderly men and women. It affects those with sun

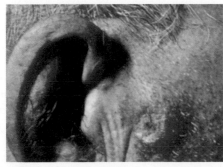

FIGURE 8-16 Squamous cell carcinoma. (Courtesy Gary Monheit, MD, University of Alabama at Birmingham School of Medicine.)

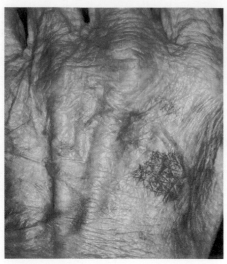

FIGURE 8-17 Lentigo, a brown macule that appears in chronically sun-exposed areas. (From Habif TP: *Clinical dermatology: a color guide to diagnosis and therapy,* ed 4, St Louis, 2004, Mosby.)

damage in the face, neck, or dorsal arms. Lesions are flat and irregular. The color is brown with variation in pigment density. They appear mottled (or washed out) and may have some areas of normal pigmentation. Later, nodules and ulceration may develop, which indicates local invasion.

Acral lentiginous melanoma (ALM) accounts for 7% of all melanomas (Habif, 2005). It is more common in men than in women and occurs mainly in older adults. It occurs mainly as a black or brown discoloration under the nails, on the soles of the feet, or on the palms of the hands. It may be an innocent-appearing, enlarging, pink-to-red papule, similar to an insect bite. It spreads superficially before it penetrates deeply (SCF, 2006), evolving over years. The lesions are similar to LM but can be amelanotic, or without color, non-pigmented; any melanoma can be amelanotic, and 2% are. It differs from the others in that it is the most common form of melanoma in the skin of Asians and blacks; it accounts for 50% of melanomas in these groups (Habif, 2005).

Nodular melanoma accounts for 10% to 15% of melanomas (Habif, 2005). It occurs in men and women equally. It can be found anywhere on the body, usually in the extremities—legs, arms, and also on the trunk of elderly people. It may occur on the scalp in men, which has a poorer prognosis. The lesions are raised, are brown to black, appear rapidly, and have papules.

Occasionally, a lesion is blue, gray, white, tan, red, or skin tone. Focal hemorrhage may occur. These lesions evolve over months and extend vertically into the skin. This type of melanoma is invasive from the time it is diagnosed and is the most aggressive of the melanomas (SCF, 2006).

Treatment depends on the risk category based on the size of the lesion. Enlarged lymph nodes will be removed. Wide local excision of the lesion often requires a skin flap or graft. Mohs' surgery is the most successful type and conserves tissue. Long-term follow-up is done at 6-month intervals. Advanced melanoma is incurable and treated palliatively. Radiation

with corticosteroids may prolong comfort. Opioids and other end-of-life measures will be necessary, and advance directives should be in place.

▲ Promoting Healthy Aging: Implications for Gerontological Nursing

The gerontological nurse caring for the older adult is in an ideal position to promote healthy aging of skin and to promote wellness in the presence of alterations in health or risk for complications.

Assessment. The usual body response to heat is to produce moisture or sweat from these glands and thus cool the skin by evaporation. Because sweating is diminished in late life (up to 70% in one study), overheating and heat intolerance are important problems. A frail elder can be encouraged to avoid spending long periods in the heat, both indoors and outdoors. The summer, in particular, poses a major threat in areas in which humidity and heat are persistently high. In these areas the death rate among the elderly from heat is high because these changes are compounded by diminished vascularity of the skin. All persons should be encouraged to wear a hat when in the sun; to wear light, cool clothing; and to drink sufficient amounts of fluid.

Deodorants and antiperspirants are often used to suppress odors from the apocrine glands in younger adults. Dusting powder with baking soda is a natural, inexpensive substance that can keep the axilla dry and free from odor in elders, if needed at all.

Interventions

Care of Dry Skin. Treatment of dry skin is focused on the relief of symptoms; the underlying problem cannot be cured. The nurse should be alert to signs of rough, scaly, flaking skin on the legs and feet, face, hands, forearms, sides of the lower trunk, and exterior and lateral aspects of the thighs. Dry skin is more common in winter months because of lower humidity of air indoors and outdoors. A complication of xerosis that occurs during these months is xerotic eczema, and when severe it is called *eczema craquelé* or *asteatotic eczema.* This disorder causes fissures and excoriations that allow the environment's irritants to penetrate skin and cause inflammation and infection (Beers and Berkow, 2000). The management of dry, itchy skin is to rehydrate the epidermis, especially the keratin, or horny layer. Elders should bathe only once a day or less often, and they should not use strong soaps or other skin cleansers that contain alcohol. Only soft material should be next to the skin (not rough woolens). The skin's only moisturizer is water. Substances may be used to enhance water's ability to stay on the skin. An emollient should be applied liberally after bathing, when the skin is moist. This is accomplished with binders (bind water to the skin) and humectants (attract moisture from the air to the skin), but other products such as oils, petrolatum, and zinc oxide keep moisture that is already in the skin from evaporating and are effective and inexpensive. Oils and ointments also are designed to coat the skin and replace the skin's natural oil barrier (sebum). Use of super-fatted soaps without hexachlorophene is most effective in helping restore the protective lipid film to the skin surface. Dove, Tone, and Caress are the most common of the super-fatted soaps used, but scented soaps and emollients should be avoided because they may irritate dry skin.

Incorporation of bath oils and other hydrophobic preparations into the bathing routine temporarily helps hold moisture and retards its escape from the skin. However, bath oil poured into the bathtub creates the potential for falls. It is safer and more effective to have the person bathe or shower, lightly towel dry, and apply the substance directly onto the moist skin; mild, water-laden emulsions are best. Light mineral oil or petrolatum rubbed in well is as effective as commercial brands and less costly.

Prescription lotions with urea or α-hydroxy acid (lactic acid) help remove scales, hydrate skin, and prevent itching. Also, a topical corticosteroid ointment containing 1% to 2% hydrocortisone will cool inflamed or itchy skin. It should be applied after bathing and at bedtime. Corticosteroid ointments should be used only for a short time and with caution because some of it is absorbed systemically and may cause further thinning of the epidermis.

Maintaining an environment with 60% humidity, alleviating mechanical irritation caused by clothing, encouraging baths and showers with water temperatures at 90° to 105° F, and applying mineral oil or other emollients after bathing help control dry skin. The need for "squeaky clean" skin is an American cultural oddity. Boxes 8-17 and 8-18 offer tips for healthy skin and care of dry skin. Use of humidifiers in the house or bedroom is helpful.

When pruritus is the result of xerosis, the most appropriate treatment is skin rehydration. If rehydration of the stratum corneum is not sufficient to control itching, cool compresses of saline solution or oatmeal or Epsom salt baths may be indicated. Use of a lotion such as Lubriderm or Nutraderm is helpful. Vigorous towel drying intensifies pruritus by overstimulating the skin and removing the needed water from the stratum corneum. Hot bath water should be avoided.

For relief of itching, use mild cleansers with low pH; rinse soap off immediately and completely; pat dry lightly; apply moisturizer cream—ammonium lactate moisturizer is suggested (American Academy of Dermatology, 2006). If the skin is open and weeping, use oatmeal soaps and antipruritic creams without steroids. Ultraviolet phototherapy has also been used; it is an antipruritic and may be tried if other measures are not successful. It is especially useful for pruritus associated with liver disease and renal disease.

Stasis Dermatitis. When caring for the person with stasis dermatitis, it is of utmost importance to protect the limb from further injury. Control of edema is paramount in avoiding or resolving the problem. Diuretics are of little use but occasionally are used. The legs should be elevated to at least heart level for 30 minutes 3 times every day to facilitate venous return (Habif, 2005).

Compressive dressings (Jobst, Venosan, Ace wraps, Unna Boots) are a mainstay of treatment; however, they must be

---

BOX 8-17   Tips for Healthy Skin

- Pay attention to any break in the skin.
- Use a humidifier if necessary to keep room humidity above 40%.
- Bathing every 2 to 3 days is sufficient.
- Use a non-deodorant mild soap with lanolin or other creams in its base.
- Do not add bath oil to water—there is a risk of slipping.
- Use a moisturizer that applies easily, leaves no greasy film, and does not stain clothing.
- Apply moisturizers as often as necessary to maintain continuous coverage.
- Choose clothing made of soft cotton or other nonabrasive materials.
- Drink several glasses of pure water every day.
- In cold and windy weather, wear a warm hat, gloves, and scarf to protect extremities.
- Wear a wide-brimmed hat to shade from the sun.
- Use a sunscreen lotion with the appropriate sun protection factor (SPF) (usually SPF 15 or higher) on all exposed areas.
- Avoid direct sunlight for extended periods.

---

used with extreme caution and are completely contraindicated in the presence of actual or suspected arterial disease.

Once the absence of arterial disease is confirmed (see Chapter 10), the nurse works with the patient and the health care provider to find a dressing that the patient can manage and tolerate. Some are one piece (thromboembolic disease [TED] hose), and others require wrapping using specific techniques; both are removed and reapplied at least daily. Others are applied by the nurse (Unna Boot) and left on for several days.

Daily compression dressings or stockings should be applied just before arising when swelling is least, and they should be checked several times during the day to ensure proper placement. Not everyone is able to put on the stockings, and they may prefer to keep using the bandages. Use of the pressure dressings or stockings should continue after the swelling appears to be gone.

Saline or silver impregnated dressings and oral antibiotics are prescribed for infection, often manifesting as yellow crusting or pustules (Flugman, 2005; Habif, 2005). For generalized dermatitis, an oral steroid is given, tapering over 3 weeks. Oral antihistamines such as hydroxyzine 10 to 25 mg every 4 to 6 hours may help control itching but can lead to serious consequences. The use of antihistamines increases the risk for falling. Bland emollients will alleviate dryness. Petroleum-based products are preferable to lotions. Avoid topical products that might result in an allergic reaction such as any product with a fragrance; also avoid bacitracin, which is overused, and neomycin ointments unless infection at the site has been demonstrated.

If ulceration is present, the nurse may find the use of hydrocolloid dressings under the compression dressing to be useful. However, the nurse must watch the wound carefully

BOX 8-18 Care of Dry Skin

To soften dry skin and keep it soft, do as little as possible to break the skin's natural protective oils; do as much as possible to maintain and replenish them.

- Take fewer and faster soaking baths. In winter, one tub or shower per week should suffice. None is OK too, for the person with dry skin. Sponge-bathe armpits, groin, and perianal areas and any other parts of the body that need daily (or more frequent) care.
- Use warm water rather than hot to bathe, whether in the tub or shower. The hotter the water, the more natural oils are washed away.
- Limit the use of soap. One lathering is enough to cleanse most of the normally moist body areas; a damp cloth without any soap is sufficient to clean extremities and body areas that stay dry. Consider using superfatted soap; it need not be expensive—Dove, especially, and Olay and Basis are superfatted and relatively inexpensive. In addition to these, one source recommends soap cleansers such as Cetaphil lotion, Oilatum-AD, and Aquanil (American Osteopathic College of Dermatology [AOCD], 2005).
- If using a deodorant soap, limit it to odorous areas such as feet, underarms, and genital area (AOCD, 2005).
- If skin is both dry and itchy, apply oil freely and often, rubbing or smoothing it into the skin. Do not use rubbing alcohol or rubs containing alcohol, because these destroy natural oils on the skin and make it dry out faster. Use hand or body oils that work on all of the dry areas, and be sure to apply immediately after bathing, while the skin is moist.
- Avoid vigorous use of the washcloth during cleansing. When toweling dry, avoid hard rubbing but pat dry so moisture remains on the skin. Then immediately apply Eucerin cream, Neutrogena Light Sesame Oil, Alpha-Keri, or Robathol.
- Avoid long periods in the sun. When going out in the sun or when staying in the sun is unavoidable, wear protective

clothing and a sun barrier oil or lotion with sun protection factor (SPF) higher than 30. Be sure to reapply after swimming. Apply 30 minutes before going into the pool and then after coming out of the pool.

- Use an oil that is affordable. The most expensive is not necessarily the best. Hydrogenated shortening (Crisco or Spry) or the least expensive mineral oil will do a good moisturizing job.
- If dry skin is a problem only in winter, consider installing an efficient, whole-house humidifier in the home heating system. Not only will it help the skin hold its natural moisture (less evaporation into dry air), but also it will help lower heat costs. Moist air feels warmer than dry; the same degree of comfort at lower temperatures will be experienced.
- If living or working in air-conditioned areas, try to keep the temperature high enough for the air to stay moist. Most air-conditioning systems reduce humidity as well as temperature; maintain temperature between 68° and 70° F.
- Take tepid baths and use bath oil afterwards so skin is not further dehydrated.
- Apply soothing creams or emollients several times daily, especially on hands, feet, and face.
- Wear soft, absorbent clothing such as cotton.
- Use the following with caution: topical steroid creams (unpredictable absorption); low-dose systemic steroids (likely to result in complications).
- Persons older than 75 years should not use antihistamines (may experience sudden, severe side effects).
- For laundry, use Tide-free, or Cheer-free, or All-free detergents. Avoid fabric softeners, especially in the dryer. Avoid irritating fabrics touching the skin. Avoid wool and other "scratchy" fabrics. Use only cotton percale sheets on the bed.

for any signs of infection or for failure to heal. Any problems should be reported to the health care provider promptly. The nurse practitioner or physician caring for the person with non-healing stasis dermatitis or ulcers should refer to the local wound clinic or wound care specialist.

Skin Cancers. Many of the changes associated with photoaging are preventable. Ideally, preventive measures should begin in childhood, but clinical evidence has shown that some improvement can be achieved by avoidance of sun exposure and regular use of sunscreens even after solar damage has occurred. Elders with sun damage appear older than those who have been protected, who have skin with pigmentation, or who have lifestyle differences.

Sunscreens offer protection from harmful ultraviolet A rays (UVA), which affect the dermis, and UVB rays, which affect the epidermis. Effectiveness of sunscreens is measured in terms of the sun protection factor (SPF). Sun-induced damage varies with skin type. Individuals who always burn, never tan, or minimally tan or who burn moderately and tan

to a light brown should be considered to have sensitive to very sensitive skin. These individuals should wear protective clothing such as light, long-sleeved shirts and a hat with a wide brim. For incidental sun exposure, these elders should wear a sunscreen that covers UVA and UVB with an SPF of 30 or higher. Because of the many years of sun exposure, the thinness of the older skin, and the damage already done to the deoxyribonucleic acid (DNA), all elders should follow the advice for those with tendency to burn. Box 8-19 offers sun protection recommendations.

Total body skin examinations should be part of the yearly assessment. Older men and middle-aged men have the worst track record for performing regular self-examinations or seeing a dermatologist (SCF, 2006). These men have the highest mortality rate from melanoma.

The nurse should ask about skin cancer prevention, teach about risk, and ask about history of sun exposure. Training in basic skin cancer triage can improve primary care providers' practice of skin cancer control measures; teach that new lesions be photographed and followed fre-

---

BOX 8-19   Sun Protection Recommendations

- Avoid getting sunburned. Persons of all skin types and races can sunburn, but fair-skinned persons burn more easily.
- Do not consider tanning healthy. Do not try to get a suntan, and avoid tanning booths.
- Avoid the midday sun (10 AM to 3 PM) when the ultraviolet radiation is most intense.
- Wear protective clothing such as a broad-brimmed hat, long sleeves, long pants; however, be aware that clothing alone does not provide complete protection.
- Use sunscreen daily (if going outside), even on a cloudy day, because clouds do not block ultraviolet radiation.
- Select and use a sunscreen with a sun protection factor (SPF) higher than 30 that is appropriate for your skin type. Apply to sun-exposed areas 30 minutes before going outside and reapply periodically after perspiring heavily or swimming. If using cosmetics on face, apply sunscreen first.
- Use a lip balm that contains a sunscreen.
- Be aware of reflection from sand, snow, and water, which will intensify the radiation.
- Avoid sun if using photosensitizing drugs.
- Avoid para-aminobenzoic acid (PABA) sunscreens if allergic to procaine, sulfonamides, or hair dyes because of cross sensitization.

Adapted from Hogstel MO: *Clinical manual of gerontological nursing,* St Louis, 1992, Mosby.

quently and referred early. Primary nurse providers should do a total body skin check at least once each year. Suspicious lesions should be referred for expert consultation by dermatologists, because research shows that primary care providers (physicians, in this case) make significantly fewer correct diagnoses of skin lesions, including malignant melanoma and BCC (NIH, 2000). The ABCDs of melanoma assessment are listed in Box 8-20.

PRESSURE ULCERS

According to the National Pressure Ulcers Advisory Panel (2007), a pressure ulcer is "localized injury to the skin and/or underlying tissue usually over a bony prominence, as a result of pressure, or pressure in combination with shear and/or friction." As tissue is compressed, blood is diverted and blood vessels are forcibly constricted by the persistent pressure on the skin and underlying structures; thus cellular respiration is impaired and cells die from ischemia and anoxia. Intervention at any point in the developing process can stop the advancement of the pressure ulcer.

Just how much pressure can be endured by tissue (tissue tolerance) is highly variable from body location to location and person to person. Tissue tolerance is inversely affected by moisture, amount of pressure, friction, shearing, and age and is directly related to poor nutritional status and low arterial pressure.

BOX 8-20   The ABCD Rules of Melanoma

Asymmetry: One half does not match the other half.
Border irregularity: The edges are ragged, notched, or blurred.
Color: The pigment is not uniform in color, having shades of tan, brown, or black, or a mottled appearance with red, white, or blue areas.
Diameter: The diameter is greater than the size of a pencil eraser or is increased, increasing in size.

Pressure ulcers are a concern for huge numbers of persons and therefore nurses. At any one time, 1.8 million elders, 10% to 23% of nursing home patients in long-term care settings (Nutrition Screening Initiative, 2001) and 10% to 29% of patients in acute care settings, have at least one pressure ulcer. The prevalence is 41% of critical care patients and about 13% of home care patients (Beers and Berkow, 2000; Cobb and Durfee, 2002). Seventy percent of pressure sores occur in persons older than 70 years (Tangalos, 2002). Reducing the proportion of pressure ulcers in the nursing home population is a national goal (Box 8-21).

Pressure ulcers can develop anywhere on the body but are seen most frequently on the posterior aspects, especially the sacrum, heels, and greater trochanters (Lyder, 2006). Secondary areas of breakdown include the lateral condyles of the knees and the ankles. The pinna of the ears is another common lateral aspect for breakdown, as are the elbows and scapulae. If one is lying prone, the knees, shins, and pelvis sustain undue pressure.

Pressure ulcers are costly to treat, with estimates up to $7.5 billion dollars a year (Lyder, 2006), and may require extended separation from friends and loved ones. For many, it can prolong recovery and extend rehabilitation. An uncomplicated wound in a person older than 60 years takes approximately 100 days to heal. The acquisition of iatrogenic complications, such as pressure ulcers and complications from them, such as the need for grafting or amputation, sepsis, or even death, may lead to legal action by the individual or his or her representative against the caregiver.

Determining Risk for Pressure Ulcers

It is difficult to predict which individuals will develop pressure ulcers, and it is even more difficult to restore skin integrity once pressure ulcers have developed. Anyone can develop pressure sores, but the normal changes to aging skin increase the risk for skin breakdown. The two most impor-

BOX 8-21   Healthy People 2010 Pressure Ulcers

Objective 1-16: Reduce the proportion of nursing home residents with a current diagnosis of pressure ulcers.
Target: 8 diagnoses per 1000 residents

From US Department of Health and Human Services: *Healthy People 2010: national health promotion and disease prevention objectives,* Washington, DC, 2000, The Department.

tant factors are severity of illness and involuntary weight loss because of poor nutritional status, especially dehydration, hypoproteinemia, and vitamin deficiencies. These account for 74% and 42%, respectively, of increased risk (Nutrition Screening Initiative, 2001). Other important indicators of increased risk are impaired sensory feedback systems so that discomfort is not noticed and impaired mobility or immobilization by restraint or sedation. Additional factors include vascular insufficiency, diabetes, anemia, lack of fat padding over bony prominences, incontinence, and some drug therapies, such as corticosteroids. Tissue breakdown is aggravated by heat, moisture, and irritating substances on the skin. The particularly high-risk groups include those hospitalized for femoral fractures, critical care patients, quadriplegic individuals, those in skilled nursing facilities, and individuals following a long surgery.

▲ Promoting Healthy Aging: Implications for Gerontological Nursing

In all settings, nurses are the persons who are the most responsible for preventing and treating pressure ulcers. Nurses identify early signs and initiate appropriate interventions to prevent further skin breakdown and to promote healing. Failure to do this jeopardizes the health and life of the elderly person. In caring for the whole person, the nurse is in a position to ensure that preventive measures are used and that prompt treatment is initiated if needed. The nurse is the person to alert the health care provider of the need for prescribed treatments, and the nurse is the one who recommends and administers treatments as well as evaluates their efficacies.

Assessment. The development of pressure ulcers is a dynamic process that requires constant vigilance and reassessment. The Braden Scale (Bergstrom et al., 1994) and the Norton Risk Assessment Scale (Norton, 1996) are risk assessment tools used frequently in the clinical setting in predicting individuals at risk for pressure sores. The Braden Scale is probably used most often. The six subscales of the Braden Scale are sensory perception, skin moisture, activity, mobility, friction and shearing, and nutritional status. Each category is rated as 1 (least favorable) to 4 (most favorable). The maximum score possible is 24 points; thus the lower the score, the more at risk a patient is for pressure sores and the greater the need for preventive interventions. The use of either the Braden Scale or another scale provides the means for a systematic evaluation and periodic reevaluation of a person's risk for pressure sores.

Assessment begins with the evaluation of risk as just noted and continues with a brief head-to-toe examination. Included in this is a review of laboratory values related to anemia and nutritional status. The nurse looks for a lymphocyte count below 1800/mm^3, body weight loss more than 15%, or serum albumin value below 3.5 g/dL—all indicative of malnutrition and positively correlated with the severity of the pressure sores (Bates-Jensen, 1996).

Visual and tactile inspection of the entire skin surface with special attention to bony prominences is essential. Inspection is best achieved by visualizing the skin in nonglare daylight or, if that is not possible, under the illumination of a 60-watt light bulb (Giger, Davidhizar, 1999). Inspection should include actual and potential areas for breakdown, with special attention directed to specific areas when an individual uses orthotic devices such as corsets, braces, prostheses, postural supports, splints, slings, or casts. Heels are a problematic site because they are particularly prone to pressure and are small surfaces that receive a high degree of pressure.

The nurse should suspect possible deep tissue injury when discolored skin or blood-filled blisters, including redness or hyperemia, is present in persons with light pigmentation. If pressure is present, it should be relieved and the area reassessed in 1 hour. In darker-pigmented persons, redness may not be present or easily visualized. Instead, it is necessary to look for induration, darkening, or a shadowed appearance of the skin and to feel for warmth or a boggy texture to the tissue compared with the surrounding tissue. Blisters or pimples with or without hyperemia should always be suspect.

Pressure ulcers are classified according to the scale developed by the National Pressure Ulcer Advisory Panel (*www.npuap.org*) ranging from a suspected injury, to stages 1 through 4 and, finally, to an unstageable wound. The ulcer is always classified by the highest stage "achieved," and reverse staging is never used. This means that the wound is documented at the stage representing the maximum damage and depth that has occurred. As the wound heals, it fills with granulation tissue composed of endothelial cells, fibroblasts, collagen, and an extracellular matrix. Muscle, subcutaneous fat, or dermis is not replaced. A stage IV pressure sore that is healing does not become a stage III and then a stage II. It remains defined as a healing (it is hoped) stage IV. Wounds that are covered in black (eschar) or yellow fibrous (slough) necrosis cannot be staged because it is not possible to see the depth until the dead tissue is removed.

Although ulcers are assessed with each dressing change, a detailed assessment is to be done on a weekly or biweekly basis to evaluate the effectiveness of the treatments and nursing interventions. Detailed assessment of each cleaned wound should include the following:

1. Location and exact size (width, depth, length)
2. Color of the wound bed
3. Condition of the surrounding tissue
4. Presence, absence, amount, odor, and color of any exudate (fluid) in the wound
5. Condition of the wound edges, for example, smooth and white; irregular and pink; undermined.

Finally, careful and detailed documentation of the condition of the skin is required. Bates-Jensen provides a detailed form that covers all aspects of assessment, but the PUSH tool (Pressure Ulcer Scale for Healing) takes less time and contains only three items. Most institutions have special forms or computer screens for recording the skin assessment. For those persons with ulcers, photographic documentation is highly recommended both at the onset of the problem and at intervals during its treatment.

Interventions.   The goal of nurses is to help maintain skin integrity against the various environmental, mechanical, and chemical assaults that are potential causes of skin breakdown. In promoting healthy aging of all persons, nurses can focus on prevention: caution with mechanical loading, actions that eliminate friction and irritation to the skin by lifting, turning, placing, and rolling (using two or more persons) the patient; reduction of moisture so that tissues can breathe and do not macerate; and displacement of body weight from prominent areas to facilitate circulation to the skin (Lyder, 2006). The nurse should be familiar with the types of supportive surfaces so that the most effective surface can be used. The nurse should assess the frequency of position change, adding pillows so that skin surfaces do not touch, and establish a turning schedule. Sitting and activity, skin care, incontinence care, and the use of heel protectors or the use of pillows to keep the heels off the bed, with or without so-called protective booties or blocks, should be used as needed. Elevating the heels off the bed with pillows or commercial products is helpful and especially important for individuals with diabetes mellitus and peripheral neuropathy.

Nutritional intake should be monitored, as well as the serum albumin level, hematocrit, and hemoglobin. Diets high in protein, carbohydrates, and vitamins are necessary to maintain and promote tissue growth. Supplements may include amino acids such as arginine, glutamine, and cysteine, although research does not yet support their effectiveness (Lyder, 2006). If appetite is lacking, appetite stimulants may be prescribed. Supplements of vitamin B help in the metabolism of carbohydrates, and pyridoxine and vitamin C assist in protein use.

Realistically, it is not always possible to prevent interruptions in skin integrity caused by overwhelming conditions, and the nurse is instrumental in both fostering and interfering with the healing process. Fortunately, the state of the science of wound care is well developed. Specific guidelines for the prevention and treatment of pressure ulcers were developed in 1994 and continue to guide practice (Lyder, 2006). Since that time, the number of products used has grown but the guidelines remain in effect. Sources of information include the National Pressure Ulcer Advisory Panel and the National Association of Wound, Ostomy and Continence Nurses.

Wounds must be kept clean, warm, moist (but not wet), and protected from further injury. Dilute skin cleansers or saline is best and the least caustic. Solutions such as alcohol, certain soaps, hydrogen peroxide, and povidone-iodine (Betadine) are contraindicated because they always damage newly formed, fragile skin (Bergstrom et al., 1994).

Common types of dressing include films, hydrogels, hydrocolloids, alginates, foams, composites, hydrofibers, and antirecalcitrant dressings. Enzymes (e.g., Santyl) may be necessary for use in débriding or removing eschar or slough. Sharp débridement and biosurgery (maggot therapy) are also used (Lyder, 2006). Dressings and treatments are selected based on the amount of exudate that needs to be absorbed and the condition of the wound bed, with the type of dressing changing as the condition of the wound changes. Dressings should be replaced as soon as the wound is cleaned to prevent cooling and slowing down the healing process. Occlusive dressing cannot be used with infected wounds. Anytime a wound shows worsening, the treatment plan must be changed. It is also reevaluated anytime a wound does not show healing during a 2-week interval. Consultation with a wound care specialist is advisable for wounds that do not follow the pattern of healing. Wound care specialists are experienced nurses or nurse practitioners who often work with wound centers or surgeons and may consult in nursing homes, offices, clinics, or home care. They can provide adjunctive therapy for recalcitrant wounds, including electrical stimulation, vacuum devices, hyperbaric oxygen, growth factor, and autologous skin (Lyder, 2006).

Human Needs and Wellness Diagnoses

Self-Actualization and Transcendence
(Seeking, Expanding, Spirituality, Fulfillment)
Seeks alternative satisfactions to compensate for any bodily limitations
Expresses creativity in personal development
Reaches beyond biological maintenance and seeks spiritual growth

Self-Esteem and Self-Efficacy
(Image, Identity, Control, Capability)
Maintains positive self-attitude
Makes decisions that facilitate maximum health achievement
Recognizes significance of self-efficacy in maintaining high-level wellness
Seeks information about current methods of augmenting biological needs

Belonging and Attachment
(Love, Empathy, Affiliation)
Accepts need for assistance of others
when necessary
Maintains broad range of significant contacts
Expresses feelings of warmth and appreciation
Respects others health habits

Safety and Security
(Caution, Planning, Protections, Sensory Acuity)
Expresses interest in maintaining a healthful lifestyle
Demonstrates ability to recognize biological needs and
attend to them appropriately
Modifies environment for ease and safety of negotiation
Seeks safe and appropriate means to care for self

Biological and Physiological Integrity
(Air, Fluids, Comfort, Activity, Nutrition, Elimination, Skin Integrity)
Makes knowledgeable decisions about body functions
Makes wise decisions about diet and is adequately nourished
Attends to all biological needs and attentive to subtle body signals

These are not all the possible wellness diagnoses that may be identified. The above
are examples of nursing diagnoses that should be considered when planning care
for the older adult.

KEY CONCEPTS

- Physical adaptation is immeasurably enhanced by good dentition, well cared for and comfortably shod feet, and soft, lubricated skin.
- The appearance, alignment, and anchoring of teeth are subject to negative effects during aging.
- Routine dental care, foods requiring vigorous chewing, and thorough brushing and flossing after meals are helpful in preventing periodontal disease and systemic disease.
- The enjoyment of food and pride in personal appearance are enhanced by care of the teeth and mouth.
- Caring for the feet and toenails is important to maintain mobility, and mobility is fundamental to independence. Foot care should not be neglected.
- Feet may reflect systemic disease or give clues to physical ailments before their actual appearance.

- Foot massage with a good lubricating lotion reduces edema, stimulates circulation, improves pedal flexibility, and tends to relax the entire body.
- Individuals with foot lesions or vascular problems of the extremities should have a qualified podiatrist care for their feet routinely. Massage only with the doctor's approval.
- The skin is the largest and most visible organ of the body; it is the direct mediator with the environment.
- Showering in warm to cool water is best for elders (but not more than two or three times weekly), followed by the use of moisturizing lotion. Avoid prolonged direct exposure to sunlight.
- Nurses are in a key position to both prevent and expertly treat pressure ulcers.

CASE STUDY: A Lifetime of Poor Teeth Care

For two reasons, Joel's teeth, like many others of those 75 years old or older, had loosened and deteriorated: he had ignored regular care, and he smoked a pipe. His teeth were stained and detracted markedly from his appearance, and because they were loosening, his ability to chew was affected. He stubbornly ignored them even though he was fastidious about his appearance and his health in every other respect. Why did he neglect his teeth? Joel grew up in a time when the dentist had a most amazing array of torture tools and knew exactly how to use them to produce the strongest reaction. Dentists were to be feared. Second, it seemed to be in God's plan that all folk lose their teeth around age 75; his parents had, his relatives had, and several of his friends had. He was, in fact, fortunate to still have his teeth and with only one bridge. He had not been to a dentist in more than a decade. He said, "Well, I'm waiting until I get these eyeglasses fitted and the hearing aids taken care of; then I'll go to the dentist." When his two lower front teeth loosened to the point that he feared swallowing them, he went to the dentist armed with the idea that dental implants would remedy the problem. After thorough discussion of the procedures and alternatives, he opted for having all his teeth removed. It seemed to him the best solution, because all his teeth and gums were ravaged by periodontal disease. There was little problem extracting the teeth. Dentures had been made before the extractions and were immediately placed in his mouth. The swelling subsided, 2 to 3 weeks elapsed, and the dentures were physically more comfortable—but then the psychosocial aspects of the situation began to predominate. Joel was adamant that he could not adapt to these horrible devices for eating. They would not stay in place, and food strayed beneath them and felt uncomfortable. He couldn't taste his food or enjoy the texture and feel of chewing. He lost interest in food and lost 15 pounds. His socialization had often centered around dining, especially going to lovely restaurants. Now he was ashamed to eat in public and thought everyone was aware of how difficult it was for him to chew. He insisted that the removal of his teeth was the most devastating thing that had ever happened to him. He did not think it amusing when one of his insensitive friends suggested that he was much better off than George Washington had been with his wooden teeth. He returned to the dentist, insisting on implants. The dentist assured him that they would consider the possibility if he was unable to adapt to the dentures within a few months. His speech was affected, and articulation was slurred. Sometimes he sounded as if he had imbibed a bit too much. He called friends who had dentures and sought their advice and support.

They assured him that he would, in time, become unaware of the dentures and they would feel very natural. They seemed not to understand that the loss of teeth was the first and most undeniable evidence that his body parts were wearing out. He was confronted many times a day with his loss of youth. Factors to consider: Eating was an important social aspect of Joel's life; Joel had been remarkably free from health problems, and this was his first confrontation with loss of bodily capacity; Joel's friends were unable to provide empathetic support; Joel felt guilty and angry that he had not taken care of his teeth because he took great pride in his appearance.

Based on the case study, develop a nursing care plan using the following procedure*:

- List Joel's comments that provide subjective data.
- List information that provides objective data.
- From these data, identify and state, using accepted format, two nursing diagnoses you determine are most significant to Joel at this time. List two of Joel's strengths that you have identified from data.
- Determine and state outcome criteria for each diagnosis. These must reflect some alleviation of the problem identified in the nursing diagnosis and must be stated in concrete and measurable terms.
- Plan and state one or more interventions for each diagnosed problem. Provide specific documentation of the source used to determine the appropriate intervention. Plan at least one intervention that incorporates Joel's existing strengths.
- Evaluate the success of the intervention. Interventions must correlate directly with the stated outcome criteria to measure the outcome success.

Critical Thinking Questions

1. How do you think this physical change has affected Joel's self-view and his self-esteem?
2. How can you assist Joel to identify and determine previous coping capacities that can help him get through this present identity crisis?
3. Discuss ways you can assist Joel to avoid a disturbance in nutritional intake.
4. Develop a teaching plan that you would like to initiate with individuals before getting dentures.
5. What anticipatory guidance might have reduced the stress in this situation?
6. What preventive strategies can you suggest to avoid loss of teeth and consequent need for dentures?

* Students are advised to refer to their nursing diagnosis text and identify possible or potential problems.

RESEARCH QUESTIONS

How frequently do older clients see their dentist?

How many old people have access to a specialist in geriatric dentistry, and how many would use these services?

Do most elders believe that dentures are an inevitable outcome of aging?

What are the common podiatric problems for which elders seek attention?

How many elders regularly have pedicures?

What percentage of elders have mobility problems related to correctable podiatric problems?

What do elders know about precancerous skin lesions?

Which ingredients in skin-cleansing agents (lotions, creams, soaps) facilitate the retention of moisture in the skin and eliminate dry skin and pruritus?

REFERENCES*

American Academy of Dermatology: *Pruritus*, 2006. (website): *www.aad.org/public/Publications/pamphlets/Pruritus.htm*. Accessed June 30, 2006.

American Cancer Society (ACS): *What are the key statistics about oral cavity and oropharyngeal cancer?* 2006a. (website): *www.cancer.org/docroot/CRI/content/CRI_2_4_2X_What_are_the-key_statistics_for....* Accessed July 1, 2006.

American Cancer Society (ACS): *Can oral cavity and oropharyngeal cancer be prevented?* 2006b. (website): *www.cancer.org/docroot/CRI/content/CRI_2_4_2X_Can_oral_cavity_and_oropharyn...* Accessed July 1, 2006.

American Cancer Society (ACS): *How is oral cavity and oropharyngeal cancer treated?* 2006c. (website): *www.cancer.org/docroot/CRI/content/CRI_2_4_2X_How_is_oral_cavity_and_oropha...* Accessed July 1, 2006.

American Cancer Society (ACS): What are the risk factors for oral cavity and oropharyngeal cancer? 2006d. (website): *www.cancer.org/docroot/CRI/content/CRI_2_4_2X_What_are_the-risk_factors_for_....* Accessed July 1, 2006.

American Geriatric Society (AGS): *Geriatric review syllabus*, ed 6, New York, 2006, The Society.

American Osteopathic College of Dermatology: *Dry skin (xerosis)*, 2005. (website): *www.aocd.org/skin/dermatologic_diseases/dry_skin.html*. Accessed July 1, 2006.

Bates-Jensen BM: *Why and how to assess pressure ulcers*. Presented at the Ninth Annual Symposium on Advanced Wound Care, Atlanta, April 20, 1996.

Beers MH, Berkow R: *The Merck manual of geriatrics*, ed 3, Whitehouse Station, NJ, 2000, Merck Research Laboratories.

Bergstrom N et al: *Treatment of pressure ulcers*. Clinical practice guideline No 15, AHCPR Pub No 95-0652, Rockville, Md, 1994, U.S. Department of Health and Human Services, Public Health Service, Agency for Health Care Policy and Research.

Bernhard JD: *Pruritus and xerosis*. American Academy of Dermatology, 2006. (website): *www.aad.org/professionsal/Residents/MedStudCoreCurr/DCPruritus-Xerosis.htm*. Accessed July 1, 2006.

Carmona RH: *Oral health problems: painful, costly, and preventable*, 2006. (website): *www.cdc.gov/nccdphp/publications/aag/oh.htm*. Accessed July 1, 2006.

Centers for Disease Control and Prevention (CDC): *CDC fact book 2000/2001*, Washington, DC, Sept 2000, Department of Health and Human Services, The Centers.

Centers for Disease Control and Prevention (CDC): *Health U.S. 2001*, Washington, DC, 2001, Department of Health and Human Services, The Centers.

Centers for Disease Control and Prevention (CDC): *Fact sheet: oral health for older Americans*, 2004. (website): *www.cdc.gov/oralhealth/factsheets/adult-older.htm*. Accessed July 1, 2006.

Cobb DK, Durfee SM: Involuntary weight loss and pressure ulcers: the role of nutrition and anabolic strategies, *Ann Long-Term Care* (suppl), May 2002.

Coleman P: Improving oral health care for frail elderly, *Geriatr Nurs* 234:189, 2002.

Crowley L: *An introduction to human disease pathology and pathophysiology correlations*, Boston, 2004, Jones & Bartlett.

Dietrich T et al: Association between serum concentrations of 25-hydroxyvitamin D3 and periodontal disease in the U.S. population, *Am J Clin Nutr* 80(1):108-113, 2004.

El-Solh A et al: Colonization of dental plaques, *Chest* 126:1575-1582, 2004.

Flugman SL: *Stasis dermatitis*, 2005. (website): *www.emedicine.com/DERM/topic403.htm*. Accessed June 30, 2005.

Fuller KE, Casparian JM: Vitamin D: balancing cutaneous and systemic considerations, *South Med J* 94(1):58-64, 2001. (website): *http://rheumatology.medscape.com/SMA/SMJ*.

Giger JN, Davidhizar RE: *Transcultural nursing: assessment and intervention*, ed 3, St Louis, 1999, Mosby.

Habif TP: *Skin disease: diagnosis and treatment*, ed 2, St Louis, 2005, Mosby.

Hardy M: Impaired skin integrity: dry skin. In Maas ML et al, editors: *Nursing care of older adults: diagnoses, outcomes, and interventions*, St Louis, 2001, Mosby.

HealthandAge: *Dental survey shows gender difference in oral hygiene*, 2004. (website): *www.healthandage.com/module/cms/cms_index/index.cfm?RequestTimeout=1500&a*. Accessed July 1, 2006.

Hochberg M et al: *Practical rheumatology*, ed 3, St Louis, 2004, Mosby.

Kagan S et al: Pressure injury and ulceration: a holistic context for advanced practice nurses. In Cotter V, Strumpf N, editors: *Advanced practice nursing with older adults*, New York, 2002, McGraw-Hill.

Knight J: Burning mouth syndrome. *Adv Nurse Pract*, 2006. (website): *http://nurse-practitioners.advanceweb.com/*. Accessed February 14, 2006.

Longley R: *Elderly pay more out of pocket for dental services*, May 4, 2004. (website): *http://usgovinfo.about.com/cs/healthmedical/a/dentalcosts_p.htm*. Accessed July 1, 2006.

Luggen AS: Oral health of older adults: problems and management, *Geriatr Nurs* 26(6):356-357, 2005a.

Luggen AS: Rapunzel no more: hair loss in older women, *Adv Nurse Pract* 13(10):28-33, 2005b.

Lyder C: Effective management of pressure ulcers, *Adv Nurse Pract* 14(7):32-40, 2006.

Mayo Clinic: *Burning mouth syndrome*, 2004a. (website): *www.mayoclinic.com/printinvoker.cfm?objectid=4E7AF27F-25B0-43D0-90383E896030/b033*. Accessed October 4, 2004.

Mayo Clinic: *Oral and throat cancer overview*, 2004b. (website): *www.mayoclinic.com/health/oral-and-throat-cancer/DS00349*. Accessed July 1, 2006.

Mayo Clinic: *Periodontitis*, 2005. (website): *www.mayoclinic.com/printinvoker.cfm?objectid=723BD56F-9C90-46D9-BD6594F6...* Accessed February 7, 2005.

Mayo Clinic: *Over-the-counter teeth whitening products: are they safe?* 2006a. (website): *www.mayoclinic.com/health/teeth-whitening/AN01231*. Accessed May 31, 2006.

Mayo Clinic: *Oral and throat cancer*, 2006b. (website): *www.mayoclinic.com/health/oral-and-throat-cancer/DS00349*. Accessed April 2, 2007.

Merck Manual of Geriatrics: *Age-related changes in skin structure and function*, 2006a. (online): *www.merck.com/mrkshared/CVMHighLight?file=/mrkshared/mmg/sec15/ch122/ch122b.jsp*. Accessed July 1, 2006.

---

* The references in this list are sources of information; some may become outdated and unavailable over time.

Merck Manual of Geriatrics: *Photoaging*, 2006b. (online): *www. merck.com/mrkshared/CVMHighLight?file=/mrkshared/mmg/ sec15/ch122/ch1*. Accessed July 1, 2006.

Momeyer A, Luggen AS: Periodontal disease in older adults, *Geriatr Nurs* 26(3):197-200, 2005.

National Cancer Institute (NCI): *Pruritus, etiology/pathophysiology*, 2006. (website): *www.cancer.gov/cancertopics/pdq/supportivecare/ pruritus/HealthProfessional/page2*. Accessed July 1, 2006.

National Institute of Diabetes and Digestive and Kidney Diseases (NIDDK): *National diabetes statistics*, 2005. (website): *http:// diabetes.niddk.nih.gov/dm/pubs/statistics/index.htm*. Accessed July 1, 2006.

National Institute on Aging: *Age page: footcare*, 2000. (website): *www.aoa.gov/aoa/pages/agepages/footcare.html*.

National Institutes of Health (NIH): *Screening for skin cancer including counseling to prevent skin cancer*, 2000. (website): *http:// text.nlm.nih.gov/temppfiles/is/tempBRPg43432.html*.

National Institutes of Health (NIH): *Counseling to prevent dental and periodontal disease*, 2004. (website): *http://nlm.nih.gov/temp- files/is/tempBrPg4342*.

National Pressure Ulcer Advisory Panel: *Pressure ulcer stages revised by NPUAP* (press release), February 2007.

National Skin Centre (NSC): *Rosacea*, 2006. (website): *www. nsc.gov.sg/cgi-bin/WB_ContentGen.pl?id=173&gid=33*. Accessed July 1, 2006.

Norton D: Calculating the risk: reflections on the Norton Scale, *Adv Wound Care* 9(6):38-43, 1996.

Nutrition Screening Initiative: *Study shows poor nutrition key cause of pressure ulcers*, Fall/Winter(33):1,4, 2001. (website): *www. aafp.org/nsi.xml*.

Reese JL: Altered oral mucous membrane. In Maas ML et al, editors: *Nursing care of older adults: diagnoses, outcomes, and interventions*, St Louis, 2001, Mosby.

Robb-Nicholson C: By the way, doctor. What's happened to my sense of taste? *Harv Womens Health Watch* 10(8):8, 2003.

Rubenstein LZ, Nahas R: Primary and secondary prevention strategies in the older adult, *Geriatr Nurs* 19(1):11, 1998.

Skin Cancer Foundation (SCF): *About melanoma; about squamous cell; about basal cell carcinoma*, 2006. (websites): *www.skincancer.org/ basal/index.php*; *www.skincancer.org/squamous/index.php*; *www. skincancer.org/melanoma/index.php*. Accessed June 28, 2006.

Sood A, Taylor J: *Pruritus*, 2002. The Cleveland Clinic (website): *www.clevelandclinicmeded.com/diseasemanagement/dermatology/ pruritus/pruritus.htm*. Accessed July 1, 2006.

Tangalos E: *Geriatric pharmaceutical care guidelines*, Covington, Ky, 2002, Omnicare.

University of Maryland (UM) Medical Center: *Skin cancer*, 2004. (website): *www.umm.edu/altmed/ConsConditions/CancerSkincc. html* Accessed June 24, 2006.

U.S. Food and Drug Administration (USFDA): *Taking care of your feet*, 2006. (website): *www.fda.gov/fdac/features/2006/206_feet. html*. Accessed July 1, 2006.

Vargas CM et al: The oral health of older Americans, *Aging Trends* March(3):1-8, 2001.

CHAPTER 9

Nutritional Needs

Ann Schmidt Luggen, Melissa Bernstein,
and Theris A. Touhy

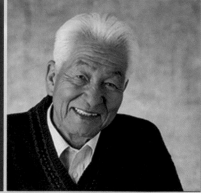
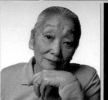

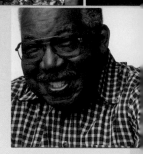

AN ELDER SPEAKS

*If I do reach the point where I can no longer feed myself, I hope that the hands holding
my fork belong to someone who has a feeling for who I am. I hope my helper will
remember what she learns about me and that her awareness of me will grow from one
encounter to another. Why should this make a difference? Yet I am certain that my
experience of needing to be fed will be altered if it occurs in the context of my being
truly known...I will want to know about the lives of the people I rely on, especially
the one who holds my fork for me. If she would talk to me, if we could laugh together,
I might even forget the chagrin of my useless hands. We would have a conversation,
rather than a feeding.*

From Lustbader W: Thoughts on the meaning of frailty,
Generations 13(4):21-22, 1999.

LEARNING OBJECTIVES

On completion of this chapter, the reader will be able to:

1. Identify the nutritional recommendations for older adults based on *Healthy People 2010*.
2. Identify factors that affect nutrition in older adults.
3. Describe the effect of chronic illnesses and other health conditions on nutrition in older adults.
4. Describe a nutritional assessment.
5. State the benefits of fiber in the diet.
6. Identify strategies to assist in ensuring adequate nutrition for older adults.
7. Delineate risk factors for malnutrition, and identify strategies for management.
8. Discuss an interventional care plan that will assist the elder in developing and maintaining good nutritional status.

Nutritional well-being is influenced by aging, nutrition, health, and lifestyle. Proper nutrition means that all the essential nutrients—carbohydrates, fat, protein, vitamins, minerals, and fluids— are adequately supplied and used to maintain optimal health and well-being. Detailed discussion of each of these nutrients can be found in textbooks devoted to nutrition. The variances in nutritional requirements throughout the life span are neither well established nor well researched in older adults. Increased amounts of calcium and vitamins A and C are needed in late life but may be deficient in the average diet of older adults or are affected by alterations in storage, use, and absorption. Total caloric intake

should decline in response to corresponding changes in metabolic rate and a general decrease in physical activity. Serious nutritional deficits may occur with metabolic disorders, psychiatric illness, and cancers and from certain drugs. Nutritional needs of the older adult and food sources of required nutrients are listed in condensed form in Table 9-1.

Healthy People 2010 addresses nutrition and considers it a leading health indicator to be used over the next 10 years to measure the health of the nation (U.S. Department of Health and Human Services [USDHHS], 2002). The objective is to increase to at least 80% the receipt of home food services by people ages 65 years and older who have

TABLE 9-1
Nutritional Needs and Food Sources of Required Nutrients

Nutrient	Comments	Major Food Sources
Fiber	Intakes are often inadequate. Increasing fiber in the diet may help prevent constipation.	Whole-grain breads (e.g., whole wheat, rye, Roman Meal, and pumpernickel); Wheatena, Ry-Krisp, and whole-wheat crackers; cereals (e.g., shredded wheat, oatmeal, four-grain, and seven-grain); whole-wheat pastas; and brown rice Fresh fruits and vegetables
Protein	The recommended level for older adults is as high as 1 g/kg body weight. Intakes are usually adequate. (Older individuals may need to be shown portion sizes that would provide the necessary protein.)	Dried peas, dried or canned beans, lentils (especially in combination with whole grains such as brown rice and whole-wheat bread), or peanut butter Cheese, milk, and nonfat dry milk Eggs Canned clams, salmon, sardines, and tuna Cottage cheese, 2% fat

Calcium	Intakes are often inadequate. Older women may need generous amounts (1-2 g daily) to protect against demineralization of the bones, leading to osteoporosis.	For those who are lactose intolerant:
		  Tofu (soybean curd)
		  All cheeses except cottage cheese
		  Corn tortillas treated in lime
		  All greens such as turnip, mustard, and collard (except spinach)
		  Sardines
		  Milk in small quantities (may be tolerated by some individuals)
		For those who are not lactose intolerant:
		  All foods listed above
		  Whole, low-fat, skim, evaporated, or dried milk
		  Yogurt, buttermilk, and cottage cheese

Iron	Intakes are often inadequate.	Dried or canned beans Cereals, whole-wheat pastas, whole-grain breads, and brown rice Liver Canned oysters
Zinc	Widespread deficiency is found in older men and women.	Legumes Whole grains Meat
Folic acid	Folic acid deficiency may be linked to dementia.	Leafy green vegetables (e.g., spinach, collard, mustard, turnip, and kale greens) Dried beans and peas, lentils, and nuts Whole-grain breads, pastas, and cereals Liver
Vitamin A	Intakes are often inadequate.	Green vegetables (e.g., spinach, turnip, mustard and collard greens, and broccoli) Carrots, winter squash, and sweet potatoes Watermelon and cantaloupe Liver
Vitamin B_6 (pyridoxine)	Intakes are sometimes inadequate. Age per se has been shown to influence blood levels, which decrease markedly with age.	Liver Vegetables Nuts and seeds, dried beans and peas Bran and whole grains Bananas, raisins, and cantaloupe
Vitamin C (ascorbic acid)	Intakes are sometimes inadequate, even in nursing home diets. Age per se influences blood levels, which decrease markedly with age. Vitamin C aids in the absorption of iron from vegetable sources.	Oranges, lemons, tomatoes, grapefruit, cantaloupe or other melon, strawberries Broccoli, cabbage, green peppers, fresh chili peppers, and dark, leafy greens Baked potatoes
Vitamin E (tocopherol)	Several researchers have demonstrated that 3-4 months of treatment with vitamin E (300-400 international units—about 30 times the recommended dietary allowance) relieves intermittent claudication (severe cramps in calf muscles during walking).	Fats of vegetable origin Some nuts and seeds Cereal products, especially whole grains Some vegetables

Compiled from Linder MC: *Nutritional biochemistry and metabolism with clinical application,* New York, 1991, Elsevier; *Recommended Daily Allowance,* ed 10, Washington, DC, 1989, National Academy Press; Roe D: *Geriatric nutrition,* ed 3, Englewood Cliffs, NJ, 1992, Prentice Hall.

difficulty in preparing their own meals or are otherwise in need of home-delivered meals. See Box 9-1 for areas of nutrition and aging in *Healthy People 2010* and Table 9-1 for the nutritional needs of older adults derived from *Healthy People 2010*.

BOX 9-1	Healthy People 2010 and Nutritional Goals: Key Recommendations for Older Adults

- Consume adequate nutrients within calorie needs.
- Consume a variant of nutrient-dense foods and drinks among the basic food groups, eliminating intake of saturated and *trans* fats, cholesterol, added sugar, salt, and alcohol.
- Meet energy needs by adopting a balanced eating pattern such as the United States Department of Agriculture (USDA) food guide (*www.usda.gov/wps/portal/usdahome*) or the Dietary Approaches to Stop Hypertension (DASH) eating plan.
- Consume vitamin B_{12} in crystalline form (fortified foods or supplements).
- Consume extra vitamin D from fortified foods and/or supplements, especially older adults with dark skin or those exposed to insufficient ultraviolet band radiation.
- Maintain body weight in a healthy range, balancing calories from foods and beverages with calories expended. At a minimum, do moderately intense cardio or aerobic activity 30 minutes/day most days of the week.
- Prevent or delay onset of hypertension. Increase potassium intake; reduce salt intake; eat a healthful diet; and engage in regular physical activity to achieve a healthy weight.
- If hypertensive or black, aim to consume no more than 1500 mg of sodium per day and meet the potassium recommendation of 4700 mg/day with food.
- To prevent or delay onset of heart disease, eat less fat. Fats that are solid at room temperature are the saturated and *trans* fats that increase risk of heart disease. Eat fewer than 10% of calories from saturated fats. Wise fat choices include fish, nuts, and vegetable oils.
- If the level of low density lipoproteins (LDLs), the dangerous lipids, are elevated, decrease saturated fat calories to fewer than 7% of total calories.
- If alcoholic beverages are consumed, take no more than two drinks/day for men and one drink/day for women. Avoid activities that require attention, skill, or coordination such as driving. Note than many medications interact with alcohol.
- Older adults are compromised immunologically. Do not eat or drink raw, unpasteurized milk or any products made from raw milk. Do not eat raw or partially cooked eggs or foods containing raw eggs or raw or undercooked meat and poultry, raw or undercooked fish or shellfish, unpasteurized juices, and raw sprouts.
- Increase or maintain fiber-rich foods to 14 g/1000 calories consumed.

(See also the American Public Health Association [APHA] Fact Sheet, Box 9-14).

From US Department of Health and Human Services: *Healthy People 2010: national health promotion and disease prevention objectives,* Washington, DC, 2000, The Department.

FACTORS AFFECTING FULFILLMENT OF NUTRITIONAL NEEDS

Fulfillment of the older person's nutritional needs is affected by numerous factors, including lifelong eating habits and ethnicity, age changes, socialization, income, transportation, housing, and food knowledge.

Lifelong Eating Habits

The nutritional state of a person reflects an individual's dietary history, as well as present food practices. Lifelong eating habits are developed out of tradition, ethnicity, and religion, all of which collectively can be termed *culture*. Food habits established in childhood may influence the intake of older adults.

Eating habits do not always coincide with fulfillment of nutritional needs. Rigidity of food habits may increase with age as familiar food patterns are sought. Ethnicity determines if traditional foods are preserved, whereas religion affects choice of foods possible. Throughout life, then, preferences for particular foods bring deep satisfaction and possess emotional significance. Such foods are called *soul food* or *comfort foods*. Preferences for soul food influence food choices and affect nutrient intake. Foods prepared or served in a special way provide "soul." Rice with every meal and homemade chicken soup given to the individual when ill are examples of what some people consider their soul food. Foods of this nature are not unique to any one group but, rather, are found all over the world. Culturally and religiously appropriate diets should be available in any institution or congregate dining program. Table 9-2 lists cultural food patterns for various ethnic groups and the dietary excesses or omissions associated with the pattern.

Lifelong habits of dieting or eating fad foods echo through the later years. Anorexia nervosa can recur in older women who experienced this in younger years. Weight loss may be more common in older people who have practiced dietary restraint throughout their life. Malnutrition may be seen in older people attempting to lower their cholesterol to prevent heart disease, a condition known as *cholesterol phobia* (Morley, 2003). Strict low-cholesterol or other rigid therapeutic diet regimens are not recommended for frail older adults in long-term care facilities and may contribute to malnutrition and other poor outcomes (Morley, 2003).

Older people, in particular, may be taken in by food fads that profess to partially or completely cure various ailments or to make one look younger or feel more vital. Skipping meals is another practice that one finds in older adults. The quantity of food eaten diminishes, and the adequacy of nutrition becomes questionable. It is difficult to reach an adequate nutritional intake if the total calories are fewer than 1200 per day. Individuals who are on self-imposed diets of 1000 calories or fewer per day are at risk for malnutrition.

TABLE 9-2

Ethnic Food Patterns

Ethnic Group	Cultural Food Patterns	Dietary Excesses or Omissions
Mexican (native)	Basic sources of protein—dry beans, flan, cheese, many meats, fish, eggs. Chili peppers and many deep-green and yellow vegetables. Fruits include zapote, guava, papaya, mango, citrus. Tortillas (corn, flour); sweet bread; fideo; tacos, burritos, enchiladas.	*Limited* meats, milk, and milk products. Some are using flour tortillas more than the more nutritious corn tortillas. *Excessive* use of lard (manteca), sugar. Tendency to boil vegetables for long periods of time.
Filipino (Spanish-Chinese influence)	Most meats, eggs, nuts, legumes. Many different kinds of vegetables. Large amounts of rice and cereals.	May *limit* meat, milk, and milk products (the latter may be because of lactose intolerance). Tend to prewash rice. Tend to fry many foods.
Chinese (mostly Cantonese)	Cheese, soybean curd (tofu), many meats, chicken and pigeon eggs; nuts; legumes. Many different vegetables, leaves, bamboo sprouts. Rice and rice-flour products; wheat, corn, millet seed; green tea. Mixtures of fish, pork, and chicken with vegetables—bamboo shoots, broccoli, cabbage, onions, mushrooms, pea pods.	Tendency among some immigrants to use *excess* grease in cooking. May be *low* in protein, milk, and milk products (the latter may be because of lactose intolerance). Often wash rice before cooking. Large amounts of soy and oyster sauces, both of which are *high in salt.*
Puerto Rican	Milk with coffee. Pork, poultry, eggs, dried fish; beans (habichuelas). Viandas (starchy vegetables; starchy ripe fruits). Avocados, okra, eggplant, sweet yams. Rice, cornmeal.	Use *large* amounts of lard for cooking. *Limited* use of milk and milk products. *Limited* amounts of pork and poultry.
Black American	Milk with coffee. Pork, poultry, eggs, dried fish; beans (habichuelas). Viandas (starchy vegetables; starchy ripe fruits). Avocados, okra, eggplant, sweet yams. Rice, cornmeal. Cereals (including grits, hominy, hot breads). Molasses (dark molasses is especially good source of calcium, iron, vitamins B$_1$ and B$_2$, and niacin).	*Limited* use of milk group (lactose intolerance). Extensive use of frying, simmering for cooking. *Large* amounts of fat: salt pork, bacon drippings, lard, gravies. May have *limited* use of citrus and enriched breads.
Middle Eastern (Greek, Syrian, Armenian)	Yogurt. Predominantly lamb, nuts, dried peas, beans, lentils. Deep-green leaves and vegetables; dried fruits. Dark breads and cracked wheat.	Tend to use *excessive* sweeteners, lamb fat, olive oil. Tend to fry meats and vegetables. *Insufficient* milk and milk products (almost no butter—use olive oil, which has no nutritive value except for calories); deficiency in fresh fruits.
Middle European (Polish)	Many milk products. Pork, chicken. Root vegetables (potatoes); cabbage; fruits. Wheat products. Sausages, smoked and cured meats; noodles, dumplings; bread; cream with coffee.	Tend to use *excessive* sweets and to overcook vegetables. *Limited* amounts of fruits (citrus), raw vegetables, and meats.
Native American (American Indian—much variation)	If acculturated, use milk and milk products. Variety of meats: game, fowl, fish; nuts, seeds, legumes. Variety of vegetables, some wild; variety of fruits, some wild, rose hips; roots. Variety of breads, including tortillas, cornmeal, rice.	*Limited* quantities of high-protein foods depending on availability (flocks) and economic situation. *Excessive* use of sugar.
Italian	Staples are pasta with sauces; bread; eggs; cheese; tomatoes and vegetables such as artichokes, eggplant, greens, and zucchini. Only small amount of meat is used.	*Limited* use of whole grains; *insufficient* servings from milk group; tendency to overcook vegetables; enjoy sweets.

From Swanson J: *Community health nursing,* Philadelphia, 1993, Saunders.

Food Fads

Elderly individuals are not immune to food faddism and may fall prey to advertisements that claim specific foods maintain youth and vitality or rid one of chronic conditions. Fad foods are often more costly than a balanced diet and can sometimes be obtained only in health food stores or by mail order. Even if the food is easily obtained in a supermarket, which is becoming common, the quantities called for may be so large that some nutrients are obtained in excess, whereas others are excluded.

Megavitamin therapy, the ingestion of large amounts of a specific vitamin or many different vitamins, can also be considered a fad. Unless the individual is severely depleted of vitamins, which can usually be obtained in an adequate diet, megavitamin therapy is nonessential and dangerous. Risks exist in megavitamin therapy: bone meal, a source of calcium, may contain lead and thus cause lead poisoning; high doses of zinc cause zinc toxicity; and kelp, with its high iodine content, can cause goiter in those with preexisting thyroid enlargement. High intake of niacin is discouraged because of a high incidence of cardiac arrhythmias, abnormal biochemical findings, and gastrointestinal (GI) problems. Excess vitamin A has two detrimental effects in elderly individuals: liver disease and bone demineralization. The

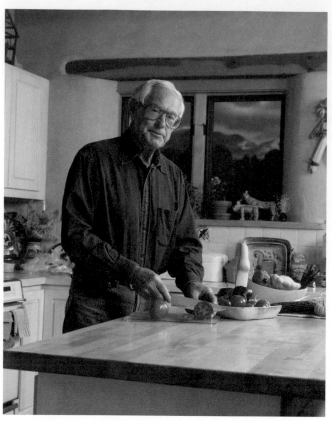

An older man preparing a meal. (Courtesy Corbis Images.)

Recommended Dietary Allowance (RDA) has recently been decreased for the desired amount of vitamin A (the retinol form, not the carotene form) by 100 mcg per day. The money spent by older people on food fads and unneeded vitamins could buy more economical foods that benefit the individual's health. Megavitamin therapy has a role in maintaining nutrition when illness, malnutrition, or excessive demands are placed on body function. Table 9-3 compares and contrasts fad diets (Russell et al., 2002).

Many older adults are lowering the cholesterol in their diets. A soy-containing diet, fatty fish (salmon, herring, mackerel, anchovies) in the diet at least four times a week, and other low-fat diets have been found to decrease total cholesterol and low-density lipoprotein (LDL) measurements. Following the Food Guide Pyramid for adults older than 70 years (see Figure 9-4 on p. 217) is best for an ideal diet, with changes based on particular problems such as hypercholesterolemia and following the primary health care provider's recommendations.

Fast foods and snack foods also constitute a substantial component of the American diet. Cross and colleagues (1995) evaluated snacking behavior among 335 community-based older adults. They found that the majority of seniors snacked at least once daily, with only 2.1% reporting that they never snack. Evening was the most common time for snacking, with the most often reported foods being salty/crunchy foods. When selecting snacks, taste outranked nutrition as a selection criterion.

TABLE 9-3
Fad Diets

Diet	Claim	Composition	Claimed Mechanism
Zone	Increased energy Decreased hunger	40% carbohydrate, 30% protein, 30% fat Restricted calories Three meals and two snacks a day Less than 400 kcal per meal	Lower insulin and eicosanoid levels are a master switch for decreasing hunger
Atkins	Carbohydrates cause obesity High protein and high fat decrease hunger	36% protein, 8% carbohydrate, 53% fat; then 24% protein, 40% fat, 31% carbohydrate No calorie restriction	Ketogenic diet does not oxidize fatty acids in the liver
Pritikin	Low fat Increases energy	8%-12% fat, 12%-15% protein, 80% carbohydrate Less than 100 mg of cholesterol per day	Reduces cholesterol (especially low-density lipoproteins) Low-fat diet carries more oxygen to the cells
Ornish	Low-fat diet lowers cholesterol Diet reverses heart disease	Less than 10% fat, 15%-20% protein, 70%-75% carbohydrate	Reduces cholesterol (especially low-density lipoproteins) Causes documented atherosclerosis regression
South Beach Diet	Excess consumption of carbohydrates increases glycemic index and causes insulin resistance syndrome Diet prevents cardiovascular disease	Three phases 1. Eat normal portions with restricted carbohydrates 2. Introduce carbohydrates, whole grains 3. Maintenance	Reduces insulin resistance Uses excess body fat Dieters lose 8-13 pounds

Adapted from Russell RM et al: *Comparison of diet claims*, 2002 (website): *www.cyberounds.com/conferences/nutrition*.

Socialization

Food and eating are behavioral and social symbols. Often, older adults may be isolated from the mainstream of life because of chronic illness, depression, and other functional limitations. When one eats alone, the outcome is often either overindulgence or disinterest in food. Misuse and abuse of alcohol are prevalent among older adults and are growing public health concerns. Excessive drinking interferes with nutrition. Drinking alcohol depletes the body of necessary nutrients and often replaces meals, thus making an individual susceptible to malnutrition. (See Chapter 25 for a discussion of alcohol use.)

Title VII of the Older Americans Act (OAA) provides funding for strategically located outreach centers or nutrition sites whose purposes are to provide at least one nutritionally sound meal daily and to facilitate congregate dining to foster social contact and relationships. No one age 60 years or older (spouses are also included) can be denied participation in the nutrition program because of his or her economic situation. Those who are able to pay for their meal do so according to their ability.

Meals-on-Wheels is another community program that encourages both the attainment of good nutrition and human contact for those who are unable to prepare meals or go out to obtain them. Most cities and rural areas throughout the United States have such programs. Delivery in the rural areas may be limited. Other congregate or group feeding programs exist through church and other community auspices such as food cooperatives, home grocery delivery services, and chore services for shopping and meal preparation. The federal government awards grants to the Congregate Housing Services Project to provide meals to elderly residents who need them to remain independent. The social essence ascribed to eating is sharing a meal, which provides a sense of belonging. We use food as a means of giving and receiving love, friendship, or belonging.

Dietary reference intakes (DRIs) and dietary guidelines (DGs) have been developed for the OAA nutrition programs, Title III and Title VI. The programs provide congregate and home-delivered meals to about 3 million older adults each year (National Resource Center on Nutrition, Physical Activity & Aging, 2006). These programs and all federal programs must comply with DGs and DRIs, which are revised every 5 years.

Anorexia of Aging

Some researchers and clinicians have suggested that diminished nutrient intake in aging individuals is a result of a decrease in metabolic rate and energy output. However, this may be exaggerated in a compromised socioeconomic situation or in the presence of depression and dementia. Functional loss can also contribute to a slow but sustained weight loss. Other age-related changed that contribute to decreased nutrient intake include diminished testosterone, leptin, cytokines, and cholecystokinin involved in appetite (McCance and Huether, 2006). Further, with the diminution of the senses of smell and taste with aging, food interest diminishes because of loss of sensory neurons, fungiform papillae on the tongue, and parageusia, which causes an unpleasant taste in the mouth that occurs occasionally in elders. See Chapter 4 on physiological changes with aging.

Income

A strong relationship exists between poor nutrition and low income (Wakefield, 2001). Poverty rates in those older than 65 years dropped to 10.2%, or 3.36 million people, in 2000 (Butler, 2001). Although it is encouraging that the rate is declining, it does not reflect the economically fragile situation of many of America's older people, especially single women and persons of color (see Chapter 17). Older adults with low incomes too often are forced to choose among needs such as food, heat, telephone bills, medications, and health care visits. Some older people eat only once a day in an attempt to make their income last through the month.

More older adults live in poverty than younger adults, according to the 2000 census (U.S. Bureau of the Census, 2001). Median household income for those older than 65 years is $22,812 compared with $40,816 for all householders. The median family income of those older than 65 years is half of that of older adults ages 50 to 64 years, reflecting the loss of income after retirement (AARP, 2004).

Many older individuals accustomed to eating meat, fish, and poultry as their main sources of protein have watched the cost climb beyond their purchasing power. Inexpensive alternative protein sources such as tofu (soybean curd) are foreign to the diets of many older people in Western society today but are slowly being accepted. Developing a taste for alternative protein sources and an understanding of what foods to mix to obtain complete dietary protein requires some knowledge and practice to ensure adequate protein intake and to prevent monotony. If possible, older adults should be encouraged to use vegetable protein sources to meet daily needs. This is a more economical form of protein that may help older people conserve their income for other necessities, medications, unexpected bills, or special treats. Combinations such as milk or cheese with bread or pasta; cereal with milk; rice and cheese or rice and bean casseroles; wheat soy or corn soy bread; wheat bread with baked beans, beans, or pea curry; tortillas and beans; and legume soup with bread are sources of protein.

Programs such as the food stamp program have the potential for increasing the purchasing power of older people who qualify, but these programs are vulnerable to federal budget cutting. Transportation may be limited and the distance too far for the older adult to travel to grocery stores or to acquire food stamps, which are sold only at designated locations in cities.

Free food programs, such as donated commodities, are also available at distribution centers (food banks, churches, senior centers) for those with limited incomes. Although this is another valuable option for older adults, use of it is not always feasible. One takes a chance on the types of food available any particular day or week; quantities distributed are frequently too large for the single older person or the older couple to use or even carry from the distribution site; the site may be too far away or difficult to reach; and the time of distribution of the food may be inconvenient.

Cafeterias and restaurants that provided special meal prices for older people have had to increase their prices as food costs have risen. Thus the previous advantages of eating out have diminished. Yet many single elders eat out for most meals. More and more are eating fast food.

Transportation

Available transportation may be limited for older people. Many small, long-standing neighborhood food stores have been closed in the wake of larger supermarkets, which are located in areas that serve a greater segment of the population. It may become difficult to walk to the market, to reach it by public transportation, or to carry a bag of groceries while using a cane. Fear is apparent in the elders' consideration of transportation. They fear walking in the street and being mugged, not being able to cross the street in the time it takes the traffic light to change, or being knocked down or falling as they walk in crowded streets. Despite reduced senior citizen bus fares, many elders are fearful of attack when using public transportation. Transportation by taxicab for an individual on a limited income is unrealistic, but sharing a taxicab with others who also need to shop may enable the older person to go where food prices are cheaper and to take advantage of sale items. For older people, convenience foods, devoid of many essential nutrients, are lighter to carry

or pull along in a cart than fresh fruits and vegetables. Many markets can be accessed on the Internet or by telephone and will make home deliveries.

Senior citizen organizations have helped provide the elderly with van service to shopping areas. In housing complexes it may be possible to schedule trips to the supermarket. Most communities have multiple sources of transportation available, but the older person may be unaware of them. Local departments of aging and senior centers are a good source of information.

Housing

Poor and near-poor older people are likely to reside in substandard housing. Some live in single rooms that lack storage space for food, a means of refrigeration, and a stove for cooking. At certain times of the year, some of the single-room dwellers use the window ledges and fire escapes to keep perishables cool for several days' use. Box 9-2 lists items suitable for the single-room occupant's pantry and items that can be purchased to be eaten the same day. Of foremost concern to the nurse is tailoring an acceptable diet. Additional factors affecting dietary intake include living arrangements, number of meals eaten daily, who cooks and shops, presence of physical impediments affecting cooking and shopping, problems with chewing, use of dentures, alcohol use, and medication use.

COMMON NUTRITIONAL PROBLEMS

Problems in nutrition are very common in older adults. Hydration, adequate fiber, lactose intolerance, weight loss, vitamin and mineral deficiencies, osteoporosis, sarcopenia, malnutrition, cardiac and renal function, dementias, infections, diabetes, arthritis and osteoporosis, and obesity are factors that affect or are affected by the nutritional status of elders. Figure 9-1 shows a Nutrition Screening Initiative checklist to determine nutritional health.

Dehydration

The older person is vulnerable to fluid and accompanying electrolyte imbalance. In children, 80% of body composition is water. In elderly people, 43% to 51% is water (Bennett, 2000). Even small decreases in fluid intake can cause more dehydration in an elder than in a child. The concentrating ability of older kidneys decreases, so urine flow is not diminished with dehydration until late. Thirst sensation diminishes or may be absent in advancing age, resulting in the loss of an important defense against dehydration (American Geriatric Society [AGS], 2006a).

Dehydration can cause altered mental status or delirium as a result of electrolyte imbalance. Adequate amounts of fluid not only prevent altered mental status associated with dehydration but also are essential for individuals who are receiving specific medications. Constipation, a common problem among elderly people, can be minimized with adequate fluid intake. Other consequences of dehydration include thromboembolism, pressure ulcers, periodontal sepsis,

---

BOX 9-2   Nonperishable Foods Suitable for Single-Room Occupant

MILK PRODUCTS
Box of dry skim or whole milk
Small can of evaporated milk
Instant cocoa
Instant pudding to use with dry milk
Small pieces of cheese (if wrapped airtight and kept in cool place)

MEAT PRODUCTS
Small can of tuna fish, sardines, or salmon
Canned potted meat
Peanut butter

FRUITS AND VEGETABLES
Small cans of any fruits and vegetables
Dried fruit (raisins, apricots, dates)
Fresh apples, oranges, seasonal fruits

MISCELLANEOUS
Instant coffee
Tea
Sugar
Condiments of choice

Read the statements below. Circle the number in the Yes column for those that apply to you or someone you know. For each "yes" answer, score the number listed. Total your nutritional score.

	YES
I have an illness or condition that made me change the kind or amount of food I eat.	2
I eat fewer than two meals per day.	3
I eat few fruits, vegetables or milk products.	2
I have three or more drinks of beer, liquor, or wine almost every day.	2
I have tooth or mouth problems that make it hard for me to eat.	2
I don't always have enough money to buy the food I need.	4
I eat alone most of the time.	1
I take three or more different prescriptions or over-the-counter drugs each day.	1
Without wanting to, I have lost or gained 10 pounds in the past 6 months.	2
I am not always physically able to shop, cook, and/or feed myself.	2

Total Nutritional Score

0-2 indicates good nutrition
3-5 moderate risk
6+ high nutritional risk

FIGURE 9-1 Nutrition Screening Initiative checklist to determine nutritional health. (From The Nutrition Screening Initiative, 1010 Wisconsin Avenue NW, Suite 800, Washington, DC 2007. The Nutrition Screening Initiative is funded in part by a grant from Ross Products Division of Abbott Laboratories, Inc.)

orthostasis, falls, and kidney stones (Morley, 2000). Use of diuretics requires that fluid intake be maintained unless specifically ordered to the contrary. Coffee has a diuretic effect that requires fluid intake to compensate for fluid loss through diuresis. Alcohol also causes diuresis. In hot weather, increased perspiration and evaporation deplete the individual of needed body fluid. Fever and upper respiratory infections cause dehydration in the older person. Older adults often have a diminished thirst sensation. Adequate fluid intake is as important to total nutrition as food. Daily fluid needs fluctuate widely in older adults and depend on general health status, medications, and activity level. To maintain water balance, eight 8-ounce servings of water, or about 2 liters, are recommended each day (Wakefield, 2000).

Standard indicators for dehydration among older people are not always reliable. In general, in mild dehydration the nurse will find diminished skin turgor, best evaluated on the forehead or sternum; dry mucous membranes, especially mucosal xerosis; and orthostatic hypotension (Beers and Berkow, 2000). Dry mucous membranes may be misleading because many elderly persons are mouth breathers. Intake and output charts are often unreliable, particularly in long-term care facilities. Other signs in the presentation of dehydration include swollen tongue, sunken eyeballs, elevated body temperature, diminished urine output, nausea and vomiting, acute renal failure, altered effects of medications, and electrolyte disturbances (Chernoff, 2006).

Tachycardia may be present, but changes in blood pressure, pulse rate, and skin turgor may not be evident early on (AGS, 2006a). Moderate dehydration causes the same signs and symptoms plus oliguria or anuria, confusion, and a resting hypotension. The older adult with severe dehydration will be in shock or near shock. The difficulty of a definitive diagnosis is that many of the signs and symptoms may be present in the older adult without volume problems. Weighing on a regular basis can be useful in assessing volume loss, and those in nursing facilities should be weighed at least monthly.

Laboratory Assessment. Urine specific gravity is not well correlated with serum biochemical parameters of hydration status. However, urinary sodium concentration is usually less than 20 mEq/L when sodium intake is reduced or the patient has vomiting or diarrhea. A urinary sodium concentration can be greater than 20 mEq/L with volume depletion. Hematocrit, blood urea nitrogen (BUN), and creatinine will be elevated. BUN/creatinine ratios are also increased (Beers and Berkow, 2000). Laboratory parameters can be used, but other conditions that can occur in elderly people can alter these laboratory findings. (See Chapter 5.)

Dehydration Management. Prevention of dehydration is essential. Gerontological nurses in long-term care facilities can identify dehydration based on poor oral intake and the occurrence of vomiting or diarrhea. Staff education to increase awareness of the need for fluids and the signs and symptoms of dehydration is encouraged. Box 9-3 is a Hydration Assessment Checklist from the Hartford Institute for Geriatric Nursing (Zembruski, 2000).

When dehydration occurs, treatment is based on the type of dehydration experienced and the amount of dehydration (Box 9-4). Oral rehydration is the first treatment approach if the patient is able to ingest fluids. Two to three liters of water or clear fluids may be necessary (Beers and Berkow, 2000). If mental status is impaired or fluid deficits are larger, intravenous therapy is required, usually with 0.9% sodium chloride. A general rule is to replace 50% of the loss within the first 12 hours (or 1 L/day in afebrile elders) or sufficient quantity to relieve tachycardia and hypotension. Further fluid replacement can be administered more slowly over a longer period. Inadequate rehydration in a reasonable time can result in complications such as renal failure, myocardial infarction, stroke, or rhabdomyolysis (Beers and Berkow, 2000). Box 9-5 lists measures to help prevent dehydration of institutionalized elders.

> **BOX 9-3** Hydration Assessment Checklist
>
> 1. Symptoms of hydration requiring immediate interventions—fever, thirst, dry and warm skin, furrowed tongue, decreased urinary output
> 2. Associated factors: older than 85 years, immobility, cognitive impairment, fluid intake less than 1500 mL, lack of awareness of thirst
> 3. Increasing vulnerability—osteoporosis, heart failure, dementia
> 4. Dietary restrictions of fluids, salt, potassium, protein
> 5. Medications—diuretics, tricyclic antidepressants, laxatives
> 6. History of dehydration, infections, difficulty swallowing
> 7. Return from a 24-hour hospitalization, dental or eye surgery, procedures that require fasting
> 8. Laboratory reports with increasing sodium, blood urea nitrogen, creatinine, hematocrit, urine specific gravity
>
> Adapted from Zembruski C: Hydration assessment checklist, *Geriatr Nurs* 18(1):20-26, 1997.

> **BOX 9-4** Estimates of Dehydration
>
> Mild dehydration: Less than 5% loss of body weight
> Moderate dehydration: 10% loss of body weight
> Severe dehydration: 15% loss of body weight
>
> Adapted from Beers MH, Berkow R: *The Merck manual of geriatrics,* ed 3, Whitehouse Station, NJ, 2000, Merck Research Laboratories.

> **BOX 9-5** Measures to Help Prevent Dehydration of Institutionalized Older Adults
>
> • Ensure a 24-hour intake of at least 1500 mL of oral fluid. (Food intake and metabolic oxidation should provide additional fluid for hydration.)
> • Offer fluids hourly during the day. Include fluids with an evening snack.
> • Ask the physician to order intravenous fluids if the elder is not able to take oral fluids.
> • Note the urine color and specific gravity.
> • Listen to bowel sounds. Note any change in activity. (Extra-soft or loose stool means losing water, and hard stool means dehydration.)
> • Be familiar with tests or examinations that the patient may have had. If they involved enemas or laxatives before the tests, there will be a fluid loss.
> • Replace fluids when nothing has been consumed orally or fluids have been lost from test preparation.
> • Obtain a drug history.
> • Provide cups, glasses, and pitchers that are not too big or heavy for older persons to handle. (Help those who cannot help themselves to fluids.)
> • Offer other fluids in addition to water. Find out the types of beverages liked and fluid temperature preferred.
> • Remember that coffee acts as a diuretic. Fluid loss by coffee should be supplemented to compensate for the fluid loss.
> • Note skin turgor and mucous membranes.
> • Note increases in pulse and respiration rates and decrease in blood pressure (suggestive of dehydration).
> • Check laboratory values for changes: sodium, blood urea nitrogen, hematocrit, hemoglobin, urine and serum osmolarity, and creatinine. Also check for signs of acidosis.
> • Weigh the patient daily at the same time and on the same scale.
>
> From Reedy DF: Fluid intake: how can you prevent dehydration? *Geriatr Nurs* 9:224, 1988.

Hyponatremia

Hyponatremia is defined as a decrease in sodium plasma concentration (<136 mEq/L) and is caused by an excess of water relative to solute. It is one of the most common causes of delirium in elderly patients. There is, in general, an age-related decrease in serum sodium without any clinical symptomatology. Dilutional hyponatremia is associated with the highest mortality rate and may be caused by nutritional supplements such as Ensure, Isocal, or Osmolite, all of which are low in sodium. Hyponatremia caused by vomiting or diarrhea, suctioning of the GI tract, and diuretics stimulates antidiuretic hormone (ADH) production, which causes retention of water but not sodium. This is usually mild, and treatment may include irrigating gastric tubes with normal saline or administering saline intravenous fluids. Hyponatremia can also occur in chronic diseases such as congestive heart failure, cirrhosis, and nephrosis (Beers and Berkow, 2000). In this instance, patients often have edema and renal ability to dilute urine is impaired.

Hypernatremia

Hypernatremia is defined as an elevated plasma sodium concentration greater than 145 mEq/L that is caused by a deficit of water relative to sodium (Desai and Isa-Pratt, 2002). Common causes include decreased water intake, increased sodium intake, and increased water loss from the GI tract and loop diuretics. Low body weight is a risk factor for hypernatremia. The mortality rate for hypernatremia is approximately 40% in older hospitalized patients, especially if it is of rapid onset and also if the sodium is higher than 160 mEq/L (Beers and Berkow, 2000). Weakness and lethargy are common symptoms, although they are not specific. If the sodium level is more than 152 mEq/L, seizures, stupor, and coma may occur. Body water deficits require hypotonic fluid replacement using 0.45% sodium chloride solution or 5% dextrose in water.

Malnutrition

The occurrence of malnutrition among the elderly has been documented in elders in acute care, long-term care, and the community. Malnutrition encompasses both overnutrition and undernutrition. It may result from inadequate intake, malabsorption, digestive disorders, or excessive intake of food

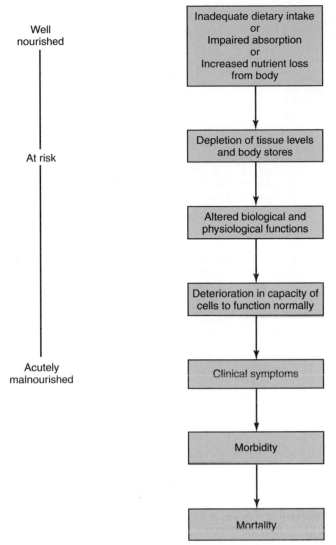

Well
nourished

At risk

Acutely
malnourished

Inadequate dietary intake
or
Impaired absorption
or
Increased nutrient loss
from body

Depletion of tissue levels
and body stores

Altered biological and
physiological functions

Deterioration in capacity of
cells to function normally

Clinical symptoms

Morbidity

Mortality

FIGURE 9-2 A trajectory for malnutrition. (Modified from Mahan LK, Arlin MT, editors: *Krause's food nutrition and diet therapy*, ed 8, Philadelphia, 1992, Saunders.)

BOX 9-6   Nutritional Factors That Potentiate Malnutrition in Older Adults

SOCIAL FACTORS

Abuse of alcohol
Poverty—inability to buy foods
Lack of help with food shopping and preparation
No socialization at meals

PSYCHOLOGICAL FACTORS

Bereavement—not eating
Confusion—not shopping, cooking, eating
Depression—not eating, efforts toward suicide

PHYSICAL FACTORS

Immobility—unable to shop or prepare foods
Inability to feed self
Poor oral hygiene
Poor dentition or ill-fitting dentures

PHYSIOLOGICAL FACTORS

Dyspnea
Decreased metabolic rate
Decreased enjoyment of foods because of diminished taste, smell, vision
Decreased feeding drive because of diminished activity of neurotransmitters, nutritional factors
Increased and early satiety because of peptide hormonal changes, stomach emptying time changes
Disease process utilizing reserves

OTHER RISK FACTORS

Decreased or limited strength and mobility with inability to open cans, lift pots and pans
Neurological deficits, arthritis, impairment of hand-arm coordination, loss of tongue strength, and dysphagia
Decreased or diminished vision or blindness
Inability to feed self
Pressure ulcers with insufficient nutrient intake
Loss of teeth, poor-fitting dentures, or chewing problems
Polypharmacy
Surgery, nothing by mouth (NPO) for extended periods, or intravenous therapy only

(Moore, 2001). Medications most frequently associated with malnutrition include digoxin, theophylline, nonsteroidal antiinflammatory drugs (NSAIDs), iron supplements, and psychoactive drugs. These can be detected in physical examinations, biochemical studies, and physiological tests. Included in malnutrition are specific nutrient deficiencies, nutritional imbalances, and obesity. Figure 9-2 provides the malnutrition trajectory. See Box 9-6 for factors that potentiate malnutrition.

Undernutrition. Undernutrition may be defined as "imbalanced nutrition: less than body requirements." About 16% of elderly people in the community eat fewer than 1000 kilocalories (kcal)/day, which is insufficient for adequate nutrition (Beers and Berkow, 2000). Undernutrition affects 17% to 65% of elders in hospitals and many of the elders in long-term care facilities. In one study by the University of Oklahoma (Rahman, 2001), 26% of ambulatory geriatric patients were identified as malnourished, with a body mass index (BMI) less than 22, unintentional weight loss more than 10% in 6 months, serum albumin less than 3.5 mg/dL, and cholesterol less than 160 mg/dL. Another 45% who had no objective signs of malnutrition were found to be at risk based on the Nutrition Screening Initiative (NSI) nutrition assessment score of higher than 2 (Figure 9-3).

A study by Thomas and associates (2000) shows that malnutrition in elders is predictive of poor clinical outcomes and risk for increased mortality. The triad of depression, impaired immune function, and unexplained weight loss of 5% or more is predictive of death within 6 months. Many medical conditions common to elders increase metabolism, thus exacerbating undernutrition. These individuals are also likely to suffer from dehydration and poor fluid intake. Persons with severe malnutrition are at higher risk for

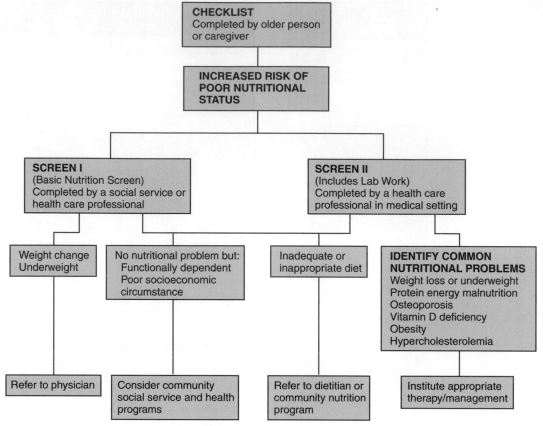

FIGURE 9-3 Nutritional assessment and approaches. (Courtesy The Nutrition Screening Initiative, Washington, DC.)

chronic medical conditions that could be prevented by early correction of reversible nutritional deficits.

The "skeleton in the nursing home closet" is the problem of malnutrition in long-term care facilities (Nutrition Screening Initiative [NSI], 2001). A clinical guideline to manage involuntary weight loss and malnutrition in nursing home residents focuses on a number of factors, including reporting of medical conditions, declines in ability to perform activities of daily living, and cognizance of delirium, depression, and mood disorders. Depression is a major cause of weight loss in long-term care residents and perhaps accounts for 36% of the residents who lose weight. The guideline recommends consultation with pharmacy on medications that may cause anorexia and medications that may stimulate appetite and reverse malnutrition.

In an effort to deal with the malnutrition in long-term care facilities, the Council for Nutritional Strategies in Long-Term Care was established. Thomas et al. (2000) provide a comprehensive structured approach to improve the management of nutritional problems in long-term care facilities that is a valuable resource for gerontological nurses and other members of the interdisciplinary team (*www.ltcnutrition.org*). A protocol for the assessment and management of eating and feeding difficulties for older people, developed by Amella and the Nurses Improving Care for Health System Elders (NICHE) faculty, is another valuable resource (Amella, 1998).

HEALTH CONDITIONS AFFECTING NUTRITION

Discussion of the effect of commonly occurring health conditions on nutrition in aging follows. For more detailed information on health conditions and chronic illness in older persons, see Chapters 7, 10, 15, 23, and 25.

Cardiac Function and Nutrition

Good nutrition is vital in primary prevention of heart disease and in management of elders with cardiac dysfunction. Some important areas for the nurse who cares for elderly clients to consider include lipids, body weight, salt intake, and exercise. The main types of cardiovascular disease (CVD) include heart disease, such as congestive heart failure and myocardial infarction, and stroke. These two types represent the first and third leading causes of death in the United States (Insel et al., 2006).

Lipid management is imperative in prevention of atherosclerosis, which includes heart disease and lower extremity arterial disease. High-fat diets are usually high in calories, leading to weight gain and obesity (Insel et al., 2006). Especially implicated in atherosclerosis are high intake of fat, saturated fat, and *trans* fat. About 65% of adults in the United States are overweight or obese, with rates climbing in children and teenagers.

TABLE 9-4
Adult Lipid Levels: Diagnosis

TOTAL CHOLESTEROL	
Desired	<200
Borderline	200-239
High	>240
HDL	
Low	<40
Desired	>45
LDL	
Optimal	<100
Near Optimal	100-129
Borderline High	130-159
High	160-189
Very High	>190
TG	
Normal	<150
Borderline High	150-199
High	200-499
Very High	>500

From National Cholesterol Eduction Program (NCEP), 2002.
HDL, High-density lipoprotein; *LDL,* low-density lipoprotein; *TG,* triglyceride.

BOX 9-7   NCEP Heart Healthy Diet (To Stay Healthy)

8%-10% total calories/day from saturated fat
30% or less total calories/day from total fats
<300 mg/day of cholesterol
<2400 mg/day of sodium
Caloric intake to achieve or maintain healthy weight and
    reduce cholesterol level

From National Cholesterol Education Program (NCEP), 2002.

Many fat calories are "hidden" and are found in take-out dinners and restaurant foods. For example, 4 oz of boiled potatoes is 97 kcal with 0.1 g of fat. Four oz of fried potatoes is 226 kcal with 9 g of fat (Insel et al., 2006). Even food that appears benign, such as green beans, are more than double in calories when a teaspoon of butter is added to a portion.

Dyslipidemia. Total cholesterol is composed of the major lipid areas of high-density lipoproteins (HDLs), low-density lipoproteins (LDLs), and triglycerides (TGs). LDLs are particularly harmful. HDLs are protective. High TG levels are associated with low HDL levels (Insel et al., 2006). See Table 9-4 for lipid levels. *Healthy People 2010* objectives (U.S. Department of Health and Human Services [USDHHS], 2002) have the target of reducing the number of adults with high cholesterol levels and

TABLE 9-5
Therapeutic Lifestyle Changes (TLC) Diet to Improve Health

Food	Recommendation
Total fat	25%-35% of total calories
Saturated fat	<7% of total calories
Polyunsaturated fat	≈10% of total calories
Monounsaturated fat	≈20% of total calories
Carbohydrates	50%-60% of total calories
Fiber	20-30 g/day
Protein	≈15% of total calories
Cholesterol	<200 mg/day

Total Calories: sufficient to achieve/maintain desirable body weight

From National Cholesterol Eduction Program (NCEP), 2002.

---

death from heart disease and stroke. The National Cholesterol Education Program (NCEP) published its final report derived from an expert panel on the detection, evaluation, and treatment of high blood cholesterol in adults.

The NCEP Expert Panel has developed population-wide dietary recommendations. The guidelines for the NCEP Heart Healthy diet is an eating plan that keeps cholesterol low and decreases risk for developing heart disease (Box 9-7). The NCEP also recommends regular moderate physical activity— 30 minutes each day for a minimum of 3 to 4 days/week. If the cholesterol level is already high and heart disease is present, this needs to be planned in collaboration with the medical provider and a lipid-lowering medication may need to be added to the regimen. Table 9-5 shows the diet recommended for elders who have hyperlipidemia, indicating the presence of heart disease.

Diabetes

Those elders with age-related weight gain and increasing adipose tissue are predisposed to insulin resistance or the inability to utilize insulin to lower blood sugar levels, which may lead to the development of diabetes (see Chapter 10).

Management of diabetes includes diet, physical activity, testing blood sugar levels, and pharmacological agents. See Box 9-8 for a healthy lifestyle plan. The goal of dietary intervention is to control fluctuations in glucose levels and to lose weight. Diets are low in saturated fats and cholesterol and contain moderate amounts of carbohydrate—preferably from whole-grain sources with high fiber content. Dietary proteins may be restricted to less than 0.8 g/kg/day to prevent progression of diabetic kidney disease. Many elders can be managed with dietary changes and exercise alone. Those who are unable to do this will be managed with medications or insulin, as well as diet.

BOX 9-8 Healthy Lifestyle for Older Adults

DIET

Eat 2 servings of fruit/day.

Eat 3 servings of vegetables/day, especially dark-green leafy ones such as broccoli and kale and orange vegetables like carrots and sweet potatoes.

Drink 3 cups of milk or equivalent/day (low-fat yogurt, cheese).

Eat 3 servings of whole grain cereals, breads, crackers, rice, pasta/day.

Eat 2-3 servings of protein (fish, poultry, beans, nuts, eggs)/ day.

PHYSICAL ACTIVITY

Check with primary health care provider before increasing activity.

Start with 5-10 minutes/activity/day; work up to 30 minutes most days of the week.

Do strength exercises (lifting weights) for flexibility, prevention of osteoporosis.

Do balance exercises to prevent falls.

From American Public Health Association, 2005 (website): *medscape.com/viewarticle/501874.* Accessed December 23, 2006.

BOX 9-9 Osteoporosis Nutrition Interventions

- Assess height and weight yearly (body mass index less than 22 is a risk factor).
- Assess bone density with dual-energy x-ray absorptiometry (DEXA) scan.
- Assess dietary intake of calcium and vitamin D and sun exposure.
- Screen for medications causing calcium or bone loss.
- Increase calcium intake to 1200 mg/day and vitamin D intake to 200-400 IU/day.
- Encourage reduction or elimination of alcohol intake.
- Encourage sun exposure 10-30 min/day.
- Consider calcium and vitamin D supplements.
- Encourage weight-bearing exercises daily if able.
- Provide analgesia to reduce pain of osteoporosis and fracture.

IU, International unit.

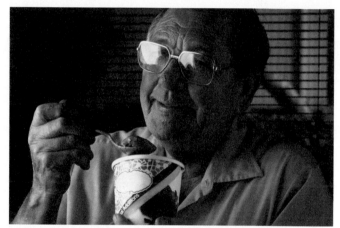

An older man eating fat-free ice cream for protein and calcium. (Courtesy Corbis Images.)

Arthritis

Arthritis and other musculoskeletal disorders are impacted by nutritional status. Obesity is a major problem for hip, knee, and ankle osteoarthritis (OA). Obesity puts considerable pressure on these major joints. Weight loss may slow the progression of disease. Hip and knee replacement surgery is not uncommon in elderly people.

The arthritic condition of gout is influenced by nutritional intake and caused in part by an excess of uric acid in the blood and crystal deposits in joints. Uric acid is a metabolite of the purines *adenine* and *guanine* (Meiner, 2002). Risk factors include obesity, high purine diet, and habitual alcohol ingestion. Foods that are high in purines include sardines in oil, liver, kidneys, anchovies, herring, mussels, and codfish. Often a rigid restriction of these foods does not prevent recurrence.

Osteoporosis

A number of minerals can impact osteoporosis and its progression. Calcium (in forms such as calcium carbonate, calcium lactate, calcium citrate, calcium gluconate, and calcium citrate maleate) helps build strong teeth and bone, especially when intake is sufficient in the bone-building years before the age of 20 years. Calcium requires phosphorus and vitamin D to be effective (Arthritis Foundation, 2005). Many experts recommend 1500 mg daily for adults older than 50 years who have inflammatory conditions and for menopausal women not taking hormone replacement therapy. A dose that is too high (2500 mg) causes bloating, constipation, kidney stones, and impaired kidney function. Calcium is found naturally in milk,

yogurt, cheese, ice cream, sardines and salmon (canned), broccoli, turnip greens, kale, bok choy, and fortified foods such as orange juice and cereals. Calcium interacts with antibiotics and calcium channel blockers used in cardiac disease management. Antacids that contain aluminum, seizure medications, corticosteroids, diuretics, and laxatives can diminish calcium levels in the blood. To prevent bone loss, elders taking corticosteroids should take calcium with vitamin D.

Box 9-9 provides osteoporosis nutrition interventions, and Box 9-10 lists causes of calcium malabsorption. Table 9-6 lists food sources for calcium.

Milk/Lactose Intolerance. The use of milk and other dairy products is a major and efficient source of protein and calcium for the elderly person. For some persons, lactose intolerance is a problem that must be considered in nutritional counseling. Lactose intolerance is thought to be a genetic characteristic occurring in 75% of African-Americans, Jews,

BOX 9-10 Causes of Calcium Malabsorption

- Inadequate vitamin D
- Lactose intolerance (causing lack of milk in the diet)
- Excessive intake of phosphorus (competes with calcium for absorption; present in meat and carbonated drinks)
- High-sodium diet (interferes with calcium absorption)
- High-protein diet
- Diet high in oxalates (spinach and very-deep-green vegetables)
- Diet high in phytates (bran and whole grains or fiber)
- Achlorhydria (calcium absorption requires acid rather than alkaline environment)
- Corticosteroids and anticonvulsants
- Smoking, moderate to high alcohol intake, and excess caffeine intake (all of which promote bone loss)

Adapted from Moore MC: *Mosby's pocket guide series: nutritional assessment and care,* ed 5, St Louis, 2005, Mosby.

Mexicans, Native Americans and in 90% of Asians and other ethnic groups for whom animal milk is not a traditional food (Cleveland Clinic, 2006). See Table 9-7 for distribution of lactose intolerance in adults worldwide. Whites of northern European descent retain the lactase enzyme in adulthood, and other whites begin to experience some degree of intolerance at about age 45 years. Even low levels of ingested lactose cause such symptoms as gas, bloating, cramping, and diarrhea.

Lactose is the sugar in milk products. The problem with lactose intolerance is a lack of lactase, the enzyme produced by the small intestine needed for digestion of lactose. Lactose intolerance resembles milk intolerance. The symptoms displayed are similar and occur when more than 8 ounces of milk is consumed. Lactose is in many dairy products such as ice cream and cheeses. It is added to foods such as bread and bakery items, cereals, salad dressings, candies, and some snacks (Cleveland Clinic, 2006). Intolerance does not always occur when other products such as hard cheese, yogurt, acidophilus milk, and buttermilk are consumed. It is difficult to know exactly if milk intolerance is a direct reflection of lactose intolerance. Lactase enzyme can be added to milk to hydrolyze the lactose to obtain the benefit of milk. Also, foods high in calcium, such as greens and dried beans, can provide essential calcium for those who are lactose intolerant or who do not like milk. It may be necessary to supplement the diet with calcium carbonate or calcium lactate, sodium fluoride, and B-complex vitamins to maintain skeletal integrity and avoid osteoporosis.

Fluoride. Fluoride is needed for strong tooth enamel and bones (Arthritis, 2005). Daily requirement for men is 4 mg; for women it is 3 mg. Intake of 10 mg will cause brown, mottled teeth. With too little, tooth decay will occur. Fluoride is found in fluoridated water, teas, and sardines and salmon (canned) with bones. It interacts with calcium supplements and antacids that contain calcium and aluminum. Stress fractures and joint pain can occur with high doses.

TABLE 9-6
Leading Calcium Sources

Food	Amount	Milligrams of Calcium
DAIRY PRODUCTS		
Low-fat milk, 1% to 2%	1 cup	310
Skim milk	1 cup	300
Whole milk	1 cup	290
Buttermilk	1 cup	290
Nonfat dry milk	2 tablespoons	105
Eggnog	1 cup	330
Ice cream	1 cup	208
Plain yogurt (whole milk)	1 cup	300
Plain yogurt (low fat)	1 cup	400
Mozzarella cheese	1 ounce	210
Parmesan cheese	1 ounce	340
Swiss cheese	1 ounce	300
Canned red salmon	4 ounces	290
Canned mackerel	4 ounces	300
VEGETABLES		
Collard greens	1 cup	360
Turnip greens	1 cup	250
Kale	1 cup	200
Bok choy	1 cup	250
Cottage cheese, 2% fat	1 cup	160
Broccoli	1 cup	150
FISH		
Canned sardines (with bone)	2 ounces	210
NUTS/SEEDS		
Sesame seeds	1 ounce	297
Almonds	6 ounces	311
MISCELLANEOUS		
Tofu	⅓ cup	581
Chocolate fudge	3½ ounces	100
Dark molasses	1 tablespoon	172
Black strap molasses	5 tablespoons	579
Seaweed, kelp, agar	3½ ounces	1093

Compiled from American Association of Retired Persons (AARP): *The state of 50+ America,* 2004, AARP Public Policy Institute (website): *ppi.aarp.org;* American Public Health Association (APHA): *Fact sheet: health lifestyle for older adults,* 2005 (website): *www.Medscape.Com/viewarticle 501874_print;* Kaiser Permanente Fact Sheet: *Women and calcium,* 1983; Sardana R: Nutritional management of osteoporosis, *Geriatr Nurs* 13(6):317, 1992; and Insel P et al: *Discovering nutrition,* ed 2, Boston, 2006, American Dietetic Association/Jones & Bartlett.

TABLE 9-7

Lactose Intolerance Worldwide

Group	% Tolerant
U.S. African Americans	95%
Caucasian Americans	12%
Native Americans	100%
Swiss	10%
Swedish	2%
Finns	18%
African Fulani	23%
African Bantu	89%
African Tussi	20%
Chinese	93%
Thais	98%
Europeans in Australia	4%
Australian Aborigines	85%

Data from Insel P et al: *Discovering nutrition*, ed 2, Boston, 2006, American Dietetic Association/Jones & Bartlett.

Phosphorus. Phosphorus helps strengthen teeth and bones (Arthritis, 2005). The RDA is 700 mg/daily. Taking too much causes upset stomach, diarrhea, and kidney damage. Excess doses are considered 4000 mg daily before age 70 years and 3000 daily after age 70 years. Phosphorus deficiency causes fatigue, loss of appetite, bone pain, susceptibility to infections, and weakness. It interacts with antacids containing aluminum, potassium supplements, and some diuretics that spare potassium. Phosphorus is contained in many soft drinks. When milk is avoided and soft drinks taken instead, a problem may occur with bone strength.

Kidney Disease

There are many nutritional and fluid issues in kidney function. Urinary tract infections (UTIs) are also common in elderly people (AGS, 2006a). Cranberry products may reduce the incidence of UTIs. A recommended dose is 300 mL of cranberry juice each day. Vitamin C tablets may be useful also since many bacteria cannot flourish in an acid environment.

Kidney stones are common in older adults. Uric acid calculi (stones) may occur in elders with gout, those with excessive supplemental calcium intake, or those unable to utilize ingested calcium. Calcium stones are common in older women, especially those who have had a surgical menopause. These women have increased bone resorption and excretion of calcium from the urinary tract. Those adults with high sodium intake increase the excretion of calcium and uric acid along with sodium excretion (Dudek, 2006). Stones containing high amounts of oxalate may occur when the elder consumes excessive amounts of foods containing oxalate. These foods are spinach, beets, nuts, chocolate, wheat bran, and strawberries. Of interest, other high-oxalate foods such as whole wheat, blackberries and gooseberries, red currants, tangerines, sweet potatoes, and cocoa do not cause development of stones. Most stones pass within 24 hours and can be very painful. Elders who are prone to this condition should consume high amounts of fluids.

Related disorders such as hypertension, heart failure, and diabetes mellitus all affect kidney function. Nearly two thirds of elders with hypertension have sodium-sensitive hypertension (AGS, 2006a). However, women are more adherent to sodium-restricted diets (Chung et al., 2006). Lifestyle management for hypertension includes weight reduction, moderation of alcohol intake, and lowered sodium, cholesterol, and saturated fat intake. Adequate intake of potassium, magnesium, and calcium is important in any hypertension regimen (AGS, 2006a).

Dysphagia

Difficulty swallowing is a common problem of older adults. Malnutrition may occur rapidly after onset of the problem, especially in instances such as stroke or Parkinson's disease (Mosqueda and Brummel-Smith, 2002). Dysphagia may also occur in elders with late-stage dementia. With poor attention and concentration, the elder often forgets to swallow (Ham et al., 2002). Other factors such as poor dentition, inadequate feeding techniques, and reduced salivation may also predispose the older adult to dysphagia. Box 9-11 presents risk factors for dysphagia.

Dysphagia is a serious problem and has negative consequences, including weight loss, malnutrition, aspiration pneumonia, and even death. More than half of the 750,000 people affected by stroke each year experience dysphagia at some point. Of these, 50% will develop pneumonia and 4.3% will die of pneumonia (Blackington et al., 2001). Dysphagia can be categorized as transfer or oropharyngeal dysphagia (difficulty moving the food from the mouth to the esophagus), transport dysphagia (difficulty passing the ingested food down the esophagus), or delivery dysphagia (the propulsion of a bolus of food to the stomach is difficult).

It is important to obtain a careful history of the elder's response to dysphagia and to observe the person during mealtime. Symptoms that alert the nurse to possible swallowing problems are presented in Box 9-12. Silent aspiration is common, and a comprehensive evaluation by a speech-language pathologist, usually including a videofluoroscopic recording of a modified barium swallow, should be considered when dysphagia is suspected (Shanley and O'Loughlin, 2000). The speech therapist will be able to assess the elder to determine the best type of food and food consistency for the swallowing problem.

Aspiration is the most profound and dangerous problem for older adults experiencing dysphagia. It is important to have a suction machine available at the bedside or in the

---

> **BOX 9-11 Risk Factors for Dysphagia**
>
> - Cerebrovascular accident (CVA, stroke)
> - Parkinson's disease
> - Neuromuscular disorders, for example, amyotropic lateral sclerosis (ALS), multiple sclerosis (MS), myasthenia gravis, dystonia
> - Anatomic abnormalities
> - Cervical osteophytes
> - Oral and oropharyngeal cancer or surgery
> - Laryngeal cancer or surgery
> - Alzheimer's disease and related dementias
> - Traumatic brain injury
> - Tracheostomy
> - Aspiration pneumonia

> **BOX 9-12 Signs and Symptoms of Dysphagia**
>
> - Difficult, labored swallowing
> - Drooling
> - Copious oral secretions
> - Aspiration
> - Coughing, choking at meals
> - Holding or pocketing of food in the mouth
> - Absence of chewing
> - Absence of swallowing
> - Excessive throat clearing
> - Difficulty swallowing medications
> - Wet or gurgling voice
> - Discomfort during swallowing
> - Sensation of something stuck in the throat during swallowing
> - Food or liquid coming out of the nose during swallowing

dining room in the institutional setting. Other interventions for dysphagia are described in Box 9-13. The gerontological nurse must work closely with other members of the interdisciplinary team, such as dietitians and speech-language pathologists, in implementing suggested interventions. A comprehensive protocol for preventing aspiration in older adults with dysphagia can be found at *www.hartfordign.org/publications/trythis/issue_20.pdf.*

Feeding Tubes. Research on the appropriate management of swallowing disorders in older people, particularly during acute illness and in long-term care facilities, is very limited (Robbins et al., 2001). Comprehensive assessment of swallowing problems and other factors that influence intake must be conducted before initiating severely restricted diet modifications or considering the use of feeding tubes, particularly in older people with dementia (Chouinard, 2000). Short-term enteral feeding may be indicated for some conditions, but the use of feeding tubes in patients with advanced dementia to prevent aspiration pneumonia, malnutrition, and infections provides few long-term benefits and may, in fact, contribute to further decline. Tube feeding has never been shown to reduce the risk of regurgitating gastric contents and cannot be expected to prevent aspiration of oral secretions (Finucane et al., 1999). Although a feeding tube may facilitate better nutrition, about one half of elderly patients will aspirate with a nasogastric or gastric tube.

When tube feeding is indicated, formulas for feedings should vary based on certain diseases such as glucose intolerance, which would entail finding a formula with low carbohydrate content, high fiber to reduce glucose response, and high monounsaturated fatty acids to reduce the risk of heart disease. Most commercial products are lactose free because of intolerance in many older adults and those with malabsorption syndromes. Most of the formulas given through

> **BOX 9-13 Interventions for Dysphagia**
>
> - Sit at 90 degrees during all oral (PO) intake.
> - Maintain 90-degree positioning for at least 1 hour after PO intake.
> - Keep suction equipment ready at all times.
> - Supervise all meals.
> - Monitor temperature.
> - Observe color of phlegm.
> - Visually check the mouth for pocketing of food in cheeks.
> - Provide mouth care every 4 hours.
> - Follow speech therapist's recommendation for safe swallowing techniques and modified food consistency.

tube feedings are concentrated, and the hydration status of the patient must be closely monitored.

Nasogastric, nasoduodenal, and nasojejunal tubes are used for short-term feedings—often indicated after a hip fracture when the serum albumin is low. The use of percutaneous endoscopic gastrostomy (PEG) feeding tubes has increased at an astonishing rate in older adults over recent years. No scientific study demonstrates improved survival, reduced incidence of pneumonia or other infections, improved function, or fewer pressure ulcers (AGS, 2006b). Few complications occur with insertion of a PEG tube; however, numerous complications occur from having a PEG tube (AGS, 2006b). Aspiration pneumonia, diarrhea, metabolic problems, and cellulitis are just a few of these complications. There is no improvement of these problems even in those severely cognitively impaired. The mortality rate has been higher in more than 5000 nursing home patients with swallowing/chewing problems who were tube-fed compared with those who were not. A prospective study needs to be done comparing tube feeding with hand feeding in comparable elderly patients.

Obesity

The American Public Health Association (APHA) has developed a fact sheet on HealthLifestyle for Older Adults (2005). It states that the prevalence of obesity among older adults increased from 12% in 1990 to 19% in 2002. Further, nearly 80% of older adults do not engage in regular leisure-time activities. The fact sheet recommendations are found in Box 9-14.

Other publications state that body fat increases until about age 50 years in women and age 40 years in men, remains steady, and then decreases after age 70 years (Beers and Berkow, 2000). Those who weigh 120% to 130% of their ideal weight are considered moderately obese; those who weigh more than 130% of their ideal weight are morbidly obese. At this time, however, the ideal body mass for elderly people has not been established.

Obesity results from decreased physical activity that frequently occurs in elderly individuals. The loss of estrogen and growth hormone (GH) contributes to obesity in women; loss of GH contributes to obesity in men. Other causes of obesity in older people include hypothyroidism, hypothalamic tumors, glucocorticoid therapy, monoamine oxidase inhibitors, and moderate dosages of phenothiazines (Beers and Berkow, 2000). Rosiglitazone, atorvastatin, and sulfonylureas are several other drugs that commonly cause weight gain (Aschenbrenner and Venable, 2006).

It has long been known that obese adults have more medical problems compared with thin and normal-weight adults, including diabetes, hypertension, and colon cancer. A study by Grabowski and Ellis (2001) supported by the Agency for Healthcare Research and Quality (AHRQ) suggests that extra weight may be protective for elderly people. Fat is a storage "organ" for excess calories and provides protection during times of acute illness (Beers and Berkow, 2000). It protects the vital organs from injury in falls, and it helps maintain the body's core temperature. Excess fat, however, causes medical complications (Box 9-15) (Beers and Berkow, 2000).

The prevalence of obesity is rising in the United States. Certain groups have classified obesity as an epidemic, including the World Health Organization and the National Heart, Lung, and Blood Institute of the National Institutes of Health. More than 70% of American adults are obese. These obese people have a BMI greater than 30.

Screening for obesity is usually done by calculating the BMI normalized for height. The National Center for Health Statistics uses the 85th percentile gender-specific values for persons ages 20 through 29 years (27.8 kg/m² or greater for men; and 27.3 kg/m² or greater for women). This was derived from the U.S. National Health and Nutrition Examination Survey (NHANES III) (National Center for Health Statistics, 2007).

Risk of mortality is increased for severely obese people, although the thinnest people also have this risk. An elevated waist/hip circumference ratio (WHR), which indicates central adiposity (fat), correlates with BMI and may be a better predictor of complications of obesity. Waist circumferences greater than 40 inches (102 cm) in men and greater than 35 inches (88 cm) in women indicate high risk. Although we can identify obese individuals from physical examination, precise methods should be used to evaluate mild to moderate obesity. The easiest and most common clinical method is the evaluation of body weight and height based on a table of "desirable" weights. The tables reflect the weight at which risk of mortality is minimized. An alternative is the calculation of BMI. Overweight is defined as a BMI of 27.8 or greater for men and 27.3 or greater for

---

BOX 9-14   American Public Health Association Fact Sheet on Older Adult Lifestyle

- >80% of elders have a poor diet.
- <33% of elders eat 51 fruits and vegetables every day.
- Elders living in poverty are less likely to eat a good diet than those living above the poverty level.
- Recommendations: eat 2+ servings of fruit every day and 31 servings of vegetables—especially dark-green, leafy ones like broccoli and kale and orange vegetables such as carrots and sweet potatoes.
- Drink 3 cups of milk or equivalent low-fat yogurt or cheese every day. These are a good source of calcium.
- Fiber: eat 3 servings of whole grain cereals, breads, crackers, rice and pasta every day.
- Protein: eat 2-3 servings every day including fish, poultry, beans, nuts, and eggs.

From American Public Health Association (APHA): *Fact sheet: health lifestyle for older adults,* Washington, DC, 2005, The Association.

BOX 9-15   Complications of Obesity

MODERATE OBESITY

Coronary artery disease
Hypertension
Osteoarthritis
Gallbladder disease
Diabetes mellitus
Colon cancer
Prostate cancer
Breast cancer
Ovarian cancer

MORBID OBESITY

Immobility
Intertrigo
Drug problems
Increased mortality rate
Increased surgical risk
All complications of moderate obesity

women. The formula is weight (kg) divided by height (m²) or, using pounds instead of kilograms, weight (lb) times 703 and then divided by height (in²).

Obesity management risk/benefit ratios should be evaluated before intervention. Excessive weight loss may be a cause of higher mortality rates (Beers and Berkow, 2000). A walking program such as mall walking may help with gradual loss of weight and can also be a social occasion. Weight-loss drugs are not recommended for older persons because the side effects may outweigh the positive effect. Orlistat (Xenical), which inhibits fat absorption, may be used in elderly obese patients, especially those with diabetes and hypertension. Orlistat can produce weight loss of 8% to 10%. It can cause soft stools and decreased absorption of fat-soluble vitamins. Stomach surgery would be considered only in those with sleep apnea and BMI greater than 40 or BMI greater than 35 with comorbid conditions.

Gastrointestinal Disorders

A number of prevalent disorders of the GI tract are influenced by nutrition. Some of these are gastroesophageal reflux disease (GERD); ulcers; lactase deficiency, which can start in older age; constipation; diarrhea; gas; diverticulosis; irritable bowel syndrome; and colon cancer (Insel et al., 2006).

Gastroesophageal Reflux Disease.

Elders with GERD should avoid peppermint, chocolate, coffee, fatty foods, alcoholic beverages, citrus juices, tomato products, and pepper (Insel et al., 2006). Eating small portions may also be helpful in avoiding the disorder. Eating low-fat meals is useful because high-fat meals delay gastric emptying. Dinner (or lunch) should be eaten 2 to 3 hours before lying down for sleep or naps so that the stomach has at least partially emptied. A primary change is elevating the head of the bed or sleeping on a wedge that elevates the esophagus in relation to the stomach so that gravity helps keep acid down. Making changes that decrease the relaxation of the esophageal sphincter is useful. Smoking cessation and weight reduction will help relieve this problem.

Peptic Ulcers.

Peptic ulcers cause a burning or gnawing pain in the mid-epigastrium. The elder may experience nausea, vomiting, loss of appetite, and weight loss (Insel et al., 2006). Most ulcers are known to be caused by a bacterium—*Helicobacter pylori* or *H. pylori* (80%-90%). Another common cause, especially in elders, is from the use of NSAIDs. This class of drug includes aspirin, ibuprofen, celecoxib, and naproxen sodium. NSAIDs interfere with GI tract ability to protect from acidic stomach digestive juices. When this occurs, ulcers develop because there are no defenses from acid.

Management of NSAID-induced ulcers is mainly stopping the use of this class of drug. Ulcers caused by *H. pylori* are managed with antibiotics and proton pump inhibitors (PPIs), which lower the stomach acidity.

Constipation.

Stool moves too slowly in the GI tract when muscle contractions in the colon are sluggish (Insel et al., 2006). The colon then absorbs too much of the water in the stool and produces hard, dry stools—constipation. The cause is usually a low-fiber diet and insufficient fluids. Elders who eat high-fiber diets rarely will experience constipation. Foods with the highest amount of fiber are split peas, lentils, kidney beans, wheat-bran flake cereal, bulgur wheat, dried plums, and apples with skin. White bread and white rice have very little fiber content.

Fiber is an important dietary component that some older people do not consume in sufficient quantities. Fiber, the indigestible material that gives plants their structure, is abundant in raw fruits and vegetables and unrefined grains and cereals.

Fiber facilitates the absorption of water, increases bulk, and improves intestinal motility. It helps control weight by delaying gastric emptying and providing a feeling of fullness (Insel et al., 2006). Fiber improves glucose tolerance by delaying movement of carbohydrate (CHO) into the small intestine. It helps prevent or reduce the incidence of constipation by increasing the weight of stool and shortening the transit time. It helps prevent hemorrhoids and diverticulosis by decreasing pressure in the colon, shortening transit time, and increasing the stool weight. Fiber reduces risk of heart disease by binding with bile (which contains cholesterol) and causes its excretion.

Various types of fiber exist, but all possess the common characteristic of indigestibility. Individuals who can chew foods well could benefit from eating increased amounts of fresh fruits and vegetables daily or combining unsweetened bran with other types of food. Those who have difficulty chewing could sprinkle oat bran on cereals or in soups, meat loaf, or casseroles. The quantity of bran used depends on the individual, but generally 1 to 2 tablespoons daily is sufficient to facilitate intestinal motility. Individuals who have not used bran should begin with 1 teaspoon and progressively increase the quantity until the fiber intake is enough to accomplish its purpose. If bran is used in larger amounts to start, bloating, gas, diarrhea, and other colon discomforts will initially occur and discourage further use of this important dietary ingredient.

Cooked dried beans are a good source of fiber. Pinto beans, split peas, red beans, and peanuts can be served in casseroles, soups, and dips. These are all relatively inexpensive and nutritious in addition to having high fiber content. See Box 9-16 for fiber choices and amounts of fiber in each (Moore, 2001). The discussion of elimination in Chapter 7 presents recipes for promoting bowel elimination. Each of these recipes has fiber agents.

Diarrhea.

Stools that are loose and watery and occur more than 3 times per day is diarrhea. It is caused by digestive products in stool moving through the large intestine too rapidly for water to be reabsorbed (Insel et al., 2006). Many disorders cause this increase in peristalsis. Stress is a major cause. Eating food that is contaminated by bacteria

BOX 9-16	Foods High in Dietary Fiber

HIGHEST

All wheat bran types
Figs
Dried peaches
Prunes (dried or cooked)

MODERATE

Oat bran
Apples with skin
Dried apricots
Whole-grain or bran English muffin
Bran muffin
Ry-Krisps
Mueslix
Beans (kidney, lima, red, northern)
Brussels sprouts
Corn
Peas
Avocados
Blackberries
Dates
Oranges
Pears

LOW

Cracked-wheat bread
Brown rice
Cornbread
Corn flakes
Cheerios
Applesauce
Grapes
Green beans
Onions
Peppers
Potatoes
Pears (canned)
French toast
Raisins
Strawberries
Pineapple
Granola
Pancakes
Grape Nuts
Cantaloupe
Blueberries
Non-bran muffins
Kiwifruit
Carrots
Cauliflower
Broccoli
Cherries
Mushrooms

Adapted from Moore MC: *Mosby's pocket guide series: nutritional assessment and care,* ed 5, St Louis, 2005, Mosby.

or viruses often causes a painful, cramping diarrhea. Other causes include gluten (in wheat) intolerance, fats, lactose intolerance, medication side effects, and intestinal irritation and damage.

Diarrhea is dangerous in the older adult and should be treated promptly. It can cause dehydration and loss of electrolytes, especially potassium.

Excessive Flatus. Flatulence is the expulsion of gas from the GI track. It may have an unpleasant odor because large intestine bacteria contain sulfur, an element that smells of rotten eggs. Air is in the stomach from swallowing or gulping it. This occurs commonly in those who eat or drink rapidly and those who chew gum, smoke, or wear loose dentures. Burping or belching releases the gas that forms in the stomach.

Gas that does not leave by burping continues through the small intestine and is partially absorbed (Insel et al., 2006). Some gas moves to the large intestine and is released via the rectum and anus. This is flatus. Its composition is related to the extent of CHO intake and the bacteria activity in the colon. Foods that contain CHO cause gas. Soft drinks and fruit drinks cause gas. Fats and proteins cause little gas. Fiber in fruits, beans, and oat bran causes gas in the large intestine as it breaks down there. Fiber in wheat bran and many vegetables produces little gas. Rice produces no gas. A study of pilots and astronauts in the 1960s found that the average person expels about one pint of gas each day (Insel et al., 2006). Some people have more gas than others do. It depends on the bacteria that predominate in the person's bowel.

Diverticulosis. Diverticulosis (see Chapter 10) occurs with higher frequency in countries that eat low-fiber diets—countries such as the United States, England, and Australia. It is rare in countries such as Asia and Africa, where mainly high-fiber vegetable diets are consumed.

Irritable Bowel Syndrome. The cause of irritable bowel syndrome is unknown. Those with this syndrome suffer abdominal pain, cramping, diarrhea, and constipation. It can be disabling. Foods that aggravate symptoms include alcohol, chocolate, milk products, beans, coffee, and animal and vegetable fats. It is generally controlled through diet and lifestyle modifications. Stress reduction is part of this management regimen.

Colon Cancer. Colorectal cancer is the second leading cause of cancer-related deaths in the United States (Centers for Disease Control and Prevention [CDC], 2004). The risk for colorectal cancer is heightened by diets high in meat, especially processed meats, and fat. Obesity increases this risk. Risk is decreased in diets high in fruits, vegetables, folate, and calcium. Exercise decreases the risk. Fiber has been thought to be protective by dilution of carcinogens in a bulky stool; however, no evidence exists to support this theory.

NEUROLOGICAL/PSYCHOLOGICAL DISORDERS AND NUTRITION

Many neurological disorders in elders affect diet. They may be caused by nutritional deficiencies, for example, in vitamin B_{12} dementia. All will affect nutritional status through decreased cognitive ability, apathy, weakness, fatigue, or hormonal dysfunction.

Depression

Depression is common in older adults and often is not diagnosed. GI complaints, poor appetite, weight loss, and weight gain often accompany depression. Weight loss is an important concern in elders with depression. The brain plays an essential role in the decision to eat or not to eat through integration of multiple hormonal signals (Smeets et al., 2006). Regulation of hunger and satiety, respiration, body temperature, and water balance all play a role in eating and drinking or not (Insel et al., 2006). Parosmia, an abnormal sense of smell, can occur with severe depression, which further causes loss of interest in eating (McCance and Huether, 2006).

Other systemic and metabolic disorders have a depression component. These include anemias, hypothyroidism and hyperthyroidism, infection, and deficiencies of omega-3 highly unsaturated fatty acids (HUFA) (Richardson, 2003). A new onset of depression may be caused by folate deficiency.

Most depressions need to be managed with medications. Unfortunately, many of these medications cause GI side effects that also affect appetite and nutrition. Selective serotonin reuptake inhibitors (SSRIs), a class of medications often used to manage depression in elders, cause nausea, anorexia, diarrhea, and dyspepsia. Weight gain is a side effect of some antidepressants (e.g., amitriptyline, doxepin, and nortriptyline in the tricyclics class) (NeighborCare, 2004) (see Chapter 12) Therapy should include more than medications and can be provided by nurses as well as psychiatrists, psychologists, and social workers. Therapy should include monitoring and promoting nutrition, elimination, sleep and rest, and physical comfort. (See Chapter 25 for a discussion of depression.)

Dementia

Dementia affects adequate nutritional intake, and in late dementia, weight loss becomes a considerable concern. The loss of weight may be the result of cognitive deficits and loss of awareness of need to eat and therefore inadequate intake of foods; depression; increased energy output caused by pacing and wandering; increased incidence of infections; and/or loss of independence for self-feeding (McCance and Huether, 2006).

One of the best strategies for managing poor intake is establishing a routine so the elder does not have to remember times and places for eating. Without this routine, anxiety and agitation may occur. Caregivers should continue to serve well-balanced foods and drinks that the older adult likes and has always eaten (Kempler, 2005). These should be served in small amounts. Attention to mealtime ambience is important, and the elder should be able to take as much time as is needed to eat the food so that hurrying does not cause anxiety. The caregiver should watch for storage of foods in the cheeks. Finger foods are a good choice because utensils may be too difficult to maneuver. Serving one dish and using one utensil at a time may also assist in promoting adequate intake. In later stages, pureed foods and liquids may be necessary as the elder forgets to swallow. The awareness of thirst may be gone, resulting in insufficient fluid intake unless strategies are in place to deal with this. Limit alcohol, colas, tea, and coffee because these contribute to dehydration. Offer small amounts of fluids between bites of foods and throughout the day. In nursing homes, refreshment stations with easy access to juices, water, and healthy snacks also promote adequate intake. (See Chapter 23 for a discussion of dementia.)

NUTRITIONAL PROBLEMS IN INSTITUTIONAL SETTINGS

Older adults in hospitals and institutional settings are more likely to experience a number of the problems that contribute to inadequate nutrition discussed earlier in this chapter. Poor oral health, swallowing disorders, lack of culturally appropriate food, depression, inadequate staffing to provide assistance with meals, and cognitive and physical impairment are some of the factors that contribute to nutritional deficiencies and are exacerbated when the person is in an institutional setting. Weight loss in institutionalized elders may be the result of a number of circumstances, both physical and emotional.

In the acute care hospital setting, it is important to give consideration, care, and attention to feeding dependent older people. Severely restricted diets, long periods of nothing-by-mouth (NPO) status, and insufficient time and staff for feeding assistance contribute to poor nutrition in this setting as well. Sufficient time should be provided to accommodate the older person who has a slow eating pace. Other suggestions are provided on p. 218.

The incidence of eating disability in long-term care is high. Approximately 50% of all residents cannot eat independently (Burger et al., 2000). Inadequate staffing in nursing homes is associated with poor nutrition and hydration, and as Kayser-Jones (1997, p. 19) states: "CNAs have an impossible task trying to feed the number of people who need assistance." She estimated that feeding impaired older adults in nursing homes with inadequate staffing could mean that each CNA would be able to spend only about 6 to 10 minutes feeding a resident. Burger et al. (2000) called for increases in staffing requirements in nursing homes, recommending the availability of one staff person for every two to three residents who need feeding assistance, thus allowing each resident about 20 to 30 minutes with the CNA. In response to concerns about the lack of adequate assistance during mealtimes in nursing homes, the Centers for Medicare and Medicaid Services (CMS) implemented a rule that allows feeding assistants 8 hours of state-approved training to help nursing home residents with eating. Feeding assistants must be supervised by the registered nurse (RN) or licensed practical/vocational nurse (LPN/LVN).

The use of restrictive therapeutic diets for frail elders in long-term care (low cholesterol, low salt, no concentrated sweets) often reduces food intake without significantly helping the clinical status of the resident and should be avoided (Morley, 2003; Tariq et al., 2001). If caloric supplements are used, they should be administered at least 1 hour before meals or they interfere with meal intake. Very little research has been conducted on the outcomes of caloric or "med-pass" nutritional supplements. Studies are warranted because these products are widely used, particularly in hospitals and nursing homes, and can be costly. One study (Kayser-Jones et al., 1998) reported that 75% of supplements ordered were dispensed and only 55% of residents consumed them as ordered.

Attention to the environment in which meals are served is important. It is not uncommon in long-term care facilities to hear over the public address system at mealtime, "Feeder trays are ready." This reference to the need to feed those unable to feed themselves is, in itself, degrading and erases any trace of dignity the older person is trying to maintain in a controlled environment. It is not malicious intent by nurses or other caregivers but rather a habit of convenience. Feeding older adults who have difficulty eating can become mechanical and devoid of conversation and feeling. The feeding process becomes rapid, and if it bogs down and becomes too slow, the meal may be ended abruptly, depending on the time the caregiver has allotted for feeding the patient. Any pleasure is destroyed that could be derived through socialization and eating, as is any dignity that could be maintained while dependent on others for food (see An Elder Speaks at the beginning of this chapter). Older adults accustomed to certain table manners may feel ashamed at their inability to behave in what they feel is an appropriate manner.

In addition to adequate staff, many innovative and evidence-based ideas can improve nutritional intake in institutions. Restorative dining programs, homelike dining rooms, individualized menu choices including ethnic foods, cafeteria-style service, kitchens on the nursing unit, availability of food around the clock, choice of mealtimes, liberal diets, finger foods, visually appealing pureed foods with texture and shape, music, touch, verbal cueing, hand-over-hand feeding, sitting while assisting a resident to eat, and many other adaptations are found in the literature (Roberts and Durnbaugh, 2002).

Federal regulations are in place in the form of the Omnibus Budget Reconciliation Act of 1987 (OBRA) that ensure nutritional standards in long-term care facilities. These standards include assessing nutritional status; ensuring maintenance of nutritional status unless the clinical state renders this impossible; and providing a therapeutic diet for nutritional problems. The Joint Commission has also set standards for nutrition (Box 9-17).

BOX 9-17 The Joint Commission Nutrition Standard

- Screen for nutritional risk.
- Provide nutritional intervention and counseling.
- Plan for nutritional care.
- Prescribe nutrition products.
- Prepare, distribute, and administer food need nutrition products.

▲ PROMOTING HEALTHY AGING: IMPLICATIONS FOR GERONTOLOGICAL NURSING

Assessment

A nutritional assessment that provides the most conclusive data about a person's actual nutritional state consists of four steps: interview, physical examination, anthropometric measurements, and biochemical analysis. The collective results can provide the nurse with data needed to identify the immediate and potential nutrition problems of the client. The nurse can then begin to establish plans for supervision, assistance, and education in the attainment of adequate nutrition for the older person. The NSI developed an algorithm for nutritional assessment and approaches (see Figure 9-3).

Interview. The interview provides background information and clues to the nutritional state and actual and potential problems of the elderly person. Questions about the individual's state of health, social activities, normal patterns, and changes that have occurred should be asked. The nurse must explore the individual's needs, the manner in which food is obtained, and the client's ability to prepare food. Information concerning the relationship of food to daily events will provide clues to the meaning and significance of food to that person. Older people who eat alone are considered candidates for malnutrition. Information about daily activities will suggest the degree of energy expenditure and caloric intake most correct for the overall activity. One's economic state will have a direct bearing on nutrition. It is therefore important to explore the client's financial resources to establish the income available for food. Knowledge of medications taken should be included

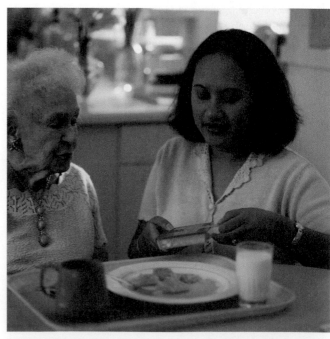

A nurse assists an older woman with a meal. (Copyright © Getty Images.)

in the nutrition history. Additional medical information should be included in the interview. The presence or absence of mouth pain or discomfort, visual difficulty, bowel and bladder function, and food intake patterns should be explored.

Diet Histories. Frequently a 24-hour diet recall compared with the Food Guide Pyramid can present an estimate of nutritional adequacy. When the older person cannot provide all the information requested, it may be possible to obtain data from a family member or another source. There will be times, however, when information will not be as complete as one would like, or the older person, too proud to admit that he or she is not eating, will furnish erroneous information. The nurse will still be able to obtain additional data from the other three areas of the nutritional assessment.

Keeping a dietary record for 3 days is another assessment tool. When one ate, what was eaten, and amounts eaten must be carefully recorded. Computer analysis of the dietary records provides information on energy and vitamin and mineral intake. Printouts can provide the older person and the health care provider with a visual graph of their intake.

Physical Examination. The second step of the nutritional assessment, the physical examination, furnishes clinically observable evidence of the existing state of nutrition. Data such as height and weight; vital signs; condition of the tongue, lips, and gums; and skin turgor, texture, and color are assessed, and the general overall appearance is scrutinized for evidence of wasting. This diminution of the number of size of muscle fibers is known as sarcopenia. Factors contributing to this age-related process include diminished exercise and physical activity, loss of motor units, and reduced skeletal muscle protein synthesis (Merck, 2007). By age 75, approximately one half of muscle mass has disappeared. Maximum isometric contraction force decreases by 50% at age 70. However, these elders can easily climb stairs, rise from a squatting position, walk a straight line, hop on one foot, and perform activities of daily living (ADLs). Debate continues in the quest to determine the appropriate weight charts for older people. Weight, however, is not the only issue; fat distribution must be considered.

Anthropometric Measurements. Anthropometric measurements are the third part of the nutritional assessment and part of the physical examination. They include height, weight, midarm circumference, and triceps skinfold thickness. These include simple body measurement procedures, which take less than 5 minutes to perform. These measurements obtain information about the status of the older person's muscle mass and body fat in relation to height and weight. In some instances, an individual is bedridden or confined to a chair or the individual has a spinal curvature preventing accurate height measurement. Unlike stature, knee height changes little with age. It should be noted that blacks have proportionally longer lower extremities and Chinese have shorter extremities than whites (Moore, 2001). An estimation of stature can be made

using knee height and a sliding broad-blade caliper, similar to the apparatus used to measure the length of an infant. This device consists of an adjustable blade attached to each end at a 90-degree angle.

Muscle mass measurements are obtained by measuring the arm circumference of the nondominant upper arm. The arm hangs freely at the side, and a measuring tape is placed around the midpoint of the upper arm, between the acromion of the scapula and the olecranon of the ulna. The centimeter circumference is recorded and compared with standard values, which can be found in most nutritional assessment and medical nutrition therapy textbooks.

Body fat and lean body mass are assessed by measuring specific skinfolds with Lange or Harpenden calipers. Two areas are accessible for measurement. One area is the midpoint of the upper arm, the triceps area, which is also used to obtain arm circumference. The nondominant arm is again used. The nurse lifts the skin with the thumb and forefinger so that it parallels the humerus. The calipers are placed around the skinfold, 1 cm below where the fingers are grasping the skin. Two readings are averaged to the nearest half centimeter. Results should be compared with standard values such as those cited in Moore (2001). If a neuropathological condition or hemiplegia after a stroke is present, the unaffected arm should be used for obtaining measurements.

There are more sophisticated methods of assessing body composition. Magnetic resonance imaging (MRI), computed tomography (CT), ultrasound, dual-energy x-ray absorptiometry (DEXA) scan, and densitometry are a few. They are becoming available in most communities but are expensive.

The BMI, discussed earlier, is a simple tool for evaluation of the appropriateness of weight to height. It does not, however, assess lean body mass or fat but does correlate well with many of the other measures of body fat content and does correlate with the risk of morbidity. It has the additional virtue of ease of assessment if accurate measures of height and weight are available (Moore, 2001).

Biochemical Examination. The final step in a nutritional assessment is the biochemical examination. A decreased albumin may indicate protein deficiency, but albumin is slow to change during malnutrition (Moore, 2001). Serum albumin of more than 4 g/dL is desired; less than 3.5 g/dL is an indicator of risk for poor nutritional status. Prealbumin level is a better indicator of protein loss because it changes rapidly in malnutrition. It also decreases in inflammatory diseases and injury situations. Transferrin, an iron transport protein, is diminished in protein malnutrition; like prealbumin, it responds quickly (diminishes) with undernutrition. However, it increases in iron deficiency anemia, which is common in older adults and those with protein calorie malnutrition, so it is not a sensitive indicator of protein calorie malnutrition. A normocytic red blood cell (RBC) anemia with low hemoglobin and hematocrit indicates protein deficiency, and a microcytic (small RBC) anemia indicates iron or copper deficiency. A macrocytic (large RBC) anemia is caused by vitamin B_{12} or folate deficiency, which is seen on the mean cell value (MCV) of the complete blood cell count (CBC).

Interventions

Interventions are formulated around the identified nutritional problem or problems. Perhaps the most significant intervention for the community-dwelling elder is nutrition education and problem solving with the elder and family members in how to best resolve the potential or actual nutritional deficit.

With the rising cost of health care, many of us are turning to the Internet or other information sources to help us understand our health needs, as well as our disease processes. Nearly 50% of adults older than 50 years have access to the Internet at home (AARP, 2004). Physicians, geriatric nurse practitioners, and other primary care health providers have less time to educate. The NSI surveyed 600 Americans older than 60 years and found that although 80% knew that nutrition played an important role in their health management, only one third reported that their physician emphasized nutrition. The vast majority said they would use nutrition strategies in their self-care if they received information from their health care provider (NSI, 2002). Effective January 1, 2002, Medicare began covering nutrition therapy for select diseases, such as diabetes and kidney disease, which creates unprecedented opportunities for older Americans to access information (Pear, 2001). (See also Box 9-18.)

Patient Education. Education in the area of reading nutritional information on labels is needed. Since 1994, the U.S. Food and Drug Administration (FDA) has required producers of processed foods to list nutrition information based on daily values. Daily values represent the maximum amounts of nutrients and fiber that are desirable in daily diets of 2000 to 2500 calories. The nutrients were chosen based on evidence suggesting that eating too much or too little of these substances has the greatest impact on one's health. FDA defines a "good source" as a food that contains 10% to 19% of the daily value per serving. The daily totals for fat, cholesterol, and sodium should be less than 100%. Balance should be emphasized as the key to a healthful diet.

Food Pyramids. Several approaches in the past few decades were applied to the education and evaluation of the nutritional status of individuals and of nations. A number of commonly used approaches in the United States are MyPyramid; the Recommended Dietary Allowances (RDA); the Dietary Guidelines for Americans 2005; the Nutrition Screening Initiative (NSI); the Healthy Eating Pyramid from Harvard School of Public Health; Oldways Preservation and Exchange Trust (a nutrition think-tank that has developed Asian, Latin, Mediterranean, and vegetarian pyramids); the American Cancer Institute and its "5-a-Day" campaign, which promotes diets that meet the Food Guide Pyramid guidelines; and the American Heart Association, which recently revised its dietary and lifestyle recommendations.

The U.S. Department of Agriculture (USDA) developed a new pyramid in 2005. The Department is mandated to develop a new pyramid every 5 years. The new pyramid is developed to help professionals and persons design their own caloric needs based on age, gender, and activity level. See Table 9-8 for the older age-groups' caloric needs.

The Modified Food Guide Pyramid for adults older than 70 years has been adapted from the USDA's Food Guide Pyramid. Adults older than 70 years need fewer calories because they are less physically active, in general, than younger adults. Older adults are susceptible to nutrient deficiencies, and the Modified Food Guide Pyramid adds vitamin and mineral supplements that should be included in the daily diet. The Modified Food Guide Pyramid provides the types and amounts of food that should be eaten to optimize nutrient intake. Figure 9-4 illustrates the Modified Food Guide Pyramid. This food pyramid emphasizes a higher ratio of nutrients to calories. Fluid is emphasized in the pyramid because elderly individuals' thirst mechanisms are less responsive than those of younger persons. With proper instruction, the Modified Food Guide Pyramid is an easy and systematic way for a person to evaluate his or her own nutritional intake and independently make corrective adjustments. Pictures can be used to transcend cultural and speech barriers and educational limitations.

TABLE 9-8
MyPyramid Food Intake Pattern of Calorie Levels

Age (in years)	Gender: Male Activity Levels			Gender: Female Activity Levels		
	Sedentary	Moderately Active	Active	Sedentary	Moderately Active	Active
56-60	2200 calories	2400	2600	1600	1800	2200
61-65	2000	2400	2600	1600	1800	2000
66-70	2000	2200	2600	1600	1800	2000
71-75	2000	2200	2600	1600	1800	2000
76+	2000	2200	2400	1600	1800	2000

Data from United States Department of Agriculture (USDA), April 2005.

TUFTS

Food Guide Pyramid for Older Adults

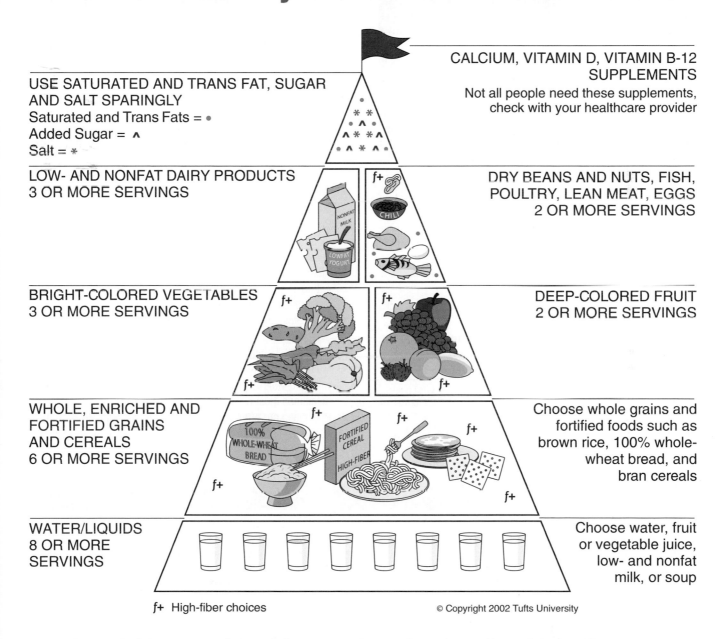

CALCIUM, VITAMIN D, VITAMIN B-12
SUPPLEMENTS
Not all people need these supplements,
check with your healthcare provider

USE SATURATED AND TRANS FAT, SUGAR
AND SALT SPARINGLY
Saturated and Trans Fats = •
Added Sugar = ⌃
Salt = *

LOW- AND NONFAT DAIRY PRODUCTS
3 OR MORE SERVINGS

DRY BEANS AND NUTS, FISH,
POULTRY, LEAN MEAT, EGGS
2 OR MORE SERVINGS

BRIGHT-COLORED VEGETABLES
3 OR MORE SERVINGS

DEEP-COLORED FRUIT
2 OR MORE SERVINGS

WHOLE, ENRICHED AND
FORTIFIED GRAINS
AND CEREALS
6 OR MORE SERVINGS

Choose whole grains and
fortified foods such as
brown rice, 100% whole-
wheat bread, and
bran cereals

WATER/LIQUIDS
8 OR MORE
SERVINGS

Choose water, fruit
or vegetable juice,
low- and nonfat
milk, or soup

f+ High-fiber choices

© Copyright 2002 Tufts University

For additional copies, visit us on the web at http://nutrition.tufts.edu.

FIGURE 9-4 Modified Food Guide Pyramid for Mature (70) Adults. (Copyright 2002 Tufts University, Medford, Mass.)

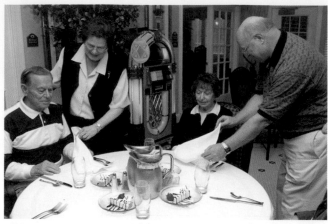

These residents are eating in the dining room. (From Sorrentino SA, Gorek B: *Mosby's textbook for long-term care assistants,* ed 5, St Louis, 2007, Mosby.)

Improving Intake. Practical suggestions for increasing intake when an older person is experiencing a poor appetite or is known to have protein calorie undernutrition can be found in Box 9-18. Other strategies for the hospital and nursing home include the following (DiMaria-Ghalili and Amelia, 2005):

- Walk around at mealtime to determine if food is being eaten or if assistance is needed.
- Take nursing breaks before or after mealtimes to ensure that all possible staff are available to help.
- Ask family members to bring food from home that they know the elder likes.
- Request that dietary service provide nutritious snacks as well as smaller frequent meals.
- Remove bedpans and urinals from the room when the patient must eat there.
- Provide analgesics and antiemetics on a schedule that provides comfort at mealtime.
- Serve meals with the patient in a chair rather than in bed when possible.
- Sit with the patient, keeping eyes at eye level and making eye contact when feeding.

- Order a late warm tray if the patient is not in the room at mealtime.
- Do not interrupt mealtimes for rounds or non-urgent procedures during mealtimes.
- Provide or help with mouth care on a regular basis during the day and evening before and after meals.

It is important for those elders who are institutionalized to receive appropriate supervision at mealtime so that they are able to eat their food, have their food cut for them (if necessary), and have any other requirements met that will enable them to meet their nutritional intake needs. Interventions are formulated around the identified nutritional problem or problems. Perhaps the most significant intervention for the community-dwelling elder is nutrition education and problem solving with the elder in how to best resolve the potential or actual nutritional deficit.

KEY CONCEPTS

- Interruptions in the basic requirements for nutrition, fluids, elimination, activity, and rest may trigger exacerbations of subclinical and chronic disorders.
- When basic needs are out of balance, it is common for the very old to demonstrate the deficiency by becoming confused.
- Recommended dietary patterns for the older adult are similar to those of younger persons, with some reduction in caloric intake based on decreased metabolic requirements.
- Adequacy of nutrition is affected by lifelong eating habits and patterns, accessibility of food, mood disorders, capacity for food preparation, and income.
- Medications may interfere with adequate food intake, absorption, digestion, and elimination. A common nutritional deficiency is calcium, especially for women.
- Making mealtimes pleasant and attractive for the older person who is unable to eat unassisted is entirely a nursing challenge; mealtimes must be made enjoyable.
- PEG tubes are often inserted in older adults with stroke and with dementia. They do not prolong survival nor do they improve quality of life.

BOX 9-18   Suggestions to Improve Intake

- Determine food preferences, including ethnic preferences.
- Ensure that the person has adequate time to eat.
- Provide snacks between meals and at night.
- Do not interrupt mealtimes with medications unless indicated.
- Encourage family members to share mealtimes for a heightened social interaction.
- If caloric supplements are given, offer between meals or with the "medication pass."
- Encourage eating in congregate dining for a more enjoyable social atmosphere.
- Recommend an exercise program, which often increases appetite.
- For those with difficulty swallowing, discourage talking during meals and remind to swallow.

- Ensure proper fit of dentures and denture use.
- Have the person wear glasses at mealtime.
- Sit while feeding a person who needs assistance, use touch, and carry on a social conversation.
- Provide music during dining.
- Use small round tables seating six to eight people in institutional living; consider tablecloths and centerpieces.
- Seat people together who have like interests and abilities, and encourage socialization.
- Utilize restorative dining programs in institutional settings.
- Evaluate the need for adaptive equipment to enhance self-feeding ability.

CASE STUDY: Nutrition

Helen, 77 years old, had dieted all her life—or so it seemed. She often chided herself about it. "After all, at my age who cares if I'm too fat? I do. It depresses me when I gain weight and then I gain even more when I'm depressed." At 5 ft, 4 in. tall and 148 lb, her weight was ideal for her height and age, but Helen, as so many women of her generation, had incorporated Donna Reed's weight of 105 lb as ideal. She had achieved that weight for only a few weeks three or four times in her adult life. She had tried high-protein diets, celery and cottage cheese diets, fasting, commercially prepared diet foods, and numerous fad diets. She always discontinued the diets when she perceived any negative effects. She was invested in maintaining her general good health. Her most recent attempt at losing 30 lb on an all-liquid diet had been unsuccessful and left her feeling constipated, weak, irritable, and mildly nauseated and experiencing heart palpitations. This really frightened her. Her physician criticized her regarding the liquid diet but seemed rather amused while reinforcing that her weight was "just perfect" for her age. In the discussion, the physician pointed out how fortunate she was that she was able to drive to the market, had sufficient money for food, and was able to eat anything with no dietary restrictions. Helen left his office feeling silly. She was an independent, intelligent woman; she had been a successful manager of a large financial office. Before her retirement 7 years ago, her work had consumed most of her energies. There had been no time for family, romance, or hobbies. Lately, she had immersed herself in reading the Harvard Classics as she had promised herself she would when she retired. Unfortunately, now that she had the time to read them, she was losing interest. She knew that she must begin to "pull herself together" and "be grateful for her blessings" just as the physician had said.

Based on the case study, develop a nursing care plan using the following procedure*:
- List Helen's comments that provide subjective data.
- List information that provides objective data.
- From these data, identify and state, using accepted format, two nursing diagnoses you determine are most significant to Helen at this time. List two of Helen's strengths that you have identified from the data.
- Determine and state outcome criteria for each diagnosis. These must reflect some alleviation of the problem identified in the nursing diagnosis and must be stated in concrete and measurable terms.
- Plan and state one or more interventions for each diagnosed problem. Provide specific documentation of the source used to determine the appropriate intervention. Plan at least one intervention that incorporates Helen's existing strengths.
- Evaluate the success of the intervention. Interventions must correlate directly with the stated outcome criteria to measure the outcome success.

Critical Thinking Questions

1. Discuss how you would counsel Helen regarding her weight.
2. If Helen insists on dieting, what diet would you recommend, considering her age and activity level?
3. What lifestyle changes should Helen make?
4. What lifestyle changes would you suggest to Helen?
5. What are the specific health concerns that require attention in Helen's case?
6. What factors may be involved in Helen's preoccupation with her weight?
7. What are some of the reasons that fad diets are dangerous?

*Students are advised to refer to their nursing diagnosis text and identify possible or potential problems.

RESEARCH QUESTIONS

What are the ideal weights for older men and women? What percentages meet this ideal?

What are the dietary patterns of older career women living alone?

What percentage of women older than 60 years are satisfied with their weight? Men?

What eating disorders are most common among older men? Women?

What is the compliance rate in regard to major dietary changes suggested for elders by nurses, dietitians, or physicians?

What percentage of men and women older than 80 years are overweight? Obese?

What nursing interventions can enhance nutritional intake of frail older adults in nursing facilities?

RESOURCES

Administration on Aging:
Nutrition services, elderly nutrition program,
   AoA network organizations
www.aoa.gov/profs/notes/docs/nutritionweb

American Dietetic Association
www.eatright.org/Public/NutritionInformation/92_nsi.cfm

American Public Health Association
Fact sheet—health lifestyle for older adults, 2005
www.medscape.com/viewarticle/501874_print

Center for Medicare and Medicaid Nursing Campaign on Nutrition and Hydration
www.medicare.gov/Nursing/Campaigns/NutriCareAlerts.asp

Consider Nutrition
www.geronurseonline.org

Council for Nutritional Clinical Strategies in Long-Term Care
www.ltcnutrition.org

Harvard School of Public Health
Food pyramids, 2005
www.hsph.harvard.edu/nutritionsource/pyramids.html

Institute of Medicine, Food and Nutrition Board
Dietary reference intakes for energy, carbohydrate, fiber, fat, fatty acids, cholesterol, protein, and amino acids. Food and Nutrition Board National Academy of Sciences, Washington DC, 2002, National Academy Press
www.iom.edu/report.asp?id=4340

Institute of Medicine, Food and Nutrition Board
Dietary reference intakes: applications in dietary planning, Washington DC, 2003, National Academy Press
www.nap.edu/books/0309088534/html/

Joint Commission Nutrition Standards
www.jointcomission.org

Kayser-Jones JS: Use of oral supplements in nursing homes: remaining questions, *J Am Geriatr Soc* 54(9):1463, 2006 (editorial).

Medicare and Medicaid Services
Centers for Medicare and Medicaid services; the Medicaid program and nutrition services; Medicaid home and community-based service.
www.cms.hhs.gov/

Mini Nutritional Assessment
www.hartfordign.org/publications/trythis/issue_9.pdf

National Heart, Lung and Blood Institute
Clinical guidelines on the identification, evaluation, and treatment of overweight and obesity in adults: the evidence report, 1998.
www.nhlbi.nih.gov/guidelines/obesity/ob_gdlns.pdf

Older Americans Act Aging Network Organizations
National Association of State Units on Aging; State Unit on Aging Nutritionist Network; National Association of Area Agencies on Aging; Meals on Wheels Association of America; National Association of Nutrition and Aging Services
www.aoa.gov/

U.S. Department of Agriculture and Health and Human Services
Dietary guidelines for Americans, 2005.
www.healthierus.gov/dietaryguidelines/

U.S. Department of Agriculture and Health and Human Services
Dietary guidelines advisory committee report
www.health.gov/dietaryguidelines/dga2005/report/

U.S. Department of Agriculture and Health and Human Services
MyPyramid, 2005
www.mypyramid.gov/

U.S. Department of Health and Human Services, Agency for Healthcare Research and Quality (AHRQ)
The pocket guide to staying healthy at 50+
AHRQ Pub No 04-IP001-A, Nov. 2003, AARP Pub No D18010
www.ahrq.gov

U.S. Government Accountability Office (GAO)
Report to Congressional Requesters, Dec 2005
Nursing homes: despite increased oversight, challenges remain in ensuring high-quality care and resident safety, GAO-09-117
www.gao.gov/cgi-bin/getrpt?GAO-09-117

REFERENCES

Amella EJ: Assessment and management of eating and feeding difficulties for older people: a NICHE protocol, *Geriatr Nurs* 19(5):269-274, 1998.

American Association of Retired Persons (AARP): *Comparing boomers and their elders wealth at midlife*, December 12, 2004.

American Geriatric Society (AGS): *Geriatrics at your fingertips*, New York, 2006a, The Society.

American Geriatric Society (AGS): *Geriatric review syllabus*, New York, 2006b, The Society.

American Public Health Association (APHA): *Fact sheet: health lifestyle for older adults*, Washington, DC, 2005, The Association.

Arthritis Foundation: *Vitamin guide*, 2005 (website): *www.arthritis.org/resources/nutrition/guide.asp.*

Arthritis (website): *org/resources/arthritistoday/2005/_archivers/2005_09_10/Vitamin_Min.* Accessed April 17, 2006.

Aschenbrenner D, Venable S: *Drug therapy in nursing*, Philadelphia, 2006, Lippincott Williams & Wilkins.

Beers MH, Berkow R: *The Merck manual of geriatrics*, ed 3, Whitehouse Station, NJ, 2000, Merck Research Laboratories.

Bennett S: Dehydration: hazards and benefits, *Geriatr Nurs* 21(2):84, 2000.

Blackington E et al: Oropharyngeal dysphagia in the elderly: identifying and managing patients at risk, *Adv Nurse Pract* 9(7): 42-49, 2001.

Burger S et al: *Malnutrition and dehydration in nursing homes: key issues in prevention and treatment*, 2000 (website): *www.cmwf.org/programs/elders/burger_mal_386.asp.* Accessed July 23, 2004.

Butler R: *Old and poor in America* (issue brief), New York, 2001, International Longevity Center—USA.

Centers for Disease Control and Prevention (CDC): *Colorectal cancer: the importance of prevention and early detection*, 2004/2005 fact sheet (website): *www.cdc.gov/cancer/colorectal/about 2004.htm.* Accessed February 4, 2006.

Chernoff R: *Geriatric nutrition: The health professional's handbook*, ed 3, Sudbury, MA, 2006, Jones & Bartlett.

Chouinard J: Dysphagia in Alzheimer's disease: a review, *J Nutr Health Aging* 4(4):214-217, 2000.

Chung M et al.: Gender differences in adherence to the sodium-restricted diet in patients with heart failure, *J Card Failure* 12(8):628-634, 2006.

Cleveland Clinic: *Digestive diseases: lactose intolerance* (website): *www.webmd.com/content/article/90/100616.htm?rp=refp_rctr_dair_osoq.* Accessed October 2, 2006.

Cross AT et al: Snacking habits of senior Americans, *J Nutr Elderly* 14(2/3):27, 1995.

Desai SP, Isa-Pratt S: *Clinical guide to laboratory medicine*, ed 2, Cleveland, 2002, Lexi-Comp.

DiMaria-Ghalili RA, Amelia E: Nutrition in older adults: intervention and assessment can help curb the growing threat of malnutrition, *Am J Nurs* 105(3):40-50, 2005.

Dudek S: *Nutrition essentials for nursing practice*, ed 5, Philadelphia, 2006, Lippincott.

Finucane TE et al: Tube feeding in patients with advanced dementia: a review of the evidence, *JAMA* 282(14):1365-1370, 1999.

Grabowski D, Ellis J: Weight goals for younger people may not be appropriate for the elderly, for whom weight may be protective, 2001, Agency for Healthcare Research and Quality (website): *www.ahrq.gov/research/oct01/1001RA14.htm.* Accessed December 28, 2006.

Ham R et al: *Primary care geriatrics*, ed 4, St Louis, 2002, Mosby.

Insel P et al: *Discovering nutrition*, ed 2, Boston, 2006, American Dietetic Association/Jones & Bartlett.

Kayser-Jones J: Inadequate staffing at mealtime: implications for nursing and health policy, *J Gerontol Nurs* 23(8):14-21, 1997.

Kayser-Jones J et al: A prospective study of the use of liquid oral dietary supplements in nursing homes, *J Am Geriatr Soc* 46(11):1378-1386, 1998.

Kempler D: *Neurocognitive disorders in aging*, Thousand Oaks, Calif, 2005, Sage.

Lustbader W: Thoughts on the meaning of frailty, *Generations* 13(4):21-22, 1999.

McCance K, Huether S: *Pathophysiology*, ed 5, St Louis, 2006, Mosby.

Meiner S: Gouty arthritis. In Lugeen A, Meinder S, editors: *Care of arthritis in the older adult*, New York, 2002, Springer.

Merck: Aging and the musculoskeletal system, *Merck manual of geriatrics* (website): *www.merck.com/mkgr/mmg/sec7/ch48/ch48e.jsp*. Accessed July 26, 2007.

Moore MC: *Pocket guide to nutritional care*, ed 4, St Louis, 2001, Mosby.

Morley JE: *Dehydration*, 2000 (website): *www.cyberounds.com/conferences/geriatrics*.

Morley JE: Anorexia and weight loss in older persons, *J Gerontol A Biol Sci Med Sci* 58(2):131-137, 2003.

Mosqueda L, Brummel-Smith K: Rehabilitation. In Ham RJ et al, editors: *Primary care geriatrics*, ed 4, St Louis, 2002, Mosby.

National Center for Health Statistics: *NHANES II* (website): *www.cdc.gov/nchs/products/elec_prods/subject/nhanesii.htm*. Accessed July 26, 2007.

National Institute of Diabetes and Digestive and Kidney Diseases. (2004). *Prescription medications for the treatment of obesity* (website): *www.win.niddk.nih.gov/publications/prescription.htm*. Accessed October 2006.

National Institute of Diabetes and Digestive and Kidney Diseases. (2006a). *Weight-control information network* (website): *www.win.niddk.nih.gov/*. Accessed October 2006.

National Institute of Diabetes and Digestive and Kidney Diseases. (2006b). *Statistics related to overweight and obesity* (website): *www.win.niddk.nih.gov/statistics/index.htm*. Accessed October 2006.

National Resource Center on Nutrition, Physical Activity & Aging (website): *http://nutritionandaging.fiu.edu/*. Accessed December 27, 2006.

National Resource Center on Nutrition, Physical Activity & Aging: *Dietary reference intakes and dietary guidelines in Older Americans Act (OAA) nutrition programs* (website): nutritionandaging.fiu.edu/SearchResourceDetail.asp?Nutrition_ID=3355. Accessed April 24, 2007.

NeighborCare. *Geriatric drug therapy handbook 2004-2005*, Hudson, OH, 2004, Lexi-Comp.

Nutrition Screening Initiative: Skeleton in the nursing home closet, *Geriatr Nurs* 22(1):46, 2001.

Nutrition Screening Initiative: *Older Americans want more information on nutrition to manage chronic disease—but many don't receive it from their doctors* (press release, January 15, 2002).

Pear R: Nutritional therapy to fall under Medicare umbrella, *New York Times*, December 31, 2001.

Rahman S: Impaired nutritional status in the geriatric population, *Geriatric Medicine Focus* 2(2):1, 2001.

Richardson A: The role of omega-3 fatty acids in behavior, cognition, and mood, *Scand J Nutr* 47(2):92-98, 2003.

Robbins J et al: Dysphagia research in the 21st century and beyond: proceedings from Dysphagia Experts Meeting, 2001, *J Rehabil Res Dev* 39:543-548, 2001.

Roberts S, Durnbaugh T: Enhancing nutrition and eating skills in long-term care, *Alzheimer's Care Q* 3:316-329, 2002.

Russell RM et al: Comparison of diet claims, 2002 (website): *www.cyberounds.com/conf/nutrition/2000-004-05/*.

Shanley C, O'Loughlin G: Dysphagia among nursing home residents: an assessment and management protocol, *J Gerontol Soc* 26(8):35-48, 2000.

Smeets P et al: Effect of satiety on brain activation during chocolate tasting in men and women, *Am J Clin Nutr* 83(6):1297-1305, 2006.

Tariq S et al: The use of a no-concentrated sweets diet in the management of type 2 diabetes in nursing homes, *J Am Diet Assoc* 101(12):1463-1466, 2001.

Thomas DR et al: Nutritional management in long-term care: development of a clinical guideline, *J Gerontol A Biol Sci Med Sci* 55A(12):M725, 2000.

U.S. Bureau of the Census: *Statistical abstract of the United States, 2000*, Washington, DC, 2001. Accessed at *www.census.gov/press-release*.

U.S. Department of Health and Human Services (USDHHS): *Healthy People 2010*, Hyattsville, Md, 2002, Public Health Service.

Wakefield B: A food pyramid for the elderly, *Women's Health In Primary Care* 3(1):36, 2000.

Wakefield B: Altered nutrition: less than body requirements. In Maas ML et al, editors: *Nursing care of older adults: diagnoses, outcomes, and interventions*, St Louis, 2001, Mosby.

Zembruski C: *Hydration checklist*, New York, 2000, Hartford Institute for Geriatric Nursing.

CHAPTER 10

Chronic Disease in Late Life

Kathleen Jett

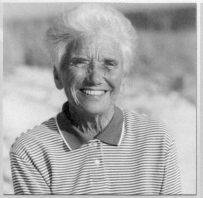

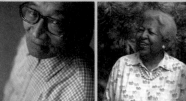

AN ELDER SPEAKS

If I'd known I was going to live this long, I'd have taken better care of myself.
Eubie Blake, on his 100th birthday

LEARNING OBJECTIVES

On completion of this chapter, the reader will be able to:

1. Identify the most common chronic disorders of late life and their sequelae.
2. Relate strategies that have been used successfully to maintain maximum function and comfort in the person with a chronic disorder.
3. Suggest nursing interventions appropriate to the care of an individual with a chronic disorder.

4. Construct nursing interventions that are consistent with a theoretical framework of maximizing wellness in the presence of chronic disease.

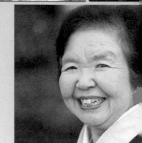

The nation's goals, as published in *Healthy People 2010*, are to increase the span of healthy life for all persons and to decrease disparities in health outcomes among population subgroups (U.S. Department of Health and Human Services [USDHHS], 2000). It is expected that these goals will or can be achieved through improved strategies to effectively treat health problems and through the increased use of preventive health strategies for all persons, regardless of ethnicity, income, and nation of origin. As a result, we have the potential to live longer and perhaps in better health than did our parents.

Life expectancy has increased considerably in the past 100 years. Persons born today may live up to 20 years longer than those who were born in the early 1900s. Life expectancy at 65 years of age is also increasing. Women have consistently had a greater longevity, with white women having the longest life expectancy (80.4 years) and black men the shortest (68.9 years) (Arias, 2006); this is translated into relative mortality by the Bureau of National Statistics (Figure 10-1).

However, at this time a longer life often means living longer with a chronic disease, especially for the longer-lived women. By the time a person has lived 50 years, he or she is likely to have at least one chronic condition. It may be slight arthritis at the site of the old football injury, hypertension or diabetes mellitus, obesity, or any one of a number of illnesses. For others, late life is faced in the presence of multiple simultaneous health problems. For older adults any chronic condition is superimposed on both the normal changes of aging and environmental hazards.

The most common chronic condition for all ages is sinusitis, whereas for persons older than 65 years it is both arthritis and hypertension (Figure 10-2). Yet for the older adult, the presence or absence of a condition is not as important as its affect on one's functioning. The effect may be as little as an inconvenience or as great as an impairment of one's ability to perform activities of daily living (ADLs) or instrumental activities of daily living (IADLs) (see Chapter 6) (Figure 10-3).

Special thanks to Catherine Hill and Ann Schmidt Luggen, the previous edition contributors, for their content contributions to this chapter.

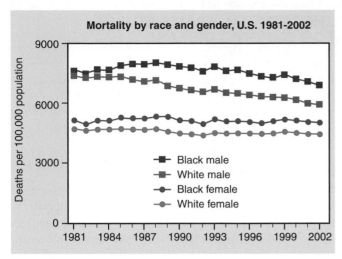

FIGURE 10-1 Mortality by race and gender (United States) 1981-2002. (Data from The National Vital Statistics System. Redrawn from the Data Warehouse on Trends in Health and Aging. [website]: *www.cdc.gov/nchs/agingact.htm.* Accessed July 1, 2006.)

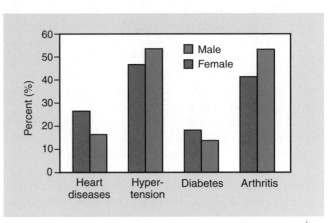

FIGURE 10-2 Percentage of persons ages 65 years and older reporting selected chronic conditions, by gender, United States, 2002-2003. (Data from National Health Interview Survey. Redrawn from the Data Warehouse on Trends in Health and Aging. [website]: *www.cdc.gov/nchs/agingact.htm.* Accessed July 1, 2006.)

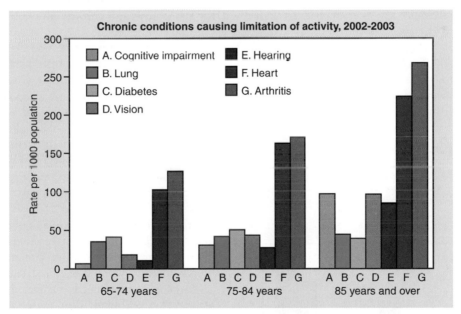

FIGURE 10-3 Chronic condition causing limitation of activity, 2002-2003. (From Centers for Disease Control and Prevention, National Center for Health Statistics, *Health,* United States, 2005, Figure 20. Redrawn from *www.cdc.gov.*)

Helping persons with chronic health problems move toward healthy aging means working toward decreasing the risk for illness whenever possible and employing strategies to reduce the incidence of acute health-related adverse events. While doing so, the gerontological nurse can contribute to the improvement of the quality of life. The gerontological nurse has the opportunity and privilege of decreasing mortality in the population of older adults worldwide. The gerontological nurse also has the opportunity and responsibility to work with older adults to minimize the potentially disabling effects of chronic disease, that is, to be instrumental in de-

creasing morbidity in older adults. And finally, the gerontological nurse can be an effective facilitator for finding ways for persons to cope effectively with the chronic disease in their lives. This chapter provides a snapshot of the most common chronic diseases found in late life and proposes strategics to promote healthy living regardless of the limitations with which one lives. We do not intend to include comprehensive medical or nursing management of these disorders but instead offer an "essentials" summary that identifies nursing responses to promote healthy aging in the presence of the chronic disease.

ACUTE VERSUS CHRONIC ILLNESS

Acute illnesses are those that occur suddenly and often without warning (e.g., stroke, myocardial infarction, hip fracture, or infection). These are usually treated aggressively when they occur. Without treatment or even with treatment, acute problems in late life can quickly become the cause of death. At other times, the sequelae of the acute episode is a new or exacerbated chronic condition.

A chronic health problem is one that is managed rather than cured. By definition, it is always present although not always visible. If not triggered by an acute event, the onset may be insidious and identified only during a health screening. Symptoms of the effects of the problem, including disabilities, may not appear for years. For example, the person with diabetes begins to have trouble with his or her vision or peripheral sensation or the person with chronic, untreated hypertension develops enough heart damage to cause an acute episode of heart failure. Or a person may complain of dull aches to hands or knees "for years" until the self-prescribed treatments no longer seem effective or the pain and stiffness interfere with usual activities.

Persons with chronic diseases often continue to work and perform their usual activities early in their diseases. Later, and with increasing age, the effects of the limitations caused by the condition increase (Figure 10-4). When the disabilities are first significant or during exacerbations in the limitations, the person may receive assistance and rehabilitation in the home or in a designated rehabilitation center. As the limitations increase further, the person at home may move to the home of another and receive informal help or into an institutional setting where formal help is available (see Chapter 17).

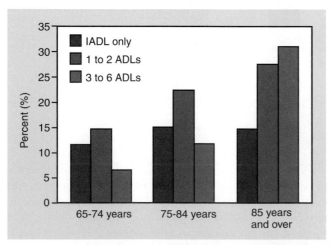

FIGURE 10-4 Percentage of Medicare beneficiaries reporting difficulty with instrumental activities of daily living (IADLs) or activities of daily living (ADLs), by age, 2002. (From Medicare Current Beneficiary Survey. The Data Warehouse on Trends in Health and Aging. [website]: *www.cdc.gov/nchs/agingact.htm.* Accessed July 1, 2006.)

THEORETICAL FRAMEWORKS FOR CHRONIC DISEASE

Two theoretical frameworks have been especially helpful in both understanding the effect of chronic illness and organizing the nurse's response to calls from persons with chronic illness: Maslow's Hierarchy of Needs and the Chronic Illness Trajectory (Corbin and Strauss, 1988; Strauss and Glaser, 1975; Woog, 1992).

Maslow's Hierarchy of Needs

Maslow's Hierarchy of Needs ranks needs from the most basic, related to the maintenance of biological integrity, to the most complex, associated with self-actualization (Figure 10-5). According to this theory, the higher levels cannot be met without first meeting the lower level needs. In other words, moving toward healthy aging is an evolving and developing process. As basic level needs are met, the satisfaction of higher level needs is possible, with ever-deepening richness to life, regardless of one's age. The nurse prioritizes care from the most essential to those things we think of as quality of life. Ensuring that the needs are met at any of the levels is significantly more complex for a person with a chronic illness than for one without a chronic condition.

As far back as Hippocrates and Galen, the basic needs of all living people were recognized as the need for air, fluids, nutrition, hygiene, elimination, activity, and skin integrity. Along with these is the basic need for comfort and relief from suffering. The gerontological nurse works to ensure that these needs are met for older adults and realizes that as these are met, higher levels of wellness are possible. The person with dementia may begin to wander or become agitated because of the need to find a toilet and not knowing where to look. Until the toileting needs are met, the nurse's attempt to comfort or redirect is likely to be ineffective and frustrating. The person who lives alone but is unable to shop or cook will be distressed until arrangements can be made for home-delivered meals, either commercially or through a friend or family member.

As people's basic needs are met, they will feel safe and secure. They will likely sleep better and feel more comfortable interacting with others. Maslow saw people as social beings with a need to belong to something outside of themselves. While interacting with others, people begin to meet their need of belonging. This need is met through memberships in churches, synagogues, mosques, and civic or social organizations and through ties to family and friends. After retirement, a person may replace belonging to a work group with belonging to a civic or special interest group. If belonging to a work group is not replaced, isolation and depressions are risks, as are common for persons who become homebound. When a person is not able to function independently and moves to live with a child in a distant city for care or into an assisted living facility or nursing home, meeting belonging needs can be especially challenging and the nurse may work with the elder to form new alliances and associations. The nurse works to create environments in which meaningful relationships and activities can remain a part of the elder's life in the presence of a chronic health problem.

A person whose basic needs are met, who feels safe and secure, and who has a sense of belonging will also have self-esteem and self-efficacy. In other words, people will accept and honor who they are and feel that they have some personal power and self-confidence; they will know that they are important as people and that they inherently have value. Self-esteem is not something someone can give to anyone else. It is, however, something that others can negatively influence through ageist attitudes and behavior. For example, anytime the nurse assumes that a patient cannot do something based solely on the person's age or pre-existing health condition or makes assumptions about abilities, he or she is being ageist and is actually belittling the individual. Unfortunately, this is commonly seen, but it can be challenged by the knowledgeable and sensitive gerontological nurse.

Finally, Maslow's highest level of wellness is that of self-actualization. Self-actualization is seen as people reaching out beyond themselves and finding meaning in their lives, a sense of fulfillment. This sense of self and meaning is often challenged with the diagnosis of a chronic condition, and as a disability develops or progresses, the sense of self may be doubted. The sensitive gerontological nurse is in the perfect position to help older adults adapt to the changes in their lives and perhaps find new joys and new meaning. For example, one of the authors (KJ) spoke to a group in a nursing home about death and dying. To her surprise, the room was not filled with staff, as she had expected, but with the frailest of elders confined to wheelchairs, bent over and silent. Instead of the usual lecture, she talked about legacies and asked the silent audience, "What do you want people to remember about you? What made your life worthwhile?" Without exception each member of the audience had something to say, from "I had a beautiful garden" to "I was a good mother" to "I designed a bridge." Meaning can be found for life everywhere—you just have to ask.

Chronic Illness Trajectory

The trajectory model of chronic illness, originally conceptualized by Anselm Strauss and Barney Glaser (1975), has long aided health care providers to better understand the realities of chronic illness. Later, Corbin and Strauss (1988) presented a view of chronic illness as a trajectory that traces a course of illness forward through eight phases. In

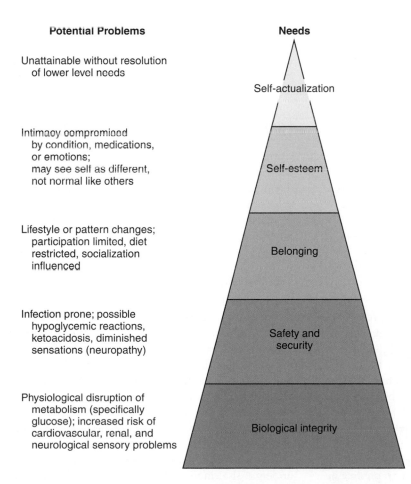

Potential Problems	Needs	Strategies to Meet Needs
Unattainable without resolution of lower level needs	Self-actualization	Growth continued within the individual's perspective
Intimacy compromised by condition, medications, or emotions; may see self as different, not normal like others	Self-esteem	Emphasis on the abilities, not the limitations, open discussion on sexuality and sex; explanation of approaches to sexual gratifications in light of drug, physical, and emotional influences
Lifestyle or pattern changes; participation limited, diet restricted, socialization influenced	Belonging	Education about normalcy in social situations such as dining out, social drinking, diet planning, and food choices; discussion and illustration about positive lifestyle pattern adjustments
Infection prone; possible hypoglycemic reactions, ketoacidosis, diminished sensations (neuropathy)	Safety and security	Rehabilitation and recovery: teach necessary skills, activities, knowledge needed to feel safe and secure—skin care, use of syringe, actions to take with signs and symptoms, ways to independently or with appropriate help accomplish necessary tasks
Physiological disruption of metabolism (specifically glucose); increased risk of cardiovascular, renal, and neurological sensory problems	Biological integrity	Treatment involvement provided with methods to control and monitor physiological state and meet needs—insulin or oral antihyperglycemic agents, urine testing, adequate balanced nutrition, exercise, etc.

FIGURE 10-5 Diabetes wellness perspective.

TABLE 10-1
The Chronic Illness Trajectory

Phase	Definition
1. Pre-trajectory	Before the illness course begins, the preventive phase, no signs or symptoms present
2. Trajectory onset	Signs and symptoms are present, includes diagnostic period
3. Crisis	Life-threatening situation
4. Acute	Active illness or complications that require hospitalization for management
5. Stable	Illness course/symptoms controlled by regimen
6. Unstable	Illness course/symptoms not controlled by regimen but not requiring hospitalization
7. Downward	Progressive deterioration in physical/mental status characterized by increasing disability/symptoms
8. Dying	Immediate weeks, days, hours preceding death

Examples of goals that nurses might establish include the following:
1. To assist a client in overcoming a plateau during a comeback phase by increasing adherence to a regimen so that he or she might reach the highest level of functional ability possible within limits of the disability.
2. To assist a client in making the attitudinal and lifestyle changes that are needed to promote health and prevent disease.
3. To assist a client who is in a downward trajectory make the adjustments and readjustments in biography and everyday life activities that are necessary to adapt to increasing physical deterioration.
4. To assist the client who is in an unstable phase to gain greater control over symptoms that are interfering with his or her ability to carry out everyday activities.
5. To assist a client in maintaining illness stability by finding a way to blend illness management activities with biographical and everyday life activities.

Goals can be broken down into specific client-oriented objectives. Built into the objectives are the criteria that will be used to evaluate the effectiveness of each intervention. What is important here is to look at what takes place in the process (the steps) of working toward a goal, as well as the end to be reached, and to be realistic about what can be achieved in what time period, taking into consideration the desires, wants, and abilities of the client and family.

Data from Woog P: *The chronic illness trajectory framework: the Corbin and Strauss nursing model,* New York, 1992, Springer.

BOX 10-1 Key Points in the Chronic Illness Trajectory Framework

- The majority of health problems in late life are chronic.
- Chronic illnesses may be lifelong and entail lifetime adaptations.
- Chronic illness and its management often profoundly affect the lives and identities of both the individual and the family members or significant others.
- The acute phase of illness management is designed to stabilize physiological processes and promote a recovery (comeback) from the acute phase.
- Other phases of management are designed primarily to maximize and extend the period of stability in the home with the help of family and augmented by visits to and from health care providers and other members of the rehabilitation and restoration team.
- Maintaining stable phases is central in the work of managing chronic illness.
- A primary care nurse is often in the role of coordinator of the multiple resources that may be needed to promote quality of life along the trajectory.

---

its entirety, a chronic illness may include a preventive phase (pre-trajectory), a definitive phase (trajectory onset), a crisis phase, an acute phase, a stable phase, an unstable phase, downward, and dying phase (Table 10-1). The shape and stability of the trajectory is influenced by the combined efforts, attitudes, and beliefs held by the elder, family members and significant others, and the involved health care providers. Key points of the model are based on the theoretical assumptions listed in Box 10-1.

The patient's perceptions of needs met and basic biological functional limitations are paramount to predicting movement along the illness trajectory (Corbin and Strauss, 1992). By using a combined approach, the gerontological

nurse may have the biggest impact on promoting the health of the person with a chronic condition. However, to do so, the nurse needs a working knowledge of the most common health problems seen in the older population. Several are covered here, and others can be found elsewhere in this text.

COMMON CHRONIC DISORDERS

Certain disorders are encountered frequently enough in late life to merit special attention. These include specific medical diagnoses of the cardiovascular, cerebrovascular, endocrine, gastrointestinal, and respiratory systems and the rheumatological disorder, giant cell arteritis. Musculoskeletal disorders are also very common and discussed in the context of their effect on mobility in Chapter 15.

Cardiovascular Disease

Cardiovascular disease (CVD) is the leading cause of death and the second most common cause of disability in all persons living in the United States and the primary diagnosis of persons admitted to long-term care facilities (Rich, 2004) (Figures 10-6 and 10-7). Persons older than 65 years make up 13% of the population in the United States yet account for 65% of all hospitalizations for CVD and over 80% of the CVD–associated deaths (Rich, 2004). These high numbers are believed to be caused from a combination of normal changes with aging in the heart (see Chapter 4) in the presence of risk factors (Box 10-2). Older adults also undergo the majority of CVD–related procedures, but treatment approaches are highly variable by ethnicity and gender (Box 10-3).

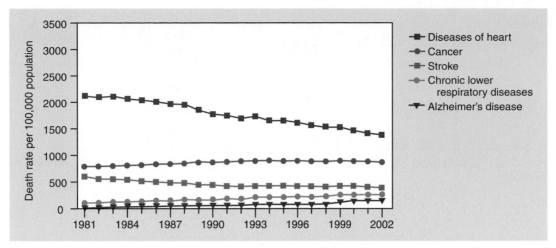

FIGURE 10-6 Leading causes of death in women older than 65 years. (Data from The National Vital Statistics System. The Data Warehouse on Trends in Health and Aging [website]: *www.cdc.gov/nchs/agingact.htm.* Accessed July 1, 2006.)

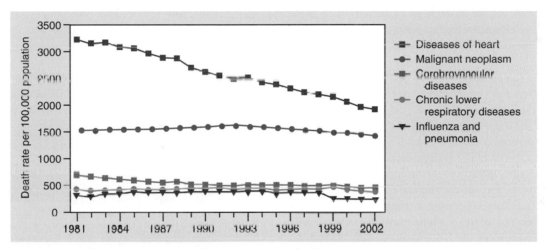

FIGURE 10-7 Leading causes of death in men older than 65 years. (Data from The National Vital Statistics System. Redrawn from the Data Warehouse on Trends in Health and Aging [website]: *www.cdc.gov/nchs/agingact.htm.* Accessed July 1, 2006.)

BOX 10-2 Risk Factors for Heart Disease

- Age (>55 years for men; >65 years for women)
- Family history of premature CHD (<55 years for men; <65 years for women)
- Microalbuminuria or estimated GFR <60 mL/min
- Hypertension*
- Cigarette smoking
- Central obesity (BMI ≥30)*
- Physical inactivity
- Dyslipidemia*
- Diabetes, IGT, or IFG*

*Components of metabolic syndrome.
CHD, Coronary heart disease; *GFR,* glomerular filtration rate; *BMI,* body mass index; *IGT,* impaired glucose tolerance; *IFG,* impaired fasting glucose.

BOX 10-3 Treatment of Chest Pain Differs by Gender and Ethnicity

The complaint of chest pain is often expressed by adult patients, especially in late life. When this chest pain is attributed to a cardiac origin, men are more likely to be diagnosed with angina (18% vs. 4%) and intermediate coronary syndrome (ICS) (21% vs. 10%) and women are more likely to be diagnosed with vague chest pain only (86% vs. 61%). Blacks received more chest pain diagnoses than whites (71% vs. 62%) with similar angina and ICS diagnoses. However, both blacks and women received fewer cardiovascular medications than white men.

Data from Hendrix KH et al: Prevalence, treatment, and control of chest pain syndromes and associated risk factors in hypertensive patients, *Am J Hypertens* 18(8):1026-1032, 2005.

| Hypertension (HTN) 50 million | Coronary heart disease (CHD) 12 million 85% of CHD deaths occur in those over age 65 | Heart failure (HF) 5 million 75% over age 65 | Cerebrovascular disease (CVD) 4 million 600,000 strokes annually 158,000 deaths annually Silent infarcts may increase the risk of dementia | Atrial fibrillation (AF) 2 million 70% between ages 65 and 85 Responsible for 15% of strokes |

FIGURE 10-8 Cardiovascular disease statistics. (Modified from U.S. Department of Health and Human Services [USDHHS]. [website]: *www.healthypeople. gov/document/tableofcontents.htm.*)

Alterations in cardiovascular functioning may be related to disease of the blood vessels or the heart wall or from prolonged effects of either. The American Heart Association identifies the major cardiovascular diseases as hypertension; coronary heart disease (CHD), including myocardial infarction and angina; and heart failure (HF) (Figure 10-8). Each of these is reviewed in this section with an emphasis on health promotion. For more detailed examination of these conditions, the reader is referred to gerontological nursing or geriatric medicine texts that are disease-based.

Hypertension. Hypertension (HTN) is the most common chronic cardiovascular disease encountered by the gerontological nurse. Both the definition of and the guidelines for treatment of HTN is provided by the Joint National Committee of the Detection, Evaluation, and Treatment of High Blood Pressure (JNC). HTN is diagnosed any time the diastolic blood pressure reading is 90 or higher or the systolic reading is 140 or higher on two separate occasions (JNC 7, 2003) (Table 10-2). Blood pressure increases with age, with a leveling off or decrease of the diastolic pressure in the 60s agegroup. Older adults most often have either isolated systolic hypertension or diastolic-systolic hypertension; they rarely have isolated diastolic hypertension (Meyyazhagan and Messinger-Rapport, 2004). During the Committee's last review in 2003, it was noted that the definition for HTN does not change regardless of age (Box 10-4). This is an important change from the former professional view of HTN in late life.

The current blood pressure goal of all persons is less than 140/90 and equal to or less than 130/80 for persons with diabetes (JNC 7, 2003).

Although often treatable and, in some cases, preventable, the rates of HTN have changed little during the last 10 years of the 1900s, and significant disparities exist among ethnic groups. As of 2003, about 50 million Americans were thought to have HTN. The prevalence is highest among black Americans and lowest among Mexican Americans (Beato, 2003).

Etiology. The etiology of HTN is primarily unknown; therefore it is called *essential hypertension*. Secondary causes are relatively rare in older adults but include pheochromocy-

---

TABLE 10-2

Blood Pressure Classification

Classification	Blood Pressure
Normal	<120 systolic and <80 diastolic
Prehypertension	120-139 systolic or 80-89 diastolic
Stage 1 HTN	140-159 systolic or 90-99 diastolic
Stage 2 HTN	>160 systolic or >100 diastolic

HTN, Hypertension.

BOX 10-4   Key Points of the JNC 7

- For persons older than 50 years, SBP is more important than DBP as a CVD risk factor.
- Starting at 115/75 mm Hg, CVD risk doubles with each increment of 20/10 mm Hg throughout the BP range.
- Persons who are normotensive at age 55 years have a 90% lifetime risk for developing HTN.
- Those with SBP 120-139 mm Hg or DBP 80-89 mm Hg should be considered prehypertensive and require health-promoting lifestyle modifications to prevent CVD.
- Thiazide-type diuretics should be the initial drug therapy either alone or combined with other drug classes unless compelling reasons are present.
- Certain high-risk conditions are compelling indications for other drug classes.
- Most patients will require two or more antihypertensive drugs to achieve goal BP.
- If BP is >20/10 mm Hg above goal, initiate therapy with two agents; one usually should be a thiazide-type diuretic.

Adapted from JNC 7: JNC 7 Express: the seventh report of the Joint National Commission of the Prevention, Detection, Evaluation and Treatment of High Blood Pressure, USHHS Pub No 03-5233, 2003. (website): *www.nhlbi.nih.gov.* Accessed July 23, 2006.
SBP, Systolic blood pressure; *DBP,* diastolic blood pressure; *CVD,* cardiovascular disease; *BP,* blood pressure; *HTN,* hypertension.

BOX 10-5   Modifiable Factors That Increase the Risk for Essential Hypertension

- Cigarette smoking or tobacco use
- Excessive alcohol intake
- Sedentary lifestyle
- Inadequate stress/anger management
- High-sodium diet
- High-fat diet

BOX 10-6   Minimizing Risk for Heart Disease

Maintain:
  Blood pressure ≤130/80
  Total cholesterol <200
  LDL <100
  HDL >40
  Triglycerides <150

LDL, Low-density lipoprotein; *HDL,* high-density lipoprotein.

---

toma, Cushing's syndrome, obstructive sleep apnea, and brain tumors (Meyyazhagan and Messinger-Rapport, 2004). Essential hypertension is most common in African-American men (Beato, 2003). Although the risk for hypertension associated with family history cannot be changed, all other factors are within control of the individual to reduce his or her risk (Box 10-5).

Signs and Symptoms. Unfortunately, HTN usually develops slowly and silently and is may not be diagnosed until some degree of end-organ damage has occurred. The person may be completely asymptomatic until suffering an acute cardiovascular event and on examination found to have extensive heart disease. Other persons are found to have HTN during health screening. It is recommended that all persons have their blood pressure screened every 2 years and more often for those at risk (U.S. Prevention Services Task Force [USPSTF], 2003). Screening may help lead to more prompt diagnosis and treatment.

Complications. The most important complication of HTN is the long-term effects of end-organ damage. Older persons with HTN have an absolute higher risk for cardiac disease such as CHD, atrial fibrillation, and heart failure, as well as acute cardiovascular and cerebrovascular events such as myocardial infarction, stroke, and sudden death. Poorly controlled HTN is also implicated in chronic renal insufficiency, end-stage renal disease, and peripheral vascular disease (Meyyazhagan and Messinger-Rapport, 2004).

Management. Accurate diagnosis is essential to any management plan. Common problems related to both the diagnosis and management of blood pressure disorders in the older adult include "white coat syndrome," postural or orthostatic hypotension, and postprandial hypotension. Because of these, it is often necessary to include ambulatory blood pressure monitoring and positional measurement in the assessment of the individual. Only when all of the information is available can a holistic plan of care be developed.

The goal of the management of HTN is to minimize the risk of complications and reduce or eliminate modifiable risk factors. This means keeping the blood pressure less than 140/90 mm Hg for otherwise healthy adults and less than 130/80 mm Hg for persons with diabetes. By doing so, many of the long-term complications (e.g., heart disease) can be

avoided, minimized, or delayed (Box 10-6 and 10-7). To accomplish this, the nurse has a responsibility to work with the elder and his or her family comprehensively to promote healthy aging.

Fortunately, the work of the American Heart Association and the JNC provides detailed evidence-based treatment guidelines for most children and adults. Unfortunately, less is known about the appropriate treatment of fragile older adults in the long-term care setting. A more careful risk-benefit analysis needs to be done related to treatment and outcomes in such situations. For someone with a limited life expectancy the significant side effects of some medications and limitations in food choices may result in an unnecessary decrease in quality of life.

Coronary Heart Disease. The beating heart, like other muscles, needs oxygen and other nutrients to provide energy for its work. Despite all the blood that passes through the heart, the muscle depends on the circulation delivered by the coronary arteries. CHD, or *coronary artery disease*, refers to a group of conditions that either completely or partially obstruct the blood flow to the heart muscle. When a complete occlusion occurs, the resultant damage from ischemia is referred to as an AMI, or acute myocardial infarction.

The overall death rate from CHD has declined dramatically in the past 20 years, from a rate of 350 per 100,000 in 1980 to 196 per 100,000 in 2000. This improvement is still far from the goal of 166 set forth in the document *Healthy People 2010.* The incidence in men exceeds the incidence in women until after menopause, at which time the rate in women accelerates. Although men die at a 40% higher rate than women, the racial disparity is even greater, with the rate for African Americans 243 per 100,000 in 2002 (Beato, 2003).

BOX 10-7   Benefits of Controlling Blood Pressure

	AVERAGE PERCENT REDUCTION IN RISK FOR NEW EVENTS
Stroke decreases	35%-40%
Myocardial infarction decreases	20%-25%
Heart failure decreases	50%

Etiology. Narrowed or blocked arterial lumina probably result from a complicated interaction of processes that may begin before birth. More than 250 genes have been proposed to be involved in CAD (Higgins, 2000). However, it is probably caused from a combination of genetic and environmental factors. The blockage in the arteries is caused by arteriosclerosis or atherosclerosis, commonly referred to as "hardening of the arteries."

Researchers have established that atherosclerosis can begin in the first year of life. The walls of the normally pliable artery thicken and stiffen. The tunica lumina undergoes a series of changes, all of which lead to a decrease in the ability of the arteries to change lumen size. Changes in lipid, cholesterol and phospholipid metabolism also occur. Although many of these changes are associated with normal aging, the sequela can be life threatening when coupled with pathophysiological conditions such as hypertension. Arteriosclerosis is considered an inflammatory condition (Figure 10-9).

Blockage may also be the result of atherosclerosis, a similar process of hardening of the arteries but caused by the accumulation of lipid-laden macrophages within the arterial wall and the formation of lesions called plaques within the vessel wall. As a result there is less capacity for oxygenation of the surrounding tissue. With complete obstruction, ischemic pain and tissue necrosis occur and death may follow. With only partial blockage, the pain may be intermittent and experienced as angina. In severe cases of complete blockage, the result is acute myocardial infarction (AMI) from tissue necrosis. Risk factors for CV events are both intrinsic and extrinsic and therefore somewhat modifiable (Figure 10-10). CHD is the specific leading cause of death for men and women.

Signs and Symptoms. Chest pain is the most common symptom of CHD and is the direct response to ischemia. The pain of cardiac origin is classically described as a pressing or squeezing, usually in the chest under the breastbone, but sometimes in the shoulders, arms, neck, jaws, or back. However, the subjective experience of ischemic pain declines with age and has been found to vary by gender. Fewer than 50% of persons older than 65 years report pain during an ischemic event and instead have what are called "silent MIs" (Rich, 2004). If any discomfort is noticed, it is more likely to be mild and may be localized to the back, abdomen, shoulders, or either or both arms. Nausea and vomiting or merely a sensation of heartburn may be the only symptom. In persons older than 80 years, even more atypical symptoms are seen, including gastrointestinal disturbances, fatigue, dizziness, syncope, or confusion. As many as 20% of persons older than 85 years have neurological complaints that are actually cardiac in origin (Rich, 2004). This array of nonspecific and atypical symptoms often leads to misdiagnosis, which delays the prompt medical intervention needed for optimal outcomes.

A definitive diagnosis of an ischemic event (AMI) usually requires the documentation of changes in biochemical markers within 24 to 72 hours of the event (see Chapter 5). In late life, many, but not all, diagnoses of CHD and cardiac events are made at the time of a screening electrocardiogram (ECG). However, because of the high numbers of nondiagnostic and false-negative ECGs, delayed recognition leads to an increased complication rate.

Complications. The potential problems and complications from CHD are either the result of long-term reduced circulation to the heart or the result of an acute event in the form of a myocardial infarction (MI). Chronic ischemic pain, known as *angina*, may be intermittent and relieved by nitroglycerine and/or nitrates or may be what is known as *unstable angina*. Unstable angina is characterized by ischemic symptoms that increase in frequency, intensity, or duration and occur with less and less provocation. Unstable angina is associated with arrhythmias, tachycardia, and ventricular fibrillation (Rich, 2004). Persons with unstable angina are at great risk for an acute MI and sudden cardiac death; there is a high variation by ethnic group, with black and white Americans still exceeding the goals of *Healthy People 2010* (Figure 10-11).

The MI can cause a small amount of damage, and the results are the same as other effects of reduced circulation;

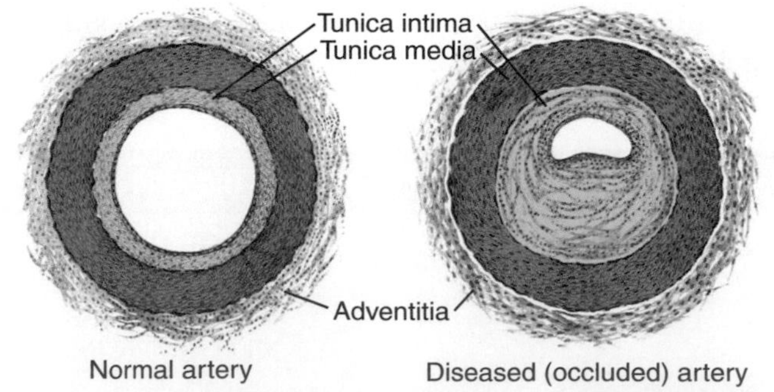

FIGURE 10-9 Arteriosclerosis. (From McCance K, Huether S, editors: *Pathophysiology: the biological basis for disease in adults and children,* ed 5, St Louis, 2006, Mosby, p. 1082.)

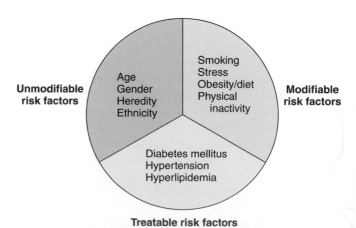

FIGURE 10-10 Risk factors for cardiovascular (CV) events. (From *www. nhlbi.gov.* From Grundy SM. *J Am Coll Cardiol* 34[4]:1348-1359, 1999.)

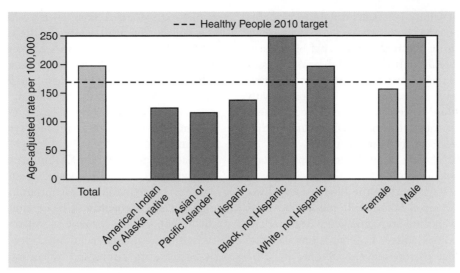

FIGURE 10-11 Coronary death rates by ethnicity. Age adjusted to the 2000 standard population. Coronary heart disease: ICD-10 codes I11, I20-I25. (Data from National Vital Statistics System—Mortality [NVSS-M], NCHS, CDC. Redrawn from *www.cdc.gov/nchs/hphome.htm.* Focus area No. 12.)

or extensive damage may occur, resulting in death if the damage is not reversed in the first several hours after the event. The acute event may be triggered by a sudden increase in myocardial oxygen demand, such as from an infection or bleeding and the arteries' inability to respond adequately or from a sudden occlusion of an artery from a blood clot or plaque passing through a narrowed vessel. Tissue death occurs quickly, and when it is extensive enough, the person will die.

In chronic CHD, the body attempts to compensate for the damage through a process called *remodeling* in which the heart enlarges and changes shape. This remodeling eventually leads to a decrease in cardiac pumping efficiency, and it can lead to a more gradual onset of heart failure months or years after the AMI.

Management. Both noninvasive (e.g., ECG, stress test) and invasive (e.g., cardiac catheterization) tests may be used in making a definitive diagnosis of CHD and the extent of damage that has occurred to the heart muscle. The selection is made thorough a collaborative decision-making process with a cardiologist. The request for consultation is the responsibility of the primary physician or nurse practitioner.

As with most chronic conditions, the management of CHD in the older adult requires a team approach and multimodal strategies. After diagnosis, pharmacological management is always required. However, the non-pharmacologic approaches are directed toward reducing risk factors and compensating for damage that has already occurred. After an acute event the person may experience depression and anxiety because of the changes in functional ability, self-image, and fear of another event. Physical therapists, occupational therapists, counselors, indigenous healers, and nutritionists work alongside the nurse, nurse practitioner, and physician.

Cardiac exercise rehabilitation programs often are the cornerstone of the plan to return the person to maximum functioning after an acute event. Cardiac rehabilitation programs for anyone should emphasize activities that build endurance and self-reliance to facilitate self-care and quality of life. Studies show that exercise training of persons with CHD increases work capacity and vagal tone and decreases resting heart rate, body weight, and percentage of body fat (Wenger, 1990). Typical programs begin with light activity and progress to moderate activity under the supervision of a nurse or physical therapist or both. For more impaired persons, it is necessary to help them identify energy conservation measures applicable to their daily tasks.

One of the major ways that care of the person with CHD differs from those with other chronic problems is that most exacerbations of CHD require hospitalization and intensive treatment, whereas many of the other chronic disorders can be managed at home. Onset of illness or exacerbation of chronic disorders may be quite different in older clients. For those with cardiac and other problems, subtle cues of potential alterations in health must be attended to minimize the likelihood of an outcome that is unnecessarily adverse (Box 10-8).

BOX 10-8 Signs of Potential Exacerbation of Illness in an Older Adult with Coronary Heart Disease

- Light-headedness or dizziness
- Disturbances in gait and balance
- Loss of appetite or unexplained loss of weight
- Inability to concentrate or shortened attention span
- Changes in personality
- Changes in grooming habits
- Unusual patterns in urination or defecation
- Vague discomfort, frequent bouts of anxiety
- Excessive fatigue, vague pain
- Withdrawal from usual sources of pleasure

Heart Failure. Heart failure is a general term used to describe several forms of cardiac dysfunction, all of which result in inadequate perfusion of the tissues with vital blood-born nutrients. It is the end result of pathological disease processes superimposed on the normal changes of aging that cause overwork of the heart muscle As more persons live longer with heart disease, more failure is seen in both men and women. Clinical heart failure is categorized as systolic failure or diastolic failure. They may occur singly or together.

Left-sided (diastolic) failure is evidenced by pulmonary symptoms, and right-sided (systolic) failure results in cardiac output that is inadequate to perfuse the vital tissues. However, long-standing left-sided failure will eventually cause right-sided failure as well. End-stage and acute heart failure is known as *congestive heart failure*. In older adults it is not uncommon to find that persons have symptoms of both-sided failure.

An individual's risk for heart failure increases with age, with the incidence increasing fourfold between the ages of 65 and 85 (Rich, 2004). Heart failure is also a common cause of hospitalization in those older than 65 years and increases with age; 77% of associated inpatient stays are of persons older than 65 years (Rich, 2004) (Figure 10-12). It is also one of the major causes of disability and hospitalization.

Although the diagnosis of heart failure is often made empirically, that is, based on presenting symptoms and examination, a definitive diagnosis requires the finding of enlargement of the heart's chambers, especially the ventricles. Such enlargement can be seen on chest x-ray film, but it can be more accurately measured using an echocardiogram or a multiple gated acquisition (MUGA) scan. After diagnosis, heart failure is classified by the impact the disease has on a person's ability to function in everyday life.

Etiology. Most heart failure is the result of end-organ damage from hypertension and coronary heart disease. These conditions are estimated to cause about 70% of the heart failure in the United States (Rich, 2003). To compensate for the damage, the heart, especially the ventricles, enlarges and dilates. In most cases, this enlargement decreases heart muscle function as the walls are remodeled but weakened. Although compensating for aging and diseases such as CHD delays the eventual loss in pumping capacity, it does not prevent it. Eventually, the heart cannot offset the lost ability to pump blood and the signs and symptoms of failure will appear.

Aside from HTN and CHD, heart failure is also associated with alcohol abuse, cocaine or amphetamine abuse, and chronic hyperthyroidism. Another common cause of the dilated cardiomyopathy of heart failure is inflammation of the heart muscle, a condition termed *myocarditis*. Myocarditis is usually caused by viral infections but also can be caused by bacterial infections and by noninfectious causes such as lupus and other inflammatory diseases. Valvular heart disease, especially aortic regurgitation and mitral regurgitation, is increasingly seen as a cause of heart failure, especially as people live longer with these underlying disorders.

Failure can appear quickly in persons who suffer simultaneous multi-vessel myocardial infarctions or more slowly in persons with long-standing and uncontrolled hypertension. Patients who suffer extensive ischemic damage with necrosis have a high risk of developing heart failure, and its onset can be acute—often within the first few hours or days after an AMI. But even patients with only a moderate amount of muscle damage can eventually advance to heart failure. For these patients, lifestyle adjustments (e.g., smoking cessation) and appropriate drug therapy can often delay or prevent the onset of heart failure. For patients with only moderate muscle damage, whether heart failure ensues depends to a large extent on the health of the remaining heart muscle.

Signs and Symptoms. Heart failure often develops slowly, and the symptoms may not appear until the condition has progressed significantly. Early in the disease,

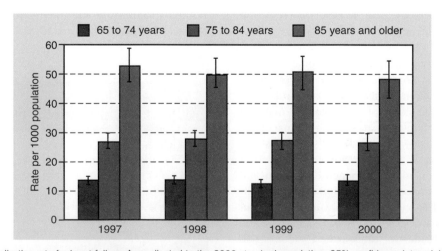

FIGURE 10-12 Hospitalization rate for heart failure. Age adjusted to the 2000 standard population; 95% confidence interval. Heart failure: ICD-9-CM code 428.0. (Data from National Hospital Discharge Survey [NHDS], NCHS, CDC. Redrawn from *www.cdc.gov/nchs/hphome.htm*. Focus area No. 12.)

symptoms are present only with exertion, but eventually the person will have symptoms at rest. The changes are in the number and intensity of symptoms in the periods of exacerbation and remission. The typical clinical pattern of a person with heart failure is periods of "baseline" symptomatology, then periods of exacerbation of symptoms that lead to hospitalization for stabilization with a return to baseline. Heart failure symptoms are ranked by activity levels (Boxes 10-9 and 10-10).

As with other disorders, atypical manifestations of heart failure in older adults often occur (Box 10-11). Common symptoms in the elderly include fatigue or shortness of breath, orthopnea, paroxysmal nocturnal dyspnea, weight gain, and lower extremity edema. However, in the older adult, symptoms of exacerbations may begin as vague complaints and general malaise. Common symptom clusters are present for right- and left-sided failure; however, because many older adults have both-sided failure, the distinction is not very helpful.

Complications. Because heart failure is the end-stage of heart disease, the complications are "limited" to exacerbations of symptoms and decline in physical functioning. Common signs of exacerbations of heart failure are often noticeable. They include tachycardia, tachypnea, S3 or S4 gallop, pulmonary crackles, and dependent edema. As the severity increases, the pulse pressure narrows and signs of impaired tissue perfusion may develop, such as cool skin and central or peripheral cyanosis. Diminished cognition, perhaps to the point of delirium, is common. Recurrent hospitalization is usually required until the point is reached when only palliative care is possible or desired. Sudden death is always a possibility, especially associated with life-threatening arrhythmias, namely ventricular tachycardia and ventricular fibrillation. In these patients, an episode of syncope should be regarded as a harbinger of sudden death.

Management. The goals of treatment and management of heart failure are to alleviate symptoms, improve functioning, and minimize exacerbations. In doing so, quality of life may be optimized and hospitalizations delayed or prevented. Whereas pharmacological management is of utmost importance in the control of the disease to prevent ventricular remodeling, non-pharmacological interventions focus on adaptation and functioning and anticipatory teaching.

Common medications include angiotensin-converting enzyme (ACE) inhibitors, beta-blockers, digitalis, and diuretics, the selection of which is guided by the type of failure. The use of antithrombotic therapy may be indicated as well. In end-stage congestive heart failure, spironolactone or other medications are often added to enhance the person's comfort. Recent research has found that the use of beta-blockers and ACE inhibitors promises to significantly improve survival in addition to strategies specifically designed to enhance coping with living with heart failure (Box 10-12).

BOX 10-9   Classification of Heart Failure by the American College of Cardiologists

STAGE A

High risk but no symptoms or structural disorder (e.g., CAD, HTN)

STAGE B

No symptoms but with structural disorder (e.g., LVH, hx MI)

STAGE C

Current or past symptoms and structural disorder
Especially dyspnea from LVSD

STAGE D

End-stage disease
Symptomatic at rest despite optimal treatment

Data from Jessup M, Brozema S: Heart failure. *NEJM,* 348: 2003, 2007-2018.
CAD, Coronary artery disease; *HTN,* hypertension; *LVH,* left ventricular hypertrophy; *hx,* history; *MI,* myocardial infarction; *LVSD,* left ventricular systolic dysfunction.

BOX 10-10   Classification of Heart Failure by the New York Heart Association

CLASS 1 MILD

No evidence of symptoms at rest or during activity

CLASS 2 MILD

Ordinary activities result in fatigue, palpitation, or dyspnea

CLASS 3 MODERATE

Less than ordinary activities cause symptoms

CLASS 4 SEVERE

Symptoms at rest, any activity increases discomfort

Data from Heart Failure Society of America: *The states of heart failure—NYHA classification,* 2002. Accessed April 18, 2007, from *www.abouthf.org.*

BOX 10-11   Atypical Symptoms of Heart Failure in Older Adults

NON-CEREBRAL

- Chronic cough
- Insomnia
- Weight loss
- Nocturia
- Syncope

CEREBRAL

- Delirium
- Falls
- Anorexia
- Decreased functional capacity

BOX 10-12 Topics of Education Related to Living with Heart Failure

1. Activities: pacing and tolerance
2. Exercise: strategizing adherence to prescribed program
3. Medications: timing, side effects, evaluation of effectiveness, obstacles to adherence
4. Disease self-management: signs and symptoms of exacerbation, intake, output and weight, when to call for help or questions, interpreting laboratory values, diet

Peripheral Vascular Disease. Peripheral vascular disease (PVD) is a cluster of disorders, all of which are the result of vascular insufficiency. That means that the ability of the blood vessels to provide the oxygen necessary for the health and sometimes survival of the surrounding tissue has been impaired. PVD affects primarily the lower extremities. That which affects the arteries is known as *peripheral artery disease (PAD)* (also called *lower extremity arterial disease [LEAD]*). Chronic venous insufficiency (CVI) of the lower extremities is a condition caused by abnormalities of the vein walls and valves, leading to obstruction or reflux of blood flow in the veins. Venous insufficiency is seen in varicose veins, deep vein thrombosis (DVT), and, when prolonged, CVI.

Age is a risk factor for PVD. PAD affects an estimated 12 million persons in the United States and more than 20% of persons older than 75 years (Begelman, 2004; Brashers, 2006a). CVI is most common in persons older than 65 years and is often associated with persons who have had DVTs (Decousus et al., 2003). Other risk factors, all of which are modifiable, include tobacco use (risk persists for >5 years after cessation), uncontrolled diabetes, uncontrolled systolic hypertension, hypercholesterolemia, and obesity.

Etiology. Arterial disease is usually the result of atherosclerosis as described previously (heart failure). As the capacity for oxygenation of the surrounding tissue lessens, pain may ensue. With complete obstruction, ischemic pain and tissue necrosis occur, and amputation may be necessary. Pain from intermittent blockage is referred to as claudication.

Venous insufficiency is the result of reduced circulation due to damaged or incompetent venous walls and valves. As thinly walled vessels, the veins depend on the compression of surrounding muscles to move the blood back to the heart. Tiny values in the veins keep the blood from flowing backward. Venous insufficiency affects the deep or superficial veins, permitting reverse flow and resulting in raised pressure in the veins during ambulation. The vein becomes engorged and the surrounding tissue becomes edematous as a result of increased hydrostatic pressure pushing plasma through the stretched wall. When movement of the extremity is reduced, the circulatory problems are exacerbated. Standing or being immobile for long periods, constricting garments, crossing the legs at the knees, and obesity all significantly increase the chance of the development of venous insufficiency. Early insufficiency is seen as varicose veins, which can progress to CVI. When the ischemia is persistent long enough, the surrounding tissue may break down, with or without trauma, producing venous stasis ulcers.

Signs and Symptoms. In early PVD, persons are often asymptomatic, with complaints noted only when the disease has progressed; early complaints may include numbness or tingling in the affected extremity. Although both arterial and venous diseases cause tissue necrosis in the end, their signs and symptoms (other than pain) are different, as is the disease management. Persons may also first present with a non-healing wound. However, the characteristics of discomfort, shape, texture, and location of the wounds help differentiate the cause. In persons with known or suspected PVD, a careful history and ankle brachial index (ABI) measurement is essential to the differentiation between PAD and CVI and to the determination of appropriate treatment. CVI is more common than PAD in older adults.

Venous insufficiency is characterized by pain with dependency, and the limb may appear a bluish purple color from the pooling of the blood. Over time, long-standing stasis of blood leads to the deposition of hemosiderin, giving the skin a dark, speckled appearance, especially in the lower calf. Varicosities of the superficial veins may be obvious. Dependent edema, dermatitis, and firm induration are common signs in CVI. As arterial disease stops the blood from flowing into a limb, the symptoms of arterial insufficiency include resting pain that is classically described as an ache, numbness, or squeezing sensation, often in the arch of the foot and toes but also in the calf, thigh, or buttock. Classically, the pain occurs when the leg is elevated and may awaken the person. It may be instantly relieved when the limb is moved to a dependent position, when gravity helps pull the blood into the compromised artery of the limb. Pain is increased with exertion as the tissue demands more oxygen, and pain is relieved by rest. When elevated, the extremity may be pale and cool, consistent with ischemia; and it may be red or purple with dependency. The skin is shiny, without hair and with thickening of nails. Buerger's sign (also called *Ratchow's sign*) is the presence of rubor with dependency and rapid blanching with elevation (Begelman, 2004).

Complications. The most common complications of CVI are pain, the development of skin ulcers, and the development of DVT. A delay in a medical diagnosis of arterial insufficiency may increase the risk of limb loss and loss of functional mobility. Wounds that result from PVD may not heal. For persons with PAD, the concern is for gangrenous infection and limb loss (Begelman, 2004).

Arterial wounds are the result of tissue necrosis. They appear distally, at the ends of the toes, between the toes, over pressure points, on the heels, and over the lateral malleolus. They are round with well-defined edges, dry, necrotic, pale at the base, and without signs of vascularity. A dense, fibrinous exudate (slough) may be present in the ulcer. Intense pain is a hallmark of ischemic ulcers.

Wounds that develop with CVI have irregular borders, are painless, and are located most often at the medial malleolus or on the adjacent tissue. Edema and the continuing increase in hemosiderin deposits make healing difficult.

Management. The primary management of PVD is in addressing the modifiable risk factors that led to the disease itself, skin care, and pharmacological intervention for pain as needed. Tight control of concurrent problems is essential (e.g., HTN, diabetes, CHD). The day-to-day management of health in the person with PVD falls largely within the scope of practice of the nurse.

For persons with **arterial insufficiency**, exercise rehabilitation and protection of the skin are paramount. Daily skin inspection and protection against the effects of pressure, friction, shear, and maceration are essential to attempt to prevent wounds. *Wearing restrictive clothing and compression stockings are specifically contraindicated.* The elder should be advised to do nothing that further limits circulation in the affected limb. Exercise rehabilitation usually includes establishing a walking program to slowly and steadily increase the pain-free walking distance. The person is asked to walk until maximum tolerable pain occurs, rest, and then continue.

Although the person with chronic **vascular insufficiency** will need intermittent courses of diuretics for severe edema, the mainstay of management is the use of customized compression stockings. Compression facilitates wound healing, reduces venous dermatitis, improves sclerotic changes, and counteracts venous hypertension. In addition to compression stockings, other devices that have been found useful to improve venous return include Unna boots, pneumatic compression pumps, and orthotic devices. Elevation of the legs above the heart for 30 minutes three to four times a day can reduce edema and improve skin microcirculation.

Although the principles of the management of PVD-related ulcers are similar to those of pressure ulcers, special care must be taken to ensure that venous stasis ulcers and arterial ulcers are differentiated and treated appropriately (Table 10-3). Because of the chronic and potentially limb-threatening nature of these ulcers, it is recommended that the nurse consult with colleagues who are wound care specialists to develop the most appropriate treatment plans.

▲ *Promoting Healthy Aging: Implications for Gerontological Nursing.* Maximizing the quality of life and health of a person with a chronic condition is one of team work. The nurse is part of an expanded network of health professionals (e.g., nurse practitioner, physical therapist, physician or physiotherapist, occupational therapist, nutritionist) who work together with the elder and his or her support persons and loved ones. In some cultures, the nurse also works with indigenous healers such as shamans, medicine men and women, and curanderas. In cross-cultural

TABLE 10-3

Comparison of Arterial and Venous Insufficiency of the Lower Extremities

Characteristics	Arterial	Venous
Pain	Sudden onset with acute; gradual onset with chronic Exceedingly painful Claudication relieved by rest Rest pain relieved by dependency (with total occlusion, no position will give complete relief)	Deep muscle pain with acute deep vein thrombosis Relieved by elevation
Pulses	Absent or weak	Normal (unless arterial disease is also present)
Associated changes in leg and foot	Thin, shiny, dry skin Thickened toenails Absence of hair growth Temperature variations (cooler if no cellulitis is present) Elevational pallor Dependent rubor Atrophy or no change in limb size	Firm ("brawny") edema Reddish brown discoloration with postphlebitic syndrome Evidence of healed ulcers Dilated and tortuous superficial veins Swollen limb Increased warmth and erythema with acute deep vein thrombosis
Ulcer location	Between toes or at tips of toes Over phalangeal heads On heels Over lateral malleolus or pretibial area over metatarsal heads, on side or sole of foot	Primarily the medial malleolus and the lower leg
Ulcer characteristics	Well-defined edges Black or necrotic tissue Deep, pale base Non-bleeding	Uneven edges Ruddy granulation tissue Superficial Bleeding

situations, the nurse may work with the help of an interpreter (see Chapter 6). The work always includes consideration of the psychosocial and physical needs of the person. Spiritual needs are often present as the person deals with the "Why me?" of chronic disease. Helping older adults to cope with chronic diseases requires that the nurse be skilled not only in hands-on care but also skilled as a teacher, advocate, consultant, and counselor.

The nurse has an active role in the promotion of cardiovascular health. This includes screening, patient education, advocacy, referral, and assistance with management. The advanced practice nurse has the added responsibility to direct management that is consistent with the available evidence-based guidelines. Both pharmacological and non-pharmacological interventions that promote a healthy lifestyle have been found to be effective in controlling HTN and minimizing the complications that can significantly interfere with quality of life. Through controlling HTN, CVD disease may be reduced or prevented (see Box 10-7).

The promotion of healthy aging in relation to CVD revolves around reducing modifiable risk factors to prevent further damage and minimize complications. Risk-reduction programs can be instituted only with a clear understanding of the person's difficulties with changing lifelong habits. Smoking, overeating, habitual anger or irritation, and a sedentary lifestyle are often deeply embedded in the personality structure and are not easily eradicated by "education." The nursing role is to provide acceptance, encouragement, resources, knowledge, and affirmation of the individual and his or her right to choose. Group programs focused on these issues have been shown to improve the motivation and perceived health status of some members (Wenger, 1990). Smoking cessation, adequate exercise, and healthy eating are the particular areas related to prevention.

Hypertension. Smoking injures blood vessel walls, increases the rate of hardening, and increases the rate of HTN and stroke. Women who smoke are two to three times more likely to have an AMI than a non-smoker. The risk of an MI decreases after 1 year of cessation (at any age) (NHLBI,

N.D.). However, assisting with smoking cessation is a very complex matter that must specifically address both physical and psychological addiction. In most cases the nurse can refer the smoker to a cessation program and support and encourage his or her participation.

There is considerable evidence regarding the importance of diet and the effectiveness of specific diet choice. A healthy diet includes control of cholesterol, sodium, and calories. Healthy eating habits have been found to irrefutably lower blood pressure. It is now recommended that persons without HTN or heart disease limit their daily sodium intake to less than 2400 mg/day. Teaching people how to read food labels can be a first step in teaching. An evidence-based DASH diet is available from the National Heart, Lung and Blood Institute at *www.nhlbi.nih.gov*. This same site has extensive information and materials that can be used by both professionals and individuals to promote health and either prevent or reduce the risk of adverse events of CVD (Table 10-4).

Heart Failure. It is still possible to promote healthy aging in a person with a life-limiting illness such as heart failure. The emphasis is not on cure but on preventing exacerbations of symptoms and maximizing both functioning and comfort. The nurse is the ideal person to work with the individual and family and often does this through specialized nurse-managed heart failure clinics and hospice (Ducharme et al., 2005). The nurse negotiates with the elder regarding the best way to adhere to the drug regimen and the lifestyle changes that may be necessary. The nurse helps the elder determine the best way to perform the desired actions while not overtaxing the heart, including the use of supplemental oxygen. The nurse teaches about the early signs of exacerbations and then works to discover the most effective approach for either stopping the exacerbation, receiving prompt medical intervention, or ensuring aggressive comfort measures (see Box 10-12).

In the long-term care setting, the nurse is the key health care provider to promote healthy aging and to advocate and secure appropriate interventions for the dependent elder. The nurse is responsible for the accurate assessment of the resident's heart sounds, pulses, jugular venous distention, and respiratory status and oxygenation, as well as the atypical signs and symptoms. The nurse is often the first to identify progressive heart failure or sudden decompensation and alerts the resident's nurse practitioner or physician about the changes. The nurse practitioner is then responsible for the prescriptive interventions that are consistent with the latest evidence-based practice.

Peripheral Vascular Disease. Preventing PVD means promoting optimal cardiovascular health as discussed earlier, especially diet, weight control, and smoking cessation. By promoting healthy aging, the nurse is astute to the condition of the extremities.

Careful assessment of the person with CVD who may have early signs of PVD includes regular palpation of the

TABLE 10-4
Relationship Between Lifestyle Change and Reduction in Systolic Blood Pressure

Lifestyle Change	Approximate Reduction in SBP
Weight reduction	Decrease of 5-20 mm Hg per 10-lb loss
Adopt the DASH diet	Decrease of 8-14 mm Hg
Lower sodium intake	Decrease of 2-8 mm Hg
Increase physical activity	Decrease of 4-9 mm Hg
ETOH in moderation	Decrease of 2-4 mm Hg

SBP, Systolic blood pressure; *DASH,* Dietary Approaches to Stop Hypertension; *ETOH,* alcohol.

peripheral pulses and examination of the color, temperature, and integrity of the extremities. It also means paying careful attention to the patient's report of pain or discomfort, especially related to activities such as walking (Box 10-13). The nurse should suspect arterial insufficiency in patients with coronary artery disease, carotid stenosis, stroke, or dystrophic toenail disease.

The sooner that potential or new problems are identified, the less the risk for complications. In persons with PVD, promoting healthy aging means carefully assessing and teaching about skin, sensation, and circulation. Persons with diabetes will need more specific instruction (see the section on diabetes in this chapter).

Cerebrovascular Disease

Cerebrovascular disease is the most commonly occurring neurological disorder. It is a group of pathological processes in cerebral blood vessels resulting in brain injury and, in some cases, brain attack. The injury may be the result of either an occlusion of the vessel lumen from a thrombus or embolus; rupture of the vessel; or an alteration in vessel permeability, such as changes in blood viscosity (Boss, 2006). Cerebrovascular disease is manifested in either a stroke or a transient ischemic attack (TIA). Because the immediate effects of the events are similar, diagnosis is geared toward identifying the specific cause of the symptoms seen and the location of the brain injury. Only when the cause is known can appropriate therapy be implemented. It has been suggested that the use of the term *cerebral vascular accident* (CVA) be discarded and replaced with more descriptive and specific terminology—*transient ischemic attack* (TIA), *ischemic stroke*, or *hemorrhagic stroke* (Kistler et al., 2003).

Cerebrovascular disease is the third most common cause of death behind heart disease and cancer. In the United States each year, about 500,000 people have a stroke, 150,000 of whom die (Boss, 2006). More than 70% of all strokes occur in persons older than 65 years and is more common in African-Americans and less common in Hispanics. The rate among African-Americans is 2.5 times higher than among their white counterparts. They also suffer more disability from the stroke and are 200% more likely to die (Figure 10-13) (Boss, 2006). The age-adjusted death rate is about equal in men and women. The death rates are highest in the "stroke belt" of the Southeastern United States and lowest in the Northeast and non-coastal Southwest (Beato 2003).

Etiology: Ischemic Events. The four main types and causes of ischemic strokes are arterial disease, cardioembolism, hematological disorders, and systemic hypoperfusion. Arterial disease in the form of the inflammatory arteriosclerosis discussed earlier is probably most common. Cardioembolism includes those caused by an arrhythmia such as atrial fibrillation, which is frequently seen in coronary heart disease. The use of antithrombotics (e.g., aspirin, warfarin) in persons with heart disease is an attempt to reduce the risk for stroke. Hematological disorders include coagulation disorders and hyperviscosity syndromes. Hypoperfusion can occur from dehydration, hypotension (including over-treatment of HTN), cardiac arrest, or syncope (Leira and Adams, 2004).

TIAs are experienced by 50,000 Americans a year and probably caused by intermittent blockage or spasms of the cerebral vessels. A TIA is clinically differentiated from an ischemic stroke in that the symptoms of a TIA begin to

NURSE CREDENTIALLING PROGRAMS
HEALTH SCIENCES DIVISION

BOX 10-13   Guidelines for Persons Living with Venous Insufficiency

GIVE LEGS A REST

Elevate the feet above heart level while sleeping and several times a day. If necessary, elevate the foot of the bed or mattress.

CHANGE POSITIONS FREQUENTLY

Avoid activities that require standing or sitting with feet on the ground for long periods.

GIVE LEGS SUPPORT

Wear professionally made compression stockings that apply even pressure from ankles to knees.
Learn how to put them on correctly.
Have at least two pairs of the compression hose available so they can be changed daily. After laundering, hang up to dry. DO NOT PUT IN DRYER.
Buy new compression hose every 6 months; after that period, the elastic is stretched.
Put hose on early in the morning; wear all day; remove at bedtime.

Avoid elastic bandages (e.g., Ace). They are difficult to wrap and exert uneven pressure.
If a compression pump has been prescribed, follow the instructions.

TAKE CARE OF THE SKIN

Wash lower legs and feet regularly with mild soap and water to avoid buildup of lotion.
Use moisturizing cream and emollients after washing.
Do NOT use lanolin- or petroleum-based creams when wearing support hose made with latex.
Avoid activities that can injure the legs or feet.
Pay attention to skin changes:
- Swelling—stays when lying down
- Discoloration—especially around ankles and lower legs
- Dryness and/or itching—around ankles and lower legs
- Any bruises or wounds that do not go away in 1 week

APPLY DRESSINGS

Follow ulcer care directions as prescribed.

Modified from San Francisco Wound Care Center, Seton Medical Center, Daly City, Calif, 1995; Staab AS, Hodges LC: *Essentials of gerontological nursing,* Philadelphia, 1996, Lippincott.

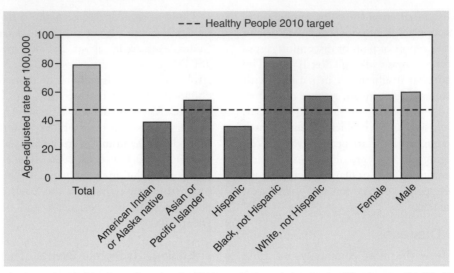

FIGURE 10-13 Stroke death rate by ethnicity. Age adjusted to the 2000 standard population. Stroke: ICD-10 codes I60-I69. (Data from National Vital Statistics System—Mortality [NVSS-M], NCHS, CDC. Redrawn from *www.cdc.gov/nchs/hphome.htm*. Focus area No. 12.)

resolve within minutes and all neurological deficits caused by the temporary ischemia resolve within 24 hours. TIAs may herald a stroke, but most strokes are not preceded by TIAs (American Stroke Association, 2002).

Etiology: Hemorrhagic Events. Hemorrhagic strokes are caused primarily by uncontrolled hypertension and less often by malformations of the blood vessels (e.g., aneurysms). Although the exact mechanism is not fully understood, it appears that the chronic hypertension causes thickening of the vessel wall, microaneurysms, and necrosis. When enough damage to the vessel accumulates, it is at risk for rupture. The rupture may be large and acute or small with a slow leaking of blood into the adjacent brain tissue. In many cases, there is a rupture or seepage of blood into the ventricular system of the brain with damage to the affected tissue through necrosis (Boss, 2006). Resolution of the event can occur only with the resorption of excess blood and damaged tissue. Hemorrhagic strokes are more life threatening but much less frequent than thrombotic strokes.

Signs and Symptoms. Both strokes and transient ischemic attacks present with acute neurological deficits that are reflective of the part of the brain affected. They are often heralded by a severe headache. In subarachnoid hemorrhages, the headache is not only sudden but also explosive, very severe, and without other neurological manifestations (Leira and Adams, 2004).

Some of the clinical signs and symptoms are suggestive of either ischemia or hemorrhage (Box 10-14). Persons with hemorrhage have more focal neurological changes and a more depressed level of consciousness than those with an ischemic stroke. If a deep unresponsive state occurs, the person is unlikely to survive (Boss, 2006). Seizures are more common in intracerebral hemorrhage. Nausea and vomiting

are suggestions of increased cerebral edema in response to the event. Focal neurological deficits include alternations in motor, sensory, and visual function; coordination; cognition; and language. The deficits are specific to the area of damage.

Diagnostics include determination of extracerebral causes, if any (e.g., infection or hypoglycemia), as well as localization of the brain damage by an un-enhanced computed tomography (CT) or magnetic resonance imaging (MRI).

Complications. Early complications of a simple TIA or stroke include extension of the amount of damage and reoccurrence. Brain edema is a problem, especially after a large infarction, and could result in obstructive hydrocephalus (Leira and Adams, 2004). After a TIA resolves, there should be no residual effect other than an increased chance of reoccurrence and the possible increased risk for stroke as noted earlier.

The long-term effects of a stroke include paralysis and hemiparesis, dysarthrias, dysphagias, and aphasias, depending on type, extent, and area affected, as well as depression. Whenever paralysis results, the development of spasticity in the affected limb(s) is a risk. Spasticity can lead to contractures if it is not managed. Iatrogenic-type complications include DVT in a flaccid lower limb, aspiration pneumonia, and urinary tract infections (Young and Hoffberg, 2001).

Management. All actual or potential cerebrovascular events are considered emergencies and should be treated as such. However, since TIAs are by their nature highly transient and resolve on their own, often before the person is even seen by a health care provider. Instead, the person reports to a primary care provider, "I think I had a small stroke last week." If the deficits and symptoms were fleeting, the diagnosis is made through the clinical interview. Management is considered preventive—to prevent recurrences and to decrease any

---

BOX 10-14 Symptoms of TIA or Stroke

- Sudden weakness or numbness on one side of the body (face, arm, or leg)
- Dimness or loss of vision in one eye
- Slurred speech, loss of speech, difficulty comprehending speech
- Dizziness, difficulty walking, loss of coordination, loss of balance, a fall
- Sudden severe headache
- Difficulty swallowing
- Sudden confusion
- Nausea and vomiting

TIA, Transient ischemic attack.

BOX 10-15 Risk Factors for Stroke/TIA

- Heart disease (and risk factors for)
- Hypertension
- Arrhythmia
- Hypercholesterolemia
- Diabetes
- Smoking
- Coagulopathies
- Brain tumor
- Family history

TIA, Transient ischemic attack.

---

risk factors possible (Box 10-15). Anticoagulant therapy has been proven to prevent recurrent cardioembolic strokes and TIAs (Leira and Adams, 2004). The person and family are also instructed in the appropriate emergency response to the return of any signs or symptoms of a stroke or another TIA. Aspirin, 30 to 325 mg/day, is the mainstay of therapy for elders with TIAs because it reduces the incidence 15% to 25% (Kistler et al., 2002). However, for those who are aspirin sensitive, clopidogrel or ticlopidine may be used. Warfarin therapy is recommended for those with atrial fibrillation.

Acute management is usually accomplished in emergency departments and intensive care units. The acute management of the stroke requires careful attention to the accuracy of the diagnosis. Reperfusion therapy (recombinant tissue-type plasminogen activator [rt-PA]) is used for occlusive strokes only if a CT scan confirms the absence of hemorrhage and is within 3 hours of the onset of the event. Administration of rt-PA is of little use if delayed more than 3 hours because 90% of the damage has probably already occurred (Saver, 2002). Most occlusive strokes are embolic. If the person actually has a hemorrhagic event and is misdiagnosed, the bleeding will be rapidly accelerated by the rt-PA, and the person will die. The initial response to the hemorrhagic stroke is to find a means to stop the bleeding rather than dissolve an occlusion.

About 90% of neurological recovery occurs within 3 months of the stroke; 10% occurs more slowly, especially after a hemorrhagic stroke (Beers and Berkow, 2000). At 18 months after the stroke, there tends to be a small decline. The inverse relationship between functional improvement and advanced age, social isolation, and emotional distress is clear. Recovery from stroke is affected by the location and extent of the brain damage. Difficulties and handicaps after stroke often involve neurological and functional deficits.

Post–ischemic stroke management begins immediately with anticoagulants or anti-platelets. Aspiration and sepsis precautions, pneumatic stocking devices, attention to bowel function, physical therapy, and early mobilization are necessary following all CVAs. A period of intense rehabilitation often takes place in a rehabilitation or skilled nursing facility setting and continues long after the person returns home or to an assisted living setting. An important role for the nurse is documenting clearly and in detail the functional capacities that are retained and those that are impaired. The assessment must be redone routinely to carefully evaluate and document areas of progress, areas of need, and signs of depression, a common sequela.

New support services are primary stroke centers. The major elements of a stroke center are patient care areas, acute stroke teams, written care protocols, emergency medical services, stroke unit, neurology service, support services, a stroke center director with support from the medical organization, neuroimaging services, laboratory services, outcome and quality improvement activities, and continuing education (Brain Attack Coalition, 2001). Specialized stroke units have been found to improve outcomes in persons after ischemic strokes (Evans et al., 2001).

Nowhere in the care of elders is the multidisciplinary team more essential than in the care of persons after a stroke. The assessment of needs after stroke is extremely complex; it requires evaluation by a team coordinated by a nurse and includes a neurologist; a physiatrist; speech, occupational, and physical therapists; an ophthalmologist; a rehabilitation specialist; and a psychologist. It also may include a spiritual advisor. It always includes the person's significant other, who may be involved with the day-to-day life and needs of the elder after a stroke.

▲ **Promoting Healthy Aging: Implications for Gerontological Nursing.** The best approach to stroke, despite new therapies and medications, is prevention and prompt intervention. Identifying high-risk or stroke-prone elders is something nurses can do in the elders' homes, in the community, or at the health facilities where the nurses work. In a quick assessment of risk factors, the nurse can work with the individual to reduce his or her risk and learn how to respond to any signs or symptoms suggestive of a stroke.

As noted previously in the section on cardiovascular disease, smoking cessation and tight control of blood pressure may be the most important of the strategies in approaching modifiable risk factors. Reducing the blood pressure 5 mm Hg in a hypertensive person reduces risk of stroke 34%; with reduction of 10 mm Hg, it is reduced 56% (Sica, 2002). Maintaining the blood pressure equal to or less than 130/85 mm Hg is recommended. Additional primary prevention includes a healthful diet, limiting salt and alcohol, and aspirin therapy unless contraindicated. Tight control of lipids, diabetes, and fibrillation has been found to be helpful, as well as regular exercise and weight-management programs.

The nurse has an active role in tertiary prevention related to the promotion of healthy aging in persons with significant functional limitations who have a history of a cerebrovascular event. The nurse works to prevent skin breakdown and falls, identifies confusion, monitors the lungs for pneumonia, and ensures and maximizes the capacity for self-care, especially related to mobility and activity, eating, maintaining adequate fluid intake, and continence. The nurse is alert for problems with sleep, constipation, and depression. The nurse acts as an advocate in the recommendation to or participation in support strokes for both the persons after a stroke and their significant others or caregivers. The gerontological nurse is challenged to take an active role in improving the quality of life of all elders, especially those with functional limitations.

Endocrine Disorders

The two endocrine disorders seen most often in the older adult are thyroid disturbances and alterations in glucose metabolism, especially diabetes.

Diabetes Mellitus. Diabetes mellitus (DM) is a syndrome of disorders of glucose metabolism resulting in hyperglycemia. The two main forms of diabetes are DM type 1 and DM type 2. Other disorders include impaired fasting glucose (IFG) and impaired glucose tolerance (IGT). Persons with problems in glucose metabolism often have other health problems as well, including problems with metabolism of lipids and proteins. When suspicions of DM are suggested by clinical signs and symptoms, the diagnosis requires specific laboratory testing. The testing will allow the differentiation between the types of impaired glucose metabolism (Box 10-16). DM is the leading cause of end-stage renal disease and blindness and is strongly related to heart disease.

The onset is usually insidious, and as many as one half of all persons with DM type 2 may be undiagnosed (Figure 10-14). They may be without treatment for a number of years while serious complications are developing. A goal of *Healthy People 2010* is to increase the number of persons who are diagnosed so that prompt treatment can be initiated (USDHHS, 2000) (Box 10-17).

DM affects approximately 8.7% of non-Hispanic whites in the United States, with this number more than doubling to 18.3% for persons older than 60 years. With more than 200,000 diabetes-related deaths per year in the United States, an estimated 21 million people are affected—14.6 million diagnosed and 6.2 million thought to be undiagnosed (NIDDKD, 2005). However, the prevalence of diabetes varies considerably for all adults by ethnicity and gender (Figure 10-15). The rate is highest among Hispanic and black men, with slightly fewer cases among Hispanic and black women. Data from other groups are less accurate. For example, for American Indians who receive their health care from one of the Indian Health Services Centers, the prevalence of diabetes for adults is an overall rate of 12.8%. However, this rate increases to 26.7% for American Indians who live in the southern United States and to 27.6% in southern Arizona. These numbers do not include information from American Indians who receive health care in other locations (NIDDKD, 2005). It is reasonable to anticipate much higher numbers for American Indians in late life.

BOX 10-16   Diagnosis of Disorders of Glucose Metabolism

Diagnosis of diabetes mellitus requires either:
  ONE random plasma glucose ≥200 mg/dL when exhibiting symptoms
  OR
  TWO of any combination of positive tests on different days:
  • Fasting plasma glucose (FPG) ≥126 mg/dL on separate occasions (**NOTE:** This is not blood glucose levels that are obtained with a fingerstick.)
  • Oral glucose tolerance test (OGTT) ≥200 mg/dL 2 hours after glucose
  • Random plasma glucose ≥200 mg/dL without symptoms

Diagnosis of impaired fasting glucose (IFG) requires:
  Fasting blood glucose between 110 and 125 mg/dL

Diagnosis of impaired glucose tolerance requires:
  Glucose between 141 and 199 mg/dL 2 hours after a glucose challenge

---

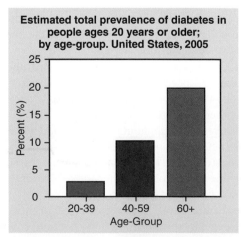

Estimated total prevalence of diabetes in people ages 20 years or older; by age-group. United States, 2005

FIGURE 10-14 Prevalence of diabetes among older adults. (Data from 1999-2002 National Health and Nutrition Examination Survey estimates of total prevalence [both diagnosed and undiagnosed] were projected to year 2005.)

A number of risk factors exist for the development of diabetes (Box 10-18). Increasing age and body mass index (BMI) and decreasing physical activity increase risk considerably.

Etiology. DM type 1 (formerly called *IDDM* or *insulin-dependent diabetes mellitus*) usually develops in early life and is a result of autoimmune destruction of the insulin-producing beta cells of the pancreas. The absolute insulinopenia and subsequent hyperglycemia is incompatible with life; without replacement of the insulin, the person will die. It is often seen in the presence of other autoimmune conditions such as vitamin B_{12} deficiencies, vitiligo, thyroid disease, and rheumatoid arthritis (Danese and Aron, 2004). It has been very rare that someone with DM type 1 lives to late life, and it is seen in only 5% to 10% of adults and much less often in adults older than 60 years.

The overwhelming number of older adults with diabetes have DM type 2 (formerly called *NIDDM* or *non–insulin-dependent diabetes mellitus*). In this case, there is a relative insulinopenia. Production of naturally occurring insulin is reduced, combined with insulin resistance in peripheral tissues. Common associated conditions include acanthosis nigricans, central obesity, hypertension, and dyslipidemia (Danese and Aron, 2004). Secondary causes of DM type 2 include pancreatic and thyroid disease, infection, and medications (diuretics, glucocorticoids, nonsteroidal antiinflammatory drugs [NSAIDs]), which may contribute to insulin resistance.

BOX 10-17 *Healthy People 2010* Objectives Related to Diabetes

OBJECTIVE 5-1

Increase the proportion of persons with diabetes who receive formal diabetes education.
Target: 60%
Baseline: 45% of persons with diabetes received formal diabetes education in 1998 (age adjusted to the year 2000 standard population)
Data source: National Health Interview Survey (NHIS), Centers for Disease Control and Prevention (CDC), National Center for Health Statistics (NCHS)

OBJECTIVE 5-10

Reduce the rate of lower extremity amputations in persons with diabetes.
Target: 1.8 lower extremity amputations per 1000 persons with diabetes per year

Baseline: 4.1 lower extremity amputations per 1000 persons with diabetes occurred in 1997 (age adjusted to the year 2000 standard population)
Data sources: National Hospital Discharge Survey (NHDS), CDC, NCHS; NHIS

OBJECTIVE 5-12

Increase the proportion of adults with diabetes who have a glycosylated hemoglobin measurement at least once a year.
Target: 50%
Baseline: 24% of adults ages 18 years and older with diabetes had a glycosylated hemoglobin measurement at least once a year (mean of data from 39 states in 1998; age adjusted to the year 2000 standard population)
Data source: Behavioral Risk Factor Surveillance System (BRFSS), CDC, National Center for Chronic Disease Prevention and Health Promotion (NCCDPHP).

From U.S. Department of Health and Human Services: *Healthy People 2010: national health promotion and disease prevention objectives,* Washington, DC, 2000, The Department.

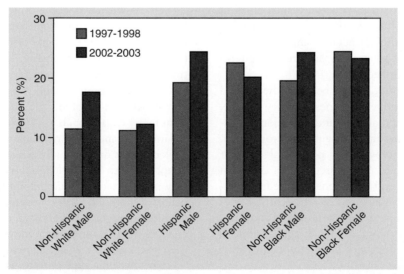

FIGURE 10-15 Percent of persons ages 65 years and older reporting diabetes mellitus, by gender and race-ethnicity. (Data from National Health Interview Survey. Redrawn from *www.cdc.gov/nchs/hphome.htm.* Focus area No. 5.)

BOX 10-18 Risk Factors for Diabetes Mellitus

- Ethnicity (see Figure 10-15)
- Increasing age
- Blood pressure ≥140/90 mm Hg
- First-degree relative (parent, sibling, child) with diabetes mellitus (DM)
- History of impaired glucose tolerance or impaired fasting plasma glucose
- Obesity: ≥120% of desirable weight or body mass index (BMI) ≥30 kg/m^2
- Previous gestational DM or having had a child with a birth weight of ≥9 pounds
- Undesirable lipid levels: high-density lipoproteins (HDLs) ≤35 mg/dL or triglycerides ≥250 mg/dL

BOX 10-19 Signs and Symptoms Suggestive of Diabetes in the Elderly

1. General symptoms such as polyphagia, polyuria, polydipsia, and occasional weight loss
2. Recurrent infections, particularly of bacterial or fungal origin, that involve the skin, intertriginous areas, or urinary tract and sores or wounds that tend to heal slowly
3. Neurological dysfunction, including paresthesia, dysesthesia, or hyperesthesia; muscle weakness and pain (amyotrophy); cranial nerve palsies; and autonomic dysfunction of the gastrointestinal tract (diarrhea); cardiovascular system (orthostatic hypotension, arrhythmias); reproductive system (impotence); and bladder (atony, overflow incontinence)
4. Arterial disease (macroangiopathy) involving the cardiovascular, cerebrovascular, or peripheral vasculature structures
5. Small-vessel disease (microangiopathy) involving the kidneys (proteinuria, glomerulopathy, uremia) and eyes (macular disease, exudates, hemorrhages)
6. Lesions of the skin, such as Dupuytren's contractures, facial rubeosis, and diabetic dermopathy
7. Endocrine-metabolic complications, including hyperlipidemia, obesity, and a history of thyroid or adrenal insufficiency (Schmidt's syndrome)
8. A family history of type 1 or type 2 diabetes and a poor obstetrical history (miscarriages, stillbirths, large babies)

Data from Andres R et al: *Principles of geriatric medicine*, New York, 1985, McGraw-Hill; Davidson MB: Diabetes mellitus and other disorders of carbohydrate metabolism. In Abrams WB et al, editors: *The Merck manual of geriatrics*, ed 2, Whitehouse Station, NJ, 1995, Merck Research Laboratories.

Signs and Symptoms. One of the reasons that the diagnosis of DM in older adults is difficult is its atypical presentation (Reed and Mooradian, 2002) (Box 10-19). Although the classic symptoms (polyuria, polyphagia, polydipsia) may be seen with plasma glucoses of more than 200 mg/dL, these may not be present with lesser elevations. The presentation in elders is more often one of dehydration, confusion, delirium, and decreased visual acuity. In severe cases, the person may be found obtunded in a nonketotic hyperglycemic-hyperosmolar coma (NKHHC) (Beers and Berkow, 2000). Glycosuria often causes incontinence. Women may present with urinary incontinence or recurrent candidiasis as the first sign. The catabolic state caused by lack of insulin causes polyphagia in younger persons but causes weight loss and anorexia in elders. Other vague signs and symptoms include fatigue, nausea, delayed wound healing, and paresthesias (Huether, 2006b). Ketosis is more common among African-American elders (McCulloch, 2002).

Complications. Acute complications of DM include myocardial infarction and stroke, with the combination of these accounting for 65% of the deaths in persons with diabetes (NIDDK, 2005). Although acute complications can and do occur in the older adult with diabetes, long-term complications are by far more common.

The long-term complications of diabetes in the United States are heart disease, stroke, blindness, kidney disease, neurological disorders, amputations, and periodontal disease. These complications are microvascular, macrovascular, or both. They include macrovascular peripheral vascular disease and neuropathies and microvascular loss of vision (diabetic retinopathy) and end-stage renal failure from diabetic nephropathy. The advancement of retinopathy correlates with nephropathy and peripheral neuropathy and duration of DM (Danaese and Aron, 2004). Wound healing is delayed, which when combined with peripheral neuropathy, may lead to amputation.

Combined macrovascular and microvascular damages also lead to sexual impotence. Impotence in men is a result of reduction in vascular flow, peripheral neuropathy, and uncontrolled circulating blood glucose. Sexual dysfunction is two to five times greater in this group than in the general population, even though interest and desire are still present.

Persons with DM commonly have problems with their feet, which can have a considerable impact on their functional status. Warning signs of foot problems include cold feet and intermittent claudication, neuropathic burning, tingling, hypersensitivity, and numbness of the extremities. Infections are common, and wounds are slow to heal.

Hypoglycemia (blood glucose <60 mg/dL) can occur from many causes, such as unusually intense exercise, alcohol intake, or medication mismanagement (Huether, 2006b). If blood sugar drops rapidly, some elders will have signs and symptoms with blood glucose greater than 60 mg/dL. These may include tachycardia, palpitations, diaphoresis, tremors, pallor, and anxiety. Later symptoms may include headache, dizziness, fatigue, irritability, confusion, hunger, visual changes, seizures, and coma. Immediate care involves giving the patient glucose either by mouth or intravenously.

Hyperglycemia appears to be well tolerated in late life. It is not unusual to find persons with fasting glucose levels of 300 mg/dL or higher. Because of this ability to tolerate high levels of circulating glucose, the risk for hyperosmolar hyperglyce-

BOX 10-20	Minimizing Cardiovascular Risk in Persons with Diabetes

- Eat a healthy diet (lower carbohydrate, lower sodium)
- Attain and maintain a healthy weight
- Get regular exercise
- Keep the BP <130/80
- Stop smoking
- Attain and maintain acceptable lipid levels
  - Cholesterol <200
  - LDL <100
  - HDL >40
  - Triglycerides <150

BP, Blood pressure; *LDL,* low-density lipoprotein; *HDL,* high-density lipoprotein.

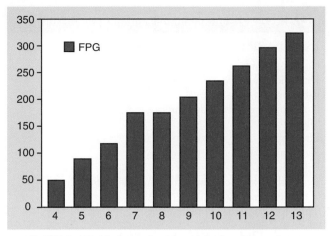

FIGURE 10-16 Comparing A1c with fasting plasma glucose.

TABLE 10-5

Maintaining Glycemic Control*

	Preprandial	Post-prandial	3 AM
Blood glucose (mg/dL)	70 120	<180	>65

Data from National Diabetes Education Program: *Diabetes: the science of control,* 2007 (website): *ndep.nih.gov/resources/presentations/diabetescontrol/.* Accessed June 13, 2007.
*Maintaining intensive control has been found to reduce the risk of eye disease (76%), kidney disease (50%), and neuropathic disease (60%).

BOX 10-21	Risk Identification for People with Diabetes

- Diabetes for longer than 10 years
- Male
- Poor glucose control
- Cardiovascular, retinal, or renal complications

Increased risk for amputation with the following:
- Peripheral neuropathy with loss of sensation
- Evidence of increased pressure (redness, bony deformity)
- Peripheral vascular disease (diminished or absent pedal pulses)
- History of ulcers
- History of amputation
- Severe nail pathology

Data from American Diabetes Association. *Diabetes Care* 25:S69, 2002.

mic nonketonic coma is present. This is especially important in persons who are otherwise medically frail and should be considered in any older adult with diabetes who is difficult to arouse. This is considered an emergency situation.

Management. DM is truly a chronic disease that, even in the best of circumstances, causes end-organ damage, especially cardiovascular disease. Therefore the goal of management is to minimize the effects of the complications (Box 10-20). To do so, glycemic control should be maintained the majority of the time. The measurements indicative of ideal glycemic control are given in Table 10-5. Maintaining the hemoglobin A1c (HbA1c) level at less than 7 is considered successful management (Cook et al., 2001) (Figure 10-16).

Management always begins with risk identification related to the assessment of end-organ damage (Box 10-21). Even mildly elevated glucose levels cause retinopathy, neuropathy, and nephropathy. A urinalysis for protein and microalbumin; blood studies of blood urea nitrogen (BUN), albumin, and creatinine level; and the calculations of creatinine clearance (see Chapter 5) and the albumin-creatinine ratio are used to screen for the presence of nephropathy. A dilated funduscopic assessment by an ophthalmologist determines the presence of microvascular retinal changes. Assessment of neuropathy requires a careful neurological examination with an emphasis

on sensation and history of functioning. Clinical guidelines suggest that the best means of testing neurological and sensory intactness is the use of the Semmes-Weinstein monofilament instrument. The measurement of blood pressure, palpation of pulses, ECG, chest x-ray examination, and possibly a stress test are included in the basic workup for the risk for heart disease.

The final part of the assessment is used to develop the plan of care related to both the treatment of the disorder and the management of everyday life. Nutrition, weight, and exercise/activity history is important to identify eating patterns, an active or sedentary lifestyle, and weight control measures, all of which can provide clues for realistic education and better adherence to a therapy regimen. Assessing economic resources helps establish the ability to purchase equipment, materials, and special foods that may be needed. Medication history of over-the-counter and prescription drugs (Box 10-22) and use of alcohol and tobacco are also factors that provide important information in the assessment of the elder. All have a direct or indirect effect on renal, circulatory, neurological, and nutritional function.

BOX 10-22   Medications Affecting Blood Sugar

INCREASE BLOOD GLUCOSE LEVELS

Corticosteroids
Diazoxide
Estrogens
Furosemide and thiazide diuretics
Glucagon
Lithium
Phenytoin
Rifampin
Sympathomimetics (antihistamines, decongestants, bronchodilators)
Thyroid replacement preparations

DECREASE BLOOD GLUCOSE LEVELS

Alcohol
Anabolic steroids
Beta-blockers (antihypertensives)
Salicylates (high doses)

INTERACTIONS WITH SULFONYLUREAS (ORAL HYPOGLYCEMICS)

Increased Effects (Lower Blood Glucose Levels Further)
Allopurinol
Beta-blockers

Clofibrate
Histamine antagonists
Imidazole antifungals
Low-dose salicylates
Monamine oxidase inhibitors
Probenecid
Tricyclic antidepressants

Drugs Not to Be Taken in Combination with Sulfonylureas
Azapropazone
Chloramphenicol
Dicumarol
Oxyphenbutazone
Phenylbutazone
Salicylates (high dose)
Sulfonamides

Decreased Effects (Hinder Hypoglycemic Action)
Barbiturates
Corticosteroids
Diuretics
Estrogens
Rifampin

Summarized from an unidentified source: handout at workshop, *Chronic disorders of the aged,* sponsored by Arizona State School of Nursing, Phoenix, Sept 1992.

In addition to the neurological assessment just discussed, additional objective data are collected, including the measurement of height, weight, and waist circumference. From the height and weight, a BMI can be calculated (Figure 10-17). The greater the BMI over 25, the greater the risk for heart disease. For the very old, BMI is less useful because of the replacement of muscle mass with adipose tissue. Additional blood studies for the person post-diagnosis are a fasting blood glucose, glycosylated HbA_{1c}, fasting lipid profile, and a thyroid panel (thyroid-stimulating hormone [TSH] and thyroxine [T_4]). Finally, the assessment includes a careful inspection of the feet, skin, and mouth for signs of injury or the presence of lesions.

Medications. One of the mainstays of the management of type 2 DM in elders is oral medication (Whitehead, 2002). Oral medications are prescribed according to the insulin deficit identified: no secretion of insulin, insulin resistance, or inadequate secretion of insulin (Table 10-6). The sulfonylureas and meglitinides increase insulin secretion. Enhanced insulin sensitivity occurs with the biguanides or thiazolidinediones, which decrease insulin resistance. One can delay or reduce the intestinal absorption of carbohydrates with alpha-glucosidase inhibitors and reduce absorption of fats with lipase inhibitors. Sulfonylureas enhance insulin secretion. These agents are used alone or in combination to achieve the desired blood glucose control. Insulin is always used with DM type 1 and is used for adjuvant therapy for DM type 2 when oral agents, exercise, and diet do not adequately control the blood sugar.

▲ **Promoting Healthy Aging: Implications for Gerontological Nursing.** Caring for the elder with diabetes centers on prevention, early identification, and delay of complications as long as possible. Gerontological nurses have great potential for helping individuals and the nation reach the goals set forth in *Healthy People 2010* (USDHHS, 2000), from conducting screenings to patient education and coaching. Screening for DM by fasting plasma and random blood glucose testing is important for early identification of potential or actual disease. Nurses participate in screenings for DM at community health fairs and in clinical settings. Medicare will pay for the annual costs of the screening for persons at risk for diabetes. Nurses also participate in community education about the need for early diagnosis and for the prompt treatment of complications. Some nurses make caring for persons with diabetes their professional focus and obtain additional preparation to become certified diabetes educators.

For persons at higher risk for DM, especially those with IFG or IGT, attention should be directed toward reducing the risk for both DM and heart disease. This means education and interventions to lower glucose, control blood pressure and blood lipids, and reduce to or maintain one's ideal body weight.

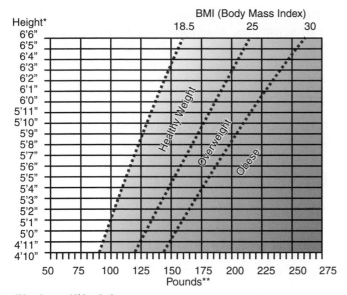

Height*

BMI (Body Mass Index)

FIGURE 10-17 Determination of body mass index (BMI). *NOTE:* For the very old, this is not useful because of the replacement of muscle mass with adipose tissue. (Source: National Institute of Diabetes and Digestive and Kidney Diseases: *Weight and waist measurement: tools for adults.* National Institutes of Health Pub No. 03-5282, Washington, DC, 2003, National Institutes of Health.)

*No shoes **No clothes

TABLE 10-6

Oral Agents in Diabetes Management

Generic Name	Brand Name	Purpose
SULFONYLUREAS		Enhance insulin secretion
Chlorpropamide	Diabinese	
Glimepiride	Amaryl	
Glipizide	Glucotrol	
Glyburide	Micronase	
Glyburide, micronized	Glynase	
MEGLITINIDES		Enhance insulin secretion
Nateglinide	Starlix	
Repaglinide	Prandin	
ALPHA-GLUCOSIDASE INHIBITOR		Decreases glucose absorption
Acarbose	Precose	
BIGUANIDE		Decreases hepatic glucose production
Metformin	Glucophage	
THIAZOLIDINEDIONES		Enhance insulin sensitivity
Rosiglitazone	Avandia	
Pioglitazone	Actos	

The goals of nursing care of persons with diabetes are to maintain the older adult with DM in the best health realistically possible and ensure that the person obtains at least the established minimum standards of care (Box 10-23).

Promoting healthy aging in the person with diabetes requires an array of interventions and usually involves persons from a number of disciplines working together with the patient and his or her family/significant others. The persons involved may include ancillary nursing staff and licensed nurses, nutritionists, pharmacists, podiatrists, ophthalmologists, physicians, nurse practitioners, certified diabetic educators, and counselors. The nurse as part of the team serves as an educator, care provider, advocate, supporter, and guide for the older person. If the person's disease is hard to control, endocrinologists are involved, and as complications develop, more specialists are called in, such as nephrologists, cardiologists, and wound care specialists. Nurses are expected to advocate for elders and encourage them to expect and receive quality care to prevent the devastating end results of poor management.

Nutrition. Adequate and appropriate nutrition is a key factor in healthy living with DM. An initial nutrition assessment with a 24-hour recall will provide some clues to the patient's dietary habits, intake, and style of eating. If a recall is not possible, have the person bring in his or her grocery list for the past week. If the elder is from an ethnic group different from the nurse, the nurse will need to learn more

BOX 10-23 Evidenced-Based Care: Minimum Standards of Care for the Person with Diabetes

- Biannual health care assessment
- Annual lipid panel
- Quarterly or biannual hemoglobin A1C
- Annual dilated funduscopic examination
- Annual foot examination

From U.S. Department of Health and Human Services (USDHHS): *Healthy People 2010*, Washington, DC, 2000, The Department.

about the usual ingredients and methods of food preparation to be able to give reasonable instructions. Ideally, all persons with diabetes should have culturally appropriate medical nutrition therapy by a registered dietitian annually. At the time of this writing, this service was covered by Medicare.

It is part of the nurse's responsibility to learn if access to food is difficult, including food preparation and shopping for food. Working with elders' dietary habits that have been formed over a lifetime may be difficult but not impossible. Control of diet (especially of portions) and weight loss may also prevent the persons with impaired fasting glucose or impaired glucose tolerance from developing DM. If the person is overweight or obese, a weight-loss plan is important. Reductions of as little as 10% in weight will improve glycemic control or be the difference between taking oral antihyperglycemic agents or insulin and controlling the DM by diet and exercise alone.

Exercise. Exercise is also an important avenue toward healthy living with DM, because exercise increases insulin production. Walking is an inexpensive and beneficial way to exercise. Exercise in conjunction with an appropriate diet may be sufficient to maintain blood glucose levels within normal levels in some cases. A more intensive exercise program should not be started until the older adult has consulted with his or her health care provider. Those who have limited mobility can still do chair exercises or, if possible, use exercise machines that enable sitting and holding-on for support.

If the person is using insulin, exercise needs to be done on a regular rather than an erratic basis, and blood glucose must be tested before and after exercise to avoid or respond promptly to hypoglycemia.

Medications. Promoting healthy aging with DM requires the elder and the nurse to develop expertise in the use of pharmacological interventions. These include the antiglycemics noted earlier, as well as preventive adjuvant therapy such as ACE inhibitors and aspirin. Both have been demonstrated to improve outcomes in persons with diabetes.

If other medications are prescribed, they are carefully reviewed. The effects of drugs on blood glucose must be seriously considered because a number of medications commonly used for elders adversely affect blood glucose levels. Therefore older adults should be advised to ask if the particular drug prescribed affects their therapy and should check with their primary care provider or endocrinologist before taking any over-the-counter medications.

Self-Care. Because of the chronicity and complexity of DM, maximum wellness is difficult to achieve without considerable self-care skills (Box 10-24). The nurse is often the professional who is responsible for working with the elder in developing such skills. In addition to diet, exercise, and medication use already discussed, self-care skills include self-monitoring of blood glucose, optimal care of the feet, "sick-day" adjustments, and knowledge about the disease and the care expected. An identification bracelet is a consideration because confusion or delirium may be a manifestation of low blood sugar and misinterpreted as dementia, which delays treatment. Self-care also includes preventive care practices for the eyes, kidneys, and feet. The nurses support the patient in obtaining the needed services related to these.

Implications for the Long-Term Care Setting. Many of the persons cared for by gerontological nurses in long-term care facilities have DM. In this setting, the nurse may be responsible for many of the activities that would otherwise fall on the patient or a home caregiver in addition to those as a professional. Meals, nutritional status, intake and output, and exercise/activity are monitored. The nurse assesses the person for signs of hypoglycemia and hyperglycemia and evidence of complications. The nurse ensures that the standards of care for the person with DM are met. The nurse monitors the effect and side effects of diet, exercise,

and medication use. The nurse administers or supervises the administration of medications. If the person requires what is called *sliding scale insulin,* wherein the dosage depends on the current glucose reading, it is the nurse who must make the determination of the dosage under "sliding scale" guidelines.

Thyroid Disorders. Although thyroid disorders are seen throughout adulthood, it is relatively common in older adults, affecting 20% or more of persons older that 65 years, especially women. Unfortunately, many of the signs and symptoms are nonspecific and frequently encountered in the older population and are incorrectly attributed to normal aging or another disorder or to side effects of medications (Shroff and Moylan, 2004). Fortunately, it is easy to diagnose either through screenings or in a diagnostic workup, which includes the simple measurement of a thyroid panel. When a patient presents with multiple symptoms without a marked change in the laboratory findings, a diagnosis of subclinical disease may be made. The TSH is elevated in hypothyroidism as the pituitary tries to stimulate the underfunctioning thyroid; the TSH is decreased in hyperthyroidism as the pituitary responds to the elevated blood levels of the thyroid hormone *thyroxine* (T_4) (see Chapter 5). The most common thyroid disturbance in older adults is hypothyroidism.

BOX 10-24 Self-Care Skills Needed for the Person with Diabetes

GLUCOSE SELF-MONITORING

Obtaining a blood sample correctly
Using the glucose monitoring equipment correctly
Troubleshooting when results indicate an error
Recording the values from the machine
Understanding the timing and frequency of the self-monitoring
Understanding the adjustments needed when ill
Understanding what to do with the results

MEDICATION SELF-ADMINISTRATION

Where Appropriate, Insulin Use
Selecting appropriate injection site
Using correct technique for injections
Disposing of used needles and syringes correctly
Storing and transporting insulin correctly

Oral Medication Use
Knowing and adhering to correct timing
Knowing drug-drug and drug-food interactions
Recognizing side effects and knowing when to report

FOOT CARE AND EXAMINATION

Selecting and using appropriate and safe footwear

HANDLING SICK DAYS

Recognizing the signs and symptoms of both hyperglycemia and hypoglycemia

Etiology. Whereas Grave's disease is the most common cause of *hyperthyroidism* in younger adults, for elders it is more often attributed to multinodular toxic goiter. It can also result from ingestion of iodine or iodine-containing substances, such as seafood, radio-contrast agents, and the medication *amiodarone*. The onset of the disease may be abrupt.

The more common *hypothyroidism* is thought to be caused most frequently by autoimmune thyroiditis. It also may be iatrogenic, resulting form radioiodine treatment, subtotal thyroidectomy, or a number of medications. It can also be caused by a pituitary or hypothalamic abnormality (Gambert and Miller, 2004).

Signs and Symptoms. Whereas younger persons with hypothyroidism report symptoms of weight gain, cold intolerance, paresthesias, and muscle cramps, these are usually absent in the older adult. These classic symptoms are often found in the older person without thyroid disturbances! Instead, the elder complains of fatigue, weakness, depression, and, in some cases, confusion. The onset of symptoms is usually insidious and subtle.

The symptoms and signs of hyperthyroidism in the older adult do not differ significantly from those in the younger adult. The person seeks attention because of a sensation of "palpitations" and may also complain of excessive perspiration and visual disturbances. The person commonly has a poor appetite, agitation, confusion, and edema. Dementia is often suspected. On examination, the person is also likely to have tachycardia, tremors, and weight loss (Gambert and Miller, 2004). Symptoms of heart failure or angina may cloud the clinical presentation and prevent the correct diagnosis.

Complications. Complications occur both as the result of treatment and in the failure to diagnose and therefore failure to treat in a timely manner. Myxedema coma is a serious complication of untreated hypothyroidism in the older patient. Because rapid replacement of the missing thyroxin is not possible because of drug toxicity, the patient must be watched carefully. Even with the best treatment, death may ensue. Because thyroid replacement is necessary to maintain life, the person has to learn to minimize the side effects, especially increased bone loss. Too high a dose can causes the complications of hyperthyroidism.

Thyroxin increases myocardial oxygen consumption; therefore the elevations found in hyperthyroidism produce significant risk for atrial fibrillation, exacerbation of angina in persons with pre-existing CHD, and may precipitate congestive heart failure. The most common complication is atrial fibrillation, which is present in 27% of elderly patients with hyperthyroidism. If the atrial fibrillation is not converted, heart failure and early death may occur (Beers and Berkow, 2000).

Management. The management of thyroid disturbances is largely one of careful pharmacological intervention and, in the case of hyperthyroidism, one of surgical or chemical ablation.

▲ **Promoting Healthy Aging: Implications for Gerontological Nursing.** Although the nurse may see little that can be done to prevent thyroid disturbances in late life, organizations like the Monterey Bay Aquarium have launched campaigns to inform consumers of the iodine and mercury found in seafood (see *www.seafoodwatch.org*) because of their association with thyroid disease. Nurses can also be involved in community screenings and should always be attentive to the possibility that the person who is diagnosed with anxiety, dementia, or depression may instead have a thyroid disturbance.

For those newly diagnosed, the nurse may be instrumental in working with the person and family to understand the seriousness of the problem and the need for very careful adherence to the prescribed regimen. If the elder is hospitalized for acute management, the life-threatening nature of both the disorder and the treatment can be made clear so that advanced planning can be done that will account for all possible outcomes.

For the person in ongoing maintenance treatment, the nurse works with the person and significant others in the correct self-administration of medications and in the appropriate timing of monitoring blood levels and signs or symptoms indicating an exacerbation.

Gastrointestinal Disorders

Because of the combination of changes related to aging, polypharmacy, co-morbid conditions, and inactivity, several chronic disorders of the gastrointestinal (GI) track are seen. Among the most common are constipation (see Chapter 7), diverticular disease, and gastroesophageal reflux disease (GERD). Diverticular disease includes both diverticulosis and diverticulitis.

Diverticular Disease. Diverticular disease is a disorder found only in industrial nations. Diverticulosis, or the presence of diverticula, has been found in more than 60% of persons older than 70 years and in nearly 80% of persons older than 80 years (Ali and Lacy, 2004; National Institutes of Health [NIH], 2005). Diverticulitis is an acute inflammatory complication of diverticulosis. Diverticular disease is primarily a "hot" illness by those persons who subscribe to the hot/cold theory of disease causation and treatment (Giger and Davidhizar, 2003). The risk factors for diverticular disease can be found in Box 10-25.

Diverticula are small herniations or saclike out-pouchings of mucosa that extend through the muscle layers of the colon

---

BOX 10-25   Risk Factors for Diverticular Disease

- Family history
- Personal history of gallbladder disease
- Low dietary intake of fiber
- Use of medications that slow fecal transit time
- Overuse of laxatives
- Obesity

wall, almost exclusive of the sigmoid colon (Huether, 2006a). They form at weak points in the colon wall, usually where arteries penetrate and provide nutrients to the mucosal layer. Usually less than 1 cm, diverticula have thin, compressible walls if empty or firm walls if full of fecal matter (Nadel, 2001). Occasionally the fecal matter in a diverticulum will become quite desiccated, even calcified.

Etiology. Although the exact etiology of diverticular disease is unknown, it is most commonly found in persons with risk factors (Box 10-25) (Melange and Vanheuverzwyn, 1990). Abnormal colonic motility, including chronic constipation and intraluminal hypertension, appears to be a contributing factor (Huether, 2006a).

Sign and Symptoms. The majority of persons with diverticulosis are completely asymptomatic, and the condition is found only when a barium enema, colonoscopy, or CT scan is performed for some other reason. About 15% to 20% of persons with diverticulosis will develop the inflammatory diverticulitis or bleeding. Persons with uncomplicated diverticulitis complain of abdominal pain, especially in the left lower quadrant, and may have a fever and elevated white blood cell count, although these latter symptoms may be delayed or absent in the older adult. The physical assessment may be completely negative. Rectal bleeding is typically acute in onset, painless, and stops spontaneously.

Complications. The complications of diverticulitis are abscess, stricture, or fistula. With any perforation, peritonitis is possible. Persons with these complications may have an elevated pulse or are hypotensive; however, in the older adult, unexplained lethargy or confusion may be seen as well or instead. A lower left quadrant mass may be palpated (Ali and Lacy, 2004).

Management. Uncomplicated diverticulitis is treated with antibiotics and a clear liquid diet and is usually managed in the outpatient setting. Complicated diverticulitis is always considered an emergency and requires hospitalization for treatment and possible surgical repair.

Gastroesophageal Reflux Disease. Gastroesophageal Reflux Disease (GERD) is the syndrome defined as the sequelae of the movement of gastric contents, especially gastric acid into the esophagus (Field, 2003). It is the most common GI disorder affecting older adults. Symptoms may affect up to 40% of the older population at some time and 7% to 10% on a daily basis (Ali and Lacy, 2004). Once any symptoms have appeared, at least 50% of those persons will either have persistent symptoms or require intervention. If GERD is left untreated, complications can develop, especially for older adults. It is often diagnosed empirically from the symptom history or the response to treatment but can be confirmed with an esophagogastroduodenoscopy (upper endoscopy) (Field, 2003).

Etiology. GERD is caused by an abnormality of the lower esophageal sphincter (LES). Normally it remains tightly closed, relaxing to allow for the movement of materials into the stomach. In GERD, the LES relaxes inappropriately, allowing the backflow of stomach contents.

Signs and Symptoms. The primary complaint of persons with GERD is indigestion. When no other symptoms are present, this is usually diagnosed as dyspepsia. When combined with sensations of heartburn and especially regurgitation or a sour or burning taste in the mouth, it is more likely to be GERD. Older adults more commonly have more atypical symptoms of persistent cough, exacerbations of asthma, laryngitis, and intermittent chest pain. Abdominal pain may occur within 1 hour of eating, and symptoms are worse when lying down with the added pressure of gravity on the LES.

Complications. Persistent symptoms have the potential to negatively affect quality of life. They also may lead to esophagitis, peptic strictures, esophageal ulcers (with bleeding), and most important, Barrett's esophagus, a precursor to cancer (Ali and Lacy, 2004). The most serious complication is the development of pneumonia from the aspiration of stomach contents.

Management. The management of GERD combines lifestyle changes with pharmacological preparations, used in a stepwise fashion. Lifestyle modifications include eating smaller meals; no eating 3 to 4 hours before bed; avoiding high-fat foods, alcohol, caffeine and nicotine; and sleeping with the head of the bed elevated (see Chapter 9). Weight reduction and smoking cessation may also be helpful (Huether, 2006a). These strategies alone may control the majority of symptoms when complications are not present. Pharmacological preparation begins with over-the-counter agents such as Tums and Rolaids and progresses to H2 blockers and then proton pump inhibitors. In severe cases of GERD, surgical tightening of the lower esophageal sphincter may be necessary.

▲ *Promoting Healthy Aging: Implications for Gerontological Nursing.* Because the etiology of both GERD and diverticular disease is unclear, prevention itself is not usually a focus with the exception of promoting healthy eating. Although neither can be prevented from developing, it may be possible to exert considerable control over exacerbation of symptoms and to have some effect on preventing complications or, at a minimum, developing awareness of the early signs of potential complications.

The nurse works with the elder to achieve lifestyle modifications. Older adults with mild GERD may report that they have no symptoms unless they eat a large meal. In an era of "super-sized" meals, the temptation to overeat is considerable. The nurse may work with the elder to identify situations that aggravate his or her GERD and come up with strategies to best deal with them. The nurse also teaches persons with GERD the alarm signs—the signs that should

BOX 10-26	Warning Signs Suggesting Possible GERD Complication

- Anemia
- Anorexia
- Dysphagia
- Hematemesis
- Odynophagia
- Weight loss

GERD, Gastroesophageal reflux disease.

receive prompt evaluation by a physician or nurse practitioner (Box 10-26).

For persons with diverticulosis, the goal is prevention of diverticulitis. High fiber diets (25 to 30 g/day) have been cited in American, European, and Asian studies as protective against diverticulosis (Rubio, 2002). In addition, persons should strive for intake of 6 to 8 glasses of fluid per day, preferably with little caffeine.

Pain may be an issue during episodes of diverticulitis. The nurse works with the individual to find effective and safe comfort strategies that include pain medication and creative non-pharmacological approaches such as massage, hot or cold packs, stretching exercises, relaxation, music, or meditation techniques.

In the promotion of healthy aging, the nurse works with the elder to analyze diet, fluid intake, and activity level to ensure adequate motility and minimal pressure within the GI tract. If the person is overweight or obese, weight loss will decrease intraabdominal pressure and decrease the risk for the development of new diverticula and exacerbations of GERD. In all cases, the nurse is responsible for patient education regarding the appropriate use of medications, the warning signs of potential problems, and the best response to the signs or symptoms. When working with an elder in a cross-cultural setting, it is especially important for the nurse to communicate effectively and incorporate cultural expectations and habits (e.g., diet) into the plan of nursing care.

Respiratory Disorders

The normal physical changes with aging in the respiratory system discussed in Chapter 4 result in a greater risk for respiratory problems, and when they occur, the mortality rate is higher in older adults than in younger adults. Diseases of the respiratory system are identified as acute or chronic and as involving the upper or lower respiratory tract. They are further defined as either *obstructive*—preventing airflow out as a result of obstruction or narrowing of the respiratory structures (e.g., chronic obstructive pulmonary disease); or *restrictive*—causing a decrease in total lung capacity as a result of limited expansion (e.g., asthma). Tuberculosis in older adults is often seen as a reactivation of a long-dormant infection and an increase in incidence in some areas of the United States.

Chronic Obstructive Pulmonary Disease. Chronic obstructive pulmonary disease (COPD) is a catch-all term used to encompass those conditions that affect airflow and include emphysema and chronic bronchitis. Chronic bronchitis is diagnosed clinically by a productive cough for 3 months in 2 consecutive years or 6 months in 1 year. It can be either obstructive or nonobstructive. Emphysema is a pathological process characterized by dilated air spaces distal to the terminal bronchiole and is associated with destruction of the alveolar wall (Rissmiller and Adair, 2004).

COPD is now the fourth leading cause of death for both older men and women in most ethnic groups; however, it is expected to be the third leading cause of death by 2020 (Figure 10-18). The death rate from COPD in women over

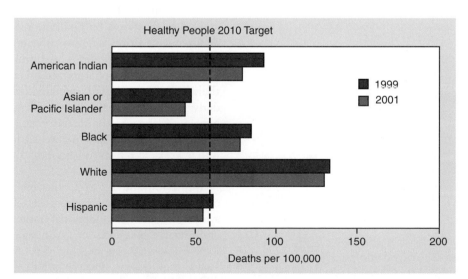

FIGURE 10-18 COPD deaths. *NOTE:* COPD is defined as ICD-10 J40-J44 and excludes asthma. Data are for ages 45 years and older and age adjusted to 2000 standard population. American Indian includes Alaska Native. Black and white exclude persons of Hispanic origin. Persons of Hispanic origin may be any race. Persons were asked to select only one race; selection of more than one race was not an option. (Data from National Vital Statistics System, NCHS, CDC. Redrawn from *www.cdc.gov/nchs/hphome.htm*. Focus area No. 24.)

45 years tripled between 1980 and 2000, with that of men increasing only 15%. Between 1999 and 2001, the overall death rate declined because of a sharp decrease in the death rate for men but with no change in the death rate for women (Beato, 2004).

COPD also contributes to activity limitations in those with the condition. For all persons older than 45 years, the activity limitation rate was 2.5% in 2002. This varies by ethnicity, with Hispanics with the lowest rate of activity limitation (1.4%) and the highest rate of limitation among non-Hispanic whites (2.6%) (Figure 10-19). However, poverty causes more disparity than race or ethnicity in COPD, with 5.7% of the poor with limitations compared with only 1.5% of the middle class (Beato, 2004).

Spirometry is indispensable in establishing the diagnosis of COPD because it is a standardized and reproducible test that objectively confirms the presence of airflow obstruction. Measurement of the diffusing capacity for carbon monoxide may help differentiate between emphysema and chronic bronchitis.

Etiology. The airway obstruction of COPD is caused from airway and lung injury but usually from the inhalation of toxins and pollutants, especially tobacco smoke—either directly or indirectly from secondhand smoke. Associated tobacco use accounts for 80% to 90% of all COPD. The smoker becomes symptomatic after 35 to 40 pack-years of exposure (Rissmiller and Adair, 2004). Additional causes include exposure to occupational pollutants such as dust, chemicals, and air pollution. In addition, the increase in the incidence in women is driven largely by cumulative and residual effects of long-term cigarette smoking and exposure to secondhand smoke (Stoller, 2002). The airflow obstruction in chronic bronchitis is caused by a combination of thickened and inflamed bronchial walls, hypertrophy of mucus glands, smooth muscle constriction, and excess mucus production, all of which cause lumen compromise, but again, stimulated by the inhalation of toxins.

Signs and Symptoms. The most common symptoms of COPD are cough, dyspnea on exertion, and increased phlegm production (Estes, 2002). However, COPD has a long presymptomatic stage, and usually about 50% of lung function has been irretrievably lost before patients become symptomatic (Stoller, 2002). Common later signs include wheezing, prolonged expiration with pursed-lip breathing, barrel chest, air trapping, hyperresonance, pale lips or nail beds, fingernail clubbing, and use of accessory breathing muscles (McCrory et al., 2001). Cough is the primary symptom of chronic bronchitis and affects the majority of smokers. Unfortunately, the cough is often dismissed by smokers as insignificant because early in the disease there is no measurable airflow obstruction. In advanced disease, cyanosis, evidence of right-sided heart failure, and peripheral edema are present.

Complications. COPD is a progressively debilitating condition characterized by exacerbations and remissions in symptoms. Acute exacerbations of COPD result in the acute worsening of the baseline signs and symptoms, generally characterized by significantly worsened dyspnea and increased volume and purulence of sputum (McCrory et al., 2001). In addition, pulsus paradoxus, marked by a decrease in blood pressure of 10 mm Hg or more during inspiration compared with expiration, may occur (Estes, 2002). Spirometry of less than 150 mL, worsening orthopnea, paroxysmal nocturnal dyspnea, and respirations greater than 30 per minute signal an emergent exacerbation of COPD. Exacerbations have numerous inciting factors, including viral or bacterial infections, air pollution or other environmental exposures, and changes in the weather. Pneumonia is a frequent and serious complication.

Exacerbations frequently precipitate the need for increased medications, hospitalization, or respiratory support. Assisted ventilation is noninvasive and is applied through a face mask. Invasive endotracheal intubation may be needed for patients with respiratory acidosis that progresses despite therapy or for those with impaired consciousness. In the elderly, decreased alertness may indicate hypoxemia or hypercapnia. Although the acute phase of an exacerbation is usually over in 10 days to 2 weeks, lung function may take 4 to 6 weeks to return to baseline.

Management. As with other chronic diseases, the goals of treatment and management of COPD are to minimize symptoms, maximize functional status, prevent exacerbation, and preserve lung function. Although the use of pharmacological interventions may increase comfort and functional status, they do not affect mortality (Rissmiller and Adair, 2004). However, the use of long-term oxygen therapy in hypoxemic patients has been shown to improve survival, and smoking cessation slows the rate of decline in lung capacity. The routine use of antibiotics is controversial because the

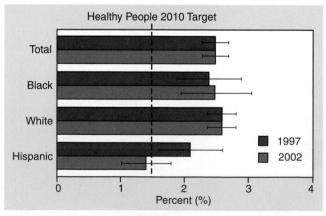

FIGURE 10-19 Activity limitation because of chronic respiratory problems. *NOTE:* Data are for ages 45 years and older and age adjusted to the 2000 standard population. Black and white exclude persons of Hispanic origin. Persons of Hispanic origin may be any race. Persons reported one or more races. Data by single race category are for persons who reported only one racial group. (Data from National Health Interview Survey, NCHS, CDC. Redrawn from *www.cdc.gov/nchs/hphome.htm.* Focus area No. 24.)

causal role of bacterial infection is often difficult to document. Antibiotics are generally indicated for patients with new pulmonary infiltrates on chest x-ray film, fever, and perhaps purulent sputum.

As for most chronic conditions, a team approach is the most useful for maximizing the quality of life for the persons with COPD. The core team includes the nurse, a pulmonologist or pulmonologist-nurse practitioner team, a respiratory therapist, and a pharmacist. Additional sources of support and guidance are an occupational or therapeutic recreation therapist to help the person adapt to declining functional capacity and a spiritual advisor and/or counselor to deal with the inherent psychological issues of an ultimately terminal illness.

Asthma. Asthma is an inflammatory airway disease that is usually closely linked to allergic mechanisms and is seen as bronchial hyperresponsiveness and inflammation resulting in bronchorestriction. It is staged from mild to severe based on the frequency of symptoms and the need for treatment. Spirometry before and after the administration of bronchodilators is used in diagnosis (National Heart Lung and Blood Institute [NHLBI], 1997).

Although the majority of asthma is diagnosed in children and those younger than 40 years, it is still seen in older adults, either as a continuation from earlier life or as new onset. However, it is often underdiagnosed and therefore undertreated in older adults. Instead, the symptoms are attributed to normal changes with aging, cardiovascular disease, or COPD. The person with asthma may have developed a tolerance to the bronchorestriction and minimizes the reports of symptoms despite the respiratory compromise actually present.

The asthma-associated death rate has decreased overall in recent years. For those older than 65 years, it went from 69.5 per million people in 1999 to 60.7 per million in 2001, close to the *Healthy People 2010* goal of 60.0 per million.

However the incidence of asthma-related deaths increases significantly in the over-65 population compared with younger adults (Figure 10-20). The rate varies further with ethnicity, with non-Hispanic blacks having the highest rate of all other groups. Women, who have a death rate nearly double that of men, also have a hospitalization rate 2½ times that of men (Beato, 2004).

Etiology. The development of asthma is influenced by genetics, environment, and lifestyle factors. A positive family history of asthma and personal history of allergies are positive predictors of asthma. Whereas males have increased risk in childhood, women seem to experience an increased risk in late life. After a susceptible person is exposed to an antigen, a cascade of reactions occurs with immediate, late, and recurrent effects. These reactions not only have direct effects on airway smooth muscle and mucus secretion but also recruit the participation of monocytes, lymphocytes, neutrophils, and eosinophils into the cells lining the airways. Repeated exposure potentiates the person's inflammatory response or desensitizes him or her to the antigen. Of interest, some age-related decline of immune system function may be helpful in minimizing the hyperresponsiveness of asthma. Common external risk factors include exposure to tobacco smoke, air pollution, viral respiratory infections, and allergens such as pet dander, fumes, and dust.

Signs and Symptoms. The presentation of asthma in the elderly is similar to that of younger adults although it may be blunted as just noted. The classic presentation is one of recurrent episodes of wheezing, shortness of breath, nonproductive cough, and chest tightness. The wheezing is characteristically limited to expiratory respirations. Symptoms are usually worse at night or in the early morning hours but may be triggered by a variety of stimuli, including emotions, cold air, pollutants, and especially infection. Symptoms provide a reliable measure of a person's need for and

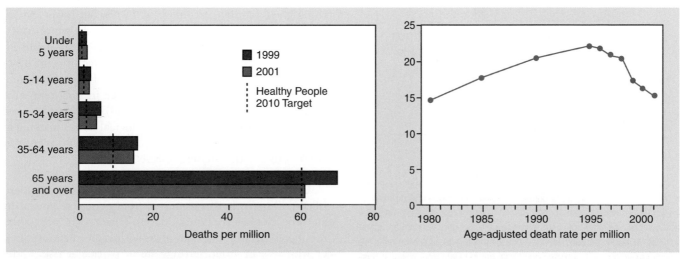

FIGURE 10-20 Asthma-related deaths. (Data from National Vital Health Statistics System, NCHS, CDC. Redrawn from *www.cdc.gov/nchs/hphome.htm.* Focus area No. 24.)

response to therapy, although differences among individuals are highly varied in regard to which symptoms are salient, how symptoms are tolerated, and how they relate to physiological alterations of lung function as measured by peak expiratory flow (PEF) meters. During periods of remissions, no symptoms may be noted.

Symptoms associated with acute asthma actually may be caused by other conditions common among the elderly, such as myocardial ischemia, GERD, CHF, or even pulmonary embolism. The assessment of episodic or acute chest symptoms in the elderly must always include the possibility of confounding causes.

Complications. Asthma can interfere with the quality of one's life, and acute or severe exacerbations may require hospitalizations, especially for women (Figure 10-21). When asthma is long-standing, especially when untreated or undertreated, structural changes to the airway can occur, resulting in thickening of the airway wall and peribronchial fibrosis.

Management. The goals of asthma management include optimizing pulmonary function, controlling cough and nocturnal symptoms, preventing exacerbations, promoting prompt recognition and treatment of exacerbations, reducing the need for emergency department visits, avoiding aggravating other medical conditions, and minimizing medication adverse effects. Each of these may be more difficult to attain for older adults.

The cornerstone to the management of asthma is control of triggers to prevent symptoms and maintain as near to normal lung function as possible (NIH, 1997). Pharmacological intervention is based on the treatment of acute and chronic manifestations of the illness. Medications include those administered on an as-needed basis using fast-acting broncho-

dilators and those with long-term agents that maintain bronchodilation and control inflammation. Inhaled medications may be taken a number of ways, including metered dose inhalers (MDIs), electric nebulizers, and dry powder inhalers. Several devices are available to facilitate effective drug administration, including spacers when coordination is limited or special devices for helping persons with hand limitations to manage the cylinders used to hold and release medications. Management of asthma in older adults is often complicated by the presence of other chronic disorders.

Tuberculosis. Tuberculosis (TB) is a communicable and infectious disease associated with one of several organisms— *Mycobacterium tuberculosis, Mycobacterium bovis,* and *Mycobacterium africanum.* The term *tuberculosis infection* refers to a positive TB skin test with no evidence of active disease. *Tuberculosis disease* refers to disease that has been documented with a positive acid-fast smear or culture for *M. tuberculosis* or radiographic and clinical presentation of TB.

It is estimated that one third of the world's population is infected with M. *tuberculosis* (Rajagopalan and Yoshikawa, 2000). M. *tuberculosis* was thought to be conquered in the 1950s with the development of the drug *isoniazid* (INH). Many of today's elders were treated after acquiring the disease during World War II. Others contracted the disease in childhood. As they become immunocompromised as a result of chemotherapy, extreme old age, or human immunodeficiency virus (HIV) infection, the bacterium could be reactivated.

The number of cases of TB in the United States has steadily decreased, with the lowest overall rate recorded in 2005, with infection found in only 4.8 persons per 100,000. However this low rate is because of the very low rate in white, natural citizens. The rate of persons born outside of the United States is 8.7 times higher. Between 2003 and 2005, 29 states and the District of Columbia reported decreased rates and 20 states reported increased rates. In absolute numbers, the most cases of TB are seen in black Americans, or 8.3 per 100,000. Asians and Pacific Islanders have the highest rate by percentage at 19.6% but lower overall numbers. In comparison, the rate is only 1.5 in white Americans (CDC, 2005b). Although these numbers are small, TB continues to be found in long-term care facilities in 42 of 52 reporting areas (50 states, District of Columbia, and New York City). The highest incidence in long-term care facilities in 2004 was in California (60), Florida (30), and Texas (35) (CDC, 2005a). Gerontological nurses working in these areas need to be particularly knowledgeable about this potentially life-threatening disease.

Etiology. As just noted, TB is an infection from an identified pathogen. It is transmitted from person to person by airborne droplets (Brashers, 2006b). Persons who are immunosuppressed, who are from areas with high infection rates, or who live in group settings are at particular risk. Older residents of congregate living settings are between two and seven times more likely to acquire the disease than those

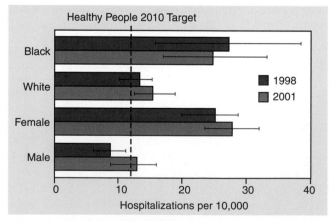

FIGURE 10-21 Asthma-related hospitalizations. *NOTE:* Data are age adjusted to the 2000 standard population. Black and white include persons of Hispanic or non-Hispanic origin. Persons were asked to select only one race category; selection of more than one race category was not an option in 1998. In 2001, persons reported one or more races. Data by race are shown for persons who reported one racial group. (Data from National Hospital Discharge Survey, NCHS, CDC. Redrawn from *www.cdc.gov/nchs/hphome.htm.* Focus area No. 24.)

who live in the community (Ferebee, 2006). The tuberculin bacilli in a person who has become infected may remain dormant for years or for life, only to be activated if the immune system becomes impaired. Although HIV is the greatest single risk factor for reactivation of the bacilli, other risk factors include cancer, renal failure, diabetes, long-term steroid therapy, and poor nutritional status (Brashers, 2006b).

Signs and Symptoms. Symptoms include unexplained weight loss or fever and a cough lasting more than 3 weeks, regardless of age-group. Night sweats and generalized anxiety may be present. In more advanced stages, the person will also have dyspnea, chest pain, and hemoptysis. Laboratory results in the elderly may show an increased sedimentation rate and lymphocytopenia. Because these signs and symptoms are associated with many disorders common in older adults, diagnosis often is during a health screening. For persons with positive skin tests, it is necessary to confirm a diagnosis with a chest film and sputum culture. The recent development of deoxyribonucleic acid (DNA) probes, polymerase chain reaction (PCR) assays, and liquid media now allows more sensitive and rapid diagnosis.

Management. The management of tuberculosis in older adults is one of ensuring the completion of a specific drug regimen. Successful completion of TB treatment in the elderly patient is complicated by a mortality of 22% during the first 3 months (Kaltenbach et al., 2001). Because of the toxicity of the medications and normal changes in the older liver and kidneys, the physiological status must be carefully evaluated before the initiation of the drug regimen, and during and afterward. For persons with TB living in the community, many municipalities require a system of direct observation of compliance. This means that a community health worker visits the person on a daily basis during the course of treatment to personally observe ingestion of the medications. Resolution of the infection is confirmed by repeat sputum culture, although bacterium are increasingly resistant to treatment.

▲ *Promoting Healthy Aging: Implications for Gerontological Nursing.* Nurses, especially public health nurses, are in the optimal position to promote healthy respiratory aging through prevention. This means playing an active role in smoking cessation education and intervention. It also means political activism with industry leaders and environmental agencies to push for clear air and water. In occupational settings, the nurse can contribute to the health of the workers by promoting healthy work environments and in some cases monitoring patients, residents, and employees for exposure to tuberculosis and treatment effectiveness for asthma. By doing these things, the nurse can decrease respiratory diseases and their associated morbidity and mortality.

The nurse can also have a large impact on the quality of life for the elder with COPD and his or her family members (Boxes 10-27 and 10-28). The nurse helps the person monitor symptoms and their effect on function and also educates

---

BOX 10-27 Suggestions in Caring for the Person with COPD

EMOTIONAL SUPPORT

Accept/encourage expression of emotions.
Be an active listener.
Be cognizant of conversational dyspnea; do not interrupt or cut off conversations.

EDUCATION

Teach breathing techniques:
- Pursed-lip breathing
- Diaphragmatic breathing
- Cascade coughing (series)

Teach postural drainage.
Teach about medications: what, why, frequency, amount, side effects, and what to do if side effects occur.
Teach use and care of inhalers and spacers and equipment.
Teach signs and symptoms of respiratory infection.
Teach about sexual activity:
- Sexual function improves with rest.
- Schedule sex around best breathing time of day.
- Use prescribed bronchodilators 20 to 30 minutes before sex.
- Use positions that do not require pressure on the chest or support of the arms.

COPD, Chronic obstructive pulmonary disease.

---

about the appropriate use of medications, oxygen, and exercise and the avoidance of triggers. The nurse encourages the person with COPD to remain as active as possible for as long as possible and to function as fully as possible within the limitations of the disease. When appropriate, the nurse can be instrumental in facilitating the services of a hospice when end-of-life care is needed.

The onset of asthma is often unavoidable. The key education needs are the identification and avoidance of triggers, the correct administration and appropriate adjustment of medications depending on the course of the disease, and the use of peak flow meters to monitor respiratory status.

Avoidance of infection for persons with either asthma or COPD is paramount to the prevention of complications, especially pneumonia. The nurse should encourage persons with these conditions to avoid persons with respiratory infections, practice good hand washing, and use preventive immunizations for influenza and pneumonia (Box 10-29).

In promoting healthy aging related to TB, the nurse has a responsibility to both the public and the individual. The nurse must be proactive in the prevention of contagious disease and in the prompt treatment of those who become or are ill. This is especially important in the long-term care setting. Elders in these settings are at higher risk because of communal living situations and the high rate of medical frailty. In 1990 the Centers for Disease Control and Prevention (CDC) recommended that every person entering a long-term care facility as a resident or an employee undergo annual testing for TB. In 2005 the guidelines were updated

BOX 10-28 Suggestions for Healthier Living with COPD

NUTRITION

Eat small, frequent, nutrient-intense meals.

Eat foods high in protein and calories.

Select foods that do not require a lot of chewing.

Have food cut in bite-size pieces to conserve energy.

Establish a plan for adequate consumption of fluid; drink 2-3 L of fluid daily (pineapple juice helps cut secretions; keep a liter of water in the refrigerator or on the kitchen counter to be consumed each day in addition to other fluids).

Weigh self at least twice a week.

EXERCISE

Walk daily all year round (in good weather, outdoors; in bad weather, go to the mall and walk indoors).

Walk up and down stairs in home (if present).

Use a stationary bicycle.

ACTIVITY PACING

Avoid high levels of exertion in early morning.

Arrange rest periods throughout day.

Allow ample time to complete activities; don't hurry.

Schedule activities in advance to reduce pressure and anxiety.

Obtain and follow prescribed exercise program for maintenance of heart/lung capacity.

ADLs

Allow ample time for bathing and dressing. Have a chair in bathroom for bathing.

Arrange toiletries within easy reach.

When buying shoes for activity and everyday wear, avoid shoes that require bending over to tie; instead, get slip-on type and use a long-handled shoehorn to assist the heel into shoe.

Select clothing with elasticized waistbands; avoid constrictive clothing; use suspenders rather than belts.

Select and wear clothing that is easy to put on and remove.

BETTER BREATHING

Attempt to keep a dust-free environment.

Minimize or eliminate use of aerosol sprays, fumes, contaminants, dander.

Place plastic covers over mattresses; use hypoallergenic pillows and blankets.

Avoid carpet and rug floor coverings.

Wear scarf over nose and mouth in cold and windy weather.

Avoid going out when air pollution is high.

Use air conditioner to filter air and make it drier; change or clean filter regularly.

Avoid situations in which you may encounter individuals with influenza or upper respiratory infections.

PREVENTIVE STRATEGIES

Obtain an annual flu vaccination unless contraindicated.

Obtain multivalent pneumococcal immunization at intervals directed by health care provider.

Notify health care provider of any temperature above 99° F.

Examine sputum; recognize and report changes to provider.

Do not use over-the-counter drugs unless approved.

ADLs, Activities of daily living.

considerably to reflect the changes in both incidence and prevalence in different geographic areas. To ensure prompt identification of persons with TB and limit its spread, especially in the long-term or extended-care facility, nurses should develop and implement an appropriate surveillance plan (Box 10-30). If such a plan is not already in place, the CDC and the state health departments are excellent sources of guidance and assistance.

TB is a reportable condition, which means that all suspected and confirmed cases are reported to the local or state health authorities (Chesnutt and Prendergast, 2006). The local public health nurses usually conduct investigations to ensure that all potentially infected people have been tested and that all persons with the disease receive treatment (Box 10-31). The nurse actively participates in health screenings that may include TB testing. As a health care provider, the nurse is also at risk for acquiring the infection and needs to be screened regularly to prevent becoming a carrier.

Nurses have a role in monitoring laboratory values, assessing for adverse drug reactions, and monitoring drug compliance in persons with TB, all of which are crucial to treatment effectiveness and the patient's well-being. The gerontological nurse in the congregate living setting partici-

pates in screening, educating regarding the seriousness of the infection, and helping persons obtain the appropriate treatment as needed.

Rheumatological Disorders

The older adult often experiences chronic rheumatological disorders, especially osteoarthritis, rheumatoid arthritis, and gout. All three have the potential to significantly affect the older adult's ability to navigate the environment. As such, they are addressed with the discussion of mobility in Chapter 15. A fourth condition, polymyalgia rheumatica (PMR), affects not only mobility but also one's overall comfort; it is addressed in Chapter 15 also. Another rheumatological disorder is giant cell (temporal) arteritis (GCA). Although it is more of an acute condition than a chronic disease, the onset can be gradual and is addressed here.

Giant Cell (Temporal) Arteritis. GCA is a granulomatous inflammation of the aorta and its branches and the cranial arteries. It affects primarily persons older than 50 years (Hellmann and Stone, 2006). The typical person with GCA is white, female, and older than 70 years (Blumenthal, 2004). It is rare in African-Americans or in those of Hispanic descent (O'Rourke, 2003). About half of those with GCA will

---

BOX 10-29 Healthy People 2010 Objectives Related to Influenza and Pneumococcal Disease Vaccines

OBJECTIVES APPLICABLE FOR NON-INSTITUTIONALIZED ADULTS AGE 65 YEARS AND OLDER*

Objective 14-29a
Increase the number of persons over 65 who receive an annual influenza vaccination
Target: 90%
Baseline (1998): 64%

Objective 14-29b
Increase the number of persons over 65 who have received a pneumococcal vaccination
Target: 90%
Baseline (1998): 46%

OBJECTIVES APPLICABLE FOR ADULTS AGE 65 YEARS AND OLDER WHO RESIDE IN LONG-TERM CARE SETTINGS†

Objective 14-29e
Increase the number of persons over 65 who receive an annual influenza vaccination
Target: 90%
Baseline (1997): 59%

Objective 14-29f
Increase the number of persons over 65 who have received a pneumococcal vaccination
Target: 90%
Baseline (1997): 25%

From U.S. Department of Health and Human Services: *Healthy People 2010: national health promotion and disease prevention objectives,* Washington, DC, 2000, The Department. Data from National Health Interview Survey (NHIS), Centers for Disease Control and Prevention (CDC) and National Center for Health Statistics (NCHS)—noninstitutionalized populations; NNHS, CDC, NCHS—institutionalized populations.
*Age adjusted to the year 2000 standard population.
†National Nursing Home Survey (NNHS) estimates include a significant number of residents who have an unknown vaccination status. See *Tracking Healthy People 2010* for further discussion of the data issues *(www.healthypeople2010.gov).*

BOX 10-30 Surveillance Guidelines for Tuberculosis in the Long-Term Care Setting*,†

- Each facility should have an individual responsible for TB infection control and an infection prevention and control plan.
- Each facility should conduct a TB risk assessment on a regularly scheduled basis that considers both patients/residents and health care workers (low moderate and high risk).
- Determine the need for TB screening based on the results of the risk assessments.
- For low risk settings:
  - Screen all new residents on admission and employees on hire for symptoms, and consider using the two-step

  TST (tuberculin skin test) or BAMT (blood assay for *M. tuberculosis*).
- Repeat annually.
- For those who test positive or have had a positive test in the past, one chest radiograph and annual review of symptoms rather than repeat of film.
- No persons with a diagnosis of TB should remain in a long-term care facility unless adequate administrative and environmental controls and a respiratory protection program is in place.

*For more details, see the CDC report Guidelines for preventing the transmission of *Mycobacterium tuberculosis* in health-care settings, 2005. *MMWR 54*(RR17): 1-141, 2005; also available on the CDC website *www.cdc.gov.*
†Each state public health unit provides guidelines and directions specific to the geographic area and the known risk estimates.

---

develop PMR (see Chapter 15). Initial diagnosis is made empirically and confirmed with a biopsy of the temporal artery.

Etiology. The cause of GCA is unknown, but studies have suggested that it is an antigen-driven disease with cell-mediated immune response to ischemia or necrosis downstream from the affected site (O'Rourke, 2003).

Signs and Symptoms. The classic local symptoms are headache and scalp tenderness. Typical systemic symptoms are fatigue, malaise, weight loss, and fever. When coupled with visual disturbances, jaw claudication, or throat pain, the situation is considered a medical emergency because of the possibility of ensuing blindness. The temporal artery may be nodular, enlarged, pulseless, and tender but also may be within normal limits. When the pulses of the arms are asymmetrical,

a new aortic murmur is heard, or bruits are heard near the clavicle, the aorta may be involved. Large vessels may become involved years after a diagnosis in about one fourth of persons with GCA. Almost half of all persons have atypical signs; these include dry cough, paralysis of the shoulder, or fever of unknown origin (FUO). GCA may account for up to 15% of all cases of FUO. People with FUO and GCA may be differentiated from those with an infection by an elevated erythrocyte sedimentation rate (ESR) and a normal white blood cell (WBC) count, but interpretation of these findings may be confounded in the older adult (see Chapter 5) (Hellmann and Stone, 2006).

Complications. The most important complication of GCA is sudden blindness, which can be prevented with prompt treatment.

BOX 10-31   **Clinical Note: Community Nursing and Persons with Tuberculosis, First Person**

As a young public health nurse, it was my responsibility to periodically check on all persons in my assigned district who were undergoing treatment for tuberculosis (TB). A new person had moved into one of the many boarding houses of this inner-city neighborhood. Mr. Jones was a pleasant, robust 60-year-old who expressed pleasure in the visit and reported that he was doing well, had plenty of medications and that they were not causing him any problems. He dashed out of the room, returned with a small suitcase, and opened it for me to assure me of his supply, and there before me were dozens of unopened bottles of isoniazid (INH), one of the staples of TB treatment. I called the medical director, who recommended that Mr. Jones be sent to the local hospital and, to make sure he got there, to deliver him forthwith. So I loaded him and his suitcase into my car and away we went; thinking of what Florence Nightingale would say, I left the windows open wide. When I returned to the health department, my first stop was for a TB test for myself and the plans for a follow-up after the incubation period. All for the sake of community well-being!

Kathleen Jett

Management. The most critical aspect of management of GCA is diagnosis. Once GCA is diagnosed, curative interventions can be initiated. The use of high-dose corticosteroids is the standard treatment (Blumenthal, 2004). Treatment may take up to 2 years.

▲ **Promoting Healthy Aging: Implications for Gerontological Nursing.** For the best outcomes, persons with GCA need prompt treatment. However, the treatment requires the long-term use of corticosteroids and between 30% and 50% of patients develop steroid-associated toxicities at some time during treatment. An important role for the nurse is to be alert for signs of the disease so that the person can get the needed treatment and for signs of complications of the treatment itself. For the frail elder, this is especially important.

COPING WITH CHRONIC HEALTH PROBLEMS

Promoting healthy aging is possible at any age, from working with teenagers to get enough calcium at they approach their peak bone mass to minimize the risk for later osteoporosis (see Chapter 15), to leading smoking cessation or clean air campaigns to minimize the eventual development of COPD. Promoting healthy aging also means being aware of special considerations that almost universally need attention and must be addressed actively by nurses and other members of the health care team. The following discussion addresses several of these, not as a comprehensive coverage of the topic but as a touchstone for further examination and discussion. Pain, which is common in some conditions, is discussed in Chapter 11.

Gender

Women typically live longer than men, more frequently live alone, and have greater financial limitations with which they must cope (see Chapter 21). Before the 1990s, the majority of research related to chronic conditions and their related medications was conducted on men (especially white men) and extrapolated to women and persons of color. Also, significantly less work was done on understanding the health issues specific to women, such as menopause and the use of hormone replacement therapy. In the landmark study of health disparities documented in the manuscript "Unequal Treatment" (Smedley et al., 2003; www.iom.gov), women were found to experience considerable disparities in health care outcomes.

We now have good evidence that women are evaluated less intensely and diagnosed and referred less frequently than men for many problems, including those of a cardiac origin. Although CVD is the number-one cause of death for both men and women, women have been found to receive fewer of the "standard interventions" than men, including thrombolytic therapy, aspirin, heparin, and beta-blockers. They are also less likely to undergo cardiac catheterization and bypass graft surgery. We also know that women may have slightly different signs and symptoms of both heart disease and other common problems (Endoy, 2004).

In April 1991, Dr. Bernadine Healy, then Director of the National Institutes of Health (NIH), attempted to address some of these issues when she launched the Women's Health Initiative (WHI) to examine the most common causes of death, disability, and impaired quality of life in postmenopausal women. This was the first multi-site study of its size specifically designed for older women. Originally scheduled for completion in 2006, in 2001 the study was interrupted temporarily because of surprising findings in the part of the study examining hormone replacement therapy (HRT). Previous studies had used observational data to suggest that HRT protected women from a number of problems, especially heart disease. The mid-study report from the WHI refuted these observations, finding that although HRT did slightly decrease a woman's risk for colorectal cancer and hip fractures, it increased her risk for coronary heart disease, stroke, and pulmonary embolism. Almost overnight the health care of postmenopausal women changed (Brucker and Youngkin, 2002). Only now are these findings and their implications being understood.

Sexuality

Sexual problems and misinformation are pervasive in society in spite of the high levels of exposure to knowledge about sex and the near constant exposure to sexuality in the media, schools, and politics. In spite of this, little attention has been paid to those who are living daily with chronic disorders that have the potential to interrupt or interfere with sexual functioning and the fundamental feelings of sexual attractiveness. In the older adult, the problem is exacerbated by the commonly held belief that older people are asexual.

Contrary to popular myth, research has shown that older couples report a steady level of interest, activity, and satisfaction with sexual activity and that the greatest impediment to sexual activity of some kind is lack of a partner, especially for women (see Chapter 19). Greater sexual activity and satisfaction are associated with open and positive attitudes toward sexuality, greater sexual knowledge, satisfaction with a relationship, supportive social networks, psychological well-being, and a sense of self-worth (Zeiss and Kasl-Godley, 2001). Much of our information on sexuality is based on research conducted with Caucasian older adults. Further research is needed related to sexuality and sexual behavior of ethnic elders and older gay, lesbian, bisexual, and transgender adults (Zeiss and Kasl-Godley, 2001).

Chronic illnesses and medical interventions can have direct and indirect effects on sexual function (Steinke, 2005). Various disorders may produce mechanical problems, erectile problems, decreased libido, and limited mobility. Certain disorders involving ostomies and incontinence may produce reticence in both partners. Discussing and assessing medication regimens, the expected dysfunctions that accompany particular diseases, and the individual's expectations are all important in promoting healthy aging. A sexual history may provide important clues regarding the individual's needs and desires. The nurse is most effective when open and accepting in discussing the person's sexuality and in providing information and resources appropriate to the situation (see Chapter 19).

Fatigue

Fatigue is a common complaint of persons living on the chronic illness trajectory, especially as the number of chronic illnesses grows. It is often variable and unpredictable and either ignored or incorrectly assumed a normal part of the aging process. Instead, fatigue may be a symptom of the illness, a side effect of a medication, or a symptom of depression, or all of these.

In promoting healthy aging, the most important intervention of the gerontological nurse may be to validate the reality and debilitating effects of the disorder if and when it occurs. It is also important to help the person differentiate a treatable depression that may be superimposed on the fatigue of chronic illness. Discussing patterns of fatigue and identifying the precipitants are important. If the elder can be engaged in keeping a log of the low points of energy, it may prove useful. It is also helpful to emphasize the wisdom of the body and balance rest and activity within limitations to help conserve energy for activities that are most important or necessary.

Energy to enjoy life's activities becomes more precious with advancing age. Chronic problems tax this existing energy level. Direct assistance by caregivers or families may be necessary to aid the older adult in exploring lifestyle adaptations that decrease energy expenditure and permit continued involvement in valued interests. Throughout this process, the older adult with a disability must remain involved in decision making on every level of need. The older adult may have different priorities from those of the caregiver. Elderly clients may relegate their health needs to a lower priority to fulfill other needs or life demands. One must understand and respect the priorities established by the elder as a competent adult. Nurses listen carefully to human needs and determine which of these are most important. People with chronic illnesses are the "experts" on managing their illnesses and lifestyle, with nurses as their collaborators.

Grieving

Grieving the loss of appearance, function, independence, and comfort may occupy much of one's time initially when adapting to and coming to terms with a chronic illness, particularly if the onset has been abrupt and the loss interferes directly with a major source of one's pleasure. As the mother with a handicapped newborn mourns the loss of the visualized "perfect" infant, the elder may begin to memorialize the "perfect" self that no longer exists. The earlier image of the self may grow far beyond the reality that existed. The nurse's function is to encourage verbalization, talk with the elder about the lost self, recognize the grief that may be occurring, and help re-frame the new self. Clearly, grief reactions will be highly individual, depending on the significance of the loss and the number of additional losses with which the individual is attempting to cope (see Chapter 26).

One may feel a sense of failure or weakness as a cause of the chronic disorder, as if it could be willed away by strength of mind, determination, and courage. Suffering in chronic illness is compounded by a sense of responsibility for remaining healthy, especially in the current wellness climate (Benner et al., 1994). There is often the persistent thought that hard work and adherence to a strict treatment regimen will bring about cure, and when that does not occur, a sense of shame develops (Doolittle, 1994). This is a serious problem that is deeply rooted in the work ethic that has been so cultivated in the older generation, and it may affect an elder's willingness to seek and accept help. However, significant cultural variations exist (Jett, 2002).

Given these tendencies, it is imperative that the nurse not overtly or covertly reinforce the elder's sense of personal failure. Living with a chronic illness is a process that is continually changing as one adapts to the grief of the lost self and learns to embrace the needs and beauty of the emerging self.

Family

Most persons share their lives in some way with persons whom they consider "family" (see Chapter 20). Families deal with changes within their members across the length of their lives and relationships. Just like the individual, the family adjusts to the chronic disease, with adjustments in roles, capabilities, resources, and identity. Families provide the majority of care to persons with disabilities. In some cultures, care-giving is an expectation; in others, it is considered a burden (Jett, 2006). Although gerontologists have extensively examined the "burden" of care-giving, the joys of care-giving are being increasingly contemplated, including the concept of a "giving back" to a loved one. This topic is dealt with in some detail in Chapter 20.

Locating Care

Although not everyone with a chronic condition will have a related disability, many will, especially as they age. Persons older than 85 years report the highest level of need of any group, both in the use of assistive devices and in the personal care related to a limitation in an ADL or IADL (Figure 10-22). More than a million elders indicate that they need and receive active assistance with bathing, dressing, and toileting. For those able to manage these basic ADLs, other need active or intermittent help with IADLs such as grocery shopping, money management, and laundry. Short and Leon (1990) reported that those who use home and community services are usually older than 85 years, female, living alone, and having difficulty with several activities.

The majority of this assistance is in the form of informal care, or that which is provided on a voluntary basis, usually within the context of the family setting (Figure 10-23). This care may be supplemented, depending on the needs and resources, by formal services such as home health, hospice, or respite care and home-delivered meals or meals provided in community adult day health centers.

When the home setting for care is not possible, group residential settings such as assisted living facilities, nursing facilities, skilled nursing facilities, and hospices are sought (Figure 10-24). Persons are also cared for in the acute care settings at the onset of a chronic condition such as after a stroke or a myocardial infarction or during exacerbations of the chronic condition. The supportive assistance of aides, therapists, and registered nurses is available in each of these settings. Regardless of the context, the goals are the same—maximizing the quality of life lived, maintaining the highest level of independence possible, and preventing exacerbations of the on-going illnesses.

The nurse's role in the promotion of healthy aging and helping elders cope with chronic illness in a variety of settings was discussed throughout this chapter. The nurse can further this approach when working with elders and their families by helping them find the right level of care in the least restrictive setting possible. This means helping them find the assistance that will facilitate independence rather than dependence. It also means helping the person and family with anticipatory planning such as living wills and durable powers of attorney (see Chapter 17).

Prevention of Iatrogenic Complications

While the nurse is working to reduce the complications of the chronic illness itself, a secondary risk increases—that of iatrogenesis (that which is a complication or by-product of the health care intervention itself). The majority of emphasis has been on control of the potential deleterious

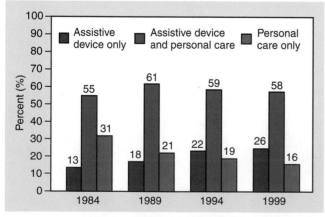

FIGURE 10-22 Distribution of Medicare enrollees ages 65 years and older using assistive devices. *NOTE:* Personal care refers to paid or unpaid assistance provided to a person with a chronic disability living in the community. Reference population: these data refer to Medicare enrollees living in the community who report receiving personal care from a paid or unpaid helper, or using assistive devices, or both, for a chronic disability. (Data from National Long Term Care Survey. Redrawn from AOA Chartbook [website]: *www.aoa.gov.*)

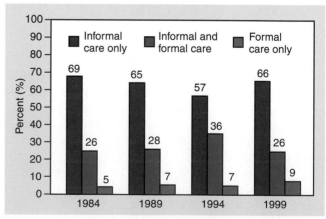

FIGURE 10-23 Distribution of Medicare enrollees ages 65 years and older receiving personal care by type. *NOTE:* Informal care refers to unpaid assistance provided to a person with chronic disability living in the community. Formal care refers to paid assistance. Reference population: these data refer to Medicare enrollees living in the community who report receiving personal care from a paid or unpaid helper for a chronic disability. (Data from National Long Term Care Survey. Redrawn from AOA Chartbook [website]: *www.aoa.gov.*)

effects of hospitalization, yet iatrogenesis can develop in any setting (Box 10-32). The person may become incontinent with the addition of a potent diuretic, not because of a new physiological problem but from the increase in urinary frequency without an increased access to toileting facilities. A new medication may cause depression, fatigue, or erectile dysfunction while improving the control of the underlying illness. Elders with some functional disabilities may find themselves completely dependent during an acute illness. The use of warfarin to prevent stroke can cause a life-ending subdural hematoma if the person has a head injury from a fall or a game of football with a grandchild.

Whenever a negative change is likely or occurs after an intervention, the nurse can be proactive in working with the care team in identifying the potential or actual effect and facilitating a cost-benefit discussion with the person and his or her significant other (Box 10-33).

Fostering Self-Care

In the day-to-day life of the person with chronic illness, self-care skills are of the greatest importance. Nurse theorist Dorothy Orem has provided us with a useful language and taxonomy for both understanding and responding to call from persons with self-care needs (1980, 1995).

According to Orem, each person has self-care needs called *universal self-care requisites*. Each person also develops self-care capacity, or the ability to meet these requisites. However, in some circumstances, the needs exceed

---

BOX 10-32   Common Iatrogenic Problems Associated with an Institutional Stay

- Loss of mobility because of insufficient ambulation
- Incontinence because of inattention when needed; sometimes becoming a permanent problem
- Confusion or delirium caused by medications, treatments, anesthesia, and translocation
- Pressure ulcers caused by immobility and reduced sensation
- Dehydration caused by limited access to fluids
- Fluid overload caused by improper use of intravenous fluids
- Nosocomial infections caused by infectious agents in surroundings
- Urinary tract infections caused by catheter usage
- Upper respiratory tract infections caused by immobility and shallow breathing and aspiration of oral secretions
- Fluid and electrolyte imbalances caused by medications and treatments
- Falls because of unfamiliar environment, weakness, and positional instability
- Impaired sleep because of treatments and environment
- Malnutrition caused by anorexia and insufficient assistance in eating

---

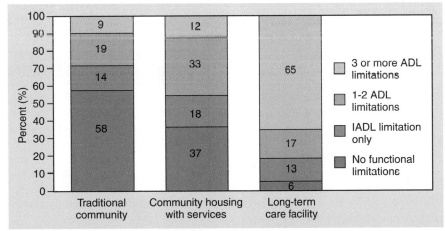

FIGURE 10-24 Percentage of Medicare enrollees ages 65 years and older with functional limitations by setting, 2002. *NOTE:* Community housing with services applies to respondents who reported they lived in retirement communities or apartments, senior citizen housing, continuing care retirement facilities, assisted living facilities, staged living communities, board and care facilities/homes, and other similar situations, AND who reported they had access to one or more of the following services through their place of residence: meal preparation, cleaning or housekeeping services, laundry services, help with medications. Respondents were asked about access to these services but not whether they actually used the services. A residence is considered a long-term care facility if it is certified by Medicare or Medicaid; or has three or more beds and is licensed as a nursing home or other long-term care facility and provides at least one personal care service; or provides 24-hour, 7-day-a-week supervision by a caregiver. Instrumental activity of daily living (IADL) limitations refer to difficulty performing (or inability to perform, for a health reason) one or more of the following tasks: using the telephone, light housework, heavy housework, meal preparation, shopping, managing money. Activity of daily living (ADL) limitations refer to difficulty performing (or inability to perform, for a health reason) the following tasks: bathing, dressing, getting in/out of chairs, walking, using the toilet. Long-term care facility residents with no limitations may include individuals with limitations in certain IADLs: doing light or heavy housework or meal preparation. These questions were not asked of facility residents. Reference population: these data refer to Medicare enrollees. (Data from Centers for Medicare and Medicaid Services, Medicare Current Beneficiary Survey. Redrawn from AOA Chartbook [website]: *www.aoa.gov.*)

the individual's capacity to meet them and a self-care deficit ensues in which an individual is unable to carry out basic functions without assistance. These deficits are primarily the result of pathophysiological disorders that impinge on neuromuscular, musculoskeletal, or sensory integrity, but they can also have a psychological or spiritual origin. They can also be the result of changes in neurological functioning or even iatrogenesis as just noted.

The appropriate nursing approach is highly individualized and may involve changing the environment, modifying the treatment, or teaching the individual strategies to compensate for the pathophysiological changes. The impact of chronic illness is also highly individual and may include identity erosion, expectation of death, dependency conflicts, and feelings of failure and fatalism.

Many of the largest health maintenance organization (HMO) providers now offer reimbursement for alternative medicine therapies such as therapeutic massage, touch therapy, acupuncture, chiropractic, biofeedback, homeopathy, and naturopathy. This trend arises from studies showing that alternative medicine is less expensive, results in fewer hospitalizations, and tends to be used by individuals who are more concerned about managing their own health in a holistic manner. Now it is possible for more individuals to direct their own care, order their own special supplies without provider approval, and, in many cases, purchase some medications over the counter. Nursing will be called on to obtain background information and to help to sort out options in self-care management. The nurse can also be instrumental in fostering self-care efficacy. Two strategies for fostering effective self-care that are receiving attention are the use of small groups and telephone/electronic follow-up.

Small Group Approaches. Small group meetings are among the most effective and economic ways of assisting clients to meet informational and psychosocial needs. They can also be designed to provide family support and counseling. Self-help groups can be seen as support systems, consumer participant systems, expressive-social influence groups, or homogeneously identified therapeutic groups. Facilitating adjustment to new roles and activities and redefinition of self and meanings constitute a large part of working with groups (Box 10-34).

Some of the most successful groups have been those in which the members identify topics and issues on which they

---

BOX 10-33   Minimizing the Effects of Institutionalization on Frail Elders

STAFF EDUCATION

Mental and functional status assessment
Management of sensoriperceptual function

MOBILITY

Environmental modifications

ORIENTATION AND COMMUNICATION

Use of cues and repetition
Discussion of condition
Providing anticipatory guidance regarding procedures
Reassurance regarding likelihood of delirium

MOBILIZATION

Getting patients up, out of bed, and out of room
Involving physical and occupational therapy in exercise

ENVIRONMENTAL MODIFICATIONS

Glasses and hearing aids available and working well.
   Calendars
Favorite programs on radio and TV available
Increased lighting, night-lights from dusk until dawn

CAREGIVER EDUCATION AND CONSULTATION

Ask families to bring in significant items; photos

MEDICATION MANAGEMENT

Review medication daily; discourage prescribers from
   ordering medications that are contraindicated in
   the older patient, especially neuroleptics and anticholinergics, which tend to exacerbate delirium
   (see Chapter 12)

DISCHARGE PLANNING

At least weekly case conferences with primary nurse,
   social worker, physical and occupational therapists,
   nutritionist, and discharge planner

BOX 10-34   Working with Small Groups Related to Health Promotion and Risk Reduction

1. Develop a therapeutic provider-participant partnership with group members.
2. Set ground rules related to confidentiality and respect.
3. Make a concerted effort to respond to the educational needs of each member of the group.
4. Do not assume that participants understand the association between certain behaviors and health.
5. Help participants identify obstacles to changing behaviors.
6. Ask participant to select one risk factor to address at a time and to commit to change.
7. Ask participant to identify measurable and realistic outcomes and an acceptable action plan.
8. Use multiple educational strategies, including counseling classes, written materials, audiovisual aids, and community resources. Individualized, personalized, and prioritized interventions are most effective.
9. Monitor progress through close follow-up in the group setting.
10. Find ways to celebrate change and accomplishments.
11. At all times, role-model healthy living.

wish to focus. The first meeting sets the tone and expectations for the group, including ground rules. The group facilitator gathers information, brochures, and other resources that may be valuable to share based on the expressed interest of the group. In addition to information, many groups related to chronic illness address psychological issues, such as the following:

1. Fears about incapacitation, pain, abandonment, isolation, and death
2. Expressions of low self-esteem and loss of confidence
3. Feelings of helplessness and uselessness; a desire to be whole and well again
4. A desire to fit into the family system once again
5. Willingness to redefine role relationships with significant others
6. A desire to face and handle public situations without fear or embarrassment

Technological Care. Fueled in part by what we have learned with heart failure clinics, in part with organizations' desire for "customer satisfaction," and in part because of cost-saving, telephone and electronic follow-up and support for patients with both acute and chronic health problems are gaining a place in the health care arena. Many organizations, including HMOs, insurance companies, and practice settings, are making telephone and e-mail/Internet contact possible. Often the first line of contact is with a nurse who consoles, supports, instructs, and refers callers or groups of callers. The caller may be the elder or a caregiver, with specific support provided as needed.

A new distance technology is the growing field of "telemedicine" including remote electronic monitoring of patients. Already found in more rural settings, this has broad usefulness to improve both the care and the timeliness of the care. A home health nurse may see a patient discharged home after an acute exacerbation of heart failure. The nurse completes a through assessment, records it on a handheld computer, and automatically transmits it to the other nurses who may respond to a call and the elder's health care provider. A specialized chair is placed in the home, and the elder is instructed to sit on it each morning. Automated blood pressure, pulse, and weight are taken at a preset time, and the information is sent automatically to the home health office and the provider's office over the patient's phone line. The home health nurse is quickly alerted to potential problems, including a missed "chair appointment," and the provider can make rapid changes to the medical plan of care as needed. A revolution in health care that may extend the lives of persons at home is underway.

Use of Adaptive and Assistive Devices

Many varieties of adaptive eating and homemaking devices are available to compensate for self-care deficits caused by arthritis, stroke, reduced hearing or vision, diminished strength, and other impairments (Figure 10-25). About 71% of all assistive devices are used by individuals older than 65 years. The most common devices used by the elderly are (in rank order) handrails (65%), canes (49%), hearing aids (38%), raised toilets (30%), hospital beds (24%), and walkers (24%). Overall, 63% of the payment for these items is out-of-pocket.

In the ideal situation, an occupational therapist conducts a comprehensive assessment of the self-care capacity and adaptive needs of the individual and matches the equipment to the person. However, not all situations are ideal and the gerontological nurse must also have a working knowledge of the most common resources available. Like that just noted, the technology in this field is changing radically; assistive devices include computerized training programs, programmed pillboxes, and robotic aids. Voice-activated computer programs are now highly developed and can assist elders who are completely disabled to accomplish many things. Speech synthesis and telecommunication devices are available for the verbally and orally handicapped. Electronic monitors can locate the person at risk for becoming lost.

Each year more training is required for families and professionals simply to use the equipment; in addition, as this equipment becomes more sophisticated, it often becomes too expensive for most elders. The challenge of the future is to make the technologically advanced equipment and services available and accessible to those who would benefit, regardless of ability to pay.

REHABILITATION AND RESTORATIVE CARE

Restorative and rehabilitative care is that which is provided under the guiding assumption that the care and services are thoughtfully designed to capitalize on the person's needs and strengths in a manner that will help him or her achieve the "highest practicable level of function" (Klusch, 1995). Rehabilitation services take place in the "acute" setting of a rehabilitation hospital and to a significantly lesser extent in skilled nursing facilities and at home. What is called "restorative care" follows the basic principles of "rehabilitative care," with the focus of the former on maintenance and the latter on improvement.

Considerations in Planning Rehabilitation Care

The rehabilitative plan often begins in the acute care setting and continues into long-term care settings, the community, and persons' homes. Rehabilitation is long term. The following issues are considered in the planning:

1. The person is in a crisis when admitted to the hospital, and personal strengths are not always visible or easily assessed.
2. Multidisciplinary discharge planning must begin on admission, and a nurse or case manager should be assigned to each client who will need rehabilitation.

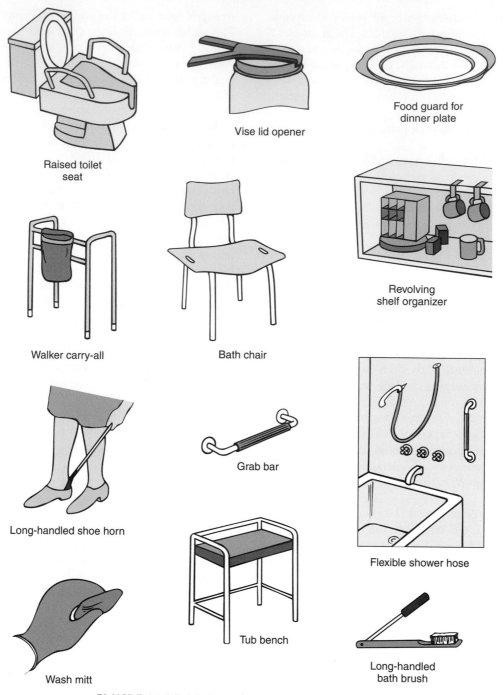

Raised toilet seat

Vise lid opener

Food guard for dinner plate

Walker carry-all

Bath chair

Revolving shelf organizer

Long-handled shoe horn

Grab bar

Flexible shower hose

Wash mitt

Tub bench

Long-handled bath brush

FIGURE 10-25 Adaptive equipment commonly used in the home.

3. Anxiety impairs learning during hospitalizations, yet some people are more motivated toward change when physical status is threatened.

4. A quick discharge to home or a nursing home will occur whenever possible; for the frail elder, this may occur sooner than he or she is ready for the level of activity required in a specialized rehabilitative setting.

Comprehensive interdisciplinary assessment is critical to the rehabilitation plan, working alongside the elder and family (Box 10-35). The total assessment includes a comprehensive bio-psycho-social history and a care plan with long- and short-term goals. Weekly interdisciplinary team/patient/family conferences are held to evaluate the person's progress, revision of goals if needed, and discharge plans.

BOX 10-35   Members of the Rehabilitation Care Team

- Rehabilitation nurse specialist
- Physical therapist
- Occupational therapist
- Speech therapist
- Social worker
- Discharge planner
- Psychologist
- Prosthetist and orthotist
- Audiologist
- Physician/nurse practitioner
- Vocational rehabilitation specialist
- Person in rehabilitation
- Person's significant others

The best of the gerontological rehabilitation units being developed now under various funding mechanisms (usually demonstration projects) are specifically designed to foster function and teach individuals how to influence their environment to adapt to whatever their disability may be. These are also the units in which health care providers become most acutely aware of the need for interdisciplinary teamwork and planning. Resnick and Fleishell (2002) report on a "restorative care unit" developed by the Department of Medicine at the University of Maryland that is designed to bridge the gap between acute care and home care. In the 6 years of the unit's existence, orthopedic procedures have been the major reason for admission to the unit. Individuals with joint replacements, fractures, stroke, amputations, and arthritis make up most of the clientele. More than 86% of the individuals are discharged to home, and 80% of those are able to remain there for 2 years or longer. Many more restorative care units are expected to emerge along the lines of this model. The National Council on the Handicapped recognizes the increasing problems of secondary and iatrogenically induced disabilities, such as pressure ulcers, contractures, and cognitive impairment, as important issues that must be considered in any future rehabilitation models.

Rehabilitation and the Future

It is estimated that 5 million severely disabled persons older than 65 years are in the United States, and this number is expected to increase as we increase the life span of the individual. Unfortunately, rehabilitative services are very expensive and face increasing restriction on who is eligible for payment for them under Medicare and other insurance plans, with the exception of the demonstration projects just noted. Instead, there is a movement toward a lowered level of care that has the potential to negatively affect elders for years to come.

Many could live independently with rehabilitative and supportive services, but because a return to employability is one of the driving forces in reimbursement, little assistance may be available when there is only slight or little expectation of improvement. Lack of education in rehabilitation among health care professionals in acute care settings has resulted in inadequate care and even further disabilities. Many health care professionals poorly understand the potential of rehabilitative care. Better education, appropriate policies and protocols, and definitions of roles in rehabilitative care for allied health professionals are needed to bring rehabilitative care into the mainstream of the health care system.

In the future, we expect wider acceptance of rehabilitation by all professionals and increased integration of its principles into all nursing, medical, and social activities. Effective rehabilitation for the older adult with disabilities is consistent with the philosophy that all persons should have the opportunity for optimal personal development and function. The result of limited accessibility to appropriate rehabilitation is increased dependence on family, nursing homes, or other care providers at an even greater personal and societal cost. The agenda for rehabilitation in the twenty-first century includes increased numbers of rehabilitation hospitals, improved reimbursement, and rehabilitation education programs.

Nurses advocating for the needs of the elderly and disabled, armed with clinical examples, anecdotal evidence, and empirical research findings, have the power to affect the character of public policy, as has been shown by the responsiveness of Congress to the lobbying power of nurses in Washington, D.C. Cost-effectiveness is the strongest argument in today's political climate. Continued emphasis on prevention of illness and disability, as evidenced by the goals of *Healthy People 2010*, is essential. As a result of such efforts, future generations of older adults may not face the consequences of chronic illness to the extent experienced today. How will their care be financed? What will happen to Medicare in the future? Will exorbitant home care costs be sustainable? Numerous questions need answers very soon.

SUMMARY

In summary, management of chronic problems in late life is an issue for the individual, the family, the nation, and the health care profession. Nurses work toward the achievement of the goals of *Healthy People 2010*. Nurses impact the quality of life for all persons with chronic diseases as they serve as resource persons, advisors, teachers, and, at times, facilitators (Box 10-36). The goals of care of persons with chronic illness are to slow decline, relieve discomfort, and support preferred lifestyle with as few restrictions as possible (Strauss and Glaser, 1975). The ability of the elder and the family to manage and cope with the problems encountered determines the need. It is necessary for those who participate in care to

---

BOX 10-36 Nurses' Role in Caring for Persons with Chronic Disease

- Assessing elder and family strengths and challenges
- Teaching related to healthy lifestyle modifications, preservation of energy, and self-care strategies
- Encouraging the reduction of modifiable risk factors
- Counseling individual in the development of reasonable expectations of self
- Providing access to resources when possible
- Referring appropriately and when needed
- Organizing and leading interdisciplinary case conferences and team meetings

---

be reoriented and re-socialized to self-care capacity in the presence of chronic illness and to recognize a different system of rewards.

The basics of the care process emphasize improving function, managing the existing illness, preventing secondary complications, delaying deterioration and disability, and facilitating death with peace, comfort, and dignity (Wells and Brink, 1980). Progress is not measured in attempts to achieve cure but, rather, in maintenance of a steady state or regression of the condition while remembering that the condition does not define the person. This thinking is essential if realistic expectations for the caregiver and the elder are to be achieved. The individual will in some manner seek to understand the meaning of the chronic disease and incorporate the old self-image with the new self-image. The nurse's involvement in this process is to ask about the meanings of the illness and to listen and learn.

Strauss and Corbin (1988) suggest that assisting individuals and their support persons to view chronic disorders as having a "trajectory" may help them cope with the ups and downs of the disorders, as well as the acute exacerbations. If they are able to better understand the phases of a disorder, they are likely to weather the difficult periods without undue discouragement. Often it must be seen as a lifetime situation that travels along a trajectory in which resources must be tailored accordingly. In summary, they suggest the following points that practitioners can consider:

1. Chronic illness must be seen through the eyes of the persons experiencing it.
2. The illness is often a lifelong course that passes through many phases.
3. Biographical, medical, spiritual, and everyday needs must be considered.
4. Collaborative rather than purely professional relationships may be most effective.

5. Lifelong support may be necessary, although the type, amount, and intensity of such support will vary.

KEY CONCEPTS

- The nation's goals include increasing the span of healthy life. The challenge to this is to help persons find ways to promote healthy aging in the presence of chronic disease.
- The effects of chronic illness range from mild to life-limiting, with each person responding to unique circumstances in a highly individualized manner.
- Coping with chronic illness can be a physical, psychological, and spiritual challenge.
- The Chronic Illness Trajectory and Maslow's Hierarchy of Needs offer useful frameworks from which to understand chronic illness and design nursing interventions.
- Cardiovascular diseases are the number-one cause of death and a frequent cause of disability in the older adult.
- The careful control of hypertension and diabetes has the potential to significantly improve health and minimize complications that have significant detrimental effects on the person.
- Most disorders that become chronic disease have atypical presentations in the older adult and may be attributed to normal aging, which delays the receipt of appropriate care and treatment.
- For most chronic diseases, optimal care includes an interdisciplinary team working closely with the elder and his or her family or significant others.
- The goals of promoting healthy aging include minimizing risk for disease, and in the presence of disease, alleviating symptoms, delaying or avoiding the development of complications including end-organ damage, and maximizing function and quality of life.
- The goals of rehabilitation are to ensure opportunity for optimal personal development and function. Though rehabilitation legislation is designed chiefly to return individuals to productive employment, this is not always compatible with the needs of the older adult.
- The gerontological nurse has the potential to serve as a leader in the promotion of health and the prevention of disease.
- The document *Healthy People 2010* serves as a guidepost for moving toward healthy aging in a healthy nation.

RESEARCH QUESTIONS

Is there any information that explains the differences in the incidence and prevalence of common chronic diseases in various ethnic groups?

Which of the chronic diseases discussed is most likely to interfere with an individual meeting his or her needs as defined by Maslow's hierarchy?

Can the trajectory model of Glaser and Strauss be used for situations other than living with a chronic disease?

Human Needs and Wellness Diagnoses

Self-Actualization and Transcendence
(Seeking, Expanding, Spirituality, Fulfillment)
Seeks meaning in illness and disorders
Surmounts impairments
Maintains values and optimism
Transcends the physical
Seeks knowledge and creative self-expression

Self-Esteem and Self-Efficacy
(Image, Identity, Control, Capability)
Exerts maximum control of self and environment
Maintains strong sense of identity regardless of impairment
Finds ways to express sexuality satisfactorily
Accepts altered body function or appearance
Maintains grooming
Copes effectively with exacerbations of disorders

Belonging and Attachment
(Love, Empathy, Affiliation)
Maintains important network of affiliations
Develops appropriate relationship with
health care providers
Keeps personal commitments
Devises ways to express reciprocity in relationships

Safety and Security
(Caution, Planning, Protections, Sensory Acuity)
Uses adaptive equipment safely
Uses mobility aids to maintain movement
Adheres to medical regimen
Monitors health and performs maintenance as needed
Demonstrates adequate health care

Biological and Physiological Integrity
(Air, Fluids, Comfort, Activity, Nutrition, Elimination, Skin Integrity)
Is attentive to shifts in bodily needs
Maintains intact skin
Has regular schedule of elimination
Has adequate fluid and fiber intake
Recognizes and responds to shifting energy demands

These are not all the possible wellness diagnoses that may be identified. The above
are examples of nursing diagnoses that should be considered when planning care
for the older adult.

CASE STUDY: Diabetes

Ms. P., an 82-year-old single woman, lives in a life-care community in her own apartment but has the reassurance of knowing her medical and functional needs will be taken care of regardless of the extent of these needs. This is the primary reason she chose to sell her home and move. She is at present independent. She has been gaining weight steadily since she moved into the community and attributes that to the fact that she eats much better now that she joins others in the congregate dining room for meals. She has diabetes, which she manages with diet, exercise, and oral medications; heart failure; and mild arthritis. Although she says she feels fine, lately she has noticed some increased fatigue and that her toes are cold and somewhat numb. The great toe on her left foot seems to be discolored. Because of the lack of feeling, she often walks around her apartment barefoot because it seems to increase the sensation in her feet. She has not needed to use the health care center and goes to the clinic only to pick up her medication. Her niece stopped by last week to see her and called the clinic and spoke with the nurse. The niece reported that her aunt seemed a little confused and lethargic. The niece accompanied Ms. P. to the clinic, where the nurses checked her blood pressure and blood sugar and found them to be 170/80 and 280 mg/dL, respectively. Ms. P. said, "Oh, I don't think it is anything to worry about! I am just a little tired."

Based on the case study, develop a nursing care plan using the following procedure*:

- List Mrs. P.'s comments that provide subjective data.
- List information that provides objective data.
- From these data, identify and state, using accepted format, two nursing diagnoses you determine are most significant to Mrs. P. at this time. List two of Mrs. P.'s strengths that you have identified from the data.

- Determine and state outcome criteria for each diagnosis. These must reflect some alleviation of the problem identified in the nursing diagnosis and must be stated in concrete and measurable terms.
- Plan and state one or more interventions for each diagnosed problem. Provide specific documentation of the source used to determine the appropriate intervention. Plan at least one intervention that incorporates Mrs. P.'s existing strengths.
- Evaluate the success of the intervention. Interventions must correlate directly with the stated outcome criteria to measure the outcome success.

Critical Thinking Questions

1. How would you explain that the number one cause of death worldwide is heart disease?
2. What risk factors do you have for heart disease, and what can you do to reduce them?
3. What thoughts do you have on the persistent disparities in health outcomes between white persons and persons of color?
4. What commonly held beliefs about aging would lead Ms. P. to believe that the changes in her health did not warrant seeking health care?
5. Of all of the symptoms that Ms. P. reports, which one should the nurse be most concerned about related to Ms. P.'s long-term health?
6. Of all of the symptoms that Ms. P. reports, which one should the nurse be most concerned about related to Ms. P.'s ability to live alone?

*Students are advised to refer to their nursing diagnosis text and identify possible or potential problems.

REFERENCES

Ali MA, Lacy BE: Abdominal complaints and gastrointestinal disorders. In Landefeld CS et al, editors: *Current geriatric diagnosis and treatment*, New York, 2004, McGraw-Hill.

American Stroke Association: *Abrupt changes in body position can trigger stroke*, 2002, Meeting report 2/08, The Association. (website): *www.americanheart.org/presenter.jhtml?identifier=3000721*.

Arias E: United States Life Tables, 2003. *National Vital Statistics Reports* 54(4). Hyattsville, MD, 2006, National Center for Health Statistics.

Beato CV: *Progress review: heart disease and stroke*, April 23, 2003, USDHHS. (website): *www.healthypeople.gov/Data/2010prog/focus12/* Accessed July 22, 2006.

Beato CV: *Progress review: respiratory diseases*, June 29, 2004, USDHHS. (website): *www.healthypeople.gov/data/2010prog/focus24/default.htm* Accessed June 22, 2006.

Beers MH, Berkow R: *The Merck manual of geriatrics*, ed 3, Whitehouse Station, NJ, 2000, Merck Research Laboratories.

Begelman SM: Peripheral vascular and thromboembolic disease. In Landefeld CS et al, editors: *Current geriatric diagnosis and treatment*, New York, 2004, McGraw-Hill.

Benner P et al: Moral dimensions of living with a chronic illness: autonomy, responsibility, and the limits of control. In Benner P, editor: *Interpretive phenomenology: embodiment, caring and ethics in health and illness*, Thousand Oaks, Calif, 1994, Sage.

Blumenthal DE: Geriatric rheumatology. In Landefeld CS et al, editors: *Current geriatric diagnosis and treatment*, New York, 2004, McGraw-Hill.

Boss B: Alterations of neurologic function. In McCance KL, Huether SE, editors: *Pathophysiology: the biological basis for disease in adults and children*, ed 5, St Louis, 2006, Mosby.

Brain Attack Coalition: *Recommendations for the establishment of primary stroke centers*, 2001, National Guideline Clearinghouse. (website):*www.guideline.gov/VIEWS/summary.asp?guideline=1784&summary_type=brief_su*.

Brashers VL: Alterations of cardiovascular function. In McCance KL, Huether SE, editors: *Pathophysiology: the biological basis for disease in adults and children*, ed 5, St Louis, 2006a, Mosby.

Brashers VL: Alteration of pulmonary function. In McCance KL, Huether SE, editors: *Pathophysiology: the biological basis for disease in adults and children*, ed 5, St Louis, 2006b, Mosby.

Brucker MC, Youngkin EQ: What's a woman to do: exploring HRT questions raised by the women's health initiative, *AWHOHN Lifelines* 6(5):406-417, 2002.

Centers for Disease Control and Prevention (CDC): *Reported TB in the U.S., 2004*, USDHHS, CDC, 2005a. (website): *www.cdc.gov/nchstp/tb*. Accessed July 26, 2006.

Centers for Disease Control and Prevention (CDC): Trends in TB—U.S., 2005b, *MMWR Weekly* 55(100):305-308.

Chesnutt MS, Prendergast TJ: Lung. In Tierney LM et al, editors: *2006 Current medical diagnosis and treatment*, New York, 2006, McGraw-Hill.

Cook CB et al: The potentially poor response to outpatient diabetes care in urban African Americans, *Diabetes Care* 24(2):209, 2001.

Corbin JM, Strauss A: *Unending work and care: managing chronic illness at home*, San Francisco, 1988, Jossey-Bass.

Corbin JM, Strauss A: A nursing model for chronic illness management based upon the trajectory framework. In Woog P, editor: *The chronic illness framework: the Corbin and Strauss nursing model*, New York, 1992, Springer.

Danese RD, Aron DC: Diabetes in the elderly. In Landefeld CS et al, editors: *Current geriatric diagnosis and treatment*, New York, 2004, McGraw-Hill.

Decousus H et al: Superficial vein thrombosis risk factors, diagnosis and treatment, *Curr Opin Pulm Med* 9(5):393-397, 2003.

Doolittle ND: A clinical ethnography of stroke recovery. In Benner P, editor: *Interpretive phenomenology: embodiment, caring and ethics in health and illness*, Thousand Oaks, Calif, 1994, Sage.

Ducharme A et al: Impact of care at a multidisciplinary congestive heart failure clinic: a randomized trial, *Can Med Assoc J* 173(1):40-45, 2005.

Endoy MP: CVD in women: risk factors and clinical presentation, *American Journal for Nurse Practitioners* 8(2), 33-40, 2004.

Estes MEZ: *Health assessment and physical examination*, Albany, NY, 2002, Delmar.

Evans A et al: Can differences in management process explain different outcomes between stroke unit and stroke-team care? *Lancet* 358:1586, 2001.

Ferebee L: Respiratory function. In Meiner SE, Luecknotte AG, editors: *Gerontologic nursing*, ed 3, St Louis, 2006, Mosby.

Field S: Detecting patients with hidden GERD, *The Clinical Advisor* April:23-24, 2003.

Gambert SR, Miller M: Endocrine disorders. In Landefeld CS et al, editors: *Current geriatric diagnosis and treatment*, New York, 2004, McGraw-Hill.

Giger JN, Davidhizar RE: *Transcultural nursing: assessment and intervention*, ed 4, St Louis, 2003, Mosby.

Hellmann DR, Stone JH: Arthritis and musculoskeletal disorders. In Tierney LM et al, editors: *Current medical diagnosis and treatment*, New York, 2006, McGraw-Hill.

Higgins M: Epidemiology and prevention of coronary heart disease in families, *Am J Med* 108(5):387, 2000.

Huether SE: Alterations of digestive function. In McCance KL, Huether SE, editors: *Pathophysiology: the biological basis for disease in adults and children*, ed 5, St Louis, 2006a, Mosby.

Huether SE: Alterations of endocrine function. In McCance KL, Huether SE, editors: *Pathophysiology: the biological basis for disease in adults and children*, ed 5, St Louis, 2006b, Mosby.

Jett KF: Making the connection: seeking and receiving help by elderly African-Americans, *Qual Health Res* 12(3):373-387, 2002.

Jett KF: Mind-loss in the African American community: a normal part of aging. *J Aging Stud* 20(1): 1-10, 2006.

JNC 7: *JNC 7 Express: the seventh report of the Joint National Commission of the Prevention, Detection, Evaluation and Treatment of High Blood Pressure*, USHHS Pub No 03-5233, 2003. (website): *www.nhlbi.nih.gov*. Accessed July 23, 2006.

Kaltenbach G et al: Influence of age on presentation and prognosis of tuberculosis in internal medicine, *Presse Med* 30(29):1446, 2001.

Kistler JP et al: *Treatment of transient cerebral ischemia*, UpToDate, 2002. (website): *www.uptodate.com*.

Kistler JP et al: Cerebrovascular disease. In Hazzard WR et al, editors: *Principles of geriatric medicine and gerontology*, ed 5, New York, 2003, McGraw-Hill.

Klusch L: *Solutions in restorative caregiving*, Des Moines, Iowa, 1995, Briggs Health Care Products.

Leira EC, Adams HP: Cerebrovascular disease. In Landefeld CS et al, editors: *Current geriatric diagnosis and treatment*, New York, 2004, McGraw-Hill.

McCrory DC et al: Management of acute exacerbations of COPD: a summary and appraisal of the published evidence, *Chest* 119:1190, 2001.

McCulloch DK: *Definition and classification of diabetes mellitus*, UpToDate, 2002. (website): *www.uptodate.com*.

Melange M, Vanheuverzwyn R: Etiopathogenesis of colonic diverticular disease: role of fiber and therapeutic perspectives, *Acta Gastroenterol Belg* 53(3):346, 1990.

Meyyazhagan S, Messinger-Rapport BJ: Hypertension. In Landefeld CS et al, editors: *Current geriatric diagnosis and treatment*, New York, 2004, McGraw-Hill.

Nadel M: *Synopsis of diverticulosis*. University of Connecticut Health Center, Pathology Department, 2001. (website): *http://esynopsis.uchc.edu/S203.htm*.

National Institute of Diabetes and Digestive and Kidney Diseases. *National Diabetes Statistics fact sheet: general information and national estimates on diabetes in the United States, 2005*. Bethesda, MD, 2005, U.S. Department of Health and Human Services, National Institutes of Health.

National Heart Lung and Blood Institute (NHLBI): *NAEPP Expert Panel Report 2: guidelines for the diagnosis and management of asthma*, Pub No 97-4051, Bethesda, Md, 1997, The Institute.

National Institutes of Health (NIH): *Second expert panel on the management of asthma, National Health Lung and Blood Institute, Highlights of the Expert Panel Report 2: Guidelines for the diagnosis and management of asthma*, Bethesda Md, 1997, NIH Pub No 97-4051A.

National Institutes of Health (NIH): *Diverticulosis and diverticulitis*, NIH Pub No 06-1163, 2005. (website): *www.niddk.gov*. Accessed July 23, 2006.

Orem DE: *Nursing: concepts of practice*, ed 2, New York, 1980, McGraw-Hill.

Orem DE: *Nursing: concepts of practice*, St Louis, 1995, Mosby.

O'Rourke KS: Myopathies, polymyalgia rheumatica and giant cell arteritis. In Hazzard WR et al, editors: *Principles of geriatric medicine and gerontology*, ed 5, New York, 2003, McGraw-Hill.

Rajagopalan S, Yoshikawa TT: Tuberculosis in the elderly, *Z Gerontol Geriatr* 33(5):374, 2000.

Reed RL, Mooradian A: Diabetes mellitus. In Ham R et al, editors: *Primary care geriatrics*, ed 4, St Louis, 2002, Mosby.

Resnick B, Fleishell A: Developing a restorative care program, *Am J Nurs* 102(7):91, 2002.

Rich MW: Heart failure. In Hazzard WR et al, editors: *Principles of geriatric medicine and gerontology*, ed 5, New York, 2003, McGraw-Hill.

Rich MW: Cardiac disease. In Landefeld CS et al, editors: *Current geriatric diagnosis and treatment*, New York, 2004, McGraw-Hill.

Rissmiller RW, Adair NE: Respiratory diseases. In Landefeld CS et al, editors: *Current geriatric diagnosis and treatment*, New York, 2004, McGraw-Hill.

Rubio MA: Implications of fiber in different pathologies, *Nutr Hosp* 17(2):17, 2002.

Saver J: Highlights from the 27th International Stroke Conference, San Antonio, Feb 7-9, 2002. Available at *Medscape Neurol Neurosurg* 4(1). (website): *www.medscape.com/viewarticle/429908*.

Short P, Leon J: *Use of home and community services by persons ages 65 and older with functional difficulties*, Pub No (PHS) 90-3466, Rockville, Md, 1990, U.S. Department of Health and Human Services, Agency for Health Care Policy and Research.

Shroff D, Moylan KC: Thyroid disease in the geriatric patient. In Moylan KC, editor: *The Washington manual: geriatrics subspecialty consult*, New York, 2004, Lippincott Williams & Wilkins.

Sica DA: ACE inhibitors and stroke: new considerations, *J Clin Hyperten (Greenwich)* 4(2):126, 2002.

Smedley B et al: *Unequal treatment: confronting racial and ethnic disparities in health care*, Washington, DC, 2003, National Academies Press.

Steinke EE: Intimacy needs and chronic illness: strategies for sexual counseling and self-management, *J Gerontol Nurs* 31(5):40-49, 2005.

Stoller JK: Acute exacerbations of chronic obstructive pulmonary disease, *N Engl J Med* 346:988, 2002.

Strauss A, Corbin J: *Shaping a new health care system*, San Francisco, 1988, Jossey-Bass.

Strauss A, Glaser B: *Chronic illness and the quality of life*, St Louis, 1975, Mosby.

U.S. Department of Health and Human Services (USDHHS): *Healthy People 2010*, Sudbury, Mass, 2000, Jones & Bartlett.

U.S. Prevention Services Task Force (USPSTF): *Screening for high blood pressure: recommendations and rationale*, 2003, AHRQ, Rockville Md. (website): *www.ahrq.gov/clinic/3rduspstf/hibloddrr.htm*. Accessed March 15, 2006.

Wells T, Brink C: Urinary continence/incontinence. Helpful equipment, *Geriatr Nurs* 1(4):264, 1980.

Wenger NK: Rehabilitation of the elderly coronary patient. In Frengley JD et al: *Practicing rehabilitation with geriatric clients*, New York, 1990, Springer.

Whitehead JB: An overview of the management of diabetes in the elderly, *Ann Long-Term Care* (suppl), 1-7, March 2002.

Woog P: *The chronic illness trajectory framework: the Corbin and Strauss nursing model*, New York, 1992, Springer.

Young MA, Hoffberg HJ: Poststroke rehabilitation, *Clin Advisor* 25-26, 31-32, Feb 2001.

Zeiss A, Kasl-Godley J: Sexuality in older adults' relationships, *Generations* 25(2):18-25, 2001.

CHAPTER 11

Pain and Comfort

Theris A. Touhy and Kathleen Jett

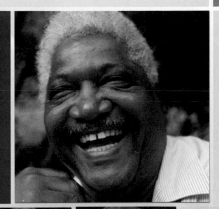
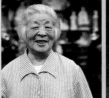

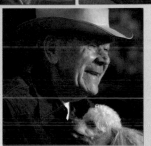

Not only degrees of pain, but its existence, in any degree, must be taken upon the testimony of the patient.

Peter Mere Latham (1789-1875),
Diseases of the Heart, Lecture XI

LEARNING OBJECTIVES

On completion of this chapter, the reader will be able to:

1. Define the concept of pain.
2. Differentiate between acute and persistent pain.
3. Identify factors that affect the elder's pain experience.
4. Identify barriers that interfere with pain assessment and treatment.
5. Describe data to include in a pain assessment.
6. Discuss pharmacological and non-pharmacological pain management therapies.
7. Develop a nursing plan of care for an elder with pain.

Comfort seems to be an intrinsic balance of the physiological, emotional, social, and spiritual essence of the individual and can be perceived as an integral component of wellness. By definition, comfort is "a state of ease and satisfaction of the bodily wants and freedom from pain and anxiety." The absence of physical pain is not always sufficient to provide comfort. The older adult may have his or her biological or bodily needs satisfied but still have emotional or spiritual pain. Conversely, physical needs may be the priority and no comfort is possible until those needs are met.

The International Association for the Study of Pain (1979, 1992) defines pain as "an unpleasant sensory and emotional experience associated with actual or potential tissue damage, or described in terms of such damage" (p. 250). Pain is a subjective response and therefore difficult to objectively assess. McCaffery's classic definition (1979) is the one most commonly used in nursing: "Pain is whatever the person experiencing pain says it is" (p. 8).

Pain is a multidimensional and totally pervasive phenomenon with sensory, physical, psychosocial, emotional, and spiritual components (Lynch, 2001). In the absence of dis-

ease, pain is not a normal part of aging. Yet the majority of older adults experience pain on a regular basis. Pain erodes personality, saps energy, and manifests itself in an ever-intensifying cycle of pain, anxiety, and anguish until the cycle is broken. Pain can evoke depression, sleep disorders, decreased socialization, impaired mobility, and increased health care costs (Fine, 2002; Jeffery and Lubkin, 2002; Morley, 2001; Thernstrom, 2001). Box 11-1 provides some of the consequences of untreated pain.

Pain is now considered the fifth vital sign. It is just as important as the other vital signs and should receive as much attention. In 1999, The Joint Commission on Accreditation of Healthcare Organizations (now The Joint Commission [TJC]) published national standards and guidelines for pain assessment and management in hospital, ambulatory care, home care, and nursing home settings. TJC guidelines were revised in 2001 (JCAHO, 2004), and failure to adequately comply with the standards can lead to an institution's loss of accreditation. TJC standards expect health care professionals working in health care settings to (1) recognize and treat pain properly, (2) make information about

Special thanks to Patricia Hess, the previous edition contributor, for her content contributions to this chapter.

both pharmacological and non-pharmacological interventions readily available, (3) promise patients attentive analgesic care, (4) define policies for using analgesic technology, and (5) continuously monitor and improve the quality of pain management (Pasero et al., 1999a). In the nursing home setting, pain is one of the quality indicators and the nurse is required to determine the presence or absence of pain when completing the Minimum Data Set (MDS) assessment (see Chapter 6). Patients have a right to have their pain adequately controlled (Box 11-2).

The American Nurses Association, in collaboration with the American Society of Pain Management Nursing, has developed *Pain Management Nursing: Scope and Standards of Practice*, and the American Nurses Credentialing Center (ANCC) offers a certification examination on pain management for nurses at the generalist level (Trossman, 2006). Trossman (2006) noted that "while evidence-based research on pain management has increased over the years, the knowledge base of most physicians, nurses, and even consumers has not" (p. 29).

The nurse has a definition or interpretation of pain, as does the patient for whom the nurse cares. These interpretations are formulated from experiences and are influenced by the unique history of the individual and the meaning ascribed to the pain. It is also important to realize that an individual responds in a way that reflects cultural expectations and acceptable behavior (Box 11-3). Values, experience with pain, and myths and stereotypes also influence both the perception of and the response to pain. Ethnically diverse responses to pain are based on years of social modeling, group-pressure influence on pain tolerance, and the observation of the family when in pain (Jeffery and Lubkin, 2002). According to Ware et al. (2006, p. 118):

> Although the relationship of minority status to pain assessment is not clearly understood, patient ethnicity may be a significant factor influencing adequate pain management. Disparity in pain assessment related to minority status is one of the most disturbing factors related to the ineffective treatment of pain in the United States.

Little research has been done examining the assessment of pain in older minority adults (Ware et al., 2006).

BOX 11-1   Consequences of Untreated Pain

- Altered immune function
- Sleep disturbance
- Malnutrition
- Physical function decline (impaired mobility and gait, delayed rehabilitation, falls)
- Impaired cognition
- Increased dependency and helplessness
- Depression, anxiety, fear
- Decline in social and recreational activities
- Increased health care utilization and costs

Data from Fine P: *Principles of effective pain management at the end of life*, 2006. (website): *www.medscape.com/viewprogram/6079_pnt;* Herr K, Decker S. *Ann Long-Term Care* 12(4):46-52, 2004.

BOX 11-2   Pain Patient's Bill of Rights

I have the right to:
- Have my pain prevented or controlled adequately
- Have my pain and pain medication history taken
- Have my pain questions answered freely
- Develop a pain plan with my health care provider
- Know the risks, benefits, and side effects of treatment
- Know what alternative pain treatments may be available
- Sign a statement of informed consent before any treatment
- Be believed when I say I have pain
- Have my pain assessed on an individual basis
- Have my pain assessed using the 0 = no pain, 10 = worst pain scale
- Ask for changes in treatment if my pain persists
- Receive compassionate and sympathetic care
- Refuse treatment without prejudice from my health care provider
- Seek a second opinion or request a pain care specialist
- Be given my records on request
- Include my family in decision making
- Remind those who care for me that my pain management is part of my diagnostic, medical, or surgical care

Modified from Cowles J: *Pain relief*, New York, 1994, MasterMedia.

BOX 11-3   Culturally Oriented Responses to Pain

- Minimizes pain with significant others
  or
- Uses pain to elicit sympathy and support from others

- Carefully controls the expression of pain (calm and unemotional)
  or
- Is vocal about pain (cries and moans, complains)

- Withdraws and wants to be alone when pain is severe
  or
- Seeks attention and presence of others

- Willingly accepts pain relief measures
  or
- Avoids pain relief measures in the belief that they indicate weakness

- Wants and expects quick pain relief
  or
- Accepts pain for long periods before requesting help

Modified from Kozier B et al: *Fundamentals of nursing*, Redwood City, Calif, 1995, Addison-Wesley; Bates MS: *Biocultural dimensions of chronic pain*, Albany, 1996, State University of New York Press; Salerno E, Willens JS: *Pain management handbook*, St Louis, 1996, Mosby.

ACUTE AND PERSISTENT PAIN

Acute pain is temporary and includes postoperative, procedural, and traumatic pain. It is easily controlled by analgesic medications. Almost everyone has experienced this type of pain and knows that it is a time-limited situation with attainable relief. Fulmer et al. (1996) provide a comprehensive protocol for management of acute pain in older adults.

Persistent pain, also called *chronic pain*, is not that simple. It has no time frame; it is continually persistent at varying levels of intensity. In the minds of providers, the term *chronic pain* may conjure up images of malingering, psychiatric problems, drug-seeking behavior, and futility in treatment. The guidelines of the American Geriatrics Society (AGS, 2002) suggest the use of the term *persistent pain* to overcome the negative images associated with the term *chronic pain*.

Persistent pain is multifactorial in nature. Lipman and Jackson (2000) note that persistent pain can manifest as depression, eating and sleeping disturbances, and impaired function. The effects of persistent pain affect physical, psychological, social, and spiritual well-being (McElhaney, 2001). Chronic, persistent pain is categorized as either of nonmalignant origin or of malignant origin. Intractable, nonmalignant pain is the most common pain in elders and erodes an individual's coping ability. Table 11-1 compares the many facets of acute and chronic or persistent pain.

Persistent pain is further classified as follows:

- Nociceptive pain is associated with injury to the skin, mucosa, muscle, or bone and is usually the result of stimulation of pain receptors. This type of pain arises from tissue inflammation, trauma, burns, infection, ischemia, arthropathies (rheumatoid arthritis, osteoarthritis, gout), nonarticular inflammatory disorders, skin and mucosal ulcerations, and internal organ and visceral pain from distention, obstruction, inflammation, compression, or ischemia of organs. Pancreatitis, appendicitis, and tumor infiltration are common causes of visceral pain. Nociceptive mechanisms usually respond well to common analgesic medications and non-pharmacological interventions (AGS, 2002; Lynch, 2001).
- Neuropathic pain involves a pathophysiological process of the peripheral or central nervous system and presents as altered sensation and discomfort. Conditions causing this type of pain include postherpetic or trigeminal neuralgia, poststroke or postamputation pain (phantom pain), diabetic neuropathy, or radiculopathies (e.g., spinal stenosis). This type of pain may be described as stabbing, tingling, burning, or shooting. These pain syndromes do not respond as well as nociceptive pain to conventional analgesic therapy. Use of antidepressant medications and anticonvulsants has been effective (AGS, 2002; Lynch, 2001).
- Mixed or unspecified pain usually has mixed or unknown causes. Examples include recurrent headaches and vasculitis. A compression fracture causing nerve root irritation, common in older people with osteoporosis, is an example of a mix of nociceptive and neuropathic pain (AGS, 2002; Lynch, 2001; McElhaney, 2001).

It is estimated that the prevalence of persistent pain is twice as high among older people as among younger individuals (Leo and Singh, 2002). The most common pain in elders is probably musculoskeletal, but a significant number also have neuropathic pain. Pain syndromes common in older adults are presented in Box 11-4. By age 50 years, nearly 90% of adults have degenerative abnormalities of the lower spine. One of the most typical is thinning of the intervertebral disks, which can eventually lead to arthritis and other painful conditions. Osteoarthritis, or the destruction of the inner joint surfaces, is one of the most common forms of joint disease and the most disabling for persons older than 65 years (see Chapter 15). Among community-dwelling elders, 66% have joint pain and 28% have back pain; among elders in long-term care facilities, 70% have joint pain, 13% have pain from old fracture sites, and 10% have neuropathic pain, much of this from postherpetic neuralgia (Ferrell, 2000).

Nearly one million cases of herpes zoster (shingles) occur each year, most often in those between ages 60 and 79 years. It has been estimated that about 50% of people who live to age 80 years will have an attack of shingles (Diamond and Urban, 2002). This may be caused by the decrease in cellular immune response to the varicella zoster antigen, which is undetected in up to 30% of previously immune healthy elders older than 60 years (Chiu, 2000). An attack of shingles can occur when the varicella virus reactivates through immunosuppression, malignancy, trauma, surgery, or local radiation.

Postherpetic neuralgia is a complication experienced because of irritation of the nerve roots that leave the spinal cord. Ophthalmic zoster causes postherpetic neuralgia when the trigeminal nerve is involved. The stinging, burning pain with or without an underlying sharp, jabbing sensation continues for weeks, months, and, for some elderly, indefinitely after the initial skin lesions have healed. Once postherpetic neuralgia is established, it is difficult to treat. Analgesics provide limited relief from the pain; codeine is often prescribed. More effective in providing relief is a combination of antiviral medications, steroids, aspirin, and topical anesthetics for pain. The U.S. Food and Drug Administration (FDA) has approved prescription medications such as acyclovir and famciclovir, which shorten the duration of persistent shingle pain but may not prevent postherpetic neuralgia. Capsaicin cream (Zostrix), an over-the-counter (OTC) topical anesthetic, or the anesthetic EMLA patch (Chiu, 2000) may be helpful in relieving postherpetic neuralgia pain. Low doses of tricyclic antidepressants (e.g., desipramine) or the newer neuropathic drugs, such as gabapentin, and nerve blocks are considered in resistant cases.

TABLE 11-1

Comparison of Acute and Persistent Pain

	Acute Pain	Persistent Pain (Nonmalignant Origin)	Persistent Pain (Malignant Origin)
Source	An event, external agent, or internal disease	A situation, state of existence Unknown, or if known, changes cannot occur or treatment is prolonged or ineffective	Usually associated with terminal disease
Onset	Usually sudden	May be sudden or insidious	Unpredictable
Duration	Hours, days, usually transient, lasting no more than 3-6 months	Prolonged for months or years	Prolonged, often for the course of the disease or in its later stages
Pain identification	Pain vs. lack of pain Areas generally well defined	Pain vs. lack of pain Areas are less well defined Intensity becomes more difficult to evaluate (change in sensation): intensity varies, may be constant or intermittent	Area(s) may be well defined or diffuse; pain may be more constant than intermittent
Associated pathological conditions	Present	Often unknown	Usually present
Associated problems	Uncommon	Depression, anxiety, secondary pain issues	Many of the same as persistent nonmalignant pain
Behavior	Typical response patterns with more visible signs: 　Facial expressions 　Crying, guarding, moaning 　Clenching teeth 　Biting lower lip 　Tightly shut eyes 　Open, somber eyes 　Involuntary movements 　Immobility of body part 　Purposeless body movement 　Rhythmical body movements, rocking, rubbing 　Change in speech and vocal pitch (anxiety) 　Slow monotone (severe pain) 　Fetal position	Response patterns vary, few overt signs (adaptation): 　Sleep disturbances 　Confusion 　Rubbing 　Stoicism 　Depression 　Inactivity 　Combativeness 　Inactivity 　Immobilizing body part or assuming an awkward body position	Response pattern similar to persistent malignant pain: 　Sleep disturbance 　Withdrawal 　Depression 　Inactivity 　Slow moving 　Anger 　Anxiety 　Fearful 　Short tempered or passive
Nerve conduction	Rapid	Slow	Slow
Autonomic system involvement (clinical signs)	Present Elevation of blood pressure Tachycardia Diaphoresis	Generally absent No change in vital signs	May be present or absent
Meaning pattern	Meaningful: Informs person something is wrong; self-limiting or readily corrected	Meaningless: person looks for meaning	May have meaning or be meaningless
Treatment	Primary: analgesic drugs	Multimodal: primary behavioral and physical therapy; drugs may be primarily adjunctive	Multimodal: analgesics usually play a major role

Compiled and modified from Karb V: Pain. In Phipps W et al, editors: *Medical-surgical nursing: concepts and clinical practice,* ed 4, St Louis, 1991, Mosby; Forrest J: Assessment of acute and chronic pain in older adults, *J Gerontol Nurs* 21:10, 1995; and Lipman AG, Jackson KC: *Use of opioids in chronic noncancer pain,* Stamford, Conn, 2000, Power-Pak Communications, Inc., Purdue Pharma LP.

BOX 11-4   Pain Syndromes Common in Older Adults

- Temporal arteritis
- Degenerative joint disease
- Rheumatoid arthritis
- Polymyalgia rheumatica
- Reflex sympathetic dystrophy
- Lumbar disk disease
- Gout
- Lumbar stenosis
- Osteoporosis and fractures
- Peripheral vascular disease
- Post-stroke syndrome
- Contractures
- Trigeminal neuralgia
- Herpes zoster
- Postsurgical intercostal neuralgia
- Postherpetic neuropathies
- Peripheral neuropathy
- Diabetic neuropathy
- Phantom limb pain
- Angina
- Postmastectomy pain
- Hiatal hernia
- Irritable bowel syndrome
- Chronic constipation
- Oral/dental

BOX 11-5   Barriers to Pain Management in Older Adults

HEALTH CARE PROFESSIONAL BARRIERS

Lack of education regarding pain assessment and management
Concern regarding regulatory scrutiny
Fears of opioid-related side effects/addiction
Belief that pain is a normal part of aging
Belief that cognitively impaired elders have less pain; lack of ability to assess pain in cognitively impaired
Personal beliefs and experiences with pain
Inability to accept self-report without "objective" signs

PATIENT AND FAMILY BARRIERS

Fear of medication side effects
Concerns related to addiction
Belief that pain is a normal part of the aging process
Belief that nothing much can be done for pain in older people
Fear of being a "bad patient" if complaining/fear of what pain may signal

HEALTH CARE SYSTEM BARRIERS

Cost
Time
Cultural bias regarding opioid use

Modified from Hanks-Bell M et al: Pain assessment and management in aging, *Online J Issues Nurs* 9(3), 2004 (website): *www.nursingworld.org/ojin/topic21/tpc21_6.htm*.

PAIN IN THE OLDER ADULT

Pain is highly prevalent and under-recognized and under-treated in the older adult population, particularly among those with cognitive impairment. "The incidence of pain more than doubles after the age of 60 with pain frequency increasing with each decade" (Hanks-Bell et al., 2004, p. 2). The prevalence of pain in the elderly who live in the community is known to be twice that of younger people and is considered to be extremely high in the long-term care setting. Estimates are that 25% to 50% of community-dwelling elders experience pain and up to 80% of long-term care residents experience substantial pain (Hanks-Bell et al., 2004; Herr and Decker, 2004).

Older people are at high risk for pain-inducing situations. They have lived longer and have a greater chance of developing degenerative and pathological conditions through disease or injury. Several conditions may be present simultaneously, so a single pain-producing condition may be overlooked in the complexity of health management. Increased susceptibility to accidents because of medications, cognitive function, or illness impacts functional abilities, which further contributes to accidents such as falls. The resultant hip fractures, sprains, and hematomas require longer time to heal and prolong the pain experience. Loneliness and emotional pain from loss of a spouse, friends, a job, and independence and the presence of boredom and depression decrease the ability to cope with physical pain. These psychosocial aspects of an elder's life are rarely self-reported because of the associated stigma.

Barriers to Pain Management in Older Adults

Despite the prevalence and consequences of pain among older adults, recognition and treatment of pain remain ineffective in this population. Hanks-Bell et al. (2004) cite the major sources of barriers to adequate pain management in older people: the patient and family, the health care community, and society at large (Box 11-5). "Patients, families, and health care professionals hold strong personal beliefs and fears about the meaning of pain and pain treatment options" (Hanks-Bell et al., 2004, p. 2). Myths about pain and the elderly further contribute to the under-diagnosis and under-treatment of pain (Box 11-6). It is critical that nurses who work with elders develop the knowledge and skill to appropriately assess and aggressively treat pain in this population.

Pain in Cognitively Impaired Elders

Older people with cognitive impairment are consistently untreated or under-treated for pain. Studies have shown that older adults who are cognitively impaired receive less pain medication even though they experience the same painful conditions as elders who are cognitively intact (AGS, 2002; Herr and Decker, 2004; Herr et al., 2006a, b; Kovach et al., 2006 a,b; Ware et al., 2006). It is best to practice under the "assumption that any condition that is painful to a cognitively intact person would also be painful to those with advanced dementia who cannot express

BOX 11-6 Fact and Fiction About Pain in the Elderly

MYTH: Pain is expected with aging.
FACT: Pain is not normal with aging. The presence of pain in the elderly necessitates aggressive assessment, diagnosis, and management similar to that of younger patients.

MYTH: Pain sensitivity and perception decrease with aging.
FACT: This assumption is dangerous! Data are conflicting regarding age-associated changes in pain perception, sensitivity, and tolerance. Consequences of this assumption are needless suffering and under-treatment of both pain and underlying cause.

MYTH: If a patient does not complain of pain, there must not be much pain.
FACT: This is erroneous in all ages but particularly in the elderly. Older patients may not report pain for a variety of reasons. They may fear the meaning of pain, diagnostic workups, or pain treatments. They may not want to be a bother, may believe suffering is necessary to atone for past sins, may fear addiction, or think pain is a normal part of aging. Cognitive and communication difficulties also may make older people unable to report pain.

MYTH: A person who has no functional impairment, appears occupied, or is otherwise distracted from pain must not have significant pain.
FACT: Patients have a variety of reactions to pain. Many patients are stoic and refuse to "give in" to their pain. Over extended periods, the elderly may mask any outward signs of pain.

MYTH: Narcotic medications are inappropriate for patients with persistent nonmalignant pain.
FACT: Opioid analgesics are often indicated in persistent nonmalignant pain.

MYTH: Potential side effects of narcotic medication make them too dangerous to use in the elderly.
FACT: Narcotics may be used safely in the elderly. Although elderly patients may be more sensitive to narcotics, this does not justify withholding narcotics and failing to relieve pain.

MYTH: Treatment of pain with narcotics can lead to addiction.
FACT: Research has shown that the actual risk of addiction to opioids is less than 1%.

MYTH: People with dementia do not feel pain.
FACT: Older adults with cognitive impairment are just as likely to experience painful illnesses. They feel pain, but changes in the brain may change the way pain is processed. They may not understand or even remember their pain or may not be able to report what they feel. Changes in behavior (agitation, aggression, calling for help, sleep pattern changes, appetite changes) are common pain behaviors in cognitively impaired elders.

Adapted from Ferrell BR, Ferrell BA: Pain in the elderly. In Watt-Watson JH, Donovan MI, editors: *Pain management: nursing perspective,* St Louis, 1992, Mosby; Herr K, Decker S: Assessment of pain in older adults with severe cognitive impairment, *Ann Long-Term Care* 12(4):46-52, 2004.

themselves" (Herr and Decker, 2004, p. 48). Research has suggested that older people with mild to moderate cognitive impairment can provide valid reports of pain using self-report scales, but people with more severe impairment and loss of language skills may be unable to communicate the presence of pain in a manner that is easily understood (Herr and Decker, 2004; Herr et al., 2006a; Kovach et al., 2006a; Ware et al., 2006).

Misconceptions and fears of older adults related to pain were discussed earlier, but lack of knowledge of the patient's family/significant other and health care providers contributes to inadequate recognition and treatment of pain in cognitively impaired older adults. Many caregivers believe that people who are cognitively impaired do not experience pain as severely as those who are cognitively intact. According to Herr and Decker (2004, pp. 47-48):

> There is no convincing evidence that peripheral nociceptor responses of pain transmission are impaired in people with dementia, although controversy does exist about central nervous system changes that influence or diminish interpretation of pain transmission. Those with dementia may have altered affective responses to pain, probably due to their inability to cognitively process the painful sensation in the context of prior pain experience, attitudes, knowledge, and beliefs.

As a result, responses to painful experiences may be different from the "typical" response of a person who is cognitively intact.

Conditions such as constipation or urinary tract infection can cause great distress in cognitively impaired older people and may lead to marked changes in behavior (agitation, falls, refusal of care) (Herr and Decker, 2004). "For the person with late stage dementia, a good deal of their discomfort comes from non-physiological sources, for example, from difficulty sorting out and negotiating everyday life activities" (Kovach et al., 1999, p. 412). Communication of pain usually occurs through behavioral responses such as agitation, aggression, increased confusion, changes in interpersonal interactions, and passive and withdrawn behaviors. Caregivers should be educated to be particularly alert for passive behaviors because they are less disruptive and may not be recognized as changes that may signal pain. Box 11-7 presents behavioral symptoms that may indicate pain in cognitively impaired elders.

Careful observation of behavior and caregiver reports need to be utilized if the person cannot reliably communicate his or her pain. "Identifying pain in the cognitively impaired older adult depends heavily on knowing the patient and paying attention to slight changes in behavior" (Hanks-Bell et al., 2004, p. 6). "Caregivers who have direct

---

BOX 11-7 Pain Cues in Older Adults

FACIAL EXPRESSION

Slight frown; sad, frightened face
Expressionless: stares or looks past you
Grimacing, wrinkled forehead; closed or frightened eyes
Rapid blinking

VERBALIZATIONS, VOCALIZATIONS

Sighing, moaning, groaning
Grunting, chanting, calling out
Repetitive vocalizations
Noisy breathing
Asking for help
Verbally abusive

BODY MOVEMENTS

Rigid, tense body posture; guarding
Fidgeting; cannot sit still
Repetitive movements
Restricted movements
Gait or mobility changes; refuses ambulation; slow, cautious
    movement
Draws up legs, fetal position
Clenched fists

CHANGES IN INTERPERSONAL INTERACTIONS

Aggressive, combative, resisting care
Striking out, pinching, hitting, biting, or scratching
Decreased social interactions
Socially inappropriate, disruptive
Withdrawn

CHANGE IN ACTIVITY PATTERNS OR ROUTINES

Refusing food, appetite change
Increase in rest periods
Sleep, rest pattern changes from baseline
Sudden cessation of common routines
Increased wandering

MENTAL STATUS CHANGES

Crying or tears
Increased confusion
Irritability or distress, complaining

Modified from American Geriatrics Society: The management of pain in older persons, *J Am Geriatr Soc* 50(suppl 6): S205-S224, 2002; McCaffery M, Pasero C: *Pain: clinical manual*, ed 2, St Louis, 1999, Mosby; Parke B: Gerontologic nurses' ways of knowing, *J Gerontol Nurs* 24(6):21, 1998.
NOTE: Some patients demonstrate little or no specific behavior associated with severe pain.

---

and long-standing relationship with the cognitively impaired person are in the best position to recognize subtle changes and communicate them to the health care provider" (Herr and Decker, 2004, p. 96). In nursing homes, the certified nursing assistants play an important role in assessment of pain.

Several instruments can be used to assist in pain assessment of persons with severe cognitive impairment, and although there is no "precise and accurate method for interpreting the expression of pain in this population, there are recommendations to guide practice decisions and provide a framework to future research in this important area" (Hanks-Bell et al., 2004, p. 6). Assessment and assessment tools are discussed on p. 279.

Pain at the End of Life

Pain is the most common and most feared symptom of people at the end of life. Pain at the end of life remains seriously under-treated, even with increased awareness of the prevalence and evidence-based protocols to guide assessment and management (Fine, 2006). The elderly, minorities, and women are at particular risk for under-treatment. Estimates are that approximately two thirds of those with advanced malignant disease experience pain, and near the end of life, 34% to 54% of people with cancer die in pain. The incidence of untreated or under-treated pain among nursing home patients is high. People dying from conditions other than cancer (cardiac failure, chronic obstructive pulmonary disease [COPD], end-stage renal disease, human immunodeficiency virus [HIV]) suffer levels of pain similar to those with malignant disease (Fine, 2006). As Fine stated (2006):

> The terminal stages of chronic, progressive diseases cause many difficult symptoms and causes of suffering. Disease-related symptoms such as pain, dyspnea, fatigue, depression, and loss of mobility intertwine and interact in a complex manner, and each one deserves attention.

Comprehensive and multifactorial assessment by an interdisciplinary team is key to appropriate management, along with the interventions described on p. 282. Chapter 26 provides additional discussion about end-of-life care.

▲ PROMOTING HEALTHY AGING: IMPLICATIONS FOR GERONTOLOGICAL NURSING

Assessment

As always, care of the elder in pain begins with assessment and continues through to the application of interventions and finally the evaluation of the interventions. Regular assessment, use of standardized tools, and consistent documentation and communication are the most important components of pain assessment (Hanks-Bell et al., 2004). The nurse is usually the first person to hear a patient's report of pain, and the ability to perform a comprehensive pain assessment is critical. The nurse is in a key position to work with the elder in the management of pain, be it acute or persistent. The nurse works with the whole person to find a solution to the problem of pain.

A comprehensive assessment of pain must include the multiple factors influencing pain and distress and includes a complete medical and surgical history, physical examination, laboratory and diagnostic procedures as indicated, a thorough pain history, and an assessment of cognition and function. Many older adults have multiple causes and locations of pain so it is important to use a comprehensive approach and allow extra time for assessment. Cognitive and sensory impairments (vision and hearing deficits) may require adaptation of communication during assessment. If the person is unable to provide a pain history or report of baseline cognitive and functional ability, information should be obtained from the formal or informal caregiver who knows the patient. The American Geriatrics Society (AGS) Panel on Persistent Pain (AGS, 2002) and the American Medical Directors Association (AMDA) (2003) have developed comprehensive guidelines for the assessment and management of older adults with persistent pain in a variety of settings.

Assessment always begins with a patient's self-report of pain. It is important to ask regularly about the presence of pain and assess it systematically. Often older people will not relate pain complaints unless directly asked specific questions such as "Do you have pain now?" "Where is your pain?" "Do you have pain everyday?" "Does pain keep you from sleeping at night or doing your daily activities?" (Frampton, 2004). In addition, older people may not use the word *pain*, so words such as *achy*, *hurt*, and *discomfort* also should be used in assessments (Frampton, 2004).

It is important to listen to patients tell you about their pain and how it affects their lives. As a result of research conducted with persons living with persistent pain, Carson and Mitchell (1998) suggested that nurses need to be more open to discover how individuals describe and live with pain so that plans of care can be developed with the person. Although accurate assessment is important, Carson and Mitchell suggest that lengthy pain assessments may interfere with the nurse's ability to understand the person's lived experience of pain. As they report (Carson and Mitchell, 1998, p. 1247):

> A sincere commitment on the nurse's part to listen, comfort and act when requested may be a more helpful approach. Pain is a ravager and people who live the anguish, the forbearance, the loss and hope of pain, are the ones who know and can teach about how to live on.

This advice may be very appropriate when working with cognitively intact elders living with conditions causing persistent pain.

Medication history, including OTC drugs and herbals, is also part of assessment. A thorough analgesic history and the effects of past treatments should also be included (Hanks-Bell et al., 2004). Screening for cognitive impairment (dementia, delirium) and depression and assessment of other quality-of-life indicators, such as functional assessment, nutrition, sleep, and involvement and enjoyment of social activities, should also be included (AGS, 2002; Herr, 2002) (Box 11-8). The Katz ADL Scale (Katz et al., 1963) and the Lawton IADL Scale (Lawton and Brody, 1969) are valid and reliable tools that can be used to assess functional abilities (see Chapter 6).

Assessment then moves to a detailed description of pain intensity, frequency, quality, location, and aggravating and alleviating factors (AGS, 2002). This information requires careful evaluation because treatment may differ based on the etiology of the complaint (Herr, 2002). Box 11-9 presents a mnemonic for pain assessment that nurses may find helpful. The McGill Pain Assessment Questionnaire (Melzack, 1975) is a comprehensive tool that is useful for initial pain

---

BOX 11-8   Additional Factors to Consider When Assessing Pain in the Elderly

Function: How is the pain affecting the elder's ability to participate in usual activities, perform activities of daily living and instrumental activities of daily living?

Alternative expression of pain: Have there been recent changes in cognitive ability or behavior, such as increased pacing, grimacing, or irritability? Is there an increase in the number of complaints? Are they vague and difficult to respond to? Has there been a change in sleep-wake patterns? Is the person resisting certain activities, movements, or positions?

Social support: What are the resources available to the elder in pain? What is the role of the elder in the social system, and how is pain affecting this role? How is pain affecting the elder's relationship with others?

Pain history: How has the elder managed previous experiences with pain? What is the perceived meaning of the past and present pain? What are the cultural factors that affect the elder's ability to express pain and receive relief?

BOX 11-9   Mnemonic for Pain Assessment

Pain is real (Believe the patient!)
Ask about pain regularly
Isolation (psychological and social problems)
Notice nonverbal pain signs
Evaluate pain characteristics
Does pain impair function?
Onset
Location
Duration
Characteristics
Aggravating factors
Relieving factors
Treatment previously tried

From *Aging Successfully* (newsletter of the Division of Geriatric Medicine, St Louis University School of Medicine; Geriatric Research, Education and Clinical Centers, St Louis Veterans Administration Medical Center; the Gateway Geriatric Education Center of Missouri and Illinois). 11(3):6, 2001.

assessment and is used as a standard in many settings. However, the tool relies heavily on verbal and cognitive capacity and may not be useful for some older people. Figure 11-1 presents an alternative initial pain assessment instrument that would cover all of the essential components.

There should also be an assessment of pain that may occur during activity, such as during physical therapy or in day-to-day nursing activities. Travis et al. (2003) use the term *iatrogenic disturbance pain (IDP)* to describe a type of pain that can be caused by the care provider. The authors suggest that, in some circumstances, tasks such as application of a blood pressure cuff, transfers out of bed, bathing, and moving and repositioning patients in the bed may cause levels of discomfort. Patients with severe physical

INITIAL PAIN ASSESSMENT TOOL

Date ______________

Patient's name ______________ Age ____ Room ______________

Diagnosis ______________ Physician ______________

Nurse ______________

I. LOCATION: Patient or nurse mark drawing.

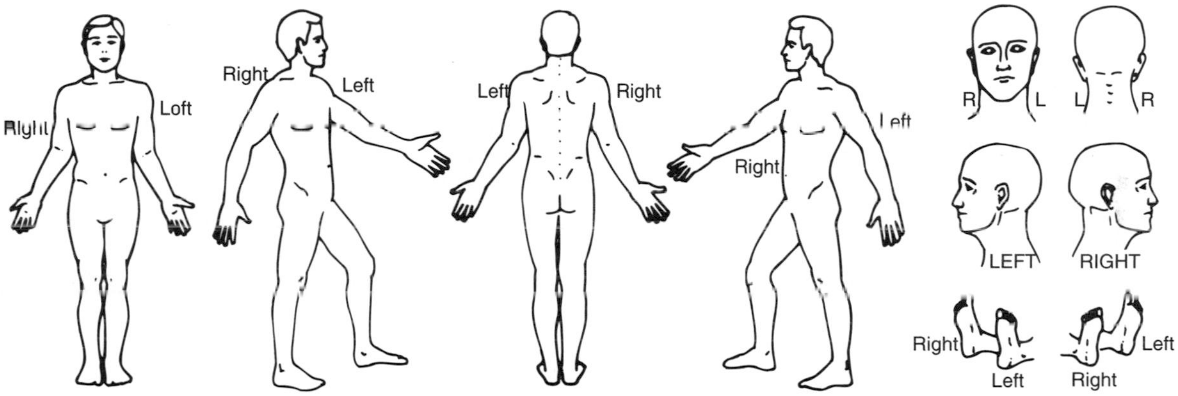

II. INTENSITY: Patient rates the pain. Scale used ______________

Present: ______________
Worst pain gets: ______________
Best pain gets: ______________
Acceptable level of pain: ______________

III. QUALITY: (Use patient's own words, e.g., *prick, ache, burn, throb, pull, sharp.*) ______________

IV. ONSET, DURATION VARIATIONS, RHYTHMS: ______________

V. MANNER OF EXPRESSING PAIN: ______________

VI. WHAT RELIEVES THE PAIN? ______________

VII. WHAT CAUSES OR INCREASES THE PAIN? ______________

VIII. EFFECTS OF PAIN: (Note decreased function, decreased quality of life.) ______________

Accompanying symptoms (e.g., nausea) ______________
Sleep ______________
Appetite ______________
Physical activity ______________
Relationship with others (e.g., irritability) ______________
Emotions (e.g., anger, suicidal, crying) ______________
Concentration ______________
Other ______________

IX. OTHER COMMENTS: ______________

X. PLAN: ______________

FIGURE 11-1 Initial pain assessment tool. (From McCaffery M, Bebee A: *Pain: clinical manual of nursing practice,* St. Louis, 1989, Mosby.)

limitations (e.g., contractures) and significant cognitive impairment and persons at the end of life may be particularly likely to experience IDP. Travis et al. (2003) suggest the use of a 5-day IDP tracking sheet for assessment and monitoring of IDP. Other suggestions provided include gentle handling, adequate staffing, appropriate lifting devices and techniques, analgesic administration before care or treatments that may cause discomfort, education of staff on proper lifting and moving techniques, and assessment of discomfort during care provision.

Brief Pain Inventory

Date _____ / _____ / _____   Time: _____

Name: _____ _____ _____
          Last   First   Middle Initial

1) Throughout our lives, most of us have had pain from time to time (such as minor headaches, sprains, and toothaches). Have you had such pain other than these everyday kinds of pain today?

    1. Yes   2. No

2) On the diagram, shade the areas where you feel pain. Put an X on the area that hurts the most.

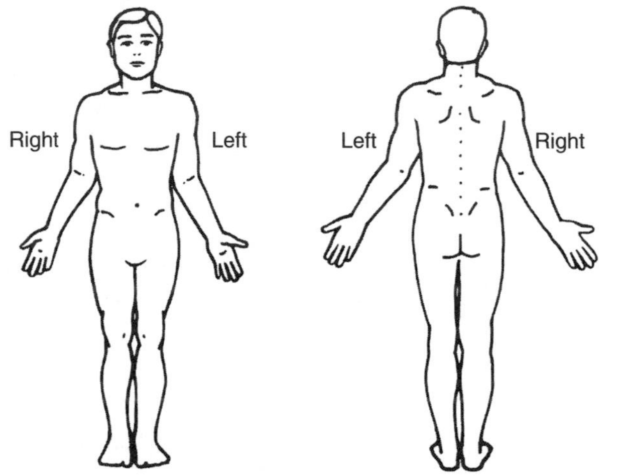

Right   Left   Left   Right

3) Please rate your pain by circling the one number that best describes your pain at its **worst** in the past 24 hours.

0	1	2	3	4	5	6	7	8	9	10
No pain									Pain as bad as you can imagine	

4) Please rate your pain by circling the one number that best describes your pain at its **least** in the past 24 hours.

0	1	2	3	4	5	6	7	8	9	10
No pain									Pain as bad as you can imagine	

5) Please rate your pain by circling the one number that best describes your pain on the **average.**

0	1	2	3	4	5	6	7	8	9	10
No pain									Pain as bad as you can imagine	

6) Please rate your pain by circling the one number that tells how much pain you have **right now**.

0	1	2	3	4	5	6	7	8	9	10
No pain									Pain as bad as you can imagine	

7) What treatments or medications are you receiving for your pain?

_____

_____

8) In the past 24 hours, how much **relief** have pain treatments or medications provided? Please circle the one percentage that most shows how much relief you have received.

0%	10	20	30	40	50	60	70	80	90	100%
No relief										Complete relief

9) Circle the one number that describes how, during the past 24 hours, pain has interfered with your:

A. General activity

0	1	2	3	4	5	6	7	8	9	10
Does not interfere									Completely interferes	

B. Mood

0	1	2	3	4	5	6	7	8	9	10
Does not interfere									Completely interferes	

C. Walking ability

0	1	2	3	4	5	6	7	8	9	10
Does not interfere									Completely interferes	

D. Normal work (includes both work outside the home and housework)

0	1	2	3	4	5	6	7	8	9	10
Does not interfere									Completely interferes	

E. Relations with other people

0	1	2	3	4	5	6	7	8	9	10
Does not interfere									Completely interferes	

F. Sleep

0	1	2	3	4	5	6	7	8	9	10
Does not interfere									Completely interferes	

G. Enjoyment of life

0	1	2	3	4	5	6	7	8	9	10
Does not interfere									Completely interferes	

FIGURE 11-2 Brief pain inventory. (Copyright Charles S. Cleeland, PhD, Houston. May be duplicated for use in clinical practice.)

Pain Rating Scales. A key component to pain assessment is the individual's rating of the intensity of pain. This rating can be used to determine the patient's level of pain at the time of the assessment and the worst, the best, and the desired level (Figure 11-2). When the same scale is used over time, it provides a reliable measure of the effectiveness of the pain-relieving interventions; thus use of the same scale is highly recommended. A variety of scales have been developed with variations for persons with or without cognitive impairment. Herr and Decker (2004) and Ware et al. (2006) note that although pain in cognitively impaired elders can be assessed using simple questions, screening tools, and direct questions about the presence of pain, challenges exist in assessing pain for those with severe cognitive decline and loss of language skills.

For cognitively intact older adults, the Numeric Rating Scale (NRS), a verbally administered 0-10 numerical rating scale, may be a good first choice, especially if the patient has limited vision (Hanks-Bell et al., 2004). The Verbal Descriptor Scale (VDS) and the Pain Thermometer, an adaptation of the VDS, are also good choices and have been shown to be effective in the older adult population (Herr, 2002). The VDS includes adjectives describing pain, such as mild, moderate, severe, worst pain imaginable. The Pain Thermometer is a diagram of a thermometer with word descriptions that show increasing pain intensities. The Faces Pain Scale (FPS) and the Faces Pain Scale-Revised (FPS-R) (Hicks et al., 2001), a series of faces each depicting a different facial expression indicating level of pain, were originally developed for children but may be effective for older adults

as well, especially for persons with poorer verbal skills. However, it may be difficult to determine if pain or mood is being measured when using the FPS (Hanks-Bell, 2004). Both the Pain Thermometer and the FPS depend on visual acuity and may need to be enlarged for the visually impaired older person. Box 11-10 presents results of a research study on the use of pain scales with older minority adults.

The Painometer, a handheld tool developed by Dr. Fannie Gaston-Johanson, incorporates many of the features of existing scales to make it a multidimensional approach. It has been clinically tested and meets the current practice guidelines. The Joint Commission on Accreditation of Healthcare Organizations (now The Joint Commission) approved its use in May 2000 with implementation beginning in 2001 (Mattson, 2000). Sample pain rating scales are presented in Figure 11-3.

Assessment of Pain in Cognitively Impaired, Noncommunicative Older Adults. Assessment of pain in older people experiencing severe cognitive impairment with loss of language skills presents many challenges. Self-report of pain is the gold standard, but in elders unable to report pain, direct observation, surrogate reports, and searching for possible causes of pain and discomfort need to be used in pain assessment (Herr and Decker, 2004). Box 11-11 presents a summary of the general recommendations for the hierarchy of assessment techniques and treatment procedures recommended in The Position Statement with Clinical Practice Recommendations for Pain Assessment in the Nonverbal Patient (Herr et al., 2006a). As noted

---

BOX 11-10 Evidence-Based Practice: Evaluation of the Revised Faces Pain Scale, Verbal Descriptor Scale, Numeric Rating Scale, and Iowa Pain Thermometer in Older Minority Adults

PURPOSE

The purpose of the study was to determine the reliability and validity of selected pain intensity scales—Faces Pain Scale Revised (FPS-R), Verbal Descriptor Scale (VDS), Numeric Rating Scale (NRS), and Iowa Pain Thermometer (IPT)—with a cognitively impaired minority sample.

SAMPLE/SETTING

A convenience sample of 68 participants, 60 years of age or older, who were admitted to acute care facilities in the South with average Mini-Mental State Examination (MMSE) score of 23. 32% males; 68% females, 74% African-Americans; 16% Hispanics; 10% Asians. 59% scored 24 or greater, indicating no cognitive impairment; 41% scored less than 24, indicating some degree of cognitive impairment with 18% having mild impairment (score 19-23); 22% with moderate impairment (score 11-18); and 1% with severe impairment (score 15).

METHOD

Participants were first screened using the MMSE and then asked to rate their present pain using the selected pain intensity scales. The majority of the sample experienced some degree of pain facilitating psychometric evaluation of the scales.

RESULTS

Older adults with and without cognitive impairment were able to use all the scales, a finding consistent with other studies with older non-minority adults. The NRS was the preferred scale in the cognitively intact group, and the FPS-R was the preferred scale for the cognitively impaired group. When race and cognitive status were considered, African-Americans and Hispanics preferred the FPS-R. Test-retest reliability at a 2-week interval was acceptable for all the scales. Somewhat low correlations existed between the FPS-R and the other scales, indicating that the FPS-R may be measuring more than the construct of pain (affective component of well-being), a finding consistent with other studies. Study limitations included the small sample size, lack of control for diagnoses in participants, limited number of cognitively impaired participants, and the fact that participants were asked only to rate their pain and not provided other words to describe the pain. The FPS-R is one tool that was preferred and useful in evaluating pain intensity in older African-Americans. Further research is indicated with larger samples, as well as research with Hispanic and Asian older adults.

Data from Ware L et al: Evaluation of the Revised Faces Pain Scale, Verbal Descriptor Scale, Numeric Rating Scale, and Iowa Pain Thermometer in Older Minority Adults, *Pain Manage Nurs* 7(3):117-125, 2006.

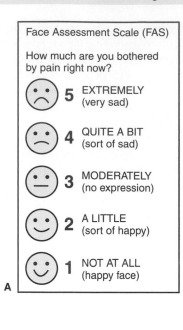

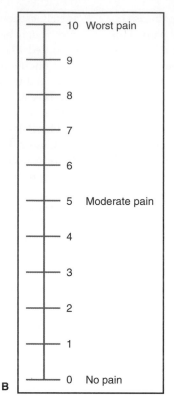

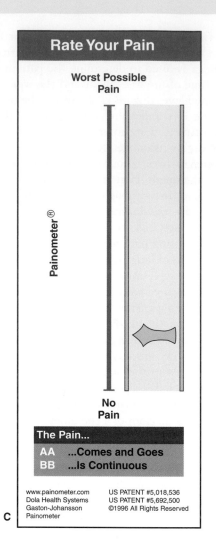

FIGURE 11-3 Examples of commonly used pain assessment scales. **A,** Face Assessment Scale (FAS). **B,** Numeric Rating Scale (NRS). **C,** The Gaston-Johansson Painometer. (**A,** Adapted from Philadelphia Geriatric Center Pain Intensity Scale. In Cramer K et al: *Philadelphia College of Pharmacy proposed guidelines for the management of chronic nonmalignant pain in the elderly LTC resident,* Feb 1988; Jacox A et al. Pub No 94-0592, Rockville, Md, 1994, Agency for Health Care Policy and Research [AHCPR], U.S. Department of Health and Human Services; Gaston-Johansson F et al. *Nursing Home Medicine* 4[11]:325, 1996; McCaffery M. *Nursing Home Medicine* 5[4]:143, 1997; Bridgeport, Conn, HealthCare Center Pain Assessment, created from pain assessment methodologies of the Joint Commission on Accreditation of Healthcare Organizations [JCAHO]; **B,** From McCaffery M, Pasero C: *Pain: clinical manual,* ed 2, St Louis, 1999, Mosby; **C,** Copyright 1996 Fannie Gaston-Johansson, Dr Med Sci, RN, FAAN, Baltimore, Md. May be duplicated for use in clinical practice.)

BOX 11-11 General Recommendations for Assessment Techniques with Noncommunicative Patients

- Attempt to obtain a self-report of pain from the patient; yes/no response acceptable.
- If unable to obtain a self-report, document why it cannot be used and further observation and investigation are indicated.
- Look for possible causes of pain or discomfort; common conditions and procedures that cause pain (e.g., arthritis, surgery, wound care, history of persistent pain, constipation, lifting/moving).
- Medicate before any procedures causing discomfort.
- Observe and document patient behaviors that may indicate pain or distress or that are unusual from the person's normal patterns and responses. Behavioral observation scales may be used but should be used consistently and with proper training.
- Surrogate reports (family members, caregivers) of pain and behavior changes as well as patients' usual patterns

and responses to pain and discomfort. This must be from a person who knows the patient well and should be combined with the other assessment techniques.

- If comfort measures and attention to basic needs (e.g., warmth, hunger, toileting) are not effective, attempt an analgesic trial based on the intensity of the pain and analgesic history. For mild to moderate pain, acetaminophen every 4 hours for 24 hours. If behaviors improve, continue and add appropriate non-pharmacological interventions. If behaviors continue, consider a single low-dose, short-acting opioid and observe effect. May titrate dose upward 25% to 50% if no change in behavior from initial dose. Continue to explore possible causes of behavior; observe for side effects and response.

From Herr K et al: Pain assessment in the nonverbal patient: position statement with clinical practice recommendations, *Pain Manag Nurs* 7(2):44-52, 2006.

earlier, identification of pain depends on intimate knowledge of the person's patterns, activity, and responses, as well as attention to slight changes in usual behavior. Older adults with cognitive impairment often present with nonspecific symptoms of pain (see Box 11-7). Figure 11-4 presents an algorithm for the assessment of pain in elders with severe cognitive impairment.

Although no instrument has strong reliability and validity for assessment of pain in cognitively impaired, non-communicative elders, several behavioral observation tools are being developed and evaluated that can be used (Hanks-Bell, 2004; Herr and Decker, 2004; Herr et al., 2006a). Tools include the Discomfort in Dementia of the Alzheimer's Type (DS-DAT) (Hurley et al., 1992); the modified DS-DAT (Miller et al.,

1996); the Checklist of Nonverbal Pain Indicators (CNPI) (Feldt, 2000) (available at *www.hartfordign.org*); the Pain Assessment in Advanced Dementia (PAINAD) (Warden et al., 2003); the Nursing Assistant–Administered Instrument to Assess Pain in Demented Individuals (NOPPAIN) (Snow et al., 2003); the Doloplus 2 (Lefebre-Chapiro, 2001); the Pain Assessment Checklist for Seniors with Limited Ability to Communicate (PACSLAC) (Fuchs-Lacelle et al., 2004); and the Serial Trial Intervention (STI) (Kovach et al., 2006a,b,c). A comprehensive systematic review of existing instruments concluded that the PACSLAC and the Doloplus 2 are the most appropriate tools currently available in terms of psychometric qualities, sensitivity, and clinical utility (Kaasalainen, 2007). A review of existing published instruments for assess-

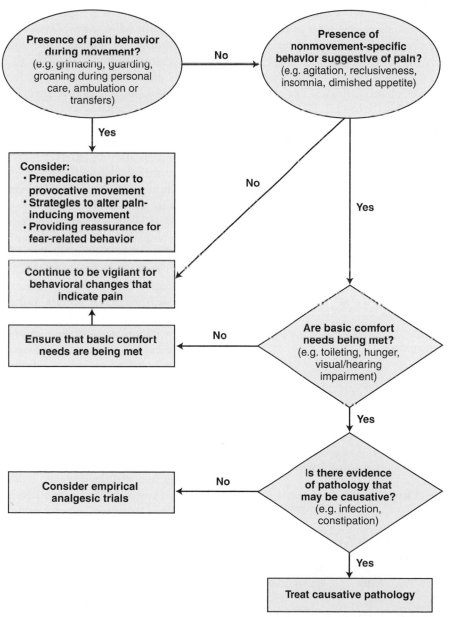

FIGURE 11-4 Algorithm for the assessment of pain in elders with severe cognitive impairment. (From Herr K, Decker S: Assessment of pain in older adults with severe cognitive impairment, *Ann Long-Term Care* 12(4):46-52, 2004; adapted from Weiner DK, Herr K: Comprehensive interdisciplinary assessment and treatment planning: an integrative overview. In Rudy T, editor: *Persistent pain in older adults: an interdisciplinary guide for treatment*, New York, 2002, Springer.)

ing pain in this population can be found at *www.cityofhope/prc/elderly.asp*. Choice of instrument will depend on appropriateness to the patient's setting, and clinicians are encouraged to obtain outcome data through quality improvement efforts (Herr et al., 2006a). Staff should receive intensive training on the use of behavioral observation tools (Kaasalainen, 2007).

Kovach et al. (2006a,b,c) developed the Serial Trial Intervention (STI), a research-based protocol to assess both physical pain, affective discomfort, and other unmet needs that may be the underlying cause of behavioral changes in people with late-stage dementia residing in nursing homes (Figure 11-5). The STI is a refinement of the original Assessment of Discomfort in Dementia (ADD) Protocol (Kovach, 2001; Kovach et al., 2006b). The three core components of the STI are behavior change identification, serial assessment, and serial treatment. "Serial assessments and treatments begin when a change in behavior is identified and basic interventions such as toileting, adjusting a hearing aid, or providing a warm sweater do not suppress behavior" (Kovach et al., 2006b, p. 19). Serial treatment may consist of either a targeted treatment or a trial of treatments, both non-pharmacological and pharmacological, depending on the need assessed. Box 11-12 describes the steps in the STI.

Use of the STI directs nurses toward careful assessment of behavior changes and possible underlying causes. This is particularly important in this population because physical conditions, particularly pain, are inadequately assessed and under-treated. Too often, psychotropic medications are given to patients with dementia who exhibit behavioral changes without adequate assessment for underlying physical problems and painful conditions. The medication may suppress the behavior but does little or nothing to relieve the underlying pain

or other physical or affective discomfort. Although further research is needed on the effectiveness of the STI, Kovach (Kovach et al., 2006b) noted that early studies "positively influenced nursing assessment, analgesic administration, and persistence of the nurse in intervening to resolve the person's troubled state" (p. 153).

Interventions

Working with the person in pain and achieving optimal pain management are especially challenging in gerontological nursing. Partly because of the experience of persistent pain and a history of poor pain control, the older adult may appear more tolerant or less vocal but is nonetheless suffering. At the least, the pain will compromise one's quality of health, and at the most, it will affect both mental and physical functioning. The knowledgeable nurse can work with the patient and significant others to achieve a high level of pain relief, with considerable effort and collaboration. Multiple modalities are available today to approach pain, and when the are used together, pain can be relieved in most cases when interventions have been individualized.

Pharmacological, non-pharmacological, and other comfort measures can relieve or minimize pain. An awareness of the totally pervasive nature of pain, as well as the multifactorial components influencing pain, requires a holistic approach in nursing interventions. Interventions include appropriate administration of pharmacological agents and use of non-pharmacological interventions with careful and systematic evaluation of response. An appreciation of the psychological and social consequences of pain includes careful listening, unconditional positive regard, ongoing support, and mobilization of resources. Pain can be minimized through gentle handling, touch, and careful observation of the person's reaction to procedures. Use of pillows for support or body positioning, appropriate and comfortable seating and mattresses, frequent rest periods, and pacing of activities to balance activity and rest are important.

Whether the pain is brief or long-standing, the anticipated result of diagnostic procedures or surgery, or related to a terminal condition, a plan for appropriate intervention should be developed and initiated. This begins with a discussion between the nurse and prescribing provider, patient, and significant others and includes how much pain is anticipated and how long it might last, how it will be treated, what alternatives will be available if the initial treatment does not adequately relieve the pain, and what level of pain is desired by the patient.

The nurse encourages elders to have a role in the management of their pain. The patient can be involved by keeping a weekly journal that includes an account of pain during the day; the times, type, and dose of medication taken; its effect; and the duration of its benefit. This type of information helps establish patterns that may be useful in improving pain management by adjusting activity, providing medications appropriately, and helping the patient feel useful and in control of some aspect of care and of their life with pain. An example of a symptom severity log can be found at *www.amda.com/clinical/chronicpain*. The diary should be reviewed

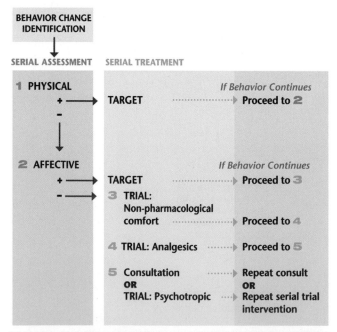

FIGURE 11-5 Illustration of the progression of nursing actions within the Serial Trial Intervention. (Reprinted by permission of Christine R. Kovach, PhD, RN, FAAN. Copyright © 2005 Christine R. Kovach.)

BOX 11-12   Steps of the Serial Trial Intervention

Behavioral symptoms are identified through appropriate assessment and knowledge of patient's usual behavior, patterns, and responses. Provide attention to basic care needs and comfort measures (e.g., warmth, hunger, toileting). If symptoms persist, the Serial Trial Intervention (STI) is initiated by the nurse and continued until behavioral symptoms decrease by 50% or more. Progression through the steps is based on results of assessments and decreases in symptoms by less than 50% in time frames that have been established for specified treatments. If the behavioral symptoms continue after completing all steps, the process is repeated. For a full discussion of the STI, see references below.

Step 1: Physical needs assessment focused on conditions that may cause discomfort (sources of physical pain such as arthritis, old fracture sites, wounds, infections, constipation/impaction). If assessment is positive, a targeted intervention is implemented or appropriate consultation is provided. If the assessment is negative or treatment does not decrease symptoms by at least 50%, move to step 2.

Step 2: Conduct affective needs assessment focusing on needs of people with dementia (stress threshold of environment; balance between sensory-stimulating and sensory-calming activity; presence of meaningful human interaction daily). If

assessment is positive, a targeted intervention is implemented and consultation with appropriate discipline initiated. If assessment is negative or fails to decrease symptoms by at least 50%, move to step 3.

Step 3: Administer a trial of non-pharmacological comfort treatments tailored to the person and found to be effective with persons with dementia who exhibit agitated behavior. A wide range of interventions have been suggested such as touch, balanced rest and activity, human contact, meaningful activities, pet therapy, exercise programs, storytelling, music therapy, reminiscence, spiritual support. If a trial of non-pharmacological comfort measures do not positively affect behavior in a time frame likely to show outcomes, move to step 4.

Step 4: Administer a trial of analgesics—use the as-needed (PRN) analgesic if ordered, or obtain an order. If there is no response to a trial course of analgesics, consider consultation or proceed to the next step.

Step 5: Consult with other disciplines or practitioners. May need to increase current analgesic or change to another. A trial of psychotropic drugs may be administered in this step if behavior continues. This must be considered carefully in light of alternatives and the risk of side effects for the particular patient.

Data from Kovach C et al: The Serial Trial Intervention: an innovative approach to meeting needs of individuals with dementia, *J Gerontol Nurs* 32(4):18-24, 2006; Kovach C et al: Effects of the Serial Trial Intervention on discomfort and behavior of nursing home residents with dementia, *Am J Alzheimers Dis Other Demen* 21(3):147-155, 2006.

by the care provider to assess the relationship between pain, medication use, and activity. A pain graph provides a visual picture of the highs and lows of the pain and provides the information needed for the appropriate adjustment of the selected intervention. The caregiver can assist in plotting the pain experience when necessary.

Pharmacological Pain Control. Generally, pharmacological pain relief is accomplished by altering the transmission of the sensation of pain from the origin to the cerebral cortex. The various pharmacological interventions available interrupt this transmission at different points in the process.

Analgesics (non-narcotic and narcotic agents) and adjuvant medications (antidepressants, anticonvulsants) are available for use and may be prescribed to the older adult. The general principles of pain control for older adults are the same as for younger adults; however, older adults may experience more adverse drug reactions related to age-associated changes in drug absorption, distribution, metabolism, and excretion (see Chapter 12). Older adults with multiple chronic illnesses requiring a number of medications are also more susceptible to drug reactions and interactions. Some medications used in younger adults, for example, meperidine (Demerol), are always contraindicated in the older adult.

Most nurses should be familiar with the essential principles of pain control as described by the World Health Organization's three-step ladder approach of pharmacological pain control (World Health Organization [WHO], 1994). The approach starts with the use of non-opioid analgesics

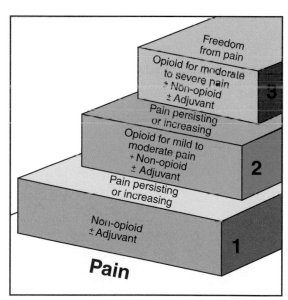

FIGURE 11-6 World Health Organization (WHO) three-step analgesic ladder. (Redrawn from World Health Organization: *Cancer pain relief,* ed 2, Geneva, 1996, WHO.)

(e.g., acetaminophen) and progresses to antiinflammatory drugs (e.g., NSAIDs), and finally, opioids (Figure 11-6). The use of this approach is also recommended for the elderly (AGS, 2002). Adjuvant drugs with analgesic effect, such as low doses of anticonvulsants and antidepressants, are particularly useful for neuropathic pain. Effective management of pain may require a combination of all these medications as indicated in the WHO ladder.

For persistent pain such as that associated with a number of terminal conditions, the nurse cannot allow the fear that frequent use of analgesic drugs will create iatrogenic addiction; the real issue is adequate pain relief. Keys to this relief are providing pain medication on time without the patient needing to ask for it and, as much as possible, erasing the memory of pain. The goal of pain management therapy, particularly for persistent pain, is to prevent the pain, not simply relieve it. The most effective way to do this is to provide around-the-clock (ATC) dosing (at the appropriate dosage) because it provides a more stable therapeutic plasma level of drugs and eliminates the extremes of over-medication and under-medication. Additional analgesics that are prescribed on an as-needed basis (PRN) should be used freely for pain that "breaks through" the ATC management (Portenoy et al., 2006). Use of opioids for long-term persistent pain control is often highly effective, and the treatment plan should be convenient, easy to administer, and initially short-acting for ease of dose adjustment. The simplest drug regimen is more likely to be effective and to be followed more easily.

Non-opioid Analgesics. The pharmacological management of pain is often discussed both in terms of the analgesic ladder and by the character of the pain, that is, mild, moderate, or severe (Figure 11-7). Non-opioid analgesics such as acetaminophen (Tylenol) are the first level and may often be adequate for mild and some moderate pain relief. If acetaminophen is used for persistent pain, around-the-clock dosing may provide adequate relief. The maximum daily dose is 4 g (4000 mg) and is reduced for people with renal or hepatic dysfunction or who drink alcohol. Although this seems like a high dose, with the availability of products such as Extra-Strength Tylenol at 1000 mg per tablet, it may be reached quickly.

If the pain is mild and acetaminophen is not effective or is not tolerated, non-acetylated salicylates (trisalicylate, choline magnesium) or one of the many NSAIDs (e.g., aspirin, ibuprofen [Advil, Motrin]) may be effective (AGS, 2002). Among older people, the use of OTC NSAIDs is common to

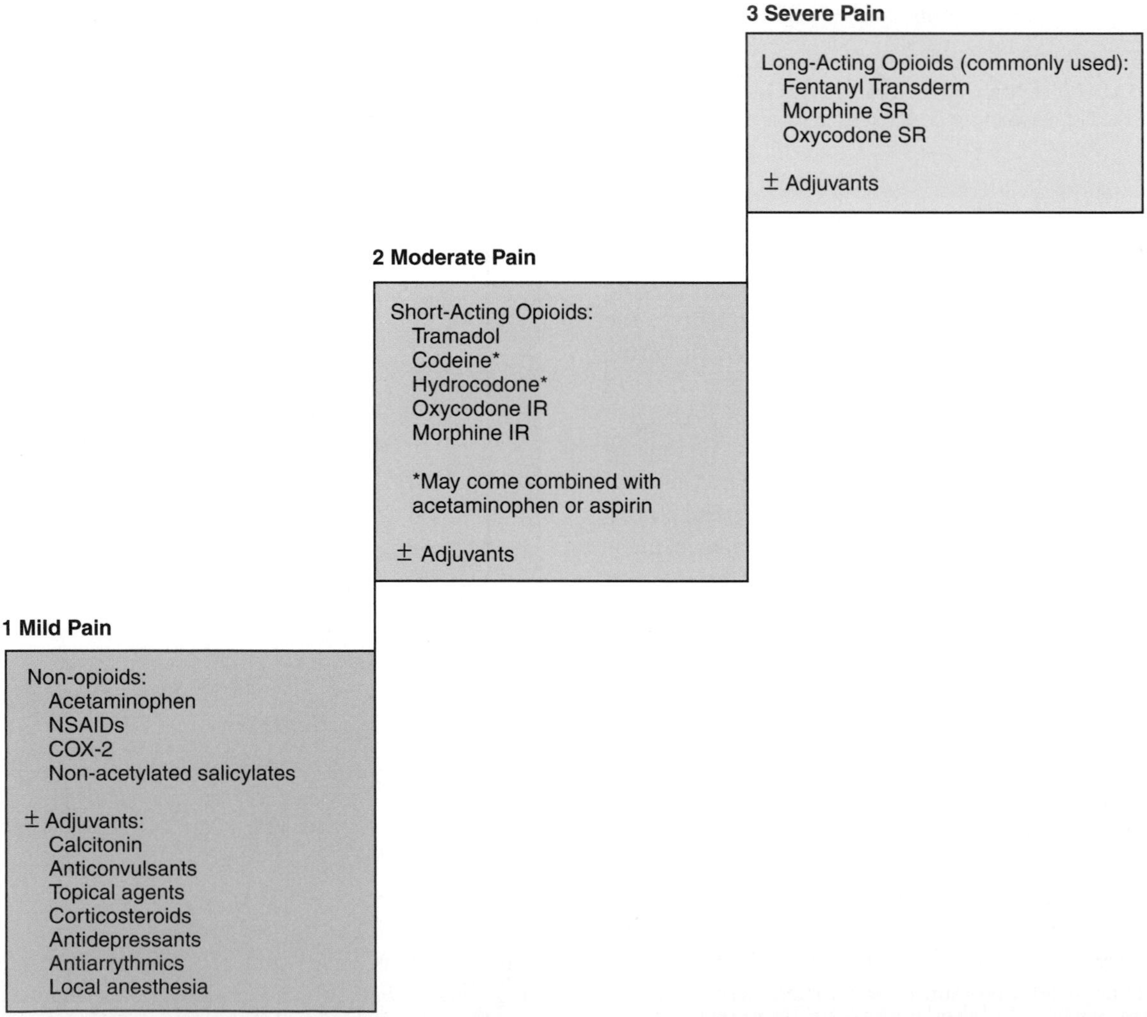

3 Severe Pain

Long-Acting Opioids (commonly used):
    Fentanyl Transderm
    Morphine SR
    Oxycodone SR

± Adjuvants

2 Moderate Pain

Short-Acting Opioids:
    Tramadol
    Codeine*
    Hydrocodone*
    Oxycodone IR
    Morphine IR

    *May come combined with
    acetaminophen or aspirin

± Adjuvants

1 Mild Pain

Non-opioids:
    Acetaminophen
    NSAIDs
    COX-2
    Non-acetylated salicylates

± Adjuvants:
    Calcitonin
    Anticonvulsants
    Topical agents
    Corticosteroids
    Antidepressants
    Antiarrythmics
    Local anesthesia

FIGURE 11-7 The ladder of frequently used drugs for pain management. (Compiled from *Acute pain management: operative or medical procedures and trauma.* Clinical Practice Guideline, Washington, D.C., 1992, U.S. Department of Health and Human Services, Public Health Service, Agency for Health Care Policy and Research; Fine PG: *Chronic pain in long-term care: assessment, management, and improvement of quality indicators,* Elder Care Summit Conference, San Francisco, April 24, 2002.;Lipman AG, Jackson KC: *Use of opioids in chronic noncancer pain,* Stamford, Conn, 2000, Purdue Pharma LP, Power-Pak, Inc.; McCaffery M, Pasero C: *Pain: clinical manual,* ed 2, St Louis, 1999, Mosby.)

relieve pain associated with osteoarthritis and degenerative joint disease. Often, older people and some nurses think that these medications are safe. However, NSAIDs bind with proteins and may induce toxic responses in elders if serum albumin levels are low. In addition, other drugs that elders routinely take compete for the same protein receptor sites and may be displaced by the NSAID, creating unstable therapeutic effects. Acetaminophen and NSAIDs must be used with caution because of increased risk of adverse effects, especially gastrointestinal bleeding and renal and hepatic impairments.

NSAIDs can potentiate and increase or decrease the effect of many prescription medications that older adults are likely to be taking. This may be intended, as with the use of non-opioids in combinations with opioids. Unintended interactions are seen most often with concurrent use of anticoagulants, oral hypoglycemics, diuretics, and antihypertensives. It is estimated that over 16,000 NSAID-related deaths occur each year among patients with osteoarthritis and rheumatoid arthritis, making it the fifteenth most common cause of death in the United States (Durrance, 2003). As cited in Durrance (2003), Mercola (2002) reported that older people taking OTC medications twice per week for 2 months were more likely to have beginning stages of chronic kidney failure. Risk for gastrointestinal bleeding is high, particularly in frail older adults with multisystem disease. Alternatives include topical therapies (e.g., capsaicin, lidocaine patch) for persons with intact skin.

The use of medications, even the non-opioids, requires careful review for potential drug interactions, monitoring for side effects and interactions, and patient teaching about safety when using OTC NSAIDs (Durrance, 2003). If long-term management of pain is necessary, the opioids may be preferred because of their lower rate of adverse reactions. Regardless of the medications used, the regimen should be convenient, easy to administer, and acceptable to the patient. Medications with the least accumulation and drug/food interactions should be sought. General guidelines for the use of non-opioids for prescribing nurses in advanced practice are provided in Box 11-13.

Opioid Analgesics. Opioid medications are used for acute pain, for both malignant (cancer) and nonmalignant persistent pain, and for transient moderate to severe pain. Opiates produce a greater analgesic effect, a higher peak, and a longer duration of effect in older adults. Sedation and impaired cognition do occur when opioid analgesics are started or doses increased. This often causes great concern from patients, families, and nurses. The AGS guidelines noted earlier state that this is to be expected and patients and caregivers should be cautioned about the potential for falls and appropriate safety precautions should be instituted. Sedation usually resolves with the development of tolerance, and if it is persistent, use of psychostimulant medications (e.g., methylphenidate [Ritalin]) might be needed (AGS, 2002; Lynch, 2001). Although there is much concern among nurses, with the appropriate use of opioids, respiratory depression is uncommon and sedation always precedes respiratory depression. In the rare cases of profound sedation or

respiratory depression, naloxone (Narcan) can quickly reverse the effects (AGS, 2002).

Opioid treatment should begin with "as needed" doses of short-acting medications and should be titrated based on the amount needed, response obtained, and side effects over a 24-hour period (Lynch, 2001). Current recommendations are to start with the lowest anticipated effective dose, monitor response frequently, and increase dose slowly to desired effect. Generally, an initial dose should be one-half to two-thirds the usual dose given to a younger person and, when needed, increased in increments of 25% (Pasero et al., 1999b). Once the amount of medication needed for relief in the 24-hour period has been determined, conversion is made to long-acting opioids to achieve a steady-state, around-the-clock effect. Additional non-opioids and adjuvant medications or short-acting opioids can then be used for break-through PRN treatment. If PRN medications are needed regularly, the long-acting opioid dosage should be adjusted accordingly. Unfortunately, too often the titration is not done (i.e., dosages are not adjusted after the original prescription) and pain relief is inadequate, especially in the long-term care setting (Hutt et al., 2006).

Side effects of opioids include gait disturbance, dizziness, sedation, falls, nausea, pruritus (itch), and constipation. Several of these will resolve on their own as the body develops tolerance to the drug. The side effects may be prevented when the prescribing provider works closely with the patient and the nurse to slowly increase the dose of the drug to a point where the best relief can be obtained with the fewest side effects.

The nurse closely observes the person's response to the medication and prevents or promptly treats side effects. Because constipation is almost universal when opioids are used in older patients, the nurse should ensure that an appropriate bowel regimen is ordered at the same time as the opioids. A daily dose of a combination stool softener and mild laxative may be very helpful, and adequate fluid intake is essential. Prophylactic use of antiemetics may be helpful for associated

---

BOX 11-13   Guidelines for the Use of Non-opioids

- Weigh risks versus benefits in selection.
- Start with a low dose to determine the patient's reaction (e.g., side effects). Increase gradually to a dose that relieves pain, not to exceed the maximum daily dose. The dose may need to be increased one to two times the starting dose.
- If maximum antiinflammatory effect is desired in addition to analgesia, allow adequate trial before discontinuing or switching. With regular doses for 1 week or longer, pain relief may improve.
- If one drug becomes ineffective but the pain is about the same, try a drug from a different chemical class.
- If the nonsteroidal antiinflammatory drug (NSAID) does not relieve pain when used alone, consider use in combination with opioids and/or adjuvant medications, but always with caution.

Adapted from McCaffery M, Pasero C: *Pain: clinical management*, ed 2, St Louis, 1999, Mosby.

nausea until tolerance develops. Lynch (2001) suggests that if nausea or vomiting continues, the provider should be asked or reminded about switching to a different drug or brand.

Opioids that can safely be used with the older adult are morphine, oxycodone, hydrocodone, hydromorphone, and transdermal fentanyl. Most are available in multiple forms. Fentanyl is available in a transdermal delivery system (Duragesic) as well as an oral transmucosal lozenge (Actiq). The transdermal form depends on absorption through body fat and should not be used in persons who are underweight or who are opioid-naïve. Unfortunately, in recent years there have been restrictions in insurance coverage of some of these, especially fentanyl.

Most of the other opioids are not recommended for use in older adults because of problems with the toxicity of metabolites (see Chapter 12). The use of meperidine (Demerol) is absolutely contraindicated. The metabolites of meperidine can quickly produce confusion, psychotic behavior, and seizure activity. The same can be said for pentazocine (Talwin), tramadol (Ultram), and methadone. Propoxyphene (Darvon) has a long half-life and a metabolite that has been associated with cardiac irregularities and pulmonary edema and is not recommended (Lynch, 2001). The nurse can refer to the Agency for Healthcare Research and Quality guidelines for acute and chronic pain management as well as the latest equianalgesic charts if they are needed (*www.ahrq.gov/guidelines*). These and other guidelines can help health care professionals improve the effectiveness of pain management for their patients (Box 11-14).

Adjuvant Drugs. Adjuvant medications have been developed for purposes other than analgesia (tricyclic antidepressants, anticonvulsants) but are thought to alter or modulate the perception of pain while also reducing the anxiety that often accompanies pain.

They may be used alone or in combination with non-opioid or opioid analgesics and are particularly effective for sharp, shooting, dull, aching, or burning pain associated with neuropathic conditions. Used in combination with analgesics, they may potentiate (enhance) the overall analgesic effects (Box 11-15). Elders frequently respond well to adjuvant pain regimens. However, it is important to remember that many adjuvant drugs have a very long half-life, which increases the plasma concentration in elders. When this group of medications is used, the nurse has to be especially diligent to watch for adverse effects or early signs of toxicity (see Chapter 12).

Non-pharmacological Measures. Nurses have a long history of comforting persons in pain through the use of non-pharmacological measures, including biological and biobehavioral techniques. Nurses are also responsible for meeting patients' education needs regarding pain management in their work with older adults, their families, and other caregivers.

Pain management entails control of not only physical pain but also emotional, psychological, and spiritual pain of the patient. The concept of pain, anxiety, and anguish cycle mentioned earlier is crucial to the successful manage-

---

BOX 11-14 Principles of Pain Management in the Elderly

- Always ask patients about pain.
- Accept the patient's word about pain and its intensity.
- Never underestimate the potential effects of persistent pain on the patient's overall condition and quality of life.
- An accurate diagnosis will lead to more effective treatment.
- Treat pain in advance of diagnostic procedures or care routines that are uncomfortable.
- Carefully observe behavior and reactions of older adults with cognitive impairment for pain. Consider pain first with a change in behavior. Involve family and caregivers in assessment of pain for cognitively impaired elders.
- Use verbal descriptor scales or visual analog scales for rating of pain intensity. Ensure that the scale is large enough for an older adult with vision impairment to read. Explain fully.
- Use a combination of pharmacological and non-pharmacological measures whenever possible.
- Give adequate amounts of drug at the appropriate frequency to control pain based on continual assessment.
- Use analgesic drugs correctly (see Figures 11-7 and 11-8).
- With opioids, start with a low dosage and increase slowly, but do increase to the desired effect or to intolerable side effects. Use around-the-clock dosing whenever possible.

- Use noninvasive route first, and try to make drug regimen as simple as possible, avoiding multiple medications and frequent dosing. Choose medications with the fewest side effects. Assess all medications, including over-the-counter drugs, for interactions.
- Anticipate and prevent common side effects:
  - Give antiinflammatory drugs with food.
  - Begin bowel regimen early to prevent constipation.
  - Be prepared to give an anti-nausea medication with narcotic analgesic drugs.
  - Anticipate some impaired balance and cognitive function with narcotic analgesic drugs.
- Consult an equianalgesic potency table when changing medication because of side effects.
- There is no role for placebos in pain management.
- Mobilize the patient physically and psychologically. Involve the patient in his or her own care.
- Anticipate and attend to anxiety and depression associated with pain syndromes.
- Reassess responses to treatment at regular intervals. Alter therapy to maximize pain relief and improve functional status and quality of life.

Modified from Ferrell BA: Pain management in elderly people, *J Am Geriatr Soc* 39:64-73, 1991; Glickstein JK, editor. *Focus Geriatr Care Rehabil* 10(3):6, 1996.

ment of pain. Reduction or relief of anxiety can be achieved by allowing the individual some control over the pain situation. Self-medication is one method. Teaching the patient about his or her medication and allowing the patient to administer the medication and keep dosage records eliminate the fear that medication will not arrive on time and that the patient may have to suffer until someone arrives to provide relief. Obviously not all patients can administer their own medications, but the potential is there, and each situation must be assessed on an individual basis. Studies have shown that effective control of pain (attention to psychological, emotional, spiritual, and physical distress) in many instances has reduced the amount of medication needed.

It has now been shown that a combination of pharmacological and non-pharmacological interventions appears to be most effective in the relief of both acute and persistent pain. The basic approach to pain management and control is one that considers that whatever has worked in the past and been effective without causing harm should be encouraged. This is particularly applicable for older adults with a lifetime of experience at managing pain with both the approaches used in Western medicine and those learned through their cultural heritages. More and more of the non-pharmacological measures are gaining acceptance by both patients and insurers such as Medicare. Several methods that elders use are compared here, but it is acknowledged that the list is far from inclusive of all those available. Table 11-2 lists and compares several of the non-pharmacological pain relief measures.

Cutaneous Nerve Stimulation. Deep and superficial stimulation of nerves for the purpose of pain relief has been practiced for centuries. Nurses have long provided massage, vibration, heat, and cold. Heat and cold temporarily interrupt the transmission of pain impulses to the cerebral pain center; however, the pathological cause of the pain should be considered and used accordingly with caution. Heat is effective for some disorders, such as the deep pain of inflammatory musculoskeletal conditions such as rheumatic conditions. Heat will increase the circulation to the area and therefore is contraindicated in occlusive vascular disease, in some types of cancer, and in non-expansive tissue such as bursae (some joints), where it may actually increase the pain. At the same time, intermittent application of cold packs is helpful in low back pain and some situations of nerve irritation. Care must be taken when applying heat and cold to the skin to prevent skin damage from extended periods of the applications. This is especially important in gerontological nursing because of the normal changes in aging skin (see Chapter 4).

Transcutaneous Electrical Nerve Stimulation. Two other methods of stimulation are transcutaneous electrical nerve stimulation (TENS) and percutaneous electrical nerve stimulation (PENS). Electrodes taped to the skin over the pain site or on the spine emit a mild electrical current that is felt as a tingling, buzzing, or vibrating sensation. The patient operates the stimulator and starts the electrical impulses, which then stimulate the dorsal column nerves that transmit impulses to close the hypothetical pain gate in the spinal cord and prevent pain signals from reaching the brain. PENS and TENS have been helpful in phantom limb pain, postherpetic neuralgia, and low back pain (Resnick, 2003). In many cases, Medicare will pay for the use of a prescribed TENS or PENS unit. Units are often available through the physical therapy department of skilled nursing facilities.

Touch. Touch is a natural form of providing comfort, although its therapeutic properties are still not clearly understood. Sometimes touch is considered a cutaneous stimulation technique, such as the specific techniques of "therapeutic touch." In this technique, developed by nurse Delores Krieger (1992), hands placed on or near the body with the concentrated intention of healing has been found to be effective in some cases but not in others (Mackey, 1995). When combined with purposeful relaxation, touch has also been found to decrease anxiety, reduce muscle tension, and help relieve pain.

Perceptual tendencies and sensory dimensions influence pain reactions and tolerance. Persons who were sensory deprived exhibited low pain tolerance, but those who received adequate or a high degree of sensory stimulation possessed a high pain tolerance. Fakouri and Jones (1987) demonstrated the positive effects of a 3-minute, slow-stroke back rub on both sides of the spinous processes from the crown of the head to the sacrum as a means of promoting relaxation. The back rub resulted in a decrease in heart rate and blood pressure and an increase in skin temperature. More recently, Meek (1993) found that slow-stroking back massage increased relaxation and produced the physiological effects of decreased blood pressure and heart rate and increased body temperature of hospice patients. No mention was made of its effect on pain. At the same time, the acceptability of touch by individual and culture varies considerably. Some touch may never be

---

BOX 11-15 Guidelines for the Use of Adjuvant Medications in Pain Management

- Avoid drugs with potent anticholinergic effects. These may result in urinary retention and subsequent urinary tract infection; constipation; blurred vision, which increases the chance for injury; dry mouth, affecting the ability to eat; and confusion.
- Neuroleptics, if used, may have the least sedating, cardiotoxic, and hypotensive effects.
- Avoid drugs that precipitate or potentiate extrapyramidal symptoms.
- Avoid tranquilizers that produce sedation and have a long half-life. Drugs with a short half-life are more suitable.
- Drugs that can cause orthostatic hypotension should be used with caution, especially when there is a preexisting cardiac condition.
- Interactions with other drugs must be monitored carefully because elders may take many medications for coexisting conditions (polypharmacy).

TABLE 11-2

Advantages and Disadvantages of Non-pharmacological Measures

Therapy	Advantages	Disadvantages

Cutaneous nerve stimulation
  Transcutaneous electrical
    nerve stimulation
    (TENS)
	Pleasurable sensations make it popular with elders
	Pain decreases during and after stimulation
	Requires little patient participation
		Some elders perceive stimulation as objectionable
		TENS or PNS requires special education and learning
		Choice may be limited by cognitive and sensory impairment

Touch	Good for those with limited mobility	
Acupuncture/acupressure	Relaxation and distraction from pain May be feasible for elders with limited income Requires limited energy expenditure Self-administration provides a sense of control	

Distraction
  Tactile, auditory, visual,
    kinesthetic
	Improved mood
	Easy to learn
	Relaxation
	Increased pain tolerance
		Lasts only as long as stimulus present

Relaxation	Decreases skeletal muscle tension Decreases anxiety Useful with chronic pain, muscle spasms, sleep loss due to pain	Must be able to understand instructions Takes time and energy to learn Ineffective with depressed or very fatigued Must be practiced daily
Biofeedback	Decreases chronic pain	Requires equipment (moderate to expensive) Time and energy to learn to administer or self-administer Must be cognitively intact

Imagery	Very simple, uses elder's imagination: may enhance
	  relaxation and distraction; may feel control over pain;
	  may perceive an escape from pain; always available
	Little or no economic or social impact for elderly
		Must be cognitively intact
		Not all health professionals able to teach it

Hypnosis	Pain relief on a long-term basis without side effects Useful for elders unable to tolerate pharmacological measures Does not alter mental function (a fear of the elderly)	May not be available in remote or small settings May be too expensive

Developed by Patricia Hess.

TENS, Transcutaneous electrical nerve stimulation; *PNS*, peripheral nerve stimulation.

acceptable, such as cross-gender touch in strict Muslim or Orthodox Jewish traditions. The culturally sensitive nurse always requests permission before touching a patient.

Acupuncture and Acupressure. Acute pain is registered as pain impulses pass through the theoretical pain gate in the spine and register the sensation in the brain, which in turn signals the central mechanism of the brain to return counter-impulses, which close the gate. Acupuncture uses tiny needles inserted along specific meridians or pathways in the body. Acupressure is pressure applied with the thumbs or tip of the index finger at the same locations as those used in acupuncture. It is thought that acupuncture and acupressure stimulate nerve clusters that cause the gate to close more quickly or that they trigger the release of the body's own opiate substances, enkephalins (endorphins). Acupuncture and acupressure have been used for thousands of years and scientific evidence of their effectiveness in the treatment of persistent pain is growing (Vas et al., 2006; Witt et al., 2006). In some cases, Medicare and some private insurance companies will pay for the cost of acupuncture treatment from a licensed acupuncturist.

Biofeedback. Biofeedback is a cognitive behavioral strategy used for a number of purposes, including pain relief. An individual can learn voluntary control over some body processes and alter them by changing the physiological correlates appropriate to them. Response to certain types of pain can be controlled with biofeedback. Boczkowski (1984) found that biofeedback decreased the persistent pain of rheumatoid arthritis. Other studies demonstrated no appreciable effect of biofeedback on migraine headaches in the elderly (Hamm and King, 1984). Training and, frequently, equipment of some type are needed to learn how to alter one's body response. Studies of the effectiveness of biofeedback have shown conflicting results. In some instances, it has proved to successfully reduce or eliminate pain.

Distraction. Distraction is a behavioral strategy that lessens the perception of pain by drawing the person's attention away from the pain and relegating it to peripheral awareness. In some instances, the individual can become completely unaware of the pain; in other instances, the intensity of pain is significantly diminished. The success of distraction can also be explained by the gate theory (see earlier Acupuncture and Acupressure section). Pain messages are slower than diversional messages; therefore the gate closes before the pain signal arrives and less pain is felt.

Mild to moderate pain responds well to distraction. At times, if an individual concentrates intently on another subject, the acute pain may be relieved. The most common forms of distraction include slow rhythmical breathing, slow rhythmical massage, rhythmical singing or tapping, active listening, guided imagery, and humor (Jeffery and Lubkin, 2002; Kozier et al., 1995). McCaffrey and Freeman (2003) found music as a form of distraction to be helpful when dealing with pain from osteoarthritis.

Relaxation, Meditation, and Imagery. As a behavioral strategy, relaxation enables the quieting of the mind and muscles, providing the release of tension and anxiety. Relaxation should be adjunctive to all pharmacological interventions. Meditation and imagery are two methods of promoting relaxation. Imagery uses the client's imagination to focus on settings full of happiness and relaxation rather than on stressful situations. Several studies using guided imagery have shown that pain perception in foot pain and abdominal pain was decreased. It was suggested that a strong image of a pain-free state effectively alters the autonomic nervous system's responses to pain (McCaffery and Pasero, 1999).

Hypnosis. Hypnosis, another behavioral strategy, can be used to alter pain perception, thus blocking pain awareness; to substitute another feeling for a painful one; to displace pain sensation to a smaller body area; or to alter the meaning of pain so that it is viewed as less important and less debilitating (Sarvis, 1995). Research has demonstrated that hypnotic analgesia reduces what are called "overreactions" to pain when apprehension and stress are apparent. Most of the population have some capacity for hypnosis and with training can increase their control in this area.

Activity. Activity can be helpful in several ways. It is thought that the less active an individual is, the less tolerable activity becomes. Anyone who becomes inactive may feel more general discomfort than the active person. However, some activities can stimulate pain. Use of analgesics in conjunction with activity may be necessary. The administration of an analgesic PRN medication 20 to 30 minutes before a specific activity may lessen or eliminate discomfort and fear of discomfort after the activity and greatly enhance the individual's capacity for that activity. The nurse should learn the patient's body tolerance for activity and work within those parameters.

Pain Clinics. Pain clinics provide a specialized, often comprehensive and multidisciplinary approach to the management of pain that has not responded to the usual, more standard approaches as described herein. The use of such pain clinics by the elderly has been limited. However, their use should be encouraged when appropriate. The number and types of pain clinics and programs have increased as a response to continued poor pain management by general health care practice. Pain center programs may be inpatient,

outpatient, or both. Pain clinics are generally one of three types: syndrome-oriented, modality-oriented, or comprehensive. Syndrome-oriented centers focus on a specific chronic pain problem, such as headache or arthritis pain. Modality-oriented centers focus on a specific treatment technique, such as relaxation or acupuncture/acupressure. The comprehensive centers tend to be larger and associated with medical centers. These centers include many services and provide a thorough initial assessment (physical, mental, psychosocial) of the person in pain. A comprehensive treatment plan is developed utilizing multiple modalities and usually a multidisciplinary team of interventionists.

The goals of pain management centers are to decrease pain intensity to a tolerable limit or eliminate it, if possible; improve functionality and activities of daily living (ADLs); increase involvement in family and social activities; decrease depression; and improve mood. This is accomplished by improving quality and frequency of assessment, improving optimal use of analgesics, assisting in minimizing analgesic adverse reactions, selecting non-pharmacological interventions, and evaluating outcomes associated with treatment. Physiological and cognitive-behavioral modalities are used to reduce or alleviate pain. The nurse should be familiar with the types of pain management clinics to provide the patient and family with necessary information to make a knowledgeable decision in selecting a center.

Evaluation

Evaluation of pain relief strategies requires repeated reassessment of the patient's status and comfort level both qualitatively and quantitatively. Qualitative indicators of better management or relief include physical indicators such as relaxation of skeletal muscles that were tense and rigid during pain. The individual no longer assumes a constricted pain posture. Behavior may reflect an increased activity level and sense of self-worth and the ability to better concentrate, focus, and increase attention span. The individual is better able to rest, relax, and sleep. In fact, the individual may sleep for what might seem like excessively long periods, but this is in response to the exhaustion that pain imposes on the body. Verbal indicators reflect the patient referring to the decrease in pain or the absence of pain during conversation.

The evaluation of pain management and relief is measured quantitatively with the same instruments used in the initial assessment for a means of comparison. Reevaluation of the frequency and intensity of pain, behavioral signs and symptoms that suggest pain, response to pharmacological and non-pharmacological interventions, and the impact of pain on mood, ADLs, sleep, and other quality-of-life measures are all included. Adjustments of treatment regimens and interventions are based on reassessment findings. Active involvement of the patient, family, and all caregivers is essential for comprehensive pain assessment, management, and evaluation. Finally, an individualized approach will optimize pain management and, in doing so, promote the health of persons at any stage of life and wellness (Box 11-16). If assessment is correct and the patient is listened to and handled gently and with care, anxiety can be controlled and interventions will prove more effective.

BOX 11-16   Guidelines for Individualizing Pain Management

1. Use a variety of pain control measures.
2. Institute pain control measures before pain becomes severe.
3. Use around-the-clock dosing for persistent pain with careful titration to achieve relief.
4. Use the lowest dose of pharmacological interventions, but use those that provide relief and those that are least invasive first.
5. Consider patients' ideas and cultural patterns in the development of pain management care plans.
6. Encourage the patient's and family's participation in the pain management plan that is educationally, culturally, and socially appropriate.

7. Listen to how patients describe the severity of pain. Physical signs and perceived severity are not predictably related, and expressions are usually culturally mediated.
8. Be aware that patients respond differently to different pain control measures. What is effective one day may not be effective the next day.
9. Be aware that persons from minority groups and older adults have been historically under-treated for pain.
10. Assess, intervene, evaluate, and repeat frequently.

Human Needs and Wellness Diagnoses

Self-Actualization and Transcendence
(Seeking, Expanding, Spirituality, Fulfillment)
Has spiritual well-being
Maintains realistic perceptions and expectations
Has control over situation
Is satisfied with self

Self-Esteem and Self-Efficacy
(Image, Identity, Control, Capability)
Maintains role
Feels appreciated and accepted in role
Makes own decisions
Has a comfortable and
appropriate demeanor

Belonging and Attachment
(Love, Empathy, Affiliation)
Does not have anxiety
Interacts with others
Expresses feelings to others

Safety and Security
(Caution, Planning, Protections, Sensory Acuity)
Manages therapeutic regimen effectively
Has intact problem-solving ability
Is coping effectively

Biological and Physiological Integrity
(Air, Fluids, Comfort, Activity, Nutrition, Elimination, Skin Integrity)
Is free of pain
Sleeps restfully
Is independent with basic needs
Has adequate assistance with basic needs when needed

These are not all the possible wellness diagnoses that may be identified. The above are examples of nursing diagnoses that should be considered when planning care for the older adult.

KEY CONCEPTS

- The absence of pain does not necessarily imply comfort. Comfort is a state of ease and satisfaction of the bodily wants and freedom from pain and anxiety.
- The nurse's response to a client's pain is influenced by the degree of ability to imaginatively identify with another and how well the other is known.
- Culture, ethnicity, family, and individual characteristics all influence one's tolerance and expressions of pain.
- Pain in older adults is under-recognized and under-treated, particularly in those with cognitive impairment and in long-term care settings.
- Older individuals with various degrees of cognitive impairment may demonstrate pain by increased levels of confusion, restlessness, agitation, or withdrawal. If behavior changes, assume pain until proven otherwise (Herr and Decker, 2004).
- Though sometimes assumed, it has not been shown that pain sensitivity and perception decrease with age.
- Pain is what the elder says it is. The nursing goal is to assist in pain relief. Some pain medications are more appropriate for use with elders than others.

- Acute pain and persistent pain require different therapeutic approaches. Persistent pain predominates in the life of many older people because of the frequency of chronic diseases.
- Various combinations of pharmacological and non-pharmacological pain control can be effective but must be individually designed with client decision making.
- Age-related pharmacokinetic and pharmacodynamic changes in the elderly influence the selection of drug therapy; drugs with a short half-life are preferred initially.

RESEARCH QUESTIONS

Do pain perceptions generally diminish as one ages?

What type of persistent pain do elders find most intolerable?

How do elders describe the pain of arthritis?

Do elders really fear the physical pain that may accompany dying?

What non-pharmacological means of pain control do elders use most frequently?

What non-pharmacological means of pain control are effective, and in what circumstances do they provide pain relief?

CASE STUDY: Pain in Elders

Ms. P. was a 66-year-old diabetic, and, after a stroke, her diabetes rapidly fulminated to uncontrollable fluctuations. Her blood sugar ranged from 20 mEq/mL to 800 mEq/mL. Some of this was caused by erratic eating habits, almost no exercise, frequent urinary tract infections, and considerable stress related to her condition and her future. She bumped her toe while being assisted into her wheelchair after occupational therapy. In a few days, the bruise had sloughed skin and an open sore was evident. In spite of the use of local ointments and various dressings, the sore became necrotic and was débrided. Within a few weeks, the débridement of necrotic tissue had removed half of her left great toe. Katy, who rarely complained, began to moan while she was sleeping and cry a lot during the day. She complained of a continuous burning sensation and said that it felt as if her toe was "on fire." One day she threw her coffee cup across the room, unable to bear the discomfort without expressing her frustration and anger. Various pain medications were given by mouth on an inconsistent basis, but the relief she experienced was minimal. She began to beg to die. The nurses thought perhaps she was right—after all, her general condition was poor, and life held little satisfaction for her. Maybe she should be allowed to die.

Based on the case study, develop a nursing care plan using the following procedure:*

- List Ms. P.'s comments that provide subjective data.
- List information that provides objective data.
- From these data, identify and state, using accepted format, two nursing diagnoses you determine are most significant to Ms. P. at this time. List two of Ms. P.'s strengths that you have identified from the data.
- Determine and state outcome criteria for each diagnosis. These must reflect some alleviation of the problem iden-

tified in the nursing diagnosis and must be stated in concrete and measurable terms.

- Plan and state one or more interventions for each diagnosed problem. Provide specific documentation of the source used to determine the appropriate intervention. Plan at least one intervention that incorporates Ms. P.'s existing strengths.
- Evaluate the success of the intervention. Interventions must correlate directly with the stated outcome criteria to measure the outcome success.

Critical Thinking Questions

1. Discuss Ms. P.'s situation and her probable prognosis.
2. What could be done, based on the information you have, to improve Ms. P.'s condition?
3. Do you think Ms. P.'s focus on pain is realistic or an avoidance mechanism?
4. What do you think impedes the nurses' understanding of Ms. P.'s pain?
5. Do you believe elders feel the pain of a necrotic (dead tissue) toe in the same degree that you would feel pain if someone cut away half of your toe?
6. Discuss the reasons for sporadic pain medication and inattention to the patient's signals and requests.
7. Do you think nurses are concerned about addiction in cases like Ms. P.'s?
8. In what situations do you believe addiction to pain medications is a priority concern?
9. Discuss issues of power and control related to pain management.

---

*Students are advised to refer to their nursing diagnosis text and identify possible or potential problems.

What are the reliable ways of assessing pain in cognitively impaired elders?

How can pain and pain relief be evaluated in the cognitively impaired?

How effective is patient-controlled analgesia (PCA) use by elders?

For whom and under what circumstances should the various modalities of pain management be used?

RESOURCES

Agency for Healthcare Research and Quality
www.ahrq.gov/guideline

American Academy of Pain Management
13947 Mono Way #A
Sonora, CA 95370
(209) 533-9744
www.aapainmanage.org

American Chronic Pain Association
PO Box 850
Rocklin, CA 95677
(800) 533-3231
www.theacpa.org

American Geriatric Society
www.americangeriatrics.org

American Medical Directors Association
www.amda.com

American Pain Foundation
201 N. Charles Street, Suite 710
Baltimore, MD 21201
www.painfoundation.org

American Pain Society
4700 W. Lake Avenue
Glenview, IL 60025
(847) 375-4715
www.ampainsoc.org

American Society of Pain Management Nursing
7794 Grow Drive
Pensacola, FL 32514
(850) 484-7766
www.aspmn.org

International Association for the Study of Pain
909 NE 43rd Street, Suite 306
Seattle, WA 98105
(206) 547-6409
www.iasp-pain.org

National Center on Complementary and Alternative Medicine
PO Box 7923
Gaithersburg, MD 20898
(888) 644-6226
www.mccam.nih.gov

Nurse Healers—Professional Associates International
Alamo Plaza, Suite 111R
4550 W. Oakey Boulevard
Las Vegas, NV 89102
(702) 870-5507
www.therapeutic-touch.org

The National Chronic Pain Outreach Association, Inc.
7979 Old Georgetown Road, Suite 100
Bethesda, MD 20814
(301) 652-4948
www.chronicpain.org

REFERENCES

American Geriatrics Society (AGS): The management of persistent pain in older persons, *J Am Geriatr Soc* 50(suppl 6):S205-S224, 2002.

American Medical Directors Association (AMDA): *Pain management in the long-term care setting,* American Medical Directors Practice Guideline, 2003. (website): *www.amda.com.*

Boczkowski JA: Biofeedback training for the treatment of chronic pain in the elderly arthritic female, *Clin Gerontol* 2:39, 1984.

Carson M, Mitchell G: The experience of living in persistent pain, *J Adv Nurs* 28(6):1242-1248, 1998.

Chiu N: Herpes zoster. In Beers MH, Berkow R, editors: *The Merck manual of geriatrics,* ed 3, Whitehouse Station, NJ, 2000, Merck Research Laboratories.

Diamond S, Urban G: Coping with postherpetic neuralgia, *Consultant* 42(5):639, 2002.

Durrance SA: Older adults and NSAIDs: avoiding adverse reactions, *Geriatr Nurs* 24(6):349-352, 2003.

Fakouri C, Jones P: Slow stroke back rub, *J Gerontol Nurs* 13:32, 1987.

Feldt KS: The checklist of nonverbal pain indicators (CNPI), *Pain Manag Nurs* 1(1):13-21, 2000.

Ferrell BA: Pain. In Beers MH, Berkow R, editors: *The Merck manual of geriatrics,* ed 3, Whitehouse Station, NJ, 2000, Merck Research Laboratories.

Fine PG: *Chronic pain in long-term care: assessment, management, and improvement of quality indicators,* Elder Care Summit Conference, San Francisco, April 24, 2002.

Fine PG: *Principles of effective pain management at the end of life,* CME/CE, 2006. (website): *www.medscape.com/viewprogram/6079_pnt.*

Frampton K: Vital sign #5: pain assessment and management in LTC requires a thorough, team-oriented care plan, *Caring for the Ages* 5(5):26, 29-30, 35, 2004.

Fuchs-Lacelle S, Hadjistavropoulos T: Development and preliminary validation of the Pain Assessment Checklist for Seniors with Limited Ability to Communicate (PACSLAC), *Pain Manag Nurs* 5(2):37-49, 2004.

Fulmer TT et al: Pain management protocol, *Geriatr Nurs* 17(5):222, 1996.

Hamm BH, King V: A holistic approach to pain control with geriatric clients, *J Holistic Nurs* 11:32, 1984.

Hanks-Bell M et al: Pain assessment and management in aging, *Online J Issues Nurs* 9(3):1-17, 2004. (website): *www.nursingworld.org/ojin/topic21/tpc21_6.htm.*

Herr K: Chronic pain challenges and assessment strategies, *J Gerontol Nurs* 28(1):20, 2002.

Herr K, Decker S: Assessment of pain in older adults with severe cognitive impairment, *Ann Long-Term Care* 12(4):46-52, 2004.

Herr K et al: Pain assessment in the nonverbal patient: position statement with clinical practice recommendations, *Pain Manag Nurs* 7(2):44-52, 2006a.

Herr K et al: Tools for assessment of pain in nonverbal older adults with dementia: a state of the science review, *J Pain Symptom Manage* 31(2):170-192, 2006b.

Hicks CL et al: The Faces Pain Scale—revised: toward a common metric in pediatric pain measurement, *Pain* 93:173-183, 2001.

Hurley AC et al: Assessment of discomfort in advanced Alzheimer's patients, *Res Nurs Health* 15(5):369-377, 1992.

Hutt E et al: Assessing the appropriateness of pain medication prescribing practices in nursing homes, *J Am Geriatr Soc*, 54(2):231-239, 2006.

International Association for the Study of Pain: Position statement, *Pain* 6:249, 1979.

International Association for the Study of Pain: Position statement, *Pain* 1992.

Jeffery JE, Lubkin IM: Chronic pain. In Lubkin IM, Larsen PD, editors: *Chronic illness*, ed 5, Boston, 2002, Jones & Bartlett.

Joint Commission on Accreditation of Healthcare Organizations (JCAHO): *Background on the development of the Joint Commission standards on pain management.* (website): *www.jcaho.org/news+room/health+care+issues/pain.htm*. Accessed July 26, 2004.

Kaasalainen S: Pain assessment in older adults with dementia: using behavioral observation methods in clinical practice, *J Gerontol Nurs*, 33(6): 6-10, 2007.

Katz S et al: The index of ADL: a standardized measure of biological and psychosocial function, *JAMA* 185:914-919, 1963.

Kovach C et al: Assessment and treatment of discomfort for people with late-stage dementia, *J Pain Symptom Manage* 18(6):412-419, 1999.

Kovach CR et al: Use of the assessment of discomfort in dementia protocol, *Appl Nurs Res* 14: 193-200, 2001.

Kovach C et al: Effects of the serial trial intervention on discomfort and behavior of nursing home residents with dementia, *Am J Alzheimers Dis Other Demen* 21(3):147-155, 2006a.

Kovach C et al: The serial trial intervention: an innovative approach to meeting the needs of individuals with dementia, *J Gerontol Nurs* 32(4):18-25, 2006b.

Kovach C et al: Deconstruction of a complex tailored intervention to assess and treat discomfort of people with advanced dementia, *J Adv Nurs* 55(6):678-688, 2006c.

Kozier B et al: *Fundamentals of nursing: comfort and pain*, Redwood City, Calif, 1995, Addison-Wesley.

Krieger D: *The therapeutic touch: how to use your hands to help or heal*, New York, 1992, Prentice-Hall.

Lawton MP, Brody EM: Assessment of older people: self-maintaining and instrumental activities of daily living, *Gerontologist* 9(3):179-186, 1969.

Lefebre-Chapiro S: The Doloplus 2 scale—evaluating pain in the elderly, *European J Palliative Care* 8(5):191-194, 2001.

Leo R, Singh A: Pain management in the elderly: use of psychopharmacologic agents, *Ann Long-Term Care* 10(2):37, 2002.

Lipman AG, Jackson KC: *Use of opioids in chronic noncancer pain*, Stamford, Conn, 2000, Purdue Pharma LP, Power-Pak, Inc.

Lynch M: Pain: the fifth vital sign: comprehensive assessment leads to proper treatment, *Adv Nurse Pract* 9(11):28-36, 2001.

Mackey RB: Discover the healing power of therapeutic touch, *Am J Nurs* 95(4):27, 1995.

Mattson JE: The language of pain, *Reflect Nurs Leadersh* 26(4):10, 2000.

McCaffery M: *Nursing management of the patient with pain*, ed 2, Philadelphia, 1979, Lippincott.

McCaffery M, Pasero C: *Pain: clinical manual*, ed 2, St Louis, 1999, Mosby.

McCaffrey R, Freeman E: Effect of music on chronic osteoarthritic pain in older people, *J Adv Nurs* 44(5):517-524, 2003.

McElhaney J: Chronic pain in older adults, *Consultant* March:337, 2001.

Meek SS: Effects of slow stroke back massage on relaxation in hospice clients, *Image J Nurs Sch* 25(1):17, 1993.

Melzack R: The McGill pain questionnaire: major properties and scoring method, *Pain* 1:277, 1975.

Mercola J: NSAIDs may harm kidneys of elderly, Sept 14, 2002. (website): *www.mercola.com/1999/may9/nsaids_may_harm_elderly_kidneys.htm*.

Miller J et al: The assessment of discomfort in elderly confused patients: a preliminary study, *J Neurosci Nurs* 28:175-182, 1996.

Morley JE: Aging successfully. In *Aging Successfully*, Division of Geriatric Medicine, St Louis University School of Medicine, 11(3):1, 2001.

Pasero C et al: JCAHO on assessing and managing pain, *Am J Nurs* 99(7):22, 1999a.

Pasero C et al: Pain in the elderly. In McCaffery M, Pasero C, editors: *Pain: clinical manual*, ed 2, St Louis, 1999b, Mosby.

Portenoy RK: Pain. In Abrams WB et al, editors: *The Merck manual of geriatrics*, ed 2, Whitehouse Station, NJ, 1995, Merck Research Laboratories.

Portenoy RK et al: Prevalence and characteristics of breakthrough pain in opioid-treated patients with chronic cancer pain, *J Pain* 7(8):583-591, 2006.

Resnick B: Managing chronic pain in the older adult, *Geriatr Nurs* 24(6):373, 2003.

Sarvis CM: *Pain management in the elderly*, Sacramento, Calif, 1995, CME Resources.

Snow AL et al: NOPAIN: a nursing assistant administered pain assessment instrument for use in dementia, *Demen Geriatr Cogn Disord* 921:1-8, 2003.

Thernstrom M: Pain, the disease, *New York Times Magazine*, December 16, 2001, p 66.

Travis S et al: Assessing and managing iatrogenic disturbance pain for frail, dependent adults in long-term care situations, *Ann Long-Term Care* 11(5):33, 2003.

Trossman S: Improving pain management: call to action, *American Nurse Today*, December:29-30, 2006.

Vas J et al: Efficacy and safety of acupuncture for chronic uncomplicated pain: a randomized controlled study, *Pain* 126(1-3):245-255, 2006.

Warden V et al: A pain assessment tool for people with advanced Alzheimer's and other progressive dementias, *J Am Med Dir Assoc* 4:9-15, 2003.

Ware L et al: Evaluation of the revised faces pain scale, verbal descriptor scale, numeric rating scale, and Iowa pain thermometer in older minority adults, *Pain Manag Nurs* 7(3):117-125, 2006.

Witt CM et al: Acupuncture in patients with osteoarthritis of the knee or hip: a randomized, controlled trial with an additional nonrandomized arm, *Arthritis Rheum* 54(11):3375-3377, 2006.

World Health Organization (WHO): *Management of cancer pain: adults.* Quick Reference Guide for Clinicians No 9, AHCPR Pub No 94-0593, Rockville, Md. 1994, U.S. Department of Health and Human Services, Public Health Service, Agency for Health Care Policy and Research.

CHAPTER 12

Geropharmacology

Gregory G. Gulick and Kathleen Jett

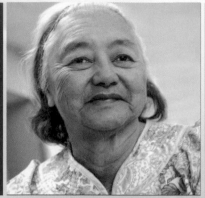
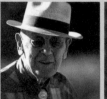
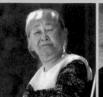

AN ELDER SPEAKS

If my social security check is late and it gets to the beginning of the month I have to make a choice: do I have my prescriptions refilled, do I buy food or do I pay my bills? I can't do it all. I can only go month by month and wait to see what happens.

Annie, age 72

LEARNING OBJECTIVES

On completion of this chapter, the reader will be able to:

1. Describe the pharmacokinetic changes that occur as a result of normal changes with aging.
2. Describe potential problems associated with drug therapy in late life.
3. Discuss the information that people should know about their medications.
4. Identify medications that are more commonly used in late life.
5. Describe medications and side effects of those more commonly used as psychotherapeutic agents in older adults, especially those residing in long-term care facilities.
6. Define inappropriate drug use and its application in gerontological nursing.
7. Identify the early signs of adverse drug reactions and strategies to prevent these.
8. Discuss barriers to medication adherence in elders.
9. Discuss the role of the health care professional in assisting elders with adherence to medication regimens.
10. Develop a nursing plan to promote safe medication practices and prevent drug toxicity.

In the United States, persons 65 years of age and older are the largest users of prescription and over-the-counter (OTC) medications. Making up only 12.7 % of the population, they consume 34% of the prescribed medications and 40% of those purchased over the counter (Randall and Bruno, 2006). It is estimated that older adults use OTC preparations 69% to 85% of the time for conditions ranging from pain to constipation to fever (Amoako et al., 2003). Because of multiple medical conditions, elders are also more likely to take multiple medications than younger adults. Elders accumulate prescriptions as they accumulate chronic diseases. In a 2003 survey conducted by the Kaiser Family Foundation (KFF), 89% of persons older than 65 years living in the community reported taking at least one medication; of these, nearly half (46%) took five or more and more than half (54%) had more than one provider prescribe for them. For those persons with at least three chronic conditions, 73% take a minimum of five medications (Kaiser Family Foundation [KFF], 2005). Elders who reside in long-term care facilities take an average of seven different medications (Gore and Mouzon, 2006). People are also taking an increasing amount of herbal preparations and supplements, referred to as *neutraceuticals* (see Chapter 13).

The most commonly prescribed and used drugs in the ambulatory older population are cardiovascular drugs, diuretics, non-opioid analgesics, anticoagulants, and antiseizure medications (Field et al., 2004). Gastrointestinal preparations, analgesics, and laxatives are the most-used OTC medications, followed by cough products, acetaminophen, nonsteroidal topical preparations, eye washes, and vitamins. The most commonly prescribed medication in the long-term care setting are psychotherapeutic agents and anticoagulants (Gurwitz et al., 2000).

Special thanks to Martha Buffum and John C. Buffum, the previous edition contributors, for their content contributions to this chapter.

Unfortunately, despite regulations and knowledge, medications deemed inappropriate for older adults continue to be prescribed in significant numbers (Table 12-1) (Simon et al., 2005). A recent increase in the inappropriate use stems in part from the increasing use of multiple providers and can lead to hospitalization or death (Randall and Bruno, 2006). Inappropriate prescription of drugs varies between Canada and the United States, with more benzodiazepines used in Ontario and opioids in the United States (Rochon et al., 2004).

More than half of all persons do not take their medications as prescribed (KFF, 2005). How elders use their prescribed medicines and their OTC products depends on many factors related to their own unique characteristics and situations. These factors include beliefs and understanding about illness, functional and cognitive status, perception about necessity of the drugs, severity of symptoms, reactions to the medications, finances, access, alternatives, and compatibility with lifestyle.

Many older adults are at risk for adverse drug events, excessive and inappropriate medication use, and nonadherence. Susceptibility to medication problems is greatly affected by physiological, functional, and social changes often seen in late life, increases in chronic disease and therefore medications, and varying levels of geriatric skills of health care providers. From the perspective of Maslow's Hierarchy of Needs, drugs impinge on many levels. When they are used appropriately, drugs can enhance one's quality of life at every level. When they are used inappropriately, they threaten all levels of the hierarchy. At times, even when drugs are used appropriately, they may adversely affect the elder's health and well-being.

This chapter includes discussions about issues and trends in health care affecting medication usage in the elderly, the basics of pharmacodynamics and pharmacokinetics, and a review of psychotherapeutics in late life, especially for persons residing in long-term care facilities. Specific strategies

TABLE 12-1
Drugs Considered Inappropriate for the Elderly

Drug	Concern
ANALGESICS	
Propoxyphene and combinations containing propoxyphene	No analgesic advantage over acetaminophen Side effects are similar to narcotics
Indomethacin	Produces the most CNS effects of all NSAIDs
Phenylbutazone	Can produce hematological effects
Pentazocine	Produces CNS effects more commonly than narcotics, including hallucinations and confusion
Meperidine	Potent metabolite, normeperidine, can accumulate in elderly, causing tremors and seizures
ANTIEMETIC	
Trimethobenzamide	Ineffective as an antiemetic Produces extrapyramidal reactions
MUSCLE RELAXANTS	
Methocarbamol, carisoprodol, oxybutynin, chlorzoxazone, metaxalone, cyclobenzaprine	Side effect profile high: anticholinergic side effects, sedation, weakness Doses of effectiveness not tolerated well in elderly
HYPNOTICS	
Flurazepam, diazepam	Long-acting benzodiazepines produce prolonged sedation, increasing fall risk and confusion risk Small doses of short- and intermediate-acting benzodiazepines may be more appropriate
Barbiturates except phenobarbital	More side effects than other sedative/hypnotics Highly addictive Use only for seizure control
ANTIDEPRESSANTS	
Amitriptyline	Strong anticholinergic and sedating properties
Doxepin	Strong anticholinergic and sedating properties
ANXIOLYTIC	
Meprobamate	Highly addictive and sedating
HYPOGLYCEMIC	
Chlorpropamide	Long-lasting, danger of hypoglycemia increased in elderly

Modified from Beers MH: Explicit data for determining potentially inappropriate medication use by the elderly, *Arch Intern Med* 157:1531, 1997; Buffum J: Geriatric dosage guidelines, 1996.

CNS, Central nervous system; *NSAIDs,* nonsteroidal antiinflammatory drugs.

Continued

TABLE 12-1
Drugs Considered Inappropriate for the Elderly—cont'd

Drug	Concern
ANTIARRHYTHMIC	
Disopyramide	May induce heart failure
	Strongly anticholinergic
ANTIPLATELET	
Dipyridamole	Causes orthostatic hypotension in elderly
	Beneficial only in artificial heart valves
ANTICOAGULANT	
Ticlopidine	No better than aspirin in preventing clots
	More toxic than aspirin in elderly
ANTIHYPERTENSIVES	
Methyldopa	May cause bradycardia
	May exacerbate depression
Reserpine	Poses danger to elderly: depression, impotence, sedation, orthostatic hypotension
CEREBRAL VASODILATORS	
Ergot mesyloids, Cyclospasmol	Not effective; not to be used for dementia or other conditions
GASTROINTESTINAL ANTISPASMODICS	
Dicyclomine, hyoscyamine, propantheline, belladonna alkaloids, clidinium-chlordiazepoxide	Highly anticholinergic, generally cause toxic effects in elderly
	Effectiveness at doses tolerated by elderly questionable
TREATMENT/PROPHYLAXIS OF DUODENAL ULCERS	
Cimetidine	Highly anticholinergic
	CNS effects: confusion, agitation, headache, fatigue
ANTIHISTAMINES (PRESCRIPTION AND NONPRESCRIPTION)	
Chlorpheniramine, diphenhydramine, hydroxyzine, cyproheptadine, promethazine, tripelennamine, dexchlorpheniramine	Potent anticholinergic properties
	For elderly, use cold and cough preparations without antihistamines in them
	Diphenhydramine should not be given for insomnia that is resistant to other sleep aids; only small doses (25 mg) for limited time should be used for allergy

Modified from Beers MH: Explicit data for determining potentially inappropriate medication use by the elderly, *Arch Intern Med* 157:1531, 1997; Buffum J: Geriatric dosage guidelines, 1996.

that gerontological nurses can use to minimize the risk for interactions and adverse events and maximize the therapeutic use of medications in the older adult are provided.

PHARMACOKINETICS

Knowledge of the basics of pharmacokinetics and pharmacodynamics will help the gerontological nurse promote healthy aging. Pharmacokinetics is the study of the movement and action of a drug in the body. Pharmacokinetics determines the concentration of drugs in the body. The concentration of the drug at different times depends on how the drug is taken into the body (absorption); where the drug is dispersed (distribution); how the drug is broken down (metabolism); and how the body gets rid of the drug (excretion). It is important for the gerontological nurse to understand how pharmacokinetics may differ in an older adult (Figure 12-1).

Absorption

For a drug to be effective, it must be absorbed, or taken into the bloodstream. The amount of time between the administration of the drug and its absorption depends on a number of factors, including the route of administration (e.g., intravenous, oral, parenteral, transdermal, rectal), bioavailability, and the amount of drug that passes through the absorbing surfaces in the body (Box 12-1). The drug is delivered immediately to the bloodstream with intravenous administration and quickly in the parenteral, transdermal, and rectal routes. Orally administered drugs are absorbed the most slowly and primarily in the small intestine. Because of these differences, a dose that is proper for one mode of administration may be inappropriate for another mode.

Drugs given orally pass through the mouth and esophagus and enter the stomach. Most solid oral drug dosage forms (e.g., tablets, capsules, powders, pills) are designed to dissolve in the stomach. Many factors affect the rate at which

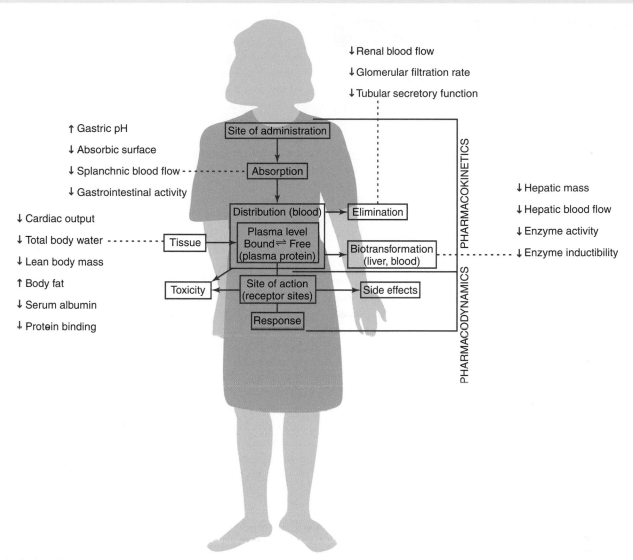

FIGURE 12-1 Physiological age changes and the pharmacokinetics and pharmacodynamics of drug use. (Data from Kane RL et al: *Essentials of clinical geriatrics,* New York, 1984, McGraw-Hill; Lamy PP: Hazards of drug use in the elderly: common sense measures to reduce them, *Postgrad Med* 76[1]:50-53, 1984; Montamat SC et al: Management of drug therapy in the elderly, *N Engl J Med* 321[5]:303-309, 1989; Roberts J, Turner N: *Clin Geriatr Med* 4[1]:127-149, 1988; Vestal RE, Dawson GW: Pharmacology and aging. In Finch CE, Schneider EL, editors: *Handbook of biology and aging,* New York, 1985, Van Nostrand Reinhold.)

a medication is dissolved. These factors include the amount of liquid in the stomach, the type of coating the tablet has, the extent of tablet compression used in making the tablet, the presence of expanders in the tablet, the solubility of the drug in the acid environment of the stomach, and the rate of peristalsis (Wilkinson, 2001). Liquid drug dosage forms for oral use come as solutions, suspensions, tinctures, and elixirs. The different forms of liquid drug administration are outlined in Box 12-2. The presence of food in the stomach may or may not delay absorption. The nurse should know the effect of food on the absorption of a medication for accurate patient education and optimal administration. This is especially true for the patient who receives artificial nutrition via a gastric or duodenum tube.

There does not seem to be conclusive evidence that the absorption process in older adults is changed appreciably. However, we do know that diminished salivary secretion

---

BOX 12-1   Routes of Medication Administration

- Oral
- Sublingual
- Rectal
- Topical
- Transdermal
- Intramuscular
- Intravenous
- Subcutaneous
- Intraarterial
- Intranasal
- Ophthalmic
- Intraperitoneal
- Intrathecal
- Inhalation
- Auricular (in the ear)

BOX 12-2   Forms of Liquid Medications

Solutions: The drug is dissolved in water.
Suspensions: The drug (generally a water-insoluble drug) is suspended in some liquid medium.
Tinctures: The drug is dissolved in an alcohol-based solution.
Elixirs: Semi–water-soluble solutions of drugs are held in solution by alcohol.

---

and esophageal motility may interfere with swallowing some medications, which could in turn lead to erosions if adequate fluids are not taken with the medications (Gore and Mouzon, 2006). Decreased gastric pH, common in the elderly, will retard the action of acid-dependent drugs. Delayed stomach emptying may diminish or negate the effectiveness of short-lived drugs that could become inactivated before reaching the small intestine. Some enteric-coated medications, which are specifically meant to bypass stomach acidity, may be delayed so long that their action begins in the stomach and may produce undesirable effects, such as gastric irritation or nausea.

Once a drug has been administered orally (or by a gastric tube), it may be absorbed directly into the bloodstream from the stomach (e.g., alcohol), but usually passes dissolved into the duodenum or small intestine (Wilkinson, 2001). The small intestine has a large surface area and is efficient at absorption. The potential changes in gastrointestinal motility in late life may also be important factors that potentially influence absorption. If the motility of the small intestine increases, drug effect is diminished because of shortened contact time and therefore decreased absorption. Conversely, slowed intestinal motility can increase the contact time and increase drug effect because of prolonged absorption (see Chapter 4). This increases the risk for adverse reactions or unpredictable effects.

During the process of absorption, the drug passes from the small intestine into the network of veins surrounding it. These veins, known as the *portal system*, drain into the portal vein, which enters the liver where the drug may undergo metabolism (see below). Drugs that pass through the liver before they reach the systemic circulation may undergo what is termed *first-pass metabolism*. Drugs that are extensively metabolized as they pass through the liver from the portal system are said to have a large first-pass effect. Drugs with a large first-pass effect usually have a much larger oral therapeutic dose than the same drug given by injection (Hall, 2003). In normal aging, both liver mass and blood flow are significantly decreased, resulting in reductions in the metabolism rate (see Chapter 4).

With sublingual administration, the drug is absorbed in the oral cavity and passes directly into the systemic circulation (Wilkinson, 2001). This route bypasses the stomach, small intestine, portal system, and liver. As a result, to the extent that the drug can be absorbed sublingually, the drug reaches the systemic circulation much faster and avoids first-pass me-

tabolism by the liver. The buccal mucosa does not have a large surface area, so it is not very efficient at absorbing anything but the most concentrated drugs. The drying of the mouth, a common side effect of many of the medications taken by older adults, may reduce or delay buccal absorption.

Rectal administration may be useful when the patient cannot tolerate oral medications (Wilkinson, 2001). Drugs absorbed by the rectum pass quickly into the portal system and the liver before reaching the systemic circulation. Like the buccal mucosa, the rectum does not have a large surface area, so it is not very efficient at absorbing drugs.

Parenterally administered drugs are absorbed the fasted in most cases, avoid the first-pass effect, and usually require a smaller dose. Intravenous administration has the fastest onset of drug effect and is the most efficient drug delivery method (Wilkinson, 2001). Drugs given intravenously should be injected slowly so as not to produce toxicity from excessive blood levels. Some drugs must be administered over 1 to 2 hours. Always check with a pharmacist or a good drug reference to find out the safe rate of drug administration before administering a drug by the intravenous route. The intramuscular and subcutaneous routes of drug administration result in a slower onset of drug action and depend on the rate of absorption from the injection site. Some drugs that are effective by intravenous administration are poorly absorbed from an intramuscular injection (e.g., phenytoin, diazepam). Drugs given by intramuscular or subcutaneous routes do not have to be given slowly.

The transdermal delivery system is the topical application of fat-soluble drugs for systemic use, usually with a patch impregnated with the medication (e.g., estrogen, clonidine, nicotine, fentanyl, nitroglycerine). The number of medications available for transdermal administration is growing rapidly, and this route of administration is sometimes thought to be more convenient, acceptable, and reliable than other routes, especially in the out-patient setting. The TDDS provides for a more constant rate of drug administration and eliminates concern for gastrointestinal absorption variation, gastrointestinal intolerance, and drug interaction. This route is indicated when a slow, timed-release delivery into the tissue and ultimately the bloodstream is desired; the skin should be tested for subcutaneous thickness and integrity before application. For the elder who is either underweight or overweight, dosing may be unreliable. Also, because of the immune changes in late life, an allergic reaction to the patch itself may be more common (Box 12-3).

Several other routes are available but are used less frequently. Very few drugs are given by the intraarterial, intraperitoneal, or intrathecal routes. Specialized training is required for safe administration using these routes. Intranasal, ophthalmic, and auricular drug administrations are usually for the purpose of delivering the drug to the site of administration, but systemic absorption may occur (Wilkinson, 2001).

Finally, the co-administration of food and medications commonly taken by older adults can also affect the absorption of other drugs. See the detailed discussion on p. 303 of food-drug and drug-drug interactions.

BOX 12-3 Guidelines for the Use of Transdermal Delivery Systems

PROPER ADMINISTRATION

1. Know the proper place for administration (some require specific anatomical placement).
2. Place on clean surface (if hairy, should be shaved).
3. Press firmly for 10 seconds for secure contact (no wrinkles or raised edges).
4. Wear gloves or wash hands after contact with patch.
5. DO NOT cut patch in half to decrease dose (this can cause evaporation or spillage of the medication and decrease adherence to skin).

SITE ROTATION

1. Do not reapply to same area for at least 7 days.

RASH MANAGEMENT

1. Rash is most common side effect (occurs in about 50% of patients because of active ingredient or adhesive).
2. If ordered, apply topical corticosteroid to site as a pretreatment or after patch is removed.

PROPER DISPOSAL

1. Fold sticky edges together.
2. Dispose in a closed garbage can to keep away from pets or children.

Modified from Fischer RG, Clark N. *Adv Nurse Pract* 2(10):15, 1994.

Distribution

Once a drug is absorbed, it must be distributed or transported to the receptor site on the target organ to have a therapeutic effect. Some drugs exert their therapeutic effect in their absorbed form, whereas others must be metabolized first.

The systemic circulation transports the drug throughout the body. The organs of high blood flow (e.g., brain, kidneys, lungs, liver) rapidly get the highest concentrations (Wilkinson, 2001). Distribution to organs of lower blood flow (e.g., skin, muscles, fat) generally occurs more slowly and results in lower concentrations of the drug in the tissues. Circulatory disease such as peripheral vascular disease could affect drug distribution.

Lipophilic (absorbed by fat) drugs pass through capillary membranes more easily than hydrophilic (absorbed by water) drugs, resulting in more rapid tissue distribution and a greater volume of distribution. Lipophilic drugs may concentrate in adipose tissue to a greater extent than in the vasculature or other tissues. Adipose tissue, or the fat content of the body, nearly doubles in older men and increases by one half in older women (see Chapter 4). Drugs that are highly lipid soluble are stored in the fatty tissue, thus extending and possibly elevating the drug effect (Masoro and Austed, 2003).

Distribution also depends on the availability of plasma protein in the form of lipoproteins, globulins, and especially albumin. Some drugs are bound to protein for distribution. Normally, a predictable percentage of the absorbed drug is inactivated as it is bound to the protein. The remaining free drug is available in the bloodstream for therapeutic effect when an effective concentration is reached in the plasma. When more than one protein-bound drug is taken (common in the polypharmacy of elders), drugs may compete with each other for binding, with the result that the drug with the stronger binding affinity may displace the other drug from the protein. This could result in the unbound drug exerting a much greater effect on the body when more unbound drug is available.

The healthy elder shows either no or only an insignificant change in plasma binding proteins. However, albumin may be significantly reduced in the ill elderly because of malnutrition, an acute illness, or a long-standing chronic condition. This potentially occurs in drugs such as lorazepam, diazepam, chlorpromazine, phenobarbital, and haloperidol (Haldol). When this occurs, there are unpredictable concentrations of free drug available that may result in toxic levels, especially for highly protein-bound medications with narrow therapeutic windows, such as lorazepam, haloperidol, and salicylates. Basic drugs (e.g., lidocaine, propranolol) will show increased protein binding and less effect, and acidic drugs (e.g., warfarin, phenytoin) will show decreased protein binding and greater effect (because of decreased plasma albumin) (O'Mahony, 2000). This is especially relevant to nurses working in long-term care settings where hypoalbuminemia is common.

Other late-life alterations in drug distribution are related primarily to changes in body composition, particularly decreases in lean body mass and increases in body fat as just noted, as well as decreases in total body water. Decreased body water leads to higher serum levels of water soluble drugs, such as digoxin, ethanol, and aminoglycosides. This would result in a higher relative volume of lipophilic drugs (e.g., diazepam, lorazepam) and a decreased volume of hydrophilic drugs (e.g., cimetidine, morphine) (O'Mahony, 2000).

Metabolism

Metabolism is the process wherein the chemical structure of the drug is converted to a metabolite that is more easily used and excreted. This process is called *biotransformation*. A drug will continue to exert a therapeutic effect as long as it remains either in the original state or as an active metabolite or metabolites. Active metabolites retain the ability to have a therapeutic effect and have the same or more chance of adverse effects as the original structure. For example, the metabolites of acetaminophen (Tylenol) can cause liver damage with doses above 4 grams in 24 hours. The duration of drug action is determined by the metabolic rate and measured in terms of half-life, the length of time the drug is active in the body. With aging, the liver activity, mass, volume, and blood flow are diminished (see Chapter 4). As a result, the half-life of many medications is extended.

The primary site of metabolism is the liver, although many other organs have metabolizing enzymes (e.g., gut, brain, lungs). Metabolism occurs in two phases—*phase I* (oxidative) and *phase II* (conjugative). Conjugation reactions primarily convert drugs and their metabolites to glucuronides. Glucuronides are very hydrophilic and are more readily excreted in the urine or bile (Wilkinson, 2001).

The oxidative metabolizing enzymes are known as the *cytochrome P450 (CYP450) monooxygenase system*. The human CYP450 system is composed of about 50 isoforms, each of which can perform a specific chemical reaction (Wilkinson, 2001). Eight to ten of these isoforms are responsible for the majority of all drug metabolism. These isoforms metabolize the parent compound by adding or subtracting a part of the drug molecule (e.g., adding an oxygen atom or subtracting a methyl group), thereby changing the molecule into a more hydrophilic (polar) compound. The drug molecule may undergo several enzymatic conversions by different CYP450 isoforms before it can be excreted by the kidney. Each CYP450 isoform has an enzymatic affinity for a uniquely different type of molecular structure (Hartshorn and Tatro, 2003).

Other drugs and certain foods can either increase or inhibit a metabolic isoenzyme. For example, grapefruit juice inhibits CYP3A3/4 in the gut and therefore the metabolism of drugs such as calcium channel blockers, whereas rifampin induces CYP3A4 metabolism of estradiol, thereby reducing its contraceptive action and perhaps the postmenopausal benefits as well. Some drugs auto-inhibit their own metabolism (e.g., fluoxetine is both a substrate and an inhibitor of CYP2D6) (Flockhart, 2000). Some drugs auto-induce their own metabolism (e.g., carbamazepine is both a substrate and an inducer of CYP3A4) (Lacy et al., 2003). Drugs with a large first-pass effect are more prone to drug interactions, because more of the parent compound reaches the systemic circulation when another drug or food inhibits its metabolism.

Several of the metabolizing enzymes (CYP450 isoforms) show genetic differences. It has been found that people from different global regions tend to metabolize at different levels of efficiency: poor metabolizers, intermediate metabolizers, extensive metabolizers, and ultrarapid metabolizers (Wilkinson, 2001). Among persons of northern European ancestry, 5% to 10% are poor metabolizers. This contrasts with persons from parts of Asia and Africa, among whom only 1% are poor metabolizers. The clinical consequence is that when poor metabolizers take codeine for pain, they may get no or little analgesic effect. This is because codeine's analgesic action depends on the 7% of the codeine that is converted to morphine by CYP2D6 isoenzymes. Concomitant administration of an inhibitor (e.g., quinine, fluoxetine) can also inhibit codeine's conversion to morphine. In an ultrarapid metabolizer, ingestion of codeine produces an exaggerated effect from the greater amount of morphine formation (Wilkinson, 2001). Because of these potential differences in people, susceptibility to adverse or unpredictable drug events varies.

Because the metabolism of drugs once they reach the liver varies considerably among individuals, it is difficult to ascribe decreased drug-metabolizing capability to increased age. Studies have shown no decrease in either conjugative metabolism or CYP450 system function as a result of age (O'Mahony, 2000). However, liver size and hepatic blood flow tend to decrease with advanced age (see Chapter 4) with resultant decreases in hepatic exposure. Drugs that undergo extensive first-pass metabolism are affected by age, whereas non–first-pass drugs are not (O'Mahony, 2000). These drugs may exhibit decreased metabolism and increased bioavailability (e.g., nalbuphine, propranolol, lidocaine) (Eddington, 1996).

Excretion

Drugs and their metabolites are excreted in sweat, saliva, and other secretions but primarily through the kidneys. They are excreted either unchanged or as metabolites (Wilkinson, 2001). A few drugs are eliminated through the lungs, as un-reabsorbed metabolites in bile and feces, or in breast milk. Very small amounts of drugs and metabolites can also be found in hair, sweat, saliva, tears, and semen.

Renal drug excretion occurs when the drug is passed through the kidney and involves glomerular filtration, active tubular secretion, and passive tubular reabsorption (Wilkinson, 2001). Glomerular filtration depends on both the glomerular filtration rate and the extent of protein binding of the drug (Wilkinson, 2001). The process is passive filtration, and only unbound drugs are filtered. Some drugs (e.g., organic cations and amphipathic anions) are actively secreted into the proximal renal tubule by way of a carrier-mediated process. Conjugated drugs and metabolites are also actively secreted into the proximal tubule.

Because kidney function declines in most older persons, so does the ability to excrete or eliminate drugs in a timely manner. Glomerular filtration rate, renal plasma flow, tubular function, and reabsorptive capacity decline. Glomerular filtration declines at a rate of about 1% per year after age 20 years, with an estimated drop of 50% between the ages of 25 and 85 years (Williams, 2002). The significantly decreased glomerular filtration rate leads to prolongation of the half-life of drugs eliminated through the renal system, resulting in more opportunities for accumulation and potential toxicity or other adverse events. Although renal function cannot be estimated by the creatinine level, it can be approximated by the calculation of the creatinine clearance. Reductions in dosages for drugs eliminated through the renal system (e.g., allopurinol, vancomycin) are needed when the creatinine clearance is reduced.

Creatinine clearance (Cl_{cr}) is a measure of renal function. The doses of many drugs eliminated through the renal system are based on the patient's measured or estimated creatinine clearance. The Cockcroft and Gault equation can be used for the calculation of Cl_{Cr} from age, serum creatinine (S_{cr}), and ideal body weight (in kg) (Cockcroft and Gault, 1976).

The estimated Cl_{cr} in milliliters per minute (mL/min) is as follows (Semla et al., 2007):

$$\text{Male} = \frac{(140 - \text{Age}) \times \text{Weight (kg)}}{72 \times S_{cr}}$$

For women, this result is multiplied by 0.85.

PHARMACODYNAMICS

Pharmacodynamics refers to the physiological processes between a drug and the body (see Figure 12-1). Specifically, pharmacodynamics describes the interaction of chemicals introduced into the body and receptors in the body. Receptors are generally specifically configured cellular proteins that, because of their shape and charge distribution, bind to specific chemicals in the medications. The receptor protein has a specific shape that fits the chemical molecule like a glove to a hand. It also has charged areas within the receptor that are opposite in charge to those of the chemical. This is known as the *ligand-binding domain* (Hohl et al., 2001). When the chemical binds to the receptor, the therapeutic effect is initiated (e.g., nerve conduction and enzyme inhibition).

Drugs are usually similar in chemical configuration or charge distribution to chemicals occurring naturally in the body such that they bind to the same receptor sites. When a drug binds to the receptor sites, it may initiate the same physiological action as the natural chemical (agonist) or it may simply occupy the receptor sites and, in doing so, block ability of the body chemical's usual physiological process (antagonist). Although the drugs are designed to bind to specific receptor sites for specific purposes, usually they will attach to various other types of receptors as well. The physiological effects that occur as a result of binding to the unplanned types may produce unwanted side effects.

Continuing to stimulate a receptor with an agonist results in desensitization or down-regulation of the receptor. Continuous blocking of a receptor with an antagonist results in sensitization or up-regulation of the receptor (Hohl et al., 2001). Consequently when a drug is given over an extended period, the dose may need to be increased to maintain the drug effect because of the change in receptor sensitivity.

The older the person gets, the more likely he or she will have an alteration or unreliable response to the drug. Although it is not always possible to explain or predict the alteration, several are known. Older adults tend to have a decreased response to beta- (β) adrenergic receptor stimulators and blockers (e.g., muscarinic acetylcholine receptors in brain, α_1-adrenergic receptors in liver, opioid receptors in brain) (Hammerlein et al., 1998). Decreased muscarinic receptors in the brain are associated with decreased memory. Consequently, if any of the muscarinic receptors are blocked with muscarinic antagonists (anticholinergic), the memory is further impaired (Vestal, 2000). The elderly are highly sensitive to anticholinergic side effects of drugs. When anticholinergics are used, in addition to the usual urinary retention and hesitancy and dry mouth, confusion may be seen as a side effect (Moore and O'Keefe, 1999). The use of benzodiazepines is associated with an increased risk for accidental injury (Briggs, 2005).

Aging is also associated with decreased sympathetic innervation of the juxtaglomerular cells of the kidney, which results in decreased plasma renin levels and decreased blood and urine aldosterone levels. Baroreceptor reflex responses decrease with age. This causes increased susceptibility to positional changes (orthostatic hypotension) and volume changes (dehydration). Drugs affecting these systems (e.g., diuretics, α_1-adrenergic blockers) have a greater effect in the elderly (Crome, 2000).

Age-related increases in sympathetic nervous system activity occur as a result of decreased myocardial sensitivity to catecholamines (e.g., norepinephrine, epinephrine) (Hammerlein et al., 1998). This is caused by decreases in the ability to activate adenylate cyclase, an enzyme necessary in the generation of cyclic adenosine monophosphate (cAMP), the second messenger for the α-adrenoceptor, rather than because of any decreases in the numbers of α-adrenoceptors (Hammerlein et al., 1998). This decreased responsiveness of the α-adrenergic system results in decreased sensitivity to β-agonists and β-antagonists (β-blockers). Because of the decreased effectiveness of β-blockers and increased sensitivity to diuretics, thiazide diuretics and not β-blockers are recommended for first-line treatment of hypertension in the elderly (Crome, 2000; National Institutes of Health [NIH], 2003).

ISSUES AND TRENDS IN MEDICATION USE

Commercialization

The biotechnology and pharmaceutical industries have provided a continuously growing number of medications; some of these are breakthroughs in treatment, and others are duplications of previously created preparations. This increase has led to intense competition among pharmaceutical companies. Instead of confining themselves to the traditional system of marketing the medications to prescribers, the consumer is now an additional target for sales. Pharmaceutical companies have recently increased targeted marketing campaigns that focus on the older adults as the number-one consumers of medication. As a result of these campaigns, many older patients now request specific medications from their health care providers, often unaware that the medication may be unnecessary or that a less-expensive alternative is available.

Polypharmacy

Polypharmacy is a situation whereby a person is taking multiple medications at the same time, especially when multiple medications are in the same class for the treatment of one or more chronic diseases (Gore and Mouzon, 2006). Simple polypharmacy may be necessary if one has multiple chronic conditions, or it may occur "accidentally" if an existing drug regimen is not considered when new prescriptions are given or any number of the thousands of OTC preparations and supplements are added to the prescribed medications.

The two major concerns with polypharmacy are the increased risk for drug interactions and the increased risk for adverse events (Gallagher, 2001). The potential for an interaction or adverse drug event is only 6% when two drugs are taken, but the risk increases to 50% with five drugs and reaches 100% with eight or more (Shaughnessy, 1992).

In the past several decades, the United States health care system has witnessed an increasing trend toward specialization. Research has found that polypharmacy in older adults is influenced by the reluctance of prescribers to discontinue potentially unnecessary drugs that have been prescribed by someone else; therefore treatments are continued longer than necessary (Randall and Bruno, 2006). Polypharmacy is too often the result of inadequate communication among specialists or between specialists and the primary care provider. As more health care providers choose to pursue specialty and subspecialty training, the result is a health care system that is becoming increasingly fragmented (Biola, 2003). In this system, patients are often managed by a collection of specialists rather than a single provider who coordinates all aspects of the patient's care. This inadequate communication results in duplicative medications, inappropriate medications, potentially unsafe dosages, and potentially preventable drug-drug interactions.

Instructing patients in the appropriate use of medications is an important part of pharmacotherapy and medication management. The prescriber should start educating the person about his or her condition and therapy when the medication is prescribed. The dispensing pharmacist should then provide specific information about the medication, educate the person about potential interactions with other medications, and instruct the patient in the proper method for administration. The nurse in any setting has the added responsibility to regularly assess the person's knowledge about all of his or her medications and to negotiate an acceptable regimen to ensure safe and appropriate medication use.

Financing Medication Use

Another current trend that affects elders' medication management is the high cost of drugs. Despite the recent implementation of Medicare Part D prescription drug benefits (see Chapter 17), many older adults are still unable to afford their medicines. Although the first few months of the annual benefit may be helpful, most reach the "donut hole" when the out-of-pocket costs may be prohibitive. Because the Medicare Modernization Act, which created Medicare Part D, also mandated that drug prices will not be negotiated, the costs were expected to skyrocket (Resnick and Jett, 2005). Fortunately, the increases in cost have not been as significant as predicted (Jett, 2006). Still, too often nurses know elders who have to decide if they will buy their medications or their groceries. This is especially true for those who are unemployed and younger than 65 years or for those recent immigrants who are ineligible for any form of governmental assistance.

Some of the new drugs differ only in subtle ways from older and less expensive alternatives. As new drugs are introduced, advantages of the newer drugs draw attention, obscuring their potential side effects. Samples provided to medical practices by drug companies are usually the more expensive and newer formulations. The tendency to believe that new is better can result in providers prescribing their older patients the newer and more expensive medications. Methods of keeping costs down include using generic drugs whenever possible, using scored tablets that could be halved for more numerous doses, and physicians and nurse practitioners prescribing older but equally effective drugs. Increasingly, elders are using pharmaceutical sources from outside the United States in an attempt to continue to be able to afford the medications they need, although they are legally prohibited.

Self-Prescribing of Medicinal Products

People of all ages frequently medicate themselves with former prescriptions, prescriptions borrowed from friends, or OTC drugs. Self-treatment includes purchasing herbal and nutritional supplements, which may be recommended by acquaintances and are thought to be harmless because they are "natural" (see Chapter 13).

According to the National Council on Patient Information and Education (NCPIE) (2002), the OTC market has more than 100,000 drug products, with 700 of them containing ingredients and dosages that would have required prescriptions 30 years ago. The many problems with OTC drug availability include excessive dose, drug interactions, adverse reactions, masking or delaying diagnosis of a serious condition, self-medicating, using analgesics and other OTC medicines to promote sleep, and OTC herbal medicines with toxic ingredients (NCPIE, 2002).

Many of the symptoms commonly experienced by older persons are amenable to OTC self-treatment, including pain and discomfort, constipation, and indigestion. Using OTC drugs often enables elders to gain relief from symptoms less expensively than using prescription drugs and enables them to obtain sufficient comfort to continue their activities of daily living (Cameron, 1996). An added benefit from purchasing OTC drugs is their accessibility at markets, drug stores and pharmacies, and on-line vendors.

However, mixing or combining medications of any kind poses potential problems. For example, OTC Tylenol (acetaminophen), if combined with other acetaminophen-containing prescribed medications such as Percocet and Vicodin, can lead to liver damage because of an excessive dose of acetaminophen. A not uncommon situation is when a patient receives prescriptions for Percocet and Vicodin on two separate occasions. The pain is chronic and bothersome, and the patient takes all the medications, including the Tylenol. Inadvertently, the patient overdoses on acetaminophen and develops liver failure. Another example is when a person is taking a prescription dosage of an antihistaminic allergy medication on a long-term basis. During a bout of insomnia, the person purchases the OTC drug *diphenhydramine*, thinking it will relieve insomnia. The anticholinergic properties are additive with another antihistamine that had been prescribed; in the elderly, smaller doses are required and cumulatively larger doses can lead to adverse effects. A sudden episode of confusion may not be attributed to the combination of medications if no one knew the patient added the diphenhydramine.

Another aspect of OTC medication self-management is the tendency to purchase combination medications. OTC cold and flu remedies that combine analgesic, antihistamine, and antitussive medications can lead to increased risk of side effects. Dosages in the "adult range," which are listed on the label, may be too high for elders. As mentioned, taking a combination medication with other drugs can lead to side effects. Further, combination medications are usually more expensive than purchasing generic versions of each type of medication (NCPIE, 2002).

Drug Interactions

Because the elderly tend to have more chronic health problems, they usually take a greater number of drugs than younger people. The more medications a person takes, either prescribed or OTC, the greater the possibility that one or more of them will interact with another one, an herbal preparation, food, or alcohol. The use of multiple medications predisposes a person to more drug-drug and drug-food interactions. When two or more medications or foods are given at the same time or closely together, the drugs may potentiate one another, that is, make one or both stronger; or antagonism may occur (when a drug or a food causes the other one or both to become ineffective).

Drug-Herbal Interactions. As a result of the increasing popularity of dietary herbal supplements, drug-herbal interactions are a real probability (Scott and Elmer, 2002; Valli and Giardina, 2002). Although much is unknown about the use of herbs and neutraceuticals, some knowledge is building that is important to the gerontological nurse. For example, *Ginkgo biloba* is a nutritional supplement touted for maintaining optimal cognitive function and treating mild forms of depression. The ingredient of St. John's wort responsible for its antidepressant effect is hyperforin, which interacts with a number of other drugs (see Chapter 13) (de los Reyes and Koda, 2002). One analysis of eight commercial St. John's wort preparations determined that the hyperforin content ranged from 0.01% to 1.89%, almost a 200-fold difference (de los Reyes and Koda, 2002). Another study of eight commercially available German St. John's wort preparations showed a range of less than 0.5 mg to 12.43 mg of hyperforin per dosage unit (a 25-fold difference), with wide variations among different batches from the same company (Wurglics et al., 2001). The lack of standardization increases the possibility of an adverse drug event or interaction. St. John's wort is known to decrease blood levels of indinavir (for treatment of human immunodeficiency virus [HIV] infection) and cyclosporin (for organ transplants) and decrease digoxin levels (Scott and Elmer, 2002).

Persons taking warfarin (Coumadin) should not take *Ginkgo biloba*, because it is known to interact with the anticoagulant effect and artificially increase the international normalized ratio (INR) used to monitor the warfarin effect. When ginkgo biloba is added to a stable anticoagulation regimen, potentially life-threatening bleeding could occur (Scott and Elmer, 2002; Valli and Giardina, 2002).

Glucosamine, a nutritional supplement touted for maintaining optimal joint function, can decrease glucose tolerance by causing increased insulin resistance (Scott and Elmer, 2002). In doing so, the use of glucosamine can interfere with the treatment of diabetes.

These interactions represent only a small fraction of the many real and potential nutritional supplement–drug interactions. Because of inadequate labeling requirements, drug interactions may not be listed on the product labels of these herbal supplements. Patients, prescribers, and nurses administering medications need to be aware of the potential interactions of the herbal preparation or nutritional supplement used. For more details on the use of herbal preparations in the older adult, see Chapter 13.

Drug-Food Interactions. Foods may interact with drugs to increase or decrease the effect of the drug. Such interactions may be pharmacokinetic or pharmacodynamic in nature (Schmidt and Dalhoff, 2002). Pharmacokinetic interactions may result in increased or decreased absorption, metabolism, or excretion. Pharmacodynamic interactions potentiate or antagonize the action of the drug.

Foods can bind to drugs, affecting their absorption. Calcium in dairy products will bind levo-thyroxine, tetracycline, and ciprofloxacin, greatly decreasing their absorption (Schmidt and Dalhoff, 2002). Lovastatin absorption is increased by a high-fat, low-fiber meal (Schmidt and Dalhoff, 2002) and saquinavir dissolution and absorption are enhanced by a high-fat meal (Lacy et al., 2003; Schmidt and Dalhoff, 2002).

Certain foods inhibit the metabolism of some drugs, whereas other foods induce the metabolism of other drugs. Grapefruit juice contains substances that inhibit CYP3A4-mediated metabolism in the gut (Greenblatt et al., 2001). Blood levels of amiodarone, lovastatin, simvastatin, and buspirone are greatly increased by concomitant administration (within 24 hours) of grapefruit juice (Greenblatt et al., 2001). Broccoli, brussels sprouts, and char-grilled meat all induce CYP1A2 metabolism (Flockhart, 2000). Because CYP1A2 mediates the major metabolic route of metabolism for both theophylline and clozapine, ingestion of those particular foods might result in sub-therapeutic blood levels (Hartshorn and Tatro, 2003).

Certain foods antagonize the therapeutic action of a drug. The vitamin K in leafy green vegetables antagonizes the anticoagulant effects of warfarin (Schmidt and Dalhoff, 2002; Lacy et al., 2003). It is recommended that patients on warfarin ingest a consistent amount of greens and not radically increase or decrease the amount they eat (Lacy et al., 2003).

Some foods greatly increase the action of a drug, which can lead to toxicity. Lithium ions (Li^+) and sodium ions (Na^+) compete for excretion in the kidney. When a person greatly decreases salt (NaCl) intake (low-salt diet) or increases salt excretion through sweating, the kidney attempts to conserve salt by tubular reabsorption. Thus when a patient on lithium carbonate decreases salt intake or increases salt excretion, the kidney stops excreting lithium, resulting in lithium toxicity (Atherton et al., 1990). Spironolactone increases potassium (K^+) reabsorption by the renal tubule. If a patient ingests a diet high in potassium (e.g., KCl salt substitute, molasses, oranges, bananas) while taking spironolactone, toxic K^+ levels could occur (Lacy et al., 2003).

Drug-Drug Interactions. Finally, drug-drug interactions may result also in altered pharmacokinetic activity or alterations in the absorption, distribution, metabolism, or excretion of one or all of the medications taken (Hartshorn and Tatro, 2003).

Within the body, absorption can be delayed by drugs exerting an anticholinergic effect. Tricyclic drugs (antidepressants) act in this manner to further decrease the age-related decrease in gastrointestinal motility and interfere with the absorption of other drugs as just noted. Several drugs may compete to simultaneously bind and occupy the binding sites needed by the other drug, creating a varied bioavailability of one or both of the drugs. Interaction may be blocked at the receptor site, preventing the drug from reaching the cells. Interference with enzyme activity may alter metabolism and cause drug deficiencies, or toxic and adverse responses may develop from altered renal tubular function. Antispasmodic drugs slow gastric and intestinal motility. In some instances this drug action may be useful, but when other medications are involved, it is necessary to consider the problem of drug absorption. Antacids and iron preparations affect the availability of some drugs for absorption by binding the drug with elements and forming chemical compounds. Calcium or other minerals may completely block thyroid preparations when taken together.

Outside the body, interactions can occur any time that two medications (or foods) are mixed before administration. An example of this is the improper preparation of more than one type of insulin for injection. Altered absorption can occur when one drug binds another drug in the small intestine to form a nonabsorbable compound (e.g., tetracycline and calcium carbonate, or ciprofloxacin and iron compounds). Separating the administration of the two drugs by 2 hours or longer can prevent some interactions.

The mechanism for altered distribution may be caused by displacement of one drug from its receptor site, from plasma albumin, or from α_1-acid glycoprotein binding by another drug. These interactions rarely cause problems clinically (Hartshorn and Tatro, 2003). However, they can become important to the older adult in the situation of lowered albumin levels, which is very common among the chronically ill frail elders often residing in long-term care facilities.

Altered metabolism can occur when one drug increases (inducts) or decreases (inhibits) the metabolism of another drug (Flockhart, 2000; Hartshorn and Tatro, 2003). Drugs may induce or inhibit the specific CYP450 isoenzymes responsible for metabolizing another drug. One drug may inhibit the metabolism of another drug if they are both substrates for the same metabolic pathway. Tables listing medications affected by those that have an effect of the CYP450 enzymes are available in most references on pharmacotherapeutics.

Altered excretion can occur when one drug changes the urinary pH such that another drug is either reabsorbed or excreted to a greater extent (e.g., sodium bicarbonate raises urinary pH, resulting in greater reabsorption of amphetamine and thereby prolonging its half-life) (Hartshorn and Tatro, 2003). Another mechanism may involve one drug increasing or decreasing the active transport in the renal tubules (e.g., probenecid decreases the active transport of penicillin, thereby prolonging its half-life) (Hartshorn and Tatro, 2003).

Pharmacodynamic drug interactions include the additive pharmacological effects of two or more similar drugs (e.g., additive central nervous system [CNS] effects of sedative-hypnotic drugs or anticholinergic drugs used simultaneously) (Hartshorn and Tatro, 2003). In pharmacodynamic interactions, one drug alters the patient's response to another drug without changing the pharmacokinetic properties. This can be especially dangerous for older adults when two or more drugs with the same effect are additive; that is, together they are more potent than they are separately.

Adverse Drug Events

When something happens that produces unwanted pharmacological effects, they are known as *adverse drug events (ADEs)*. These range from a minor annoyance to death and include adverse drug reactions (ADRs) and allergic reactions. Some ADRs are the result of drug interactions just noted, but many are the result of medication errors. The number of ADEs associated with errors in nursing homes has been estimated to exceed 800,000 per year (Stefanacci, 2006). In another study, 50% of the elderly patients (older than 65 years) treated in an emergency department were found to have an adverse drug-related event (Hohl et al., 2001).

ADEs can also be from a single drug. Sometimes an ADR can be predicted from the pharmacological action of the drug (e.g., bone marrow suppression from cancer chemotherapy; bleeding from warfarin [Coumadin]). A lesser number are unpredictable and have nothing to do with the action of the drug (e.g., hives from penicillin and bone marrow suppression from methimazole). These reactions may be caused by allergic or autoimmune processes.

Adverse Drug Reactions. It is no surprise that with the increased use of medications and OTC preparations, the older one is, the more likely one is to have an ADR (Crome, 2000). Women older than 80 years and ethnic elders are the most likely to experience an ADR (Field et al., 2004). The costs associated with preventable reactions is estimated at $1983 per event (Field et al., 2005).

The particularities of the ADR vary by setting. In a study of two large nursing homes, 42% of the events were preventable. Most were the result of errors at ordering or monitoring. The drug categories for those most likely to cause an ADR were (in order of importance) anti-psychotics, anticoagulants, diuretics, and antiepileptics (Gurwitz et al., 2005). In a study conducted in an ambulatory multi-specialty practice, 27.6% of the patients had an ADR in the year of the study. Thirty-eight percent of these were classified as serious, life-threatening, or fatal, and many (42.2%) were considered preventable (Gurwitz et al., 2003). In the same study, patients taking anticoagulants, antidepressants, antibiotics, cardiovascular drugs, diuretics, hormones, and corticosteroids were at increased risk. Those most at risk for a preventable ADR were patients taking non-opioid analgesics (especially nonsteroidal antiinflammatory drugs [NSAIDs] and acetaminophen), anticoagulants, diuretics, and antiepileptics (Field et al., 2004).

Hospitalization is a common result of an ADR in the older adult. Although the figures vary from study to study, they probably represent between 20% and 40% of all admissions. Chan et al. (2001) reviewed unplanned admissions of persons older than 75 years to an Australian hospital. The presenting complaints were falls from hypotension (24.1%), heart failure (16.9%), and delirium (14.5%). About one third (30.4%) were the result of ADRs, many of these attributed to a single medication (46%). Like those ADRs just noted, over half (53.4%) were considered preventable.

ADRs that are extensions of the drug's pharmacological activity may be predictable, and others may be unexpected. An elderly patient who is well controlled on a stable dose of a drug may undergo a change in his or her environment such that the relationship with the drug is altered. Changes in diet can have a profound impact on drug regimens. Some drugs interfere with the body's ability to regulate temperature such that hot weather can lead to heat stroke (e.g., antipsychotics, stimulants) (Semla et al., 2007). Other drugs are photosensitizing, and an increase in sun exposure can lead to sunburn more quickly than expected (e.g., sulfa drugs, antidepressants) (Semla et al., 2007) (Box 12-4). Elderly patients who decrease their fluid intake because of illness or inadequate intake during hot weather may become volume depleted and develop increased sensitivity to the orthostatic hypotensive effects of alpha-blockers (e.g., phenothiazines, terazosin) (Lacy et al., 2003).

More predictable ADRs can occur when a patient is started on a drug at a dose that is inappropriately high or one that requires laboratory monitoring that is not done. A good example of this is the elderly hypertensive patient (older than 80 years) started on hydrochlorothiazide (25 mg) for blood pressure control. Within a month the patient came to the emergency department with mental status changes and severe hyponatremia (Buffum, 2003). The recommended starting geriatric dose of hydrochlorothiazide is 12.5 to 25 mg daily with close monitoring of the patient's serum sodium (see Chapter 5) (Semla et al., 2007).

Another example of inappropriate dosing is the case of a 75-year-old man admitted to an orthopedic ward for a procedure. Because of the man's high level of anxiety about being in the hospital, he was given a total of 20 mg of diazepam over a 12-hour period. The following day the man wandered off the ward and was not seen again until he came to the emergency department with sore feet, 5 days later. He had been wandering the streets with no idea of where he was or how he got there (Buffum, 2003). Valium is not recommended for use in older adults. It is associated with delirium and anterograde amnesia. The half-life of Valium in a younger person is about 37 hours, but in an older adult this

---

BOX 12-4 Drugs with Potential for Causing Photosensitivity*

DRUG CLASSES

Anticancer agents
Antidepressants
Antihistamines
Antihyperlipidemics
Antimicrobials
Antiparasitics
Antipsychotics
Antiseizure agents
Diuretics
Hypoglycemics
NSAIDs

INDIVIDUAL DRUGS

Amiodarone
Atorvastatin
Benzocaine
Captopril
Chlordiazepoxide
Diltiazem
Disopyramide
Enalapril
Estazolam
Estrogen
Fluvastatin
Gold sodium thiomalate
Hexachlorophene
Lovastatin
PABA
Pravastatin
Quinidine
Saquinavir
Selegiline
Simvastatin
Zolpidem

From Semla TP et al: *Geriatric dosage handbook,* ed 11, Cleveland, 2007, Lexi-Comp, Inc.
NSAIDs, Nonsteroidal antiinflammatory drugs; *PABA,* para-aminobenzoic acid.
*These classes of drugs contain specific medications that can increase sensitivity to ultraviolet light. (For specific drugs under these classes, consult the most recent edition of the *Geriatric Dosage Handbook.*)

---

may be extended up to 82 hours, with potentially dangerous problems of accumulation (Ray et al., 1989).

Age-related pharmacokinetic and pharmacodynamic changes may mean that the older adult should be prescribed lower dosages of several of the drugs commonly needed, especially when starting a drug regimen. To minimize the likelihood of an ADR, the dose can be slowly increased until it safely reaches a therapeutic level. A common adage related to drug dosing in older adults is, "Start low, go slow, but go." The annually updated *Geriatric Dosage Handbook* (Semla et al., 2007) is considered a classic standard of geriatric care. It is now also available in a PDA format. Regular use of drug interaction programs may lead to the prevention of some ADRs (Tatro, 2003).

Drug Allergy. One type of ADE is an allergic reaction. An allergic reaction to a drug can occur after prior or continuous exposure to the drug. This can happen if the drug or its metabolite is an antigen or combines with an endogenous protein to form an antigenic complex (Klaassen, 2001). The antigen or antigenic complex can induce the development of antibodies in 1 to 2 weeks. When the patient is exposed to the drug again or if exposed continuously, an antigen-antibody reaction may occur, with resultant allergic response.

It is noteworthy that most of these reactions subside within 1 to 3 weeks after discontinuing contact with the offending irritant. Allergic reactions have been classified as four different types, as shown in Box 12-5.

It has been estimated that about 1% to 1.5% of hospitalized patients have an adverse drug reaction that may be allergic or immunological in nature (Gruchalla, 2000). There are no specific statistics on how many of these occur in the elderly. The elderly make up a greater percentage of the hospitalized patient population and the elderly are exposed to more drugs, so a disproportionate share of allergic reactions seems likely.

Misuse of Drugs

Drug misuse includes overuse, underuse, erratic use, and contraindicated use. The more drugs taken, the more likely misuse will occur. Misuse can occur for any number of reasons from inadequate skills of the nurse or the prescriber, to misunderstanding of instructions, to inadequate funds to purchase prescribed medications.

As early as 1994, Willcox and others (Willcox et al., 1994) identified 20 drugs that were inappropriately prescribed for elders, including controversial cardiovascular agents (propranolol, methyldopa, reserpine). Since that time, Beers (1997) has worked further to identify drugs that have higher-than-usual risk when used in older adults. These have been now transferred to a "do not use" list for residents in nursing facilities. When one is prescribed without documentation of the overwhelming benefit of its use, it can be considered a form of drug misuse by the prescribing practitioner. See Table 12-1 for a list of some of the medications that should not be prescribed for or used by the older adult because of their potential for adverse events.

Misuse by patients may be accidental, such as with misunderstanding, or deliberate, such as with trying to make a prescription last longer for financial reasons or because of beliefs about drug dosing (Hughes, 2004). Even most health care professionals would admit to having some leftover medications, especially antibiotics, in their medicine cabinet, which is evidence of drug misuse. When the misuse is on the part of the patient, the derogatory term of *noncompliance* is often used.

Noncompliance/Nonadherence

The term *nonadherence* to medication regimens is considered less pejorative than is *non-compliance*. It still means that medications are not taken as prescribed, but it is hoped that it implies that there may be multiple reasons for this, some of which may be reasonable and even predictable. The rate of medication nonadherence ranges between 20% and 70% in community-dwelling elders (Barat et al., 2001). The term *adherence* also connotes patient collaboration with the treatment regimen. Adhering to treatment can prevent relapses of symptoms of serious illnesses such as diabetes, heart failure, schizophrenia, depression, asthma, and pain.

There are multiple reasons for nonadherence. A person may have considerable difficulty complying with a medication regimen that is inconsistent with his or her established life pattern. The more frequently a medication needs to be taken, the less anyone will comply. For example, the individual cannot follow the instruction to take medication three times per day with meals if he or she eats only two meals each day. With more medications coming in once-daily dosing rather than three or four times each day, we can expect people to adhere to the instructions more often.

Memory failures associated with nonadherence or the misuse of medications are of two general types: forgetting the way to correctly take medications, and "prospective" recall failure (failing to remember to take medication at the correct times) (Leirer et al., 1991). This problem can be greatly exacerbated when the medications prescribed have the potential to negatively affect cognition (Box 12-6).

Problems with health literacy also limit the older person's ability to correctly follow instructions. Limitations in vision will interfere with reading instructions, especially of

---

BOX 12-5   Coombs and Gell Classification of Allergic Response
Type I. Immediate hypersensitivity reactions, characterized by anaphylaxis and urticaria and mediated by IgE antibodies (e.g., penicillin). These subside within a few days after discontinuing the drug.
Type II. Cytolytic reactions, characterized by destruction of cells in the circulatory system and mediated by IgG and IgM antibodies (e.g., cephalosporin-induced hemolytic anemia). These subside within several months after discontinuing the drug.
Type III. Arthus reactions or serum sickness, characterized by skin eruptions, arthralgia or arthritis, lymphadenopathy, and fever and mediated by IgG (e.g., sulfonamides). These subside within 6 to 12 days after discontinuing the drug.
Type IV. Delayed hypersensitivity reactions or contact dermatitis, characterized by an inflammatory skin reaction and mediated by sensitized T lymphocytes and macrophages (e.g., poison oak).

From Gruchalla R: Understanding drug allergies, *J Allergy Clin Immunol* 105(6 pt 2): S637, 2000; Klaassen C: Principles of toxicology and treatment of poisoning. In Hardman J et al, editors: *Goodman and Gilman's the pharmacological basis of therapeutics,* ed 10, New York, 2001, McGraw-Hill.

bottle labels. The practice of giving rapid-fire directions is not effective in addressing the person with hearing impairments or the normal age-related need for slightly slower verbalizations; and the use of ambiguous terms such as "slowly increase" or "only in moderation" leads to further difficulties.

It is also common to explain the treatment and give directions concerning medications when the patient is physically uncomfortable or as the person is about to be discharged, to explain in English even when the person has limited English proficiency, or to explain in a noisy or busy place.

Some elders alter the dose or stop taking a drug because they cannot afford it, think that it has been ineffective or not necessary, dislike the side effects, believe they have had enough medication, want to avoid feeling stigmatized (e.g., antidepressants), want some control over their own lives, have difficulty adapting the regimen to their lifestyle, or have poor understanding of instructions. Patients who think the medications are not necessary are not likely to comply (Horne and Weinman, 1999). Factors that further contribute to noncompliance include elders' depression (Ciechanowski et al., 2000), poor cognitive ability (Barat et al., 2001), low educational level (Aljasem et al., 2001), living alone (Barat et al., 2001), greater severity of illness (Aljasem et al., 2001), longer number of years with the illness (Aljasem et al., 2001), poor knowledge of the medications (Lowe et al., 1995), and larger number of medications and greater dosing frequency (Barat et al., 2001). A busy and active lifestyle has also been attributed to forgetting to take medicines (Park et al., 1999). On the other hand, experiencing pain may promote adherence to analgesics if persons learn how to take the medication properly (Edworthy and Devins, 1999).

One study found that patients' adherence reports differed from what their physicians believed. Of a random sample of 348 persons with a mean age of 75 years, patients disagreed with their physicians' prescriptions (22%), doses (71%), and regimens (66%). The message for nurses is clear—adherence must be approached from a collaborative process, building on the relationship between the prescriber, the nurse, and the patient.

An innovative hypothesis has been proposed that past trauma from medical illness is related to nonadherence with treatment for that medical illness. Shemesh and colleagues (2001) followed 102 patients with an average age of 61 years who had survived myocardial infarction (MI) for their adherence post-MI up to 1 year. They found that nonadherence to medication (i.e., captopril) was associated with adverse outcome during the first year and that nonadherence was associated with posttraumatic stress disorder symptoms. The authors suggest that patients avoided medication because it reminded them of the MI trauma.

Patients' beliefs about their capacity to adhere, conceptualized as self-efficacy, is also theorized to predict adherence (Bandura, 1977). A person's self-judgments reflect his or her beliefs about his or her own ability to practice healthy self-care behaviors (Bandura, 1982; O'Leary, 1985). The self-efficacy theory has been used in an exploratory study of 309 persons with type 2 diabetes. The researchers found from patients' self-reports that greater self-efficacy was predictive of diabetic self-care behaviors that included diet, exercise, frequent blood glucose testing, less-frequent omission of medication, and less binge eating (Aljasem et al., 2001). A clinical implication of this study for the nurse in working with elders includes asking patients whether they believe they can (i.e., ability, desire) follow a particular regimen.

A Conceptual Framework for Understanding Medication Adherence. Kutzik and Spiers (1993; Spiers and Kutzik, 1995) developed a multidimensional framework for medication use that looks at the barriers to adherence for elders. The framework suggests that there is a simultaneous branching out among the three stages (initial instruction, regimen establishment, and self-management) and the three levels (individual, provider-treatment, and social support network). The integration of the stages and levels provides a reasonable approach to understanding the dynamics of elder adherence (Table 12-2).

The individual must first comprehend and be committed to the treatment. The care provider must be able to communicate the information in a way that compensates for physical-sensory and cognitive changes so that the individual understands and is willing to follow the treatment plan.

The elder must be able to use what has been learned so as to "operationalize" this information (obtain the medication, apply the instructions, adjust to the regimen). The influence of the health professional is relatively strong to this point. Social context has a less direct influence on the drug regimen. However, it is affected by medical knowledge in the elder's cultural/belief system (see Chapter 21).

Finally, strong social network factors are more important because of the shrinking network that elders have available to them. Success at this level depends on the number of persons in the elder's support network who are able to assist the elder, if necessary, with integrating or reintegrating the regimen and monitoring adherence.

BOX 12-6   Drugs with the Potential to Cause Intellectual Impairment

- Alcohol
- Analgesics
- Anticholinergics
- Antidepressants
- Antipsychotics
- Antihistamines
- Antiparkinsonian agents
- Beta-blockers
- Cimetidine
- Digitalis
- Diuretics
- Hypnotics
- Muscle relaxants
- Sedatives

Data from Lamy PP: Drug interactions and the elderly, *J Gerontol Nurs* 12(2):36-37, 1986; Lamy PP: Adverse drug effects, *Clin Geriatr Med* 6(2):293-307, 1990; Nolan L, O'Malley K: Prescribing for the elderly. Part I: sensitivity of the elderly to adverse drug reactions, *J Am Geriatr Soc* 36(2):142-149, 1988.

TABLE 12-2

A Multidimensional Framework for Medication Adherence

	Individual	Provider-Treatment	Social Support Network
Stage 1: Initial instructions	Comprehension Commitment to treatment	Communication effectiveness Number of providers	Community medical education Cultural benefits
Stage 2: Regimen establishment			
Attaining medications	Mobility Finances Beliefs (e.g., medication sharing) Motivation	Medication cost Number of medications needed	Accessibility to pharmacies Financial aid
Application	Ability to reconstruct instructions Regimen strategy	Complexity of regimen Container design Label readability	Administration aid
Adjustment	Perception of effectiveness Self-manipulation of dosage/regimen	Rx manipulation Rx monitoring	Level of emotional/functional support
Stage 3: Self-management			

Integration/reintegration	Emotional adjustment to long-term
	   medication dependence
	Regimen "routinization" and synthesis
	Response to challenges/change
		Lifestyle change required by regular
		   medication taking
		Regimen changes
			Response to individual change
			Stability of support network/living
			   situation

Monitoring	Ability to self-monitor for change	Degree of comprehensive Rx review	Support network vigilance

From Spiers MV, Kutzik DM: *A multidimensional framework for understanding medication adherence in the elderly: prescription for rethinking,* Unpublished paper, 1995.
Rx, Prescription.

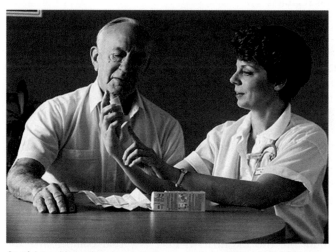

Careful teaching using demonstration and return demonstration increases the possibility of successful learning by the patient. (From Lewis SM et al: *Medical-surgical nursing: assessment and management of clinical problems,* ed 6, St Louis, 2004, Mosby; courtesy Rick Brady, Riva, MD).

▲ Promoting Healthy Aging: Implications for Gerontological Nursing

The gerontological nurse is a key person in ensuring that the medication use is appropriate, effective, and as safe as possible. The knowledgeable nurse is alert for potential drug interactions and for signs or symptoms of adverse drug effects. The nurse promotes the actions necessary to prevent drugs from becoming toxic and to treat toxicity promptly should it occur (Table 12-3). Nurses in the long-term care setting are responsible for monitoring the overall health of the residents, including fluid and dietary intake, and for being alert for the need for laboratory tests and other measures to ensure correct dosage. They are responsible for prompt attention to changes in the patient's or resident's condition that are either the result of the medication regimen or affected by the regimen, such as potassium level. The nurse is often the person to initiate assessment of medication use, evaluate outcomes, and provide the teaching necessary for safe drug use and self-administration. In all settings, a vital nursing function is to educate patients and to ensure that they understand the purpose and side effects of the medications and to assist the patient and family in adapting the medication regimen to functional ability and lifestyle.

An evidence-based guideline for improving the medication management for older adults has recently been published by the University of Iowa College of Nursing Gerontological Nursing Intervention Research Center and can be purchased from *www.nursing.uiowa.edu* (Bergman-Evans, 2006).

Assessment. The initial step in ensuring that drug use is safe and effective is conducting a comprehensive drug assessment. Although in some settings a clinical pharmacist interviews patients about their medication history, more often it is completed through the combined efforts of the licensed nurse and the health care provider (e.g., a physician or a nurse practitioner).

The gold standard of assessment begins with a "brown bag approach," in which the person is asked to bring in a bag of all medications he or she is taking, including OTCs, herbals, and

TABLE 12-3

Toxic Characteristics of Specific Drugs Prescribed for the Elderly

Drugs	Signs and Symptoms
Benzodiazepines Diazepam (Valium) Lorazepam (Ativan)	Ataxia, restlessness, confusion, depression, anticholinergic effect
Cimetidine (Tagamet)	Confusion, depression
Digitalis (digoxin)	Confusion, headache, anorexia, vomiting, arrhythmias, blurred vision or visual changes (halos, frost on objects, color blindness), paresthesia
Furosemide (Lasix)	Electrolyte imbalance, hepatic changes, pancreatitis, leukopenia, thrombocytopenia
Gentamycin (Garamycin)	Ototoxicity (impaired hearing and/or balance), nephrotoxicity
Levodopa (L-dopa)	Muscle and eye twitching, disorientation, asterixis, hallucinations, dyskinetic movements, grimacing, depression, delirium, ataxia
Lithium (Eskalith, Lithane)	Confusion, diarrhea, drowsiness, anorexia, slurred speech, tremors, blurred vision, unsteadiness, polyuria, seizures, muscle weakness
Nonsteroidal antiinflammatory drugs (NSAIDs) Ibuprofen (Advil, Motrin, Nuprin, Rufen) Indomethacin (Indocin) Fenoprofen (Nalfon)	Photosensitivity, fluid retention, anemia, nephrotoxicity, visual changes, bleeding
Phenylbutazone (Butazolidin) Piroxicam (Feldene) Sulindac (Clinoril) Tolmetin (Tolectin)	Confusion plus all the above
Phenothiazines	Tachycardia, arrhythmias, dyspnea, hyperthermia, postural hypotension, restlessness, anticholinergic effects
Phenytoin (Dilantin)	Ataxia, slurred speech, confusion, nystagmus, diplopia, nausea, vomiting
Procainamide (Pronestyl, Procan Promine)	Arrhythmias, depression, hypotension, SLE syndrome, dyspnea, skin rash, nausea, vomiting
Ranitidine (Zantac)	Liver dysfunction, blood dyscrasias
Sulfonylureas—first generation Chlorpropamide (Diabinese) Tolbutamide (Orinase)	Hypoglycemia, hepatic changes, heart failure, bone marrow depression, jaundice
Theophylline (Theo-Dur, Elixophyllin, Slo-Bid)	Anorexia, nausea, vomiting, gastrointestinal bleeding, tachycardia, arrhythmias, irritability, insomnia, seizures, muscle twitching
Tricyclic antidepressants Amitriptyline (Elavil, Endep) Doxepin (Sinequan, Adapin) Imipramine (Tofranil)	Confusion, arrhythmias, seizures, agitation, tachycardia, jaundice, hallucinations, postural hypotension, anticholinergic effects

Data from Semla TP et al: *Geriatric dosage handbook,* ed 12, Cleveland, 2007, Lexi-Comp, Inc.
SLE, Systemic lupus erythematosus.

neutraceuticals or dietary supplements. As each product container is removed from the bag, the necessary information can be obtained. To determine possible misunderstandings or misuse, it is best to ask the person how he or she actually takes the medicine rather than depending on how the label is written. An alternative method is a 24-hour medication history, such as, "Tell me everything you have taken in the past 24 hours." Two final approaches are associated with the review of systems or problems. These questions will be something like, "What do you take for your heart? Circulation? Breathing?" Or, if you know the person's major health problems, you may say, for example, "What do you take for headaches?" or "What do you use for indigestion?" Without the bag of medications or a list of some kind, patients often answer some of these questions with descriptions (e.g., "a little blue pill" or "a bad-tasting one"), but it is a start. In the nursing home setting, all the medications prescribed are reviewed monthly by the consulting pharmacist and questions and concerns expressed to the nurse and health care provider.

As the nurse learns the herbs, supplements, and OTC and prescribed medications that are taken, the assessment can continue. Much information is needed, but it is vital to promoting the health of the person and healthy aging. See Box 12-7 for details of the information needed in a comprehensive medication history for all substances taken. Through this assessment, the nurse can learn of discrepancies between the prescribed dosage and the actual dosage, potential interactions, and potential or actual ADRs.

Good interviewing and communication skills will help the nurse taking the drug history to obtain correct information. Open-ended questions should be used, such as "What do you take for headaches?" and "What do you use for indigestion, or bowels?" The purpose of open-ended questions is for the elder to engage in discussion, and the nurse can ascertain motivation and beliefs concerning the taking of medications. Discussions about addictive drugs, illicit drugs, or drugs obtained from others' prescriptions require sensitivity and a nonjudgmental attitude. Patients should be encouraged to ask questions and to learn about interactions between drugs, regardless of prescription status.

Another part of the assessment is obtaining information about possible drug allergies. Taking an adequate food and drug allergy history plays a great role in preventing allergic reactions. Some patients will state that they are allergic to a drug because they became nauseated or vomited after taking it. Such a reaction would be drug intolerance rather than an allergy. If a true allergic reaction has occurred (rash, respiratory distress, swelling, anaphylaxis), it is essential to record the type of allergic reaction the patient had, when the patient had it, how long it lasted, and how it was treated. It is important to ask about food allergies such as eggs, shellfish, tomatoes, strawberries, dairy products, and nuts. Because of the common presence of latex in the clinic or hospital environment, latex allergy should be assessed as well. Allergy information should be entered into the patient's chart, on the front of the patient's chart, and into the patient's computerized record.

The nurse who collects the data regarding the patient's drug use is also the same person who analyzes the findings (Box 12-8) and initiates interventions as needed. In the nursing home or hospital setting, communicating with the interdisciplinary care team is important in eliminating unnecessary or inappropriate medications, establishing safe usage, assessing the patient's cognitive ability, and motivating to adhere to a recommended medication regimen. The nurse should focus the discussion on the need for the drug, any side effects from taking it, any interactions with it, and any deficiencies it may be causing, such as dehydration or malnutrition. Ideally, the nurse should know what resources are available for teaching about medications, such as the clinical pharmacist. The nurse is well situated to coordinate care, learn about the patient's

---

BOX 12-7 Components of a Comprehensive Medication Assessment

- Medication names, doses, and frequency, prescribed and taken
- Diagnosis associated with each medication
- Belief regarding medication
- OTC preparations, with doses, frequency, and reason taken
- Herbals, with doses, frequency, and reason taken
- Neutraceutical supplements, with doses, frequency, and reason taken
- Medication-related problems, such as side effects
- Ability to pay for prescription medications
- Ability to obtain medications
- Persons involved in decision making regarding medications
- Use of other drugs, such as tobacco or nicotine in gum or patch
- Use of social drugs such as alcohol and caffeine
- Drugs obtained from others
- Recently discontinued drugs or "leftover" prescriptions
- History of allergies, interactions, and adverse drug effects
- Strategies used to remember when to take drugs
- Identification of malnutrition and hydration status
- Recent drug blood levels as appropriate
- Recent measurement of liver and kidney functioning
- Frequency of visits to primary care providers or specialists
- Level of sensory, memory, and physical disability

OTC, Over the counter.

BOX 12-8 Analysis of Assessment Findings Related to Medication Use

1. Is the drug working to improve the patient's symptoms?
   a. What are the therapeutic effects of the drug? (What symptoms are targeted?)
   b. What is the time frame for the therapeutic effects?
   c. Have the appropriate drug and dose been prescribed?
   d. Has the appropriate time been tried for therapeutic effects?
2. Is the drug harming the patient?
   a. What physiological changes are occurring?
   b. What laboratory values are changing?
   c. What mental status changes are occurring?
   d. What functional changes are occurring?
   e. Is the patient experiencing side effects?
   f. Is the drug interacting with any other medication?
3. Does the patient understand the following?
   a. Why he or she is taking the drug
   b. How the drug is supposed to be taken
   c. How to identify side effects and drug interactions
   d. How to reduce or manage side effects
   e. Limitations imposed by taking the drug (e.g., sedative effects)

goals, learn what the patient needs for understanding his or her medications, and arrange for follow-up care to determine outcome of medication teaching.

Education for Safe Medication Use. Nurses have an opportunity to improve treatment outcomes through patient education. Education begins with the assessment of the patient's readiness to learn, ability to comprehend, and functional capacity to incorporate lifestyle adaptations for medication management. In a collaborative process, the nurse works with the elder to provide medication information. If needed or requested, the educational process includes the person or persons who assist the elder with medication management. In doing this, it is important not to assume that the person accompanying the elder to an appointment or hospital is this person.

Education relating to the safe use of drugs can be accomplished on an individual basis or in small groups. The persons can be empowered to ask questions and know what they are taking, how it will affect them, and the alternatives available to them (Box 12-9). Pamphlets and booklets written in lay terms and in appropriate language and reading level should be available. If the patient's reading level is unknown, the materials provided should be written at no higher than the 8th-grade level. If there are no appropriate materials, the nurse can be creative and develop a booklet or information sheet that will meet the drug information needs of the patient. Information is best presented in bulleted line fashion rather than in paragraph form. Written information should be in large, boldface type. Audiovisual aids are available for health teaching, but if they are too expensive, the nurse may consider devising some. The use of commercially prepared patient education materials, such as those from pharmaceutical companies, should be used with caution. Often the reading level of these is higher than the 5th- or 8th-grade level recommended for general use. The nurse may use the SMOG calculation to determine the reading level of all materials provided to patients (Box 12-10).

Ideally, the nurse empowers the person to participate fully in self-care related to medication use (Box 12-11). However, because of the complex needs of the older patient, education can be particularly challenging. The following tips may be helpful when the goal of the nurse is to promote healthy aging related to medication use:

- **Key persons:** Find out who, if anyone, manages the person's medications, helps the person, or assists with decision making; and with the elder's permission,

---

BOX 12-10 SMOG Calculation of Reading Level of Written Materials

- Choose 10 consecutive sentences in the beginning, middle, and end of the document (e.g., booklet)
- Count the number of 3-syllable words in the 30 sentences
- Obtain the nearest square root of that number
- Add three to the square root

The sum of the square root plus three is the reading level of the document.

From McLaughlin GH: SMOG grading: a new readability formula, *J Reading* 12(8): 639-646, 1969.

BOX 12-9 Empowering the Patient for Safe Medication Practices: What Elders Should Ask and Know About Safe Medication Use

- What is the name of each drug?
- What is the purpose of each drug?
- What is the dose per administration?
- What is the number of doses every day?
- What is the best time to take the medication?
- How should the medication be taken?
- Can the medication be taken with other drugs?
- Which medications can and cannot be taken together?
- Are any special techniques, devices, or procedures necessary to administer the medication?
- For how long should the medication be taken?
- What are the common side effects?
- If side effects occur: What should the elder do? What changes in administration are necessary? When should the drug be stopped? When should the physician or pharmacist (or both) be called?
- What can be done at home to monitor for a therapeutic drug response?
- What should be done if a dose is missed?
- How many refills are allowed and necessary?
- How should the medication be stored?

- What are the nonprescription (OTC) preparations, including herbs and supplements, that should not be used with the present drug therapy?
- Take all medications prescribed unless the physician states otherwise.
- Stop taking the medication and report any new or unusual problems such as shortness of breath, nausea, diarrhea, vomiting, sleepiness, dizziness, weakness, skin rash, or fever.
- Never take medication prescribed for another person.
- Do not take any medication more than 1 year old or past the expiration date on the container.
- Store medications in a safe place, preferably the kitchen, rather than the bathroom, where moisture from bathing, especially showers, may affect the medicine.
- Do not keep medicines, especially sedatives and hypnotics, on the bedside stand, because when you are sleepy, you may forget that you have already taken the medication earlier.
- Do not place different medicines in the same container.
- Take a sufficient supply of all medicines in their individual containers when traveling away from home.
- Use a chart to keep track of medications.

OTC, Over the counter.

BOX 12-11   Empowering Patients for Self-Care Related to Medication Use

Elders and family members can be encouraged to do the following:

- Ask the provider or nurse about the specific signs and symptoms to watch for as early warnings for adverse drug reactions.
- Be aware of changes in usual health and functioning, especially when starting a new medication or treatment.
- Ask when the changes should be reported and to whom.
- Be honest and open with nurse and provider about all other substances taken, including over-the-counter medications, herbal remedies, and nutritional supplements.
- Make sure that the correct medications are received from the pharmacy each time a prescription is refilled; when in doubt, ask questions or seek clarification.
- Ask for written information about any new medication: name, reason given, dosage, precautions with self-administration (e.g., possible food or drug interactions) and if it needs to be refilled.
- Question each new prescription, especially if seeing more than one prescribing provider.
- Inform the nurse or provider any time the elder feels that he or she should stop a medication and why.

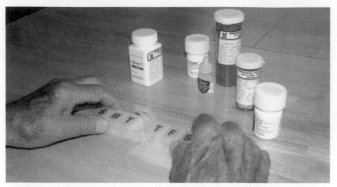

The use of commercially prepared storage boxes may be helpful. (From Monahan F et al: *Phipps' medical-surgical nursing: health and illness perspectives,* ed 8, St Louis, 2006, Mosby.)

make sure that the helper is present when any teaching is done.

- **Environment:** Minimize distraction, and avoid competing with television or others demanding the patient's time; make sure the person is comfortable and is not hungry, thirsty, tired, too warm or too cold, in pain, or in need of the toilet.
- **Timing:** Provide the teaching during the best time of the day for the person, when he or she is most engaged and energetic. Keep the education sessions short and succinct.
- **Communication:** Ensure that you will be understood. Make sure the elders have their glasses or hearing aids on if they are used. Use simple and direct language, and avoid medical or nursing jargon (e.g., "intake"). Remain respectful at all times, and do not allow negative stereotypes to cloud the communication. Encourage questions. If the person is blind, braille instructions may be available from the pharmacy. If the person has limited language proficiency in the country in which care is delivered, a trained medical interpreter is recommended.
- **Reinforce teaching:** Provide memory aids to reinforce teaching. Have actual medications or containers handy to visually illustrate directions. For persons who can read, use written charts and lists with large letters and simple language. For persons who cannot read but can see, charts with pictures of the medications and symbols for times of the day or color coding can be used. If the person cannot see, alternative forms of communication will be necessary. If food is required with the medication or must be avoided, this should be indicated on the charts. Weekly calendars with pockets for

medications indicating day, time, and date can be used; or a daily tear-off calendar to remind the elder to take daily medication can be used. Clear envelopes or sandwich bags containing the medication can be affixed to the dated square on a daily basis; each envelope or bag should state the name of the drug, dose, and times to be taken that day. Commercial drug boxes are available for single or multiple doses by the day, week, or month, and some have alarms. After discharge from a hospital or nursing home, a follow-up phone call can help with assessing accurate medication usage or other problems with medications. A nurse's home visit to patients at high risk for problems, such as those with cognitive deficits or those with many medications for new conditions, could reinforce medication information and provide assessment information.

- **Evaluate teaching:** Have the patient repeat back instructions, including names of medications, purposes, side effects, times of administration, and method for remembering to take the medicines and to mark off their ingestion. For example, a strategy is to turn the medication bottle upside down once the dose has been taken for the day. A combination of interventions over an extended period has been shown to be the most effective approach (Haynes et al., 1987). Computer-assisted medication teaching has demonstrated effectiveness for improving medication knowledge, adherence, and clinical outcome when given to older patients with osteoarthritis (Edworthy and Devins, 1999).
- **Avoiding drug interactions and reactions:** Patients should be taught to obtain all their medications from the same pharmacy if possible. This will allow the pharmacist to monitor for drug duplications and interactions. When elders have no prescription drug coverage, they may need to shop around for the best prices, and this does increase the risk for problems.

Medication Administration. Most elders self-administer their medications; others receive them from family, friends, or health care professionals. In long-term care settings, the administration of medications to residents occupies nearly all of some nurses' time. Several skills are needed for safe administration.

Because of the high rate of arthritis and other debilitating conditions, it may be difficult or impossible for the person to remove a cap or break a tablet. If no children have access to the medications, the patient can request alternative bottle caps that are easier to open. Either the person or nurse can also ask the pharmacist to pre-break the pills or dispense a smaller dose.

Most medications are taken orally. Many tablets and capsules are difficult to swallow because of their size or because they stick to the buccal mucosa. Some people have difficulty swallowing capsules. The person can be advised to place capsules on the front of the tongue and swallow a fluid; this should wash it to the back of the throat and down. Other persons do better with pills or capsules when taken with a semisolid food, such as applesauce, chocolate, or peanut butter—as long as the substances do not interact.

Administration of a drug in liquid form is sometimes preferable and allows flexibility; concentrations can be varied so that quantities of solution can be prepared and taken by the teaspoon, tablespoon, or ounce—simple and commonly used household measurements. Because household spoons vary greatly in actual volume, the nurse should ensure that the client is using an accurate measure. Crushing tablets or emptying the powder from capsules into fluid or food should not be done unless specified by the pharmaceutical company or approved by a pharmacist, because it may interfere with the effectiveness of the drug (either underdose or toxicity) or create problems in administration, as well as injure the mouth or gastrointestinal tract.

Enteric-coated, extended-release, or sustained-released products are all used to allow absorption at different places in the gastrointestinal tract. These should never be crushed, broken, opened, or otherwise altered before administration. When in doubt, the patient or the nurse should refer to a drug book, the package insert, or the pharmacist. Even the most basic pharmacology text or reference will provide a complete listing of medications that cannot be crushed or opened.

When the transdermal delivery system (TDDS) is used, patients and caregivers must be cautioned not to touch the "skin side" of the patch, to never cut or bend it, and to remove the old patch before adding a second.

General suggestions for improving medication adherence are provided in Box 12-12.

Evaluation of Effectiveness of the Nursing Intervention. How does the nurse know the education was effective? Observing the patient while teaching will provide information about the patient's alertness and interest. Facial expression and body language will demonstrate tension, confusion, anxiety, or suggestions of comprehension and eagerness to learn. Questions to ask oneself include the following: Did the elder appear to be listening during the teaching? Did the elder ask relevant questions? Could the person repeat the instructions, purpose, and side effects to watch for? Did the person participate in planning the medication regimen? Does the person appear motivated to com-

---

BOX 12-12 Suggestions to Improve Medication Adherence

SIMPLIFY THE MEDICATION ADMINISTRATION PROCESS*

Memory aids
- Calendars
- Day, week, month pill containers
- Voice-mail reminders

Convenient medication refills
Easy-to-open medication containers
Reduce number of doses daily when possible
Reduce number of medications when possible
Reduce frequency per day by grouping compatible medications together
Tailor medication regimen to lifestyle

DISSEMINATE DRUG INFORMATION

Audiovisual information
Individual or group instruction (including family, caregiver, significant other)
Written instructions
- Information sheets, leaflets in bold type
- Reasonably large print

Periodic review of drug information

TEACH PROPER MEDICATION MANAGEMENT SKILLS

Medication administration and training program
Self-care instruction

*Use lay terms: for example, *twice each day* instead of *bid*.

---

ply with the regimen? How did the patient perform in recalling instructions? In demonstrating procedure? What are the impairments? What does the person need? What type of follow-up should be done to reinforce the patient's learning? How did we (the patient and the nurse) respond to each other? What was the quality of our communication? The LEARN Model described in Chapter 21 can also be useful.

Another significant part of the responsibilities of the gerontological nurse is to monitor and evaluate the effectiveness of prescribed treatments and observe for signs of problems or side effects (Table 12-4). Monitoring and evaluating involve making astute observations and documenting those observations, noting changes in physical and functional status (e.g., vital signs, performance of activities of daily living, sleeping, eating, hydrating, eliminating) and mental status (e.g., attention and level of alertness, memory, orientation, behavior, mood, emotional display and affect, content and characteristics of interactions). Monitoring also means ensuring that blood levels are measured as they are needed, such as regular thyroid-stimulating hormone (TSH) levels for all persons taking thyroid replacement, INRs for all persons taking warfarin, or periodic hemoglobin A1c levels for all persons with diabetes (see Chapter 10). Care of a patient also means that the nurses promptly communicate their findings of potential problems to the patient's nurse practitioner or physician. Accurate monitoring requires that

TABLE 12-4

Determining Whether the Drug Is Working: Monitoring Parameters and Common Side Effects of General Drug Categories

Class of Drug	Monitoring Activity	Common Side Effects
Antibiotics and antivirals	Improvement of infection: symptom reduction Takes complete prescription	Change in normal flora: yeast infections in mouth or vagina, diarrhea
Antihyperlipidemics	Lipid profile (specific drug is matched to lipid profile) Observation for lifestyle changes (exercise, smoking cessation), dietary alterations (decreased fat intake, elimination of trans-fat products), gradual improvement in low-density lipoprotein (LDL) and high-density lipoprotein (HDL) levels, see change within 2-4 weeks Monitor liver function and blood glucose	Statins: muscle weakness, aches Niacin: muscle weakness, aches; flushing, elevations in blood glucose or signs/symptoms of elevation
Cardiac medications	Measurement of heart rate and rhythm	Mental status change, visual changes Bradycardia Fever, chills
Anticoagulants	Clotting times (international normalized ratio [INR], prothrombin time)	Bleeding, bruising, blood in stool
Anticonvulsants	Blood levels Seizure activity	Sedation Mental status changes
Antihypertensives	Measurement of blood pressure Central nervous system (CNS) effects Intake and output Weight	Diuretics: postural hypotension, bradycardia, hypokalemia Beta-blockers: bradycardia, hypotension, chest pain, constipation, diarrhea, nausea, mental status changes (insomnia, confusion, depression, lethargy)
Hypoglycemics	Blood glucose	Hypoglycemia, allergic reactions to beef or pork insulin
Antineoplastics	Cancer activity Bone marrow suppression, laboratory values (e.g., white blood cell [WBC] count)	Nausea, vomiting, diarrhea, signs of infection, hair loss, fatigue
Antihistaminics	Relief from allergy symptoms such as rhinitis	Drowsiness, blurred vision, confusion
Antiarthritics	Relief from arthritis symptoms such as pain and inflammation	Gastrointestinal (GI) problems, depression, personality disturbance, irritability, toxic psychoses
Antiparkinsonians	Improved functional status Less visible immobility; improved mobility	Nausea, hypotension, dyskinesia, agitation, restlessness, insomnia
Cholinergic agents (antidementia medications)	Improved mental status in mildly and moderately demented patients	Nausea, diarrhea, anorexia, weight loss, bradycardia, hypotension, headache, fatigue, depression
Analgesics	Improved symptoms of pain and inflammation	Nonsteroidal antiinflammatory drugs (NSAIDs): GI distress Opiates: constipation, sedation, confusion, decreased respiration

From Semla TP et al: *Geriatric dosage handbook,* ed 12, Cleveland, 2007, Lexi-Comp, Inc.

the nurse has information about the treatments and medications that are administered.

PSYCHOTHERAPEUTICS IN LATE LIFE

The gerontological nurse, especially one working in a long-term care setting, is likely to care for older adults who are receiving psychoactive drugs for the treatment of psychiatric concerns, especially depression, anxiety, and psychosis. The rate of depression for elderly persons living in the community is estimated at about 20% but increases to about 50% for those living in long-term care settings (Pollock and Reynolds, 2000). Anxiety is also common, and when it is treated with benzodiazepines, it is always a cause for concern because of the

propensity for adverse effects and drug interactions. Unfortunately, the use of psychotherapy is very limited—first, because of the rarity of persons with a specialty training in gerontological psychiatry or counseling; and second, because of the very low reimbursement rates established by Medicare.

A small group of elders in the community and a growing number of those residing in long-term care facilities, especially those with neurological conditions or dementia, may develop psychotic symptoms at some time in their illnesses. Psychosis is also seen in delirium from an infection or from an adverse drug effect and in the few elders with schizophrenia (Arunpongpaisal et al., 2004). Persons with psychosis are often treated with antipsychotics that require special attention and skills from the gerontological nurse.

TABLE 12-5

Classes and Side Effects of Antidepressants Available in the United States

Class	Examples	Side Effects
Tricyclic antidepressants (TCAs)	Amitriptyline, doxepin, imipramine, clomipramine	Dry mouth, constipation, urinary retention, orthostasis, sedation. Contraindicated for use of depression in the elderly
	Nortriptyline, desipramine	Less of above side effects
Selective serotonin reuptake inhibitors (SSRIs)	Fluoxetine, sertraline, paroxetine, fluvoxamine, citalopram	Nausea, vomiting, dry mouth, headache, sedation, nervousness, anxiety, dizziness, insomnia, sweating, sexual dysfunction
Serotonin-norepinephrine reuptake inhibitors (SNRIs)	Venlafaxine	Nausea, dry mouth, headache, dizziness, nervousness
Other antidepressants	Trazodone, bupropion, mirtazapine, duloxetine	Sedation, orthostasis, nausea, dizziness, headache

Data from Kaplan HI, Sadock BJ: *Pocket handbook of psychiatric drug treatment,* ed 2, Baltimore, 1996, Williams & Wilkins; Schatzberg AF: Course of depression in adults: treatment options, *Psychiatr Ann* 26(6):336-341, 1996; Semla TP et al: *Geriatric dosage handbook,* ed 12, Cleveland, 2007, Lexi-Comp, Inc.

Psychotropic medications are drugs that alter brain chemistry, emotions, and behavior. They include antipsychotics or neuroleptics, antidepressants, mood stabilizers, antianxiety agents, and sedative-hypnotics. Because each individual experiences symptoms in a unique way, several types of drugs may be prescribed to any one patient. This section of the chapter provides an overview of psychotropic medications used to treat symptoms that occur in disorders of behavior, cognition, arousal, and mood in the gerontological population. A section is devoted to treating the movement disorders that may occur as a side effect from the use of neuroleptics.

In 1987 the Health Care Finance Administration mandated that the residents of long-term care settings may be prescribed psychotropic drugs only for specific diseases or symptoms and that the use be monitored, reduced, or eliminated when possible (Omnibus Budget Reconciliation Act [OBRA], 1987). Prescribing physicians and nurse practitioners may exceed the recommended doses only if documentation reasonably explains the rationale for the benefit of the higher dose in restoring function or preventing dangerous behavior (Stoudemire and Smith, 1996) (see Chapters 23 and 25).

A patient should be prescribed a psychotropic medication only after thorough medical, psychological, and social assessments are done and non-pharmacological interventions have been found to be inadequate or ineffective. Nursing assessment before medication intervention contributes knowledge and baseline information that can optimize the patient's medical and psychological improvement. Issues to consider include the patient's medical status, other medications that might interact with psychotropics, mental status, ability to carry out activities of daily living, ability to participate in social activities and maintain satisfying relationships with others, and the potential for patient or caregiver compliance with any pharmacological or non-pharmacological treatment plan.

Antidepressants

Antidepressants, as the name implies, are drugs to treat depression. In the past, the major drugs used were monoamine oxidase (MAO) inhibitors and tricyclic antidepressants (TCAs), especially amitriptyline (Elavil) and doxepin (Sinequan). These drugs required high doses to be effective and have a significant number of side effects and adverse effects, especially related to their anticholinergic properties. Since the development of newer drugs, especially the selective serotonin reuptake inhibitors (SSRIs), the MAO inhibitors and TCAs are no longer indicated in most cases.

The SSRIs and the new serotonin reuptake inhibitors (SRIs) have been found to be highly effective with minimal or manageable side effects and are the drugs of choice for use in older adults. Most of these cause initial problems with nausea, dry mouth, or sedation. However, both these and other side effects usually resolve over time (Table 12-5). One side effect of the SSRIs, if experienced, that does not resolve with time is sexual dysfunction. The nonselective SRIs and other antidepressants, such as venlafaxine (Effexor), bupropion (Wellbutrin), and trazodone, are less likely to cause this problem and may be preferred by persons who are or who expect to be sexually active.

Most older adults are sensitive to the SSRIs and may find significant relief from depression at low doses. Although it sometimes takes time to find the most optimal dose, the nurse can help the elder monitor target symptoms and advocate for continued dose adjustments or changes of medication until relief is obtained. See Chapter 23 for a discussion on depression in late life.

Stimulants

In extreme cases of depression that are resistive to pharmacological intervention, very low doses of stimulants have been found to be effective with some elders who have what are called *vegetative symptoms* (severe lethargy) or are profoundly withdrawn and apathetic. These symptoms may respond to central nervous system stimulants, such as amphetamine or methylphenidate, although their use is controversial.

Methylphenidate (Ritalin) and dextroamphetamine (Dexedrine) should be administered only in the morning and early afternoon to prevent insomnia at night. Side effects include tachycardia, mild blood pressure increases, agitation, restlessness, and confusion. Methamphetamine (Desoxyn) has similar effects. Patients taking these medications should be encouraged to resume all daily activities. Responses should include motivation, interest, attention, and a sense of well-being.

Anxiolytic Agents

Drugs used to treat anxiety are referred to as *anxiolytics* or *antianxiety agents*. These agents include benzodiazepines, buspirone (BuSpar), and beta-blockers. Antihistamines, especially diphenhydramine (Benadryl), are often used but are not recommended for use in older adults because of their anticholinergic effects. The decision to treat anxiety pharmacologically is based on the degree to which the anxiety interferes with the person's ability to function and subjective feelings of discomfort. See Chapter 23 for a discussion of anxiety in late life.

The most frequently used agents are benzodiazepines. Although benzodiazepines have been available for almost 30 years, only minimal research has been done in the elderly (Madhusoodanan and Bogunovic, 2004). What we do know is that older adults metabolize these drugs slowly so they persist in the bloodstream for long periods and can easily reach toxic levels. Side effects include drowsiness, dizziness, ataxia, mild cognitive deficits, and memory impairment. Signs of toxicity include excessive sedation, unsteady gait, confusion, disorientation, cognitive impairment, memory impairment, agitation, and wandering. Because these symptoms resemble dementia, persons can easily be misdiagnosed once they start taking benzodiazepines.

Benzodiazepines are highly addicting yet very popular because of their quick sedating effects for the person who is experiencing acute anxiety. However, because of the problems just noted, they should be avoided except in extreme cases. If necessary, lorazepam (Ativan) appears to be the least problematic when prescribed in very low doses and for short periods. It has the shortest half-life of the benzodiazepines with no active metabolites. Benzodiazepines are specifically excluded from coverage in the Medicare Part D drug plans (Resnick and Jett, 2005) (see Chapter 17). It will be interesting to see if this restriction deceases their use.

Buspirone is a safer alternative. Although a side effect is dizziness, this is often dose related and resolves with time. Buspirone is not addicting and has an additive effect to some of the SSRIs so lower doses can be used. No effect is felt by the patient or observed by the nurse for 5 to 7 days, and the drug may be inappropriately discontinued for apparent lack of effect. Buspirone is used for chronic anxiety and is not effective for acute relief.

Antipsychotics (Neuroleptics)

Psychosis covers a range of thinking and behavioral characteristics that are based on responses of the ill person to a private reality—a reality that may be distressing and problematic for the patient and those around him or her. Characteristically, psychosis occurs in schizophrenia but can occur also in mania, depression, delirium, dementia, and paranoid states. Psychosis manifests itself as delusional thinking and hallucinations, both of which can cause extreme anxiety and bizarre behavior. Antipsychotics, formerly known as *major tranquilizers* and now known as *neuroleptics*, are drugs used to treat psychotic symptoms.

Unfortunately neuroleptics are often misused by caregivers and health care providers in an attempt to control troublesome behaviors, and too often they are used without a careful assessment of the underlying cause of the behavior. Inappropriate use of antipsychotic medications may mask a reversible cause for the psychosis, such as infection, dehydration, fever, electrolyte imbalance, an adverse drug effect, or a sudden change in the environment (Bullock and Saharan, 2002).

When used appropriately and cautiously in true psychosis, antipsychotics can provide a person with relief from what may be frightening and distressing symptoms. When used, drugs with the lowest side effect profile and at the lowest dose possible should be prescribed by the patient's health care provider. In most states, the use of antipsychotics in long-term care settings is carefully monitored.

There are different classes and potencies of antipsychotics. Strong antipsychotics (high potency), such as haloperidol (Haldol), are less sedating but cause more extrapyramidal reactions. The elderly are susceptible to developing extrapyramidal reactions, particularly neuroleptic-induced parkinsonian symptoms. Weak antipsychotics (low potency), such as chlorpromazine (Thorazine), are sedating and cause orthostatic hypotension, thereby precipitating falls. Further, the anticholinergic properties in the weaker antipsychotics can cause dry mouth, constipation, urinary retention, hypotension, and confusion. Table 12-6 compares sedative, anticholinergic, extrapyramidal, and hypotensive side effects of the different potencies of antipsychotics. Careful nursing observation is essential for monitoring side effects and drug interactions whenever any of these medications are administered.

The overuse of the atypical antipsychotic medications to treat behavioral responses is of concern in light of the side effects of such medications. None of these medications have been approved for use in the treatment of behavioral responses in dementia, and a recent study reported that the benefits of such medications are uncertain and that the adverse effects offset any advantages (Schneider et al., 2006).

Antipsychotics impair the body's hypothalamic, dopaminergic, thermoregulatory pathways. Hence patients taking neuroleptics cannot tolerate excess environmental heat. Even mild elevations of core temperature can result in liver damage called *neuroleptic malignant syndrome*. The problem is more likely to occur during hot weather. The nurse or caregiver must protect the elder from hyperthermia by making sure the environment is cool enough. Appropriate interventions include adequate hydration, relocation to a cooler area away from direct sunlight, and use of a fan or sponge bath. The patient may or may not share his or her discomfort about the heat, so assessment of body temperature is essential. Any circumstance resulting in dehydration greatly increases the risk of heatstroke. Diuretics, coffee, alcohol, lithium, and uncontrolled diabetes may decrease vascular

TABLE 12-6

Comparison of Side Effects of Antipsychotics

Generic Name	SIDE EFFECTS			
	Sedative	Anticholinergic	Extrapyramidal	Hypotensive
LOW POTENCY				
Chlorpromazine	High	High	Low	IM: High PO: Low
Thioridazine	High	High	Low	Moderate
INTERMEDIATE POTENCY				
Perphenazine	Moderate	Moderate	Moderate	Low
Loxapine succinate	Moderate	Moderate	Moderate	Low
Molindone HCl	Moderate	Moderate	Moderate	—
HIGH POTENCY				
Haloperidol	Low	Low	High	Low
Thiothixene	Low	Low	High	Moderate
Fluphenazine HCl	Low	Low	High	Low
Trifluoperazine HCl	Moderate	Low	Moderate	Low
NEWER ANTIPSYCHOTICS				
Risperidone	Low	Low	Dose related	Low
Clozapine	High	High	Low	High
Olanzapine	Moderate	Moderate	Low	Moderate

Modified from Bloom HG, Shlom EA: *Drug prescribing for the elderly,* New York, 1993, Raven; Jenike MA: *Geriatric psychiatry and psychopharmacology: a clinical approach,* St Louis, 1989, Mosby; Semla TP et al: *Geriatric dosage handbook,* ed 12, Cleveland, 2007, Lexi-Comp, Inc.

IM, Intramuscularly; *PO,* orally.

volume, thereby decreasing the body's ability to sweat. Anticholinergics inhibit sweating and lead to further heat retention (Lazarus, 1989). Heatstroke in late life is associated with very high mortality and morbidity rates.

Movement Disorders. Although neuroleptic malignant syndrome is not commonly seen, the most significant potential side effects of antipsychotics in older adults are movement disorders, also referred to as *extrapyramidal syndrome (EPS) reactions.* These include acute dystonia, akathisia, parkinsonian symptoms, and tardive dyskinesia.

Acute Dystonia. An acute dystonic reaction may occur hours or days after antipsychotic medication administration or after dosage increases. The reaction may last minutes to hours. An acute dystonic reaction is observed as an abnormal involuntary movement consisting of a slow and continuous muscular contraction or spasm. Involuntary muscular contractions of the mouth, jaw, face, and neck are common. The jaw may lock (trismus), the tongue may roll back and block the throat, the neck may arch backward (opisthotonos), or the eyes may close. In an oculogyric crisis, the eyes are fixed in one position. Often this creates a feeling of needing to look up constantly without the ability to make the eyes come down. Dystonias can be painful and frightening.

Akathisia. Akathisia refers to the compulsion to be in motion and may occur at any time during therapy. Patients describe feeling restless, being unable to be still, having an unrelenting desire to move, and feeling "like crawling out of my skin." Often this symptom is mistaken for worsening psychosis instead of the adverse drug reaction that it is. Pacing, aimless walking, fidgeting, shifting weight from one leg to the other, and marked restlessness are characteristic behaviors for a person experiencing akathisia.

Parkinsonian Symptoms. The use of neuroleptics may cause a collection of symptoms that mimic Parkinson's disease. A bilateral tremor (as opposed to a unilateral tremor in true Parkinson's), bradykinesia, and rigidity may be seen, which may progress to akinesia, or the inability to move. The patient may have an inflexible facial expression and appear bored and apathetic and be mistakenly diagnosed as depressed. More common with the higher-potency antipsychotics, parkinsonian symptoms may occur within weeks to months of initiation of antipsychotic therapy.

Caregivers or others unfamiliar with these EPS reactions often become alarmed. Although frightening, acute dystonia is not usually dangerous and is quickly relieved by anticholinergic medication, such as benztropine (Cogentin), trihexyphenidyl (Artane), or diphenhydramine (Benadryl), providing relief within minutes if given intravenously, within 10 to 15 minutes if given intramuscularly, and within 30 minutes if given orally. These medications should be readily available to treat an EPS reaction for all persons taking antipsychotics. Although they are not recommended for use in the elderly, anticholinergics and amantadine (Symmetrel), a dopamine agonist, are sometimes prescribed to prevent dystonic reactions, but because of slow onset of action, they are not used for acute treatment.

The same drugs are used to counteract akathisia and parkinsonian symptoms; however, their effectiveness is less predictable in these situations. Propranolol and clonidine have also been used for complaints of akathisia. However, hypotension and sedation are often unacceptable side effects and can be dangerous in the elderly.

Tardive Dyskinesia. When neuroleptics have been used continuously for at least 3 to 6 months, patients are at risk for the development of the irreversible movement disorder of tardive dyskinesia (TD). Both low- and high-potency agents are implicated (Bullock and Saharan, 2002; Goldberg, 2002). TD symptoms usually appear first as wormlike movements of the tongue; other facial movements include grimacing, blinking, and frowning. Slow, maintained, involuntary, twisting movements of the limbs, trunk, neck, face, and eyes (involuntary eye closure) have been reported.

No treatment reverses the effect of TD; therefore it is essential that the nurse is attentive for early detection so that the health care provider can make prompt changes to the psychotropic regimen. Response to treatment is the most important consideration when gerontological patients are

Human Needs and Wellness Diagnoses

Self-Actualization and Transcendence
(Seeking, Expanding, Spirituality, Fulfillment)
Seeks knowledge regarding medications and alternatives
Recognizes certain alterations of mentation with some medications
Seeks to transcend ego needs

Self-Esteem and Self-Efficacy
(Image, Identity, Control, Capability)
Exerts maximum control of self on environment
Copes effectively with acute and chronic health disorders
Makes wise choices regarding medication usage
Avoids reliance on medications to manage life problems
Makes self aware of possible medication interactions

Belonging and Attachment
(Love, Empathy, Affiliation)
Maintains important network affiliations
Keeps personal commitments
Expresses appreciation when appropriate

Safety and Security
(Caution, Planning, Protections, Sensory Acuity)
Maintains healthy skepticism
Inquisitive regarding effects of medications
Demonstrates body awareness and self-monitoring ability
Follows directions but questions untoward effects
Routinely reports to provider all medications being taken

Biological and Physiological Integrity
(Air, Fluids, Comfort, Activity, Nutrition, Elimination, Skin Integrity)
Modifies lifestyle as necessary to avoid unnecessary reliance on medications
Reports changes in basic biological functions that may be a result of medications
(e.g., thirst, appetite, sleep patterns, comfort activity, skin reactions)

These are not all the possible wellness diagnoses that may be identified. The above
are examples of nursing diagnoses that should be considered when planning care
for the older adult.

taking psychotropics. Subjective patient comments about feelings and symptoms and objective observations about the patient's behavior are important data for evaluating the effectiveness of a drug.

Mood Stabilizers

Although bipolar disorders are not common in the older population, some elders do suffer from them. Often this is something that has been a lifelong problem. Mood stabilizers are the group of agents used for the treatment of bipolar disorders. However, mood stabilizers, especially valproic acid (Depakene) and the newer agent Lamictal (also indicated for seizure activity), have also been found useful for some persons with depression. Symptoms of the manic phase include confusion, paranoia, labile affect, pressured speech and flight of ideas, morbid or depressive content of thought, increased psychomotor activity resembling agitated depression, a long period between the depressive episode and the appearance of mania, and altered orientation and attention span. In older adults it is essential to combine both non-pharmacological and pharmacological approaches to optimize wellness (Lantz, 2003).

The nurse who is caring for a patient with a bipolar disorder or for one who is taking a mood stabilizer should seek guidance from the person's psychiatrist regarding specific strategies to enhance the person's quality of life. The nurse should also be proactive in ensuring that serum concentrations of all mood stabilizers are monitored frequently and correctly.

If the patient is taking lithium, close monitoring by nurses is especially important. Lithium interacts with other medications and certain foods. For example, a low-salt diet will elevate the lithium level and a high-salt diet will decrease it. Likewise, thiazide diuretics and NSAIDs will elevate the serum lithium level. Side effects include the following: confusion, disorientation, and memory loss; flattening of T waves on the electrocardiogram; polyuria and polydipsia; nausea, vomiting, and diarrhea; fine resting tremor; benign goiter; and ataxia.

▲ PROMOTING HEALTHY AGING: IMPLICATIONS FOR GERONTOLOGICAL NURSING

All the medications presented in this section of the chapter have indications, side effects, interactions, and individual patient reactions. The nurse's advocacy role includes education for the patient and family or caregiver. Further, the nurse must determine whether side effects are minimal and tolerable or serious (Table 12-7). Asking the patient produces subjective data; and observing the patient's interactions, behavior, mood, emotional responses, and daily habits provides objective data. From this compilation of data, patient problems can be delineated, nursing diagnoses developed, outcome criteria planned, and interventions initiated.

Medications occupy a central place in the lives of many older persons: cost, acceptability, interactions, untoward side effects, and the need to schedule medications appropriately all combine to create many difficulties. Although nurses, with the exception of advanced practice nurses, do not prescribe medications, we believe that a full understanding of medications is needed by nurses working with elders.

TABLE 12-7

Determining Whether the Drug Is Working: Monitoring Parameters and Common Side Effects of Psychiatric Drug Categories

Class of Drug	Monitoring Activity	Common Side Effects
Anxiolytics	Decreased anxiety Immediate effect Habit-forming	Sedation, confusion, gait disturbances, disinhibition
Mood stabilizers	Blood levels: gradual behavior change based on blood level Lithium: avoid salt restriction; maintain adequate hydration Ensure adequate renal function Decreased hyperactivity, explosive outbursts, mania	Sedation, confusion, tremors
Antidepressants	Dose titration depends on side effects; start with low dose and increase dosage slowly Gradual effect; patient does not usually see early improvement of depression	Tricyclics: dry mouth, blurred vision, constipation, sedation, confusion, urinary retention, orthostatic hypotension SSRIs: restlessness, insomnia, irritability, sexual dysfunction
Antipsychotics	Decreased agitation Immediate response Use lowest possible dose, and eliminate medication as soon as possible	Sedation, confusion, dyskinesia, akathisia, extrapyramidal effects, parkinsonian reactions, somnolence
Hypnotics	Nighttime sleep improvement Habit-forming Taper (rebound on withdrawal from those causing decrease in rapid eye movement [REM] sleep)	Daytime drowsiness, hangover, worsening dementia, confusion, hypotension, delirium, depressed respirations

From Semla TP et al: *Geriatric dosage handbook*, ed 12, Cleveland, 2007, Lexi-Comp, Inc.
SSRIs, Selective serotonin reuptake inhibitors.

KEY CONCEPTS

- Individuals older than 75 years cannot be expected to react to medication in the way they did when they were 25 years old.
- Any medication has side effects. The therapeutic goal is to reduce the targeted symptoms without undesirable side effects. Drug-drug, drug-herb, and drug-food incompatibilities are an increasing problem of which nurses must be aware.
- Polypharmacy reactions are one of the most serious problems of elders today and are usually the first area to investigate when untoward physiological events occur.
- Drug misuse may be triggered by prescriber practices, individual self-medication, physiological idiosyncrasies, altered biodegradability, nutritional and fluid states, and inadequate assessment before prescribing.
- Nurses must investigate drugs immediately if a change in mental status is observed in an individual who is normally alert and aware. Many drugs cause temporary cognitive impairment in older persons.
- Nonadherence of clients with medication regimens is a constant concern among health professionals. Look for possible reasons. One cannot comply with a prescription or treatment when incompatibilities interfere with the practicalities of life or are distressful to the individual's well-being or when actual misinformation or disability prevents compliance.

- Biochemical processes in the brain influence all activities, including behavior, emotion, mood, cognition, and movement.
- The side effects of psychotropic medications vary significantly; thus these medications must be selected with care when prescribed for the older adult.
- The response of the elder to treatment with psychotropic medications should show reduced distress, clearer thinking, and more appropriate behavior.
- It is always expected that pharmacological approaches augment rather than replace non-pharmacological approaches.
- Older adults are particularly vulnerable to developing movement disorders (extrapyramidal symptoms, parkinsonism symptoms, akathisia, dystonias) with the use of antipsychotics.
- The Health Care Financing Administration and the congressional Omnibus Budget Reconciliation Act (OBRA) have severely restricted the use of psychotropic drugs for the elderly unless they are truly needed for specific disorders and to maintain or improve function. Then they must be carefully monitored.
- Any time a behavior change is noted in a person, reversible causes must be sought and treated before psychotropic medications are used.
- Antidepressant medications must be tailored to the elder with careful observation for side effects.
- Dosage levels of psychotropics must be carefully titrated for elders and their responses accurately and consistently recorded.

CASE STUDY: At Risk for an Adverse Event

Rose was a 78-year-old woman who lived alone in a large city. She had been widowed for 10 years. Her children were grown, and all were successful. She was very proud of them because she and her husband had immigrated to the United States when the children were small and had worked very hard to establish and maintain a home. She had had only a few years of primary education and still clung to many of her "old country" ways. She spoke a mixture of English and her native language, and her children were somewhat embarrassed by her. They thought she was somewhat of a hypochondriac because she constantly complained to them about various aches and pains, her knees that "gave out," her "sugar" and "water" problems, and her heart palpitations. She had been diagnosed with mild diabetes and congestive heart failure. She was a devout Catholic and attended mass each morning. Her treks to church events, to the senior center at church, and to her various physicians (internist; orthopedic, cardiac, and ophthalmic specialists) constituted her social life. One day the recreation director at the senior center noticed her pulling a paper bag of medication bottles from her purse. She sat down to talk with Rose about them and soon realized that Rose had only a vague idea of what most of them were for and tended to take them whenever she felt she needed them.

Based on the case study, develop a nursing care plan using the following procedure*:

- List Rose's comments that provide subjective data.
- List information that provides objective data.

- From these data, identify and state, using accepted format, two nursing diagnoses you determine are most significant to Rose at this time. List two of Rose's strengths that you have identified from data.
- Determine and state outcome criteria for each diagnosis. These must reflect some alleviation of the problem identified in the nursing diagnosis and must be stated in concrete and measurable terms.
- Plan and state one or more interventions for each diagnosed problem. Provide specific documentation of the source used to determine the appropriate intervention. Plan at least one intervention that incorporates Rose's existing strengths.
- Evaluate the success of intervention. Interventions must correlate directly with the stated outcome criteria to measure the outcome success.

Critical Thinking Questions

1. When you are given a prescription for medication, what do you ask about it?
2. As a nurse visiting the center for a 6-week student assignment, how would you begin to help Rose?
3. What factors about Rose's probable medication misuse would be most alarming to you?
4. What aspect of Rose's situation related to medications do you think are common among elders?
5. Who should be responsible for teaching and monitoring medication use in Rose's case? In any case?

*Students are advised to refer to their nursing diagnosis text and identify possible or potential problems.

RESEARCH QUESTIONS

Do you think most elders seek adequate information about their medications before taking them?

Where would you obtain sufficient drug information for persons with limited English proficiency (LEP)?

What symptoms do elders self-treat with OTC and herbal medicines?

What are nursing roles in preventing adverse events in elders?

Among the following three teaching strategies, which works the best: computer-assisted medication teaching, telephone teaching, and in-person medication teaching?

Mrs. J. a patient of yours in a long-term care setting, is calling out repeatedly for a nurse; other patients are complaining, and you simply cannot be available for long periods to quiet her. Considering the setting and the OBRA guidelines, what would you do to manage the situation?

REFERENCES

Aljasem L et al: The impact of barriers and self-efficacy on self-care behaviors in type 2 diabetes, *Diabetes Educ* 27(3):393, 2001.

Amoako EP et al: Self-medication with over-the-counter drugs among elderly adults, *J Gerontol Nurs* 29(8):10-15, 2003.

Arunpongpaisal S et al: Anti-psychotic use for the treatment of elderly people with late onset schizophrenia, *The Cochrane Library (Oxford)* 2:ID No CD004162, 2004.

Atherton JC et al: Lithium clearance in healthy humans: effects of sodium intake and diuretics, *Kidney Int Suppl* 28:S36, 1990.

Bandura A: Self-efficacy: toward a unifying theory of behavioral change, *Psychol Rev* 84:191, 1977.

Bandura A: Self-efficacy mechanism in human agency, *Am Psychol* 37:122, 1982.

Barat I et al: Drug therapy in the elderly: what doctors believe and patients actually do, *Br J Clin Pharmacol* 51.615, 2001.

Beers M: Explicit criteria for determining potentially inappropriate medication use by the elderly, *Arch Intern Med* 157:1531, 1997.

Bergman-Evans B: Evidenced-based guideline: improving medication management for older clients, *J Gerontol Nurs* 32(7):6-14, 2006.

Biola H: The U.S. primary care physician workforce: persistently declining interest in primary care medical specialties, *Am Fam Physician* 68(8):1484, 2003.

Briggs GC: Geriatric issues. In Younkgin E et al, editors: *Pharmacotherapeutics: a primary care guide*, Upper Saddle River, NJ, 2005, Prentice-Hall.

Buffum J: Unpublished data, 2003.

Bullock R, Saharan A: Atypical antipsychotics: experience and use in the elderly, *Int J Clinic Prac* 56(7):515-525, 2002.

Cameron K: *Nonprescription medicines: new opportunities and responsibilities for self care*, Washington, DC, 1996, United Seniors Health Cooperative.

Chan M et al: Adverse drug events as a cause of hospital admission in the elderly, *Intern Med J* 31(4):199-205, 2001.

Ciechanowski P et al: Depression and diabetes: impact of depressive symptoms on adherence, function, and costs, *Arch Intern Med* 160:3278, 2000.

Cockcroft DW, Gault MH: Prediction of creatinine clearance from serum creatinine, *Nephron* 16(1):31, 1976.

Crome P: Adverse drug reactions. In Crome P, Ford G, editors: *Drugs and the older population*, London, 2000, Imperial College Press.

de los Reyes GC, Koda RT: Determining hyperforin and hypericin content in eight brands of St. John's wort, *Am J Health Syst Pharm* 59(6):545, 2002.

Eddington N: Pharmacokinetics. In Roberts J et al, editors: *Handbook of pharmacology of aging*, ed 2, Boca Raton, Fla, 1996, CRC Press.

Edworthy S, Devins GM: Improving medication adherence through patient education distinguishing between appropriate and inappropriate utilization. Patient Education Study Group, *J Rheumatol* 26(8):1793, 1999.

Field TS et al: Risk factors for adverse drug events among older adults in the ambulatory setting, *J Am Geriatr Soc* 52(8):1349-1354, 2004.

Field TS et al: The costs associated with adverse drug events among older adults in the ambulatory setting, *Med Care* 43(12):1171-1176, 2005.

Flockhart DA, Oesterheld JR: Cytochrome P450-mediated drug interactions, *Child Adolesc Psychiatr N Am* 9(1):43-76, 2000.

Gallagher LP: The potential for adverse drug reactions in elderly patients, *Appl Nurs Res* 14(4):221-224, 2001.

Goldberg RJ: Tardive dyskinesia in elderly patients: an update, *J Am Med Dir Assoc* 3(3):152-161, 2002.

Gore VF, Mouzon M: Polypharmacy in older adults: front line strategies, *Adv Nurse Pract* 14(9):49-52, 2006.

Greenblatt DJ et al: Drug interactions with grapefruit juice: an update, *J Clin Psychopharmacol* 21(4):357, 2001.

Gruchalla R: Understanding drug allergies, *J Allergy Clin Immunol* 105(6 pt 2):S637, 2000.

Gurwitz JH et al: Incidence and preventability of adverse drug events in nursing homes, *Am J Med* 109(2):87-94, 2000.

Gurwitz JH et al: Incidence and preventability of adverse drug events among older persons in the ambulatory setting, *JAMA* 289(9):1107-1116, 2003.

Gurwitz JH et al: The incidence of drug events in two large academic long-term care facilities, *Am J Med* 118(3):251-258, 2005.

Hall KE: Effect of aging on gastrointestinal function. In Hazzard WR et al, editors: *Principles of geriatric medicine and gerontology*, ed 5, New York, 2003, McGraw-Hill.

Hammerlein A et al: Pharmacokinetic and pharmacodynamic changes in the elderly: clinical implications, *Clin Pharmacokinet* 35(1):49, 1998.

Hartshorn E, Tatro D: *Principles of drug interaction, drug interaction facts 2003*, St Louis, 2003, Facts and Comparisons.

Haynes RB et al: A critical review of interventions to improve compliance with prescribed medications, *Patient Educ Couns* 10:155, 1987.

Hohl CM et al: Polypharmacy, adverse drug-related events, and potential adverse drug interactions in elderly patients presenting to an emergency department, *Ann Emerg Med* 38(6):666, 2001.

Horne R, Weinman J: Patients' beliefs about prescribed medicines and their role in adherence to treatment in chronic physical illness, *J Psychosom Res* 47(6):555, 1999.

Hughes CM: Medication nonadherence in the elderly: how big is the problem, *Drugs Aging* 21(12):793-811, 2004.

Jett KF: Medicare D: a new drug benefit in its first year, *Adv Nurs* 26(8) (serial online): *http://nursing.advanceweb.com*.

Kaiser Family Foundation (KFF): *Prescription drug coverage and seniors: findings from a 2003 national survey*, 2005. (website): *www.kff.org*. Accessed November 25, 2006.

Klaassen C: Principles of toxicology and treatment of poisoning. In Hardman J et al, editors: *Goodman and Gilman's the pharmacological basis of therapeutics*, ed 10, New York, 2001, McGraw-Hill.

Kutzik D, Spiers M: *Drug therapy adherence among elderly: barriers to successful self management.* Paper presented at the Gerontological Society of America, San Francisco, November 21, 1993.

Lacy C et al: *Drug information handbook 2003-2004,* Cleveland, 2003, Lexi-Comp, Inc.

Lantz MS: Bipolar disorders in the older adult, *Clinical Geriatr* 11(7):18, 20, 21-22, 2003.

Lazarus A: Differentiating neuroleptic-related heatstroke from neuroleptic malignant syndrome, *Psychosomatics* 30(4):454-456, 1989.

Leirer VO et al: Elders' nonadherence: its assessment and medication reminding by voice mail, *Gerontologist* 31(4):514-520, 1991.

Lowe C et al: Effects of self-medication programme on knowledge of drugs and compliance with treatment in elderly patients, *BMJ* 310(6989):1229, 1995.

Madhusoodanan S, Bogunovic OJ: Safety of benzodiazepine use in the geriatric population, *Expert Opin Drug Saf* 3(5):485-493, 2004.

Masoro EJ, Austed SN, editors: *Handbook of biology and aging,* ed 5, San Diego, 2003, Academic Press.

Moore AR, O'Keefe ST: Drug induced cognitive impairment in the elderly, *Drugs Aging* 15(1):15-28, 1999.

National Council on Patient Information and Education (NCPIE): *Attitudes and beliefs about the use of over-the-counter medicines: a dose of reality,* Bethesda, Md, 2002, Harris Interactive. (website): *www.harrisinteractive.com.*

National Institutes of Health: *Seventh report of the Joint National Committee on Prevention, Detection, Evaluation, and Treatment Of High Blood Pressure* (JNC 7 Express). National Institutes of Health Publication No 03-5233, May 2003.

O'Leary A: Self-efficacy and health, *Behav Res Ther* 23:437, 1985.

O'Mahony S: Pharmacokinetics. In Crome P, Ford G, editors: *Drugs and the older population,* London, 2000, Imperial College Press.

Omnibus Budget Reconciliation Act (OBRA) of 1987, Washington, DC, 1987, US Government Printing Office. House of Representatives, 100th Congress, 1st Session, Report 100-391.

Park D et al: Medication adherence in rheumatoid arthritis patients: older is wiser, *J Am Geriatr Soc* 47(2):172, 1999.

Pollock G, Reynolds CF III: *Depression in late life.* Harvard Mental Health Letter, Harvard Health Online, 2000. (website): *www.health.harvard.edu/medline/Mental/M0900b.html.*

Randall RL, Bruno SM: Can polypharmacy reduction efforts in an ambulatory setting be successful? *Clin Geriatrics* 14(7):33-35, 2006.

Ray WA et al: Benzodiazepines of long and short elimination half-life and the risk of hip fracture, *JAMA* 262(23):3303-3307, 1989.

Resnick B, Jett K: *The Medicare Modernization and Improvement Act: The Medicare Part D drug benefit,* 2005 (website): *www.hartfordign.org.* Accessed May 11, 2007.

Rochon PA et al: Potentially inappropriate prescribing in Canada relative to the US, *Drugs Aging* 21(14):939-947, 2004.

Schmidt LE, Dalhoff K: Food-drug interactions, *Drugs* 62(10):1481, 2002.

Schneider LS et al: Effectiveness of atypical antipsychotic drugs in patients with Alzheimer's disease, *N Engl J Med* 355(15):1525-1538, 2006.

Scott GN, Elmer GW: Update on natural product–drug interactions, *Am J Health Syst Pharm* 59(4):339, 2002.

Semla TP et al: *Geriatric dosage handbook,* ed 12, Cleveland, 2007, Lexi-Comp, Inc.

Shaughnessy AF: Common drug interactions in the elderly, *Emerg Med* 24(21):21, 1992.

Shemesh E et al: A prospective study of posttraumatic stress symptoms and nonadherence in survivors of a myocardial infarction (MI), *Gen Hosp Psychiatry* 23:215, 2001.

Simon SR et al: Potentially inappropriate medication use by elderly persons in the U.S. Health Maintenance Organizations, 2000-2001, *J Am Geriatr Soc* 53(2):227-232, 2005.

Spiers MV, Kutzik DM: *A multidimensional framework for understanding medication adherence in the elderly: a prescription for rethinking,* Unpublished paper, 1995.

Stefanacci RG: Preventing medication errors, *Ann Long-Term Care* 14(10):15-17, 2006.

Stoudemire A, Smith DA: OBRA regulations and the use of psychotropic drugs in long-term care facilities: impact and implications for geropsychiatric care, *Gen Hosp Psychiatry* 18:77, 1996.

Tatro D: *Drug interaction facts 2003,* St Louis, 2003, Facts and Comparisons.

Valli G, Giardina EG: Benefits, adverse effects and drug interactions of herbal therapies with cardiovascular effects, *J Am Coll Cardiol* 39(7):1083, 2002.

Vestal RE: Clinical pharmacology. In Hazzard W et al, editors: *Principles of geriatric medicine and gerontology,* New York, 2000, McGraw-Hill.

Wilkinson G: Pharmacokinetics. In Hardman J et al, editors: *Goodman and Gilman's the pharmacological basis of therapeutics,* ed 10, New York, 2001, McGraw-Hill.

Willcox SM et al: Inappropriate drug prescribing for the community-dwelling elderly, *JAMA* 272(4):292-296, 1994.

Williams CM: Using medication appropriately in older adults, *Am Fam Physician* 66(10):1917-1924, 2002.

Wurglics MK et al: Comparison of German St. John's wort products according to hyperforin and total hypericin content, *J Am Pharm Assoc (Wash)* 41(4):560, 2001.

CHAPTER 13

The Use of Herbs and Supplements in Late Life

Ellis Quinn Youngkin

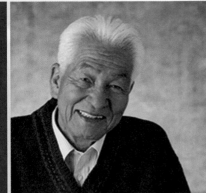
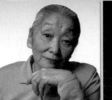

AN ELDER SPEAKS

I would like to take the medicines that the nurse practitioner gives me but I can't always afford them, so I ask my friend what I should do because she knows a lot about teas and other treatments. They really help sometimes and maybe that is all I need!

Jean-Marie, age 65

LEARNING OBJECTIVES

On completion of this chapter, the reader will be able to:

1. Identify the legal standards that affect herb and supplement use.
2. Describe the altered effects of herbs and supplements on the older adult.
3. Discuss the information that older adults should know about the use of select herbs and supplements.
4. Discuss the role of the gerontological nurse when assisting the older adult who uses herbs and supplements.
5. Describe the effects of select commonly used herbs and supplements on the older adult.

6. Develop a nursing care plan to prevent adverse reactions related to herb or supplement use.
7. Identify the important aspects of client education related to the use of herbs and supplements with the older adult.
8. Describe the effects of herbal supplements on the older adult with chronic disease.
9. Describe the effects of herbal supplements on the older adult who is experiencing altered health conditions.

USE OF HERBS AND SUPPLEMENTS IN THE UNITED STATES

Herbs have been used by humans for thousands of years to treat illness, but during most of the past century in the United States, they took a back seat to the burgeoning increase in prescription and over-the-counter (OTC) standardized drugs (Israel and Youngkin, 2005). Then an interesting phenomenon occurred. In the last decades of the twentieth century, alternative therapy use resurged. Today, herbal and other supplement products make up one of the largest groups of alternative pharmaceuticals used by millions of Americans, especially those who are 65 years of age or older (Keller and Lemberg, 2001;Yoon and Schaffer, 2006). Some supplements, such as vitamins and minerals, are approved by the Federal Drug Administration (FDA), but others, including most herbs and many other non-herbal

supplements, are not regulated. Several popular examples of non-herbal supplements used by older adults that fall into this category are melatonin for sleep, Co-Q10 sometimes advised for strengthening the heart, and glucosamine, often used for painful joints. Herbs are considered dietary supplements. Yeh et al. (2006) reported on the 2002 National Health Interview Survey that examined the use of complementary and alternative medicine (CAM) for cardiovascular disease. The most common CAM therapies used were herbal and mind-body therapies. Echinacea, garlic, ginseng, *Ginkgo biloba*, and glucosamine with or without chondroitin were the herbs/supplements used most often.

A 1999 to 2000 National Health and Nutrition Examination Survey assessed the prevalence of dietary supplement use (Radimer et al., 2004). Non-Hispanic white, older, normal-to-underweight women with more education were found to use these supplements more than any other racial/

Special thanks to Dianne Thames, the previous edition contributor, for her content contributions to this chapter.

ethnic, age, or gender groups. Weng and associates (2004) surveyed 318 people in a retirement community about supplement use. They found that 20% of both men and women used herbal supplements, and most (97%) used vitamin and mineral supplements. More than half said that they received information related to supplement use from physicians or nurses.

The increasing use of herbs and supplements by older adults is related to their hopes of preventing illness, promoting health, treating a particular health problem, or replacing some currently missing dietary component (Bruno and Ellis, 2005; Eskin, 2001; Yoon and Horne, 2001; Yoon et al., 2004). Older adults with chronic conditions are more likely to use herbal supplements in addition to their traditional therapies (Stupay and Sivertsen, 2000).

Yoon and Horne (2001), after studying community-dwelling women 65 years of age and older over a year's period, found that more than 40% used an average of 2.5 herbs, and 85% of these herbal remedies were used continuously. In addition, the study noted that these women used an average of 3.2 prescribed medications and 3.8 OTC supplements and medications. Typically, the women did not tell their health care providers about the use of such alternative therapies. This finding has been supported by other research. A large national survey found that 49% of older adults taking herbs never reported them to the provider (Bruno and Ellis, 2005). More than half of individuals using alternative therapies in another survey did not tell their providers, although a conflicting study found that those older than 50 years were more likely than younger persons to share information about their use of supplements with their providers (Durante et al., 2001; Israel and Youngkin, 2005).

In a study of white Hispanic and non-Hispanic adults 65 years of age and older by Zeilmann and associates (2003), herb use within the past year was reported by 49%. Yoon (2006) found no differences in reported herb use between white American and African-American women 65 years of age and older. Use of both herbs and non-prescribed medications was significantly associated and was more complementary than used in place of other therapies.

Use of alternative therapies is increasing because people perceive that herbs or other supplements will give them more control of their health and bodies. Gerontological nurses must accept that older clients may use a variety of alternative therapies, including herbs and supplements, as well as prescribed and OTC drugs. The nurse has a significant obligation to ask the right questions and obtain specific information related to use—reason, form, frequency, duration, dose, any side/adverse effects, plans for continuing, and communication with providers about use (see Chapter 12).

Lack of Standards in Manufacturing

Many Americans believe that herbs and supplements are derived from harmless "natural" plants or substances, but nurses must remind clients that any substance that is consumed and that affects the body should be considered a drug and can be potentially harmful (Israel and Youngkin, 2005).

Before 1962, all herbs were regarded as medications. That year, the FDA began to require that all medications be evaluated for safety and efficacy. In response, herbal manufacturers decided to label herbs as foods (Youngkin and Israel, 1996). As such, herbs became regulated by the Dietary Supplement Health and Education Act (DSHEA) of 1994 and ordered to be called *dietary supplements*.

Herbs and other supplements may not be labeled for prevention, treatment, or cure of a health condition but may state effects on the body. Also, the label must state that FDA review has not occurred (Israel and Youngkin, 2005). Of the well over 1400 identified herbs, only a handful are FDA-approved, such as aloe, psyllium, capsicum, witch hazel, cascara, senna, and slippery elm. Nevertheless, these herbs may be hazardous if improperly used, as may be any substance. An herb or supplement must be reported as dangerous to the FDA before it will investigate the product for possible removal from the market (Allen and Bell, 2002).

Because herbs are not typically under the protection of patent laws, companies have been less inclined to participate in clinical trials to determine their effectiveness, although the market for herbs and supplements is growing so fast that some companies now are undertaking more scientific study of their safety and efficacy. However, the lack of consistency among the methods different companies use to produce herbal products makes analytical analyses of them difficult (Allen and Bell, 2002). Despite the fact that very few dietary supplements are FDA-approved, not every such product is unsafe or ineffective for use (Israel and Youngkin, 2005).

The World Health Organization (WHO) and regulatory agencies of individual countries across the world are answering the call for safety and efficacy information based on scientific evaluation (Blumenthal et al., 2000; Israel and Youngkin, 2005). Increasing and valuable scientific information is available to consumers from numerous sources, such as from the National Center for Complementary and Alternative Medicine (NCCAM); however, more systematic scientific trials and reviews are needed (Israel and Youngkin, 2005).

Thus the consumer must be alert to possible adverse effects and risks from use. Risks include the product containing the wrong parts of the herb, containing no or so little active ingredient that it is ineffective, or being adulterated with one or more unaccounted-for substances that may be dangerous. Mixed herbal-supplement therapies, such as some of the weight-loss products that can cause hazardous effects on blood pressure and heart rate and rhythm, are particularly risky because actually knowing what the product contains may be difficult. For example, bitter orange (citrus aurantium), now widely used to replace ephedra in many weight-loss products since it was removed from the general market by the FDA in 2004, is found in many products and is reported to cause serious cardiac effects. Bitter orange has synephrine (epinephrine-like) effects that can lead to cardiac arrest and ventricular fibrillation (Swanson, 2006).

Nurses must maintain current knowledge about herbs and other supplements so that when they assess older clients about their drug and substance intake, potential and actual harmful effects may be recognized. Consideration of each product's intended use, dose, possible adverse effects, and possible interactions with other substances based on the person's health or illness conditions is required. Fortunately, many manufacturers today have heeded the call to standardize production and labeling of herb and supplement products and independent testing of products for purity and marketing honesty is occurring. Nevertheless, nurses should urge their clients to be wary and purchase products only from reputable distributors (Brodeur, 2002).

HERB FORMS

Different parts of an herb may have uses and actions that are unrelated. The bulb of the garlic contains the active essence, whereas the leaf of the chamomile is used (Israel and Youngkin, 2005). Herbs are manufactured in several forms; most popular are capsules, extracts, oils, tablets, salves, teas, and tinctures. Efficacy varies depending on the form of the herb that is used and how it is prepared. An extract is a fluid or solid form of the herb that is concentrated. It is made from mixing the crude herb with alcohol, water, or some other solvent that is then distilled or evaporated (Libster, 2002; Skidmore-Roth, 2005). Oils are found in two forms. *Essential oils* are aromatic, volatile, and can be derived from various parts of the fresh plant. To be therapeutic, they are usually diluted. *Infused oils*, on the other hand, are developed when the volatile oil of one herb is mixed with that of another. Herbal oils are often used in massage therapy or aromatherapy (Libster, 2002; Skidmore-Roth, 2005).

When an herb is soaked in water, alcohol, vinegar, or glycerin for a specific time and the liquid is then strained to dispose of the plant remains, a tincture is formed. The liquid is used therapeutically at a concentration of 1:5 or 1:10 (Libster, 2002; Skidmore-Roth, 2005). A salve is a type of ointment—a semisolid substance that is used topically. Salves and ointments can be purchased or prepared by "simmering two tablespoons of the herb in 220 grams of a petroleum-based jelly for about ten minutes" (Eliopoulos, 1999, p. 103) or by using herbal-infused oil or plain oil with drops of the essential oil or some other wax base and the essential oil (Libster, 2000).

Teas

The consumer should be advised that teas are both foods and herbs, are not regulated, may be highly concentrated if grown at home, and may be mixed with other substances. An example is *Ginkgo biloba* added to Snapple tea by manufacturers to boost sales (Barnes and Winter, 2001; Israel and Youngkin, 2005). Tea is consumed by millions across the world, second only to water, and newly reported research indicates that some teas may have very positive effects, especially related to cardiovascular disease. Researchers found that drinking three cups of green tea daily was associated with a decreased mortality risk (Kuriyama et al., 2006). Women and nonsmokers seemed to benefit the

most from green tea. The consumer does need to remember that tea is generally safe but in excess may be harmful. For instance, senna leaf tea may cause serious consequences of fluid and electrolyte imbalance if used in excess and for a prolonged period (Israel and Youngkin, 2005). Consumption of more than the recommended amounts of certain teas may cause illness and possible death. For example, comfrey tea has been linked with serious liver disease (Youngkin and Israel, 1996).

SELECT COMMONLY USED TEAS, HERBS, AND SUPPLEMENTS

Chamomile

Chamomile (*Matricaria recutita* or *Chamomilla recutita*), also known as *German chamomile* or *Hungarian chamomile*, is usually taken in tea form (Jellin et al., 2006). Its primary uses are as an antiinflammatory and antispasmodic, said to relax smooth muscle (Israel and Youngkin, 2005). Jellin and his research team (2006) report that this form of chamomile, when combined with several other herbs, including peppermint leaf, is associated with improvement in dyspepsia (acid reflux, pain in epigastrium, nausea, cramping, vomiting). However, it has mixed and less clear results in the scientific literature (Basch and Ulbricht, 2005). It may cause gastrointestinal (GI) upset in large doses, and contact dermatitis and hypersensitivity reactions have been reported. It should be used cautiously with clients who report allergies to ragweed, asters, or chrysanthemums. Use with benzodiazepines and other sedative-causing drugs is not advised, and it may inhibit some cytochrome P450 substrates (see Chapter 12). A dose of the commercial combination product, Enzymatic Therapy, of 1 mL three times daily is suggested for oral use for dyspepsia (Jellin et al., 2006). Chamomile capsules or tablets taken alone are in divided doses of 400 to 1600 mg orally daily or, if used as a tea, 1 to 4 cups daily made from tea bags is suggested (Basch and Ulbricht, 2005). Another type of chamomile, Roman chamomile (*C. nobile*), is available and its use is similar to that of German chamomile (Basch and Ulbricht, 2005; Jellin et al., 2006). German chamomile is thought to be somewhat stronger in effect.

Echinacea

Echinacea (*Echinacea angustifolia*, *E. purpurea*, *E. pallida*), also known as *Sampson root* and *purple coneflower*, is used for cold and flu therapy. Annual sales in the United States are in the $20 million range, second only to garlic (Jellin, 2006a). Study results are mixed as to its efficacy in the past (Basch and Ulbricht, 2005; Ernst, 2002; Jellin et al., 2006). Researchers, reporting at the American College of Clinical Pharmacy in September 2006 on a meta-analysis of randomized controlled trials, found that using the purple coneflower extract when a cold first begins and before symptoms become "full-blown" reduced the incidence of colds by 58% and the duration by 1.9 days (Kerr, 2006). Jellin (2006a,b) indicates modest improvement with the use of this herb at the start of symptoms.

Echinacea has immune stimulant qualities and is usually taken in tea form, but it can be used also as a tincture. Jellin and colleagues (2006) report some adverse reactions, including fever, sore throat, allergic reactions, diarrhea, nausea and vomiting, and abdominal pain, but indicate that the herb is tolerated without incident. Persons allergic to daisy family plants or who have human immunodeficiency virus/acquired immunodeficiency syndrome (HIV/AIDS) or an autoimmune disease should use this herb with caution (Jellin et al., 2006). It may interfere with the clearance of drugs eliminated by CYP3A or CYP1A2 in the liver (Gorski et al., 2004). When used as a tea, the dose ranges from 0.3 to 1 g (Israel and Youngkin, 2005; Scorza, 2002). In tablet form, it is advised three times daily and should contain 6.78 mg of the crude extract when the herb content equals 95% (Jellin et al., 2006). Begun at the first sign of a cold or flu, it is taken for 5 to 14 days and should not be continued longer than the package directions advise (Basch and Ulbricht, 2005; Israel and Youngkin, 2005; Jellin et al., 2006).

Garlic

Garlic (*Allium sativum* bulb), also known as *clove garlic*, is thought to protect against stroke and atherosclerosis. Garlic is composed of more than 200 chemicals. And one, a sulfur called *allicin*, is thought to be a primary active health ingredient (Garlic, 2006). When the garlic clove is crushed, chewed, or chopped, allicin is released. Benefits of garlic are reported to be many, but scientific evidence is mixed (Basch and Ulbricht, 2005; Jellin et al., 2006). Use is associated with decreased blood clots by keeping platelets from sticking together. It has been shown to reduce low-density–lipoprotein cholesterol but does not alter high-density–lipoprotein cholesterol (Basch and Ulbricht, 2005). Small decreases in blood pressure have been seen with garlic use, and it also may have some anti-cancer activity (Garlic, 2006). Persons with diabetes should watch their blood sugar carefully if they consume garlic because it has been shown to lower glucose levels (Israel and Youngkin, 2005). It may cause allergic reactions, and consuming more than five cloves a day could lead to heartburn and to increased flatulence. Persons taking aspirin or other drugs or supplements with anticoagulant properties, such as Coumadin or fish oil, should not ingest large amounts of garlic because it may cause excessive bleeding, which makes it especially risky for many older adults (Garlic, 2006; Israel and Youngkin, 2005). Persons with peptic and reflux disease should avoid garlic because it may irritate the upper GI system lining, causing nausea and heartburn. Topical garlic preparations can cause skin irritation (Scorza, 2002). There is actually no standard dose or accepted standard for which form is best—oil, powder, or deodorized extract (Garlic, 2006). Many supplements labeled to contain high-potency garlic do not, according to Consumerlab.com testing (Garlic, 2006). The suggested dose is 600 to 1200 mg divided into three doses daily (Jellin et al., 2006). Cooking garlic decreases its effectiveness (Keller and Lemberg, 2001).

Ginkgo biloba

Ginkgo (*Ginkgo biloba* leaf abstract), also known as *maidenhair tree, fossil tree, Asiatic ginseng, Chinese ginseng,* and *wonder of the world,* comes from the oldest living tree species (Jellin et al., 2006; Waddell et al., 2001). It is prepared in capsule, extract, and tablet form. The usual dose varies, but 120 to 240 mg per day of ginkgo leaf extract in 2 or 3 divided doses is frequently prescribed (Jellin et al., 2006).

Jellin and colleagues (2006) report that ginkgo may somewhat improve cognitive function associated with mild or moderate memory impairment in some older persons but will not help older persons with normal mental ability and will not aid forgetfulness. It also seems to be helpful in treating vertigo, intermittent claudication, and some visual impairments (Jellin et al., 2006). It is believed by many to work by preventing oxidative damage, by increasing blood flow to the brain and the rest of the body, and by its effects on coagulation, but results of research remain controversial (Jellin et al., 2006).

A serious side effect of taking ginkgo is spontaneous bleeding. Persons taking anticoagulants, such as warfarin or aspirin, should not take ginkgo. Those who take ginkgo should be taught to report bleeding, bruising, dizziness, headache, and blurred vision to their health care provider (Kuhn, 2002). Post-surgery bleeding may result if ginkgo is not stopped well before surgery. Other herbs increase the risk of bleeding, such as Panax ginseng, ginger, garlic; and preparations containing ergotamine-caffeine (Jellin et al., 2006; Kuhn, 2002).

Side effects of taking ginkgo include GI upset, headache, hypersensitivity, palpitations, dizziness, and constipation (Israel and Youngkin, 2005; Jellin et al., 2006). Significant and serious interaction effects of ginkgo are reported with certain drugs and herbs, such as with St. John's wort, melatonin, and monoamine oxidase (MAO) inhibitors, to name only a few, and some health conditions are worsened by its use. For example, ginkgo seeds can be toxic (Allen and Bell, 2002), and consumption is associated with lowering the seizure threshold (Jellin et al., 2006). Clients who use this herb must be carefully assessed for complications. Acetaminophen, not usually associated with causing bleeding, is recommended for headache or other pain.

Ginseng

Ginseng (*Panax ginseng,* a Chinese perennial herb), also known as *Asian ginseng, Chinese ginseng,* and *Korean ginseng,* may be of special interest to older adults. It is best known for its use to improve well-being and help with stress adaptation, although research results are mixed (Jellin et al., 2006). It has been found to be possibly effective in improving some cognitive functions, such as abstract thinking, math skills, and how quickly one reacts but not effective in improving memory as single-use product (Basch and Ulbricht, 2005; Jellin et al., 2006). It may reduce fasting blood glucose and hemoglobin A_{1c} in persons with type 2 diabetes (Basch and Ulbricht, 2005; Jellin et al., 2006). It is associated with improvement in erectile dysfunction in some men (Hong et al., 2002).

Ginseng root provides the most active constituents, ginsenosides or panaxosides, but contains other constituents that may also play a role (Jellin et al., 2006). The most common preparations are capsules, extracts, and tinctures. Insomnia is the most often reported adverse effect. However, among the more common serious complaints, especially for the elderly, are tachycardia, hypertension, hypotension, edema, and diarrhea. Thus clients with hypertension, cardiac problems, or diabetes must use ginseng with significant caution. Ginseng may interact with other herbs such as fenugreek, which further reduces blood glucose, or with drugs such as anticoagulants, hypoglycemic agents, and insulin, further altering their effects. The usual dose for individuals with type 2 diabetes is 200 mg daily. For erectile dysfunction, 300 mg three times daily has been used (Jellin et al., 2006).

American ginseng and Siberian ginseng are two distinct types of ginseng not to be confused with *Panax ginseng*. American ginseng is said to decrease blood glucose levels in type 2 diabetes and also may help decrease the risk of upper respiratory infections, such as cold or flu in older adults. Siberian ginseng may be helpful in decreasing herpes type 2 infections. There is not enough evidence to support its use for improving memory, feelings of well-being, hyperlipidemia, arrhythmias, or stroke outcomes, as some resources suggest (Jellin et al., 2006).

Glucosamine Sulfate

Glucosamine sulfate, also known as *chitosamine*, is used orally for glaucoma and as an antiinflammatory and antiarthritic and therefore is commonly used by persons in late life (Jellin et al., 2006). Numerous studies support that glucosamine sulfate helps reduce pain and improve function with osteoarthritis of the knee, acting similarly to nonsteroidal antiinflammatory drugs (NSAIDs). However, glucosamine hydrochloride and chondroitin sulfate are frequently used together for joint pain, and the results of the Glucosamine/chondroitin Arthritis Intervention Trial (GAIT) found that neither of these drugs together or alone was more effective than placebo, except in one small subgroup with moderate-to-severe pain who had a 20% improvement in pain (Clegg et al., 2006). The nurse should advise the older person that this latter combination may not be as effective as the glucosamine sulfate alone, though none of the glucosamine alternatives may be particularly effective with severe osteoarthritis that is long-standing. The nurse also should warn of interaction effects with multiple drug use (prescribed, OTC—particularly NSAIDs, and supplements) (Burks, 2005). The dose varies, but glucosamine sulfate is usually prepared in capsule, tablet, and liquid form. The usual dose is 1500 mg daily in one dose or in divided doses such as 500 mg three times daily (Jellin et al., 2006). GI upsets have been reported with glucosamine sulfate use. Increased insulin resistance or decreased production of insulin has been reported, but generally, this drug is well tolerated by older adults (Jellin et al., 2006). Nonetheless, persons with diabetes, asthma, or a shellfish allergy should take glucosamine with caution.

Hawthorn

Hawthorn (*Crataegus monogyna, Crataegus laevigata*) is known by names such as *maybush, maythorn,* and *whitethorn*. Believed to have positive effects on congestive heart failure and coronary circulation, hawthorn may work by increasing cardiac output, and it also has effects as an antispasmodic, diuretic, sedative, and anxiety reducer (Jellin et al., 2006). It is generally believed safe if taken orally and short-term up to 16 weeks. Vertigo and dizziness are the most common adverse effects and are of particular concern in the elderly who have an increased incidence of serious falls. GI upsets, allergic response with rash, palpitations, fatigue, and sweating are among less-common side effects. Hawthorn may interact with cardiovascular drugs, such as antihypertensives, causing hypotension, and can alter blood sugar levels (Allen and Bell, 2002; Jellin et al., 2006). Although used as an extract or tea, it is often taken as a capsule. The standard dose for heart failure is 160 to 180 mg in divided doses daily for 4 to 8 weeks (Jellin et al., 2006).

St. John's Wort

St. John's wort (*Hypericum perforatum*) is also called *amber, demon chaser, goatweed, Johnswort,* and *klamath weed*. St. John's wort (SJW) is commonly used to treat mild or moderate depression and seasonal affective disorder (SAD), and research indicates that it also may have antiviral properties (Israel and Youngkin, 2005; Jellin et al., 2006; Lawvere and Mahoney, 2005). It is one of the most popular herbs used today, known to be well tolerated. However, based on major clinical trials, SJW is not effective for treatment of major depression (Sego, 2006). Thus its use could endanger the individual with that level of serious depression because of inadequate effect. In such a situation, the risk of suicide could be increased.

Common side effects may include photosensitivity, dermatitis, GI upset, restlessness, anxiety, and headache. Occasionally, hypomania has been reported with bipolar disorder. Other cytochrome P450 enzyme inducers, such as certain other drugs, red wine, broccoli, and cigarette smoke, should be used cautiously with SJW, and the list of possible drug-drug, drug-herb, herb-disease, and anesthesia interactions is long (Jellin et al., 2006).

SJW is contraindicated with other antidepressants, especially selective serotonin reuptake inhibitors (SSRIs) (Israel and Youngkin, 2005) (see Chapter 15). Individuals taking SSRIs should wait at least 2 weeks after discontinuing them before beginning SJW. Because of possible photosensitivity, persons taking SJW should be careful about their exposure to the sun. When taking this herb, clients should be warned not to take medications containing monoamines, such as medications for nasal decongestants, hay fever, and asthma, because this combination can cause hypertension (Waddell et al., 2001). The gerontological nurse must be familiar with these concerns in counseling the older client. The usual dose is 300 mg three times daily or 450 mg twice daily (Israel and

TABLE 13-1

Select Commonly Used Herbs and Recommended Dosages

Herb/Supplement	Form	Recommended Dosage*
Chamomile	Capsule or tablet	400-1600 mg in divided doses
	Fluid extract	1-4 mL three times daily
	Tea	1-4 cups from tea bags daily
	Tincture	15 mL three to four times daily
Echinacea	Capsule	500 mg-1 g three times a day
	Tea	2 tsp steeped in cup boiling water for 10-15 minutes
	Tincture	0.75-1.5 mL two to five times a day Gargle, then swallow
Garlic	Capsule or tablet	600-1200 mg daily divided into three doses
	Extract	4 mL daily
	Fresh	4 g daily
	Oil	4-12.3 mg daily
	Tincture	2-4 mL three times daily
Ginkgo	Capsule or tablet	80-240 mg two to three times daily
	Extract	80 mg three times daily
Ginseng	Capsule or tablet	100-200 mg one to two times daily
	Extract	1-2 mL daily
	Tincture	5-10 mL daily
Glucosamine	Capsule or tablet	500 mg three times daily
Hawthorn	Extract LI 132	100-300 mg three times daily
	Extract WS 1442	60 mg three times daily or 80 mg twice daily
St. John's wort	Capsule	300 mg three times daily (maintenance 300-600 mg daily)
Saw Palmetto	Capsule	160 mg one to two times daily
	Suppository	640 mg once daily

Adapted from Basch E, Ulbricht C: *Natural standard herb & supplement handbook: the clinical bottom line,* St Louis, 2005, Mosby; Jellin JM et al: Natural Medicines Comprehensive Database, 2006 (website): *www.naturaldatabase.com/.* Accessed November 15, 2006; Skidmore-Roth L: *Mosby's handbook of herbs and natural supplements,* St Louis, 2005, Mosby.

* Readers are advised to follow the most up-to-date dosage and duration-of-use recommendations from expert sources for any herb or supplement.

Youngkin, 2005). It may take up to 6 weeks for SJW to reach its full effect; it should be discontinued slowly (Jellin et al., 2006; Stupay and Sivertsen, 2000).

Saw Palmetto

Saw palmetto, a fruit-bearing palm tree, grows wild in southern U.S. states and is said to offer mild to modest symptom improvement for benign prostatic hyperplasia (BPH) (Israel and Youngkin, 2005; Jellin et al., 2006). BPH symptoms, commonly seen in the elderly, include urinary frequency, dysuria, urgency, hesitancy, and nocturia. Bent et al. (2006), however, found that saw palmetto did not improve BPH in men who had moderate to severe symptoms. Other studies show mixed results in outcomes for BPH symptoms. Thus it may not be as effective as the prescription medication *finasteride,* as promoted in the past. The saw palmetto essential oils used for treating mild BPH are in many standardized

products today. Dosing of 160 mg two times a day or 320 mg once a day is advised (Jellin et al., 2006). Adverse reactions are reportedly mild, such as dizziness, headache, and GI upset. Saw palmetto may prolong bleeding time, so use with anticoagulant/antiplatelet drugs, supplements, or herbs is advised with caution.

Table 13-1 lists select commonly used herbs and supplements and their recommended dosages.

USE OF HERBS AND SUPPLEMENTS FOR SELECT CONDITIONS

Organ Transplantation

Although it is unusual for a person over 65 years to receive a transplant, advances in technology are making it more likely that persons who received an organ transplant earlier in life will live into late life.

TABLE 13-2

Select Herbs and the Transplant Client

Herb	Claim	Interactions/Contraindications
Echinacea	Stimulates the immune system	Contraindicated with some infections, autoimmune disease, and use of immunosuppressants
Garlic	Decreases cholesterol, triglycerides, and blood pressure	May interact with antiplatelet drugs, may increase bleeding time
Ginger	Prevents nausea and vomiting	May interact with antiplatelet drugs
Ginkgo	Has antioxidant actions and increases blood flow	Slows body's ability to metabolize some drugs
Ginseng	Acts as either stimulant or relaxant; may enhance immunity	Slows drug metabolism; interacts with antiplatelet drugs
St. John's wort	Used to treat depression	Reduces blood levels of cyclosporine

From Allen D, Bell J: Herbal medicine and the transplant patient, *Nephrol Nurs J* 29(3):269, 2002.

As with any other patient, transplant patients will often speak with their health care provider about the use of prescribed medications but may forget to mention herbal products. Research indicates that significant drug-herb interactions can occur when persons are taking medications for immunosuppression. This puts patients with renal transplants at significant increased risk (Dahl, 2001). Liver transplant patients frequently use alternative medication products, with 19% using herbal therapies (Neff et al., 2004). Side effects, such as elevation of liver enzymes in liver transplant patients, symptoms of rejection in any transplant patient, and other complications may be more difficult to identify. In addition, immunosuppressive agents have a very narrow window of therapeutic effectiveness (Allen and Bell, 2002). Again, the literature emphasizes the need for transplant team members to educate patients on hazards of herb and supplement use. Select herbs with specific effects on the transplant patient's immune function are listed in Table 13-2.

Hypertension

Hypertension is a common problem in late life (see Chapter 10). Hawthorn has been used as a treatment for hypertension for years. A British study found that people with diabetes type 2 who were taking medications for the diabetes had a significant reduction in diastolic blood pressure when randomized to take hawthorn (Walker et al., 2006). However, the nurse must realize that a reduction in blood pressure for persons already taking beta-blockers or calcium channel blockers may precipitate dangerous hypotension (Jellin et al., 2006). Because therapeutic levels are not established, over-treatment and under-treatment can occur when used alone. Caution is urged with concomitant use of erectile dysfunction drugs, like Viagra, with hawthorn because hypotension may result (Hong et al., 2002). Obviously, overdose of hawthorn may result in hypotension. Garlic also may decrease blood pressure but only modestly after a month of treatment (Jellin et al., 2006). Health care providers are urged to provide up-to-date information on the use of herbs, including garlic, when counseling patients who have hyper-

tension (Edwards et al., 2005). (See the Garlic and Hawthorn sections earlier in this chapter.)

Human Immunodeficiency Virus–Related Symptoms

Persons with HIV–related symptoms are known to use a number of alternative therapies, including herbs, to assist with symptoms. Eller et al. (2005) found that herbal therapies were among the self-care strategies used by 92% of subjects studied related to symptoms of depression and HIV disease. SJW is commonly used for depression, as discussed earlier. However, research indicates a lowered blood level of antiretroviral medications when taken with SJW (Jellin et al., 2006). Some studies of the use of herbal medicines with HIV/AIDS patients in Thailand and Africa indicate significant improvement in health overall and quality of life, suggesting a need for further study (Sugimoto et al., 2005; Tshibangu et al., 2004).

Gastrointestinal Disorders

A number of factors make gastrointestinal disorders common in late life (see Chapter 10). Elders who have GI problems are likely to use alternative therapies, including herbs (Tillisch, 2006). One example of use is with irritable bowel syndrome (IBS). The Chinese have used herbal therapies for thousands of years to treat IBS. A search of the literature by Liu et al. (2006) found that 75 random trials for IBS had been done and IBS was improved by some of the herbal therapies, indicating a need for further quality research. Psyllium (*Plantago ovata* and *P. ispaghula*), well known to assist the older client with constipation, is used as a bulk laxative and may assist with IBS though results are conflicting (Basch and Ulbricht, 2005). Also, see the Chamomile section earlier in this chapter for use with GI problems. Chronic alcohol-induced and fulminate hepatitis have both been positively affected by the use of milk thistle (Basch and Ulbricht, 2005; Jellin et al., 2006). Misuse of some herbs may cause physical harm, such as liver damage, or delay the client from seeking appropriate traditional health care. Comfrey, kava kava, and chaparral are examples of herbs that may be toxic to the gastrointestinal system (Jellin et al., 2006).

Cancer

Cancer is the second leading cause of death among persons over 65 years (see Chapter 10). In the United States, many herbs have the potential to be used in the treatment of cancer but none has met the goals for use in biomedicine. Cancer patients often use alternative therapies in self-care. In a descriptive study of adults receiving chemotherapy for various cancers, herbal treatments, specifically green mint tea and garlic, were used by subjects (Williams et al., 2006). Garlic is possibly effective for colorectal and gastric cancer in decreasing risk according to population studies (Jellin et al., 2006). Hann et al. (2006) found that older women with early-stage breast cancer were less likely to use complementary therapies with chemotherapy. The authors suggested that women who used more alternative therapies might be more dissatisfied with their medical care and that better communication between the patient and the provider about such therapies is needed.

Claims are often made that a substance or an herb will "cure" or help the cancer patient, even though no data support such claims. Clients and their families may become desperate in an effort to "do something" to help. Gerontological nurses must be sensitive to this situation and work with all concerned to provide the most appropriate care possible.

Alzheimer's Disease

Kales et al. (2004) found that among 82 elderly veterans with dementia and depression, nearly one fifth of the veterans and their caretakers used herbs and supplements. Ginkgo is often used by older persons with dementia because it increases blood supply to the brain. There is some realistic scientific support for modest improvement in Alzheimer's and dementia symptoms (Jellin et al., 2006). The improvement is comparable to a delay in disease progression of about 6 months. Doses of 120 to 240 mg daily in divided doses of ginkgo leaf extract for 3 to 6 months has a "small but significant effect on cognitive function in patients with Alzheimer's disease" (Jellin et al., 2006; Waddell et al., 2001, p. 52). Primarily memory and attention are improved. In an Iranian double-blind, randomized, placebo controlled trial, sage (*Salvia officinalis*) significantly improved cognitive outcomes as measured by the cognitive subscale of the Alzheimer's Disease Assessment Scale and on the Clinical Dementia Rating Scale in 42 adults ages 65 to 80 years with mild to moderate Alzheimer's disease (Akhondzadeh et al., 2006). Further study is advised based on these outcomes in use of sage with dementia and Alzheimer's disease.

Diabetes

Herbal approaches to diabetes management were in place before the discovery of insulin in 1921. Approximately 400 different plants affect blood glucose, and many are still in use. Fenugreek (*Trigonella foenum-graecum*), a seed powder, when consumed as a cup of tea three times daily or taken orally in a capsule, can induce a hypoglycemic response (Basch and Ulbricht, 2005; Jellin et al., 2006). However, it may cause diarrhea and flatulence and it may increase anticoagulant activity of other drugs the person is taking. Caffeinated coffee has recently gotten much press for significant reduction in the risk of type 2 diabetes development (Jellin et al., 2006). The greater the dose, the greater the risk reduction. Drinking 6 or more cups daily lowers the risk by about 54% to 61% in men and 29% to 30% in women. The downside of drinking this much coffee is that it can cause a number of side effects, including headache, insomnia, and nervousness. Cinnamon is another herb that has been linked with lowering blood glucose, but the research evidence is mixed at this date (Jellin et al., 2006). One teaspoon daily for 40 days has been suggested. Other herbs linked with possibly lowering blood glucose are bilberry, banaba, bitter lemon, and glucomannan, but evidence is not yet sufficient to support that these are effective in treating or reducing development of diabetes type 2 (Jellin et al., 2006). If any of the aforementioned herbs or others are used by clients for diabetes management, the nurse needs to be sure to urge careful and regular blood glucose monitoring with concurrent indicated prescribed medication dose adjustments.

HERB AND SUPPLEMENT INTERACTIONS WITH STANDARDIZED DRUGS

Many herb and supplement products do interact with prescription or OTC medications, foods, and/or other herbs and supplements (see also Chapter 12). When an interaction occurs with a standardized medication, which is usually more pharmacologically active than the herb, the medication is typically the cause. This chapter will address only select herb-drug interactions especially relevant to the older adults because of the extensive nature of such interaction issues. The reader is referred to the references at the end of the chapter for further information on interactions.

The more herbs and other drugs that the client is taking, the more likely it is that an interaction will occur (see Chapter 12) (Kuhn, 2002). Yoon and Schaffer (2006) reviewed the interaction prevalence of drugs reported in a study of 58 women who were 65 years of age and older. Nearly 75% of the women took herbs, prescription drugs, and/or OTC drugs that could interact at a moderate- or a high-risk level. Sixty-three percent of the total interactions involved NSAIDs. The authors found this very worrisome, since older adults are at risk for bleeding even when NSAIDs are taken properly.

Clients taking medications that have a narrow therapeutic index should be especially discouraged from using herbal remedies. Interactions include absorption-type, such as with aloe or rhubarb, that usually binds to a medication, such as digoxin or warfarin, reducing the effectiveness of the medication. In these cases, the drug should be taken at least 1 hour before the herb. Herbs that are more likely to cause a distribution-type interaction may increase the possibility of adverse effects. For example, meadowsweet and black willow may interact with warfarin and carbamazepine. When taken together, the adverse effects of the medications are amplified. Metabolism-type interactions may increase or decrease the effectiveness of the medication, depending on the herb and the medication. The action of digoxin is increased in the presence of St. John's wort, whereas the action of corticosteroids is decreased in the presence of black licorice. Also, additive-type interactions may occur, such as with

ginkgo increasing the possibility of bleeding when the client takes warfarin (Kuhn, 2002).

Because the content of active herb or herbs in products by different manufacturers varies considerably, the therapeutic outcome and potential for herb-drug interactions varies greatly. Table 13-3 lists the interactions between some commonly used herbs and select medications. Complications and nursing actions that can promote healthy aging are also listed.

TABLE 13-3
Select Herb-Medication Interactions

Herb	Medication	Complication	Nursing Action
Garlic	Warfarin sodium, or any anticoagulant or antiplatelet drug NSAIDs such as ketoprofen Anti-clot drugs such as streptokinase and urokinase	Risk of bleeding may increase	Advise client not to take without provider approval
	Antimetabolite such as cyclosporine	Risk of less effective response	Advise against use
	Insulin or oral hypoglycemic agent such as pioglitazone or tolbutamide	Serum glucose control may improve, requiring less antidiabetic medication	Monitor blood glucose levels
Ginkgo	Aspirin Heparin sodium Warfarin sodium	Risk of bleeding may occur	Teach client not to take without approval of provider
	Antidiabetic drugs Insulin Glimepiride, metformin, and other oral drugs for DMT2	May alter blood glucose levels	Monitor blood glucose closely
	Antidepressants MAOIs, SSRIs	May cause abnormal response or decrease effectiveness	Advise not to take with these drugs
	Antihypertensives Nifedipine	May cause increased effect	Monitor blood pressure
Ginseng	Insulin and oral antidiabetic drugs	Blood glucose levels may be altered	Monitor blood glucose levels; monitor for hyperglycemia, hypoglycemia
	Anticoagulants and antiplatelet drugs	May increase bleeding	Advise use with caution
	MAOIs	Headaches, tremors, mania	Advise against use
	Immunosuppressants	May interfere with action	Advise against use
	Stimulants	May cause additive effect	Advise against use
Green tea	Warfarin sodium	May alter anticoagulant effects	Advise against use
	Stimulants	May cause additive effect	Advise to use with care
Hawthorn	Digoxin	May cause a loss of potassium, leading to drug toxicity	Monitor blood levels
	Beta-blockers and other drugs lowering blood pressure and improving blood flow	May be additive in effects	Monitor blood pressure meticulously; advise that this concern holds true for erectile dysfunction drugs also
St. John's wort	Triptans such as sumatriptan, zolmitriptan	May increase risks of serotonergic adverse effects, serotonin syndrome, cerebral vasoconstriction	Advise against use
	HMG-CoA reductase inhibitors	May decrease plasma concentrations of these drugs	Monitor levels of lipids
	MAOIs	May cause similar effects as with use with any SSRI	Advise against use

Adapted from Basch E, Ulbricht C: *Natural standard herb & supplement handbook: the clinical bottom line,* St Louis, 2005, Mosby; Jellin JM et al: Natural Medicines Comprehensive Database, 2006. (website): *www.naturaldatabase.com/.* Accessed November 15, 2006; *NDH pocket guide to drug interactions,* Philadelphia, 2002, Lippincott, Williams & Wilkins; Wilson BA et al: *Nurses drug guide,* Upper Saddle River, NJ, 2004, Pearson Prentice Hall; Yoon SL, Schaffer SD: Herbal, prescribed, and over-the-counter drug use in older women: prevalence of drug interactions, *Geriatr Nurs* 27(2):118-129, 2006.

Continued

TABLE 13-3

Select Herb-Medication Interactions—cont'd

Herb	Medication	Complication	Nursing Action
St. John's wort—con't	Digoxin	Decreases the effects of the drug	Advise against use
	Alprazolam	May decrease effect of drug	Advise against use
	Amitriptyline	May decrease effect of drug	Advise against use
	Efavirenz and other anti-HIVs	May decrease drug level	Advise against use
	Ketoprofen	Photosensitivity	Advise sun block use
	Tramadol and some SSRIs	May increase risk of serotonin syndrome	Advise against use
	Olanzapine	May cause serotonin syndrome	Advise against use
	Paroxetine	Sedative-hypnotic intoxication	Advise against use
	Theophylline Albuterol	Increases metabolism; decreases drug blood level	Monitor drug effects
	Warfarin	May decrease anticoagulant effect	Advise against use
	Amlodipine	Lowers efficacy of calcium channel	Advise against use
	Estrogen or progesterone	May decrease effect of hormones	Advise that this effect may occur

Adapted from Basch E, Ulbricht C: *Natural standard herb & supplement handbook: the clinical bottom line,* St Louis, 2005, Mosby; Jellin JM et al: Natural Medicines Comprehensive Database, 2006. (website): *www.naturaldatabase.com/.* Accessed November 15, 2006; *NDH pocket guide to drug interactions,* Philadelphia, 2002, Lippincott, Williams & Wilkins; Wilson BA et al: *Nurses drug guide,* Upper Saddle River, NJ, 2004, Pearson Prentice Hall; Yoon SL, Schaffer SD: Herbal, prescribed, and over-the-counter drug use in older women: prevalence of drug interactions, *Geriatr Nurs* 27(2):118-129, 2006.

MISUSE OF HERBAL AND DIETARY SUPPLEMENTS

As discussed earlier, patients often do not reveal their use of herbs and supplements to their provider. This failure to share important health information can severely jeopardize the client because many of these products may have serious consequences of misuse based on actions or interactions with the individual's current health status. In a study of older clients with a mean age of 84.8 years who lived in assisted living facilities in Oregon and Washington State, 84.4% were using self-prescribed OTC medications and dietary supplements (Lam and Bradley, 2006). Nutritional supplements (vitamins and minerals) were used by 32%, gastrointestinal products by 17%, products to relieve pain by 16.3%, and herbal products by 14.4%. Other products used included topicals and cough and cold drugs. Misuse was found in 51% of the participants, including duplication of the active ingredients, drug-illness-food interactions, and inappropriate use. Most thought the products were helping them. In a study of differences in the perceptions of older users and nonusers of herbal supplements in relation to supplement safety and satisfaction with their current medical care, those who used herbal supplements perceived supplements to be safe and were not as satisfied with their medical care as those who did not use herbal supplements (Shahrokh et al., 2005). An example of an issue associated with herb misuse was described in relation to the complex naming of herbs in the Chinese culture (Wu et al., 2006). A similar issue can be projected with the use of ginseng as discussed earlier because a number of types of ginseng might be easily misunderstood and misused, including *Panax pseuodoginseng,* not discussed in the prior section because no reliable information exists about its main reported effectiveness to stop bleeding.

▲ PROMOTING HEALTHY AGING: IMPLICATIONS FOR GERONTOLOGICAL NURSING

One of the most important aspects of the role of the nurse working with an older adult who is using herbs and/or supplements is distinguishing the reliable data from the unproven claims. Maintaining a sound knowledge base is an ongoing responsibility of any health care professional. Second is the importance of developing a rapport with and listening to the older client, so that when collecting data about drugs and supplements, the person may be more willing to share such information. A British survey noted that because older people often do not report use of herbs and supplements, it behooves the health professional to encourage sharing this information for safety sake (Canter and Ernst, 2005). Third, becoming an educator is significantly important. Facilitating learning is an essential role in assisting the older adult to use herbs and supplements safely and effectively.

Assessment

As part of the comprehensive nursing assessment, the nurse needs to determine the abilities of the client—cognitive, motor, sensory—that would come into play with self-management of any medication (Curry et al., 2005) (see Chapter 12). Then, the questions about current and past medications that the client is taking or took should be asked, including all prescribed, OTC, and complementary therapies. Because clients may consider herbal remedies insignificant, they may not mention them unless specifically asked. These questions should be asked in a non-confrontational manner, remembering that it may take several interviews to complete the data (Stupay and Sivertsen, 2000).

If there is a beneficial rationale for the client to continue to use the herb(s) and/or supplement(s), the health care provider should continue to assess the situation. An important part of the planning phases is a review of the client's health condition; the medications that have been prescribed and possible side effects; the herbs, supplements, and any OTC standardized medications the client is taking; and possible adverse interactions (Stupay and Sivertsen, 2000). It is helpful to know what the person hopes to accomplish by using the herb/supplement. Reinforcing the positive effects and reviewing the costs of using the products may assist him or her to relax and open additional lines of communication. Any verbal or nonverbal action from the provider that may block this openness may lead to incomplete and potentially dangerous lack of assessment data.

Perioperative Assessment. Including herbal remedies in the perioperative assessment is an important aspect of total care. The reader is advised to see the article by Messina (2006) for risks associated with the use of 10 herbs by the patient who is to have surgery. Hypertension, excessive and prolonged bleeding, and the increased chance for interactions between the herb and other drugs are discussed. Herbs that affect bleeding and clotting time, such as garlic, ginger, ginkgo, and ginseng, should be especially noted and reported to the surgical team. Several select herbs and their perioperative effects are listed in Table 13-4. Patients should be told to stop the herbal treatments as advised before the scheduled surgery. Patients having emergency surgery should be questioned about the use of herbal remedies so that accommodations can be made or potential adverse events monitored.

Interventions

When planning care, the nurse should know that for many elders from other cultures, the traditional form of health care in the United States is foreign and raises suspicions, decreasing willingness to share personal information (Spector, 2000). The main reasons given for use of alternative therapies by elders from areas outside the country of service (especially United States and Canada) are (1) dissatisfaction with traditional medicine (too impersonal, too high tech, not effective, produces adverse effects, too costly); (2) need for more autonomy and control in one's own health care; and (3) incongruence with one's meaning of health and illness (philosophy derived from cultural beliefs) (Spector, 2000). In many cultures it is expected that family members are included in the planning and decision-making process (O'Hara and Zhan, 1994; St. Hill et al., 2003).

If the elder is using an herb or supplement in an inappropriate manner, the goal is to discontinue use or to use only the advised dosage for a specific condition. This can be done by providing needed information and asking the individual to consider the correct use of the product. The client may be willing to show the specific herb or supplement to the health care professional and discuss safer and better ways to use it. Whatever the selected strategy, the assistance of the family or a close friend could prove to be invaluable (Stupay and Sivertsen, 2000).

If it is unclear whether the herb is beneficial or harmful to the elder, it is the health care professional's responsibility to inform the person about this (Stupay and Sivertsen, 2000). The health care professional may also observe the placebo effect with clients who are taking herbs and supplements. That is, the taking of the product and not the action of the herb or supplement itself may produce a positive effect on the client. In this instance, if the herb or supplement causes no harm, it may be continued. However, the safe or unsafe use of a certain herb or supplement in a particular person is often difficult to determine.

Important interventions of the gerontological nurse in the promotion of healthy aging include education; checking for side effects, adverse reactions, and interactions among herbs, supplements, medications, foods, and the illness; and urging discontinuance of possibly harmful products or referring to the person's usual health care provider. Remaining sensitive to the client's situation is essential. Whether it is a need for additional information about a particular herb or supplement or assessment for side effects and interactions, the nurse must be alert for opportunities to intervene on the elder's behalf. In instances in which an adverse reaction or harmful interaction is suspected, the client must be urged to stop taking the herb or supplement and to see his or her prescribing health care provider. Teaching information about side effects and interaction possibilities in realistic and understandable ways may be the most useful intervention.

TABLE 13-4
Select Herbs and the Perioperative Patient

Herb	Perioperative Issue	Preoperative Discontinuation
Echinacea	Allergic reactions; decreased effectiveness of immunosuppressants	No time advised in data
Garlic	Potential for increased bleeding	1 to 2 weeks before surgery
Ginkgo	Potential for increased bleeding	2 weeks before surgery
Ginseng	Hypoglycemia; potential for increased bleeding	1 to 2 weeks before surgery
St. John's wort	Potential for increased sedation with anesthetics	5 days before surgery*

Adapted from Basch E, Ulbricht C: *Natural standard herb & supplement handbook: the clinical bottom line,* St Louis, 2005, Mosby; Jellin JM et al: Natural Medicines Comprehensive Database, 2006. (website): *www.naturaldatabase.com/.* Accessed November 15, 2006; Norred CL, Brinker F: Potential coagulation effects of preoperative complementary and alternative medicines, *Altern Ther Health Med* 7(6):58, 2001.

*Clients taking St. John's wort for depression must be advised not to stop herb abruptly and to discuss with physician when to stop before surgery. A washout period of 3 weeks may be needed.

Evaluation

The review of herb-supplement-medication-drug-food inter-actions specifically is an essential component of the evaluation phase. Outcomes of all teaching should be evaluated, as well as the effectiveness of herbs and supplements used in select conditions. In evaluating the outcomes of client goals, the health care professional must discuss and consider the client's condition from a holistic view and the important effects that culture may have in the outcomes.

Education

Patient education is one of the most important roles that the gerontological nurse has when working with older adults who are taking any herb or supplement. Education can occur in a variety of formats and includes assessing the client's readiness and ability to learn (Curry et al., 2005). See Chapter 12 for detailed information related to medication-related patient education. *Healthy People 2010*'s goal related to medication teaching includes receipt of written information. Thus the nurse needs to provide specific information in a way that the individual can understand, with particular emphasis on what to do in an emergency.

One-on-one teaching sessions are useful, as is the use of written materials. Education could occur in the home, at the clinic or office, or in the senior citizen center (see Chapter 12). Scientific data and information on the safe use of herbs must be provided based on the client's age and particular learning needs. Follow-up is essential. Just because it says "natural" on the label does not mean that it is healthy for every client. Cli-

Human Needs and Wellness Diagnoses

Self-Actualization and Transcendence
(Seeking, Expanding, Spirituality, Fulfillment)
Educates self about numerous transcendent possibilities for bodily control
Recognizes importance of spiritual elements in achieving health
Understands significance of humor, music, and placebo effects

Self-Esteem and Self-Efficacy
(Image, Identity, Control, Capability)
Makes carefully considered choices of herbs and supplements
Recognizes need to maintain control of unusual treatments
Maintains independence and judgment
Avoids undue expectations of herbs and supplements
Seeks knowledge about adjunctive health strategies

Belonging and Attachment
(Love, Empathy, Affiliation)
Discusses treatment possibilities with
trusted friends and affiliates
Considers effects of personal interactions
on treatment successes
Places appropriate levels of trust in providers

Safety and Security
(Caution, Planning, Protections, Sensory Acuity)
Carefully considers possible interactions of
medications with herbal treatments
Maintains healthy skepticism
Carefully monitors purity and strength of substances
Investigates accuracy of claims made of successful treatments

Biological and Physiological Integrity
(Air, Fluids, Comfort, Activity, Nutrition, Elimination, Skin Integrity)
Is moderate in use of herbal and nutritional supplements
Understands that herbs are foods and considers nutritional implications
Is attuned to subtle body signals

These are not all the possible wellness diagnoses that may be identified. The above
are examples of nursing diagnoses that should be considered when planning care
for the older adult.

ents may switch from one harmful product to another without talking with their health care provider (Stupay and Sivertsen, 2000). The provider must seek the motivation for the use of herbs or supplements to provide significant help.

Several additional issues do need to be addressed with persons who are taking herbs and supplements:

- Elders should be helped to understand the importance of reporting the use of all herbs and supplements to their health care provider. They should be encouraged to speak with their health care provider before beginning an herb or supplement for the first time. Persons should use only the herbs and supplements recommended by the health care provider and only for the time prescribed. The emphasis is on the fact that herbs and supplements are still drugs.
- (1) There is no standardization among manufacturers, so the amount of active ingredients per dose among brands is inconsistent; (2) herbs and supplements should be purchased from reputable sources; (3) herbs are available in different forms, making accurate dosing difficult; (4) research is inadequate on both the untoward effects and the benefits of most herbs and supplements, making recommendations about specific herbs and supplements difficult; and (5) persons who have allergies to certain plants may have allergies to herbs in the same plant family.
- If side effects occur within an hour or two of taking the supplement, the supplement should be discontinued immediately. If the side effects continue or worsen, the client should report them to the health care provider or go to the emergency department nearest him or her if the provider is unavailable. Because older adults may react differently to supplements, health care providers may need to prescribe less than the recommended dose. Herbs and supplements taken with other such products may cause unpredictable effects (Stupay and Sivertsen, 2000).
- A fact of life for nurses today is that many older clients do take herbs and supplements along with prescribed and OTC medications. Thus the approach to the client must be open and encouraging for effective assessment, evaluation of risks, and appropriate teaching-learning applications, intervention, and monitoring. The gerontological nurse today must be knowledgeable and continue to seek out the latest information on herbs, supplements, OTC medications, prescribed medications, and interactions.

KEY CONCEPTS

- Older adults who are diagnosed with chronic conditions are more likely to take herbs and other supplements.
- Many individuals continue their traditional therapies in addition to herb and supplement therapies.
- The renewed interest in herbal therapies is based in part on the focus of preventing illness. Herbs are often used by individuals who want to be more involved in their own health care or who are unable to afford prescription medications.

CASE STUDY: Common Use of Herbs and Supplements

Anna is an 80-year-old woman who lives with her 83-year-old husband in the suburbs of a large city. They have been married for 57 years and have two grown children, six grandchildren, and five great-grandchildren. Anna is very proud of all of them. Anna taught high school English for 20 years but was raised with many of the "old country" traditions, speaking French for most of her formative years. As part of her background, she would rather use herbs and "home treatments" than prescribed "pills." She has been diagnosed with hypertension, diabetes mellitus, and arthritis. She often complains of symptoms that are related to these chronic conditions, but she refuses to consistently follow her diet or take any prescribed medications. Anna attends mass daily and, with her husband, takes part in community activities. While accompanying her husband on a visit to his health care provider, she mentions the use of herbal supplements. After some discussion, the nurse realizes that Anna has little information about herbal supplements and has some incorrect assumptions about them.

Based on the case study, develop a nursing care plan using the following procedure*:

- List Anna's comments that provide subjective data.
- List information that provides objective data.
- From these data, identify and state, using accepted format, two nursing diagnoses that you determine are most

significant to Anna at this time. List two of Anna's strengths that you have identified from the data.

- Determine and state outcome criteria for each diagnosis. These must reflect some alleviation of the problem identified in the nursing diagnosis and must be stated in concrete and measurable terms.
- Plan and state one or more interventions for each diagnosed problem. Provide specific documentation of the source used to determine the appropriate intervention. Plan at least one intervention that incorporates Anna's existing strengths.
- Evaluate the success of the intervention. Interventions must correlate directly with the stated outcome criteria to measure the outcome success.

Critical Thinking Questions

1. How would you begin your discussion with Anna regarding her knowledge of herbal supplements?
2. What information would you be especially interested in obtaining regarding herbal supplements and each of Anna's medical diagnoses?
3. How would you prepare Anna should she need surgery?
4. Prepare a teaching plan for Anna to include the effective use of herbal supplements.

---

* Students are advised to refer to their nursing diagnosis text and identify possible or potential problems.

- The U.S. government has no standards in place to control the quality of herbs or herbal products or other supplements.
- Nurses and other health care providers should always ask about the use of herbs and supplements when conducting a health interview.
- Nurses and other health care providers should teach clients to ask about the concurrent use of herbs, supplements, and medications, both prescribed and OTC.
- Patients should be told to stop the herbal treatments for the prescribed period of time before scheduled surgery and should be told why.
- Whichever educational strategy is chosen, follow-up is essential to determine that instructions are being followed and that the client is aware of the situation.

RESEARCH QUESTIONS

Interview a member of your health care community who recommends the use of herbs along with traditional strategies. How does this individual decide which herbs to use? How does he or she ensure standardization among products?

Tour a local health food store. Read the labels of the more commonly used herbal supplements. Do the labels list the information you expected? How would you make sure that your clients have the necessary information?

Visit a senior citizen center. Talk with members about their use of herbal supplements. Keep track of the more commonly used herbs and the reasons for their use. How did the older adults find out the herbal action?

Are older adults aware of possible negative effects of herbs and supplements?

What questions do older adults ask before taking an herbal or non-herbal supplement?

What information do older adults need before considering taking an herbal or non-herbal supplement?

What are the rewards (positive factors) versus the costs (negative factors) of using herbal and non-herbal supplements?

What strategies should health care providers use to bridge the gap between herb/supplement remedies and traditional health care?

Why do older adults choose to use herbs and supplements?

REFERENCES

Akhondzadeh S et al: *Salvia officinalis* extract in the treatment of patients with mild to moderate Alzheimer's disease: a double blind, randomized and placebo-controlled trial, *J Clin Pharm Ther* 28(1):53-59, 2006.

Allen D, Bell J: Herbal medicine and the transplant patient, *Nephrol Nurs J* 29(3):269, 2002.

Barnes JE, Winter G: Supplemental products growing, *The New York Times*, In *The Sun Sentinel*, May 27, 2001, p. 4A.

Basch E, Ulbricht C: *Natural standard herb & supplement handbook: the clinical bottom line*, St Louis, 2005, Mosby.

Bent S et al: Saw palmetto for benign prostatic hyperplasia, *N Engl J Med* 354:557-566, 2006.

Blumenthal M et al: *Herbal medicine: expanded commission E monographs*, Newton, Mass, 2000, Integrative Medicine Communications.

Brodeur MA: Understanding dietary supplement regulation, *AWHONN Lifelines* 6(2):106-109, 2002.

Bruno JJ, Ellis JJ: Herbal use among U.S. elderly: 2002 National Health Interview Survey, *Ann Pharmacother* 39:643-648, 2005.

Burks K: Osteoarthritis in older adults: current treatments, *J Gerontol Nurs* 31(5):11-19, 2005.

Canter PH, Ernst E: Herbal supplement use by persons aged over 50 years in Britain: frequently used herbs, concomitant use of herbs, nutritional supplements and prescription drugs, rate of informing doctors and potential for negative interactions, *Drugs Aging* 21(9):597-605, 2005.

Clegg DO et al: Glucosamine, chondroitin sulfate, and the two in combination for painful knee osteoarthritis, *N Engl J Med* 354:795-808, 2006.

Curry LC et al: Teaching older adults to self-manage medications: preventing adverse drug reactions, *J Gerontol Nurs* 31(4):32-42, 2005.

Dahl NV: Herbs and supplements in dialysis: panacea or poison? *Semin Dial* 14(3):186-192, 2001.

Durante KM et al: Use of vitamins, minerals and herbs: a survey of patients attending family practice clinics, *Clin Invest Med* 24(5):242-249, 2001.

Edwards Q et al: What's cooking with garlic: is this complementary and alterative medicine for hypertension? *J Am Acad Nurse Pract* 17(9):381-385, 2005.

Eliopoulos C: *Integrating conventional and alternative therapies: holistic care for chronic conditions*, St Louis, 1999, Mosby.

Eller L et al: Self-care strategies for depressive symptoms in people with HIV disease, *J Adv Nurs* 51(2):119-130, 2005.

Ernst E: The risk-benefit profile of commonly used herbal therapies: ginkgo, St. John's wort, ginseng, echinacea, saw palmetto, and kava, *Ann Intern Med* 136:42-53, 2002.

Eskin SB: Dietary supplements and older consumers, *Data Digest* 66:1-8, AARP Public Policy Institute, Washington, DC, 2001.

Garlic: Allicin wonderland? *University of California, Berkley Wellness Letter* 23(1):1-2, 2006.

Gorski J et al: The effect of echinacea (*Echinacea purpurea* root) on cytochrome P450 activity in vivo, *Clin Pharmacol Ther* 75(10):89-100, 2004.

Hann D et al: Use of complementary therapies during chemotherapy: influence of patients' satisfaction with treatment decision making and the treating oncologist, *Integ Cancer Ther* 5(3):224-231, 2006.

Hong B et al: A double-blind crossover study evaluating the efficacy of Korean red ginseng in patients with erectile dysfunction: a preliminary report, *J Urol* 168:2070-2073, 2002.

Israel D, Youngkin E: Herbal therapies for common health problems. In Youngkin E et al: *Pharmacotherapeutics: a primary care guide*, ed 2, Upper Saddle River, NJ, 2005, Pearson Prentice Hall.

Jellin J: *Natural database eUPDATE and eCE*, Natural Medicines Comprehensive Database, 2006a. (website): *www.naturaldatabase.com/*. Accessed November 15, 2006.

Jellin J: *Natural medicines in the clinical management of cold and flu*, Natural Medicines Comprehensive Database, 2006b. Received 10/21/06 from Natural Database eUPDATE and eCE (Florida Atlantic University Libraries Database).

Jellin JM et al: Natural Medicines Comprehensive Database, 2006 (website): *www.naturaldatabase.com/*. Accessed November 15, 2006.

Kales HC et al: Herbal products and other supplements: use by elderly veterans with depression and dementia and their caregivers, *J Geriatr Psychiatry Neurol* 17(1):25-31, 2004.

Keller KB, Lemberg L: Herbal or complementary medicine: fact or fiction, *Am J Crit Care* 10(6):438, 2001.

Kerr M: *Echinacea cuts cold incidence*, Reuters Health Information, 2006. (website): *www.medscape.com/viewarticle/544846*. Accessed October 3, 2006.

Kuhn M: Herbal remedies: drug-herb interactions, *Crit Care Nurse* 22(2):22, 2002.

Kuriyama S et al: Green tea consumption and mortality due to cardiovascular disease, cancer, and all causes in Japan: the Ohsaki study, *JAMA* 296(10):1255-1265, 2006.

Lam A, Bradley G: Use of self-prescribed nonprescription medications and dietary supplements among assisted living facility residents, *J Am Pharm Assoc* 46(5):547-581, 2006.

Lawvere S, Mahoney MC: St. John's wort, *Am Fam Physician* 72:2249-2254, 2005.

Libster M: *Delmar's integrative herb guide for nurses*, Albany, NY, 2002, Delmar Thompson.

Liu J et al: Herbal medicines for treatment of irritable bowel syndrome, 2006. *Cochrane Database Syst Rev*, Jan 25 (1): CD004116.

Messina BA: Herbal supplements: facts and myths—talking to your patients about herbal supplements, *J Perianesth Nurs* 21(4):268-278, 2006.

Neff G et al: Consumption of dietary supplements in a liver transplant population, *Liver Transpl* 10(7):240-241, 2004.

O'Hara EM, Zhan L: Cultural and pharmacologic considerations when caring for Chinese elders, *J Gerontol Nurs* 20(10):11, 1994.

Radimer K et al: Dietary supplement use by U.S. adults. Data from the National Health and Nutrition Examination Survey, 1999-2000, *Am J Epidemiol* 160(4):339-349, 2004.

Scorza E: *Use of herbal and nutritional supplements*. Paper presented at National Conference of Gerontological Nurse Practitioners, Chicago, 2002.

Sego S: Alternative meds update: St. John's wort, *Clin Advisor* July:134,137, 2006.

Shahrokh LE et al: Elderly herbal supplement users less satisfied with medical care than nonusers, *J Am Diet Assoc* 105(7):1138-1140, 2005.

Skidmore-Roth L: *Mosby's handbook of herbs and natural supplements*, St Louis, 2005, Mosby.

Spector RE: *Cultural diversity in health & illness*, ed 5, Upper Saddle River, NJ, 2000, Prentice Hall.

St. Hill PF et al: *Caring for women cross-culturally*, Philadelphia, 2003, Davis.

Stupay S, Sivertsen L: Herbal and nutritional supplement use in the elderly, *Nurse Pract* 25:56, 2000.

Sugimoto N et al: Herbal medicine use and quality of life among people living with HIV/AIDS in northeastern Thailand, *AIDS Care* 17(2):252-262, 2005.

Swanson B: Beware bitter orange, *ADVANCE for Nurses* (September 4):43, 2006.

Tillisch K: Complementary and alternative medicine for functional gastrointestinal disorders, *Gut* 55(5):593-596, 2006.

Tshibangu K et al: Assessment of effectiveness of traditional herbal medicine in managing HIV/AIDS patients in South Africa, *East Afr Med J* 81(10):499-504, 2004.

Waddell DL et al: Three herbs you should get to know, *Am J Nurs* 101(4):48, 2001.

Walker A et al: Hypotensive effects of hawthorn for patients with diabetes taking prescription drugs: a randomized controlled trial, *Br J Gen Pract* 56(527):437-444, 2006.

Weng YL et al: Herbal and vitamin/mineral supplement use by retirement community residents: preliminary findings, *J Nutr Elderly* 23(3):1-13, 2004.

Williams P et al: Cancer treatment, symptom monitoring, and self-care in adults: pilot study, *Cancer Nurs* 29(5):347-355, 2006.

Wu KM et al: Complexities of the herbal nomenclature system in traditional Chinese medicine (TCM): lessons learned from the misuse of Aristolochia-related species and the importance of the pharmaceutical name during botanical drug product development, *Phytomedicine* 14(4):273-279, 2007.

Yeh G et al: Use of complementary therapies in patients with cardiovascular disease, *Am J Cardiol* 98(5):673-680, 2006.

Yoon SL: Racial/ethnic differences in self-reported health problems and herbal use among older women, *J Natl Med Assoc* 98(6):918-925, 2006.

Yoon SL, Horne CH: Herbal products and conventional medicines used by community-residing older women, *J Adv Nurs* 33:51-59, 2001.

Yoon SL, Schaffer SD: Herbal, prescribed, and over-the-counter drug use in older women: prevalence of drug interactions, *Geriatr Nurs* 27(2):118-129, 2006.

Yoon SL et al: Herbal product use by African American older women, *Clin Nurs Res* 13(4):271-288, 2004.

Youngkin EQ, Israel DS: A review and critique of common herbal alternative therapies, *Nurse Pract* 21(10):39, 1996.

Zeilmann C et al: Use of herbal medicine by elderly Hispanic and non-Hispanic white patients, *Pharmacotherapy* 23(4):526-532, 2003.

CHAPTER 14

Sensory Function

Theris A. Touhy

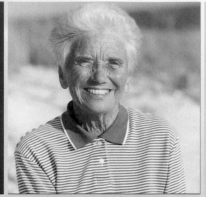
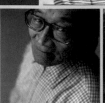
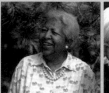

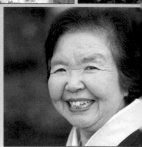

A STUDENT SPEAKS

During the years I worked as a food server I grew accustomed to waiting on older people. They can't always read the menu, they complain that the lighting in the restaurant is too low, they like their dinner experience to be slower, they can't find their silver when they need it, the soup is never hot enough and the cup of coffee is never full enough. They would yell at me because they could not hear me. It used to make me mad, but now I understand they are just real people experiencing growing old. Yes, they may have problems like losing some of their senses and other physical changes, but in actuality they are the same as me.

Debbie, age 27

AN ELDER SPEAKS

One of the great frustrations is the matter of eyesight. One can get used to large print and hope for black letters on white paper but why do modern publishers seem to prefer the shiny, slick off-white paper and pale ink in miniscule print? And, my new prescription glasses have not restored my ability to cut my own toenails without danger of wounding myself. I find myself wishing for some treatment for incipient cataracts. Please researchers, let's get rid of this scourge of the elderly.

Lyn, age 85

LEARNING OBJECTIVES

On completion of this chapter, the reader will be able to:

1. Identify several sensory changes accompanying aging that alter the perceived world of older adults.
2. Explain changes in the aging system that impair sensation.
3. Relate sensory changes to perceptual and environmental insecurity.
4. Describe several conditions that affect sensory function and awareness.
5. Discuss the appropriate use of various assistive devices that assist the older adult with sensory deficits.
6. Identify nursing responses that enhance sensory function and perceptual integration.
7. Develop a nursing care plan appropriate to the care of an elder experiencing a sensory deficit.

THE SENSORY APPARATUS

The common view is that sensory organs are our windows on the world. Less poetically, the senses are the primary interface with the environment. The senses seem to put boundaries and order into our lives, and when they are understimulated or overloaded, the structure weakens. We rely on our senses to perceive the environment and to enjoy the plea-

sures of life. Most sensory losses are irreversible but occur gradually so that function is maintained.

Appreciation of Sensory Changes

All senses gradually lose their acuity with age. Although normal changes of aging do not result in an abrupt awareness of sensory loss, the accumulated atrophy of sensory receptors in the eyes, ears, nose, buccal cavity, and peripheral afferent

Special thanks to Ann Schmidt Luggen, the previous edition contributor, for her content contributions to this chapter.

nerves substantially reduces the vividness of environmental impressions. Events no longer alert the nervous system with such clarity as in youth. When the senses are impaired, the sense of self is altered.

The issues of concern to nurses are assessing age-related sensory changes versus disease; devising methods to keep the senses functional enough to negotiate the environment safely and effectively; supplementing sensory loss with additional pleasures to the remaining senses; and providing touch, color, and variety. The sensory environment is to be revered and cultivated. Therein lie many problems. Old age subjects one to decreased appreciation of the environment through drugs, machines, treatments, paresthesias, presbyopia, presbycusis, agnosia, and other factors. Life may be more cautiously sampled. Stored experiences often come to the rescue, and older people remember things they can no longer perceive.

When describing the capacities and changes in the various sensory apparatus, we must understand that they all work in consensus. The senses are tightly interwoven in forming the perceptual base of our world. Possibly the "sixth sense" (intuition, or the power of perception that goes beyond that of the five senses) is really the consensus of all the senses in an acutely aware individual. In some cases, a disorder of one of the senses may stimulate the others in a compensatory manner. No one has studied this in older adults, but anecdotally some elders have experienced and described enhancement of the sense of hearing when sight was poor or vice versa.

Age-related declines are variable and cannot be generalized to all sensory systems or to all older individuals. Personal hardiness and an orderly, meaningful environment contribute in ways yet unidentified to good perceptual processing and high-level functioning. It is not uncommon that elders are thought to be cognitively impaired when, in fact, attention to enhanced sensory function through an adapted environment and appropriate assistive devices reveal much higher functional levels. General perceptual organization and efficiency are modified by health status, frailty of aging, illness, medications, fatigue, and stress and anxiety.

This chapter focuses on the normal age-related alterations and the most commonly experienced problems of the major sensory organs. How these affect the individual and his or her ability to successfully negotiate the environment is the nurse's concern. The task is to augment and maximize sensory experiences when senses are diminished and to help design a colorful, rewarding environment that fits the needs and abilities of the individual (Table 14-1).

TABLE 14-1
Age-Related Sensory Changes, Outcomes, and Health Promotion, Prevention, and Maintenance Approaches

Age-Related Sensory Changes	Outcomes	Health Promotion, Prevention, and Maintenance
VISION		
Lid elasticity diminishes	Pouches under the eyes	Use isotonic eye drops as needed
Loss of orbital fat	Excessive dryness of eyes	
Decreased tears		
Arcus senilis becomes visible		
Sclera yellows and becomes less elastic		
Yellowing and increased opacity of cornea	Lack of corneal luster	
Increased sclerosis and rigidity of the iris		
Decrease in convergency ability	Presbyopia	Have eyes examined at least once a year
Decline in light accommodation response	Lessened acuity	Use magnifying glass and high-intensity light to read
Diminished pupillary size	Decline in depth perception	Increase light to prevent falls
Atrophy of ciliary muscle	Diminished recovery from glare	Clip on sunglasses, visors, sun hat, nonglare coating on prescription glasses/sunglasses
Night vision diminishes	Night blindness	Do not drive at night; keep night-light in bathroom and hallway; paint first and last step of staircase and edge of each step between with a bright color
Yellowing of lens	Diminished color perception (blues and greens)	Use warm colors such as reds and oranges
Lens opacity	Cataracts	Surgical removal of lens
Increased intraocular pressure	Rainbows around lights	Have a yearly eye examination including tonometer testing
Shrinkage of gelatinous substance in the vitreous	Altered peripheral vision	

Continued

TABLE 14-1

Age-Related Sensory Changes, Outcomes, and Health Promotion, Prevention, and Maintenance Approaches—cont'd

Age-Related Sensory Changes	Outcomes	Health Promotion, Prevention, and Maintenance
VISION—cont'd		
Vitreous floaters appear		
Ability to gaze upward decreases		
Thinning and sclerosis of retinal blood vessels		
Atrophy of photoreceptor cells		
Degeneration of neurons in visual cortex		
HEARING		
Thinner, drier skin of external ear		
Longer and thicker hair in external ear canal		
Narrowing of auditory opening		
Increased cerumen		Check ears for wax or infection
Thickened and less resilient tympanic membrane		
Decreased flexibility of basilar membrane	Difficulty hearing high-frequency sounds (presbycusis)	Formal hearing test
Ossicular calcification		
Diminished neuron, endolymph, hair cells, and blood	Gradual loss of sound	Consultation for proper hearing and speaking tone–shouting distorted
Degeneration of spiral ganglion and arterial blood vessels		
Weakness and stiffness of muscles and ligaments		
SMELL		
Decreased olfactory cells	Decreased appetite; decreased protection from noxious odors and tainted food	Encourage social dining; be around cooking aromas
TASTE		
Possible decrease in size and number of taste buds	Lowered ability to distinguish between the four components of taste: sweet, sour, bitter, salty; poor nutrition, decreased appetite	Nutritional supplementation; use of stronger flavors, spices, and herbs
TOUCH		
Diminishes with age, especially with diseases such as diabetes	Injuries, pressure ulcers, touch deprivation, loss of thermal sensitivity	Tactile stimulation, teach injury prevention, monitor for injury and skin breakdown

Alteration in Sensory Experience

The normal gradual diminution of the senses during the aging process is usually well accommodated by experience. We are all subject to alterations in our sensory experience, and with increasing age it is likely that these circumstances will occur more frequently and perhaps be more devastating.

Alterations in sensory input may contribute to increased anxiety in older adults. When the senses are grossly underloaded or overloaded, perception and reactions are distorted. The world becomes an alien, confusing place. Fear and anxiety increase, or one withdraws into a fabricated world that provides security. Altered sensory experience will affect one's view of self and one's ability to relate to others (Figure 14-1). Isolation and loneliness may be the result. Emotional responses to altered sensory input include boredom, diminished concentration, incoherent thoughts, anxiety, fear, depression, lability of affect, delusions, and even hallucinations. Clear and sometimes repetitive data about the environment must be given when perceptions are impaired. Manipulating the environment to reduce demands and enhance sensory function should decrease these symptoms, although studies show that signs may persist for several days.

Significant research on elders' varied adaptations to sensory losses is limited. The assumption of increasing loss of

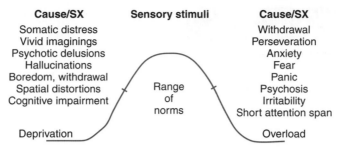

FIGURE 14-1 Reaction to sensory and environmental alterations. (Illustration by Joseph Pierre.)

acuity of all senses and the importance of well-designed and well-fitted assistive devices make up the bulk of attention given to the topic. Adequate input is essential to continued cognitive development.

Sensory Deprivation. There are at least three types of sensory deprivation: (1) reduced sensory capacities, (2) elimination of patterns and meaning from input, and (3) restrictive, monotonous environments. Prisoners, astronauts, and solitary explorers have made the public aware of the effects of isolation from ordinary environmental stimulation. Psychological and physiological effects of such situations have been reported through personal accounts and from studies of artificial situations constructed for the express purpose of studying sensory deprivation. None of the natural or laboratory experiences demonstrated the particular significance of age variables. It has been more or less assumed that older people who are isolated from adequate stimuli by failing sensory organs or reduced environmental variation react with the same symptoms as younger adults. Certain effects thought to be "confusion" or "old age" may arise from sensory deprivation. Box 14-1 summarizes some effects of sensory deprivation. Any situation lacking varied environmental stimuli deprives the senses of adequate material for perceptual integrity.

Common contributors to sensory deprivation in older people are altered sensory capacities and restrictive environments. Problems such as poor vision, decreased energy, poor hearing, extended periods in a supine position, debilitating illness and chronic disorders, few pleasant sounds, and limited meaningful contact with others often result in *disorientation*. Late afternoon may aggravate the deprivation if daylight is diminished and indoor lighting is inadequate. Simple nursing responses can enhance the environment. Open drapes and open the window a crack; sights, sounds, and smells of outdoors and life can be enjoyable and reassuring. Encourage sitting outside enjoying nature. Turn on lights; raise the head of the bed or assist the person to a chair bolstered comfortably with pillows; bring a flower to the room; sit down; speak, touch, and listen to the person's feelings. Discuss the person's interests; radio, television, computers, books, puzzles, and handicrafts may all amuse the solitary person. It is essential to plan with them, not for them.

When the ambiance is one of monotony, even a small stimulus may trigger a strong response. Knowing this makes

---

BOX 14-1 Effects of Sensory Deprivation

- Sensory deprivation tends to amplify existing personality traits.
- Perceptual disorganization occurs in visual/motor coordination, color perception, apparent movement, tactile accuracy, ability to perceive size and shape, and spatial and time judgment.
- Sensory deprivation alters mechanisms of attention, consciousness, and reality testing (similar to brain anoxia).
- Marked behavior changes, such as an inability to think and solve problems, affectual disturbance, perceptual distortions, hallucinations and delusions, vivid imagination, poor task performance, increased anxiety and aggression, somatic complaints, temporal and spatial disorientation, emotional lability, and confusion of sleep and waking states.
- Monotony disrupts the capacity to learn and the ability to think.
- In the absence of varied stimulation, brain function lessens.
- Illness often increases perceptual confusion, particularly in older adults.

---

it easier to understand the overreactions displayed when a routine is interrupted. One lady became extremely upset when a large sign was hung above her bed; another refused to return to her room after it had been rearranged. People are more sensitive to changes of any sort when changes are so few and they feel deprived of control. Gradual environmental enrichment evokes a good response. Rapid increases and overstimulation may produce anxiety, fear, and confusion. The benefits of orderly, gradual environmental enrichment geared to individual personality and interests are yet to be thoroughly studied.

Sensory Overload. Neuroexcitability and secretion of stimulating neurotransmitters decrease as one ages. Overarousal is usually from abrupt, unexpected environmental change such as accident or hospitalization. These are situations of sensory overload precipitated by actual or perceived environmental demands. Sensory overload is a contributing factor to the development of delirium in older adults who are hospitalized. An individual with marginal adaptation and

BOX 14-2   *Healthy People 2010* Goals and Objectives: Vision and Hearing

GOAL: Improve the visual and hearing health of the Nation through prevention, early detection, treatment, and rehabilitation
- Increase the number of persons who have dilated eye examinations at appropriate intervals
- Reduce visual impairment due to diabetic retinopathy, glaucoma, and cataracts
- Increase vision rehabilitation
- Increase the number of persons who have had a hearing examination on schedule
- Increase the number of persons who are referred by their primary care physician for hearing evaluation and treatment
- Increase the use of appropriate ear protection devices, equipment, and practices
- Increase access by hearing-impaired persons to hearing rehabilitation services and adaptive devices, including hearing aids, cochlear implants, or tactile or other assistive or augmentative devices

cognitive decrements is particularly vulnerable. Sensory overload is a highly individual matter, often related to cognitive capacity. It can be recognized by certain symptoms: thoughts may race, and attention scatters in many directions. People find it difficult to sit still. Aberrant thoughts or actions may occur. Evidences of anxiety are present.

The amount of stimuli necessary for healthy function varies with each individual; relevance and familiarity of stimuli may be more important than amount. Biorhythms are another important consideration. Individuals may be more subject to environmental overload at one time than another. Sensations are generally most acute in the late afternoon when cortisol levels are highest, although effects on the older person have not been established. Sensory overload cannot always be avoided, but when one is extremely stressed and bombarded with adaptive demands, time must be arranged for peacefulness and frequent rest periods. It is often helpful to sit quietly with the person, saying very little, or to engage him or her in a nondemanding repetitive activity that will help focus attention on something that provides security and reduces stress. Walking can be beneficial. Careful assessment of behavior is important to determine both the internal and external precipitants for changes.

Healthy People 2010 contains goals and objectives that relate to sensory problems of older adults (*Healthy People 2010*, 2002). Box 14-2 presents some of these objectives.

VISION AND VISION IMPAIRMENT

According to the Centers for Disease Control and Prevention (CDC) (2002), 1.8 million community-dwelling elders report difficulty with activities of daily living because of visual impairment. *Visual impairment* is considered vision loss that cannot be corrected by glasses or contact lenses. Snellen wall chart readings of 20/40 or worse with corrective lenses is considered visual impairment. Snellen chart readings of 20/200 or more are considered legal blindness or severe visual impairment. About 2.7 million elderly adults have severe visual impairment. About 27% of elderly men 85 years of age and older are visually impaired. Women are more visually impaired than men; 33% of women 85 years of age and older report visual impairment compared with 27% of men over 85 years of age. African-Americans are twice as likely to be visually impaired as whites of comparable socioeconomic status. Hispanics, who have three times the risk of developing type 2 diabetes as whites, have a higher risk of visual complications (*Healthy People 2010*, 2002). Blindness increases with age. It peaks at about 85 years and occurs in 2.4% of the population (CDC, 2002). Visual impairment and blindness are caused by cataracts, age-related macular degeneration, glaucoma, and diabetic retinopathy. Age-related changes in the eye are described in Chapter 4.

Presbyopia

The condition of vision in which the normally flexible lens of the eye gradually loses elasticity, affecting the refractive ability of the eye, is *presbyopia* (see Chapter 4). It affects the ability of the eyes to accommodate to close and detailed work. Usually, it is noticed when one has difficulty reading close up and begins holding reading materials farther away. Presbyopia begins in the fourth decade and continues throughout the rest of one's life. It affects everyone, and there is no known prevention. Nearly everyone between the ages of 40 and 45 years requires glasses for close vision. For most individuals, the reading lens must be increased in strength every 2 or 3 years after age 45 years. Presbyopia occurs earlier in individuals who live in warm climates where there is much sun exposure and later in individuals who are nearsighted (myopia).

For those who are "farsighted" (hyperopic), the presbyopia tends to occur earlier than for the "nearsighted" (myopic—a condition that occurs early in life). As lens opacity increases, some refractive power increases at the same time that accommodation, or lens resilience, decreases. The result is a temporary shift toward myopia and improved close vision. Thus some individuals at 60 or 70 years of age develop better vision in that they can again read without glasses, which they may have used since childhood.

Dry Eye

Tear production normally diminishes as we age. The condition is termed *keratoconjunctivitis sicca*. It occurs most commonly in women after menopause. There may be age-related changes in the mucin-secreting cells necessary for surface wetting, in the lacrimal glands, or in the meibomian glands that secrete surface oil, and all of these may occur at the same time (Beers and Berkow, 2000). The older person will describe a dry, scratchy feeling in mild cases (xerophthalmia). Marked discomfort and decreased mucus production may be present in severe situations.

Medications can cause dry eye, especially antihistamines, diuretics, beta-blockers, and some sleeping pills. The problem is diagnosed by an ophthalmologist using a Schirmer tear test in which filter paper strips are placed under the lower eyelid to measure the rate of tear production. A common treatment is artificial tears, but dry eyes may be sensitive to them because of preservatives, which can be irritating. The ophthalmologist may close the tear duct channel either temporarily or permanently. Other management methods include keeping the house air moist with humidifiers, avoiding wind and hair dryers, and using artificial tear ointments at bedtime. Vitamin A deficiency can be a cause of dry eye, and vitamin A ointments are available for treatment. Sjögren's syndrome is a cell-mediated autoimmune disease in which decreased lacrimal gland activity is part of the syndrome and can occur in elderly people. Systemic manifestations that occur in the autoimmune disease include Raynaud's phenomenon, polyarthritis, interstitial pneumonitis, vasculitis, psychiatric manifestations, and loss of exocrine functions (Beers and Berkow, 2000).

Diseases Affecting Vision

For elders with visual impairments, the consequences for functional ability, safety, and quality of life can be profound. The major diseases affecting vision are glaucoma, cataracts, macular degeneration, and diabetic retinopathy. With appropriate eye care, these diseases are readily diagnosed, but many older people, particularly ethnically and culturally diverse elders, do not receive necessary care. It is estimated that 40% of blindness and visual impairment is treatable or preventable. The problem of undiagnosed visual disorders is increasing, and the number of blind and visually impaired elders is expected to double in the next three decades (Rowe et al., 2004). Impaired vision is a serious condition among nursing home residents, with estimates of impairment ranging from 21% to 52%. Women completely lose vision more frequently than men, and in both genders it is common to have better vision in one eye than in the other. The following section discusses the major causes of vision impairment in older adults.

Glaucoma. Glaucoma is a major public health problem in the United States. It affects an estimated 3 million Americans, with 120,000 who are blind because of this condition. Even if people with glaucoma do not become blind, their vision can be severely impaired. Glaucoma is a chronic progressive disease involving increased intraocular pressure, usually bilaterally, that can lead to permanent damage of the optic nerve. There are several types of glaucoma: primary open-angle glaucoma (more than two thirds of cases); normal-pressure glaucoma; and *acute angle-closure glaucoma, which is an emergency*. An acute attack of angle-closure glaucoma is characterized by a rapid rise in intraocular pressure (IOP) accompanied by redness and pain in and around the eye, severe headache, nausea and vomiting, and blurring of vision. It occurs when the path of the aqueous humor is blocked and intraocular pressure builds to greater than 50 mm Hg. If untreated, blindness can occur in 2 days. An iridectomy, however, can ease pressure.

Primary open-angle glaucoma accounts for 80% to 90% of glaucoma cases. It is asymptomatic until very late in the disease, when there is a noticeable loss of peripheral vision, causing tunnel vision (Cotter and Strumpf, 2002; O'Neil, 2002). Glaucoma has been described as the "silent thief" because it will steal vision without warning (Higginbotham et al., 2004). However, if detected early, glaucoma can usually be controlled and serious vision loss prevented.

Although the etiology of glaucoma is variable and often unknown, the problem occurs when the natural fluids of the eye are blocked by ciliary muscle rigidity or an overproduction of aqueous humor and the buildup of pressure, which damages the optic nerve (Figure 14-2). Age is the single most important predictor of glaucoma, and older women are affected twice as often as older men. A family history of glaucoma, diabetes, and past eye injuries have been noted as risk factors for the development of glaucoma. Glaucoma accounts for 19% of all blindness among African-Americans compared with 6% of whites (Higginbotham et al., 2004). African-Americans develop glaucoma at younger ages and have almost three times the age-adjusted prevalence of glaucoma than whites. Factors contributing to the increased prevalence of glaucoma in African-Americans include an increased incidence of diabetes, later detection of the disease, and economic and social barriers to treatment (Boyd-Monk, 2005). Mexican-Americans and persons of Asian descent also are at higher risk (National Eye Institute, 2004). Many drugs with anticholinergic properties or those that cause papillary dilation, including antihistamines, stimulants, vasodilators, clonidine, and sympathomimetics, are particularly dangerous for patients predisposed to angle-closure glaucoma (Table 14-2).

Management of glaucoma involves medications (oral medications or topical eye drops) to decrease IOP and/or laser surgery. Medications lower eye pressure either by decreasing the amount of aqueous fluid produced within the eye or by improving the flow through the drainage angle. Beta-blockers are the first-line therapy for glaucoma, and the patient may need combinations of several types of eye drops. Usually medications can control glaucoma, but laser surgery treatments (trabeculoplasty) may be recommended for some types of glaucoma. Surgery is usually recommended only if necessary to prevent further damage to the optic nerve. Statins and other cholesterol-lowering medications may be associated with a reduced risk of glaucoma, particularly among those with cardiovascular and lipid diseases (McGwin et al., 2004). Further research is warranted.

Screening. It is recommended that adults older than 65 years be evaluated annually and those with medication-controlled glaucoma be examined at least every 6 months. Annual screening is also recommended for African-

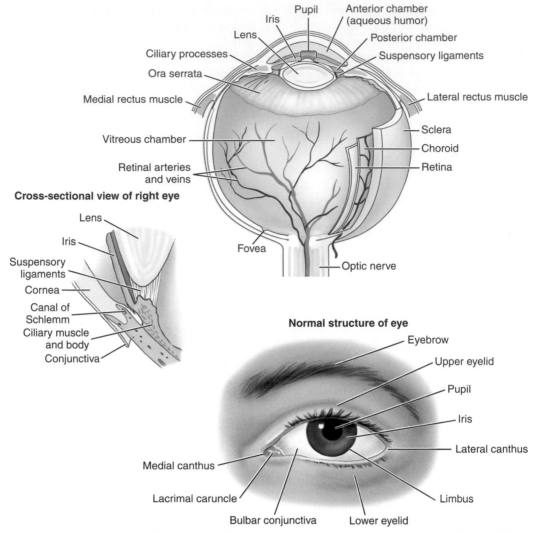

Cross-sectional view of right eye

Normal structure of eye

FIGURE 14-2 Cross-sectional view of right eye. (From Drain CB: *Perianesthesia nursing: a critical care approach,* ed 4, St Louis, 2003, Saunders; and from *Mosby's medical, nursing, and allied health dictionary,* ed 2, St Louis, 1986, Mosby.)

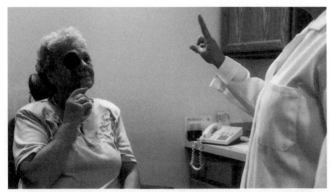

Client counting fingers during determination of visual acuity. (From Ignatavicius DD, Workman ML: *Medical-surgical nursing: critical thinking for collaborative care,* ed 5, St Louis, 2006, Saunders.)

Americans and other individuals with a family history of glaucoma who are older than 40 years. A dilated eye examination and tonometry are necessary to diagnose glaucoma. These procedures can be performed by a primary care provider, optometrist, or nurse practitioner, who will then refer the person to an ophthalmologist if glaucoma is suspected. Medicare began paying for annual screening in January 2002 but only in high-risk patients. Normal IOP is between 11 and 20 mm Hg. Glaucoma is present when the pressure is greater than 20 mm Hg; there is nerve head atrophy, optic cupping, and loss of peripheral visual fields in all types of glaucoma (Reuben et al., 2002). No symptoms are present in the early stages, and about 20% of loss of visual fields is found in elders *at diagnosis* (Luggen, 2001). Many elders have undiagnosed glaucoma that has not been screened or evaluated. Figure 14-3 simulates vision loss from glaucoma.

Cataracts. Cataracts are a prevalent disorder among older adults caused by oxidative damage to lens protein and fatty deposits (lipofuscin) in the ocular lens. By age 80 years, more than half of all Americans either have a cataract or have had cataract surgery. When lens opacity reduces visual acuity to 20/30 or less in the central axis of vision, it is considered a cataract. Cataracts are categorized according to their location within the lens and are usually bilateral. They are virtually universal in the very old but may be only minimally

TABLE 14-2

Drugs That Are Contraindicated or Must Be Used with Caution in the Presence of Glaucoma or Prodromal Signs of Glaucoma

Generic Name	Trade Name*	Generic Name	Trade Name*
Albuterol	Proventil Ventolin	Lorazepam	Ativan
Aminophylline or theophylline with ethylenediamine	Aminophyllin Corophyllin	Loxapine succinate	Daxolin Loxitane
Amitriptyline hydrochloride*	Amitril Elavil	Mesoridazine	Serentil
		Methamphetamine hydrochloride	Desoxyn
Amyl nitrate*		Nitroglycerin	Nitrostat
Atropine*		Nortriptyline hydrochloride*	Pamelor
Carbamazepine	Tegretol	Orphenadrine citrate	Norflex
Chlorpheniramine maleate	Chlor-Trimeton preparations	Papaverine	Pavabid
Chlorphenoxamine hydrochloride	Phenoxene	Pentaerythritol tetranitrate	Peritrate
Chlorpromazine*	Thorazine	Perphenazine	Etrafon Trilafon
Chlorprothixene	Taractan	Phenylephrine hydrochloride	Neo-Synephrine Tear-Efrin
Clemastine fumarate	Tavist		
Clonazepam	Klonopin	Prochlorperazine	Compazine Stemetil
Clorazepate dipotassium	Tranxene		
Cyclobenzaprine hydrochloride	Flexeril	Promethazine hydrochloride*	Phenergan
Cyproheptadine hydrochloride	Periactin	Protriptyline hydrochloride	Vivactil
Desipramine hydrochloride*	Norpramin Pertofrane	Pseudoephedrine hydrochloride*	Actifed Sudafed
Diazepam*	Valium	Succinylcholine chloride	Anectine
Dimenhydrinate	Dramamine	Tetrahydrozoline hydrochloride	Murine Visine
Diphenhydramine hydrochloride*	Benadryl		
Doxepin hydrochloride*	Adapin Sinequan	Theophylline*	Theo-Dur Uniphyl
Epinephrine	Bronkaid mist Primatene mist	Thioridazine hydrochloride	Mellaril
		Thiothixene hydrochloride	Navane
Fluphenazine hydrochloride*	Prolixin	Trifluoperazine hydrochloride	Stelazine
Glutethimide	Doriden	Trihexyphenidyl*	Artane
Glycopyrrolate*	Robinul	Trimeprazine tartrate	Panectyl
Haloperidol*	Haldol	Tripelennamine hydrochloride	Pyribenzamine
Hydrocodone bitartrate	Hycodan	Tropicamide	Mydriacyl
Hydroxyzine	Atarax	Zinc sulfate	Op-Thal-Zin
Imipramine hydrochloride*	Impril Tofranil		
Isopropamide iodide	Darbid		
Isosorbide dinitrate	Isordil		
Levodopa*	Bendopa Dopar Levopa		

*Multiple trade names not listed.

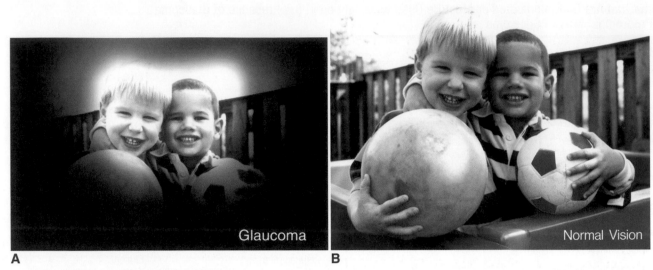

FIGURE 14-3 **A,** Simulated vision with glaucoma **B,** Normal vision. (From National Eye Institute, National Institutes of Health, 2004.)

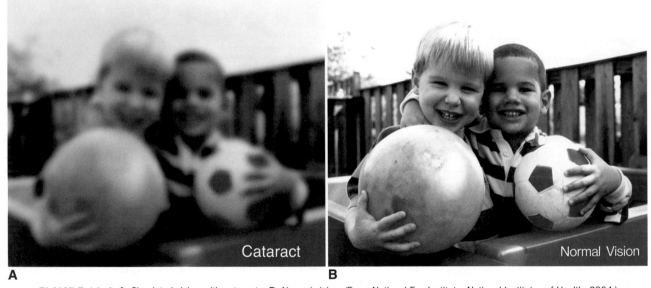

A   B

FIGURE 14-4 **A,** Simulated vision with cataracts. **B,** Normal vision. (From National Eye Institute, National Institutes of Health, 2004.)

visible, particularly in individuals with pale irises. Cataracts are recognized by the clouding of the ordinarily clear ocular lens; the red reflex may be absent or may appear as a black area. The cardinal sign of cataracts is the appearance of halos around objects as light is diffused. Other common symptoms include blurring, decreased perception of light and color (a yellow tint to most things), and sensitivity to glare (Figure 14-4 simulates vision loss from cataracts).

The most common causes of cataracts are hereditary and advancing age. They may occur more frequently and at earlier ages in individuals who have been exposed to excessive sunlight or who have poor dietary habits, diabetes, hypertension, kidney disease, eye trauma, or history of alcohol intake and tobacco use.

Cataract surgery is considered whenever the visual disturbance becomes an impediment in the individual's daily life and is the most common surgery performed in the United

States (Ham et al., 2002). Usually cataract surgery involves only local anesthesia and is one of the most successful surgical procedures, with 95% of patients reporting excellent vision after surgery (Tumosa, 2001). The surgery involves removal of the lens and placement of a plastic intraocular lens (IOL). If the plastic lens is not inserted, the patient may wear a contact lens or glasses. This is not commonly done because the older adult may have difficulty placing and removing the contact lens, and the glasses would be very thick.

Unfortunately, cataracts and other related eye diseases such as maculopathy, diabetic retinopathy, or glaucoma often occur simultaneously, which complicates the management of each. Individuals who have had cataract surgery are less likely to be surgically treated effectively for glaucoma. The nursing role is to prepare the individual for significant changes in vision and adaptation to light and to be sure the individual has received adequate counseling regarding realistic postsurgical expectations. Postsurgical teaching includes avoidance of heavy lifting, straining, or bending at the waist. Eye drops may be prescribed to aid healing and prevent infection. If the person has bilateral cataracts, surgery is performed on one eye with the second surgery a month or so later to ensure healing (Tabloski, 2006).

Diabetic Retinopathy. Some visual disabilities are acquired through the deleterious effects of elevated blood sugar caused by diabetes, which creates microaneurysms in retinal capillaries that cause impairment of oxygen and nutrients to the eye. These are the source of diabetic retinopathy. Because of vascular and cellular changes accompanying diabetes, other pathological vision conditions worsen rapidly as well. Diabetic retinopathy is the third leading cause of blindness in the United States, and the incidence curves upward abruptly with increased age (Tumosa, 2001). In the United States, approximately 4.1 million adults 40 years of age and older have diabetic retinopathy; 1 of every 12 persons with diabetes in this age-group has advanced, vision-threatening retinopathy (National Eye Institute, 2004). Most diabetic patients will develop diabetic retinopathy within 20 years of diagnosis.

There is little to no evidence of retinopathy until 3 to 5 years or more after the onset of diabetes. Early signs are seen in the funduscopic examination and include microaneurysms, flame-shaped hemorrhages, cotton wool spots, hard exudates, and dilated capillaries (Tumosa, 2001). Constant, strict control of blood glucose, cholesterol, and blood pressure and laser photocoagulation treatments can halt progression of the disease (Ham et al., 2002). Laser treatment can reduce vision loss in 50% of patients. Annual dilated funduscopic examination of the eye is recommended beginning 5 years after diagnosis of type I diabetes and at the time of diagnosis of type 2 diabetes.

Macular Degeneration. Age-related macular degeneration (AMD) is the leading cause of vision loss and blindness in Americans 65 years of age and older. The prevalence of AMD increases drastically with age, with more than 15% of Caucasian women older than 80 years having the disease. AMD is far more prevalent among whites than among black persons. With the projected increases in the number of older adults over the next 20 years, AMD has been called a growing epidemic (Bressler et al., 2004).

AMD is a degenerative eye disease that affects the macula—the central part of the eye responsible for clear central vision. The disease causes the progressive loss of central vision, leaving only peripheral vision intact. It usually starts in one eye, but there is a high risk (>40%) that the disease will affect the other eye within 5 years (Bressler et al., 2003). AMD results from systemic changes in circulation, accumulation of cellular waste products, tissue atrophy, and growth of abnormal blood vessels in the choroid layer beneath the retina. Fibrous scarring disrupts nourishment of photoreceptor cells, causing their death and loss of central vision. Although etiology is unknown, risk factors are

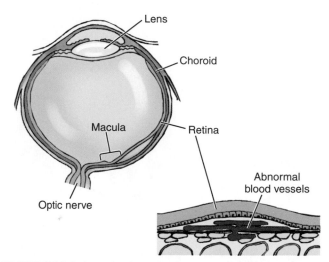

FIGURE 14-5 Age-related macular degeneration (AMD) results if abnormal blood vessels grow in the choroid layer beneath the retina or if any part of the retina fails to receive proper nutrients. (From Macular degeneration, *Mayo Clinic Health Letter* 8[9]:5, 1990.)

thought to include genetic predisposition, smoking, and excessive sunlight exposure.

The two forms of macular degeneration are the "dry" form and the "wet" form. Dry AMD accounts for the majority of cases, rarely causes severe visual impairment, but can lead to the more aggressive wet AMD (Figure 14-5). With wet AMD, the severe loss of central vision can be rapid and many people will be legally blind within 2 years of diagnosis. Peripheral vision usually remains normal, but the person will have difficulty seeing at a distance or doing detailed work such as sewing or reading. Faces may begin to blur, and it becomes harder to distinguish colors. Figure 14-6 simulates vision loss from AMD. An early sign may be distortion that causes edges or lines to appear wavy. An Amsler grid is used to determine clarity of central vision (Figure 14-7). A perception of wavy lines is diagnostic of beginning macular degeneration, and vision loss can occur in days. In the advanced forms, the person may begin to see dark or empty spaces that block the center of vision.

Patients in the early stage of the disease may attribute the vision problems to normal aging or cataracts. Early diagnosis is the key, and individuals older than 50 years should have an eye examination at least every 2 years. The Age-Related Eye Disease Study (AREDS) found that a combination of antioxidants and zinc can reduce the risk of developing AMD (Sackett and Bressler, 2001). Treatment of wet AMD includes photodynamic therapy (PDT) and laser photocoagulation (LPC). Lucentis and Avastin (anti-VEGF therapy) are biological drugs that stop the growth of abnormal blood vessels and have been shown to preserve or restore sight in newly diagnosed patients. These drugs are injected into the eye as often as once a month. For more information, see the National Eye Institute website (*www.nei.nih.gov*).

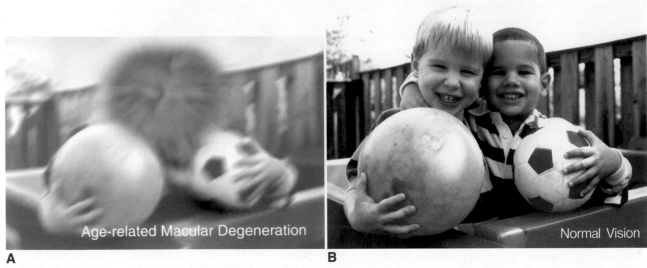

FIGURE 14-6 **A,** Simulated loss of vision with age-related macular degeneration (AMD). **B,** Normal vision. (From National Eye Institute, National Institutes of Health, 2004.)

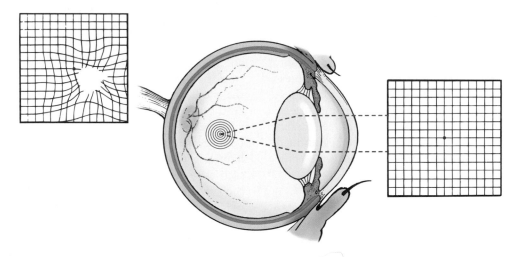

FIGURE 14-7 Macular degeneration: distortion of center vision; normal peripheral vision. (Illustration by Harriet R. Greenfield, Newton, Mass.)

▲ Promoting Healthy Aging: Implications for Gerontological Nursing

Assessment of Vision. The Snellen chart is commonly used by nurses to test for distance vision. Testing the older person should be done in good light and with the bulb shielded to prevent glare. If the 20/40 line on the chart cannot be read, looking through a pinhole in a piece of cardboard should improve vision. If it does improve, that is indication for a change in eyeglass prescription. Gross visual field deficits, or confrontation, can be determined by displaying a wide arc with outstretched arm and noting when the individual no longer detects the moving finger of the nurse's

arm. These are superficial assessments and are not meant to replace more thorough examination by an ophthalmologist. Near vision can be evaluated using a book or newspaper or a Rosenbaum chart about 12 to 14 inches away and asking the elder to read several lines. This is an excellent way to assess the need for change of glasses and a more sophisticated evaluation.

Color vision is evaluated using an Ishihara chart, which is a plate with multiple colors in the background. Results are determined by the number of plates identified correctly. This examination is sensitive for red/green blindness but not for blue, which is more common in older adults. This examina-

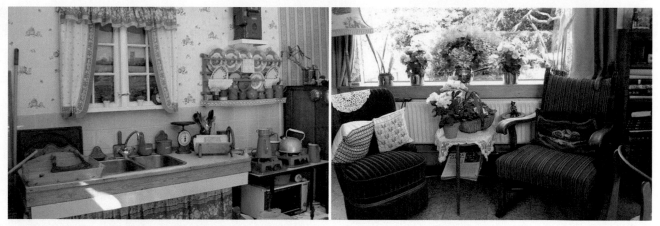

FIGURE 14-8 Sitting room. Højdevang Sogns Plejecenter, Copenhagen Denmark. Reminiscence Kitchen, Activity Room, Højdevang Sogns Plejecenter, Copenhagen, Denmark. (Photos courtesy Christine Williams, PhD, RN.)

BOX 14-3   Signs and Behaviors That May Indicate Vision Problems

INDIVIDUAL MAY REPORT

Pain in eyes
Difficulty seeing in darkened area
Double vision/distorted vision
Migraine headaches coupled with blurred vision
Flashes of light
Halos surrounding lights
Difficulty driving at night
Falls or injuries

HEALTH CARE STAFF MAY NOTICE

Getting lost
Bumping into objects
Straining to read or no reading
Stumbling/falling
Spilling food on clothing
Social withdrawal
Less eye contact
Placid facial expression
TV viewing at close range
Decreased sense of balance
Mismatched clothes

Modified from McNeely E et al: Teaching caregivers to recognize diminished vision among nursing home residents, *Geriatr Nurs* 13(6):332-335, 1992.

---

tion is used when taking a driver's license test to determine if the older adult is able to discriminate red from green.

Observation of the retina and optic nerve disc via funduscopy reveals important systemic, circulatory, and vision information, but pupillary constriction and clouding of the vitreous and lens often hamper the eyeground ophthalmological examination of an older person. One must be cautious because pupil dilation with a mydriatic for the purposes of examination may precipitate an acute attack for those predisposed to angle-closure glaucoma.

Because visual impairment affects most daily activities, such as driving, reading, maneuvering safely, dressing, cooking, and social activities, assessing the effect of vision changes on functional abilities, safety, and quality of life is most important. Decreased vision has also been found to be a significant risk factor for falls. Certain signs and behaviors of visual problems that should alert the nurse to action are noted in Box 14-3.

General principles in caring for the elder with visual impairment include the following: use warm incandescent lighting; increase intensity of lighting; control glare by using shades and blinds; suggest yellow or amber lenses to decrease glare; suggest sunglasses that block all ultraviolet light; select colors with good contrast and intensity; and recommend reading materials that have large, dark, evenly spaced printing.

Interventions to Enhance Vision

Use of Contrasting Colors. Color contrasts are used to facilitate location of items. Sharply contrasting colors assist the partially sighted. For instance, a bright towel is much easier to locate than a white towel hanging on a beige wall. When choosing color, use warm and intense colors such as reds and oranges rather than blues and beiges. Figure 14-8 illustrates the use of color in a nursing home. Most visually impaired people have enough residual vision to use their eyesight with proper aids or training to read, write, and move around safely. Unfortunately, many older persons with serious visual impairments consider themselves blind and are usually treated as if they are. Adequate training in using residual vision can prevent partially sighted older persons from falling into unnecessarily dependent lifestyles. Box 14-4 provides further suggestions for communicating and caring for the visually impaired elder.

Low-Vision Assistive Devices. Technology advances in the past decade have produced some low-vision devices that may be used successfully in the care of the visually impaired elder. People with severe visual impairment may qualify for disability and financial and social services assistance through government and private programs including vision rehabilitation programs. An array of low-vision assistive devices are now available, including insulin delivery systems and glucose-monitoring equipment, talking clocks

---

BOX 14-4 Suggestions for Communicating with and Caring for Visually Impaired Elders

- Remember, there are many degrees of blindness; allow as much independence as possible.
- Assess your position in relation to the individual. One eye or ear may be better than the other.
- When in the presence of a blind person, speak promptly and clearly identify yourself and others with you. State when you are leaving to make sure the person is aware of your departure.
- Make sure you have the individual's attention before you start talking.
- Speak descriptively of your surroundings to familiarize the blind person, and state the position of the people who are in the room.
- Speak normally but not from a distance; do not raise or lower your voice, and continue to use gestures if that is natural to your communication. Do not alter your vocabulary; words such as *see* and *blind* are part of normal speech. When others are present, address the blind person by prefacing remarks with his or her name or a light touch on the arm.
- Try to minimize the number of distractions.
- Use the analogy of a clock face to help locate objects. Describe positions of food on the plate in relation to clock positions (e.g., 3 o'clock, 6 o'clock).

- Check to see that the best possible lighting is available.
- Try to keep the individual between you and the window; you will appear as a dark shadow.
- Whenever possible, choose bright clothing with bold contrasts.
- Do not change the room arrangement or arrangement of personal items without explanation.
- Speak before handing a blind person an object.
- Keep color and texture in mind when buying clothes.
- When walking with a blind person, offer your arm. Pause before stairs or curbs; mention them. In seating, place the person's hand on the back of the chair. Let him or her know the position in relation to objects.
- Blind people like to know the beauty that surrounds them. Describe flowers, scenery, colors, and textures. People who have been blind since birth cannot conceive of color, but it adds to their appreciation to hear full descriptions. Older people most frequently have been sighted and can enjoy memories of beauty stimulated by descriptive conversation.
- Use some means to identify residents who are known to be visually impaired.
- *Be careful about labeling a resident as confused.* He or she may be making mistakes as a result of poor vision.

---

and watches, large-print books, magnifiers, computers with low-vision devices, and the low-vision enhancement system (Goldzweig et al., 2004). This last device uses tiny cameras to place an enlarged image on a video screen in front of the eyes. This is worn as a headset and can be used for distance viewing, as well as reading. Persons with reduced visual acuity should be encouraged to consider some of these sophisticated aids because severe visual deficits may result in mobility restrictions and create cognitive, sensory, and behavioral disturbances.

Magnifying lenses are available in many forms in addition to those commonly found in spectacle frames. These can be recommended in relation to the use for which they are desired. The most complex of the low-vision devices are telescopes that can be focused at various distances, thus increasing the number of tasks that can be performed. In addition, closed-circuit television magnifying units are available that can enlarge written characters up to 45 times.

Another method of magnification is through the use of a standard copying machine that has magnifying capabilities. One need not buy one of these but only make use of those available to the public. By repeatedly magnifying printed words or images, even small print can be made as large as desired.

Eyeglasses, once heavy and bulky, are now cosmetically appealing. Many also incorporate prismatic lenses that expand the visual field. Sunglasses are designed to filter out ultraviolet rays that may be harmful to sensitive retinas. Some eyeglasses adjust to light source and become darker in the sun. Magnifiers have been redesigned for ease of changing batteries and bulbs, positioning, and grasping. Telescopic lens

eyeglasses are smaller, are easier to focus, and have a greater range. It is now possible to electronically magnify video- and computer-generated text. Some software converts text into artificial voice output. All these resources must be considered when attempting to help the visually impaired elder achieve the visual activities that are important to his or her quality of life. Because individual needs are unique, it is recommended that before investing in any of these vision aids, the client be advised to consult with a low-vision center or low-vision specialist. See the Resources section at the end of the chapter for additional information.

Orientation Strategies for the Nonsighted. Methods to assist those individuals with total lack of sight are not generally included in nursing curricula. Methods in common use include the following: (1) the clock method, in which the individual is simply told where the food or item is as if it were on a clock face; (2) the sighted guide, in which a companion guides the visually impaired and enables safe mobility; (3) the cane sweep, which encounters obstacles; (4) varied textured surfaces; (5) sound signals, for example, at street crossings; and (6) guide dogs.

Sighted Guide. Ask the blind person if he or she would like a sighted guide. A strong element of dependency and trust is necessary in this method, and many people would rather manage on their own. Initially, as a person is adjusting to blindness, it can be helpful. If assistance is accepted, offer your elbow or arm. Instruct the person to grasp your arm just above the elbow. If necessary, physically assist the person by guiding his or her hand to your arm or elbow.

Walk one-half step ahead and slightly to the side of the blind person. The shoulder of the person should be directly behind your shoulder. If the person is frail, place his or her hand on your forearm. With this modified grasp, the person will be positioned lateral to your body. Relax and walk at a comfortable pace. Tell the person when you are approaching doorways, uneven surfaces, or a narrow space.

Cane Sweep. White canes, sometimes called "long canes," are used by about 109,000 persons in the United States. The person sweeps the space in front of him or her with the cane just before forward movement and in doing so alerts others to his or her presence as a nonsighted person and alerts the blind person of obstacles in the space ahead (All About Vision, 2001).

Sound Signals. In some U.S. cities and most European and Japanese cities, intermittent sound signals alert the person with limited vision when it is safe to cross the street—a simple solution, surprisingly not common in the United States. As nurses become more involved in political activist groups, this would be an area on which to focus federal and state lawmakers' attention.

Varied Textures. Those elders who have been blind for some time have developed hypersensitivity to textural variations. This sensitivity can be incorporated into the environment in numerous ways to assist the blind person.

Guide Dogs. There are 14 guide dog schools in the United States, and about 10,000 persons use guide dogs to assist them in mobility. Trained guide dogs are matched to individuals' needs and personalities, and those elders who have guide dogs have had several during the course of their adult years. Each dog becomes a companion, as well as a guide. It is important to avoid petting or otherwise interacting with the guide dog while it is "working" to allow the dog to maintain focus.

HEARING AND HEARING IMPAIRMENT

Oliver Sacks, author of the well-known book *Awakenings* (on which a popular film was based), wrote *Seeing Voices* (Sacks, 1989) to elucidate "a journey into the world of the deaf." Sacks presents a view that blindness may in fact be less serious than loss of hearing because of the interference with communication with others and the interactional input that is so necessary to stimulate and validate. One elderly man said that a great annoyance of hearing loss is in the subtle aspects of living with a partner, who most probably has a hearing loss as well. "You must often repeat what you say, and in lovemaking, whispering sweet words becomes a gesture for yourself alone." Perhaps Helen Keller was most profound in her expression: "Never to see the face of a loved one nor witness a summer sunset is indeed a handicap. But I can touch a face and feel the warmth of the sun. But to be deprived of hearing the song of the first spring robin and the laughter of children provides me with a long and dreadful sadness" (Keller, 1902).

Today in the United States more than one third of all community-dwelling elders are hearing impaired (Desai et al., 2001). It is estimated that 50% of persons older than 85 years have a hearing problem, and the occurrence is as high as 90% among the institutionalized older people. In all age-groups, elderly men are more likely than women to be hearing impaired. Further, white men and women report hearing loss more than blacks. As a review, the anatomy of the ear is shown in Figure 14-9. Age-related changes, auditory changes, and changes in the ear are discussed in Chapter 4.

Like visual impairment, hearing impairment diminishes the quality of life. Hearing loss contributes to decreased function, miscommunication, increased social isolation, depression, falls, and loss of self-esteem (Crews and Campbell, 2004). Older people are initially unaware of hearing loss because of the gradual manner in which it usually develops. They may believe others are mumbling, and they may become irritated at individuals around them who they perceive as not speaking up. Impaired hearing increases isolation and suspicion that sometimes progresses to what appears to be paranoia. Because older people with a hearing loss may not understand or respond appropriately to conversation, they may be inappropriately diagnosed with dementia. It is essential that appropriate assessment and testing be done to determine the nature of the loss, how much it interferes with communication, whether it is treatable, and whether a hearing aid will be useful. Recent advances in hearing aid technology make it possible to find appropriate hearing aids for some who have not found them satisfactory in the past.

Hearing impairment is underdiagnosed and undertreated in older people. For example, only 25% of people with hearing loss receive hearing aids and fewer than 10% of internists offer hearing tests to their patients older than 65 years. Assessment of hearing loss and hearing aides have not been covered under Medicare and other health plans, contributing to the problem of unremediated age-related hearing loss (Ham et al., 2002).

Presbycusis

The two major forms of hearing loss are *conductive* and *sensorineural*. Sensorineural hearing loss (presbycusis) is related to aging and is the most common cause of hearing loss in the United States. Sensorineural hearing loss is treated with hearing aids. Conductive hearing loss usually involves abnormalities of the external and middle ear, such as otosclerosis, perforated eardrum, fluid in the middle ear, or cerumen accumulations.

Presbycusis affects primarily individuals older than 50 years but is not a universal change, and although age-related, it may really be more reflective of environmental conditions and lifestyle. The influence of genetics, noise exposure, cardiovascular status, central processing capacity, certain medications, smoking, diet, personality, and stress have all been implicated to varying degrees in the etiology of hearing impairment. Presbycusis is a bilateral and symmetrical sensorineural hearing loss that also affects the ability to understand

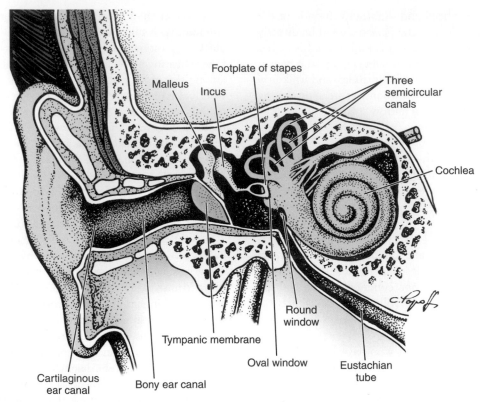

FIGURE 14-9 External auditory canal, middle ear, and inner ear. (From Malasanos L et al: *Health assessment,* ed 4, St Louis, 1991, Mosby.)

speech. Men seem to experience more severe presbycusis then women of the same age. Changes in the middle and inner ear make many elders intolerant of loud noises and incapable of distinguishing among some of the sibilant consonants such as *z, s, sh, f, p, k, t,* and *g*. People often raise their voice when speaking to a hearing-impaired person. When this happens, more consonants drop out of speech, making hearing even more difficult. Without consonants, the high-frequency–pitched language becomes disjointed and misunderstood. Consider the simple sentence, "How are you today?" To the individual with presbycusis it might sound like "hOw arE yOU tOdAy?"

Older people with presbycusis have difficulty filtering out background noise and often complain of difficulty understanding women's and children's speech and conversations in large groups. The condition progressively worsens with age. The environment is teeming with distracting sounds and noises, such as traffic, television, appliances, crowds, and noisy restaurants and shopping malls. Institutions in which elders may be patients are also noisy with many distracting sounds that make communication difficult for sensory and cognitively impaired elders—intercoms or pagers, clattering equipment, meal and medication carts, and "canned music." Use of rapid speech when conversing with an elder with a hearing impairment will make sounds garbled and unintelligible, and even though the problem is related to presbycusis, it is one that is easily remedied. The common but treatable problem of cerumen in the ear canal, particularly seen with hearing aid use, intensifies hearing difficulties for the person with presbycusis.

Prelingual Deafness

Reading and writing skills may be impaired in the person with prelingual deafness. Even though the intelligence of prelingually deaf persons may be normal, they may not have had the common educational opportunities of their cohort. This is thought to be related to the early orientation to signing and lip reading. For these individuals, signing is their first language and English their second. Subtleties of verbal communication may be lost to them, though they often compensate and become extremely alert to nonverbal cues and feelings. At times, a certified interpreter who is well enmeshed in the world of the deaf will be needed. For additional information in this regard, the reader might contact the National Center of Deafness at Gallaudet University (800 Florida Avenue NE, Washington, DC 20002; [202] 651-5051).

It is often incorrectly assumed that an elder can read lips; however, it is more likely that body language and the context of a situation clue an elder to words being said. In addition, it seems common to overlook the fact that vision may also be fading, thus impinging on lip-reading ability. Some elders become dependent on vision for understanding speech at the same time their vision is becoming compromised. Nurses will need to seek resources appropriate to augment vision to the greatest degree possible in these individuals.

Cerumen Impaction

Cerumen impaction is the most common and easily corrected of all interferences in the hearing of older people. Cerumen interferes with the conduction of sound through

<table>
<tr><td>

BOX 14-5   Protocol for Cerumen Removal

- Assess for ear pain, traumas, abnormalities, drainage, surgeries, or perforations. These or any other unusual findings should be referred to an otolaryngologist.
- When aural examination reveals cerumen impaction with no other abnormalities, the nurse may irrigate for cerumen removal using the following techniques:
  1. Carefully clip and remove hairs in ear canal.
  2. Instill a softening agent such as slightly warm mineral oil 0.5 to 1 mL twice daily or ear drops such as Cerumenex, Debrox, or Murine ear drops for several days until wax becomes softened. Allergic reactions to Cerumenex have been noted if used for longer than 24 hours.
  3. Protect clothing and linens from drainage of oil or wax by placing small cotton ball in each external ear canal.
  4. When irrigating the ear, use hand-held bulb syringe, 2- to 4-ounce plastic syringe, or otologic syringe (20- to 50-mL syringe equipped with an Angiocath or Jelso catheter rather than a needle) with emesis basin under ear to catch drainage; tip head to side being drained.
  5. Use solution of 3 ounces of 3% hydrogen peroxide in quart of water warmed to 98° to 100° F; if client is sensitive to hydrogen peroxide, use sterile normal saline.
  6. Place towels around neck; empty emesis basin frequently, observing for residue from ear; keep client dry and comfortable; do not inject air into client's ear or use high pressure when injecting fluid.
  7. If the cerumen is not successfully washed out, begin the process again of instilling a softening agent for several days.

</td></tr>
</table>

Modified from Meador JA: Cerumen impaction in the elderly, *J Gerontol Nurs* 21(12):43-45, 1995.

air in the eardrum. The reduction in the number of cerumen-producing glands and activity of the glands results in a tendency toward cerumen impaction. Long-standing impactions become hard, dry, and dark brown. This can be removed and must be before accurate audiometry can be done. Many older people admit to using foreign objects to clean their ears. Some have perforated the tympanic membrane in the process, resulting in severe hearing loss in the injured ear. Individuals at particular risk of impaction are African-Americans and older men with large amounts of ear canal tragi (hairs in the ear) that tend to become entangled with the cerumen, which prevents dislodgment. A protocol for removal is outlined in Box 14-5. Irrigation is contraindicated if the tympanic membrane has been perforated, because it may induce an infection. Cautions are also necessary for those with especially sticky cerumen, which can damage the mechanism of a hearing aid and involve costly repairs.

Others who may develop excessive cerumen are those who habitually wear hearing aids, those with benign growths that narrow the external ear canal, and those who have a predilec-

tion to cerumen accumulation. More commonly, older adults will have less cerumen and dryer cerumen because of a greater amount of keratin present (Maas et al., 2001).

Tinnitus

Tinnitus, or ringing in the ear, may also manifest as buzzing, hissing, whistling, crickets, bells, roaring, clicking, pulsating, humming, or swishing sounds. The most common type is high-pitched tinnitus with sensorineural loss; less common is low-pitched tinnitus with conduction loss such as is seen in Ménière's disease (Dinces, 2001). The sounds may be constant or intermittent and are more acute at night or in quiet surroundings.

Tinnitus generally increases over time. It is a condition that afflicts many older people and can interfere with hearing, as well as become extremely irritating. It is estimated to occur in nearly 11% of elders with presbycusis. Approximately 50 million people in the United States have tinnitus, and 12 million people are estimated to have tinnitus to a distressing degree (American Tinnitus Association, 2002). The incidence of tinnitus peaks between ages 65 and 74 years (about 11%), is higher in men than in women, and then seems to decrease in men.

Tinnitus can be caused by loud noises, excessive cerumen or auditory canal obstruction, disorders of the cervical vertebrae or the temporomandibular joint, allergies, an underactive thyroid, cardiovascular disease, tumors, conductive hearing loss, anxiety, depression, degeneration of the bones in the middle ear, infections, or trauma to the head or ear. In addition, more than 200 prescription and nonprescription medications list tinnitus as a potential side effect, aspirin being the most common.

Assessment. Tinnitus may be described as pulsatile (matching the beating of the heart) or nonpulsatile (unilateral, asymmetric, or symmetric). Tinnitus may be subjective (audible only to the person) or objective (audible to the examiner). Subjective tinnitus is more common. Objective tinnitus is rare and is frequently caused by a vascular or neuromuscular condition. The mechanisms of tinnitus are unknown but have been thought to be analogous to cross-talk on telephone wires, phantom limb pain, or transmission of vascular sounds such as bruits, and they are sometimes hallucinatory.

A Tinnitus Handicap Questionnaire developed by Newman et al. (1995) measures physical, emotional, and social consequences of tinnitus. It can be used also to assess the changes the individual experiences with treatment. Some persons with tinnitus will never find the cause; for others, the problem may arbitrarily disappear. Hearing aids can be prescribed to amplify environmental sounds to obscure tinnitus, and a device is available that combines the features of a masker and a hearing aid, which emits a competitive but pleasant sound that distracts from head noise. Therapeutic modes of treating tinnitus include transtympanal electrostimulation, iontophoresis, biofeedback, tinnitus masking with alternative sound production (white noise), dental treatment, cochlear implants, and hearing aids. Some have found hypnosis, acupuncture, chiropractic, naturopathic, allergy, and drug treatment effective.

Nursing actions include discussions with the client regarding times when the noises are most irritating and having the person keep a diary to identify patterns. Some evidence exists that caffeine, alcohol, cigarettes, stress, and fatigue may exacerbate the problem. Assess medications for possible contribution to the problem. Discuss lifestyle changes and alternative methods that some have found effective. Also, refer clients to the American Tinnitus Association for research updates, education, and support groups.

The Hospitalized Hearing-Impaired Person

Hospitalization in a new facility can be very difficult for a hearing-impaired elder. The gerontological nurse can apply a number of supports to ease the process:

- Note on the patient's chart that he or she is hearing impaired.
- Place a sign in a prominent place in the patient's room.
- Determine from the patient or family the most effective way to communicate with the patient.
- If the patient "signs," try to avoid restrictions of arms and hands.
- Use visual aids (charts, models) to explain procedures.
- Ensure good lighting in the patient's room.
- Encourage the use of the patient's hearing aid, and ensure the safety of the hearing aid at night.
- Obtain a certified sign language interpreter for obtaining consent for any procedure. It is essential that the patient understand possible risks and outcomes.

Assessment. Assessment of a hearing disability may be done in a superficial manner by almost any observant health care professional. However, the responsibility for the initial

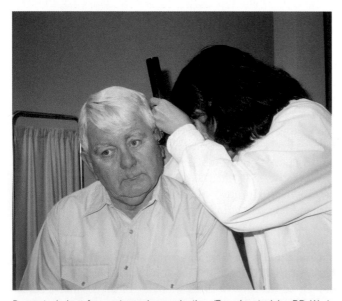

Proper technique for an otoscopic examination. (From Ignatavicius DD, Workman ML: *Medical-surgical nursing: critical thinking for collaborative care,* ed 5, St Louis, 2006, Saunders.)

identification of hearing problems usually falls on the nurses, and therefore rapid, reliable, effective screening methods must be available to them. Few elders have had audiometric testing even though a great many elders older than 75 years have hearing impairment. Screening should include the use of the Hearing Handicap Inventory for the Elderly-Screening (HHIE-S), visual inspection of the ear, pure-tone screening, and the client's history (Demers, 2001).

Because many elders are very sensitive about admitting losses, they may be reluctant to share such information. It can best be obtained by first establishing rapport with the person and then proceeding to open interviewing with a comment such as "Many people have difficulty hearing in certain situations. Have you experienced any difficulty? Describe these situations for me." If friends and relatives have insisted that the older person needs a hearing evaluation, he or she may be doubly resistant. Nurses are reminded that the older person is the best judge of adequate hearing capacity, based on his or her own evaluation (Figure 14-10). However, older persons are often unaware of mild to moderate hearing loss because of the gradual manner in which it usually develops.

Otoscopic examination allows for visualization of the ear canal and tympanic membrane for possible discovery of cerumen impaction or a perforated eardrum. Weber's test, placement of a tuning fork on the forehead of the individual, will determine the presence of unilateral conductive hearing loss. This is a screening test and does not measure bilateral hearing loss. The Rinne test screens for difficulty in air and bone conduction. A simple "whisper test" can be helpful in determining hearing capabilities until more extensive testing can be done by an audiologist. The audioscope (similar to the ear thermometer) is used to determine the frequency range of hearing (Figure 14-11). Human speech is usually heard below the 2000- to 3000-hertz (Hz) range. Those who have used the audioscope find it a highly valid screening instrument. It is a simple, fast, and accurate method of screening for hearing loss. Audiometry is still needed for more precise information. Each elder is entitled to a complete and thorough audiometric examination if there is any doubt about adequate hearing capacity. Early detection of hearing loss often depends on a nurse's observational assessment. Box 14-6 presents assessment and interventions for hearing-impaired elders.

Interventions. Physical examination, interview, self-assessment, relative or friend assessment, and audiometric findings are all necessary to arrive at a meaningful recommendation for the hearing-impaired older person. Counseling includes specific information regarding the problem, encouragement that sensorineural loss (nerve deafness) can often be partially counteracted by a hearing aid, assistance in the adjustment phase of wearing a hearing aid, and work with family members to improve their communication techniques.

Hearing Aids

A hearing aid is a personal amplifying system that includes a microphone, an amplifier, and a loudspeaker. The appearance and effectiveness of hearing aids have greatly improved

Hearing Handicap Scale

Rating:
Always—1 or 2
Frequently—3 or 4
Never—5

Scoring:
Raw score — 29 x 1.25 = %

Scores:

No handicap	0% to 20%
Mild hearing handicap	21% to 40%
Moderate hearing handicap	41% to 70%
Severe hearing handicap	71% to 100%

	Score
1. At 2 to 4 meters from radio or television, do you understand speech?	
2. Can you converse on the telephone easily?	
3. Can you carry on conversation comfortably when in a noisy place?	
4. Can you understand speech when in a noisy bus, on an airplane, at a movie, on the street corner?	
5. Can you understand a person when seated beside him and you cannot see his face?	
6. Can you understand speech if someone is talking to you while chewing crunchy foods?	
7. Can you understand a whisper when you cannot see a person's face?	
8. Can you carry on conversation across a room when someone speaks in normal tone of voice?	
9. Can you understand women when they talk?	
10. Can you carry on conversation outdoors when it is reasonably quiet?	
11. When in a meeting or at a large dinner would you know what the speaker said if lips were not moving?	
12. Can you follow conversation at a large dinner or in a small group?	
13. When seated under the balcony of a theater or auditorium, can you hear what is going on?	
14. When in a church, lodge meeting, or lecture hall, can you hear if the speaker does not use a microphone?	
15. Can you hear the telephone ring when it is located in another room?	
16. Can you hear warning signals such as automobile horns, railway crossing bells, or emergency vehicle sirens?	
17. Can you carry on conversation in a car with the windows open?	
18. Can you carry on conversation in a car with the windows closed?	
19. Can you hear when someone calls from another room?	
20. Can you understand when someone speaks to you from another room?	
21. Can you carry on conversation with someone who speaks quietly?	
22. When you ask for directions, do you understand what is said?	
23. When you are introduced, do you understand the name the first time it is spoken?	
24. Can you hear adequately when conversing with more than one person?	
25. When seated in the front of an auditorium, can you understand most of what is being said?	
26. Can you carry on everyday conversations with family members without difficulty?	
27. When seated in the rear of an auditorium, can you understand most of what is said?	
28. When in a large formal gathering, can you hear what is said if the speaker uses a microphone?	
29. Can you hear night sounds, such as dogs barking, distant trains, bells, trucks passing, etc.?	

FIGURE 14-10 Hearing Handicap Scale. (Modified from High WS et al: Scale for self-assessment of hearing handicap, *J Speech Disord* 29:215, 1964.)

in recent years. Hearing aids have been miniaturized, but the small size may present difficulties for older people with visual deficits, loss of sensation, or arthritic hands. A recent advance has been the introduction of a remote-control device that contains an on/off switch and volume device. There are approximately 50 different manufacturers of hearing aids, and thus the informed consumer has a broad selection from which to choose. Hearing aids generally improve hearing by about 50%, and it is important that hearing-impaired elders understand that the goal is to improve communication and quality of life, not to restore normal hearing (Karev and Bartz, 2001).

Telephones are required to be compatible with hearing aids. Hearing aids with a telecoil can be set on "T" to receive the signal from the magnetic coil in the telephone (Beck and Roe-Beck, 2000).

Although hearing aids have improved considerably, only 20% of older adults with hearing impairment purchase and

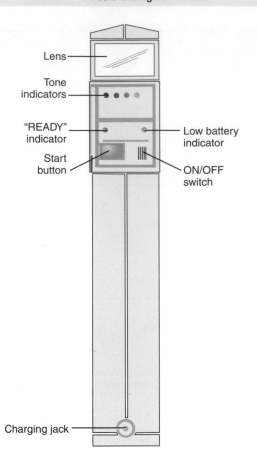

Lens

Tone indicators

"READY" indicator

Low battery indicator

Start button

ON/OFF switch

Charging jack

1. Turn on the instrument by sliding up the ON/OFF switch.

2. Inform the client that he or she will hear some faint tones, and ask the client to raise the index finger each time the sound is heard.

3. Gently pull the ear canal up and back, and then carefully insert the audioscope into the ear canal using the largest ear speculum that can be comfortably inserted into the ear canal.

4. The tip is positioned so that the tympanic membrane is visualized.

5. Depress the start button.

6. The tone indicators illuminate sequentially (with a red light) as each tone is presented to the client for 1.5 seconds.

7. Repeat the same procedure in the opposite ear.

NOTE: Occluding the opposite eardrum does not appear to influence the accuracy of the test results.

FIGURE 14-11 The audioscope. (From Campbell S: The audioscope: a valuable hearing assessment tool, *J Gerontol Nurs* 12[12]:28, 1986.)

consistently wear them (Fozard and Gordon-Salant, 2001). Many factors may influence a person's ability and willingness to wear a hearing aid. If the person has been taught to use an aid gradually and correctly and yet does not do so, the nurse should attempt to discover the reasons: the appearance of having an infirmity, the difficulty manipulating a small object, poor vision, inadequate training and support, lack of energy, uncomfortable fit, forgetfulness, and cost. In this era of highly sophisticated, personalized, and computerized hear-

ing aids, most individuals can obtain some hearing enhancement. Hearing aids have changed dramatically in recent years, both in effectiveness and appearance, but many individuals who tried one a number of years ago have decided against using them.

The law requires that audiologic testing be preceded by an examination by a physician to rule out ear, nose, and throat (ENT) disorders. Before a hearing aid can be purchased, medical clearance consisting of a signed waiver from a physician is mandatory, stating that none of the following conditions exist:

1. Visible congenital or traumatic deformity of the ear
2. Active drainage from the ear within the past 90 days
3. Sudden or progressive hearing loss within the past 90 days
4. Acute or chronic dizziness
5. Unilateral sudden hearing loss within the past 90 days
6. Visible evidence of significant cerumen accumulation or a foreign body in the ear canal
7. Pain or discomfort in the ear
8. Audiometric air-bone gap equal to or greater than 15 decibels (dB)

Many ENT specialists have an audiologist and audiologic testing available in the office. Audiologists may favor certain models, and it is wise for a client to shop around for fit and sound regardless of what the physician and audiologist recommend. The investment in a good hearing aid is considerable, and a good fit is crucial. Hearing aids can range in price from about $500 to several thousand dollars a piece.

Styles. Numerous hearing aids and assistive devices are available to improve hearing. The behind-the-ear hearing aid looks like a shrimp and fits around and behind the ear. It is less commonly used now than the small, in-the-ear aid, which fits in the concha of the ear (Figure 14-12). This type of hearing aid is used for elders with moderate, severe, or profound hearing loss. Also, a larger version is available that is custom-made to fit the entire external auricular cavity. This type of hearing aid is the most visible and least expensive. It is usually recommended for elders with mild or moderate hearing loss. The analog hearing aids are designed to be worn at all times; other devices are designed to solve specific problems. Some products are designed to overcome the effects of noise and distance. These transform sound waves to a different energy spectrum, such as infrared or electromagnetic waves that are then transmitted from the microphone to the receiver and delivered as a clear signal directly to the person's ear. Digitally programmed hearing aids that have more than 1 million different settings from which to select are becoming available. These are matched to the individual's hearing loss.

In the past 5 years a miniaturized computer with a memory chip has been integrated into a hearing aid that eliminates many major hearing aid problems, such as adjustment levels, background noise, and whistling. These aids automatically electronically separate incoming sound without

BOX 14-6   Assessment and Interventions for Hearing-Impaired Elders

ASSESSMENT

History

In the past 3 months, have you had discharge from your ears?

In the past 3 months, have you experienced dizziness (not related to sudden changes in position)?

In the past 3 months, have you had pain in your ears?

In the past 3 months, have you noticed a sudden or rapid change in your hearing?

Have you ever experienced tinnitus, vertigo, or sudden or gradual hearing loss?

In which situations do you have difficulty hearing?

In the past, have you experienced ear infections, surgery, treatment, or hearing aid use?

Is there a family history of hearing loss?

What drugs have you used or are you now using (note particularly toxic levels of streptomycin, neomycin, or aspirin)?

Observations by Family and/or Caregiver

Does the person often seem inattentive to others?

Does the person respond with inappropriate anger or irritation when spoken to?

Does the person believe people are talking about him or her?

Does he or she lack a movement response to sounds in the environment?

Does the person have difficulty following clear directions?

Is he or she withdrawn and alone much of the time?

Does the person frequently ask to have something repeated?

Does he or she tend to turn one ear toward a speaker?

Does the person have a monotonous or unusual voice quality?

Is speech unusually loud or soft?

INTERVENTIONS

General

Never assume hearing loss is from age until other causes are ruled out (infection, cerumen buildup).

Inappropriate responses, inattentiveness, apathy may be symptoms of a hearing loss.

Face the individual, and stand or sit on the same level.

Gain the individual's attention before beginning to speak.

You may need to sit or stand closer to decrease interpersonal space. Assess the individual's comfort with this, and make sure individuals know you are there before touching them or when coming from behind.

If a hearing aid is used, make sure it is on, is clean, and has batteries.

Speakers need to keep hands away from their mouth and project their voice by controlled diaphragmatic breathing.

Avoid conversations in which the speaker's face is in glare or darkness.

Avoid "elderspeak" (overly patronizing, rising baby talk, assuming the elder will not understand unless simplified).

Careful articulation and moderate speed of speech are helpful.

Avoid eating, chewing, or smoking while speaking.

Facial and hand expressions used liberally facilitate understanding.

Pause between sentences or phrases to confirm understanding.

Restate with different words when you are not understood.

When changing topics, preface the change by stating the topic.

Provide visual cues to locate noise direction, since there appears to be an age-related deficit to picking up directional cues.

In most cases there is a better ear.

Reduce background noise.

If paranoia has developed, the individual may not respond well to touch. A handshake is a benign gesture and will signal acceptance or rejection of your efforts to communicate.

The Hospitalized or Institutionalized Hearing Impaired

Note on the intercom button and the patient's chart whether the patient is deaf.

Note the most effective way to communicate with the patient.

Never restrict arm movement of deaf patients who use sign language as the primary means of communication.

Use charts, pictures, or models to explain medications and procedures.

Do not shout.

Talk TO a hard-of-hearing person, not ABOUT him or her.

In group situations, speak one at a time.

Use assistive devices such as pocket talkers (audio-amplified units).

Adequate lighting is essential.

If the patient has a hearing aid, encourage its use and make sure it is fitted properly and in good working order.

Obtain a certified sign language interpreter for obtaining consent for any procedure. It is essential that the patient understand possible risks and outcomes.

Be PATIENT.

---

the need to adjust the volume. Although these can offer great benefit, they may be prohibitively expensive for many. Because of the rapidly developing technology, it behooves the hearing-impaired individual to be thoroughly evaluated in an audiologic center that is not marketing specific hearing aids. Many hospitals and health centers have such services and may have dozens of models an individual can try until the most suitable one is found.

In most states, the purchase of a hearing aid comes with a 30-day trial during which time the purchase price is fully refundable. For programmable devices, the purchaser must be seen a number of times during the month until an optimal adjustment is found. If problems occur during that time, the person should return to the audiologist for assistance. Recent federal regulations have influenced hearing aid manufacturers toward more careful marketing and fitting procedures. It is important to advise older people that charges for hearing aids are not paid for by Medicare or private insurance. Suggestions for using and caring for a hearing aid are given in Box 14-7. It is important for nurses, particularly those working in hospitals and long-term care facilities, to be knowledgeable about the care and maintenance of aids.

Sound amplifiers are on the market that fit in a pocket or are worn on the belt and are inexpensive, walkabout-style hearing boosters. Their appearance is similar to that of a portable personal audio player such as Walkman. These are particularly useful for individuals with conductive hearing loss and in situations in which background noise is inevitable. The amplifying microphone can be attached to the television or telephone or clipped on a friend's collar. In situations where a primary sound source is desirable, these devices are ideal. Headsets with small or large earphones are available. Thus amplification of desired sounds is available without the use of a hearing aid. The receiver is a custom-made clear plastic ear mold in the ear canal and attached to the unit by a wire. This type of hearing aid is used for those with profound hearing loss. It is less esthetically pleasing compared with the other types.

Cochlear Implants

Cochlear implants are increasingly used for older adults who are profoundly deaf as a result of sensorineural loss. Considerable refinement has been achieved, and implants have shown the most success for those elders who have not been deaf for long and have a strong desire to hear. Unlike hearing aids that magnify sound, the cochlear implant converts sound waves into electrical impulses and transmits them to the inner ear. A cochlear implant is surgically implanted in the mastoid bone behind the ear and electrically stimulates the primary hearing organ, the cochlea, setting the cilia in motion and transmitting impulses along the auditory nerve to the brain's hearing center (Figure 14-13). For people whose hearing loss is so severe that amplification is of little or no benefit, the cochlear implant is a safe and effective method of auditory rehabilitation. Most insurance plans cover the cochlear implant procedure (Ham et al., 2002). The implant carries some risk because the surgery destroys any residual hearing that remains. Therefore cochlear implant users can never revert back to using a hearing aid. Individuals with cochlear implants need to be advised not to undergo magnetic resonance imaging (MRI) because the implanted devices are not compatible with MRI (Miller, 2004).

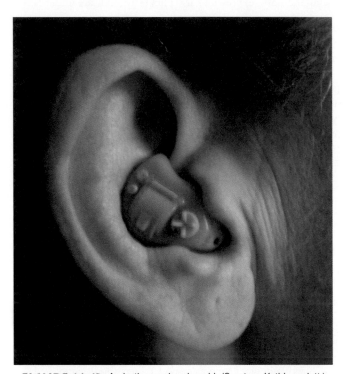

FIGURE 14-12 An in-the-ear hearing aid. (Courtesy Kathleen Jett.)

BOX 14-7   Care and Use of Hearing Aids

HEARING AID USE

Initially, wear aid 15 to 20 minutes daily.
Gradually increase time until 10 to 12 hours.
Hearing aid will initially make client uneasy.
Insert aid with canal portion pointing into ear, press and twist until snug.
Turn aid slowly to ⅓ to ½ volume.
A whistling sound indicates incorrect ear mold insertion.
Adjust volume to a level comfortable for talking at a distance of 1 yard.
Do not wear aid under heat lamps or hair dryer or in very wet, cold weather.
Do not wear aid while bathing or perspiring heavily.
Concentrate on conversation; request repeat if necessary.
Sit close to speaker in noisy situations.
Continue to be observant of nonverbal cues.
Be patient with self and realize the process of adaptation is difficult but ultimately will be rewarding.

CARE OF THE HEARING AID

Insert battery when hearing aid is turned off.
Store hearing aid in a dry, safe place.
Remove or disconnect battery when not in use.
Batteries last 1 week with daily wearing 10 to 12 hours.
Common problems include switch turned off, clogged ear mold, dislodged battery, twisted tubing between ear mold and aid.
Ear molds need replacement every 2 or 3 years.
Check ear molds for rough spots that will irritate ear.
Avoid exposing aid to excess heat or cold.
Clean batteries occasionally to remove corrosion; use a sharpened pencil eraser and gently scrape.

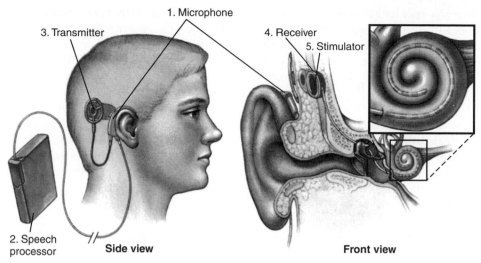

1. Microphone

3. Transmitter

4. Receiver

5. Stimulator

2. Speech processor

Side view

Front view

FIGURE 14-13 How cochlear implants work: A microphone *(1)* picks up sound. The sound travels through a thin cable to a speech processor *(2)*. The processor can be worn on a belt or in a pocket. The processor converts the signal into an electrical code and sends the code back up the cable to a transmitter *(3)* fastened to the head. The transmitter sends the code through the skin to a receiver-stimulator *(4 and 5)* implanted in bone directly beneath the transmitter. The stimulator sends the code down a tiny bundle of wires threaded directly into the cochlea (snail-shaped primary hearing organ). Nerve fibers are activated by electrode bands on this bundle of wires. The auditory nerve carries the signal to the brain, which interprets the signal. (From Cochlear implants, *Mayo Clinic Health Letter* 9[11]:4, 1991.)

Assistive Listening and Adaptive Devices

Assistive listening devices (also called *personal listening systems*) should be considered as an adjunct to hearing aids or in place of hearing aids for people with hearing impairment. These devices are available commercially and can be used to better understand speech in large rooms such as theaters and auditoriums, use the telephone, and listen to television. Text messaging devices for telephones and closed-caption television, now required on all televisions with screens 13 inches or larger, are other examples. Alerting devices, such as vibrating alarm clocks that shake the bed or activate a flashing light and sound lamps that respond with lights to sounds such as doorbells, telephones, babies crying, or other noises, are also available. Assistive devices, such as pocket talkers (audio-amplified units), are helpful in health care situations in which accurate communication and privacy are essential. Some very innovative people have developed ideas and products to enrich the lives of the hearing impaired. Music especially for the profoundly hearing impaired that is focused only in the low-frequency cycles (which are most easily heard) has been recorded. Assistive listening and adaptive devices can be purchased from hearing aid dealers, telephone companies, electronic and appliance shops, and catalogs. In some states, a monthly surcharge is included on all users' phone bills that pays for free phones with adjustable volume controls for all persons with documented hearing losses. Resources for hearing assistance are in the Resources section at the end of this chapter.

A program called *Hearing Dogs for the Deaf* has gained recognition. Seventeen locations in the United States train hearing dogs. In some locations the Society for the Prevention of Cruelty to Animals (SPCA) trains shelter dogs; some dogs are especially bred and raised to be hearing dogs, and in some locations the individual's own dog is trained appropriately. Hearing dogs serve to warn the hearing impaired of impending danger, audible signals, phones ringing, fire and smoke alarms, emergencies, and intruders. Although other electronic means of dealing with many of these problems are available, persons who have hearing dogs consistently comment on the alleviation of the sense of isolation that often accompanies hearing impairment. With a hearing dog companion, elders may experience renewed courage, confidence, and freedom.

Any facility that receives financial aid from Medicare is required by the Americans with Disabilities Act to provide equal access to public accommodations. Such facilities are required to have sign language interpreters, telecommunication devices for the deaf (TDDs), flashing alarm systems, and telecaptioning devices on televisions for the deaf. Unfortunately, these are seldom seen.

In old age, when people have transcended work and have more time to communicate for pleasure, they often develop hindrances to the communication process. When interactions are thwarted by sensory disturbances and motor disabilities, isolation and withdrawal soon follow. However, some people are able to transcend the limitations amazingly well. One very deaf elderly woman remained responsive and warm, often carrying the conversation by sharing her life experiences and observations. The conversation was one-sided but enjoyable to those who listened. She was very aware of verbal and nonverbal cues, which encouraged her to continue or to cease sharing. Health care professionals may need to focus on ability rather than disability and not assume a deaf person does not wish or is not able to talk. The ability to communicate verbally is gratifying to most persons. One older man said he missed hearing conversations around him almost as much as the ability to comfortably converse. Listening and talking can be comforting, enlightening, and reassuring, particularly for those who may have been surrounded by conversation for most of their lives.

▲ Promoting Healthy Aging: Implications for Gerontological Nursing

When vision and hearing are diminished, the elder has lost major sensory input, which has a direct effect on his or her everyday life. Decreases in these senses can potentiate isolation, depression, withdrawal, and loss of self-esteem; raise personal safety issues; and affect health. Inadequate communication with deaf or hearing-impaired patients can also lead to misdiagnosis and medication errors. In interviews with hearing-impaired patients about their communication concerns during medical visits and procedures, interviewees described not understanding therapeutic regimens, not understanding medication doses and side effects, and not knowing what to expect during physical examinations and procedures. Some suggestions to improve communication included using lights as signals for required actions such as holding one's breath during a mammogram and finding alternatives to lengthy phone message menus, such as e-mail or fax. Health care staff should be able to use telecommunication devices and receive training in communication with the hearing impaired (Iezzoni et al., 2004).

To promote healthy aging and quality of life, gerontological nurses in all settings must be knowledgeable about the impact of hearing and vision changes on the functional abilities and quality of life of older adults, vision and hearing assessment, prevention and treatment of diseases affecting vision and hearing, effective communication techniques, and ways to assist the individual in adapting to and compensating for these losses.

TASTE AND SMELL

Age-related losses of smell and fine taste normally begin in the sixth decade. These senses intertwine to provide links to the environment. They allow appreciation of good tastes and smells and also serve as a warning of environmental hazards (Wharton, 2000). Four basic tastes have been identified (sweet, sour, salty, and bitter), conveyed by approximately 9000 taste buds. Scientists believe more are yet to be identified and an unknown number of basic and subtle odors. The senses of taste and smell (chemosenses) can provide great pleasure, as well as protection from harm. Fine taste, such as the subtle differences between turkey and chicken, is an olfactory function; crude taste, such as sweet and sour, depends on the taste buds. It is thought that there is about a 75% decrement in smell (hyposmia) by age 80 years and a 50% loss of taste buds (hypogeusia) by age 60 years that accelerates after age 70 years (Wharton, 2000). (Chapter 4 discusses age-related changes in smell and taste.)

The senses of taste and smell play an important role in eating behaviors and in the maintenance of health (Maas et al., 2001). The enjoyment of taste is really the totality of the experience of temperature, texture, smell, appearance, and flavors. The sense of smell is affected by aging more than the sense of taste. It is important, then, to identify foods that appeal to the changed senses of smell and taste. Colors and textures may compensate for diminished sensory appeal of foods (O'Neill, 2002). Many older people, particularly those in institutions, no longer cook and never have the experience of smelling food cooking, an important appetite stimulant. Many long-term care institutions have adapted kitchens and dining rooms so that the residents can smell the food cooking and even participate in the preparation of food as a way of increasing interest and enjoyment of food.

When dealing with canned foods, older persons should be cautioned to check for bulges in the can and to discard any that are suspicious (Wharton, 2000). Stored foods should be dated and checked for spoilage. Defrosted foods should be used right away because thawing and refreezing significantly affects flavor and texture. Significant, rapid, and noticeable changes in smell or taste may be the result of medication, disease processes, or, in rare situations, hallucination. Gustatory and olfactory hallucinations are danger signals of brain lesions or head and neck cancers and should be immediately suspect.

Diseases that affect taste and smell are numerous. Among them are allergic rhinitis (23% suffer loss of smell), Alzheimer's disease, asthma, cancers, epilepsy, diabetes, liver disease, Parkinson's disease (an early sign), chronic renal failure, viruses, vitamin deficiencies, and zinc deficiency (Luggen, 2001). Drugs affecting taste and smell include many antibiotics, anticonvulsants, antidepressants, antihistamines, antihypertensives, antiinflammatories, beta-blockers, bronchodilators, calcium channel blockers, lipid-lowering agents, and vasodilators—all drugs commonly used by elderly persons.

Taste

Taste acuity is at least two thirds dependent on the olfactory sense. Tasting depends on an intact nerve supply (cranial nerves VII [facial] and IX [glossopharyngeal]) (Luggen, 2001). However, it is not only taste but also the sensual aspects of food that are enjoyable. The pleasure of eating comes more from masticating than from the taste buds or the hunger center in the hypothalamus. This knowledge can be important in preparing food for older people.

Taste buds that seem most affected by aging are those for sweet and salty at the tip of the tongue. These supposedly are exposed to more contact and thus may deteriorate slightly. This theory is based on the knowledge that taste buds begin to atrophy and diminish in number in midlife, for some as early as age 40 years, and the observation that many elders tend to salt and sweeten their foods more than when they were younger. This can be a problem for those with diabetes. Bitterness, located at the very back of the tongue, seems to remain a strong sensation at all ages, and in fact, older persons may experience an increased sensitivity to bitterness, with the resulting complaint that foods taste bitter or sour (Wharton, 2000).

Individuals have varied levels of taste sensitivity that seem predetermined by genetics and constitution, as well as age variations. Comparatively little interest has been demonstrated in studying these differences. Many denture wearers say they lose some of their satisfaction in food, possibly because texture is such an important element in food enjoyment and possibly because mastication is less enjoyable. The sensory pleasure of food and the symbolic nurturance inherent in eating and feeling satiated are important ways one maintains a sense of security. Indeed, when feeling insecure, many people begin to eat compulsively. Difficulties measuring flavor appreciation come from individual variables such as smoking, olfactory sensitivity, attitude toward food and eating, and the presence of moistening secretions. Also, aberrations in flavor sensations are caused by certain medications and by viruses, for example, colds.

Assessment. Detailed and meaningful gustatory evaluations are difficult to administer. Assessing taste, especially salty, sweet, sour, and bitter, is part of the complete physical assessment examination. Individuals complaining of *dysgeusia* (unpleasant taste in the mouth) should be evaluated for dental disease and dental hygiene, medication side effects, head trauma, upper respiratory disease, and cranial nerve integrity. If these screening procedures are inadequate, the individual may need to be referred to an otolaryngologist for more intensive testing.

There are no known therapies for primary gustatory dysfunction. If all secondary causes have been eliminated, the most useful approach to the client is simply being concerned and supportive. Help the person experiment with various herbs, spices, flavor extracts, and sugar and salt substitutes and identify foods that are most enjoyable (Wharton, 2000).

Encourage smokers to refrain from smoking. Do not burden them with a bland, soft, or liquid diet unless it is essential. They may enjoy the sensations of the food appearance and chewing even if their taste for flavors is not acute.

Olfaction

One of every two persons older than 65 years has lost some sense of smell, and women are more likely than men to experience such loss (Luggen, 2001). Most people, however, lose some olfactory discriminatory capacity, resulting in a lowered capacity for enjoyment of scents and fragrances and a stronger reliance on texture and visual cues. Smell losses outnumber taste problems. The sense of smell requires an intact cranial nerve I.

A decreased sensitivity to odors may be dangerous for the older person, such as when one may fail to detect the odor of leaking gas, a smoldering cigarette, or tainted food. The loss of smell may also present social problems. We all experience habituation to and unawareness of our own body odor. Some elders are unaware that the odor of urine accompanies them even though they have only slight leakage. This particular sensory reduction can be an alienating factor unless attended to. Perfumes may be overused and be overwhelming and offensive to others (Wharton, 2000).

Three causes can explain 60% of the problems with loss of smell: nasal sinus disease that results in obstruction of passages, thereby interfering with odors reaching the smell receptors; repeated injury to olfactory receptors through viral infections (Figure 14-14); and head trauma that results in bleeding into the nasal mucous membrane (least common cause). In the elder, it is more likely that a viral infection will result in permanent changes to the sense of smell. Abrupt loss of the sense of smell may occur after a viral nasal

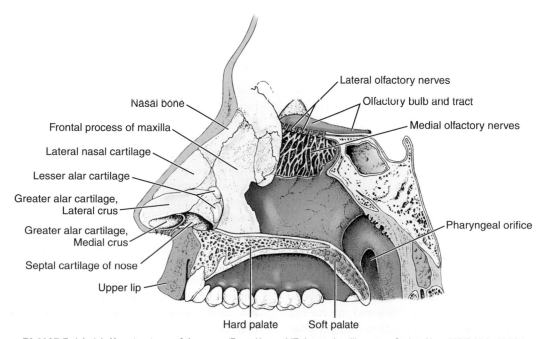

FIGURE 14-14 Key structures of the nose. (From Knapp MT: A rose is still a rose, *Geriatr Nurs* 10[6]:290, 1989.)

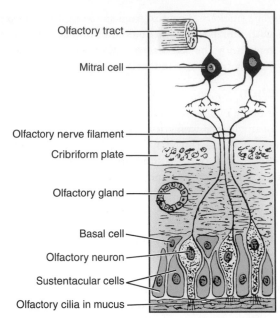

Olfactory tract

Mitral cell

Olfactory nerve filament

Cribriform plate

Olfactory gland

Basal cell

Olfactory neuron

Sustentacular cells

Olfactory cilia in mucus

FIGURE 14-15 Scheme of cell and fiber arrangement in olfactory epithelium. (From *Mosby's medical, nursing, and allied health dictionary,* ed 2, St Louis, 1986, Mosby.)

infection, although usually it will not be total loss (anosmia); this requires immediate attention because it could signal a serious disorder.

Exposure to medications and environmental agents affects chemosensation, especially in men and particularly those who have worked in factories. The accumulation of noxious agents over time results in an impaired sense of smell, especially from acid fumes, lead, or cocaine, a growing problem (Springhouse, 2001). Olfactory dysfunction can be among the first signs of Parkinson's disease and may in fact be a preclinical indication of the disease.

Olfactory nerve cells are thought to be the only sensory nerves capable of regeneration (Figure 14-15); however, if the sense of smell has been absent for 6 months or more, it is likely to be permanent, indicating destruction of the olfactory nerve (cranial nerve I) or olfactory neuroepithelium (Springhouse, 2001).

Assessment. A reliable and easy odor recognition tool is the University of Pennsylvania Smell Identification Test, a prepackaged scratch-and-sniff test that can be done with ease in any setting. *Dysosmia* (the sensation of unpleasant smell) may be individually idiosyncratic. For example, one woman found a particular incense nauseating; others are repelled by certain perfumes.

The practitioner will want to check the nose for swelling of the mucous membranes. It is important to look for polyps, which may be obstructive. Assess hydration. Ask about smoking and past viral infections. Sinusitis and rhinitis are major causes of loss of smell and taste. Box 14-8 presents assessment of the nose.

BOX 14-8   **Assessing the Nose**

- Visually inspect the nose. Note any asymmetry that could interfere with breathing or smell. Expect that the nose will be relatively long and broad because of the ongoing formation of cartilage through the years. Examine the color and texture of the surface of the nose. Diffuse redness, papules, pustules, and dilated venules can signal excess alcohol intake.
- Palpate the nose. Feel for raised bumps along the frontal bone at the base and hard nodes in the cartilage. Note any frontal bone depression suggesting nose fracture in the past.
- With an otoscope, look inside the vestibule of each naris. With age, nasal hair becomes coarser and thicker. Inspect the base of the hairs for signs of irritation or infection caused by clipping the hairs too close. Examine the nasal mucosa: Is it moist and intact? Or dry and broken? With age, the mucosa becomes fragile and easily broken. A smooth, shiny membrane with engorged turbinates is a sign of vasomotor rhinitis. Check the anterior septum and note whether it appears straight or deviates to the left or right of the columella separating the nares. At least a mild degree of septal deviation is common in adults.
- Occlude each nostril, one at a time, and ask the person to close his mouth and breathe through the open nostril. Note whether both nostrils are patent.
- Test olfactory nerve function by asking the person to identify various smells: Nerve fibers in the olfactory bulb decline at a rate of about 1% per year, which may account for a decreased ability to recognize or distinguish smells with age.
- Palpate the paranasal sinuses to detect swelling or any sign of tenderness that may indicate sinusitis or postnasal drip.

From Knapp MT: A rose is still a rose, *Geriatr Nurs* 10(6):290, 1989.

PERCEPTUAL ORGANIZATION

Perception arises from the integration of sensory signals into percepts that give meaning to raw data. Perception depends on sensations and experience. An older person has a wealth of experience to draw from when interpreting data, but at times the sensation is incomplete or experience distorts the present reality. When this happens, we may label the person "confused." *Confusion* is a term that is frequently misplaced. It often refers to the nurse as much as the client. When nurses are confused, they need more data. When clients are confused, nurses need to find out the specific source and limits of their data. The terms *confusion* and *disorientation* are sometimes used synonymously, although "confusion" is a catchall diagnosis of unexplained symptoms whereas "disorientation" can be highly specific. For thorough understanding we recommend *Confusion: Prevention and Care* (Wolanin and Phillips, 1981). It is the classic work on this subject. Disorientation and illusions usually have an organic base. Hallucinations may be organic or functional in origin. Chapter 23 discusses altered mental status in more depth.

Disorientation

Thoreau (1946, p. 285) said, "If a man does not keep pace with his companions, perhaps it is because he hears a different drummer." When people are disoriented, they are listening to a different drummer in another time or place but the beat is uneven and the impulses disquieting. Following their inner drummer brings insecurity and uncertainty. Sensory impressions are confusing and disconnected rather than intermingling in the subtle manner necessary for integration and accurate perception.

Perception of Time. The first level of disorientation to emerge is often related to timing of events. Being unclear about time measurement puts one out of step with the world at large and subject to an altered sense of linear time. Time orientation is evidence of a personal organization and structure and is somewhat more subjective in the old than in the young. It is the first level of individual awareness to be distorted by stressful circumstances, monotonous environments, or altered awareness. Illness, loss, and crises are frequently accompanied by an expanded, contracted, or muted sense of time passage. Keeping track of time requires attention, devices, and interest; all of these are easily diverted by biological, psychological, and sociological disruption. When stress is severe enough, personal time may remain out of synchronization with the world of clocks and dates or become totally submerged. Widows often move in slow motion for several weeks after the spouse's death. People in these major crises are preoccupied and experience sensory distortion. This kind of reaction has important implications for caregivers. When the world is perceived as threatening and chaotic, we must attempt to move slowly and patiently to restore order.

Elderly persons in monotonous environments who lack contrasting events and experiences that mark progression in most peoples' lives eventually lose interest and pay little attention to the flow of time. Organic impairment usually produces disorientation toward recent events such as whether the last meal was lunch or breakfast. It is difficult for the individual with physiological disturbance in cerebral function to focus attention or to remember events.

In these situations, our interventions are aimed toward capturing the elderly person's attention by direct, personalized communication and through provision of cues in the form of cards, name tags, calendars, clocks, reality boards, and schedules. Daily living patterns should remain as constant as possible. Meaningful stimulating events introduced into a consistent supportive atmosphere may produce improved client affect and function.

Some clients experience time disorientation of multiple origins: organic impairment, personal crises and loss, and colorless and boring environments. These are the clients whose time sense is likely to be most profoundly impaired.

Perception of Place. The second level of orientation is interrupted when a person is uncertain of territory. At this time we will explore the internal perception of placement. Distortion of perception relating to one's place usually occurs following translocation. It seems as if one's subconscious lends itself toward establishing security. An individual will perceive characteristics in the environment that relate to previous life experiences; for example, "Did you hear that ringing? It must be the trolley going by," or "What kind of hotel is this? I can't find the bar." Misconceptions of the environment are intensified by poor lighting, intercoms, and room transfers.

Frequently an individual is disoriented toward time and place; usually the older person slips into the security of the familiar past; for example, "I heard the clattering pans and thought Mother would call me for breakfast any minute." The nurse who responds with, "Mr. Jones, this is a hospital and it will soon be lunchtime," is listening and assessing on a most superficial level. It would be far more useful to sit with the client for a few moments, ask about his remembrance of breakfast when he was a child, note the strange noises that disturb one's rest in the hospital, and ask if the client may have been dreaming about a time that was more comfortable and secure.

The nurse will recognize themes of dependence, fears, unfamiliar expectations, and pain. All these commonly expected reactions to illness and hospitalization may be exacerbated by medications, lying in bed (alters perceptions), and slipping from waking to dozing state and states of reverie. If the client consistently insists that he or she is not in the place he or she should be or repeatedly calls for someone who is not there, the following interventions aimed toward increasing security and orientation may be helpful:

1. Gear activity to client level and reduce or increase stimulation toward a more normal range because either extreme will increase psychological stress and the need to hold onto delusion.
2. See the client frequently, introduce yourself each time, and explain what you would like to do.
3. Obtain some objects that provide comfort or familiarity, for example, pictures or sentimental objects. If the client has no family, find out comfort routines, for example, a glass of warm water with lemon before breakfast, a spread carefully folded on the foot of the bed, or a particular brand of toothpaste or denture cleanser on the nightstand. In long-term care situations, it is imperative to alter the environment toward personalization.

Perception of Person. The third level of disorientation is to person and often is closely tied to confusion about one's whereabouts. A patient who believes he or she is at home may expect a family member to enter the room. Often health care personnel resemble a significant person in a client's past and are believed to be that person. Sometimes it is not disorientation but rather longing that precipitates identity confusion. One older man wandered the halls of a nursing home calling his wife's name toward the backs of departing female patients. This phenomenon is not limited to the old. Younger people also sometimes imagine they see a dead loved one.

Disorientation regarding one's identity is the most profound insecurity. Even stuporous patients will usually give some response to their own name. Standing very close to a comatose patient, holding the hand firmly but gently, and calling the patient by name close to his or her ear may bring a flicker of recognition.

Perception of Space

In old age certain changes occur in total body awareness (proprioception) that affect one's sensorium. Reaction time increases and movement decreases steadily after 20 years of age. Psychomotor slowing seems to be related to four central nervous system processing factors: (1) functional neuron loss reduces signal strength and processing capacity, (2) an increase in random neural activity creates "noise" interference in processing, (3) reconstitution after neural activity takes longer, and (4) arousal levels are diminished. Some people find natural ways to stimulate vestibular function and movement integration. Perhaps old people rock frequently in response to a subliminal need for body movement.

When a patient has been bedridden for some time, it is important for the nurse to alert the patient to unfamiliar environmental sensations and support the patient as he or she regains upright bearings. The patient is in fact seeking navigational bearings to reorient himself or herself, just as a sailor develops "sea legs" and must adapt to the feel of the land again. An older person is particularly vulnerable to this disorientation because the sensory/spatial body systems do not reintegrate as quickly as in youth. Both physical support and psychological support are necessary as older persons regain strength and movement.

Touch Sensitivity

A significant amount of vestibular stimulation, information, and sensual gratification comes about through touching. Touch is used for awareness and protective responses. Touch intensifies bonding and defines boundaries of self. Those who have visual and hearing impairments often compensate by cultivating the sense of touch to a high degree. Touch is often lacking in the older person's environment, which can contribute to a diminishing sensorium (Wharton, 2000).

BOX 14-9   Evidence-Based Practice: Effects of Hand Massage on Comfort of Nursing Home Residents

PURPOSE

To test the effectiveness of hand massage (HM) as an intervention that affects nursing home residents' comfort and satisfaction

SAMPLE/SETTING

50 residents of two nursing homes located in the Midwest. Residents were alert, oriented, able to understand English, and had a projected stay of at least 3 weeks or more.

METHOD

Quasi-experimental design was used to measure differences in comfort and satisfaction between treatment and comparison groups. Treatment group received 6 HM interventions over a 5-week period and comparison group received only 1 HM at the end of the study. Data was collected at three times: Time 1 (baseline); Time 2 (2½ weeks after baseline); and Time 3 (approximately 2½ weeks after Time 2). Comfort was measured using the General Comfort Questionnaire adapted for use in the study. Satisfaction with care was evaluated with a single question asking participants to rate satisfaction with their care on a 6-point scale drawn horizontally on a 10-cm line, with 1 being low satisfaction and 6 high satisfaction. Qualitative and anecdotal data was also evaluated to determine the feasibility of using HM as an intervention during routine care.

FINDINGS

Multivariate analysis of variance results showed no significant findings on group differences for comfort levels. Significant differences in comfort between treatment and comparison groups occurred at Time 2 measurements with the treatment group having higher comfort levels. Mean satisfaction with care was significantly higher at Time 3 for both treatment and comparison groups. Although the treatment group had a greater increase in mean satisfaction over time, the finding was not statistically significant.

IMPLICATIONS

HM may provide comforting and caring effects within a short period of time and may also facilitate connections between the person administering the massage and the recipient. Social interaction between data collectors administering HM may have an effect on comfort and satisfaction scores, making it difficult to determine the unique contribution of HM. Nursing assistants were trained in HM and were to deliver the intervention. However, no staff participated and nursing students were utilized instead. Students felt that HM helped them get to know the resident and was helpful in overcoming their own communication barriers when caring for nursing home residents. HM is easily learned, noninvasive, simple to administer, and enhances satisfaction with care. Encouraging this comfort intervention as a part of daily care by nursing assistants may be beneficial to quality of care.

Data from Kolcaba K et al: Effects of hand massage on comfort of nursing home residents, *Geriatr Nurs* 27(2):85-91, 2006.

Little research has been done on the sense of touch, the physiological and psychological benefits of touch, and the use of touch with older people (Gleeson and Timmins, 2004). Although it varies in individuals, it is believed that touch sensitivity diminishes with aging (Wharton, 2000). Many of the losses of this sensitivity are caused by disease processes; for example, diabetes mellitus causes peripheral neuropathy and the loss of light touch in the extremities. Changes predispose older people to skin damage, particularly the development of pressure ulcers. Loss of sensitivity to hot and cold, or thermal sensitivity, predisposes the elder to burns and hyperthermia and to frostbite and hypothermia. Degenerative changes in Meissner's corpuscles on the hands and feet result in diminished sensitivity of the palms and soles (not on hairy areas) (Wharton, 2000). This may cause

a decrease in reaction time when stepping on a sharp object or touching the burner on the stove.

Less obvious is the deprivation of tactile senses. Introducing texture (e.g., textured upholstery, very soft blankets) into the elder's environment can enhance tactile input and contribute to safety. Some research has suggested that the use of expressive, caring touch by nurses with older people in long-term care settings may be beneficial. Further research is needed to explore the older person's view of touch, particularly the effect of touch with cognitively impaired clients. Box 14-9 presents a recent study investigating the effects of touch in the form of hand massage as a comforting, caring intervention for residents of long-term care (Kolcaba et al., 2006). Chapter 19 discusses touch and the use of touch with older people.

Human Needs and Wellness Diagnoses

Self-Actualization and Transcendence
(Seeking, Expanding, Spirituality, Fulfillment)
Becomes more attuned to inner voices
Recognizes sensory decline as heralding transcendence
Values spiritual aspects of existence
Recognizes sensory apparatus as filters of the universe adapted to
basic levels of human existence

Self-Esteem and Self-Efficacy
(Image, Identity, Control, Capability)
Assertive in obtaining appropriate
assistive devices
Takes responsibility for augmenting
hearing and vision as necessary
Attends carefully to grooming

Belonging and Attachment
(Love, Empathy, Affiliation)
Recognizes need for sensory stimulation
and social interaction
When necessary, seeks alternative modes
of expressing self in relationships
Affiliates with others with similar afflictions when helpful
Accepts assistance graciously when needed

Safety and Security
(Caution, Planning, Protections, Sensory Acuity)
Seeks and accepts augmentation for sensory decline
Recognizes normal changes of aging
Seeks evaluation of abnormal sensory changes
Modifies activities to maintain safety

Biological and Physiological Integrity
(Air, Fluids, Comfort, Activity, Nutrition, Elimination, Skin Integrity)
Recognizes increased energy demands of adaptation to sensory change
Aware of declining sensations and adapts appropriately

These are not all the possible wellness diagnoses that may be identified. The above
are examples of nursing diagnoses that should be considered when planning care
for the older adult.

▲ PROMOTING HEALTHY AGING: IMPLICATIONS FOR GERONTOLOGICAL NURSING

Throughout this chapter we have examined the older person's communication with the environment through the senses and perceptual organizational processes. These factors are fundamental to the maintenance of safety and security. When in disorder, these limitations hinder one's ability to obtain what is needed from the environment. Many older people rely on devices to assist them in this process. Those most frequently used to facilitate environmental contact are hearing aids, glasses, wheelchairs, dentures, canes, and crutches. The nurse's presence in the environment provides a lighthouse to those running aground in their perceptual storms. Here our goal has been to increase the nurse's understanding of how one may assist an older person to effectively negotiate and make meaning of the personal environment, using all capacities to an optimal level.

KEY CONCEPTS

- The sensory apparatus all lose some degree of acuity in the aging process; hearing is the most prevalent loss.
- The importance of cerumen removal is frequently overlooked and often greatly improves hearing.

CASE STUDY: Hearing Impairment

Sonya is a 66-year-old high school nurse/consultant. She retired from the Army Nurse Corps with an officer's rank after serving 20 years, much of it in the Korean conflict with heavy exposure to shelling in the early part of her career. She became aware of hearing loss at about age 45 years, and by age 55 years it had become severe. While in the service she had considerable assistance from noncommissioned personnel and functioned very well. When she entered civilian life, it became more difficult for her to manage but she was unwilling to admit to others her major hearing deficit. During those years she simply attempted to cover it as much as possible, and some of her co-workers thought she was rather obtuse; others suspected her deafness. When she took the position with the school district, she was involved with three high schools, numerous faculty members, and students, and interpersonal communication was a major aspect of her position. When she was evaluated at the end of the first year, it was pointed out that feedback indicated she was inattentive. She did then admit her hearing problem and was advised to get hearing aids. She said, "I've known several people over the years who have hearing aids, and none of them were really satisfied with them. I guess that is why I have not gotten them before now." She complied but, after a few weeks, rarely wore them. The personnel officer of the school board, after hearing several more complaints of inappropriate communication, told her she must wear the hearing aids if she wished to continue in her position. Sonya knew that hearing aids were essential, not only for communication but also for safety—she had almost been hit by a car while walking because she simply did not hear it coming. Yet she did not want to go back to the audiology clinic, because they did not seem to know what they were doing, and each time she saw someone, the person gave her different information. She tried three different types of aids that seemed of little help. She lost confidence in her ear, nose, and throat specialist because he had been unable to help her resolve the ringing in her ears. Now her school district had contracted with a health maintenance organization, and she was not even sure which health care provider she should see.

Based on the case study, develop a nursing care plan using the following procedure*:
- List Sonya's comments that provide subjective data.
- List information that provides objective data.

- From these data identify and state, using accepted format, two nursing diagnoses you determine are most significant to Sonya at this time. List two of Sonya's strengths that you have identified from data.
- Determine and state outcome criteria for each diagnosis. These must reflect some alleviation of the problem identified in the nursing diagnosis and must be stated in concrete and measurable terms.
- Plan and state one or more interventions for each diagnosed problem. Provide specific documentation of the source used to determine the appropriate intervention. Plan at least one intervention that incorporates Sonya's existing strengths.
- Evaluate the success of the intervention. Interventions must correlate directly with the stated outcome criteria to measure the outcome success.

Critical Thinking Questions

1. What are some of the possible reasons Sonya suffered severe hearing loss at so young an age?
2. Discuss the stigma of hearing loss and hearing aids.
3. Obtain a "hearing aid loaner." Instruct students to wear it for several hours and report their reactions in writing. List difficulties experienced.
4. How would you advise Sonya if you were her nurse/friend?
5. Discuss the various kinds of hearing aids and how they differ.
6. Discuss reasons Sonya may have discontinued wearing her hearing aids.
7. What might you suggest that would be helpful in adapting to wearing a hearing aid?
8. What are some of the options you would discuss with Sonya?
9. Which of the various sensory/perceptual changes of aging would you find most difficult to cope with?
10. Discuss the meanings and the thoughts triggered by the student's and elder's viewpoints expressed at the beginning of the chapter. How do these vary from your own experience?

---

*Students are advised to refer to their nursing diagnosis text and identify possible or potential problems.

- Those with hearing impairment often find it difficult to adapt to hearing aids. If they have not recently been to a certified audiologist, they should do so. Many improvements have recently been made, and a proper assessment is essential to obtain a recommendation for the most appropriate hearing aid.
- The loss of vision is greatly feared by many elders. However, vision impairment is only one-third as common as hearing loss, and total loss of vision is rare and caused by pathological processes rather than aging per se.
- When working with the visually impaired, announcing your presence and describing surroundings in vivid detail are usually greatly appreciated.
- Some believe that the "sundowner's" confusion is magnified by sensory impairment and that all experiences of confusion and illusion are magnified by sensory losses.
- Many stimuli in the environment are not perceived within the narrow parameters of the human sensory equipment. Therefore we may sometimes "sense" things that are not clearly discerned by the senses. Some of these may be labeled *intuition, paranormal phenomenon,* or *extrasensory perception.* These would be an area of fruitful investigation with older people.
- Environments and environmental changes have major effects on the sensory input available to elders.
- Environmental sensory deprivation may have seriously disorienting consequences for the elderly.
- Sensory overload when individuals are physically depleted by illness may cause behavioral disturbances and great anxiety. Maintaining a quiet and peaceful environment allows healing energies to be applied toward recovery.

RESEARCH QUESTIONS

How frequently is cost a factor that prohibits elders from using eyeglasses or hearing aids?

Does participation in simulated experiences of sensory loss change a provider's attitudes toward these losses in older people?

What environmental hazards are most detrimental to hearing?

What percentage of older individuals are troubled by tinnitus (ringing or other internally generated sounds)?

What methods are most effective for reducing the interference of tinnitus?

Which sensory losses are elders most aware of experiencing?

Do older individuals who grew up in urban/industrial cities experience sensory losses earlier in their life span than those individuals from a more pastoral environment?

Are there distinct cohort differences in the types and degrees of sensory loss older individuals experience?

How many elders are aware of the specific sensory/perceptual changes that occur with the use of certain medications?

What assistance is most commonly sought for hearing impairment and tinnitus, and is satisfaction obtained?

What is the effect of caring touch on older people with Alzheimer's disease or other dementia-type disorders?

RESOURCES

Visual Impairment
American Foundation for the Blind
11 Penn Plaza, Suite 300
New York, NY 10001
(800) 232-5463
e-mail: afbinfo
www.afb.org

The Choice Magazine Listening Program
(A free service providing tape-recorded articles from more than 100 publications)
www.choicemagazinelistening.org
(888) 724-6423

The Glaucoma Foundation
116 John Street, Suite 1605
New York, NY 10038
(212) 651-1888
e-mail: info
www.glaucomafoundation.org

Glaucoma Research Foundation
490 Post Street, Suite 1427
San Francisco, CA 94102
(800) 826-6693
e-mail: info
www.glaucoma.org

Health information for older adults in large print and "talking" function that reads text aloud
www.nihseniorhealth.gov

Lions Clubs International
300 West 22nd Street
Oakbrook, IL 60523-8842
(630) 571-5466
www.lionsclubs.org

National Association for Visually Handicapped
22 West 21st Street
New York, NY 10010
(212) 889-3141
www.navh.org

National Eye Institute
31 Center Drive, MSC 2510, Building 31, Room 6A32
Bethesda, MD 20892-2510
(301) 496-5248
www.nei.nih.gov

See for Yourself: Vision and Older Adults Program
www.nei.nih.gov/nehep/seeforyourself.asp

Vision Simulator
(to experience visual impairments)
http://visionsimulator.com

Hearing Impairment
American Tinnitus Association
PO Box 5
Portland, OR 97207-0005
(800) 634-8978
www.ata.org

AUDIENT: An Alliance for Accessible Hearing Care
Northwest Lions Foundation for Sight and Hearing
(877) AUDIENT

International Hearing Dog, Inc.
5901 E. 89th Avenue
Henderson, CO 80640
(303) 287-3277
www.ihdi.org

National Institute on Deafness and Other Communication Disorders
National Institutes of Health
31 Center Drive, MSC 2320
Bethesda, MD 20892-2320
e-mail: nidcdinfo
www.nidcd.nih.gov

Self-Help for Hard of Hearing People
7910 Woodmont Avenue, Suite 1200
Bethesda, MD 20814
(301) 657-2248 voice; (301) 657-2249 TTY
www.shhh.org

Stay Tuned: The Challenge of Hearing Loss
(Stories and comments from people with hearing impairments)
Available from:
Communication Sciences Program
City University of New York
Hunter College
425 E. 25th Street
New York, NY 10010-2590

Assistive and Adaptive Equipment
Independent Living Aids, Inc.
PO Box 9022
Hicksville NY 11802-9022
(800) 537-2118
e-mail: can-do
www.independentliving.com

REFERENCES

All About Vision: *Slow or prevent vision loss for AMD*, 2001. (website): *www.allaboutvision.com.*

American Tinnitus Association: *Information about tinnitus*, Portland, Ore, 2002, The Association.

Beck D, Roe-Beck B: Hearing loss. In *Merck manual of geriatrics*, 2000. (website): *www.merck.com.*

Beers MH, Berkow R: *The Merck manual of geriatrics*, ed 3, Whitehouse Station, NJ, 2000, Merck Research Laboratories.

Boyd-Monk H: The eyes have it: understanding problems of the aging eye, *Am J Nurs* 3(5):34-45, 2005.

Bressler NM et al: Potential public health impact of Age-Related Eye Disease Study results: AREDS report no. 11, *Arch Ophthalmol* 121(11):1621-1624, 2003.

Bressler NM et al: Age-related macular degeneration is the leading cause of blindness, *JAMA* 291(15):1900-1901, 2004.

Centers for Disease Control and Prevention (CDC): *Trends in vision and hearing among older Americans*, March 2002. (website): *www.cdc.gov.* Accessed June 24, 2006.

Cotter VT, Strumpf N: *Advanced practice nursing with older adults*, New York, 2002, McGraw-Hill.

Crews JE, Campbell VA: Vision impairment and hearing loss among community-dwelling older Americans: implications for health and functioning, *Am J Public Health* 94(5):823-829, 2004.

Demers K: Hearing screening, *J Gerontol Nurs* 27(11):8-9, 2001.

Desai M et al: *Trends in vision and hearing among older Americans. Aging trends no. 2*, Hyattsville, Md, 2001, Centers for Disease Control and Prevention, U.S. Department of Health and Human Services.

Dinces EA: *Tinnitus. Up-to-date*, 2001. (website): *www.uptodate.com.*

Fozard J, Gordon-Salant S: *Handbook of the psychology of aging*, San Diego, 2001, Academic Press.

Gleeson M, Timmins F: The use of touch to enhance nursing care of older persons in long-term mental health care facilities, *J Psychiatr Ment Health Nurs* 11:541-545, 2004.

Goldzweig CI et al: Preventing and managing visual disability in primary care: clinical applications, *JAMA* 291(12):1497-1502, 2004.

Ham R et al: *Primary care geriatrics*, ed 4, St Louis, 2002, Mosby.

Healthy People 2010: Vision and hearing, 2002. (website): *www.health.gov/healthypeople/document/html./volume2/28vision.htm.*

Higginbotham EJ et al: The Ocular Hypertension Treatment Study: topical medication delays or prevents open-angle glaucoma in African American individuals, *Arch Ophthalmol* 122(6):813-820, 2004.

Iezzoni L et al: Communicating about health care: Observations from persons who are deaf or hard of hearing, *Ann Intern Med* 140(5): 356-362, 2004.

Karev M, Bartz S: Hearing aids. In Mezey MD, editor: *The encyclopedia of elder care*, New York, 2001, Springer.

Keller H: *The story of my life*, Garden City, NY, 1902, Doubleday.

Kolcaba K et al: Effects of hand massage on comfort of nursing home residents, *Geriatr Nurs* 27(2):85-91, 2006.

Luggen AS: Sensory problems. In Luggen A, Meiner S, editors: *NGNA core curriculum for gerontological nursing*, ed 2, St Louis, 2001, Mosby.

Maas ML et al: *Nursing care of older adults: diagnoses, outcomes, and interventions*, St Louis, 2001, Mosby.

McGregor D: Driving over 65: proceed with caution, *J Gerontol Nurs* 28(8):22-26, 2002.

McGwin G Jr et al: Statins and other cholesterol-lowering medications and the presence of glaucoma, *Arch Ophthalmol* 122(6):822-826, 2004.

Miller C: *Nursing for wellness in older adults*, ed 4, Philadelphia, 2004, Lippincott Williams & Wilkins.

National Eye Institute: *Don't lose sight of glaucoma*, 2004. (website): *www.nei.nih.gov.* Accessed June 24, 2006.

Newman CW et al: Retest stability of the tinnitus handicap questionnaire, *Ann Otol Rhinol Largyngol* 104(9 pt 1):718-723, 1995.

O'Neill PA: *Caring for the older adult: a health promotion perspective*, Philadelphia, 2002, Saunders.

Reuben D et al: *Geriatrics at your fingertips*, New York, 2002, Blackwell.

Rowe S et al: Preventing vision loss from chronic eye disease in primary care: scientific review, *JAMA* 291(12):1487-1495, 2004.

Sackett K, Bressler S: *Age-related eye disease study results*, 2001. (website): *www.nei.nih.gov*. Accessed June 25, 2006.

Sacks O: *Seeing voices: a journey into the world of the deaf*, Berkeley, 1989, University of California Press.

Springhouse: *Signs and symptoms*, ed 3, Springhouse, Penn, 2001, Springhouse.

Tabloski P: *Gerontological nursing*, Upper Saddle River, NJ, Pearson Prentice Hall, 2006.

Thoreau HD: *Walden XVIII, Conclusion*, New York, 1946, Dodd, Mead.

Tumosa N: *Aging and the eye*. In The Merck manual of geriatrics online, 2001. (website): *www.merck.com/pubs/mm_geriatrics*.

Wharton MA: Environmental design: accommodating sensory changes in the elderly. In Guccione AA, editor: *Geriatric physical therapy*, ed 2, St Louis, 2000, Mosby.

Wolanin MO, Phillips LRF: *Confusion: prevention and care*, St Louis, 1981, Mosby.

CHAPTER 15

Mobility

Theris A. Touhy

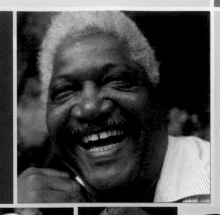

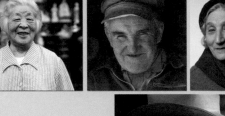

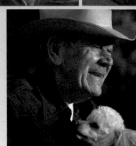

A STUDENT SPECULATES

The thought of needing someone to help me shower and dress and transfer me from a chair to bed requires more acceptance than I have ever had to muster. I'm very good at making the best out of a bad situation, but somehow adapting to something like never walking again cannot be equated with a "bad situation." It is permanent, and it is the sacrifice of my precious independence. I was born on Independence Day! Thinking about these things overwhelms me with sadness.

Holiday, age 22

AN ELDER SPEAKS

I hate to have the family see me like this. You know, I was a military man. I took pride in the way I marched...or just stood at attention. I never imagined a time when I wouldn't be able to walk without assistance.

Jerry, age 78

LEARNING OBJECTIVES

On completion of this chapter, the reader will be able to:

1. Describe age-related changes in bones, joints, and muscles that may predispose older adults to falls and accidents.
2. Discuss the effects of impaired mobility on general function and quality of life.
3. Discuss risk factors for impaired mobility.
4. Discuss factors that increase vulnerability to falls.
5. Describe the effects of restraints, and discuss alternative safety interventions.
6. Describe assessment measures to determine gait and walking stability.
7. Enumerate several measures to reduce fall risks, and identify those at high risk.
8. Discuss the effect of osteoporosis, rheumatic diseases, and Parkinson's disease on mobility, and discuss nursing responses to enhance functional ability.
9. Develop a nursing care plan appropriate to an elder at risk of falling.
10. Consider the impact of available transportation and driving in relation to independence.

Mobility is the capacity one has for movement within the personally available microcosm and macrocosm. In infancy, moving about is the major mode of learning and interacting with the environment. In old age, one moves more slowly and purposefully, sometimes with more forethought and caution. Throughout life, movement remains a significant means of personal contact, sensation, exploration, pleasure, and control. Movement is integral to the attainment of all levels of need as conceived by Maslow. Pride, maintaining dignity, self-care, independence, social contacts, and activity are all

needs identified as important to elders, and all are facilitated by mobility. Thus, in terms of Maslow's Hierarchy and the needs identified by elders, maintaining mobility is an exceedingly important issue.

This chapter focuses on maintaining maximum mobility in health and in the presence of various disorders, the assessment of gait and mobility status, the effects of restraints and immobility, risk factors related to falls, preventive actions that nurses may take to reduce the risks, and aids and interventions that are useful when mobility is impaired. Although

Special thanks to Ann Schmidt Luggen and Catherine Hill, the previous edition contributors, for their content contributions to this chapter.

a number of common chronic diseases are addressed in Chapter 10, osteoporosis, rheumatic diseases, and Parkinson's disease are specifically related to potential challenges to mobility and are discussed in this chapter. Also included are transportation and driving as essential aspects of environmental mobility.

Mobility and comparative degrees of agility are based on muscle strength, flexibility, postural stability, vibratory sensation, cognition, and perceptions of stability. Aging produces changes in muscles and joints, particularly of the back and legs. Strength and flexibility of muscles decrease markedly; endurance decreases to a somewhat lesser extent, especially if activity diminishes as one ages. Movements and range of motion (ROM) become more limited. Normal wear and tear reduce the smooth cartilage of joints. Movement is less fluid as one ages, and joints change as regeneration of tissue slows and muscle wasting occurs. Sarcopenia, a condition prevalent in older people and a marker of frailty, contributes to mobility impairments and disability (Janssen, 2006; Morley, 2002). Some normal gait changes in late life include a narrower standing base, wider swaying when standing, slowed responses, a greater reliance on proprioception, diminished arm swing, and increased care in gait. Steps are shorter and with a decreased stepping motion. These changes are less pronounced in those who remain active and at a desirable weight. Exercise and strength training, even for frail elders, improve mobility and function. Chapter 4 discusses age-related changes in the musculoskeletal system. Chapters 3 and 7 discuss the benefits of exercise to health and wellness of older adults.

Inappropriate clothing may also hinder mobility. Fitted, back-closing, or knee-length clothing is not comfortable for persons confined to wheelchairs, those with limited ROM, or those who require catheters or prosthetic devices. Elders living alone have no one to help them button or zip the back of clothing. This can make dressing and undressing a time-consuming and frustrating experience. Adaptive fashions have been designed to facilitate easy or independent dressing and include features such as back and side openings, Velcro front openings, raglan sleeves, and cape-styled clothing. Slacks with front flaps or extra room in back or longer skirts are helpful. The fabric should be chosen for comfort, durability, attractiveness, and ease of laundering.

Various degrees of immobility are often the temporary or permanent consequences of illness. Falls and fractures often produce periods of immobility. Consequences of immobility are shown in Box 15-1.

On a broader scale, elders frequently have limited environmental mobility because of lack of transportation or loss of driver's license. On the most personal level, some elderly are immobilized by the fear of falling. In summary, many normal and abnormal changes affect the fluidity and comfort of movement and the capacity for involvement with surroundings. Impairment of mobility is highly associated with poor outcomes in older people (Morley et al., 2003).

BOX 15-1   Consequences of Immobility

- Dehydration
- Bronchial pneumonia
- Contractures
- Constipation
- Pressure ulcers
- Incontinence
- Hypothermia
- Iatrogenic complications
- Disability
- Institutionalization
- Loss of independence
- Isolation and depression

BOX 15-2   Goals and Objectives *Healthy People 2000/2010:* Mobility and Safety

- Reduce deaths from falls
- Reduce hip fractures among older adults
- Eliminate racial disparities in the rate of total knee replacement
- Prevent illness and disability related to arthritis and other rheumatic conditions and osteoporosis
- Decrease the proportion of all adults with chronic joint symptoms who have difficulty in performing two or more personal care activities thereby preserving independence
- Increase the proportion of adults ages 18 and older with arthritis who seek help if they experience personal and emotional problems
- Increase the proportion of adults who have seen a health care provider for chronic joint symptoms
- Increase the proportion of persons with arthritis who have had effective, evidence-based arthritis education as an integral part of the management of their condition
- Increase the mean number of days without severe pain among adults who have chronic joint symptoms
- Reduce the proportion of adults with osteoporosis
- Reduce the proportion of adults who are hospitalized for vertebral fractures associated with osteoporosis

From U.S. Department of Health and Human Services: *Healthy People 2010: national health promotion and disease prevention objectives,* Washington, DC, 2000, The Department.

HEALTHY PEOPLE 2000/2010

Healthy People 2010 contains goals and objectives that relate to mobility and safety concerns for older adults. Box 15-2 presents some of these objectives.

DISORDERS AFFECTING MOBILITY

Common conditions that accompany the normal changes of aging, as well as disorders that occur more frequently in the elderly, merit special attention. Such disorders are orthopedic impairments and significantly impede older people. Osteoporosis, gait disorders, Parkinson's disease, strokes, and arthritic conditions markedly affect movement and functional capacities. Mobility may be limited by paresthesias;

TABLE 15-1

Activity Limitations: People Over 65 in the United States

Activity Limitations	Men (in percent)	Women (in percent)
Total (one or more limitations)	**57.7**	**70.5**
Very difficult/unable to walk a quarter of a mile (about 3 city blocks)	16.8	28.3
Very difficult/unable to stand/be on one's feet for 2 hours	16.0	27.4
Very difficult/unable to climb 10 steps without resting	11.9	21.8
Very difficult/unable to sit for 2 hours	3.8	5.8
Very difficult/unable to reach over one's head	5.5	8.3
Very difficult/unable to use one's fingers to grasp or handle small objects	3.2	4.9
Very difficult/unable to lift/carry something as heavy as 10 pounds (such as a full bag of groceries)	7.4	19.1
Very difficult/unable to push/pull large objects (such as a living room chair)	13.1	27.9

From National Center for Health Statistics, 2002c, Table 19.
NOTE: The reference population for these data is the civilian noninstitutionalized population.

hemiplegia; neuromotor disturbances; fractures; foot, knee, and hip problems; and illnesses that deplete one's energy. All these conditions are likely to occur more frequently and have more devastating effects as one ages. Many elders in later years have some of these impairments, with women significantly outnumbering men in this respect. Mobility-related tasks may be difficult for some elderly men and women to accomplish (Table 15-1).

FALLS: CAUSES AND CONSEQUENCES

Falls are one of the most important geriatric syndromes and the leading cause of morbidity and mortality for people older than 65 years (Cesari et al., 2002). A fall has been defined in the literature as unintentionally coming to rest on a lower area such as the ground or floor (Buchner et al., 1993). A recent study (Zecevic et al., 2006) comparing the definition of a fall and reasons for falls among seniors, health care providers, and the research literature suggested that the word *fall* is interpreted in many different ways. Often, the terms *slips*, *trips*, and *falls* are used interchangeably, and *near falls*, *mishaps*, or *missteps*, not usually reported, may be important in assessing fall risk. Exactly what constitutes a fall for reporting procedures in institutions is also problematic and can lead to inconsistencies in data (Zecevic et al., 2006). Therefore it is important to define a fall in words that seniors understand and to use an operational definition of falls in all research and fall-reporting data. Further recommendations from the study included asking older people about falls that did not result in injury and assessing the circumstances of a fall, near fall, mishaps, or missteps as important information for prevention of future falls.

Falls are a significant public health problem, and the federal government and many aging groups have made fall risk reduction a major initiative. All falls in the nursing home setting are considered sentinel events and must be reported to the Centers for Medicare & Medicaid Services (CMS). The Joint Commission (TJC) has established national patient safety goals for fall reduction in hospitals, assisted living

and long-term care facilities, and home care. The National Center for Injury Prevention and Control and the National Resource Center for Safe Aging provide valuable information on falls and fall risk reduction programs useful to older people and professionals. Additional resources are listed in the Resources section at the end of this chapter. Following are some statistics about falls and fall-related concerns:

- Injury as a result of falls is the leading cause of death in older adults.
- The fall-related mortality rate increases with advanced age.
- Of those who fall and require hospitalization, 50% will die within 1 year.
- One third of people older than 65 years fall at least one time each year, and about half of those fall repeatedly. After the age of 75 years, the rates are higher (American Geriatrics Society, 2001).
- Falls account for 40% of nursing home admissions annually (Tideiksaar, 2005).
- Of those who fall, 20% to 30% suffer moderate to severe injuries such as hip fractures or head traumas that reduce mobility and independence and increase the risk of premature death (National Center for Injury Prevention and Control [NCIPC], 2006).
- Up to 20% of hospitalized patients and 45% of those in long-term care facilities will fall. In these settings, injury rates are considerably higher with 10% to 25% of institutional falls resulting in fracture, laceration, or the need for hospital care (American Geriatrics Society, 2001).
- Direct care costs related to falls are estimated at more than $20 billion and projected to rise to over $34 billion by 2020 (Chang et al., 2004; Quigley, 2005).

Falls are a symptom of a problem, although they become the focus of the problem when they occur. The etiology of falls is multifactorial; falls may indicate neurological, sensory, cardiac, cognitive, medication, and musculoskeletal problems or impending illness. A fall is usually an interaction between an environmental factor, such as a wet floor, and an intrinsic factor, such as limited vision, cognitive impairment, or gait problems. In institutional settings, iatrogenic factors such as limited staffing, lack of toileting programs, and restraints and side rails also interact to increase fall risk. Frail older people with mobility and functional limitations are at the greatest risk for falls (Tideiksaar, 2005).

Falls are rarely benign in older people. Incomplete diagnosis of reasons for a fall can result in repeated incidents. Post-fall assessments are essential to prevention of future falls and implementation of risk-reduction programs, particularly in institutional settings (Gray-Micelli et al., 2005). If the elder cannot tell you about the circumstances of a fall, information should be obtained from staff or witnesses. Having an older person keep a fall diary documenting the circumstances of the fall may be helpful. The American Geriatrics Society provides a patient education tool "Story of Your Falls" (*www.americangeriatrics.org*) that can be completed by the older person and brought to the health care provider (Box 15-3). Institutions may also consider a fall diary as a way of evaluating patterns of falling and organizing information from post-fall assessments. Wagner et al. (2005) reported significant improvement in accurate documentation of falls, as well as "near misses" not usually reported, in the nursing home setting with the use of a computerized falls menu-driven incident–reporting system (MDIRS). Box 15-4 provides information for a post-fall assessment that can be used in health care institutions.

Drop attacks, a condition first described in 1948, are characterized by a sudden and unexpected fall to the ground without loss of consciousness in an otherwise healthy individual (Rich, 2005). The syndrome is reported to occur more frequently in older women and was thought to be the result of brainstem ischemia caused by impaired vertebral artery blood flow. Older people may attribute the fall to "their legs giving way under them." Drop attacks can cause hip trochanter cracks, femur fractures, or both. Possible causes may be osteoporotic bone erosion that accompanies aging and that, in some women with a high-risk profile, reaches pathological proportions. When osteoporosis of this magnitude occurs, the bone can no longer bear the weight of the individual in walking. It is difficult to determine whether the fall creates the fracture or the fracture creates the fall. Some older adults may think falls and drop attacks are just part of growing older. Providing education about falls and proper assessment and treatment to prevent falls is an important nursing intervention.

The prevalence, etiology, and prognosis of drop attacks are relatively unknown because it can be difficult to differentiate this syndrome from falls attributable to other identifiable causes. However, in a recent study by Parry and Kenny (2005), an attributable diagnosis was found in 90% of drop attack cases. The primary causes of most falls were found to be cardiovascular (vasovagal syncope, orthostatic hypotension, carotid sinus hypersensitivity), followed by neurological causes (primarily vestibular disorders), gait and balance disturbances, and drug-related causes. Older people experiencing drop attacks should have a thorough history and physical examination, especially cardiovascular evaluation, to determine existing conditions contributing to the fall. Cardiovascular abnormalities are being recognized as a significant fall risk factor (American Geriatrics Society, 2001; Nnodim and Alexander, 2005).

Factors Contributing to Falls

Falls are generally classified as extrinsic (related to environmental factors), intrinsic (related to host factors), or iatrogenic (related to treatment factors). After age 65 years, individuals fall most frequently because of external reasons; however, with increasing age, internal and locomotor reasons become increasingly prevalent. Fall risk factors that increase proportionally as one ages are disturbances in visual acuity, cognitive impairment, postural hypotension, cardiac arrhythmias, uncontrolled diabetes, depressive symptoms, lower extremity weakness, gait disturbances, and the use of four or more prescription medications (particularly psychotropics) (Tinetti, 2003). Abnormal gait affects 20% to 50% of people older than 65 years and increases susceptibility to

---

BOX 15-3 Story of Your Falls

- When was this fall? Date and time of day?
- Where were you when you fell?
- Think about the items listed below. Then in the box below, write down everything you can remember about your fall.
- What were you doing before you fell?
- How did you feel just before?
- How did you feel going down?
- What part of your body hit?
- What did it strike?
- What was injured?
- Anything else you recall?
- Do you think you passed out?
- Where were you when you fell?
- What were you doing when you fell?

Answer the following questions about how you felt before this fall:

Were you dizzy?	Yes ___	No ___
Did the room spin around?	Yes ___	No ___
Did your vision blur?	Yes ___	No ___
Did your heart skip?	Yes ___	No ___
Did you feel weak?	Yes ___	No ___
Did you pass out?	Yes ___	No ___
Did you feel like you might pass out?	Yes ___	No ___
Were you wearing shoes?	Yes ___	No ___
Was it dark where you fell?	Yes ___	No ___
Were you going to the bathroom when you fell?	Yes ___	No ___

If you have had other falls or near falls different from this fall, describe those, too.

Adapted from *Story of your falls*, American Geriatrics Society. (website): *www.americangeriatrics.org*. Used with permission from the American Geriatrics Society.

BOX 15-4 Post-Fall Assessment Suggestions

HISTORY

Description of the fall from the resident or witness
Resident's opinion of the cause of the fall
Circumstances of the fall (trip or slip)
Person's activity at the time of the fall
Presence of co-morbid conditions, such as a previous stroke, Parkinson's disease, osteoporosis, seizure disorder, sensory deficit, joint abnormalities, depression, cardiac disease
Medication review
Associated symptoms, such as chest pain, palpitations, light-headedness, vertigo, fainting, weakness, confusion, incontinence, or dyspnea
Time of day and location of the fall
Presence of acute illness

PHYSICAL EXAMINATION

Vital signs: postural blood pressure changes, fever, or hypothermia
Head and neck: visual impairment, hearing impairment, nystagmus, bruit
Heart: arrhythmia or valvular dysfunction
Neurological signs: altered mental status, focal deficits, peripheral neuropathy, muscle weakness, rigidity or tremor, impaired balance
Musculoskeletal signs: arthritic changes, range of motion (ROM), podiatric deformities or problems, swelling, redness or bruises, abrasions, pain on movement, shortening and external rotation of lower extremities

FUNCTIONAL ASSESSMENT

Observe and inquire about the following:
  Functional gait and balance: observe resident rising from chair, walking, turning, and sitting down
  Balance test, mobility, use of assistive devices or personal assistance, extent of ambulation, restraint use, prosthetic equipment
  Activities of daily living: bathing, dressing, transferring, toileting

ENVIRONMENTAL ASSESSMENT

Staffing patterns, unsafe practice in transferring, delay in response to call light
Faulty equipment
Use of bed, chair alarm
Call light within reach
Wheelchair, bed locked
Adequate supervision
Clutter, walking paths not clear
Dim lighting
Glare
Uneven flooring
Wet, slippery floors
Poor-fitting seating devices
Inappropriate footwear
Inappropriate eye wear

---

fall. Arthritis of the hip and knee and deformities of the foot are common causes of gait disturbances and instability (Rubenstein and Trueblood, 2004).

Declines in depth perception, proprioception, vibratory sense, and normotensive response to postural changes are important factors although the majority of falls occur in individuals with multiple medical problems. The month after hospital discharge and episodes of acute illness or exacerbations of chronic illness are also times of high fall risk (Tinetti, 2003). A relationship may exist also between urinary tract infections (UTIs) and falls, particularly in nursing home patients with dementia. One study noted insomnia as a fall risk factor in institutionalized elders who may get out of bed during the night while drowsy and fall (Avidan et al., 2005). Box 15-5 presents fall risk factors.

Fall Risk Assessment. A variety of fall risk assessment instruments are available, and those that have been evaluated for reliability and validity should be used in institutional settings rather than creating new instruments. Fall risk assessments provide general information about a person's risk factors but need to be combined with additional individual assessment so that appropriate fall risk reduction interventions can be developed and modifiable risk factors identified and treated. Capezuti (2004) suggested that ad-

ditional research is needed to develop valid, reliable instruments to differentiate levels of fall risk in various settings. The Morse et al. (1989) Fall Scale (*www.nursing.upenn.edu/centers/hcgne/gero_tips/PDF_files/Morse_Fall_Scale.htm*) and the Hendrich II Scale (Hendrich et al., 2003) (*www.hartfordign.org/publications/trythis/issue08.pdf*) are commonly used fall risk instruments in acute and long-term care. The presence of dementia may call for specific risk assessment and fall risk reduction interventions. Further research is needed in this area.

Fear of Falling. Even if a fall does not result in injury, falls contribute to a loss of confidence that leads to reduced physical activity, increased dependency, and social withdrawal (Rubenstein et al., 2003). Fear of falling (fallophobia) may restrict an individual's life space (area in which an individual carries on activities). Fear of falling is an important predictor of general functional decline and a risk factor for future falls. Frequent falls contribute significantly to the downward spiral in frail older people (Morley, 2002). Resnick (2002) suggests that nursing staff may also contribute to fear of falling in their patients by telling them not to get up by themselves or by using restrictive devices to keep them from independently moving about. More appropriate nursing responses are to assess fall risk and design individual in-

BOX 15-5 Fall Risk Factors for Elders

CONDITIONS

Diabetes
Female or single (incidence increases with age)
Maternal history of hip fracture
Sedative and alcohol use, psychoactive medications
Previous falls, unsteadiness, dizziness
Acute and recent illness
Pathological conditions, drop attacks
Cognitive impairment, disorientation
Weakness of lower extremities
Abnormalities of balance and gait
Foot problems
Depression, anxiety
Decreased vision or hearing
Fear of falling
Postural hypotension
Postprandial drop in blood pressure
Terminal drop (dies in following 1-2 years)
Skeletal and neuromuscular changes that predispose to weakness and postural imbalance
Acute and severe chronic illness, debilitation
Functional limitations in self-care activities
Multiple disorders and medications
Wheelchair bound
Sensory deficits
Decreased weight
Inability to rise from a chair without using the arms
Slow walking speed
Predisposing physiological and psychological conditions
Preoccupation with stressors
Anxiety related to previous falls

Four or more medications, especially psychotropics
History of fractures
Dehydration

SITUATIONS

Urinary urgency, particularly nocturia
Environmental hazards
Recent relocation, unfamiliarity with new environment
Inadequate response to transfer and toileting needs
Assistive devices needed for walking
Inadequate or missing safety rails, particularly in bathroom
Poorly designed or unstable furniture
Low stools
High chairs and beds
Uneven floor surfaces
Glossy, highly waxed floors
Wet, greasy, icy surfaces
Inadequate lighting
General clutter
Pets that inadvertently trip an individual
Electrical cords
Loose or uneven stair treads
Reaching for a high shelf
Changing positions (sitting to standing or transferring to or from a bed or wheelchair)
Inability to reach personal items, lack of access to call bell or inability to use
Side rails, restraints
Lack of access to bathrooms
Lack of staff training in fall risk reduction techniques

Data from Rubinstein I et al. *Clin Geriatr* 11(1):52-61, 2003; Tinetti ME et al: Risk factors for falls among elderly persons living in the community, *N Engl J Med* 319(26):1701-1707, 1988.

terventions and safety plans that enhance mobility and independence and decrease fall risk.

A falls efficacy scale, an instrument to measure fear of falling based on self-perceived ability to avoid falls during nonhazardous activities of daily living (ADLs), may be useful in predicting functional decline based on limitations induced by fear (Tinetti et al., 1990, 1994). In research with this instrument, elderly individuals named activities they most avoided because of fear of falling as follows: reaching into cabinets or closets, taking a bath or shower, walking around the house, and getting in and out of bed. The bedroom and bathroom are the most common areas for falls in the home (Tanner, 2003). When performing a functional or home assessment, these activities should be assessed and suggestions provided for ways the person can alter the activities and feel more secure. Home safety assessment is discussed further on p. 380 and in Chapter 16. The following scenario depicts the possible consequences of a fear of falling:

Mr. W. was a sprightly 83-year-old widower, the son of an immigrant laundry worker. He had lived in San Francisco's Chinatown all his life. He hurried about in the crowded area and bartered with the market vendors for his fresh vegetables and other needs. He tripped and fell one day for no known reason and suffered shoulder contusions and a mild concussion. After an examination and thorough radiographic studies, he was released from the emergency department with the physician's warning, "Be careful, you are an old man." Gradually Mr. W. began to believe this and slowed his pace, carefully watching the ground to see that there was nothing to trip him. He began to shuffle rather than walk. All of this was so gradual that it was a year before his family realized he was not leaving his room very often. In deference and respect, they did not interfere until, during a surprise visit, they discovered he had no food in his flat, dirty clothes were heaped about, and it appeared that he rarely left his bed. He had obeyed the physician.

▲ Promoting Healthy Aging: Implications for Gerontological Nursing

Assessment. Patients who fall present a complex diagnostic challenge to physicians and nurses. The American Geriatrics Society *Guideline for the Prevention of Falls in Older Persons* (2001) recommends that all persons older than 65 years be asked at least once a year about falls. A history of falls is an important predictor of future falls, and any older person who reports a fall should be observed using the get-up-and-go test (Mathias et al., 1986). If unsteadiness or difficulty is observed during this test, the person should have further assessment. An older person who is seen after a fall, who demonstrates abnormalities of gait and/or balance, or who has had recurrent falls should have a comprehensive fall evaluation (CFE).

Assessment must be multifactorial and should include the following (Tinetti, 2003):

- Review and possible reduction of medications
- Balance and gait
- Postural pulse and blood pressure
- Cardiovascular (heart rate and blood pressure responses to carotid sinus stimulation if appropriate), neurological, and musculoskeletal systems
- Foot deformities, pain, or limitations in ROM
- Vision and hearing
- Muscle strength
- Lower extremity peripheral nerves
- Proprioception
- Reflexes
- Cortical, extrapyramidal and cerebellar function
- History of falls
- Acute or chronic medical problems
- Urinary urgency and incontinence
- Dehydration and anemia
- Cognition
- Nutrition

Assessment of mood is also important because depression has been found to be a risk factor for falls in some studies (Cesari et al., 2002). Box 15-6 provides fall assessment and management recommendations.

Appropriate assessment of postural changes in pulse and blood pressure is important. Clinically significant postural hypotension (orthostasis) is detected in up to 30% of older people (Tinetti, 2003). Postural hypotension is considered a decrease of 20 mm Hg (or more) in systolic pressure or a decrease of 10 mm Hg (or more) in diastolic pressure. Irvin and White (2004) suggested that assessment of postural hypotension in everyday nursing practice is often overlooked or assessed inaccurately. Postural hypotension is more common in the morning so assessment should occur then (Morley, 2002). Box 15-7 provides recommendations for the measurement of postural hypotension. All older persons should be cautioned against sudden rising from sitting or supine positions, particularly after eating. Postprandial hypotension (PPH) occurs after ingestion of a carbohydrate meal and may be related to the release of a vasodilatory peptide. PPH is more common in people with diabetes and Parkinson's disease but has been found in approximately 25% of persons who fall (Morley, 2002).

The nurse is more likely to have had extended opportunities to observe the elder's function whether in the community or in an institution. Families' observations also provide important data. Older people may be reluctant to share information about falls because of fear of losing independence,

so it is important to use judgment and empathy in eliciting information about falls, assuring the person that many modifiable factors can increase safety and maintain independence. The following sections discuss assessment and interventions in greater detail.

Assessing Balance and Gait. Balance and gait assessment may be the single best predictor of fall risk (Schneider and Mader, 2002). Many studies report that the velocity of walking decreases with age (Howe and Oldham, 2001), and although gait varies widely among elders, often a gait pattern may be seen. The mean stride length of men is 89% of their height when young and 79% of their height at age 80 years. Women's stride length also is reduced. Because balance diminishes with increasing age, there is a compensating increase in stride width and angle of the feet. The double stance is the most stable phase of gait, and elders spend more time in this phase. The swing phase of gait is a vulnerable time because only one foot is in contact with the ground (Table 15-2).

Balance disorders may result from arthritis, stroke, Parkinson's disease, diabetic neuropathy, cardiac disease, and deconditioning. Elders who have spent much time in bed or at rest can become deconditioned in a very short time. Balance may be tested in the clinical or home setting. Inability to perform the test indicates increased risk of falling. See Box 15-8 for balance assessment tests.

Interventions. If the elder appears unstable, further assessment is necessary. A physical therapy evaluation is also a good option. The physical therapist can instruct the elder on strengthening exercises, as well as balance exercises, or prescribe assistive devices with training. Fall risk reduction and safety education should also be provided. If the elder is institutionalized, a fall risk reduction and safety plan of care should be in place.

Gait Disorders

Gait disorders make one vulnerable to tripping and falling. In addition, they impede activity and increase anxiety in the elder who is aware of instability in gait. At least 20% of older adults living in the community have problems walking. This increases to approximately 50% in adults 85 years and older (American Geriatrics Society, 2006). Given the magnitude of this problem, routine examination of the elderly should include not only gait but also postural assessment (Box 15-9). Normal gait involves the vestibular system of balance, proprioception (sensitivity to body in motion), neurophysiological integrity, and vision.

Arthritis of the hip, the knee, and especially the foot is a common cause of instability. Arthritis of the knee may result in ligamentous weakness and instability, causing the legs to give way or collapse. Foot deformities and ill-fitting shoes also contribute to gait problems, so it is important to inspect the feet and footwear. Muscle weakness is often experienced in hyperthyroidism and hypothyroidism, hypokalemia, hyperparathyroidism, osteomalacia, and hypophosphatemia, and in some cases it is brought on by various medications.

BOX 15-6 Recommended Components of Clinical Assessment and Management for Older Persons Living in the Community Who are at Risk for Falling

ASSESSMENT AND RISK FACTOR	MANAGEMENT
Circumstances of previous falls*	Changes in environment and activity to reduce the likelihood of recurrent falls
Medication use High-risk medications (e.g., benzodiazepines, other sleeping medications, neuroleptics, antidepressants, anticonvulsants, or class IA antiarrhythmics)*,†,‡ Four or more medications‡	Review and reduction of medications
Vision* Acuity <20/60 Decreased depth perception Decreased contrast sensitivity Cataracts	Ample lighting without glare; avoidance of multifocal glasses while walking; referral to an ophthalmologist
Postural blood pressure (after ≥5 minutes in a supine position, immediately after standing, and 2 minutes after standing)‡ ≥20 mm Hg (or ≥20%) drop in systolic pressure, with or without symptoms, either immediately or after 2 minutes of standing	Diagnosis and treatment of underlying cause, if possible; review and reduction of medications; modification of salt restriction; adequate hydration; compensatory strategies (e.g., elevation of head of bed, rising slowly, or dorsiflexion exercises); pressure stockings; pharmacological therapy if the previous strategies fail
Balance and gait†,‡ Patient's report or observation of unsteadiness Impairment on brief assessment (e.g., the Get-Up-and-Go Test or performance-oriented assessment of mobility)	Diagnosis and treatment of underlying cause, if possible; reduction of medications that impair balance; environmental interventions; referral to physical therapist for assistive devices and for gait and progressive balance training
Targeted neurological examination Impaired proprioception* Impaired cognition* Decreased muscle strength†,‡	Diagnosis and treatment of underlying cause, if possible; increase in proprioceptive input (with an assistive device or appropriate footwear that encases the foot and has a low heel and thin sole); reduction of medications that impede cognition; awareness on the part of caregivers of cognitive deficits; reduction of environmental risk factors; referral to physical therapist for gait, balance, and strength training
Targeted musculoskeletal examination: examination of legs (joints and range of motion) and examination of feet*	Diagnosis and treatment of the underlying cause, if possible; referral to physical therapist for strength, range-of-motion, and gait and balance training and for assistive devices; use of appropriate footwear; referral to podiatrist
Targeted cardiovascular examination† Syncope Arrhythmia (if there is known cardiac disease, an abnormal electrocardiogram, and syncope)	Referral to cardiologist; carotid-sinus massage (in the case of syncope)
Home-hazard evaluation after hospital discharge†,‡	Removal of loose rugs and the use of nightlights, nonslip bathmats, and stair rails; other interventions as necessary

From Tinetti M: Preventing falls in elderly persons, *N Engl J Med,* 348(1), 42-49, 2003.
*Recommendation of this assessment is based on observational data that the finding is associated with an increased risk of falling.
†Recommendation of this assessment is based on one or more randomized controlled trials of a single intervention.
‡Recommendation of this assessment is based on one or more randomized controlled trials of a multifactorial intervention strategy that included this component.

Diabetes, dementia, alcoholism, and vitamin B deficiencies may cause neurological damage and resultant gait problems (Resnick et al., 2001).

Vestibular dysfunction causes unsteadiness in walking and listing to one side or the other when the eyes are closed. The individual cannot focus well on a fixed target while moving or on a moving object while standing still. Some elders experience dizziness, unsteadiness, and light-headedness. Postural instability increases and is exacer-

bated by some medications. Extrapyramidal symptoms produce a shuffling gait in some individuals taking psychotropic medications and in those who have Parkinson's disease or parkinsonian symptoms. Postural reflex impairment occurs with aging, and postural sway, forward and backward, can be observed when an individual stands still. Mobility aids such as canes and walkers can take the load off painful joints and increase balance and stability and provide a sense of security. Even lightly touching firm surfaces like

---

BOX 15-7   Assessment of Orthostatic (Postural) Hypotension

- Assessment should be done in the morning.
- Have the patient lie supine for 10 minutes and obtain blood pressure and heart rate.
- Take blood pressure and heart rate immediately after the patient arises and ask about dizziness. (Dizziness may be more clinically important than change in pressure reading. The patient may not be experiencing postural hypotension but may have short periods of dizziness and imbalance related to baroreceptor response time. This is important for teaching about fall prevention and the importance of changing positions slowly.)
- After the patient maintains an upright position for 3 minutes, obtain blood pressure and heart rate again.

From Irvin D, White M: The importance of accurately assessing orthostatic hypotension, *Geriatr Nurs* 25(2):99-101, 2004.

TABLE 15-2

Gait Changes in Aging

Factor	Aging Effect
Velocity	Decreases
Length of step	Decreases
Length of stride	Decreases
Width of stride	Increases
Steps per minute (cadence)	Decreases or changes little
Double stance phase of walking	Increases
Rotation of hip	Increases
Rotation of trunk	Decreases
Ankle movement	Decreases
Toe clearance	Decreases

Adapted from Howe T, Oldham JA: Posture and balance. In Trew M, Everett T, editors: *Human movement*, ed 4, St Louis, 2001, Mosby.

BOX 15-8   Balance Assessment Tests

1. Get up from an armchair, walk about 10 feet, turn around, walk back to the chair, and sit down (get-up-and-go test). If this can be done in less than 20 seconds and there is no staggering when turning and no need to hold onto something or someone, balance is very good.
2. A variation on the get-up-and-go test is to rise from the armchair without using hands, walk about 10 feet, turn around, walk back to the chair, turn, and sit down (no time frame). Watch for smooth motion, deviation from the walking path, and smooth turns.
3. Put one foot directly in front of the other (heel to toe). Hold position for 30 seconds.
4. Stand on two feet; close eyes. Hold a steady position for 15 seconds.
5. Bend down to pick up an object from the floor; retrieve the object within 5 seconds.
6. Stand with eyes open, placing feet together as closely as possible. For safety, have another person stand behind the elder. Touch or nudge the elder's chest on the sternum with enough gentle force to cause imbalance. The appropriate response is to stretch out one's arms to the front to compensate and possibly take a step backward.

---

vocate for proper and thorough assessment and diagnosis. Nurses are the most likely providers to observe gait disturbances. A guide nurses can use for gait and balance problem descriptions is provided in Box 15-10. The Tinetti Balance and Gait Evaluation is precise and has been tested for validity and reliability (Tinetti, 1986) (see Appendix 15-A). A number of tests may need to be ordered to discover the cause of the gait disorder. These include x-ray examination and computed tomography (CT) of the cervical spine to assess for a cervical myelopathy; electromyography and nerve conduction studies for peripheral neuropathies; laboratory tests, including thyroid, vitamin B_{12}, folate, complete blood count (CBC), electrolytes, and liver function; CT of the head for normal-pressure hydrocephalus or stroke or tumor; lumbar puncture for infection or amyotrophic lateral sclerosis (ALS); and electrocardiogram (ECG) for arrhythmias and cardiac events (Resnick et al., 2001).

Interventions. Well-fitting shoes, canes, leg braces, pain relief, handrails, or walkers may improve mobility status. The nurse is responsible for initial assessment of gait disturbance and gaining appropriate professional consultation for prostheses, orthotic and orthopedic shoes, and gait training. Rehabilitative specialists are usually responsible for teaching gait training to patients, but nurses must understand concepts and specific methods because they will assist the patient to carry out correct procedures on a daily basis. A complete analysis of gait patterns and characteristics requires special equipment and expertise, but simple gait observation by nurses can yield valuable information. In most gait disturbances, nervousness or anxiety aggravates the condition.

walls or "furniture surfing" while walking can help with balance (American Geriatrics Society, 2001).

Assessment. The get-up-and-go test is a practical assessment tool for elderly people and can be conducted in any setting (Resnick et al., 2001). The client is asked to rise from a straight-back chair, stand briefly, walk forward about 10 feet, turn, walk back to the chair, turn around, and sit down. Performance is graded on a 5-point scale from 1 (normal) to 5 (severely abnormal). The quality of the movement is assessed for impaired balance. A score of 3 or higher suggests high risk of falling. Gait speed and agility have been found to correlate well with functional level. Marked gait disorders are not normally a consequence of aging alone but are more likely indicative of an underlying pathological condition.

Investigation of gait disorders in elderly people is a complex issue, and it is important that nurses recognize and ad-

BOX 15-9 Gait Disorders

ATAXIA

Wide-based gait with frequent side-stepping

NORMAL PRESSURE HYDROCEPHALUS

Step height reduced, shuffling gait as if feet stuck to floor; short steps, unsteady speed, and ataxia

PARKINSON'S DISEASE

Stooped posture; short, rapid, shuffling gait; uncontrollable propulsion or retropulsion; "freeze" walk when feet abruptly halt while body continues to move forward

SPONDYLOTIC CERVICAL MYELOPATHY

Spastic, shuffling gait; deep tendon reflexes below level of compression increase muscle tone; sometimes nonspecific, e.g., "clumsy feet," "legs gave way"

SENILE GAIT

Associated with stooped posture; hip and knee flexion; diminished arm swing; stiffness in turning; broad-based, small steps with poor gait intention

HEMIPLEGIA

Poor arm and leg swing, affected limb does not bend at knee; ankle fixed and inverted as leg swings in wide circle; foot tends to drag

OSTEOMALACIA

Ill-defined skeletal pain; pain on weight bearing; unstable, waddling gait

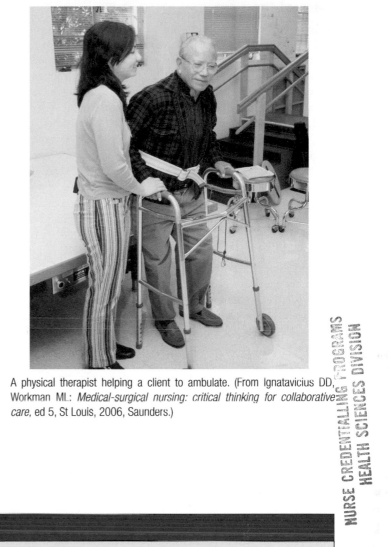

A physical therapist helping a client to ambulate. (From Ignatavicius DD, Workman ML: *Medical-surgical nursing: critical thinking for collaborative care*, ed 5, St Louis, 2006, Saunders.)

BOX 15-10 Gait Description and Assessment

Pain in back and lower limbs	Antalgic gait; short steps flexed toward affected side
Contracture or ankylosis	Short-leg gait; wide outward swing of affected side, unaffected knee flexed, and body bent forward
Foot deformities	Loss of spring and rhythm in step, toes inward or outward bilaterally or unilaterally
Footdrop	Foot slap heard caused by knee raised higher than usual
Gluteus medius weakness	Waddle gait; drop and lag in swing phase of unaffected side, seen in osteomalacia and senile gait in women
Stroke	Wide, open, flinging foot on affected side, uncoordinated
Cerebroarteriosclerosis	Bilateral involvement manifested by extremely short steps
Parkinsonism	Festinating gait; short, hurried, often on tiptoe, or rigid, tremorous, slow, tends toward retropulsion, mincing
État lacunaire	Similar to Parkinson's gait, irregular footsteps
Dementia	Slow, shuffling, apraxic, short steps
Peripheral neuropathy	Difficulty lifting feet, stumbles easily
Subdural hematoma	Ataxia, prominent feature is gait disturbance
Cerebellar ataxia	Staggering, unsteady, irregular, wide-based gait; inappropriate foot placement
Vitamin B_{12} deficiency	Paresthesias, unsteadiness, foot dragging
Endocrine disorders	Gait ataxia, particularly with hypothyroidism
Medications	Ataxia, parkinsonian gait, imbalance

NURSE CREDENTIALLING PROGRAMS HEALTH SCIENCES DIVISION

Care of the Feet

Care of the feet is an important aspect of mobility, comfort, and a stable gait and one that is often neglected. Some older persons are unable to walk comfortably, or at all, because of neglect of corns, bunions, and overgrown nails. Other causes of problems may be traced to loss of fat cushioning and resilience with aging, diabetes, ill-fitting shoes, poor arch support, excessively repetitious weight-bearing activities, obesity, or uneven distribution of weight on feet. As many as 35% of persons living at home may have significant foot disability that goes untended. Foot problems and assessment and care of the feet are discussed in Chapter 8.

Feet and footwear should be inspected as a part of assessment and proper foot care taught to older people and their caregivers. Podiatric referral should be available to older people in both home and institutional settings. Well-fitting walking shoes with low heels and a relatively thin, firm sole (leather) and interior are recommended. Rubber-soled shoes such as sneakers, often recommended for older people, can increase the risk of stumbling while walking, particularly if the person is not accustomed to this type of shoe. This type of shoe may provide too much "sway" and may not promote good balance (American Geriatrics Society, 2001). Orthotic and orthopedic shoes may be indicated for certain foot problems and can greatly enhance mobility and comfort.

Assessment of the Environment

Environmental (extrinsic) factors require modification for safety. In the home, look at the floor and the position of furniture. If you need to walk around furniture, it is hazardous. Remove throw rugs, or use double-sided tape or a non-slip backing so the rugs will not slip. Pick up items on the floor and stairs. Coil or tape cords and wires next to the wall so you cannot trip over them. If you have stairs, fix loose or uneven steps. Use an overhead light at the top and bottom of the stairs with a switch at the top and bottom as well. Light switches that glow are helpful. Make sure the carpet is attached to every step, or remove carpet and attach non-slip rubber treads to the stairs. Fix loose handrails, and make sure they are on both sides of the stairs and are as long as the stairs. Paint a contrasting color on the top edge of all steps so you can see the stairs better. In the kitchen, keep items you use often on the lower kitchen shelves. Never use a chair as a stepstool. If you must use a stepstool, get one with a bar to hold on to. For bathroom safety, put a non-slip rubber mat or self-stick strips on the floor of the tub and shower. Put grab bars inside the tub and next to the toilet. Consider a raised toilet seat, a hand-held shower device, and a shower chair. Place a lamp close to the bed and a nightlight so you can see where you are walking. Wear shoes both inside and outside the house, and avoid going barefoot or wearing slippers. Improve the lighting in your house. Put in brighter bulbs (at least 60 watts); florescent bulbs are bright and cost less to use. Have uniform lighting in a room, add lighting to dark areas, and hang curtains or shades to reduce glare. Keep emergency numbers in large print near a phone. Have a cordless phone or put a phone near the floor in case you fall and cannot get up. Think about wearing an alarm device that will bring help if you fall and cannot get up (NCIPC, 2006). Chapter 16 further discusses home safety.

In institutional settings, hallways and rooms should be free of clutter and personal objects positioned within easy reach. Patients should be assessed for fall risk and individualized fall risk reduction plans instituted. Proper equipment to maintain safety is essential and may include bed or chair alarms, motion sensors, proper assistive devices, and low beds. The Minimum Data Set (MDS) requires information about a history of falls and hip fractures within the past 180 days, balance assessment, and the fall resident assessment protocol (RAP) provides an excellent overview of fall risk and fall assessment (Box 15-11).

Environmental barriers often discourage ambulation among persons in various settings. In the outer environment, steps and curbs may be too high. Buses, subway trains, elevators, revolving doors, and escalators may move too rapidly for the slow-moving elderly person to enter and exit comfortably. Traffic congestion may make crossing streets difficult and hazardous. Thus the individual may find the interactional world gradually shrinking because of factors that are unintentional. Fortunately, in the past two decades government has made a concerted effort to encourage the elimination of environmental barriers for the disabled, and this has had a beneficial effect on the elderly as they negotiate the environment.

BOX 15-11   Fall Resident Assessment Protocol Triggers Identified on the MDS 2.0

- Alzheimer's disease or other dementia
- Arthritis
- Cane, walker, crutch
- Cardiac arrhythmia
- Cardiovascular, psychotropic, diuretic medications
- Decline in cognition
- Decline in functional status
- Delirium
- Device or restraint
- Dizziness, vertigo, syncope
- Fracture of hip, history of falls
- Incontinence
- Hemiplegia or hemiparesis
- Hypotension
- Impaired hearing or vision
- Joint pain
- Loss of arm or leg movement
- Manic depression
- Missing limb
- Osteoporosis
- Pacemaker
- Parkinson's disease
- Seizures
- Unstable chronic or acute condition
- Unsteady gait
- Wandering

Adapted from Buckwalter K et al. II: Guide to the prevention and management of falls in the elderly, *CNS Long-Term Care* 3(2):31, Spring 2004.

Restraints and Side Rails

Restraints have been used historically for the "protection" of the client and for the security of the client and staff. Restraints may be physical or chemical. A physical restraint is defined as "any manual method or physical or mechanical device, material or equipment attached or adjacent to the individual's body that the individual cannot remove easily which restricts freedom of movement or normal access to one's body" (*www.cms.gov*). Chemical restraints have come under careful scrutiny, legal and ethical, in recent years. Chemical restraints are considered the use of medication, particularly psychotropics, under any of the following conditions (Tideiksaar, 1998):

- Given without specific indications
- Given in excessive doses affecting functioning
- Used as sole treatment without using behavioral interventions
- Administered for the convenience of staff

Physical restraints were originally used to control the behavior of individuals with mental illness considered to be dangerous to themselves or others (Evans and Strumpf, 1989). Some common reasons for restraining patients today include prevention of falls, altered mental status, prevention of harming self or others, wandering, agitation, and prevention of interference with treatment. The problem of restraint usage was first brought to the forefront of nursing attention by a request from Doris Schwarz, one of the pioneer gerontological nurses, for information from practicing nurses regarding their observations and concerns about restraint usage. In the intervening time, and largely through the efforts of Schwartz, her colleagues, and substantial nursing research, the use of restraints has been drastically reduced.

To date, there is no evidence in the literature documenting the efficacy of physical restraints in maintaining safety, preventing disruption of treatment, or controlling behavior. In fact, research over the past 20 years has repeatedly demonstrated that physical restraints, intended to prevent injury, do not protect patients from falling, wandering, or removing tubes and other medical devices. Physical restraints may actually exacerbate many of the problems for which they are used and can cause serious injury and emotional and physical problems. Physical restraints are associated with higher mortality rates, injurious falls, nosocomial infections, incontinence, immobility, contractures, pressure ulcers, agitation, and depression. Although prevention of falls is most frequently cited as the primary reason for using restraints, restraints do not prevent serious injury and may increase the risk of injury and even death.

Restrictions on restraint usage dictated by the Omnibus Budget Reconciliation Act (OBRA) provide specific guidelines for restraint use in long-term care facilities. All long-term care facilities must comply with statements from the *Federal Register* (1991) that relate to physical and chemical restraints and abuse in order to receive Medicare licensure (Box 15-12). Research over the past 15 years, primarily in the long-term care setting, has shown the practice of physical restraint to be ineffective and hazardous. The combination of

> ### BOX 15-12   Statements on Use of Restraints and Abuse
>
> - The resident has the right to be free from any physical or chemical restraints imposed for purposes of discipline or convenience, and not required to treat the resident's medical symptoms. The resident has the right to be free from verbal, sexual, physical, and mental abuse; corporal punishment; and involuntary seclusion.
> - The facility must develop and implement written policies and procedures that prohibit mistreatment, neglect, and abuse of residents.
> - The facility must ensure that the resident environment remains as free of accidental hazards as is possible, and that each resident receives adequate supervision and assistance devices to prevent accidents.

From *Federal Register* (V56187), Sept. 26, 1991, p. 48825.

research-based clinical evidence, increased knowledge about restraint alternatives, advocacy groups' efforts, and changed standards and regulations concerning restraints has contributed to a significant reduction in restraint use (Eliopoulos, 2005). Restraint-appropriate care is now the standard of practice and an indicator of quality care in all settings although transition to that standard is still in progress, particularly in acute care settings (Stone et al., 1999; Sullivan-Marx, 2001; Park and Hsiao-Chen Tang, 2007).

With the move toward freedom from restraints and the promotion of the least restrictive environment, the establishment of safety plans is essential. Removing restraints without careful attention to safety promotion and effective alternatives can jeopardize safety. Many of the suggestions on safety and fall risk reduction in this chapter can be used to promote a safe and restraint-free environment. Implementing best practice nursing in restraint-appropriate care requires recognition, assessment, and intervention for physical and psychosocial concerns contributing to patient safety, knowledge of restraint alternatives, interdisciplinary team work, and institutional commitment. The use of advanced practice nurse consultation in combination with education is most effective in implementing restraint-appropriate interventions (Bourbonniere and Evans, 2002; Capezuti, 2004).

The use of side rails is also coming under scrutiny through nursing research. Historically, side rails have been used to prevent falling from the bed, but this practice is being replaced by careful evaluation of the need and benefits of side rails. Side rails are no longer viewed as simply attachments to a patient's bed but may be considered restraints with all the accompanying concerns just discussed. When side rails impede the person's desired movement or activity, they meet the definition of a restraint. Evaluation of the proper use of side rails is required in long-term care. Elizabeth Capezuti, a gerontological nurse researcher, has extensively studied the use of side rails and bed-related fall outcomes, as well as individualized safety interventions (Capezuti et al., 2002). Fall risk reduction and restraint alternative strategies are presented in Boxes 15-13 and 15-14.

BOX 15-13   Fall Risk Reduction and Restraint Alternative Strategies

- Work with the interdisciplinary team; nurses cannot manage these complicated challenges alone.
- Lower the bed to the lowest level, or use a bed that is especially designed to be low to the floor.
- Use concave mattress.
- Use bed boundary markers to mark edges of bed such as mattress bumpers, rolled blanket, or "swimming noodles" under sheets.
- Place soft floor mat or a mattress by the bed to cushion any falls.
- Use water mattress to reduce movement to edge of bed.
- Have person at risk sleep on mattress on the floor.
- Remove wheels from bed.
- Clear the floor of debris, excessive furniture; make sure it is not wet or slippery.
- Place call bell within reach, and make sure the patient can use it—attach call bell to garment.
- Provide visual reminders to encourage the patient to use call bell.
- Use night lights in room and bathroom.
- Use identification bracelet or door sign to indicate patients at risk for falling.
- Inform all staff of fall risk, and put fall risk and fall risk reduction interventions on care plan.
- Involve family and all staff in fall risk reduction education and activities.
- Identify on Kardex and call bell console those patients at high risk.
- Assess ambulation ability; refer to physical therapy for walking/strengthening.
- Have ambulation devices within reach, and make sure patient knows how to use properly.
- Use bed, chair, or wrist alarms (the best alarm tells you only that there is an emergency; still need frequent checks, supervised areas). Apply patient-worn sensor (lightweight alarm worn above the knee that is position sensitive).
- Keep in supervised area or room within view of the nursing station.
- Check for orthostasis (systolic drop greater than 20 mm Hg systolic and/or greater than 10 mm Hg after 3-5 minutes of standing).
- Know that a history of falls is predictive of future falls: "Once a faller, always a faller." Assess the patient for history of falls.
- If the patient is able, walk at every opportunity possible. If the patient walked in or could walk before hospitalization, make every effort to keep the patient walking during hospitalization.

- Establish toileting plan, and take to toilet frequently.
- Have patient use bedside commode.
- Make sure patient knows the location of the bathroom—leave door open so he or she can see the toilet, or put a picture of a toilet on the door; clear path to bathroom.
- Know sleeping patterns—if usually up during the night, get up in a chair and keep at nursing station.
- Use bolsters, lap buddies.
- Minimize medication, especially sleepers, sedating or anticholinergic medications.
- Do frequent bed checks, especially in evening and night.
- Be especially alert at change-of-shift times.
- Understand that very few people spend all day in bed; activity is necessary.
- Use upper ½ side rails only.
- Provide diversional activities (catalogues, puzzles, busy box).
- Wedge cushions in wheel chairs or materials that promote sitting in an upright position without restraints (occupational therapy can be helpful in this area).
- Have patients sit in reclining geriatric (geri) chairs or geri chairs with trays, chairs with deep seats, bean bag chairs, rockers—keep close to nurses' station in the chair.
- Arrange for family/sitter with patient, especially at high-risk times.
- If patient has glasses, hearing aid, dentures, toupee, see that they are worn.
- Have purse (empty or without harmful items or important papers/money) in bed with patient if woman.
- Have patient sleep with shoes on or rubber-soled slippers.
- Ensure that pain is well managed.
- If patient is (or has been) married, line spouse's side of the bed with pillows or bolsters.
- Place non-slip strips on floor next to bed; ensure that floors are non-slip.
- Provide trapeze to enhance mobility in bed.
- Provide grab bars in bathroom and shower, shower chair with suction bottom.
- Provide elevated toilet seat.
- Have patient wear clothing that is easy to pull down for toileting.
- Create a grid with masking tape on floor in front of doorway, use black half rug, and camouflage exit doors with wallpaper, window treatments, etc. if patient is wandering or trying to exit.
- Place stop sign on exit door.
- Use a behavior log to track when patient is trying to get up, when he or she seems agitated.
- Provide hip protectors, helmets, arm pads.

For suggestions on how to maintain safety without restraints, see the *Hartford Institute for Geriatric Nursing Try This* best practice guidelines, which can be found at *www. hartfordign.org/resources/education/tryThis.html*. The *RN+ Safe-T-Net* online newsletter provides helpful information about fall safety and restraint reduction (*www.rnplus.com*). Every facility should have structured fall risk assessment and fall risk reduction programs and maintain fall rates for quality control and management. Box 15-15 presents an innovative fall risk reduction program in an acute care facility.

Fall Risk Reduction Interventions

The goal of fall risk reduction intervention programs is to eliminate or reduce remediable risk factors (Nnodim and Alexander, 2005). The most successful approaches to fall risk reduction are multifactorial assessment followed by in-

---

BOX 15-14 | Restraint Alternatives: Dealing with Tubes, Lines, and Other Medical Devices

- Preoperative teaching and showing the tubes and explaining may be effective in decreasing anxiety about devices.
- Use guided exploration and a mirror to help patient understand what is in place and why.
- Provide comfort care to the site—oral/nasal care, anchoring of tubing, topical anesthetic on site.
- First question: "Is the device really necessary?" Remove as soon as possible. Foley catheters should be used only if patient needs intensive output monitoring or has an obstruction.
- Weigh risks and benefits of restraint versus therapy. Are alternatives available—replace intravenous (IV) tubing with heparin lock, deliver medications intramuscularly (IM), intermittent administration.
- Use camouflage: clothing or elastic sleeves, temporary air splint (occupational therapy [OT] can be helpful), skin sleeves to prevent IV tube dislodgement.
- Use mitts instead of wrist restraints; roll belts instead of vest restraints.
- Use diversional activity aprons (zipping/unzipping, threading exercises, dials and knobs), busy box, or therapeutic activity kit (*www.hartfordign.org/trythis*).

- Hide lines by placing in unobtrusive place; place tubing behind patient out of his or her view; have patient wear long sleeves or double surgical gowns with cuffs to prevent access.
- Hang IV bags behind the patient's field of vision.
- Nasogastric (NG) tubes—replace with percutaneous endoscopic gastrostomy (PEG) tube if necessary but obtain comprehensive speech therapy (ST) swallowing evaluation. If NG tube is used, use as small a lumen as possible to minimize irritation; consider taping with occlusive dressings.
- Cover PEG tube or abdominal incisions and other tubes with abdominal binder, sweat pants.
- For men with Foley catheters—shave area just above pubis, and tape catheter to pubis. NEVER secure catheter to leg (causes discomfort and can cause a fistula). Run tubing around back and down leg to a leg bag. Patient should wear underpants and pajama pants.
- Take restraints off while working with patient.
- Use modified soft collar for tracheotomy protection.

BOX 15-15 | The Ruby Slipper Fall Intervention Program

Nurse Ginny Goldner of St. Joseph's Hospital in Tucson, Arizona, started the "Ruby Slipper" program to identify patients at risk for falling and to help prevent falls in elderly patients. Patients at risk for falls wear red socks with non-slip treads so that anyone from a housekeeper to a head nurse who sees them walking around or trying to get out of bed will know to stay with them until they are safely back in bed. Education on fall risk reduction, identification of patients at high risk, and Ruby Slipper rounds on high-risk patients to see if they need anything, such as to go to the bathroom, are included in the program as well. The program has reduced patient falls by nearly 75%. Ginny was awarded the March of Dimes Arizona Innovation and Creativity Nurse of the Year Award for the program.

Data from Arizona Hospital and Healthcare Association, *www.azhha.org*. For information, contact Ginny Goldner RN, MS at (520) 873-3722 or email vgoldner@carondelet.org.

terventions directed at the identified risk factors. These approaches have been shown to reduce the occurrence of falling by 25% to 39% (Tinetti, 2003). Capezuti (2004, p. 461) cautions against a "one size fits all" approach to fall risk reduction, and further research is needed to determine the type, frequency, and timing of interventions best suited for specific populations (e.g., community-living older adults, institutionalized elders, women, men, ethnically diverse elders) (Quigley, 2005). The American Geriatrics Society Panel on Falls Prevention (2001) recommends the following interventions:

- For community-living elders, interventions should include gait training and correct use of assistive devices, medication review (particularly psychotropics), exercise programs that include balance training, assessment and treatment of postural hypotension and cardiovascular disorders, and environmental hazard modification.
- For elders in long-term care and assisted-living facilities, interventions should include staff education, gait training, correct use of assistive devices, and medication review (particularly psychotropics).

Evidence is insufficient to recommend specific types of interventions for acute care, but a multifactorial approach targeted to specific risk factors in this setting may also be useful. Further research is needed in both acute and subacute settings.

Exercise. The relationship between exercise and fall risk reduction is strong, particularly combined with balance training for elders in the community. Although the best type, duration, and intensity of exercise have not been determined, exercise must be at least 10 weeks in duration, must be individualized, and must include balance training for benefit. Group exercises may also be effective. Further research is needed to evaluate the effect of exercise in long-term care settings, as well as the effect of programs such as tai chi chuan (see Chapter 3).

Environmental Modifications. Environmental modifications alone have not been shown to reduce falls, but when included as part of a multifactorial program, they may be of benefit in prevention. However, a home safety assessment conducted by an occupational therapist after hospital discharge resulted in significant fall risk reductions in a group of older patients. A facilitated home safety assessment for all older patients at risk for falls is recommended on hospital discharge (American Geriatrics Society, 2001).

Medication Review. Reduction of medications is an important component of effective fall-reducing interventions in both community-based and long-term care studies. Medications, including over-the-counter (OTC) and herbals, should be reviewed and limited to those absolutely essential. Risk of falls increases with the use of four or more medications, particularly the use of neuroleptics, benzodiazepines (both long- and short-acting), and antidepressants.

Behavior and Educational Programs. As a single strategy, behavior and education programs do not reduce falls but are recommended as part of multifactorial intervention programs. Information should be provided to the older person and to caregivers on fall risk factors and fall risk reduction strategies.

Assistive Devices. Research on multifactorial interventions including the use of assistive devices (bed alarms, canes, walkers, hip protectors) has demonstrated benefits in fall risk reduction. It is important to provide instruction and supervision on the correct use of assistive devices. If you think your client could benefit from an assistive device, consult specialists and rehabilitation therapists. Assist your client in obtaining a written prescription from the appropriate therapist because Medicare may cover up to 80% of the cost of the device if this is done; other insurance coverage varies.

Many devices are available that are designed for specific benefits (Figure 15-1). Developments in assistive technology hold the potential to significantly improve functional ability and independence for older people. Chapter 16 discusses assistive technology.

When the correct device is obtained, the client will need assistance in learning to use it correctly. This, again, should be taught by specialists in physical therapy. In general, the following principles should be observed:

- Place your cane firmly on the ground before you take a step, and do not place it too far ahead of you. Put all of your weight on your unaffected leg, and then move the cane and your affected leg at a comfortable distance forward. With your weight supported on both your cane and your affected leg, step through with your unaffected leg.
- Always wear low-heeled, nonskid shoes.
- When using a cane on stairs, step up with the stronger leg and down with the weaker leg. Use the cane as support when lifting the weaker leg. Bring the cane up to the step just reached before climbing another step. When descending, place the cane on the next step down, move the disabled leg down, and then move the good leg down.

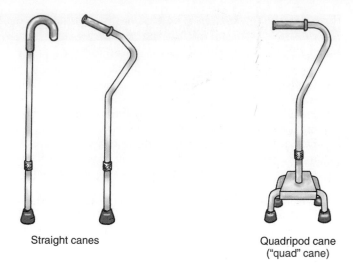

Straight canes   Quadripod cane ("quad" cane)

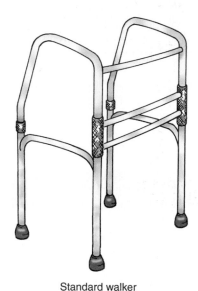

Standard walker

FIGURE 15-1 Assistive devices for ambulation. (From Ignatavicius DD, Workman ML: *Medical-surgical nursing: critical thinking for collaborative care,* ed 5, St Louis, 2006, Saunders.)

- When using a walker, stand upright and lift or roll the walker with both hands a step's length ahead of you. Lean slightly forward, and hold the arms of the walker for support. Step toward it with the weaker leg, and then bring the stronger leg forward. Do not climb stairs with a walker.
- Every assistive device must be adjusted to individual height; the top of the cane should align with the crease of the wrist.
- Choose a size and shape of cane handle that fits comfortably in the palm; like a tight shoe, it will be a constant irritant if it is not properly fitted.
- Cane tips are most secure when they are flat at the bottom and have a series of rings. Replace tips frequently because they wear out and a worn tip is insecure.

Wheelchairs are a necessary adjunct at some level of immobility. These can be used in a healthful way and without demeaning the individual. The various types of motorized chairs can be handled with ease and provide a great deal of independence for wheelchair users. It is important that a professional evaluate the wheelchair for proper fit and provide training on proper use and safety.

Other potential interventions include assessment and treatment of osteoporosis to reduce fracture rates. Older people with osteoporosis are more likely to experience serious injury from a fall. Interventions for osteoporosis (calcium and vitamin D supplements, bisphosphonates) and the use of hip protectors can reduce the risk of falling and sustaining a hip fracture by one third (Tinetti, 2003). The use of hip protectors for prevention of hip fractures in high-risk individuals is strongly supported through research although adherence has been a concern (Capezuti, 2004). Formal vision assessment is also an important intervention to identify remediable visual problems. Although a significant relationship exists between visual problems and falls and fractures, little research has been done on interventions for visual problems as part of fall risk reduction programs. Poor visual acuity, reduced contrast sensitivity, decreased visual field, cataract, and non-miotic glaucoma medications have all been associated with falls (American Geriatrics Society, 2001).

▲ Promoting Healthy Aging: Implications for Gerontological Nursing

Gerontological nurses need to be knowledgeable about fall risk factors and fall risk reduction interventions in all settings. Health promotion interventions to maintain fitness and mobility; appropriate assessment of fall risk; teaching older adults, their caregivers, and staff about fall risk factors; fall risk reduction interventions; and restraint-appropriate care are important nursing responses. For community-dwelling older adults, nurses need to have knowledge of home, community, and environmental safety factors, assistive devices and technology, environmental modifications, and resources to aid in maintaining independence and functional abilities. In institutions, working as members of the interdisciplinary team, nurses bring expert knowledge of patient activities, abilities, and needs from a 24 hr/day, 7 day/wk perspective to help the team implement the most appropriate interventions and evaluate outcomes. Accidents and injuries among older adults in all settings are significant in terms of morbidity and mortality, and utilizing evidence-based practice can ensure improvement of many modifiable and preventable injuries, as well as mobility limitations and functional decline. Maintenance of mobility and safety for older adults is one of the most important components of gerontological nursing.

OSTEOPOROSIS

Osteoporosis means "porous bone." Primary osteoporosis is associated with the normal changes of aging. A gradual, continual loss of cortical bone (the outer shell of a bone and 80% of the skeleton) and trabecular bone (the spongy mesh-work inside the bone and 20% of the skeleton) occurs in both men and women as they age (Thorndyke, 2001). Secondary osteoporosis, accounting for 15% of cases, is caused by another disease state or medications (hyperthyroidism, hyperparathyroidism, gastrointestinal [GI] disorders, neoplasms, alcoholism). Long-term use of corticosteroids, methotrexate, aluminum-containing antacids, phenytoin, and heparin can cause secondary osteoporosis (Meiner and Lueckenotte, 2006). Both primary and secondary osteoporosis are characterized by low bone mass (or bone mineral density) and subsequent deterioration of the bone structure.

Epidemiology

Osteoporosis (OP) is a major medical, economic, and social health problem in the United States. It results in significant pain, loss of function, suffering, and mortality. OP affects about 55% of people older than 50 years in some way. Ten million people have OP, and another 34 million have a lesser (but perhaps precursor) condition of bone loss called osteopenia. Of those affected by osteoporosis, 80% are women. Thin, white, postmenopausal women of Northern European descent are at the highest risk. Of non-Hispanic black women older than 50 years, 5% are estimated to have OP and an additional 35% have low bone mass. Of Hispanic women older than 50 years, 10% are estimated to have osteoporosis and 49% have low bone mass. OP is under-recognized and under-treated in Caucasian, African-American, and Hispanic women.

The most serious health consequence of OP is the fall-related morbidity and mortality. One in two women and one in four men ages 50 years and older will have an osteoporotic-related fracture in his or her lifetime, and the sequelae of pain and long-term disability are devastating. Osteoporotic fractures in women have a greater incidence than the incidence of heart attack, breast cancer, and stroke combined (Zarowitz, 2006). The primary sites for fractures are the vertebrae (700,000), hip (300,000), wrist (250,000), or other site (300,000), with a cost of $18 billion in 2002 (National Osteoporosis Foundation, 2003).

Causation and Pathophysiology

Osteoporosis is a silent condition, and a person may have no symptoms of any kind ever or for years. In the normal process of growth, the bones build up mass (formation) and strength while they are also losing both through resorption. Before the age of 25 years, the formation is greater than the resorption; bone strength and density peak and then begin to decline. At first the loss of bone mineral density (BMD) is quite minimal, but then it speeds up. For women, the fastest overall loss of BMD is in the 5 to 7 years immediately after menopause, with losses up to 20% (National Institutes of Health [NIH], 2004).

The dual-energy x-ray absorptiometry (DEXA) scan provides the most reliable measurement of bone integrity. The U.S. Prevention Task Force recommends that all persons older than 64 years and those with more than one risk factor have at least one screening DEXA scan, which is covered by

Medicare (U.S. Prevention Services Task Force [USPSTF], 2002). DEXA scans have low radiation exposure. Other screening devices, such as heel or wrist scans done at malls and health fairs, do not give an accurate picture of the bone density in all areas of the body. One area, such as the heel, may be normal, but the vertebrae may be osteoporotic.

The results are a calculated comparison "T-score," the density of the bone scanned compared with that of a 30-year-old healthy man or woman. If the bone loss is between −1 and −2.5 standard deviations from that of a healthy 30-year-old, it is called *osteopenia*. If the bone loss is greater than −2.5 standard deviations, the person is diagnosed with *osteoporosis*.

Risk Factors for Osteoporosis

The amount of bone mass one has as a young adult and the rate at which it is lost as one ages determine risk for OP (Arthritis Foundation, 2000). Other areas of risk that should be a part of any nursing assessment of an elder include both modifiable and nonmodifiable factors. Risk factors for osteoporosis are presented in Box 15-16.

Assessment

A person with osteoporosis may be without symptoms until a fracture occurs. Some of the outward signs that identify a history of OP are a loss of height of more than 3 cm or kyphosis, the development of a C shape to the cervical vertebrae (see Figure 4-3). The nurse may be the one to identify the changes to the spine or realize that the person had a fracture or unexplained back pain but has not received a medical diagnosis. In the nursing home setting, the MDS includes indicators of OP that will assist in assessment of this patient population. Without a diagnosis, it is unlikely that the person will have access to the full treatments that are available. It is important to assess the person's risk factors and urge both formal screening and lifestyle changes to minimize risk and enhance prevention.

BOX 15-16   Risk Factors for Osteoporosis

NON-MODIFIABLE FACTORS

Female gender
Caucasian race
Northern European ancestry
Advanced age
Family history of osteoporosis

MODIFIABLE FACTORS

Low body weight (underweight)
Low calcium intake
Estrogen deficiency
Low testosterone
Inadequate exercise or activity
Use of steroids or anticonvulsants
Excess coffee or alcohol intake
Current cigarette smoking

Prevention and Management

Prevention of OP must begin in the teen years. As women increasingly live into their 80s and 90s, the treatment of OP is becoming more important. Preventive measures include weight-bearing, physical activity and exercise, nutrition, and lifestyle changes that reduce risk factors. Education and fall risk reduction must also be considered. Awareness of OP in all age-groups remains low. A study of community-dwelling woman who experienced a hip fracture showed that only 13% received adequate treatment according to the guidelines of the National Osteoporosis Foundation (Bellantonio et al., 2001).

Weight-bearing and resistance-training exercises help maintain bone mass. Brisk walking and working with light weights provide mechanical force and spinal and long bone movement. Muscle-building exercises help maintain skeletal architecture by improving muscle strength and flexibility. Avoiding smoking and excessive alcohol intake can also help prevent OP.

Nutrition, especially the adequate intake of calcium and vitamin D, is the cornerstone to all other treatments. The diet during adolescence is probably a key to healthy bones later. A balanced diet that includes food sources of calcium is best. Calcium carbonate is the least expensive form of calcium and should be taken with meals to enhance absorption. Patients should be advised to start with one supplement daily and build up gradually to the recommended dosage to minimize GI problems that can occur. Persons older than 50 years, including nursing home residents, should take in 1200 mg of calcium per day, which can come from combined dietary and supplementary sources. Most diets contain less than 600 mg/day. If using supplements, the doses are best when spread over the course of the day (e.g., 400 mg of calcium in the morning, diet with 400 mg during the day, and another 400 mg of calcium in the evening). Several drugs may decrease absorption of calcium and calcium also interferes with absorption of some medications, so patient teaching is important.

Vitamin D deficiency is common in older people, with up to 60% of patients with hip fractures having some deficiency (Burke, 2004). Unless the person gets 15 minutes of sunshine each day, vitamin D supplementation is also necessary. Daily doses of 400 to 800 international units are sufficient and should not be exceeded (Jett and Lester, 2004). Patient teaching includes discussion of the factors that inhibit calcium absorption (e.g., excess alcohol, protein, or salt); excretion enhancers (e.g., caffeine, excess fiber, phosphorus in meats, sodas, and preserved foods); and the influence of the body's response to stress (decreased calcium absorption, increased excretion of calcium in the urine). Management interventions are presented in Figure 15-2. See Chapter 9 for further discussion of OP and nutrition.

Patient teaching also includes other key aspects of the prevention and treatment of OP. Education about the sites most vulnerable to fracture through accidents, falls, back strain, and poor posture should be provided. Fall risk assessment and fall risk reduction measures should also be included in patient

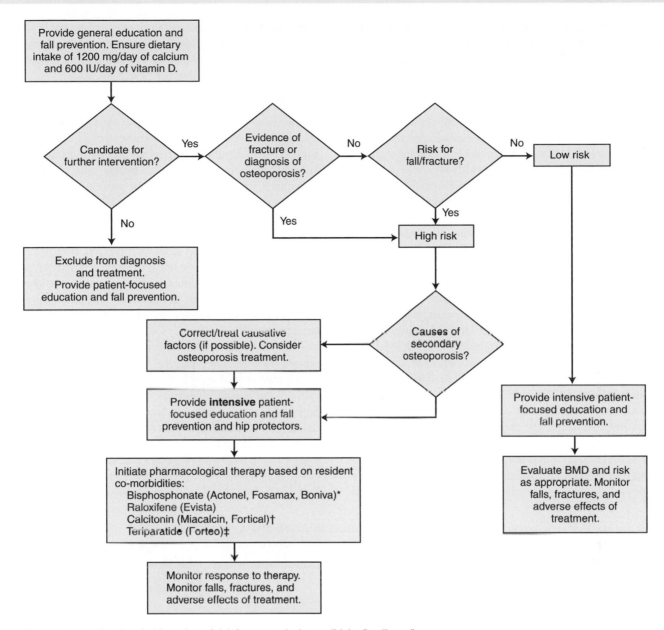

There is no precise threshold number of risk factors to designate "higher" or "lower."

*Bisphosphonates are preferred due to fracture reduction in both vertebral and nonvertebral sites.
†Calcitonin is only FDA indicated for osteoporosis.
‡Teriparatide is a parenteral agent that is indicated only for treatment of osteoporosis in individuals at high risk for fracture potential; benefits vs. risks of treatment should be considered before initiating therapy; use of teriparatide beyond 2 years is not recommended.

FIGURE 15-2 Osteoporosis management. (From Zarowitz B: Management of osteoporosis in older persons, *Geriatr Nurs* 27[1]:16-18, 2006. Adapted and reproduced with permission from Omnicare Inc. © Copyright 2007. All rights reserved. The final choice of drug therapy is a decision made by the prescriber based on the individual patient circumstances and clinical situation.)

teaching. Hip protectors should be recommended for older adults with OP. Other fall risk reduction interventions and safety measures were discussed earlier in this chapter.

Pharmacological Interventions

Considerable progress has been made in the past decade in the development of pharmacological treatments for both the prevention and treatment of osteoporosis. The currently available medications include bisphosphonates, calcitonin, selective estrogen receptive modulators (SERMs), estrogen,

and parathyroid hormone. Adequate intake of calcium and vitamin D is required for all the prescribed treatments currently available.

Estrogen had been the primary treatment prescribed for many years. However, the Women's Health Initiative found that although estrogen is an excellent means to prevent bone loss, it also increased the rate of breast cancer, colon cancer, and thrombotic events (Brucker and Youngkin, 2002). Because of these findings, estrogen is not usually prescribed for osteoporosis, and if it is, it is for a limited period.

The SERM *raloxifene* is a good substitute for estrogen and may have a protective effect against breast cancer, but it can cause hot flashes and coagulation disorders so it is contraindicated for someone with a history of deep vein thrombosis (DVT) or someone who is taking warfarin (Coumadin).

The most common treatments that are seen in older adults are the bisphosphonates *alendronate (Fosamax)*, *risedronate (Actonel)*, and *ibandronate (Boniva)*. Fosamax and Actonel are available as a pill in daily and weekly doses. Boniva is available as a pill in a monthly dose and as an intravenous injection administered every 3 months. Bisphosphonates are the drug class of choice, and evidence suggests that they reduce bone loss and increase bone mass at the hip, spine, and total body as early as 3 months into therapy, as well as reduce fractures (Zarowtiz, 2006). Oral forms of these medications must be used by the patient and administered by the nurse with caution. They must be taken on an empty stomach (when first awake), with a full glass of water, and the person must remain in an upright position for at least ½ hour and not eat or drink for at least 30 minutes. Side effects include heartburn, nausea, and severe esophageal erosions. It should not be given to patients who are not able to follow these instructions exactly, often limiting its use in frail nursing home residents.

Another medication that is quite useful is calcitonin (Miacalcin). Although the mechanism is not known, for some it not only slows bone resorption but also reduces osteoporosis-related pain and may be particularly useful in the treatment of vertebral fractures. It is given either subcutaneously or as a nasal spray. Parathyroid hormone (PTH) is also approved for the treatment of OP with treatment limited to 2 years. Safety of long-term administration has not been established, and it should be used only for persons who cannot receive other forms of therapy (Zarowitz, 2006).

Complications

Fractures are common in elders with OP. Osteoporotic-related hip fractures have the most serious consequences. Rate of hip fracture is increasing among men and among Hispanic women, and men have nearly twice the mortality of women after a hip fracture, as well as higher rates of certain complications (Hawkes et al., 2006). Women with a hip fracture are at a fourfold risk of a second fracture (National Osteoporosis Foundation, 2003). A striking 24% of persons older than 50 years with hip fractures die within 1 year. Half of all people with hip fractures will be unable to walk without assistance and one fourth of those who were ambulatory before the fracture will need long-term care. Box 15-17 presents an exercise program for older women post–hip fracture.

Vertebral fractures are the most common osteoporotic-related fracture. They may be "silent" or extremely painful with paravertebral muscle spasms and radiation of pain because of nerve root compression (Thorndyke, 2001). Vertebral fractures are often not recognized by clinicians or the radiologist when an elder has back pain (Watts, 2001). It is suggested that any patient with height loss have a spinal x-ray examination and obtain lateral spine imaging. Quality of life is greatly impaired with vertebral deformities because they have been shown to limit activity and increase days of

---

BOX 15-17   Evidence-Based Practice: Exercise Plus Program for Older Women Post–Hip Fracture

PURPOSE

This study explores the experiences of older women after hip fracture who were involved in a home-based motivational intervention.

SAMPLE/SETTING

70 community-living older women (mean age 80.9) who had some type of surgical repair of a hip fracture and had completed the Exercise Plus Program. The program was implemented by certified exercise trainers and consisted of five exercise sessions (strength training and aerobic) of 30 minutes duration each. The program was 1 year in duration.

METHOD

A naturalistic or constructivist inquiry with single open-ended interviews. Basic content analysis was used to analyze data.

RESULTS

The following efficacy enhancement components of the program facilitated motivation:
- Confidence gained from repeatedly exercising and recognizing positive outcomes (e.g., exercise was good for me,

exercise builds bone density), importance of a regular schedule
- Verbal encouragement from the trainers (warmth, kindness, and caring from trainers)
- Self-modeling and cues from written materials provided (knowing exactly what exercises to do and how and when to do them; visual cues and the exercise booklet helped)
- Eliminating unpleasant sensations associated with exercise (anxiety, fear of falling, fatigue, pain)

IMPLICATIONS

In setting up exercise programs, specific motivational interventions to encourage continuation of a regular exercise program are important. Focus for exercise programs should be on the benefit of exercise and should provide simple and clear guidelines for what exercise activity to engage in, individualized goals should be established, on-going encouragement and reinforcement of progress toward goals provided in a supportive and caring manner, and ways to overcome barriers to exercise should be explored. Interventions such as these will help older women to initiate and remain engaged in exercise over time.

Data from Resnick B et al: The Exercise Plus Program for older women post hip fracture: participant perspectives, *Gerontologist* 45:539-544, 2005.

bedrest. Further, history of fracture is an additional risk for another fracture. Treatment of these fractures can be with nonsteroidal antiinflammatory drugs (NSAIDs) if osteoarthritis is in the area of the fracture, use of heat or cold for pain, and gentle massage if muscle spasms are present (Neyhart and Gibbs, 2002). Effective pain management will allow early mobilization and prevent complications. Calcitonin may be useful in pain relief.

Newer treatments with vertebroplasty and kyphoplasty may be considered in those with continued pain (Lesley, 2002). Usual therapy is bedrest, with variable success and the possible complications of DVT, pneumonia, and further bone loss; fixation surgery, which has a high failure rate because of weakened bone foundation; and analgesics. Percutaneous polymethylmethacrylate vertebroplasty (PPV) is the percutaneous injection of a cement into the affected vertebral body. PPV is performed under local anesthesia with conscious sedation as an outpatient procedure. PPV is usually performed after a trial of conservative therapy. The elder is able to walk within 2 to 4 hours and usually has dramatic or complete pain relief (Lesley, 2002; Syed et al., 2006).

Much remains to be done in preventing OP. Young women must be taught preventive measures to forestall the development of OP and reduce the enormous cost of osteoporotic fractures and the painful disability and discomfort to the individual (see Appendix 15-B).

RHEUMATIC DISEASES OF OLDER ADULTS

Arthritis is the term used to refer to more than 100 diseases that affect more than 15% of the U.S. population, young as well as old, and includes disorders of joints and connective tissue throughout the body. Almost 60% of people older than 65 years report arthritis or chronic joint symptoms. Arthritis is the leading cause of disability and the number-one reason for activity limitations from middle age on (Callahan and Jonas, 2002). A number of rheumatic disorders occur in older adults; some of these are bursitis, polymyalgia rheumatica, gout, rotator cuff tears, tendinitis, frozen shoulder, low back pain, acute disk herniation, chronic disk de-

generation, lumbar spinal stenosis, rheumatoid arthritis, osteoarthritis, and many others (Reuben et al., 2002). Because of space considerations and because management and nursing care are similar in some of these disorders, we highlight the most common.

Osteoarthritis

Definition. Osteoarthritis (OA) is a degenerative joint disorder (DJD) that affects at least 20 million Americans. It was previously thought to be a normal consequence of aging that had no cure, and many older people still believe this to be true (Kalunian and Brion, 2002). However, it is now known that OA results from a complex interplay of many factors, including increased age, genetic predisposition, obesity, cellular and biochemical processes, and repetitive use or trauma to the joint. Most persons older than 65 years will have x-ray evidence of OA even if they have no symptoms. Native Americans have the highest prevalence of OA, and Asians and Pacific Islanders have the lowest. Whites and African-Americans have similar rates of arthritis, but African-Americans have greater rates of activity limitation (*www.healthypeople.gov*).

The osteoarthritic joint is one in which the normal soft and resilient cartilaginous lining becomes thin and damaged. This causes the joint space to narrow and the bones of the joint to rub together, causing destruction of the joint. Bone spurs (osteophytes) may develop in the spaces (Figure 15-3). In classic OA, stiffness with inactivity and pain with activity that is relieved by rest occur (Concoff, 2002). The stiffness is greatest in the morning after the disuse of sleep but should resolve within 20 to 30 minutes. As the disease advances, pain with little activity and at rest is present as more and more joints become involved. Joint instability may occur, and crepitus may be felt or heard. This crepitation is an indication of the deterioration of the synovial covering of the joints. Physiologically, there is bony growth of osteophytes and joint space narrowing from loss or destruction of cartilage; inflammation of the synovium lining the joint may occur. The joint will enlarge, and ROM will be reduced. The most common locations for OA are the knees, hips, neck (cervical spine), lower back (lumbar spine), fingers, and thumbs (Figure 15-4).

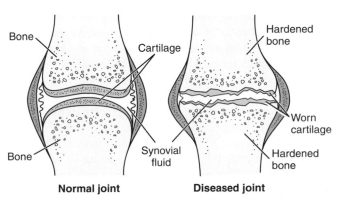

FIGURE 15-3 Normal joint and diseased joint.

What Areas Does Osteoarthritis Affect?

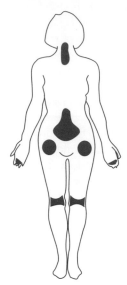

FIGURE 15-4 Common locations for osteoarthritis. (Source: National Institutes of Health [NIH]: *Handout on health: osteoarthritis,* Washington, DC. [website]: *www.niams.nih.gov/hi/topics/arthritis/oahandout.htm.* Accessed July 29, 2004.)

OA is a condition that cannot be cured without a joint replacement. Many elders elect this procedure for hips and knees, and the nurse is involved in the perioperative period and active in the rehabilitation process when the person is learning to use the new joint.

Assessment. The diagnosis of OA is made clinically; there are no laboratory tests to confirm the diagnosis. The history will reveal a gradual onset of joint pain and stiffness that worsens with activity and is relieved at rest. Weather appears to aggravate symptoms. Spinal involvement occurs most commonly at C5, T8, and L3, areas of greatest flexibility. Osteophytes (bony outgrowths) in the lumbar region can become spinal stenosis if encroaching in the foramina and spinal cord and can result in radiating low back pain.

When assessing the musculoskeletal system, the nurse examines the joints for tenderness, swelling, warmth, redness, subluxation (partial dislocation of a joint), and crepitus (a crackling sound). Crepitus indicates the loss of a smooth, articulating surface and joint effusion. Effusions may be large and hinder movement so that aspiration is needed for relief. The hands are examined for the presence or absence of osteophytes. Osteophytes in the distal joints of the fingers are called *Heberden's nodes,* and those in the nodes in the proximal joints are called *Bouchard's nodes.* If present, they are often accompanied by deformities in the flexion of these joints. Heberden's nodes are thought to have a hereditary component. X-rays are highly insensitive to OA, especially early OA (Concoff, 2002).

Both passive ROM and active ROM are evaluated. How far can the person reach and bend all joints without assistance, and what are the reach, flexion, and extension with assistance? The testing of passive ROM must go only to the point of discomfort and never to induce pain. Test the functional ability of the arms by asking the person to touch the back of the head with both hands. Test the flexibility of the hands by surveying the movements as the individual uses eating utensils. Assessment should also focus on activities of daily living. Assess comfort in walking, cooking, bathing, dressing, using the toilet, and performing household chores (Agency for Healthcare Research and Quality, 2002a). Arthritis limits the major activities of nearly one of every five persons with the disease. Assess changes in social activities, exercise, and mood. Arthritis, like other chronic pain conditions, has a negative effect on a person's mental health. Assessment and rating of pain are also components of assessment.

Interventions. The goals of intervention and management of OA are to control pain and minimize disability. The nurse is very involved with both of these in terms of pain assessment, medication administration, evaluation, and patient teaching. Pain management and the minimization of disability are interconnected. To minimize disability, the joint must be used, strengthened, and protected. Exercises will not be done if they cause pain. Balancing pain relief with appropriate and safe exercise is important.

Pharmacological Interventions. Pharmacological management is usually necessary, and acetaminophen (Tylenol) remains the drug of choice for the treatment of pain associated with mild arthritis (Jett and Lester, 2004). When this is not effective, the next choice is one of the NSAIDs, such as aspirin or ibuprofen; however, these are not without significant risk for GI problems such as bleeding, as well as cardiovascular side effects. To minimize this risk, the NSAID can be taken with a protecting agent such as a proton pump inhibitor (e.g., omeprazole [Prilosec]) or in a combination drug such as misoprostol (Arthrotec). Celecoxib (Celebrex) is the only COX-2 inhibitor still on the market for treatment of arthritis. Other COX-2 inhibitors have been withdrawn because of the cardiovascular side effects (heart attack and stroke) and the well-known risk of potentially life-threatening GI bleeding. The Food and Drug Administration (FDA) has requested manufacturers of all NSAID drugs and celecoxib to revise the labels to include boxed warnings stating an increased risk of cardiovascular events and GI adverse events. Patients taking NSAIDs must be taught about the risks and monitored closely. A recent study suggested that risedronate, used for the treatment of OP, may also be useful in reducing cartilage degradation and bone resorption and may be beneficial in OA.

As the disease progresses or during exacerbations, stronger medications may be necessary to help control pain and the nurse may need to act as a patient advocate to ensure that the pain is satisfactorily addressed. Tramadol is used for moderate to severe pain. Although it is not an opioid, the effect may be similar. It can cause nausea and vomiting and should be started in very low doses and increased very slowly to avoid these side effects. Codeine and other opiates can be used for moderate to severe pain, with a bowel regimen.

The goals of intervention and management of OA are to help the elder prevent or control pain, to minimize disability, and to ensure optimal medical management. For older persons with persistent pain, the nurse should be less concerned about the addictive quality of the medications and strive for pain relief adequate enough to allow the person to function at as high a level as possible. The recognition and management of pain in elders, particularly those with dementia or those who are nonverbal, is inadequate and causes a great deal of needless suffering. Chapter 11 discusses pain management in more detail.

For persistent and disabling pain in the knees, joint injections may be helpful. Either cortisone or the chemical *hyaluronic acid* (a derivative of hyaluronan) is used. In some cases, these provide at least temporary and sometimes instantaneous relief. Repeated injections may be necessary (especially for hyaluronic acid), but there is a limit to how many injections can be done. The nurse should be aware that even after an injection the joint will still need protection and support.

Other pharmacological agents often used in OA management include topical capsaicin made from pepper plants and available over the counter in two strengths. It becomes effective after several days of use. Approximately one half of the individuals who use capsaicin cream experience local burning sensations. This sensation diminishes over time (Agency for Healthcare Research and Quality, 2007). Menthol and aspirin creams are also useful and preferred by many elders.

Surgical Interventions. For disabling pain in the knees, hips, shoulders, elbows, and fingers, surgical replacement of the joint (arthroplasty) may be highly successful and restore the person to his or her previous level of functioning. Surgical replacements are recommended for even the very old. Nearly twice as many females as males have joint replacements, and over 60% of all joint replacements are in individuals older than 65 years. The Well Elderly Study found that elderly people report better quality of life, less pain, and better physical function after knee replacement surgery (Agency for Healthcare Research and Quality, 2002b).

The acute postsurgical care is designed to restore the physiological functions (maintenance of fluids, movement, and nutritional adequacy) and to prevent complications such as infection. Pain management is critical to ensure that the individual will move about as necessary and is essential to achieve maximal recovery. It cannot be overstated that ongoing therapy from accredited physical therapists is essential for restoration of full movement. During the recovery period, weight loss (if the person is overweight) and muscle building are highly recommended. In many cases, the increased ease and enhancement of the activities of daily living become highly motivating. Outcomes depend on the timing of surgery; the number of procedures that the surgeon and the hospital have to their credit; and the patient's

medical status, perioperative and postoperative management, and rehabilitation.

▲ *Promoting Healthy Aging: Implications for Gerontological Nursing.* To provide holistic care to the person with OA, the nurse works with a number of nonpharmacological approaches and teaches these to the person to enable and empower self-care. These approaches include the use of heat and cold, joint support and protection, exercise, and diet.

The use of heat and cold is well known for management of pain. Patient preference is important, but cold usually works best for an acute process, using cold packs that decrease muscle spasm, decrease swelling, and relieve inflammatory pain. Heat may be applied superficially or deep; either works well (Lozada and Altman, 2001). Ultrasound provides deep heat. Hot packs, hydrotherapy, and radiant heat provide superficial heat. A recent device available for prolonged heat application is ThermaCare, which is a band applied to the affected area (e.g., neck, lower back, abdomen) and lasts for 8 to 12 hours. It is available without a prescription and can be worn under clothing throughout the day.

Devices and techniques are available that relieve some of the pressure to the joints and protect the joints from further stress and, in doing so, may decrease pain and improve balance. Canes, crutches, walkers, collars, shoe orthotics, and corsets are such devices. A cane can relieve hip pressure by 60%. A shoe lift can improve lumbar pain. A knee brace is useful for knees, especially if there is lateral instability (the knee "gives out"). If the hands are affected, the person can resist carrying packages by the fingers or use adaptive devices on utensils and household equipment to make a larger grip surface. A variety of adaptive equipment is available to make daily activities less problematic. The Resource section at the end of this chapter provides more information. Avoiding exposure of the affected joints to cold temperatures also may help. The person is encouraged to wear leggings, gloves, or scarves when outside in cold climates.

A careful exercise plan should be strongly encouraged. Working with a skilled physical therapist or rehabilitation nurse specialist may improve clinical outcomes. Regular exercise can improve flexibility and muscle strength, which in turn support the affected joints, reduce pain, improve function, and reduce falls (Brion and Concoff, 2002). Exercise can also improve coordination, endurance, and ability to perform daily activities; increase energy; reduce fatigue; prevent depression; control weight; and lead to improved self-esteem. Exercise should include flexibility (stretching, ROM) exercises, strengthening (resistance) exercises, and cardiovascular (aerobic) exercises. Water exercise is recommended for people with arthritis and is a gentle way to exercise joints and muscles. Water supports joints and lessens stress on them to encourage free movement and also may act as resistance to build muscle strength. The Arthritis Foundation (*www.arthritis.org*) offers a water exercise program for people with arthritis, as well as other information on appropriate exercise programs. Resnick (2001) provides suggestions for an exercise program for older adults with arthritis, as well as a seven-step approach to assist in motivation for exercise.

Attention should also be given to diet. With the decreases in activity associated with pain, it is easy for the person to gain weight. Excess weight significantly increases the pressure and wear and tear of the joints, leading to less activity and more weight gain. Weight reduction should be considered for all persons who are overweight (body mass index [BMI] >25). The nurse can work with the person to identify weight and caloric goals and develop meal plans that are culturally acceptable but still balanced and healthy. The nurse can also refer the person to a registered dietitian and then lend support and encouragement. Figure 15-5 illustrates management of OA from a wellness perspective.

A number of complementary and alternative interventions show promise in contributing to pain relief for persons with arthritis. Pharmaceutical grade glucosamine hydrochloride (1500 mg/day) plus chondroitin sulfate (1200 mg/day) may reduce moderate to severe pain. The Food and Drug Administration (FDA) does not regulate these supplements; therefore the purity of these supplements may vary (Agency for Healthcare Research and Quality, 2007). McCaffrey and Freeman (2003) found a significant reduction in arthritic pain for persons who listened to music. Others have found the ancient techniques of acupuncture and acupressure also effective in some cases (Gaylord and Crotty, 2002; Roberts, 2003). Massage, progressive relaxation, meditation, and guided imagery may be helpful in managing stress and pain. Baird (2003), in a qualitative study to understand the lived experience of OA in older women, suggested that learning more about OA and self-care behaviors and strategies may assist in

successful management. Health care providers need to assess individual strengths, problems, and knowledge of self-care interventions when working with older adults with OA.

People with arthritis should be encouraged to participate in self-management courses such as the Arthritis Self-Help Course developed by nurse researcher Dr. Kate Loring, offered through the Arthritis Foundation. The course covers problem solving, decision making, and communicating with one's physician, as well as arthritis-specific content on exercise and relaxation techniques. Long-term outcomes include reduction of pain and physician visits for people who take the course (American Society on Aging, 2004; Newman, 2001). Information about the course and other arthritis information can be found at both the Arthritis Foundation and the National Institutes for Health websites (*www.arthritis.org*; *www.niams.nih.gov*). Arthritis education and outreach activities, particularly to culturally, ethnically, and socially diverse people, are essential and have been facilitated by funding to the Centers for Disease Control and Prevention (CDC) from the government through the public health system at the national and state levels (American Society on Aging, 2004). Box 15-18 summarizes nursing interventions for osteoarthritis.

Rheumatoid Arthritis

Definition. Rheumatoid arthritis (RA) is a chronic, systemic inflammatory joint disorder. It is considered an autoimmune disease in which an inflamed synovium (lining of the joint) invades and destroys the cartilage and bone within the joint. The cause is unknown, and RA may be one disease or several different diseases with common features (*www.arthritis.org*). Approximately 2.1 million people

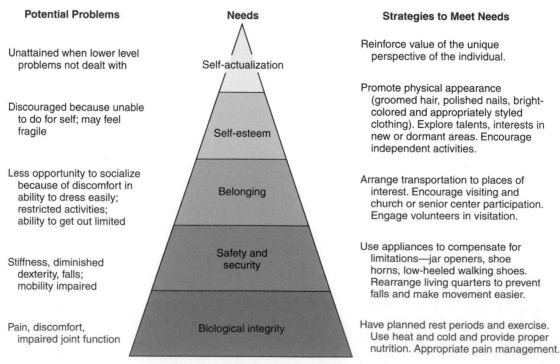

Potential Problems	Needs	Strategies to Meet Needs
Unattained when lower level problems not dealt with	Self-actualization	Reinforce value of the unique perspective of the individual.
Discouraged because unable to do for self; may feel fragile	Self-esteem	Promote physical appearance (groomed hair, polished nails, bright-colored and appropriately styled clothing). Explore talents, interests in new or dormant areas. Encourage independent activities.
Less opportunity to socialize because of discomfort in ability to dress easily; restricted activities; ability to get out limited	Belonging	Arrange transportation to places of interest. Encourage visiting and church or senior center participation. Engage volunteers in visitation.
Stiffness, diminished dexterity, falls; mobility impaired	Safety and security	Use appliances to compensate for limitations—jar openers, shoe horns, low-heeled walking shoes. Rearrange living quarters to prevent falls and make movement easier.
Pain, discomfort, impaired joint function	Biological integrity	Have planned rest periods and exercise. Use heat and cold and provide proper nutrition. Appropriate pain management.

FIGURE 15-5 Osteoarthritis wellness perspective.

BOX 15-18	Nursing Interventions for Osteoarthritis

COMFORT

Behavioral-cognitive pain control (imagery, relaxation, distraction)
Analgesic medications
Localized applications of heat

EXERCISE

Range of motion initially, progressing to aerobic exercise as tolerated or prescribed
Exercise alternated with rest
Avoiding prolonged rest periods

DIET

Weight loss if obese
Balanced, nutritious diet

JOINT PROTECTION

Avoiding high-impact activities in affected joints
Good body mechanics
Assistive devices: canes, commode extenders, Velcro-fastened clothing

PSYCHOSOCIAL PARAMETERS

Assessment of coping strategies, self-efficacy beliefs, social support

EDUCATION

Nature of osteoarthritis disease process
Purpose of prescribed interventions

From Kee CC et al: Perspectives on the nursing management of osteoarthritis, *Geriatr Nurs* 19(1):19-26, 1998.

in the United States have RA, and it can affect anyone, including children. RA affects more women than men (3:1). Onset usually occurs between ages 40 and 60 years (Anderson, 2004). About 1% of adults older than 65 years have RA, and the onset may be more sudden than in younger adults. Large joints may be more affected, and fatigue, weakness, and fever may be presenting signs (Meiner and Lueckenotte, 2006). Risk of mortality with RA is increased compared with a non-RA population, especially from GI problems and cardiac deaths, as well as hematological, respiratory, and infectious causes (Gornisiewicz and Moreland, 2001). Atherosclerosis may be accelerated somewhat in RA (Van Doornum et al., 2002).

RA is characterized by symmetrical polyarticular pain and swelling, morning stiffness lasting longer than 30 minutes, and malaise (Gornisiewicz and Moreland, 2001). Whereas morning stiffness in OA lasts less than 30 minutes, in RA it is longer than 30 minutes. The joints are warm and tender (Gornisiewicz and Moreland, 2001). It normally affects the small joints of the wrist, knee, ankle, and hand, although it affects large joints as well. As the inflammatory changes of the disease progress, joint deformities occur, with more than 10% developing hand deformities within 2 years. Older

people who have had RA for many years may present with multiple deformities, especially of the hands and feet, and may have undergone joint replacement surgeries (Tabloski, 2006). The natural course of RA is highly variable, with remission and exacerbations. The disease may be unremitting, with continuing progression, disability, and death, or it may be a remitting (rare) disease.

Early diagnosis is important because of the significant and irreversible destruction of affected joints within 1 to 2 years of onset. Nearly one half of those affected are disabled within 10 years (Luggen, 2003). Symptoms in late life tend to be acutely uncomfortable and spread throughout the joints in the body. Sometimes the disorder affects systems other than joints. An elevated rheumatoid factor (RF) combined with an elevated erythrocyte sedimentation rate (ESR) are most suggestive of RA. RA is classified as seropositive or seronegative; about 80% of people with RA are RF antibody positive. This is associated with a more severe and progressive course, with a reduced life expectancy of 10 to 15 years (Luggen, 2003). Elders who have seronegative RA may become seropositive.

Assessment. The American College of Rheumatology has established criteria for the diagnosis of RA (Luggen, 2002):
- Morning stiffness lasting longer than 1 hour (and present for 6 weeks)
- More than three of the following joints are involved: proximal interphalangeal (PIP), metacarpophalangeal (MCP), wrist, elbow, knee, ankle, and metatarsophalangeal (MTP) (for 6 weeks)
- Arthritis of the wrist, MCP joint, or PIP joint (for 6 weeks)
- Joint involvement is symmetrical (for 6 weeks)
- Presence of rheumatoid nodules
- Positive serum rheumatoid factor (up to 50% are false positive at age 80 years)
- X-ray examination changes such as erosions, bone decalcification (localized in or adjacent to the involved joints)

No one test is necessary to confirm the diagnosis of RA; in some patients all tests will be normal. On the other hand, elderly patients who have a number of other chronic illnesses may have many positive tests that confuse and confound the diagnosis. For instance, a positive RF is often present in older smokers (Gornisiewicz and Moreland, 2001).

A baseline assessment should include subjective data from the elder. Ask about stiffness, joint pain, fatigue, and function. Ask about activities the client is no longer able to do. In the physical examination, note the tender and swollen joints and any deformities present. Assess for depression because this is a common component of RA.

Systemic Manifestations. RA is a systemic disease and affects many organ systems in addition to the joints. Rheumatoid nodules may arise within tendons or ligaments and can cause rupture or joint dysfunction (Gornisiewicz and Moreland, 2001). They can also occur (less often) in the lungs, the sclera, and the vocal cords. About 15% of people with RA develop Sjögren's syndrome, which, in addition to RA, includes dry eyes and dry mouth, Raynaud's phenomenon, vasculitis, and erythema. Many elders develop dry eyes and xerostomia without having RA, thus confusing the diagnosis. Other manifestations include scleritis of the eyes, a serious problem requiring regular ophthalmological examinations. Pulmonary involvement can occur as interstitial lung disease or pleurisy with or without effusions; this occurs in about 70% of RA patients. The heart may be involved, with pericarditis or pericardial effusion. Felty's syndrome occurs mainly in older adults with RA. This syndrome is the triad of neutropenia, splenomegaly, and severe RA. The client may have recurrent bacterial urinary tract and pulmonary infections.

Interventions. In the past, NSAIDs were the drugs of choice for early disease. It was thought that these would reduce the swelling and therefore the damage to the joints, as well as address pain. However, it has been found that the disease is most aggressive in the first 2 years and that prompt efforts must be made to halt or slow the damage as much as possible (Anderson, 2004). Persons diagnosed with RA are usually cared for by rheumatologists, and treatment involves the use of aggressive therapy using a class of drugs called *disease-modifying antirheumatic drugs (DMARDs)*. Other medications that may be prescribed include cortisone, biological response modifiers, and analgesic drugs. Protein-A immunoadsorption therapy, a blood filtering therapy that removes antibodies and immune complexes that promote inflammation, may also be used. All the DMARDs are potentially toxic and must be prescribed by a physician and administered (by a registered nurse) with care. The DMARD *methotrexate* has been the standard for treatment of RA. Recent studies suggest that DMARDs, in combination with another drug, particularly the biological response modifiers, may be a more effective treatment, especially for people who have built up resistance to methotrexate or another drug alone. The biological response modifiers are injected or given intravenously and are costly (*www.arthritisfoundation.org*).

In RA, the management goals are to decrease pain, prevent and control joint damage, and prevent loss of function (American College of Rheumatology, 2002). Additional goals are maintaining normal physical, social, and emotional function and the capacity to do work and perform ADLs (Gornisiewicz and Moreland, 2001). As in OA, it is necessary to decrease the pain and inflammation of RA to manage the disease and to work with the person to prevent deformity. It is important that the elder understand the nature of this disease and that the care prescribed must be followed to prevent the pain, deformity, and disability that are the natural course.

▲ *Promoting Healthy Aging: Implications for Gerontological Nursing.* All the non-pharmacological nursing interventions discussed in the section on OA apply here. However, the use of dietary supplements cannot be

---

BOX 15-19 Goals of Nursing Management and Intervention in Arthritis

GOALS

Pain management and promotion of comfort
Exercise and rest interspersed
Psychological support
Reduction of swelling and inflammation
Prevention of deformity
Promotion of optimal lifestyle

SUGGESTED INTERVENTIONS

Provide realistic information.
Teach client self-care to promote comfort.
Assist client in modifying lifestyle appropriately.
Prescribe exercises for muscle maintenance.
Promote participation in weight reduction program if necessary.
Have client balance rest and activity.
Teach relaxation and stress reduction.
Teach client to avoid bending painful joints and to splint when joints are inflamed.
Teach client to maintain body alignment when standing, sitting, and lying down.

Data from Heckheimer EF: *Health promotion of the elderly in the community,* Philadelphia, 1989, Saunders.

---

recommended because of their potential and unknown interactions with the complex drug regimen. In helping the patient manage the associated pain and other symptoms, expert nursing care must be provided. See the discussion of pain management in Chapter 11 and the suggested interventions in Box 15-19.

Self-management and education and support groups may increase feelings of self-efficacy and sense of control and may promote more positive outcomes even in the presence of increasing debilitation. In addition to the physical management of RA are the consequences of RA and the management of these. The practitioner should look for and treat problems such as depression, anxiety, poor coping strategies, learned helplessness, cognitive changes, and impaired self-efficacy (Callahan and Jonas, 2002). These problems are associated with poor outcomes and increased use of health care services. It takes great courage to learn to live fully despite a certain degree of constant discomfort.

Rest is as important as exercise in RA. For many years it was thought that people with RA should rest only their joints to protect them from damage; however, both rest and exercise are necessary. In terms of rest, this may be resting the particular affected joint, such as a hand or wrist, or total body rest. Therapeutic exercise programs are designed to help maintain or improve the ability to do ADLs. Even a warm, inflamed joint should be given ROM exercises to maintain movement in the joint. A physical or occupational therapist should be consulted for developing a program of rest and exercise. Splints and assistive devices, as well as occupational therapy consultation to enhance self-care ability, are important interventions.

Environmental modifications are often necessary for elders with RA. Zipper pulls and Velcro closures on clothing are two practical measures. Book holders, chairs to sit on while preparing foods, light switch changes, and secure stair railings are other measures. An on-line database, ABLEDATA (*www.abledata.com*), sponsored by the National Institute on Disability and Rehabilitation Research, lists more than 25,000 available assistive devices.

Polymyalgia Rheumatica

Polymyalgia rheumatica (PMR) is one of the more common inflammatory diseases seen in older adults, and patients with PMR also may have coexistent OA. Although it is sometimes difficult to differentiate PMR from OA, it is important since PMR is potentially reversible and requires different treatment. PMR is a chronic inflammatory disease characterized by severe stiffness and pain in the muscles of the neck, shoulders, lower back, buttocks, and thighs.

Epidemiology. The average age of onset of PMR is 65 to 70 years and occurs more often in older women than in men (2:1) and more in whites in the United States and Europe; it is uncommon in blacks (Spiera and Spiera, 2004). The etiology is unknown, but a genetic predisposition may exist (Kennedy-Malone and Enevold, 2001).

Clinical Signs and Symptoms. PMR usually has an acute onset, and pain usually begins in the neck and upper arms and may evolve to involve the pelvic and pectoral girdles. Fatigue and low-grade fever may occur. Nocturnal pain, especially in the shoulder, interferes with sleep and there may be difficulty when trying to stand after sitting for awhile or when getting out of a car or bathtub (gelling phenomenon). Pain is usually greatest at night and in the early morning, but usually no joint inflammation is present. If swelling and joint inflammation are present, RA is more likely.

An elevated ESR (>50 mm/hr) is common, as well as mild normocytic or normochromic anemia. Diagnosis can be difficult because infection, fibromyalgia, and other diffuse connective tissue diseases may share similar symptoms. Temporal arteritis (discussed in Chapter 8) is found in approximately 10% to 30% of people with PMR. Temporal arteritis needs immediate treatment or it can result in irreversible blindness (Kennedy-Malone and Enevold, 2001). Patients on statin medications may present with myalgias, and it is important to discontinue these drugs before diagnosing PMR to see if pain remits (Spiera and Spiera, 2004).

Treatment. The mainstay of therapy is glucocorticoids (typically prednisone 15 mg/day or another glucocorticoid such as methylprednisolone). Pain and stiffness may be gone within days, ESR decreases to normal, and anemia resolves in several weeks. Treatment may continue for 2 to 3 years; however, some may be able to stop drug treatment in several months. The side effects of steroid therapy can be problematic, especially osteoporosis, myopathy, increased blood glucose levels, and cholesterol elevation. Blood pressure and fluid retention must be monitored (Spiera and Spiera, 2004). Efforts should be made to lower the dose to the optimal level to suppress symptoms. Relapse is common if therapy is lowered too quickly. If the elder has diabetes, careful monitoring is important. Bisphosphonates should be given to prevent bone loss and fractures.

Bursitis and Tendinitis

These disorders are known as *soft tissue rheumatic syndromes* and become more common with aging. They cause pain, swelling, and inflammation around joints and in the tissues and structures such as ligaments, tendons, bursae, and muscles. Because the problem is so near a joint, it is often confused with arthritis.

Pathophysiology. Bursae are closed sacs lined with a membrane, resembling synovium, that secretes and absorbs fluid from the bursa (Reginato and Reginato, 2001). This provides a gliding mechanism between two musculoskeletal structures (muscle over muscle or tendon over bone). There are about 150 bursae in the body. Adventitious bursae may develop at pressure points, for example, bunions or Baker's cysts. Inflammation of a bursa can be deep (popliteal) or superficial (elbow, shoulder) and is common in older adults.

Tendinitis refers to inflammation of the tissues or synovial sheaths around a tendon (*tenosynovitis*). It usually occurs from overuse, unaccustomed activity, or exercise (Reginato and Reginato, 2001).

Bursitis occurs with repetitive physical stresses. It occurs mainly in subacromial bursae (shoulder) and olecranon bursae (elbow). In the lower extremity, it occurs in the trochanteric, prepatellar, gastrocnemius-semimembranosus, and anserine bursae. Inflammation may cause rupture of the bursa, for example, Baker's cyst. Pain is usually described as deep, aching discomfort. Bursitis can occur because of RA and gout.

Hand and wrist tendinitis may exhibit as Dupuytren's contracture. This is a fibrous thickening of the palmar fascia (Reginato and Reginato, 2001). It occurs mainly in middle-aged men and elders of Northern European descent. It is an inherited trait and is associated with tobacco smoking, diabetes mellitus, local trauma, alcohol abuse, and long-term use of epileptic medications. It is usually bilateral. As it progresses, there is contracture of the MCP and PIP joints. Ring and little fingers are often involved. This disorder is associated with "trigger finger" (inflammation causing a popping sound when extending the trigger finger), carpal tunnel syndrome, lateral epicondylitis, and frozen shoulder. Surgical correction is the only treatment and is not curative.

Shoulder problems are common in elderly patients. Many joints may be affected, including the acromioclavicular, sternoclavicular, glenohumeral, and scapulothoracic muscular joints (Reginato and Reginato, 2001). Often the problem is caused by bursitis, RA, or pseudogout. Pseudogout is a microcrystalline arthritis associated with calcification of hyaline and fibrous cartilage, often in the knee or shoulder in elders (Beers and Berkow, 2000). It begins in the late 50s, women are more affected than men, and there may be a history of hypothyroidism. Elders with subacromial bursitis often awaken at night with severe pain when they turn to the affected shoulder. It radiates in the C5 dermatome. Rotator cuff tears are common in elderly people. They may be acute or chronic and full or partial thickness. They cause severe dysfunction because of the pain. These are best diagnosed by magnetic resonance imaging (MRI) and treated with analgesics, steroid injection, and exercise for the weakness that occurs with disuse. Surgical treatment is necessary if conservative management fails.

Gout

Gout is another form of inflammatory arthritis that results from accumulation of uric acid crystals (tophi) in a joint. Gout may be a one-time acute illness, or it may become a chronic condition with acute attacks. The joint of the great toe is the most typical site of an attack. Sometimes the ankle, knee, wrist, or elbow is involved. Men between 40 and 50 years of age are most commonly affected, but the prevalence increases significantly with age. In older people, gout may present insidiously and acute attacks of gout are less commonly seen. Gout is often misdiagnosed as RA because symptoms of arthritis and subcutaneous tophi deposits on toes, fingers, and elbows may appear (Tabloski, 2006).

Gout typically starts with an acute attack. The person complains of what is called *exquisite pain* in the affected joint, often starting in the middle of the night during sleep. The joint is bright red, hot, and too painful to touch. Fever, malaise and chills may also be present. Gout may be exacerbated by drugs commonly taken by older people, particularly thiazide diuretics and salicylates (even in small doses). A laboratory test finding of elevated uric acid is possible, but the uric acid level also may be normal.

The first goal of treatment during an attack is pain relief. This may include NSAIDs, colchicines, and sometimes injection of long-acting steroids into the joint. The nurse ensures that the person takes in enough fluids to help flush the uric acid through the kidneys (2 L/day if not contraindicated). During drug therapy, the person should not take salicylates, which may inhibit drug effectiveness (Meiner and Lueckenotte, 2006).

After the acute attack, the medical goal is to prevent another attack, systemic spread of the disease, and the development of chronic gout. This may be done by avoiding drugs or foods that are high in purine and alcohol, both of which increase uric acid levels, and by taking medications to either decrease uric acid production (e.g., allopurinol) or increase its excretion (probenecid). Weight reduction if the patient is overweight is also encouraged (Jett and Lester, 2004).

The nurse's role includes teaching the person how to decrease the likelihood of another attack by employing preventive measures. In administering gout-related medications, the nurse pays close attention to renal function and notifies the physician or nurse practitioner of any impairment so that dosages can be adjusted.

PARKINSON'S DISEASE

Definition and Epidemiology

Parkinson's disease (PD) is a progressive disease of the basal ganglia (corpus striatum) and involves the dopaminergic nigrostriatal pathway. This type of disorder produces a syndrome of abnormal movement called *parkinsonism* that leads to difficulty with mobility (Miller, 2002). PD affects more than 1.5 million people in the United States with estimates of 60,000 new cases each year and costs of over $20 billion annually (Swantek, 2002). PD appears to be slightly more common in men than in women, and the average age of onset is about 60 years. Prevalence and incidence increase with age, but 15% of those diagnosed are younger than 50 years. Early onset of the disease is often inherited, and some have been linked to specific gene mutations. All races and ethnicities throughout the world appear to be affected; however, a number of studies have found a higher incidence in developed countries. It is speculated that this might be related to the use of pesticides or other toxins. PD is the second most common neurodegenerative disease (stroke is the first). It was first described in 1817 in a paper by Dr. James Parkinson, a British physician, who described "the shaking palsy" and presented the major symptoms of the disease.

PD is the most common form of parkinsonism, a group of disorders with similar features and symptoms. PD is a clinical syndrome characterized by the following: bradykinesia (slow movement); resting tremor; rigidity; abnormalities of posture, balance and gait; and deficiency of the neurotransmitter *dopamine*. Parkinson's disease is called either *primary parkinsonism* or *idiopathic*. Idiopathic is a term describing a disorder for which a cause has not yet been found. In other forms of parkinsonism, either the cause is known or the disorder occurs as a secondary effect of another disorder causing loss or interference with the action of dopamine in the basal ganglia (e.g., head trauma, postencephalitic parkinsonism, stroke, tumors, and toxin- and drug-induced parkinsonian syndrome). Older people are especially prone to the development of Parkinson's-like symptoms as a side effect of antipsychotic medications, and any older adult receiving these medications should be routinely screened for extrapyramidal symptoms (EPS). Box 15-20 lists symptoms of PD.

Pathophysiology

The pathogenesis is unknown. Epidemiological data suggest genetic, viral, and toxic (pesticide exposure) causes. In more than one half of those with PD, atrophy and neuronal loss are found (Boss, 2002). The main feature is degeneration of the neurons of the substantia nigra. Lewy bodies and intracytoplasmic eosinophilic inclusions are found in those neurons remaining in the substantia nigra. The severity of PD is associated with the degree of neuron loss and the reduction of dopamine receptors in the basal ganglia. PD is progressive, and symptoms grow worse over time. Symptoms vary and the intensity of symptoms also varies from person to person; some become severely disabled, and others experience only minor motor disturbances. The progression of symptoms may

BOX 15-20   Primary Symptoms of Parkinson's Disease (PD)

RESTING TREMOR

Occurs in approximately 50% to 75% of all PD patients and is often the initial symptom

Affects mainly hands and feet but may also involve the head, neck, face, lips, tongue, or jaw

Appears regular and rhythmic; approximately four to six beats per second

RIGIDITY

Sustained muscle contractions; often mistaken for common stiffness or achiness

Walking with arms held stiffly at the sides (rather than swinging naturally)

Most common types include:
- Cogwheeling: muscles move in a series of short jerks
- Lead-pipe: muscles move smoothly, yet stiffly

May affect breathing, eating, swallowing, and speech

BRADYKINESIA   SLOW (BRADY) MOVEMENT (KINESIA)

Slowing of ordinary movements, such as walking, sitting down, and getting dressed

Reduction in semiautomatic gestures, such as crossing the legs or scratching

Reduction of spontaneous facial movements, resulting in masklike stare

Handwriting begins large and becomes smaller as patient fatigues

Voice may become soft and trail off

POSTURAL INSTABILITY

Difficulty maintaining balance when walking or standing

Leans forward in an effort to maintain center of gravity

May result in injuries from frequent falls

From The American Parkinson Disease Association, Inc., 60 Bay Street, Staten Island, NY 10301.

take 20 years or more. Older age at onset and the presence of rigidity/hypokinesia as an initial symptom may predict a more rapid rate of motor progression (American Academy of Neurology [AAN], 2006a). In late stages of the disease, complications such as pressure ulcers, pneumonia, aspiration, and falls can lead to death.

Clinical Signs

By the time a person becomes overtly symptomatic, 80% to 90% of the dopamine-producing cells are lost (Burke and Laramie, 2000). PD has such an insidious onset that it is very difficult to diagnose, particularly in the early stages. Diagnosis is one of exclusion, ruling out other possible causes of symptoms. Classic signs of PD are (1) tremor at rest, (2) rigidity (stiff muscles), (3) akinesia (poverty of movement), and (4) postural abnormalities. The American Academy of Neurology (AAN) recommends olfactory testing and administration of a levodopa or apomorphine and evaluating effect on symptoms (challenge test) as useful in confirming the diagnosis if there is doubt (AAN, 2006a). Early falls, poor response to levodopa, symmetry of motor symptoms, lack of tremor, and early autonomic dysfunction may be useful in distinguishing PD from other parkinsonian syndromes (AAN, 2006a).

The most conspicuous sign is the tremor—an asymmetrical, regular, rhythmic, low-amplitude tremor. It disappears briefly during voluntary movement. It can occur in the leg, but the arm is more commonly involved. Rarely is the head involved. All tremors are increased with stress and anxiety. Tremor is a minor part of the clinical picture. It is not present during sleep and when present is a pill-rolling movement. A greater cause of disability is the rigidity and slow movements and postural instability. Other signs include soft-spoken voice, little facial animation (masked facies), infrequent blinking, restless legs, and greasy skin (Miller, 2002). The characteristic gait is called *festination* and consists of very short steps and minimal arm movements. Turning is difficult and may require many steps. If off balance, correction is very slow, so falls are common. Other clinical signs include sleep difficulties (up at night, sleeping all day), constipation, fatigue, excessive salivation, pain, loss of smell, depression, visual disturbances, psychosis, seborrhea, sweating, and hypotension, which is a considerable problem in PD and with the medications used to treat PD.

Recent studies have suggested that impulse-control disorders such as pathological gambling and hypersexuality may occur in an estimated 3% to 5% of people with PD. These may be related to some anti-parkinsonian drugs or to factors yet unknown. Screening for the presence of these disorders and early recognition and treatment are important (Dodd et al., 2005; Parkinson Disease Foundation, 2005). Further research is needed in this area.

Rigidity impedes passive and active movement. It is a state of involuntary contraction of all skeletal muscles. Severe muscle cramps may occur in the toes or hands. On examination, a limb may exhibit "lead pipe" resistance during passive movement. Akinesia (absence or poverty or movement) is an often overlooked symptom. All the striated muscles in the extremities, trunk, ocular area, and face are affected, including the muscles of mastication (chewing), deglutition (swallowing), and articulation. Handwriting is small (micrographia). The elder with PD will sit for long periods or lie motionless with few shifts in position. The patient has difficulty initiating movement. "Freezing" is a common problem and may be precipitated by trying to move, turning, or initiating tactile and visual contact. Postural reflexes are lost. The elder will have involuntary flexion of the head and neck, a stooped posture, and a tendency to fall backward.

Management

Many treatment options to manage the symptoms and the consequences of PD are available. The AAN has published comprehensive clinical practice guidelines related to PD, as well as excellent patient information tools (*www.aan.com*). Drug therapy focuses on replacement, mimicking, or slowing dopamine breakdown. Typically, individuals are maintained on a combination of carbidopa and levodopa (Sinemet), which are dopamine precursors. The AAN recommends either levodopa or a dopamine agonist (Parlodel) to treat initial symptoms. Selegiline (monoamine oxidase [MAO] inhibitor) also may be of mild benefit as an initial treatment (AAN, 2006d). Sinemet loses effectiveness as the amino acid L-dopa competes with other amino acids for absorption at both the intestinal wall and the blood-brain barrier. It also has a higher risk of dyskinesia side effects.

Other medications useful in management include the dopamine agonists; dopaminergics; catechol O-methyltransferase (COMT) inhibitors; MAO inhibitors; antihistamines; and anticholinergics (for tremor relief). Medications may be used in combination and for specific effects. Most recently, rasagiline (Azilect) was approved as a single drug therapy and also to be used in combination with levodopa in advanced disease. The action of Azilect is to block the breakdown of dopamine. People taking this medication must avoid food or drinks that contain tyramine because of interactions causing sudden and severe rises in blood pressure causing stroke or death. Neupro (Rotigotine Transdermal System) has been recently approved for treatment of early-stage PD (U.S. Food and Drug Administration, 2007).

Medication therapy is complicated and should be closely supervised by a neurologist. The medications used to treat PD are not without serious side effects. Hypotension is a problem, as are dyskinesias, dystonia, end-of-dose deterioration, and the on-off phenomenon. Medications also cause hallucinations and sleep disorders, as does PD. Sinemet must be taken 1 hour before or 2 hours after a meal to minimize GI side effects, and it must also be given routinely and on time to prevent fluctuations in symptoms.

Anxiety and depression frequently occur in PD. Currently, selective serotonin reuptake inhibitors (SSRIs) such as venlafaxine are used. Bupropion, sertraline, paroxetine, trazodone, and mirtazapine also are used. For patients with PD and psychosis, antipsychotics may be required and should be those with the least anticholinergic effects. The AAN (2006b) recommends clozapine and quetiapine. Agranulocytosis that may be fatal is a side effect of clozapine, and close monitoring of neutrophil count is essential. Approximately 20% of patients with PD will develop dementia, usually after the age of 70 years. The etiology of dementia in PD is not clearly understood, and it may be a specific type of dementia or diffuse Lewy body (DLB) dementia. Lewy bodies (protein deposits in the nerve cells) characterize this dementia, and presentation is different from that of Alzheimer's disease and includes changes in alertness, withdrawal, loss of problem-solving skills, and lack of flexibility in thinking. Patients with DLB are intolerant of neuroleptic agents (particularly risperidone). The AAN recommends the use of the cholinesterase inhibitors *donepezil* and *rivastigmine* for PD patients with dementia to improve cognitive function. Chapter 23 discusses dementia in more depth.

Surgical procedures include ablation (pallidotomy/thalamotomy), deep brain stimulation (DBS), and trans-plantation. DBS is the most commonly performed surgery for PD and is used in patients who have not responded to drug therapy or have intractable motor fluctuations, dyskinesias, or tremor. Transplantation is in the experimental stage. Research is ongoing and has shown promising results for both DBS and transplantation. However, the AAN (2006d) states that evidence is insufficient to support or refute DBS at this time.

Non-pharmacological interventions such as exercise, relaxation, stress management, education, and self-care management may be beneficial in helping people cope with PD. Music therapy is being researched as a therapeutic intervention for people with PD, investigating the use of different rhythms to assist in movement (*www.pdtrials.org*). At this time, the AAN (2006c) does not recommend any vitamin or food additive or other treatment such as acupuncture, biofeedback, or manual therapy as effective treatment of PD. Exercise therapy and speech therapy for patients with dysarthria should be considered.

BOX 15-21   Having Parkinson's Disease

Parkinson is the name of the disease we got
It can strike anyone when it's cold or when it's hot
You might get tremors that cause you to shake
But living with them is a piece of cake
Stiffness of the body occurs in some
And you shuffle your feet like some old bum
Slurring of your speech makes others think you're drunk
But faith keeps you going and you gotta have spunk
Sometimes when you're walking you freeze and cannot move
And people who are watching think you've missed the groove
Penmanship is a thing of the past
In a handwriting contest you'd come in last
Simple little movements like getting in a car
Turn into big projects like draining a reservoir
You get going walking and fell like you're falling
If you weren't so stubborn you'd feel like bawling
Frequent naps are a plus if you like to sleep
But along comes your caregiver and your sleep isn't deep
Your instant response to an act that calls for action
Is harder to do than figuring out a fraction
Sharing your problems with others like you
For yourself is the best thing you can do
You meet with your cohorts in a support group
And you're with people that also have your droop
You're all in the same boat you are all afflicted
You take so many pills you think you're addicted
It's not all bad no matter what you say
You make new friends most every day
And you'll still live to a ripe old age
And no one will put you away in a cage
So don't you worry that I'm not going to fret
I'm still on this earth fighting for all I can get
For all your tribulation and what you gotta do
Chin up comrades learn to laugh at "YOU"

Author: Ken Weber, Sheboygan Wisconsin, 1987. Poem appeared in a Parkinson's Foundation newsletter.

BOX 15-22   Nursing Interventions for Parkinson's Disease

EXERCISE

- Flexibility exercises, gentle stretching or yoga
- Range of motion twice a day
- Walking at least 4 times a day. Bring your toes up with every step you take. Use a wide base (legs 12-15 inches apart when walking); swing your arms freely when walking; if legs feel frozen or "glued" to the floor, a lift of the toes eliminates muscle spasm; if walking with a helper, have them walk by your side, never pull from the front; wear shoes with a firm sole (no rubber or crepe-soled)
- Practice sitting down and getting up. Sit down slowly with your body bent sharply forward until you touch the seat; when getting up, try rising as quickly as possible; use a lift chair
- Balance exercises (tai chi)
- Proper use of assistive devices
- Try exercise in pool or in bed, or try crawling if balance is poor

EATING AND NUTRITION

- Small, frequent meals
- Drink ample water—drink by the clock to ensure intake of at least 6-8 cups/day
- Cut foods in smaller portions
- Exercise your face and jaw—blow kisses or read aloud; sing with forceful lip and tongue motion; practice making faces in the mirror; recite the alphabet (try these with your grandchildren)
- For upset stomachs linked to medication, try eating an oatmeal cookie or pretzel

- Chew food hard and move food around in the mouth; avoid just swallowing
- Eat sitting up, and remain upright for at least 30 minutes after eating
- Allow adequate time for meals; keep food at proper temperature (insulated cups, warming trays)
- Try non-slip china, swivel or weighted utensils, or wrist weights

CONTINENCE AND CONSTIPATION

- Routine toileting
- Consider bedside commode
- Use raised toilet seat and grab bars
- Wear clothing that is easy to remove
- Drink 6-8 cups of water every day; seltzer water adds air and moisture to the bowel and can increase intestinal motility
- Increase fruits and vegetables in diet
- Weak hot tea or hot water with lemon first thing in the morning or prune juice with pulp can stimulate the bowel
- Medications such a stool softener; avoid stimulant laxatives and bulk/fiber laxatives (unless you drink at least 48 ounces of water/day)

SLEEP DIFFICULTIES

- Try relaxation exercises, meditation, music
- Medication for pain or discomfort if present
- Avoid sleeping medications
- Use body pillows or bolsters for comfort in bed
- Satin sheets to aid turning

Adapted from Parkinson Handbook, National Parkinson Foundation; Imke S: *Nutritional guidelines for people with Parkinson's disease and bowel hygiene: curing the GI blues*, presented at NCGNP Conference, 2005, Cleveland, Ohio; *Parkinson disease: signs and symptoms*. (website): *www.helpguide.org*; Bonifazi W: *A question of balance*, Nursing Spectrum, June 19, 2006. (website): *www.nursingspectrum.com*.

▲ Promoting Healthy Aging: Implications for Gerontological Nursing

Treatment focuses on relieving symptoms with medication, increasing functional ability, preventing excess disability, and decreasing risk of injury. Persons with PD experience great functional problems in mobility, communication, and ADLs, and nursing interventions can contribute greatly to quality of life and functional ability. Comprehensive functional assessments with attention to self-care abilities in ADLs and nutritional assessment are important, as well as fall assessment and risk reduction interventions. Nurses who care for people with PD in the hospital setting must be knowledgeable about functional abilities and interventions to maintain function during episodes of acute illness. The goal of treatment is to preserve self-care abilities and prevent complications. Support system encouragement and information about the disease are essential if the family and the person are to cope with the losses associated with PD. Whitney (2004), in an analysis of the stories of older adults with PD, suggested that learning what gives persons purpose and meaning in life and helping them understand what is happening to their bodies can assist in coping with the loss of prior abilities. Listening to stories is a wonderful way to come to know the person and individualize interventions to meet expressed needs, so ask your patients to tell you their story (Box 15-21).

Exercise, walking, ROM, and balance work need to begin early in the course of PD, and physical therapy evaluation and treatment are important. Rigidity of facial muscles and bradykinesia affect eating ability, nutrition, swallowing, and communication. Occupational therapy can assist with adaptive equipment such as weighted utensils, non-slip dinnerware, and other self-care aids. Speech therapy is beneficial for dysarthria and dysphagia, and patients can be taught facial exercises and swallowing techniques. Regular pain assessments and appropriate management are also essential to address the often unnoticed problem of pain related to rigidity, contractures, dystonias, and central-pain syndromes of the disease itself, which may cause unexplained uncomfortable sensations. Other important interventions are assessment and treatment of postural hypotension, continence, GI distress, depression and anxiety, sleep disturbances, and constipation. Box 15-22 provides some suggestions for nursing interventions. Many resources are available for people with PD to provide practical information about living with the disease, as well as information related to new developments and treatment. The Resources section at the end of this chapter provides further information that the nurse can use for referral.

Because of the slow progression of the disease and the disability that accompanies PD, individuals experience a change in roles, activities, and social participation. Tremors may produce embarrassing moments. The expressionless face, slowed movement, and soft, monotone speech

TABLE 15-3

Items in the Sickness Impact Profile (SIP) Endorsed by a Third or More of Patients with Parkinson's Disease (PD)*

SIP Category	SIP Item	Percent (no.) of PD Patients Endorsing Item	Percent (no.) of Controls Endorsing Item
Ambulation	I walk more slowly.	59 (26)	30 (13)
Body care and movement	I move my hands or fingers with some limitation or difficulty.	39 (17)	11 (5)
	I dress myself but do so very slowly.	46 (20)	9 (4)
Mobility	I stay home most of the time.	50 (22)	7 (3)
Emotional behavior	I act nervous or restless.	43 (20)	30 (13)
Social interaction	I am going out less to visit people.	50 (22)	14 (6)
	I am doing fewer social activities with groups of people.	50 (22)	27 (12)
	My sexual activity is decreased.	61 (27)	16 (7)
Alertness behavior	I have more minor accidents, drop things, trip and fall, bump into things.	46 (20)	14 (6)
	I forget a lot, for example, things that happened recently, where I put things, appointments.	36 (16)	25 (11)
Communication	I am having trouble writing or typing.	75 (33)	14 (6)
	I often lose control of my voice when I talk; for example, my voice gets louder or softer, trembles, changes unexpectedly.	41 (18)	2 (1)
	I do not speak clearly when I am under stress.	52 (23)	5 (2)
Sleep and rest	I sit during much of the day.	41 (18)	27 (12)
	I lie down more often during the day to rest.	34 (15)	16 (7)
	I sleep less at night, for example, wake up too early, do not fall asleep for a long time, awaken frequently.	46 (20)	25 (11)
Home management	I do work around the house only for short periods or rest often.	41 (26)	23 (10)
	I am doing *less* of the regular daily work around the house than I would usually do.	59 (26)	25 (11)
	I am not doing *any* of the maintenance or repair work that I would usually do in my home or yard.	39 (17)	11 (5)
	I have difficulty doing handwork, for example, turning faucets, using kitchen gadgets, sewing, carpentry.	39 (17)	9 (4)
	I am not doing heavy work around the house.	48 (21)	23 (10)
Recreation and pastimes	I do my hobbies and recreation for shorter periods.	43 (19)	18 (8)
	I am going out for entertainment less often.	43 (19)	32 (14)
	I am cutting down on *some* of my usual physical recreation or activities.	46 (20)	30 (13)

*Patients are instructed to endorse those items that apply to themselves and are related to their health.

may give the impression of apathy, depression, and disinterest and discourage others who might otherwise be social. Others, observing these symptoms, may feel that the person is unable to participate in activities and relationships and may even think the person is cognitively impaired. A sensitive nurse is aware that the visible symptoms produce an undesired façade that may hide an alert and responsive individual who wishes to interact but is trapped in a body that no longer responds. It is important to see beyond the disease to the person within and provide nursing interventions that enhance hope and promote the highest quality of life despite disease. The Sickness Impact Profile (SIP) is a useful tool that can be used by nurses to determine problems most troublesome from the client's perspective (Table 15-3).

TRANSPORTATION

Even though one is physically able to move about, there may be many hindrances to full use of public space. Available transportation is a critical link in the ability of the elderly to remain independent and functional. The lack of accessible transportation may contribute to other problems, such as social withdrawal, poor nutrition, or neglect of health care. Even when municipal transportation service is available, elders may not use it. Urban buses and subways not only are physically hazardous but also are often dangerous. A "crisis in mobility" exists for many older people because of the lack of an automobile, an inability to drive, limited access to public transportation, health factors, geographical location, and economic considerations. Culturally and ethnically diverse older people may experience more difficulty getting around than older whites, and rural residents may experience more difficulty than urban residents.

Older people may desire increased contact with other people, particularly relatives; however, even more crucial is the need to reach medical services, shopping areas, and service agencies. If mobility is hampered, both security and the sense of belonging to the mainstream of society may be blocked. The emphasis on a "barrier-free" (structurally revised) transportation system and reduced fares has been helpful to many older people, but some cannot avail themselves of public transportation because of physical disability or residence in a high-crime area. County, state, or federally subsidized transportation is being provided in certain areas to assist older people in reaching social services, nutrition sites, health services, emergency care, medical care, recreational centers, mental health services, day care programs, physical and vocational rehabilitation, continuing education, and library services. Although transportation can often be found for special needs, it is virtually impossible to locate transportation for pleasure or recreation. Senior centers offer a wide range of activities for older people, as well as transportation services. Nurses can refer older people to local social service and aging organizations, such as area agencies on aging, for information on resources and financial assistance for services.

AUTOMOBILES AND OLDER PEOPLE

Driving is one of the instrumental activities of daily living for most elders because it is essential to obtaining necessary resources for those individuals who live in rural and suburban areas. Assessments of functional capacities often neglect this important activity. We should evaluate whether an individual can drive, feels safe driving, and has a driver's license. Giving up mobility and independence afforded by driving one's own car has many psychological ramifications, as well as inconveniences. The following scenario illustrates:

> When Maury had a stroke, his physician told him he could no longer drive. He had been an auto addict all of his adult life and found his major pleasures behind the wheel of the new car that he would buy each year. As a young man, having an auto was a major status symbol because few teenagers owned a car in 1935. Driving was much more than a means of transportation for him.

As a group, older drivers are some of the United States' safest drivers. Older drivers drive fewer miles than younger drivers and tend to drive less at night, during adverse weather conditions, or in congested areas. Fewer older drivers speed or drive after drinking alcohol than drivers of other ages. However, when compared with younger age-groups, people older than 70 years are more likely to be involved in a crash and more likely to die in that crash. The leading cause of accidental death among persons older than 65 years is a motor vehicle accident; for those older than 75 years, motor vehicle accidents are the second leading cause of death after falls. Age-related changes in driving skills, including vision changes, cognitive impairment, and various medical illnesses and functional impairments, are all factors related to driving safety for older adults.

To help ensure the safety of older drivers, driver's license renewal procedures vary from state to state and may include accelerated renewal cycles, renewal in person rather than electronically or by mail, and vision and road tests (*www.iihs.org/laws/state_laws/older_drivers.html*). Many older people depend on driving to maintain their basic needs, and the inability to drive can cause depression and isolation. For many, alternate transportation is not readily available and, consequently, they may continue driving beyond the time it is safe. The issues of driving in the older adult population are the subject of a great deal of public discussion. Many older drivers and their families struggle with issues related to continued safety in driving, and families struggle with when and how to tell older people they are no longer safe to drive.

Health care providers should encourage open discussion of issues related to driving with the older person and his or her family and should identify impairments that affect safe driving, correct them when possible, and offer alternatives for transportation. Vehicle adaptations, sensory aids, elder driving training, and driving assessment programs are helpful in promoting safe driving (Gilfillan and Schwartzberg, 2005; Perkinson et al., 2005). Jett et al. (2005) provide useful strategies for driving counseling for people with dementia from a qualitative study involving guided interviews with

---

BOX 15-23 Action Strategies Used to Bring About Driving Cessation

IMPOSED TYPE	INVOLVED TYPE
Report person to division of motor vehicles for possible license suspension	All family members and individual meet, discuss the situation, and come to a mutual agreement of the problem
Use of deception or threats such as false keys, disabling the car, saying car was stolen	Dialog is ongoing from the earliest signs of cognitive impairment about the eventuality of the need to stop driving
Attempts to order or control, such as provider writing a prescription, commands from children to stop driving	Arrangements are made for alternative transportation plans that are available when needed and acceptable to the individual

From Jett K et al: Imposed versus involved: different strategies to effect driving cessation in cognitively impaired older adults, *Geriatr Nurs* 26(2):111-116, 2005.

Human Needs and Wellness Diagnoses

Self-Actualization and Transcendence
(Seeking, Expanding, Spirituality, Fulfillment)
Finds inspiration in creative pursuits
Plans adventures within capacities
Seeks transcendence of physical incapacities
Demonstrates spiritual growth and satisfaction

Self-Esteem and Self-Efficacy
(Image, Identity, Control, Capability)
Has strong sense of personal identity
Has the ability to tolerate limitations
Takes active role in seeking compensatory activities
Is assertive in obtaining services and assistive devices
Maintains independence to greatest degree possible considering impairments

Belonging and Attachment
(Love, Empathy, Affiliation)
Copes with mobility restrictions by increased
reliance on phones, letters, and e-mail
Maintains important personal connections
Demonstrates capacity for intimacy and affection

Safety and Security
(Caution, Planning, Protections, Sensory Acuity)
Monitors shifting capacities for function and
comfort and adapts appropriately
Uses adaptive devices effectively for maintaining mobility
Drives carefully and gives up license when necessary
Modifies environment to facilitate safe use of assistive devices

Biological and Physiological Integrity
(Air, Fluids, Comfort, Activity, Nutrition, Elimination, Skin Integrity)
Exercises regularly to capacity
Uses physical capacities to maximize comfort zone
Maintains sufficient circulation
Avoids the obesity of inactivity
Protects skin from abrasions due to rubbing of devices

These are not all the possible wellness diagnoses that may be identified. The above
are examples of nursing diagnoses that should be considered when planning care
for the older adult.

BOX 15-24   Driving Skills Quiz

If you answer "yes" to one or more of the following questions, you may want to limit your driving or take steps to improve a problem.

If you answer "yes" to most of the questions, it may be time to consider letting someone else do your driving for you.

The quiz is based in part on an American Association of Retired Persons publication.

- Does driving make you feel nervous or physically exhausted?
- Do you have difficulty seeing pedestrians, signs, and vehicles?
- Do cars frequently seem to appear from nowhere?
- At night, does the glare from oncoming headlights temporarily "blind" you?
- Do you find intersections confusing?
- Are you finding it harder to judge the distance between cars?
- Do you have difficulty coordinating your hand and foot movements?
- Are you slower than you used to be in reacting to dangerous situations?
- Do you sometimes get lost in familiar neighborhoods?
- Do other drivers often honk at you?
- Have you had an increased number of traffic violations, accidents, or near-accidents in the past year?

From Mayo Foundation for Medical Education and Research. *Mayo Clin Health Lett* 14(7):7, 1996.

participants (Box 15-23). A mnemonic, SAFE DRIVE, addresses key components to screen for in older drivers. The components include the following: Safety record, Attention skills, Family report, Ethanol, Drugs, Reaction time, Intellectual impairment, Vision or visuospatial function, and Executive functions (McGregor, 2002). The American Medical Association, in partnership with the National Highway Traffic Safety Administration, provides the *Guide to Assessing and Counseling Older Drivers* with step-by-step plans for assessing older driver safety (see Box 15-24 for a self-test of driving adequacy). See other resources in the Resources section at the end of this chapter.

In summary, the capacity to move about, on two legs, horses, and wheeled vehicles, has been portrayed from the earliest recorded time. The nurse can be significant in facilitating this most fundamental human need, to assist our patients to maintain independence, preserve autonomy, and move as far as their reach extends and as far as the imagination will allow.

KEY CONCEPTS

- Mobility provides opportunities for exercise, exploration, and pleasure and is the crux of maintaining independence.
- Changes in bones, muscles, and ligaments affect one's balance and gait as one ages and increase instability.
- Ease of mobility is thought to be the most visible measure of one's overall health and survival capacity.

- Muscle weakness must be investigated because it is often a result of reversible problems such as endocrine imbalances, particularly hypothyroidism, or medication reactions.
- Gait disorders are often the obvious indexes of systemic problems and should be investigated thoroughly.
- A thorough nursing assessment must include descriptions of gait and mobility patterns, as well as fall risk factors.
- Restraint-appropriate care is the standard of practice in all settings, and knowledge of restraint alternatives and safety measures is essential for nurses.
- Many illnesses that may accompany aging affect mobility and safety. Nursing interventions to enhance functional ability, prevent excess disability, and promote safety are essential.
- Transportation for the elderly is critical to their physical, psychological, and social health.
- Driving safety for older people is an important issue, and health care professionals must be knowledgeable about assessment, safety interventions, and transportation resources.

STUDY QUESTIONS

Discuss the meanings and the thoughts triggered by the student's and elder's viewpoints expressed at the beginning of the chapter. How do these vary from your own experience?

List all of the risk factors in your home that may contribute to falls.

Discuss psychosocial and physiological issues that affect mobility.

List five hazards of immobility in old age, and discuss the effects on an elder's health and function.

Spend 30 minutes in a shopping mall observing older individuals, and identify as many types of gait disorders and mobility assistive devices as possible.

Enumerate and discuss the reasons that falls increase in frequency as one ages.

What are some of the practical tips you would give an elder to prevent falls?

Discuss concerns you have about falling now. What do you think your concerns will be when you are 80 years old?

Discuss the reasons you would avoid applying restraints.

Identify several alternatives to restraint use.

Work with a partner and take turns restraining each other in a chair with soft restraints. Leave the restrained individual alone for 20 minutes, and after both have experienced this, discuss your thoughts and feelings.

What are some of the ways that older individuals could be assisted to drive safely? What criteria would you use to deny an individual a driver's license?

RESEARCH QUESTIONS

Osteoporosis

Compare the accuracy and expense of the various methods of measuring bone density.

What remedial measures have produced the best results in slowing or stopping bone deterioration?

What is the earliest age at which it is possible to detect bone resorption and to predict osteoporosis?

CASE STUDY: Osteoporosis

Maude was a small woman, barely 5 feet tall, weighed nearly 100 pounds, and was 73 years old. She had retired from a position as manager of the marketing department of a telephone company in a major U.S. city. She had been active socially and involved in numerous political causes and campaigns. She was known as a dynamo, often working 12 to 14 hours a day and so intensely involved she would forget to eat. And when discussing nutrition, she said, "Milk! You must be kidding—my diet is cigarettes and coffee." When she fell from a stool and braced herself with her right hand, her wrist swelled terribly but was not extremely painful. The bruise extended over the palm of her hand and up her forearm. After several days, the pain increased and she went to see a physician, a member of a preferred providers organization (PPO) of physicians to which she had belonged through her employment. She was very surprised to find that her wrist was broken. She had always climbed about and done whatever she wished with little concern for safety. When the physician cast her wrist, he told her she might have osteoporosis. She usually gave little thought to her physical status, but she began to worry about her bones. She knew that she could manage whatever came along, as she always had, but she wanted to know exactly what her future might hold in relation to osteoporosis and the possibility of broken bones. To reassure herself regarding the integrity of her bone structure, she called the PPO to schedule an evaluation. You are the advanced practice nurse whom she will see initially to determine her need for follow-up.

Based on the case study, develop a nursing care plan using the following procedure*:
- List Maude's comments that provide subjective data.
- List information that provides objective data.
- From these data, identify and state, using accepted format, two nursing diagnoses you determine are most significant to Maude at this time. List two of Maude's strengths that you have identified from data.
- Determine and state outcome criteria for each diagnosis. These must reflect some alleviation of the problem identified in the nursing diagnosis and must be stated in concrete and measurable terms.
- Plan and state one or more interventions for each diagnosed problem. Provide specific documentation of the source used to determine the appropriate intervention. Plan at least one intervention that incorporates Maude's existing strengths.
- Evaluate the success of the intervention. Interventions must correlate directly with the stated outcome criteria to measure the outcome success.

Critical Thinking Questions

1. What characteristics put one at risk for osteoporosis?
2. How would you evaluate Maude regarding risk of developing osteoporosis?
3. Discuss lifestyle changes that you would suggest to Maude.
4. What do you imagine her internist will do to determine her propensity for osteoporosis?
5. What ideally should have been done for Maude, or what should she have done for herself?

*Students are advised to refer to their nursing diagnosis text and identify possible or potential problems.

CASE STUDY: Rheumatoid Arthritis

Marilou is a devout Southern Baptist African-American woman who developed rheumatoid arthritis in her early 60s. She learned to manage the pain fairly well, but as she neared 70 years of age, the combination of rheumatoid arthritis and the "wear and tear" of osteoarthritis had created deformities and pain that restricted her movement considerably. She could no longer move her arms in positions above her chest, and her shoulders felt stiff. She found it difficult to twist jar lids and to open containers. It was particularly difficult to climb the stairs to her bedroom. Sometimes a soak in a hot tub, a heating pad, or ice packs would bring relief. She often prayed for relief and usually felt better afterward. She tried to keep active by walking her dog every morning, but she was becoming discouraged and depressed and said, "It upsets me that I never know whether I'm going to have a good day or a bad day." She sometimes found herself tempted to try some of the "miracle cures" that she knew were probably fraudulent but seemed to offer some hope.

Based on the case study, develop a nursing care plan using the following procedure*:
- List Marilou's comments that provide subjective data.
- List information that provides objective data.
- From these data, identify and state, using accepted format, two nursing diagnoses you determine are most significant to Marilou at this time. List two of Marilou's strengths that you have identified from data.
- Determine and state outcome criteria for each diagnosis. These must reflect some alleviation of the problem identified in the nursing diagnosis and must be stated in concrete and measurable terms.
- Plan and state one or more interventions for each diagnosed problem. Provide specific documentation of the source used to determine the appropriate intervention. Plan at least one intervention that incorporates Marilou's existing strengths.
- Evaluate the success of the intervention. Interventions must correlate directly with the stated outcome criteria to measure the outcome success.

Critical Thinking Questions

1. Describe the differences between rheumatoid arthritis and osteoarthritis.
2. Discuss Marilou's lifestyle and beliefs as they may affect her arthritis. What are some of the modifications in her activities that might be useful? How would you incorporate her beliefs into a care plan?

*Students are advised to refer to their nursing diagnosis text and identify possible or potential problems.

Has the incidence of osteoporosis decreased in particular geographical areas where fluorides have been added to drinking water?

Does the condition of dentition have any correlation with the condition of skeletal bones?

Rheumatoid Arthritis

What factors predispose one to osteoarthritic changes?

What types of alternative comfort measures are sought and used by sufferers of arthritis?

What do elders say reduces the discomfort of arthritis?

What aspects of arthritis cause most distress for elders?

What do demographical comparisons reveal about the geographical, ethnic, cultural, gender, and age distribution of arthritis?

Further Research Questions

What types of gait disorders trigger falls and in what situations?

What activities and exercises are most useful in maintaining mobility in elders?

What are the psychological reactions of elders to the use of assistive devices for ambulation?

What factors in the institutional environment induce immobility?

What factors outside home and institution (in the community) are most hazardous for the mobility of elders? Where do the most falls occur?

How does a new environment affect mobility? Is the incidence of falls higher in the first few weeks of adaptation to a new environment as compared with later?

How does obesity affect agility and mobility?

Does obesity predispose one to falling?

How often and in what circumstances are falls precipitated by the distractions or actions of another individual?

What interventions would increase adherence to wearing hip pads?

RESOURCES

ABLEDATA
www.abledata.com

Alzheimer's Association—Driving Checklist
www.alz.org/care/safetyissues/driving.asp

American Association of Retired Persons (AARP)
Driving courses and driver safety information
330 Independence Ave., SW
Washington, DC 20201
(202) 619-7501
www.aoa.gov

American Automobile Association (AAA)
Driving courses and driver safety information; includes on-line
 driver safety course
1000 AAA Drive
Heathrow, FL 32746
(407) 444-7000
www.aaa.com

American Geriatrics Society
Tool kit on falls and practice guidelines for prevention of falls in
 older persons
The Empire State Building
350 Fifth Avenue, Suite 801
New York, NY 10018
(212) 308-1414
www.americangeriatrics.org/education/falls.shtml

American Parkinson Disease Association
1350 Hylan Blvd., Suite 4B
Staten Island, NY 10305
(800) 223-2732
www.apdaparkinson.org

Arizona Technology Access Program
Comprehensive list of resources for older adults with disabilities
Jill Sherman, Project Director, AzTAP
Institute for Human Development
Northern Arizona University
4105 N. 20th St., Suite 260
Phoenix, AZ 85016
(800) 477-9921
www.nau.edu/ihd/aztap

Arthritis Foundation
1314 Spring St. NW
Atlanta, GA 20309
(800) 283-7800
www.arthritis.org

Arthritis National Research Foundation
200 Oceangate, Suite 830
Long Beach, CA 90802
(800) 588-2873
www.curearthritis.org

Dependable Acceptable Technology Solutions
Information on adaptive environments, assistive technology,
 home modification, safety and risk assessments
www.gdewsbury.ukideas.com

Hartford Insurance Company: Warning Signs for Older Drivers
www.thehartford.com/talkwitholderdrivers

Institute for Clinical Systems Improvement
Practice guidelines for osteoporosis diagnosis and treatment
www.icsi.org

Motivating Moves for People with Parkinson's
Video/DVD on exercise
Available from Parkinson's Disease Foundation
www.pdf.org

National Center for Injury Prevention and Control
Tool kit to prevent senior falls
Mailstop K65
4770 Buford Highway NE
Atlanta, GA 30341-3724
(800) 232-4636
www.cdc.gov/ncipc/pub –res/toolkit/toolkit.htm

National Center for Patient Safety
Department of Veterans Affairs
PO Box 486
Ann Arbor, MI 48106-0486
(734) 930-5890
www.patientsafety.gov

National Council on Aging, Center for Healthy Aging
300 D Street, SW
Suite 801
Washington, DC 20024
(202) 479-1200
www.healthyagingprograms.org/

National Fire Protection Association
Remembering When: A fire and fall prevention program for older adults
1 Batterymarch Park
Quincy, MA 02169-7471
(617) 770-3000
http://nfpa.org

National Institute on Aging Senior Health
National Institute on Aging
Building 31, Room 5C27
31 Center Drive, MSC 2292
Bethesda, MD 20892
www.nihseniorhealth.gov/

National Institute of Health
Office of Alternative Medicine
Building 31, Room 5C27
31 Center Drive, MSC 2292
Bethesda, MD 20892
www.altmed.od.nih.gov

National Institute for Health and Clinical Excellence
Practice guidelines for Parkinson's disease diagnosis and management in primary and secondary care
www.nice.org/uk

National Osteoporosis Foundation
1232 22nd Street NW
Washington, DC 20037-1292
(202) 223-2226
www.nof.org

National Parkinson Foundation, Inc.
1501 NW 9th Avenue/Bob Hope Rd.
Miami, FL 33136
(800) 327-4545
www.parkinson.org

National Resource Center for Safe Aging
San Diego State University
6505 Alvarado Rd., Suite 211
San Diego, CA 92120
(619) 594-0986
www.safeaging.org

Rehabilitation Engineering and Assistive Technology Society of North America
1700 N. Moore St., Suite 1540
Arlington, VA 22209-1903
(703) 524-6686
www.resna.org

The Arthritis Foundation
Arthritis Foundation
PO Box 7669
Atlanta, GA 30357-0669
(800) 283-7800
www.arthritis.org

The Michael J. Fox Foundation for Parkinson's Research
Grand Central Station
PO Box 4777
New York, NY 10163
(800) 708-7644

The Parkinson's Disease Foundation
710 W. 168th St.
New York, NY 10032
(800) 457-6676
www.pdf.org

Wheelchair Information
www.wheelchairnet.org

REFERENCES

Agency for Healthcare Research and Quality: *Managing osteoarthritis, helping the elderly maintain function and mobility*, Research in Action, issue 4, 2002a. (website): *www.ahrq.gov/research/osteoria/osteoria.htm.*

Agency for Healthcare Research and Quality: *AHRQ research has improved OA management*, 2002b. (website): *www.ahrq.gov/research/osteoria/osteoria.htm.*

Agency for Healthcare Research and Quality: *Choosing non-opioid analgesics for osteoarthritis.* AHRQ Publication Number 06(07)-Eltc009-3, January 2007. (website): www.effective healthcare. ahrq.gov.

American Academy of Neurology (AAN), Practice Parameter: *Diagnosis and prognosis of new onset Parkinson disease* (an evidence based-review), 2006a. (website): *www.aan.com.*

American Academy of Neurology (AAN), Practice Parameter: *Evaluation and treatment of depression, psychosis, and dementia in Parkinson disease* (an evidence-based review), 2006b. (website): *www.aan.com.*

American Academy of Neurology (AAN), Practice Parameter: *Neuroprotective strategies and alternative therapies for Parkinson disease* (an evidence-based review), 2006c. (website): *www. aan.com.*

American Academy of Neurology (AAN), Practice Parameter: *Treatment of Parkinson disease with motor fluctuations and dyskinesia* (an evidence-based review), 2006d. (website): *www. aan.com.*

American College of Rheumatology: Recommendations for the medical management of OA of the hip and knee, *Arthritis Rheum* 46(2):328, 2002.

American Geriatrics Society: *Guideline for the prevention of falls in older persons*, May 2001, National Guideline Clearinghouse. (website): *www.american_geriatrics.org.*

American Geriatrics Society. (website): *www.healthinaging.org/agingintheknow/chapters_ch_trial.asp?ch=22.* Accessed July 3, 2006.

American Society on Aging: *CDC new backgrounder: Arthritis and elders.* May 6, 2004. Accessed 6/27/06 from *www.asaging/org/media/pressrelease.cfm?id=57.*

Anderson DL: TNF inhibitors: a new age in rheumatoid arthritis treatment, *Am J Nurs* 104(2):60-68, 2004.

Arthritis Foundation: *Osteoporosis*, Atlanta, 2000, Arthritis Foundation.

Avidan A et al: Insomnia and hypnotic use, recorded in the minimum data set, as predictors of falls and hip fractures in Michigan nursing homes, *J Am Geriatr Soc* 53(6):955-962, 2005.

Baird CL: Holding on: self-caring with arthritis, *J Gerontol Nurs* 29(6):32-39, 2003.

Beers MH, Berkow R: *Merck manual of geriatrics*, ed 3, Whitehouse Station, NJ, 2000, Merck Research Laboratories.

Bellantonio S, Fortinsky R, Prestwood K: How well are community-living women treated for osteoporosis after hip fracture? *J Am Geriatr Soc* 49(9):1197-1204, 2001.

Boss BJ: Alterations in neurologic function. In McCance KL, Huether SE, editors: *Pathophysiology: the biologic basis for disease in adults and children*, ed 4, St Louis, 2002, Mosby.

Bourbonniere M, Evans LK: Advanced practice nursing in the care of frail older adults, *J Am Geriatr Soc* 50:2062-2076, 2002.

Brion PH, Concoff AL: *Nonpharmacologic therapy of osteoarthritis*, UpToDate, 2002. (website): *www.uptodate.com*.

Brucker MC, Youngkin EQ: What's a woman to do? Exploring HRT questions caused by the women's health initiative, *AWHOON Lifelines* 6(5):208-417, 2002.

Buchner DM et al: Development of the common data base for the FICSIT trials, *J Am Geriatr Soc* 41(3):297-308, 1993.

Burke M: Osteoporosis: a neglected but treatable disease, *Ann Long-Term Care* 12(9):20-24, 2004.

Burke MM, Laramie JA: *Primary care of the older adult: a multidisciplinary approach*, St Louis, 2000, Mosby.

Callahan LF, Jonas BL: Arthritis. In Ham RJ et al, editors: *Primary care geriatrics: a case-based approach*, ed 4, St Louis, 2002, Mosby.

Capezuti E: Building the science of falls-prevention research, *J Am Geriatr Soc* 52(3):461-462, 2004.

Capezuti E et al: Side rail use and bed-related fall outcomes among nursing home residents, *J Am Geriatr Soc* 50(1):90-96, 2002.

Cesari M et al: Prevalence and risk factors for falls in an older community-dwelling population, *J Gerontol A Biol Sci Med Sci* 57(11):M722-726, 2002.

Chang J et al: Interventions for the prevention of falls in older adults: systematic review and meta-analysis of randomised clinical trials, *BMJ* 328(20):680-684, 2004.

Concoff AL: *Clinical manifestations of osteoarthritis.* UptoDate 10(1):2002. (website): *www.uptodate.com*.

Dodd M et al: Pathological gambling caused by drugs used to treat Parkinson disease, *Arch Neurol* 62(9):1377-1381, 2005.

Eliopoulos C: *Gerontological nursing*, Philadelphia, 2005, Lippincott Williams & Wilkins.

Evans L, Strumpf N: Tying down the elderly: a review of literature on physical restraint, *J Am Geriatr Soc* 37:65, 1989.

Federal Register (V56187), Sept 26, 1991, p 48825.

Gaylord S, Crotty N: Enhancing function with complementary therapies in geriatric rehabilitation, *Top Geriatric Rehab* 18(2):63-79, 2002.

Gilfillan C, Schwartzberg J: Addressing the at-risk older driver, *Clin Geriatr* 13(8):27-34, 2005.

Gornisiewicz M, Moreland LW: Rheumatoid arthritis. In Robbins L, editor: *Clinical care in the rheumatic diseases*, ed 2, Atlanta, 2001, Association of Rheumatology Health Professionals.

Gray-Micelli D et al: A stepwise approach to a comprehensive post-fall assessment, *Ann Long-Term Care* 13(12):16-24, 2005.

Hawkes W et al: Gender differences in functioning after hip fracture, *J Gerontol* 61A(5):493-499, 2006.

Hendrich AL, Bender PS, Nyhuis A: Validation of the Hendrich II Fall Risk Model: a large concurrent case/control study of hospitalized patients, *Appl Nurs Res*, 16(1): 9-21, 2003.

Howe T, Oldham JA: Posture and balance. In Trew M, Everett T, editors: *Human movement*, ed 4, St Louis, 2001, Mosby.

Irvin D, White M: The importance of accurately assessing orthostatic hypotension, *Geriatr Nurs* 25(2):99-101, 2004.

Janssen I: Influence of sarcopenia on the development of physical disability: the cardiovascular health study, *J Am Geriatr Soc* 54:56-62, 2006.

Jett KF, Lester PB: Musculoskeletal disorders. In Youngkin EQ et al, editors: *Pharmacotherapeutics*, ed 2, Upper Saddle River, NJ, 2004, Prentice-Hall.

Jett K et al: Imposed versus involved: different strategies to effect driving cessation in cognitively impaired older adults, *Geriatr Nurs* 26(2):111-116, 2005.

Kalunian KC, Brion PH: Classification and diagnosis of osteoarthritis, UptoDate 10(1), 2002. (website): *www.uptodate.com*.

Kennedy-Malone L, Enevold G: Assessment and management of polymyalgia rheumatica in older adults, *Geriatr Nurs* 22(3):152-155, 2001.

Lesley WS: Osteoporotic compression fractures and treatment with vertebroplasty, 2002. (website): *www.cyberounds.com/conferences/ge...rics/conferences/current/conference.html*.

Lozada CJ, Altman RD: Osteoarthritis. In Robbins L, editor: *Clinical care in the rheumatic diseases*, ed 2, Atlanta, 2001, Association of Rheumatology Health Professionals.

Luggen AS: Rheumatoid arthritis. In Luggen AS, Meiner S, editors: *Care of the older adult with arthritis*, New York, 2002, Springer.

Luggen AS: Arthritis in older adults: current therapy with self-management as centerpiece, *Adv Nurse Pract* 11(3):26-35, 2003.

Mathias S et al: Balance in elderly patients: the "get-up-and-go" test, *Arch Phys Med Rehabil* 67(6):387-389, 1986.

McCaffrey R, Freeman E: Effects of music on chronic osteoarthritis pain in older people, *J Adv Nurs* 44(5):517-524, 2003.

McGregor D: Driving over 65: proceed with caution, *J Gerontol Nurs* 28(8):22-26, 2002.

Meiner S, Lueckenotte A: *Gerontological nursing*, ed 3, St Louis, 2006, Mosby.

Miller JQ: Parkinson's disease. In Ham RJ et al, editors: *Primary care geriatrics: a case-based approach*, ed 4, St Louis, 2002, Mosby.

Morley J: A fall is a major event in the life of an older person, *J Gerontol* 57A(8):M492-M495, 2002.

Morley JE et al: Geriatricians, continuous quality improvement, and improved care for older persons, *J Gerontol A Biol Sci Med Sci* 57(8):M492-M495, 2003.

Morse J, Morse R, Tylko S: Development of a scale to identify the fall-prone patient, *Can J Aging*, 8:366-377, 1989.

National Center for Injury Prevention and Control (NCIPC), Centers for Disease Control and Prevention: *Falls and hip fractures in older adults*, Atlanta, 2006. (website): *www.cdc.gove/ncipc/factsheets/falls/htm*. Accessed July 5, 2006.

National Institutes of Health (NIH): *Fast facts on osteoporosis*, 2004. (website): *www.nih.gov*.

National Osteoporosis Foundation: *Physician guide to osteoporosis prevention and treatment*, Washington DC, 2003.

Newman A: Self-help care in older African Americans with arthritis, *Geriatr Nurs* 22(3):135-138, 2001.

Neyhart B, Gibbs LM: Osteoporosis. In Ham RJ et al, editors: *Primary care geriatrics: a case-based approach*, ed 4, St Louis, 2002, Mosby.

Nnodim J, Alexander N: Assessing falls in older adults, *Geriatrics* 60(10):24-29, 2005.

Park M, Hsiao-Chen Tang J: Evidence-based guideline: changing the practice of physical restraint use in acute care, *J Gerontol Nurs* 33(2):9-16, 2007.

Parkinson Disease Foundation: *Gambling, sex and Parkinson disease*, 2005. (website): *www.pdf.org*.

Parry S, Kenny R: Drop attacks in older adults: systematic assessment has a high diagnostic yield, *J Am Geriatr Soc* 53(1):74-78, 2005.

Perkinson M et al: Driving and dementia of the Alzheimer type: beliefs and cessation strategies, *Gerontologist* 45(5):676-685, 2005.

Quigley P: Research agenda on the risk and prevention of falls: 2002-2007, *J Rehabil Res Dev* 42(1):vii-x, 2005.

Reginato AM, Reginato AJ: Periarticular rheumatic diseases. In Robbins L, editor: *Clinical care in the rheumatic diseases*, ed 2, Atlanta, 2001, Association of Rheumatology Health Professionals.

Resnick B: Managing arthritis with exercise, *Geriatr Nurs* 22(1):143-152, 2001.

Resnick B: In Henkel G: Beyond the MDS: team approach to falls assessment, prevention and management, *Caring for the Ages* 3(4):15-20, 2002.

Resnick B et al: Gait and balance disorders. In Adelman AM, Daly MP, editors: *Twenty common problems in geriatrics*, New York, 2001, McGraw-Hill.

Resnick B et al: The Exercise Plus program for older women post hip fracture: participant perspectives, *Gerontologist* 45:539-544, 2005.

Reuben DB et al: *Geriatrics at your fingertips*, Malden, Mass, 2002, American Geriatric Society/Blackwell.

Rich M: Drop attacks revisited: yet another manifestation of cardiovascular disease, *J Am Geriatr Soc* 53(1):161, 2005.

Roberts D: Alternative therapies for arthritis treatment, 2, *Orthop Nurs* 22(6):412-420, 2003.

Rubenstein L, Trueblood P: Gait and balance assessment in older persons, *Ann Long-Term Care* 12(2):39-46, 2004.

Rubenstein T et al: Evaluating fall risk in older adults: steps and missteps, *Clin Geriatr* 11(1):52-61, 2003.

Schneider DC, Mader SL: Falls. In Ham RJ et al, editors: *Primary care geriatrics: a case-based approach*, ed 4, St Louis, 2002, Mosby.

Spector T et al: Effect of risedronate on joint structure and symptoms of knee osteoarthritis: results of the BRISK randomized, controlled trial, *Arthritis Res Ther* 7(3):R625-R633, 2005.

Spiera R, Spiera H: Inflammatory disease in older adults: polymyalgia rheumatica, *Geriatrics* 59(11):39-43, 2004.

Stone J et al: *Clinical gerontological nursing*, Philadelphia, 1999, Saunders.

Sullivan-Marx E: Achieving restraint-free care of acutely confused older adults, *J Gerontol Nurs* 27(4):56-61, 2001.

Syed M et al: Vertebroplasty: the alternative treatment for osteoporotic vertebral compression fractures in the elderly, *Clin Geriatr* 14(2):20-23, 2006.

Swantek SS: *Medical comorbidities in older patients*, American Association for Geriatric Psychiatry, 15th Annual Meeting. (website): *www.medscape.com/viewarticle/430712*. Accessed June 27, 2002.

Tabloski P: *Gerontological nursing*, Upper Saddle River, NJ, 2006, Pearson Prentice Hall.

Tanner E: Assessing home safety in homebound older adults, *Geriatr Nurs* 24(4):250-255, 2003.

Thorndyke L: Osteoporosis. In Adelman AM, Daly MP, editors: *Twenty common problems in geriatrics*, New York, 2001, McGraw-Hill.

Tideiksaar R: *Falls in older adults*, Baltimore, 1998, Health Professions Press.

Tideiksaar R: *Falls in older persons: prevention and management*, ed 3, Baltimore, 2005, Health Professions Press.

Tinetti M: Performance oriented assessment of mobility problems in elderly patients, *J Am Geriatr Soc* 34:199, 1986.

Tinetti M: Preventing falls in elderly persons, *N Engl J Med* 348(1):42-49, 2003.

Tinetti M et al: Risk factors for falls among elderly persons living in the community, *N Engl J Med* 319(26):1701, 1988.

Tinetti M et al: Falls efficacy as a measure of fear of falling, *J Gerontol* 45(6):239, 1990.

Tinetti M et al: Fear of falling and fall-related efficacy in relationship to functioning among community-living elders, *J Gerontol* 49(3):M140, 1994.

U.S. Food and Drug Administration: *FDA News, FDA approves Neupro patch for treatment of early Parkinson's disease*, May 9, 2007. (website): *www.fda.gov/BBS/topics/news/2007/new01631. html.* Accessed July 7, 2007.

U.S. Prevention Services Task Force (USPTF): *Screening for osteoporosis*, 2002. (website): *www.acpr.gov.*

Van Doornum S et al: Accelerated atherosclerosis: an extraarticular feature of rheumatoid arthritis? *Arthritis Rheum* 46(4):862, 2002.

Wagner L et al: Impact of a falls menu-driven incident-reporting system on documentation and quality improvement in nursing homes, *Gerontologist* 45:835-842, 2005.

Watts N: *Pharmacologic therapy provides long-lasting fracture risk reduction in postmenopausal women with osteoporosis.* Presentation at 2001 Annual Meeting of the Endocrine Society, August 2001.

Whitney CM: Maintaining the square: how older adults with Parkinson's disease sustain quality in their lives, *J Gerontol Nurs* 30(1):28-35, 2004.

Zarowitz B: Management of osteoporosis in older persons, *Geriatr Nurs* 27(1):16-18, 2006.

Zecevic A et al: Defining a fall and reasons for falling: comparisons among the views of seniors, health care providers, and the research literature, *Gerontologist* 46(3):367-376, 2006.

Tinetti Balance and Gait Evaluation

Balance

Instructions: Subject is seated in a hard, armless chair. The following maneuvers are tested.

1. Sitting balance
   0 = Leans or slides in chair
   1 = Steady, safe
2. Arise
   0 = Unable without help
   1 = Able but uses arms to help
   2 = Able without use of arms
3. Attempts to arise
   0 = Unable without help
   1 = Able but requires more than one attempt
   2 = Able to arise with one attempt
4. Immediate standing balance (first 5 seconds)
   0 = Unsteady (staggers, moves feet, marked trunk sway)
   1 = Steady but uses walker/cane or grabs other object for support
   2 = Steady without walker or cane or other support
5. Standing balance
   0 = Unsteady
   1 = Steady but wide stance (medial heels >4" apart) or uses cane/walker or other support
   2 = Narrow stance without support
6. Nudge (subject at maximum position with feet as close together as possible. Examiner pushes lightly on subject's sternum with palm of hand 3 times)
   0 = Begins to fall
   1 = Staggers, grabs but catches self
   2 = Steady
7. Eyes closed (at maximum position #6)
   0 = Unsteady
   1 = Steady
8. Turn 360°
   0 = Discontinuous steps
   1 = Continuous steps
   0 = Unsteady (grabs, staggers)
   1 = Steady
9. Sit down
   0 = Unsafe (misjudged distance, falls into chair)
   1 = Uses arms or not a smooth motion
   2 = Safe, smooth motion

/16 BALANCE SCORE

Gait

Instructions: Subject stands with examiner. Walks down hallway or across room, first at his/her usual pace, then back at a "rapid but safe" pace (using usual walking aid such as cane/walker).

10. Initiation of gait (immediately after told "go")
    0 = Any hesitancy or multiple attempts to start
    1 = No hesitancy
11. Step length and height (right foot swing)
    0 = Does not pass L. stance foot with step
    1 = Passes L. stance foot
    0 = R. foot does not clear floor completely with step
    1 = R. foot completely clears floor
12. Step length and height (left foot swing)
    0 = Does not pass R. stance foot with step
    1 = Passes R. stance foot
    0 = L. foot does not clear floor completely with step
    1 = L. foot completely clears floor
13. Step symmetry
    0 = R. and L. step length not equal (estimate)
    1 = R. and L. step length appear equal
14. Step continuity
    0 = Stopping or discontinuity between steps
    1 = Steps appear continuous
15. Path (estimated in relation to floor tiles, 12 inches wide. Observe excursion of one foot over about 10 feet of course.)
    0 = Marked deviation
    1 = Mild/moderate deviation or uses a walking aid
    2 = Straight without walking aid
16. Trunk
    0 = Marked sway or uses walking aid
    1 = No sway but flexion of knees or back or spreads arms out while walking
    2 = No sway, no flexion, no use of arms, and no walking aid
17. Walk stance
    0 = Heels apart
    1 = Heels almost touching while walking

/12 GAIT SCORE
/28 TOTAL MOBILITY SCORE (BALANCE AND GAIT)

From Brady R et al: Geriatric falls: prevention strategies for the staff, J Gerontol Nurs 19(9):26, 1993. Reprinted with permission, Mary Tinetti, M.D.

Osteoporosis Functional Disability Questionnaire

The osteoporosis functional disability questionnaire was developed as a specific instrument to measure disability in several domains: feelings of adequacy, comfort, mood, activities of daily living, instrumental activities of daily living, and social activities. Self-evaluation of impairment (on a Likert scale 1-5 indicating frequency and/or severity of problems) provides information for designing and planning self-care and supportive activities.

Motivation and need for participation in therapeutic regimens and exercise programs are evaluated by the following indications.

Indicate in degrees of 1 (good) to 5 (poor) your estimation of your general health aside from your osteoporosis. _____

Indicate in degrees of 1 (no difficulty) to 5 (very difficult) any problems meeting your financial commitments in the following areas.

Housing _____
Food _____
Personal expenses _____
Transportation _____
Medical expenses _____
Other _____

Indicate in degrees of 1 (least) through 5 (most) items below that are of most concern related to your osteoporosis.

Pain _____
General health _____
Appearance _____
Interferes with social activities _____
Interferes with work _____
Other _____

Mark in degrees of 1 (least) through 5 (most) the organizations or groups of importance to you that you are hindered from enjoying because of your osteoporosis.

Church _____
Job related _____
Recreational _____
Fraternal _____
Civic/political _____
Other _____

Indicate by numbers 1 (least) through 5 (most) the intensity/frequency of feelings you have experienced in the past week.

I was bothered by things that usually don't bother me. _____
I did not feel like eating; my appetite was poor. _____
I was unable to shake off the blues even with help from family and friends. _____
I felt I was just as well off as other people. _____
I had trouble keeping my mind on what I was doing. _____
I felt depressed. _____
I felt as if everything I did was an effort. _____
I felt hopeful about the future. _____
I thought my life had been a failure. _____
I felt fearful. _____
My sleep was restless. _____
I was happy. _____
I talked less than usual. _____
I felt lonely. _____
People were unfriendly. _____
I enjoyed life. _____
I had crying spells. _____
I felt sad. _____
I felt that people disliked me. _____
I could not get going. _____

Indicate by numbers 1 (unable) through 5 (independent) your ability to accomplish the following activities without assistance.

Get in and out of bed _____
Use the toilet _____
Bathe yourself _____
Dress yourself _____
Put on your shoes _____
Cut your toenails _____
Prepare light meals _____
Prepare meals for family or entertainment _____
Wash the dishes _____
Do laundry _____
Do light housework _____
Do your vacuuming _____
Do heavy housework _____
Go shopping _____

Go on social outings _____
Walk around your house _____
Climb stairs _____
Walk down stairs _____
Hold a book to read _____
Walk outdoors for over 15 minutes _____
Board a bus _____
Drive an automobile _____
Do gardening _____

Bend down _____
Reach overhead _____
Sit down and get out of chair _____

Ideally, this self-evaluation tool should be used before and after program interventions.

Modified from Helmes E et al: A questionnaire to evaluate disability in osteoporotic patients with vertebral compression fractures, *J Gerontol* 50A(2): M91, 1995. Copyright © The Gerontological Society of America. Reproduced by permission of the publisher.

CHAPTER 16

Environmental Safety and Security

Theris A. Touhy

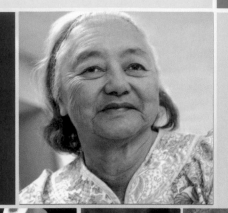

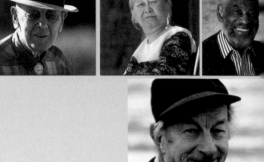

A STUDENT LEARNS

My client during the community nursing experience decided to stay in her own home in spite of being barely able to shuffle around. The state gave a homemaker a small sum each month to provide a few hours of assistance on a daily basis. She had to rely on the goodwill of neighbors when the budget for those services was discontinued. She wants so much to remain in her own home. I worry about her but don't know what I should do.

Jennifer, age 24

AN ELDER SPEAKS

I have been in my home for 50 years and widowed for 25 of those 50. The upkeep on my home is expensive and my resources are limited. I'm hoping I can manage to re-main here, but I need some modifications to make it safe and I really don't know how to go about getting assistance to make the necessary changes.

Esther, age 79

LEARNING OBJECTIVES

On completion of this chapter, the reader will be able to:

1. Identify interactions of intrapersonal, interpersonal, geographical, economic, and health factors that influence environmental safety and security for older adults.
2. Discuss the effects of declining health, reduced mobility, reloca-tion, isolation, and unpredictable life situations on the older adult's perception of security.
3. Explain the underlying vulnerability of older adults to effects of extreme temperatures, and identify actions to prevent and treat hypothermia and hyperthermia.
4. Define strategies and programs designed to prevent, detect, or alleviate crimes against older adults.
5. Discuss the use of assistive technologies to promote self-care, safety, and independence.

FEELING SECURE AS ONE AGES

Feeling secure in one's environment surpasses the need for physical safety and freedom from crime or violence. It in-volves sensing an identity with one's personally significant space, whether that is a home or a tiny cubicle in a care facil-ity. Feelings of security as one ages also depend on the per-ceived familiarity and predictability of the life-space in which one moves or interacts. Having personal items brought in to make a new location "one's own" is an effort to restore identity and mark one's personal space. Reminiscence ther-apy is sometimes an effective approach to restoring a con-nection to the familiar and reducing feelings of isolation for older adults in a new adult day program or residential com-munity (Pittiglio, 2000). Anxiety and insecurity increase when situations and conditions become unpredictable, whether they are geographically, economically, health, or time related. In addition, these perceptions induce stress-related responses or agitation that can threaten comfort and quality of life. Relocation stress syndrome describes the con-fusion resulting from a move to a new environment and is discussed more fully in Chapter 24.

Perceptions of security and feeling safe are strongly influ-enced by cognitive capabilities and ability to problem solve.

Special thanks to Barbara J. Holtzclaw, the previous edition contributor, for her content contributions to this chapter.

Even simple forgetting tends to make a person feel less confident in carrying out daily tasks. Nurses can encourage older persons to participate in steps to organize their environment, use reminders and calendars to gain greater control over time, and create simple maps to outline the "territory" in which they expect to move. Promoting feelings of environmental security in persons with dementia is a more complex challenge because, as memory fades, one's sense of identity, as well as location, becomes fragmented. Heightened feelings of fear, insecurity, and inconsolable loss often affect comfort and alter behavior. These dynamics are discussed further in Chapter 23. Helping caregivers, both professional and family, understand reasons for behavior from the person's perspective will enhance well-being and feelings of safety. Efforts to preserve privacy and periphery in one's personal space will help restore pattern, order, and environmental predictability. This, in turn, will promote feelings of safety and security.

Healthy People 2000/2010

According to *Healthy People 2010*, more than 400 Americans die each day from injuries. Motor vehicle accidents, firearms, falls, and fires are responsible for many of these deaths. Violent crime is also a concern and *Healthy People 2010* uses the homicide rate as an indicator of all violent crime. The following are some of these objectives that relate to driving and fire safety and crime prevention for older adults:

- Reduce deaths caused by motor vehicle crashes
- Reduce homicides

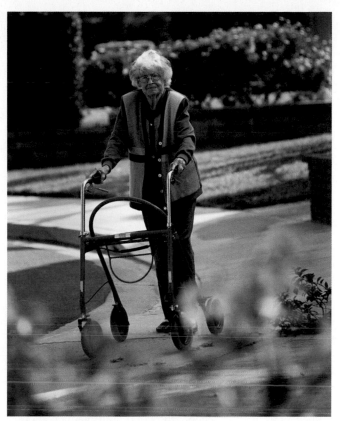

Maintaining ambulation and safety with appropriate assistive devices. (Courtesy Corbis Images.)

INFLUENCES OF CHANGING HEALTH AND DISABILITY ON SAFETY AND SECURITY

Physical Vulnerability

Vulnerability to environmental risks and mistreatment by others increases as people become less physically or cognitively able to recognize or cope with real or potential hazards. Aging itself does not necessarily bring about failing health or disease, yet some physical changes can be anticipated in all body systems. These changes occur at varying rates among older people and depend on genetic, immunological, and general systemic health factors. Older adults are able to learn about these changes and take precautions to avoid risks of unsafe behaviors and situations. Many healthy older adults are also able to share responsibility for maintaining a healthy lifestyle that includes exercise, adequate nutrition and hydration, avoidance of temperature extremes, reduction of environmental hazards, and protection from crime and violence. In teaching about risk reduction, it is important to emphasize the strong influence of stress, whether it is physical, emotional, mental, or spiritual in nature. Stress affects cognitive awareness and vigilance while influencing visual acuity, thirst, and hormonal release. (See Chapter 24 for further discussion of stress-related influences.) This, in turn, makes the older adult more vulnerable to distraction, falls, fatigue, and criminal assault.

Physical activity is known to improve mobility, balance, and muscle strength, even among frail and very old adults. Therefore such activities as walking, stretching, and gardening help improve the strength and stability—factors important to preventing falls and physical injuries. These factors are discussed more fully in Chapters 3, 7, and 15. Helping the older person be vigilant about hazardous surroundings includes offering suggestions for adequate lighting, placement of furniture and rugs, and markings on sidewalks and steps and providing information on crime prevention. Sensory deficits, whether visual, auditory, or olfactory, reduce the individual's ability to detect dangerous conditions or imminent threats. Tactile or neurosensory impairment raises the risk of tissue injury from burns, pressure, or beginning inflammation that escapes the person's awareness.

Home safety assessments must be multifaceted and individualized to the areas of identified risks. An evidence-based home safety assessment tool has been developed by Tanner (2003) and includes fall and injury risk, as well as fire and crime risk assessment (Box 16-1). Hurley et al. (2004) describe a home safety injury model for persons with Alzheimer's disease and their caregivers that addresses the physical environment and caregiver competence. Special home modifications for persons with Alzheimer's disease have also been

---

BOX 16-1 Evidence-Based Practice: Assessing Home Safety in Homebound Older Adults

PURPOSE

The study explored safety risks for vulnerable homebound elders.

SAMPLE/SETTING

208 homebound adults (60 years of age and over), living in rural areas in northern Alabama, were assessed for safety risks within their own homes.

METHOD

Registered nurse students conducted the home safety assessments in two 1-hour home visits over a 4-week period using a 57-item home safety assessment instrument modified from several existing tools. Subscales of the instrument were: risk for falls (external and internal factors); history of falls; risk for injury; use of personal precautions; risk and preparation for fire and disasters; and risk for crime. Individual item responses were analyzed based on frequency of responses. Total subscale analyses were examined with an ordinal scale range of no, low, moderate, and high risk.

RESULTS

The subscale with the highest level of risk was risk for falls (external) with 44% of the participants scoring at moderate to high risk levels for falls. 49% had experienced a fall, and 50% or more reported previous falls and the use of medications that cause dizziness. 41% of the participants did not have grab bars around the shower/bath and toilet in the bathroom, an important safety feature to prevent falls. 28% were poorly prepared to respond to fire or disaster; 11% had been a victim of crime at home, and 34% considered themselves a moderate to high risk for crime.

IMPLICATIONS

Conducting home safety assessments to prevent injury is an important nursing responsibility. Home safety assessments should be multifaceted and include internal and external risk for falls, history of near and past falls, use of personal precautions, risk and preparation for fire and disasters, and risk for crime. Following identification of risks, specific plans to minimize risk must be implemented and evaluated.

Data from Tanner E: Assessing home safety in homebound older adults, *Geriatr Nurs* 24(3):250-254, 256, 2003.

---

described (Warner, 2000). Chapter 23 discusses safety and dementia as well. A recent study of a multimedia computer touchscreen CD-ROM suggested this type of format as an effective and economically feasible way to provide information on home safety and accident prevention to older adults (Sweeney and Chiriboga, 2003). Table 16-1 provides suggestions for assessment of the home environment.

Vulnerability to Environmental Temperatures

Given the nation's growing problems with supply and costs of energy, many older adults are exposed to temperature extremes in their own dwellings. Environmental temperature extremes impose a serious risk to older persons with declining physical health. Preventive measures require attentiveness to impending climate changes, as well as protective alternatives. Early intervention in extreme temperature exposure is crucial because excessively high or low body temperatures further impair thermoregulatory function and can be lethal.

To be vigilant or aware of elders at risk, it is important to understand the basis of thermal vulnerability. A decline in thermoregulatory responsiveness to temperature extremes as one ages is well documented, yet these changes vary widely among individuals and are related more to general health than to age. The susceptibility to lose or gain heat during extreme temperature changes depends more on the person's physiological and behavioral coping defenses against transient heat exchange than it does on how old the person is.

Healthy people of all ages have body temperatures that range above and below the level of 37° C (98.6° F) and yet are considered "normal" basal temperatures. Studies of elders show that basal body temperature declines with advancing age. The delicate equilibrium required to maintain thermal balance at any age involves the generation or replacement of body heat at about the same rate as heat is lost to the environment. A number of physiological changes associated with aging affect heat generation, distribution, and conservation. Heat conservation is especially affected by changes in body density, water content, and insulation that accompany old age. Circulatory impairment and changes in vascular responsiveness affect the distribution of heat carried by blood. Thermoregulatory sensitivity declines with age, and both cooling and warming responses appear to be blunted (Kramer et al., 1989; Wongsurawat et al., 1990). In addition, many older persons complain of "feeling cool," whether or not their actual body temperatures are lower.

These neurosensory changes tend to delay or diminish the older person's awareness of temperature changes and may impair behavioral and thermoregulatory responses to dangerously high or low environmental temperatures. Many of the drugs taken by older people affect thermoregulation by affecting ability to vasoconstrict or vasodilate, both of which are thermoregulatory mechanisms. Other drugs inhibit neuromuscular activity (a significant source of kinetic heat production), suppress metabolic heat generation, or dull awareness (tranquilizers, pain medications). Alcohol is notorious for inhibiting thermoregulatory function by affecting vasomotor responses in either hot or cold weather.

Economic, behavioral, and environmental factors may combine to create a dangerous thermal environment in which older persons are subjected to temperature extremes from which they cannot escape or that they cannot change. Caretakers and family members should be aware that persons are vulnerable to environmental temperature extremes if they are unable to shiver, sweat, control blood supply to the skin, take in sufficient liquids, move about, add or remove clothing, adjust bedcovers, or adjust the room temperature.

TABLE 16-1

Assessment and Interventions of the Home Environment for Older Persons

Problem	Intervention
BATHROOM	
Getting on and off toilet	Raised seat; side bars; grab bars
Getting in and out of tub	Bath bench; transfer bench; hand-held shower nozzle; rubber mat; hydraulic lift bath seat
Slippery or wet floors	Nonskid rugs or mats
Hot water burns	Check water temperature before bath; set hot water thermostat to 120° F or less Use bath thermometer
Doorway too narrow	Remove door and use curtain; leave wheelchair at door and use walker
BEDROOM	
Rolling beds	Remove wheels; block against wall
Bed too low	Leg extensions; blocks; second mattress; adjustable-height hospital bed
Lighting	Bedside light; night-light; flashlight attached to walker or cane
Sliding rugs	Remove; tack down; rubber back; two-sided tape
Slippery floor	Nonskid wax; no wax; rubber-sole footwear; indoor-outdoor carpet
Thick rug edge/doorsill	Metal strip at edge; remove doorsill; tape down edge
Nighttime calls	Bedside phone; cordless phone; intercom; buzzer; lifeline
KITCHEN	
Open flames and burners	Substitute microwave; electrical toaster oven
Access items	Place commonly used items in easy-to-reach areas; adjustable-height counters, cupboards, and drawers
Hard-to-open refrigerator	Foot lever
Difficulty seeing	Adequate lighting; utensils with brightly colored handles
LIVING ROOM	
Soft, low chair	Board under cushion; pillow or folded blanket to raise seat; blocks or platform under legs; good armrests to push up on; back and seat cushions
Swivel and rocking chairs	Block motion
Obstructing furniture	Relocate or remove to clear paths
Extension cords	Run along walls; eliminate unnecessary cords; place under sturdy furniture; use power strips with breakers
TELEPHONE	
Difficult to reach	Cordless phone; inform friends to let phone ring 10 times; clear path; answering machine and call back
Difficult to hear ring	Headset; speaker phone
Difficult to dial numbers	Preset numbers; large button and numbers; voice-activated dialing
STEPS	
Cannot handle	Stair glide; lift; elevator; ramp (permanent, portable, or removable)
No handrails	Install at least on one side
Loose rugs	Remove or nail down to wooden steps
Difficult to see	Adequate lighting; mark edge of steps with bright-colored tape
Unable to use walker on stairs	Keep second walker or wheelchair at top or bottom of stairs
HOME MANAGEMENT	
Laundry	Easy to access; sit on stool to access clothes in dryer; good lighting; fold laundry sitting at table; carry laundry in bag on stairs; use cart; use laundry service
Mail	Easy-to-access mailbox; mail basket on door

Modified from Rehabilitation Engineering Research Center on Aging (RERC-Aging), Center for Assistive Technology, University at Buffalo.

Continued

TABLE 16-1

Assessment and Interventions of the Home Environment for Older Persons—cont'd

Problem	Intervention
HOME MANAGEMENT—cont'd	
Housekeeping	Assess safety and manageability; no-bend dust pan; lightweight all-surface sweeper; provide with resources for assistance if needed
Controlling thermostat	Mount in accessible location; large-print numbers; remote-controlled thermostat
SAFETY	
Difficulty locking doors	Remote-controlled door lock; door wedge; hook and chain locks
Difficulty opening door and knowing who is there	Automatic door openers; level doorknob handles; intercom at door
Opening and closing windows	Lever and crank handles
Cannot hear alarms	Blinking lights; vibrating surfaces
Lighting	Illumination 1-2 feet from object being viewed; change bulbs when dim; adequate lighting in stairways and hallways; night-lights
LEISURE	
Cannot hear television	Personal listening device with amplifier; closed captioning
Complicated remote	Simple remote with large buttons; universal remote control; voice control–activated remote control; clapper
Cannot read small print	Magnifying glass; large-print books
Book too heavy	Read at table; sit with book resting on lap pillow
Glare when reading	Place light source to right or left; avoid glossy paper for reading material; black ink instead of blue ink or pencil
Computer keys too small	Replace keyboard with one with larger keys

Modified from Rehabilitation Engineering Research Center on Aging (RERC-Aging), Center for Assistive Technology, University at Buffalo.

Economic conditions often play a role in this vulnerability, such as when an older person cannot afford air conditioning or adequate heating. During winter months, the older person may try using little or no room heat to either reduce or eliminate high cost of fuel. Although most of these problems occur in the home setting, older adults with multiple physical problems residing in institutions may be especially vulnerable to temperature changes. Fear of unsafe neighborhoods in some urban areas prompts many elders to keep doors and windows bolted throughout the year.

More older people die from excessive heat than from hurricanes, lightening, tornadoes, floods, and earthquakes combined (CDC, 2006). In 2003, a record heat wave in Europe claimed an estimated 30,000 lives; 14,000 people died in France alone (Sykes, 2005; Schwartz et al, 2006). Trends toward global warming will increase the risks of extreme heat-related events in the future. Local governments and communities must coordinate response strategies to protect the older person. Strategies may include providing fans, opportunities to spend part of the day in air-conditioned buildings, and identification of high-risk older people.

Hyperthermia. When body temperature increases above normal ranges because of environmental or metabolic heat loads, a clinical condition called *heat illness,* or *hyperthermia,* develops. Recognizing that heat illnesses tend to follow a continuum (Table 16-2), beginning with mild heat strain

and ending with the potentially fatal heat stroke, makes it imperative to assess hyperthermia quickly and appropriately. Heat exhaustion is an early stage of heat illness that is characterized by water or salt depletion (or both), usually accompanied by circulatory abnormalities, such as rapid pulse, falling blood pressure, diminished superficial blood flow, clammy skin, and disorientation. Body temperature is generally high, above 38° C (100.4° F). The person usually has lost considerable amounts of sodium in heavy sweating (Horowitz and Hales, 1998). Diuretics and low intake of fluids exacerbate fluid loss and can precipitate the onset of heat exhaustion in hot weather. Medical attention is necessary to prescribe necessary fluid replacement and determine the extent of heat illness present, because heat exhaustion is part of a continuum that leads to heat stroke.

Heat stroke, the most serious form of heat illness, is a medical emergency that usually arises from failure of normal body-cooling mechanisms to cope with extremely high environmental heat or humidity. Heat stroke affects the hypothalamic thermoregulatory center and impairs the ability to sweat or lose heat by vasodilation. This condition can quickly lead to death unless treated, and rising core temperatures above 40° C (104° F) increase the likelihood of irreversible brain damage. Elders with cardiovascular disease, diabetes, neurological disorders, and peripheral vascular disease and those taking certain medications (anticholinergics, antihistamines, diuretics, beta-blockers, antidepressants,

TABLE 16-2

Hyperthermia

Illness	Causes	Symptoms	Treatment
Heat stroke	Breakdown of body's cooling system	Hot and dry skin, fever (106° F), rapid pulse, nausea, hypotension, headache, dizziness, syncope	Move patient to shade, wrap in wet sheet, call for emergency equipment, and give fluids
Heat exhaustion	Loss of fluid and sodium; often follows heavy exertion and precedes heat stroke	Fatigue, giddiness, elevated temperature, muscle cramps, delirium, cold and clammy skin	Have patient lie down away from source of heat and keep feet elevated, give cold fluids with 1 teaspoon of salt per liter, and wrap in cold, wet towels
Heat syncope	Sudden exertion or sudden exposure to unusual heat	Dizziness, lower-than-usual blood pressure, slowed pulse, sudden fainting, cool and sweaty skin	Get patient out of the sun, put head between knees, and have patient drink fluids

antiparkinson drugs) are at risk. Preexisting conditions such as neurological disorders, alcohol use, and use of atropine-containing drugs make the elder more susceptible to heat stroke by affecting heat loss mechanisms. In addition, alcohol consumption contributes to dehydration, a condition often preexisting in elders. Dehydration increases serum osmolality and reduces circulatory volume. Both of these conditions raise body temperature and make the body more vulnerable to thermal stress (Morimoto and Itoh, 1998). High humidity interferes with the ability of sweat to evaporate and cool the body.

Hyperthermia requires active cooling and fluid replacement by caregivers. Early treatment includes actively cooling to reduce core body temperature by means of a conductive cooling blanket, until core temperatures drop to levels below 40° C (104° F) to avoid risk of neurological damage. Because hyperthermia induces loss of thermoregulatory control, caregivers must monitor temperature closely to avoid inducing hypothermia. Concern for skin protection and comfort during cooling procedures makes it prudent to wrap extremities before application of the cooling blanket. It is also an effective measure to suppress shivering and other warming responses. Parenteral fluids and electrolytes are given to improve circulation, restore deficits, and promote heat loss from skin. In cases of heat stroke and heat exhaustion, when appropriate action is taken to restore fluids and stabilize body temperature for several hours, thermoregulatory ability is often remarkably restored. Box 16-2 presents interventions to prevent hyperthermia when the ambient temperature exceeds 90° F (32.2° C).

Hypothermia. Hypothermia is a medical emergency requiring comprehensive assessment of neurological activity, oxygenation, renal function, and fluid and electrolyte balance. The term *hypothermia* literally means "low heat," but it is used clinically to describe core temperatures below 35° C (95° F). During cold weather, two situations tend to produce hypothermia: (1) when exposure involves a healthy individual in severely cold environmental conditions for a prolonged period; or (2) when exposure involves a person with

---

BOX 16-2   Interventions to Prevent Hyperthermia

- Drink 2 to 3 L of cool fluid daily.
- Minimize exertion, especially during the heat of the day.
- Stay in air-conditioned places, or use fans when possible.
- Wear hats and loose clothing of natural fibers when outside; remove most clothing when indoors.
- Take tepid baths or showers.
- Apply cold wet compresses, or immerse the hands and feet in cool water.
- Evaluate medications for risk of hyperthermia.
- Avoid alcohol.

---

impaired thermoregulatory ability in room temperature without protection. The more severe the impairment or prolonged the exposure, the less able are thermoregulatory responses to defend against heat loss. The elderly are particularly predisposed to hypothermia because the opportunity for heat loss frequently coexists with the decline in heat generation and conservation responses. Such coexistence occurs frequently among persons who are homeless or cognitively impaired, those injured in falls or from trauma, and persons with cardiovascular, adrenal, or thyroid dysfunction. Other risk factors include excessive alcohol use, exhaustion, poor nutrition, inadequate housing, and use of sedatives, anxiolytics, phenothiazines, and tricyclic antidepressants.

Unfortunately, a dulling of awareness accompanies hypothermia, and persons experiencing the condition rarely recognize the problem or seek assistance. For the very old and frail, environmental temperatures below 65° F (18° C) may cause a serious drop in core body temperature to 95° F (35° C). Factors that increase the risk of hypothermia are numerous, as shown in Box 16-3.

Under normal temperature conditions, heat is produced in sufficient quantities by cellular metabolism of food, friction produced by contracting muscles, and the flow of blood. Paralyzed or immobile persons lack ability to generate significant heat by muscle activity and become cold

---

BOX 16-3   Factors That Increase the Risk of Hypothermia in the Elderly

THERMOREGULATORY IMPAIRMENT

Failure to vasoconstrict promptly or strongly on exposure to cold

Failure to sense cold

Failure to respond behaviorally to protect oneself against cold

Diminished or absent shivering to generate heat

Failure of metabolic rate to rise in response to cold

CONDITIONS THAT DECREASE HEAT PRODUCTION

Hypothyroidism, hypopituitarism, hypoglycemia, anemia, malnutrition, starvation

Immobility or decreased activity (e.g., stroke, paralysis, parkinsonism, dementia, arthritis, fractured hip, coma)

Diabetic ketoacidosis

CONDITIONS THAT INCREASE HEAT LOSS

Open wounds, generalized inflammatory skin conditions, burns

CONDITIONS THAT IMPAIR CENTRAL OR PERIPHERAL CONTROL OF THERMOREGULATION

Stroke, brain tumor, Wernicke's encephalopathy, subarachnoid hemorrhage

Uremia, neuropathy (e.g., diabetes, alcoholism)

Acute illnesses (e.g., pneumonia, sepsis, myocardial infarction, congestive heart failure, pulmonary embolism, pancreatitis)

DRUGS THAT INTERFERE WITH THERMOREGULATION

Tranquilizers (e.g., phenothiazines)

Sedative-hypnotics (e.g., barbiturates, benzodiazepines)

Antidepressants (e.g., tricyclics)

Vasoactive drugs (e.g., vasodilators)

Alcohol (causes superficial vasodilation; may interfere with carbohydrate metabolism and judgment)

Others: methyldopa, lithium, morphine

From Worfolk JB: Keep frail elders warm, *Geriatr Nurs* 18(1):7-11, 1997.

BOX 16-4   Factors Associated with Low Body Temperature in the Elderly

AGING

Increases risk of thermoregulatory dysfunction.

Increases risk of acute and chronic conditions that predispose to hypothermia.

LOW ENVIRONMENTAL TEMPERATURE

Risk of hypothermia increased below 65° F.

THINNESS AND MALNUTRITION

Very thin people have less thermal insulation, higher surface area/volume ratios.

Prolonged malnutrition can decrease the metabolic rate by 20% to 30%.

POVERTY

Increases risk of thinness and malnutrition, inadequate clothing, low environmental temperature secondary to poor housing conditions and inadequate heat.

LIVING ALONE

Associated with poverty, delayed detection of hypothermia, delayed rescue if person falls.

NOCTURIA/NIGHT RISING

Associated with falls; if rescue delayed and person lies immobilized for a long time, hypothermia may develop as heat is conducted away from the body to the cold floor.

ORTHOSTATIC HYPOTENSION

An indicator of autonomic nervous system impairment; dizziness and postural instability are associated with falls.

From Worfolk JB: Keep frail elders warm, *Geriatr Nurs* 18(1):7-11, 1997.

even in normal room temperatures. Persons who are emaciated and with poor nutrition lack insulation, as well as fuel for metabolic heat-generating processes, so they may be chronically mildly hypothermic. Box 16-4 lists factors that may induce low basal body temperatures in elders. When exposed to cold temperatures, healthy persons conserve heat by vasoconstriction of superficial vessels, shunting circulation away from the skin where most heat is lost. Heat is generated by shivering and increased muscle activity, and a rise in oxygen consumption occurs to meet aerobic muscle requirements. Circulatory, cardiac, respiratory, or musculoskeletal impairments affect either the response to or function of thermoregulatory mechanisms. Elderly persons with some degree of thermoregulatory impairment, when exposed to cold temperatures, are at high risk for hypothermia if they undergo surgery, are injured in a fall or accident, or are lost or left unattended in a cool place. At brain temperatures below 20° C (68° F), all thermoregulatory ability is lost. This condition, called *poikilothermy*, is potentially lethal if untreated because body temperatures fall to levels incompatible with life. All body systems are affected by hypothermia, although the most deadly consequences involve cardiac arrhythmias and suppression of respiratory function.

Recognition of clinical signs and severity of hypothermia is an important nursing responsibility. Nurses are responsible for keeping frail elders warm for comfort and prevention of problems. It is important to closely monitor body temperature in older people and pay particular attention to lower-than-normal readings compared with the person's baseline. The potential risk of hypothermia and its associated cardiorespiratory and metabolic exertion makes prevention important and early recognition vital.

BOX 16-5 Nursing Interventions to Prevent Cold Discomfort and the Development of Accidental Hypothermia in Frail Elders

DESIRED OUTCOMES

- Hands and limbs warm
- Body relaxed, not curled
- Body temperature >97° F
- No shivering
- No complaints of cold

INTERVENTIONS

- *Maintain a comfortably warm ambient temperature* no lower than 65° F. Many frail elders will require much higher temperatures.
- *Provide generous quantities of clothing and bedcovers.* Layer clothing and bedcovers for best insulation. Be careful not to judge your patient's needs by how you feel working in a warm environment.
- *Limit time patients sit by cold windows* to short periods in which they are warmly dressed.
- *Provide a head covering* whenever possible—in bed, out of bed, and particularly out-of-doors.

- *Cover patients well during bathing.* The standard—a light bath blanket over a naked body—is not enough protection for frail elders.
- *Cover naked patients with heavy blankets for transfer to and from showers;* dry quickly and thoroughly before leaving shower room; cover head with a dry towel or hood while wet.
- *Dry wet hair quickly* with warm air from an electric dryer. Never allow the hair of frail elders to air-dry.
- *Use absorbent pads* for incontinent patients rather than allow urine to wet large areas of clothing, sheets, and bedcovers. Avoid skin problems by changing pads frequently, washing the skin well, and applying a protective cream.
- *Provide as much exercise as possible* to generate heat from muscle activity.
- *Provide hot, high-protein meals and bedtime snacks* to add heat and sustain heat production throughout the day and as far into the night as possible.

From Worfolk JB: Keep frail elders warm, *Geriatr Nurs* 18(1):7-11, 1997.

Detecting hypothermia among home-dwelling elderly is sometimes difficult, because unlike in the clinical setting, no one is measuring body temperature. For persons exposed to low temperatures in the home or the environment, confusion and disorientation may be the first overt signs. As judgment becomes clouded, a person may remove clothing or fail to seek shelter, and hypothermia can progress to profound levels. For this reason, regular contact with home-dwelling elders during cold weather is crucial. For those with preexisting alterations in thermoregulatory ability, this surveillance should include even mildly cool weather. Specific interventions to prevent hypothermia are shown in Box 16-5.

Vulnerability to Natural Disasters

Natural disasters such as hurricanes, tornadoes, floods, and earthquakes claim the lives of many people each year. In addition, human-made or human-generated disasters include chemical, biological, radiological, and nuclear terrorism and food and water contamination. The events of September 11, 2001, have prompted much thought and planning related to human-generated disasters. Older people are at great risk during and after disasters, and nurses must participate in disaster planning to support older people during these times. Older people may be less likely to seek formal or informal help than younger people during disasters and may not get as much assistance as younger individuals. The tragedies that occurred during Hurricane Katrina in 2005 highlighted the serious consequences of disasters on elderly people, both those in the community and those living in institutions. More than 60% of those who died or suffered medical problems during Hurricane Katrina were frail older adults (American Association of

Retired Persons [AARP], 2006). Gerontological nurses must be knowledgeable about disaster preparedness and assist in the development of plans to address the unique needs of older adults, as well as educate fellow professionals and older adult clients about disaster preparedness. Excellent information about disaster planning considerations for older populations is presented by Lach et al. (2005). AARP's Public Policy Institute Report, *We Can Do Better: Lessons Learned for Protecting Older People in Disasters*, and *Recommendations for Best Practices in the Management of Elderly Disaster Victims* also provide guidelines for preparation and responding to disasters affecting older people. See the Resources section at the end of this chapter for disaster preparedness information for elderly and disabled individuals.

EFFECTS OF CHANGING LIFE SITUATIONS

Change is usually stressful, regardless of whether the change is perceived as positive or negative. Advancing age may make a change in residence necessary or even desirable for some persons who wish to live closer to remaining family members, medical facilities, or provision sources. Changing life situations for the older adult can affect safety and security by posing unfamiliar routes, routines, and persons in the environment. Different locations for finding essential resources often present a stressful distraction that contributes to "getting lost," becoming fearful, and straying into unsafe areas of a town or city. These problems are not limited to large metropolitan areas. The Federal Interagency Forum on Aging-Related Statistics has documented continued social activity of older adults as a key indicator for successful aging. Persons who continue to interact with others tend to be physically and mentally healthier than persons who become socially isolated. Friends and family interactions provide emotional, social, and practical support to elders that can reduce the need for formal health care services and possibly enable them to remain in the community longer (Federal Interagency Forum on Aging-Related Statistics, 2000). Conversely, relocation may erode security because of loss of familiar faces and places.

Auto Safety

A factor that often contributes to feelings of isolation for older adults is the decision, sometimes imposed by others, to give up one's driver's license and no longer drive. These decisions are often instigated by automobile accidents, growing feelings of insecurity about driving, failing health, and the influence of family and friends. Finding and navigating public transportation may be a challenge when no willing friends or relatives are available to drive the older person. Losing one's orientation in any area can be frustrating and exhausting, and it may contribute to an elder's vulnerability to injury or crime. Uneven terrain, varying heights of curbs, and busy congested streets in unfamiliar areas increase the chance of stumbling, tripping, or falling. An older person may also have impaired sight and less energy and may appear to be an easy target for a pickpocket or purse snatcher. One cannot assume that persons living in rural areas have greater difficulty finding transportation or locating health care because they lack public conveyances. Although rural dwellers may have fewer agency supports, they often have strong social supports sustained through family, church, and neighbors. Older urban dwellers, on the other hand, may not have formed a neighborhood network of persons willing or able to provide needed social support, such as transportation or assistance in seeking health care. They may find available public transportation difficult and unsafe to navigate, particularly when they are ill or frail. Neighborhood networks promoted through churches, volunteer service organizations, community agencies, merchants, and health care providers can improve social support for older persons. Community aids in the form of Meals-on-Wheels, shopping assistance, and volunteer transportation to senior centers and health care facilities are among some of the services provided. Key referrals to these networks come from nurses, social workers, neighbors, and home care providers. Safe driving tips are provided in Box 16-6, and Chapter 15 discusses transportation and issues related to driving safety and driving cessation in more detail.

Neighborhood Security

The idea of neighborhood is a smaller concept than community and is more attuned to the convenience and friendliness of daily contacts. Nine blocks roughly corresponds to the size of most neighborhoods. As social factors or disability shrinks the geographical area in which a person moves, the neighborhood becomes smaller. The neighborhood commonly includes the corner grocery, the newspaper stand, the mail carrier, small cafes, barbershops, the church

---

BOX 16-6   Safe Driving Tips

- Plan your travel route in advance, and carry a map of your area.
- Wear your seat belt.
- Keep your eyes on the road.
- Avoid distractions. If you have to use your car phone, pull over at a convenient place first.
- Follow the 4-second rule when following.
- Obey traffic and motor vehicle laws, signs, and signals.
- Adjust your speed to the road and weather conditions.
- Drive with doors locked and windows rolled up.
- Park your car in a visible, well-lighted area.
- Expect the unexpected and always drive defensively.

From Leahy L. *Home Health Focus* 3(4):27, 1996.

---

or synagogue, and, ideally, the clinic or health care provider one uses. This network of contacts may provide informal surveillance of people and activities that can serve as an alert system for neighbors in need. The availability of this network to monitor situations out of the ordinary often points the way to emergency intervention, crime detection, or social services. Low morale and isolation are inversely correlated with one's sense of having a "neighborhood." The neighborhood seems to be a most important environmental unit for the elderly. The character of a neighborhood may be an important source of satisfaction or alienation. Many older people who once belonged in their neighborhood have been left behind by migration to the suburbs and find themselves in a neighborhood that has evolved into an alien and often frightening place. A significant contributor to fear of crime among the elderly is the socioeconomic deterioration of the neighborhood and loss of neighbors. See Chapter 3 for discussion of elder-friendly communities.

CRIMES AGAINST OLDER ADULTS

Risks and Vulnerability

Older individuals share many of the same fears about violent crime held by the rest of the population, but they may feel more vulnerable because of frailness or disability. Living alone, memory impairments, and loneliness may make elders more susceptible to crime. U.S. Department of Justice statistics show that elderly persons experienced less violence and fewer property crimes than younger people between 1993 and 2002 (*www.ojp.usdoj.gov*). Property crime is the most common crime against persons ages 65 years and older. Older people are more likely to be victims of consumer fraud and scams that include telemarketing fraud, e-mail scams, and undelivered services. Older people are defrauded at twice the rate of the rest of the population and also experience rising problems with identity theft (National Association of Triads, n.d.)

Several crime-prevention programs for the elderly have been established through combined efforts of agencies and provide information about crime prevention for seniors (Na-

---

BOX 16-7 Crime-Reduction Suggestions

- Do not wear flashy jewelry in public places or carry deadly weapons.
- Purse and wallet snatchers are usually not interested in injuring anyone. You are less likely to get hurt when accosted if you hand over your purse or wallet readily.
- Carry only a little money and personal items in your wallet or purse. Keep your car keys, larger amounts of money, and credit cards in an inside pocket of clothing.
- Some people wear a small police whistle around their neck or carry mace.
- Identify police and security personnel that are available in high-risk areas.
- Institute informal surveillance agreements by tenants to increase security.
- Receive a home security check by police, and follow through on their security suggestions.
- Attend a crime-prevention program.
- Keep doors locked, install deadbolt locks, and choose locks that you can easily manipulate. If key is lost or if you move, have locks replaced. Do not attach ID tag to key ring.
- Use peephole (install one if necessary). Confirm authenticity of a service person's ID by calling that service agency before opening the door. Never open doors to strangers or let them know you are alone.

- Lock windows. Get fire department–approved grates put on ground floor/fire escape windows. Keep all hidden entries locked (e.g., garage, basement, roof). Draw curtains and blinds at night.
- Protect valuables:
  Keep money and securities in a bank.
  Have Social Security pension check deposited directly to your account.
  Mark all valuables with Social Security number, record serial numbers.
- Beware of phone tricks.
  Hang up on (and report) nuisance callers.
  Do not give any information to strangers over phone.
- Consider a pet. A dog—even a small one—can provide excellent protection and good company if you are willing to care for one.
- Organize a buddy system. Neighbors can watch out for each other, go to basement/laundry room together, and so on.
- Keep alert to stories and coverage of fraud, bogus schemes, and protective actions on the news media.
- Take advantage of self-defense courses, public awareness programs.

---

tional Association of Triads [website]: *www. nationaltriad. org*). The National Crime Prevention Council also offers information on prevention of crime for older people (see Resources section at the end of this chapter.

Community-centered projects have shown the effectiveness of neighborhood crime prevention networks, public education in self-protective measures, avoidance of fraudulent schemes, community safety inspection programs, security advice in homes, and civic and organizational assistance in obtaining security devices and escort services. In some instances, elderly volunteer peer counselors provide support and counseling to elderly victims of crime and violence. Strategies for promoting security-conscious behaviors among elders are aimed at decreasing vulnerability to criminal victimization and playing a role in self-protection. Nurses can be instrumental in reducing fear of crime and assisting elders in exploring ways they may protect themselves and feel more secure. Box 16-7 offers suggestions for crime-reduction activities.

Fraudulent Schemes Against Elders

Fraud against elders ranges from solicitations from seemingly worthwhile charities to requests for a cash deposit to win a nonexistent prize. Trusting elderly persons may be duped into giving money to pen pals, Internet acquaintances, phony religious causes, or new acquaintances who "need help." Attractive prices of fraudulent door-to-door contractors, who offer services the older adult cannot perform, may entice a substantial cash outlay. According to the Internal Revenue Service (IRS), every year impersonators swindle

vulnerable taxpayers out of thousands of dollars by posing as IRS agents. Elderly people are often targets of these frauds. Scams may involve announcements that they have won a large cash sweepstakes that requires payment of taxes before the prize is delivered. Other IRS impersonators have called on widows or widowers to pay the "back taxes" owed by their deceased spouse. These abuses often go unpunished because the older person waits too long to report the fraud or feels embarrassment at having been taken in. Several key precautions should be shared with those at risk for fraud from IRS impersonators:

- All IRS employees carry identification and are required to show it to taxpayers when visiting a home or office.
- All citizens can obtain an IRS office address in their local telephone directory or call the national IRS directory number at 1-800-829-1040 to find its location.
- No check should ever be made payable to an IRS employee. Checks for federal taxes should be made payable to the Internal Revenue Service, not IRS; spelling out the full name makes it more difficult for criminals to alter the check.

Medical fraud is another serious type of fraud that affects older citizens on a national scale. Medical supplies and equipment delivered to homes by various suppliers have either been grossly overpriced or charged for but never received by the client. Scams to defraud Medicare beneficiaries for the new Medicare Part D benefit have also been reported. Callers ask for bank information and use the account numbers to electronically withdraw money for a Medicare card and drug plan that is not legitimate. The Centers for Medicare and Medicaid Services (CMS) has offices to inform Medicare and Medicaid beneficiaries of ways to avoid fraud and also provides toll-free numbers to report suspected fraud. National agencies have combined forces to bring about reform. CMS offers the following advice for seniors:

- No one should come to your house uninvited.
- No one can ask for personal information during his or her marketing activities.
- Keep personal information safe, including your Medicare number, and do not give out any information about bank accounts or credit cards to marketers.
- Legitimate Medicare drug plans will not ask for payment over the telephone or Internet and must send a bill to the beneficiary for the monthly premium (Centers for Medicare and Medicaid Services [CMS], 2006.)
- Most states offer the volunteer program *Seniors Health Information Needs of Elders (SHINE)*, which offers assistance on Medicare and health insurance–related concerns, and local area agencies on aging often offer assistance to older people on completion of tax returns.

FIRE SAFETY FOR ELDERS

Risk Factors for Elders

A number of factors predispose the older person to fire injuries. In home-dwelling elders, economic or climatic conditions may promote the use of ill-kept heating devices. Attempts to cook over an open flame while wearing loose-fitting clothing or inability to manage spattering grease from a frying pan can often start a fire from which the elder cannot escape. Those living in apartment dwellings are often at the mercy of cluttered wooden buildings and the careless behaviors of others. Many older people living in their own homes cannot afford home repairs, placing them at risk for fire (Tanner, 2003). Failing vision can contribute to an elderly person's setting a cook-top burner, heating pad, or hot plate at too high a temperature, resulting in fire or thermal injury.

According to the U.S. Fire Administration, people older than 65 years are one of the groups at highest risk of dying in a fire. In the United States, 1200 persons older than 65 years die each year in fires. Fire-related mortality rates are three times higher in people older than 80 years than in the rest of the population. The risk of injury during a fire is greater if medication or illness slows response time or decision making and if help is not available to contain the fire and help the person escape. In a study of 228 homebound elders, Tanner (2003) reported that only 69% of participants at moderately low risk for fires were prepared to respond to a fire in the home.

Most fires occur at home during the night, and deaths are attributed to smoke injury more often than burns. Smoking materials are the most common sources of residential fires. Fire-related deaths are more common among men than women,

BOX 16-8 Measures to Prevent Fires and Burns
<ul><li>Do not smoke in bed or when sleepy.</li><li>When cooking, do not wear loose-fitting clothing (e.g., bathrobes, nightgowns, pajamas).</li><li>Set thermostats for water heater or faucets so that the water does not become too hot.</li><li>Install a portable hand fire extinguisher in the kitchen.</li><li>Keep access to outside door(s) unobstructed.</li><li>Identify emergency exits in public buildings.</li><li>If you consider entering a boarding or foster home, check to see that it has smoke detectors, a sprinkler system, and fire extinguishers.</li><li>Wear clothing that is nonflammable or treated with a permanent fire-retardant finish. Fabrics of animal hair, wool, and silk are less flammable.</li><li>Use several electrical outlets rather than overloading one outlet.</li></ul>

which may be related to higher incidence of smoking and alcohol consumption. Plastic articles and other synthetics can produce noxious fumes that are deadly, particularly to persons with preexisting respiratory disorders. Even flame-retardant garments have been linked to noxious fume release when burned, and therefore they are a possible hazard to elders. Specific fire prevention guidelines for elders appear in Box 16-8. The National Fire Protection Association offers a fire prevention program for older adults (see Resources section).

Reducing Fire Risks in Group Residential Settings

Residents of institutional settings, such as nursing homes or assisted living facilities, are particularly vulnerable to fire because of the high numbers of frail or immobilized elderly. Activities to promote a fire-safe institutional environment include use of noncombustible building materials, sprinkler systems, smoke detectors, closed air spaces, written fire procedures, orientation of personnel, and assessment of environment by fire prevention officials. Nurses are in a position to ensure familiarity of personnel with fire safety procedures and evacuation protocol and also to report or remove any potential fire hazards. Personnel protocols should address these issues:

1. Predetermined staff members should be given specific duties and posts.
2. Notification procedures for fire department and personnel should be clearly described.
3. Management of exit maneuvers should be assigned and specifically described.

Reducing Fire Risks at Home

Practical suggestions that should be practiced by nurses personally and used to educate patients in home safety are presented in Box 16-9.

A number of potentially hazardous substances are found in most homes and should be surveyed regularly. In cases where the substance is rarely or never used, it is prudent to

BOX 16-9   Reducing Fire Risks in the Home

1. When you smell smoke, see flames, or hear the sound of fire, evacuate everyone in the house before doing anything else.
2. Use normal exits unless blocked by smoke or flame. Never use elevators during fire evacuation.
3. Stay near the floor because gases and smoke collect near the ceiling.
4. In a high-rise apartment, remain in room with doors and hall vents closed unless smoke is in your apartment. Open or break a window to obtain fresh air.
5. Define and discuss evacuation plans with other residents of the building.
6. Home fire alarm systems and smoke detectors should have a label indicating Underwriters' Laboratories (UL) approval. Smoke detectors should be installed outside each sleeping area, at the top of the basement stairs, in the bedroom of smokers, and in all levels of the house. Do not install a smoke detector too near a window, door, or forced-air register, where drafts could interfere with the detector's operation; do not install a smoke detector within 6 inches of where walls and ceilings meet, because air is less likely to circulate smoke to the alarm.
7. Rehearse what to do: If clothing catches fire, do not run; lie down, and then roll over and over ("stop, drop, and roll"). If someone else's clothing is burning, smother the flames with the handiest item, such as a rug, a coat, a blanket, or drapes.

BOX 16-10   Fire Hazards in the Home

- Flammable liquids (e.g., gasoline, acetone, lacquer thinner)
- Combustible liquids (e.g., lighter fluid, kerosene, turpentine)
- Gas leaks
- Rubbish and trash stored near stove, water heater, or furnace
- Christmas trees and tree lights that are frayed or poorly insulated
- Smoking in bed or discarding burning cigarettes
- Overloaded or worn electrical systems

eliminate it from the home. Some elderly persons may have kept old bottles and cans of hazardous materials in their garage or shed for decades and should be assisted in having them discarded in acceptable reception sites. A local fire department can give instructions regarding where flammable or combustible substances can be taken. Box 16-10 presents suggestions for a survey of a home's fire hazards.

ROLE OF ASSISTIVE TECHNOLOGY

Advancements in all types of technology hold promise for improving quality of life, decreasing the need for personal care, and enhancing independence and the ability to live safely at home. Assistive technology is any device or system that allows a person to perform a task independently or that makes the task easier and safer to perform. Health care technologies, telemedicine, mobility and activities-of-daily-living (ADL) aids, and environmental control systems (smart houses) are some examples of assistive technology. *Gerotechnology* is the term used to describe assistive technologies for older people and is expected to significantly influence how we live in the future.

Assistive technology is decreasing the number of older people who depend on others for personal care in ADLs (Freedman et al., 2006). In hospitals and long-term care facilities, devices such as wireless pendants to track people's movements, load cells built into beds to create an alert when the residents get out of bed as well as monitor patients' weights and sleep patterns, and bed lifts that allow persons to go from lying down to standing up with the push of a button are being used (Mason, 2005). The Alzheimer's Association, with Intel Corporation, sponsors the Everyday Technologies for Alzheimer grant program to study technology for people with Alzheimer's disease and their caregivers.

Telemedicine offers exciting possibilities for managing medical problems in the home or other setting, reducing health care costs, and promoting self-management of illness. Smart medical homes (*www.futurehealth.rochester.edu*) are being studied as a way to aid in the prevention and early detection of disease through the use of sensors and monitors; these devices keep data on vital signs and other measures such as gait, behavior, and sleep and provide an interactive medical-advising system. It is estimated that over 200 telemedicine programs are in the United States (Edwards and Patel, 2003). The number of programs is increasing and offer exciting possibilities for nurses, particularly advanced practice nurses.

The Arizona Technology Access Program (AzTAP) (*www.nau.edu*) gave the following examples of assistive technologies that are already available or will soon be on the market:

- A controller woven into the fabric of clothes or worn as a pin that will turn lights on and off, open doors automatically, and control the thermostat
- A universal controller operated by hand or voice that will operate any household appliance
- Voice recognition computers
- Body monitors that automatically call an emergency number when a person falls
- Laser-guided canes for people who are blind

As the "baby boomers" and future generations age, comfort with technology will be increased and people will seek options for better, safer, and more independent ways not yet imagined (Knecht, 2006). At this time, assistive technologies can be cost prohibitive for many older people, but with more development they may be more accessible and affordable for more people. See the Resources section for further information.

In summary, security and safety of elders should be of utmost importance in priorities for families, care providers, communities, and community agencies. These concerns go

Human Needs and Wellness Diagnoses

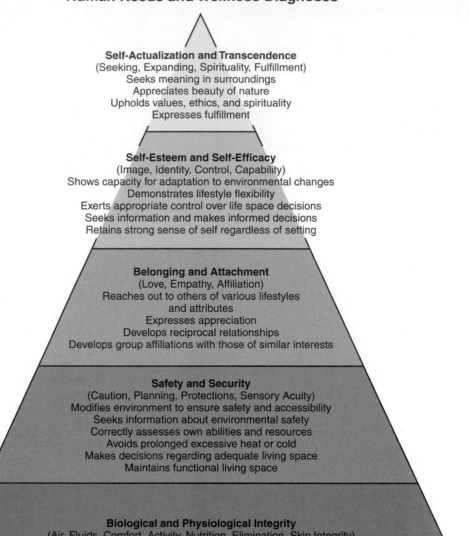

Self-Actualization and Transcendence
(Seeking, Expanding, Spirituality, Fulfillment)
Seeks meaning in surroundings
Appreciates beauty of nature
Upholds values, ethics, and spirituality
Expresses fulfillment

Self-Esteem and Self-Efficacy
(Image, Identity, Control, Capability)
Shows capacity for adaptation to environmental changes
Demonstrates lifestyle flexibility
Exerts appropriate control over life space decisions
Seeks information and makes informed decisions
Retains strong sense of self regardless of setting

Belonging and Attachment
(Love, Empathy, Affiliation)
Reaches out to others of various lifestyles
and attributes
Expresses appreciation
Develops reciprocal relationships
Develops group affiliations with those of similar interests

Safety and Security
(Caution, Planning, Protections, Sensory Acuity)
Modifies environment to ensure safety and accessibility
Seeks information about environmental safety
Correctly assesses own abilities and resources
Avoids prolonged excessive heat or cold
Makes decisions regarding adequate living space
Maintains functional living space

Biological and Physiological Integrity
(Air, Fluids, Comfort, Activity, Nutrition, Elimination, Skin Integrity)
Ensures environment will meet all basic needs
(e.g., air purity, nutrition, shelter, comfort, and rest)

These are not all the possible wellness diagnoses that may be identified. The above
are examples of nursing diagnoses that should be considered when planning care
for the older adult.

beyond simply providing a safe physical environment and freedom from violence and crime. It is clear that declining health and limited mobility erode the older person's perceptions of security, provide a source of stress, and contribute to depression and self-neglect. Of paramount importance are older persons' connections with the world outside themselves. In this respect, the need is apparent for new "neighborhoods" of contacts and resource people when older persons must relocate to other surroundings. The need for ongoing observation of elders living alone is particularly important during temperature extremes, when dangers of thermoregulatory problems increase, or during natural disasters such as hurricanes. Assisting the older person to keep his or her home environment uncluttered and free of hazardous materials also helps avoid possible injuries from falls, fires, or exposure to danger. Several strategies and programs have been successful across the United States in providing key resources to elders. Enabling the community to become the good neighbor to older citizens provides mutual benefits to all who are involved.

KEY CONCEPTS

- Feelings of security are generated from within an individual and are related to stability of inner drives and convictions.
- With increasing age and dependency, the environment becomes a larger factor in maintaining a sense of security.
- Anxiety and insecurity increase when situations and conditions become unpredictable.
- Sensory deficits increase feelings of insecurity and uncertainty in the environment.
- Because of declining thermoregulatory mechanisms in older adults, extremes of heat and cold must be avoided.

- Severe hypothermia and hyperthermia are medical emergencies and may result in death if not properly attended.
- Changing living situations may result in deterioration of function for some elders.
- Unavailable or inappropriate transportation considerably reduces an elder's life space.
- Neighborhoods change over the years, and long-term dwellers may find themselves in dangerous or crime-ridden areas as they age.
- Elders are often targets of fraud and deception.
- Reducing fire hazards is essential to feelings of security.
- A familiar and comfortable environment allows an elder to function at his or her highest capacity.

CASE STUDY: Changing Life Situations and Environmental Vulnerability

Ethel had lived in one home for all her married life, but when her husband died her children worried about her safety being alone in a big home. She could fall and lie undiscovered to die of hypothermia, the deteriorating neighborhood was no longer considered safe, and she could no longer drive so was limited in her ability to get around. They convinced her to move to a community in Phoenix near them.

They were able to find a suitable apartment that she could afford. For a while they visited her each week, but each visit became more depressing for them as she continually talked about her old home, old friends, old furniture, old priest; everything old. Their visits became less frequent. She called them faithfully each morning but detected their urge to get off the phone and on with their lives. One morning she called her daughter Gladys and said, "I'm so sick! Yesterday I walked outside and I swear I saw my friend Rose from the old neighborhood getting on the bus, but she didn't see me. I was so disappointed but managed to make it home, then couldn't find the key to my apartment so finally had to call 911 for help. They were really irritated with me when I said I had lost my key. I want to go back to Detroit. I know how things work there." After a family conclave, they found a nice place in assisted living for her and were much relieved. Ethel said, "I don't know where I am anymore. Seems I bounce around like a rubber ball." She seldom left her room except for meals, and soon she needed meals brought to her. Last week she wandered out and, when found, had suffered a serious case of heat stroke.

Based on the case study, develop a nursing care plan using the following procedure*:

- List Ethel's comments that provide subjective data.
- List information that provides objective data.
- From these data, identify and state, using accepted format, two nursing diagnoses you determine are most significant to Ethel at this time. List two of Ethel's strengths that you have identified from data.
- Determine and state outcome criteria for each diagnosis. These must reflect some alleviation of the problem iden-

tified in the nursing diagnosis and must be stated in concrete and measurable terms.
- Plan and state one or more interventions for each diagnosed problem. Provide specific documentation of the source used to determine the appropriate intervention. Plan at least one intervention that incorporates Ethel's existing strengths.
- Evaluate the success of the intervention. Interventions must correlate directly with the stated outcome criteria to measure the outcome success.

Critical Thinking Questions

1. Locate low-cost housing in your area, and assess for convenience and safety.
2. Are purse snatching and mugging of elders commonplace in your city?
3. What resources are available to prevent or assist those who may be vulnerable to attack?
4. Discuss how you would assist your parents in making a decision regarding a change in living situations as they become increasingly disabled and unable to care for themselves.
5. List several aspects of your environment that are important to you, and discuss their significance.
6. Discuss housing options that would be most suitable and feasible for you if you were unable to get around without the assistance of a walker.
7. Discuss the meanings and the thoughts triggered by the student's and elder's viewpoints expressed at the beginning of the chapter. How do these vary from your own experience?
8. Make a plan for assistance to your elderly parents when they are no longer able to fully care for themselves. Discuss the signals that will let you know they are insecure in their environment.
9. What are your city's and state's plans for disaster preparedness for disabled and older people living in the community and institutions?

---

* Students are advised to refer to their nursing diagnosis text and identify possible or potential problems.

RESEARCH QUESTIONS

What criminal activities are of most concern to older people?

What percentage of major cities or states have crime victimization programs in place?

What environmental safety factors are most frequently neglected by older people?

What home safety factors most frequently cause trouble for older people?

What have proved to be the most effective crime stoppers in relation to protecting older people from victimization?

What are the geographical distribution and incidence of hypothermia and hyperthermia in the United States?

What are the most frequent causes of fires among elders?

Survey a group of elders and determine what they most fear in their environment.

Survey the homes of elders you are serving in your clinical practice for the presence or absence of safety features.

What are the barriers to the use of assistive technology in institutions and personal homes?

RESOURCES

American Association of Retired Persons
Operation Take Charge (fighting fraud)
www.aarp.org

American Association of Retired Persons
Public Policy Institute Report: We Can Do Better: Lessons Learned for Protecting Older People in Disasters
www.aarp.org/katrina

American Red Cross
Preparing for people with disabilities and other special needs
www.redcross.org/services/disaster

Arizona Technology Access Program
(Comprehensive list of resources for older adults with disabilities)
Jill Sherman, Project Director, AzTAP
Institute for Human Development
Northern Arizona University
4105 N. 20th St., Suite 260
Phoenix, AZ 85016
(800) 477-9921
www.nau.edu/ihd/aztap

Center for Aging Services Technologies and American Association of Homes and Services for the Aging
Imagine the Future of Aging
A DVD that looks at new technology solutions to improve health care and preserve independence for older people
www.agingtech.org

Center for Future Health
University of Rochester
601 Elmwood Ave., Box CFH
Rochester, NY 14642
(585) 275-1332
www.futurehealth.rochester.edu

National Association of Home Builders
(Certified aging-in-place specialist program)
1201 15th St., NW
Washington, DC 20002
(800) 368-4242
www.nahb.org

The National Association of Triads, Inc.
1450 Duke St.
Alexandria, VA 22314
www.nationaltriad.org

National Crime Prevention Council
1000 Connecticut Ave., NW, 13th Floor
Washington, DC 20036
(292) 466-6272
www.ncpc.org

National Fire Protection Association
Remembering When: A Fire and Fall Prevention Program for Older Adults
www.nfpa.org

National Institute on Aging Senior Health
National Institute on Aging
Building 31, Room 5C27
31 Center Drive, MSC 2292
Bethesda, MD 20892
Age Page: Hyperthermia, hypothermia, crime and older people
www.nihseniorhealth.gov/

National Resource Center for Supportive Housing and Home Modification
Andrus Gerontology Center, University of Southern California
3715 McClintock Ave.
Los Angeles, CA 90089-0191
(213) 740-7069
www.homemods.org

Recommendations for Best Practices in the Management of Elderly Disaster Victims
Dr. Carmel Bitondo-Dyer
carmel_dyer@hchd.tmc.edu

Technology for Long-Term Care
Polisher Research Institute
Madlyn and Leonard Abramson Center for Jewish Life
1425 Horsham Rd.
North Wales, PA 19454-1320
(440) 256-1880
www.techforltc.org

United States Department of Justice, Office of Justice Programs, Bureau of Justice Statistics
www.ojp.usdoj.gov

REFERENCES

American Association of Retired Persons (AARP): Disaster management report, *J Gerontol Nurs* 32(8):5, 2006.

Centers for Disease Control and Prevention: Heat-related deaths—United States, 1999-2003, *MMWR* 55(29):796-798, 2006.

Centers for Medicare and Medicaid Services (CMS): Medicare fights against new schemes to defraud beneficiaries (website): *www.cms.hhs.gov/apps/media/press/release.asp?Counter=1882.* Accessed June 16, 2006.

Edwards M, Patel A: Telemedicine in the State of Maine: a model for growth driven by rural needs, *Telemed J E Health* 9(1):25-39, 2003.

Federal Interagency Forum on Aging-Related Statistics: Older Americans: Key indicators of well-being, 2000 (website): *www.agingstats.gov/chartbook2000/healthrisks.html*. Accessed August 30, 2002.

Freedman V et al: Trend in use of assistive technology and personal care for late-life disability, 1992-2001, *Gerontologist, 46*: 124-127, 2006.

Horowitz M, Hales JRS: Pathophysiology of hyperthermia. In Blatteis CM, editor: *Physiology and pathophysiology of temperature regulation*, River Edge, NJ, 1998, World Scientific.

Hurley A et al: Promoting safer home environments for persons with Alzheimer's disease: the home safety/injury model, *J Gerontol Nurs* 30(6):43-51, 2004.

Knecht B: *Aging baby boomers want smart houses for their golden years* (website): *http://archrecord.construction.com*. Accessed July 11, 2006.

Kramer MR et al: Mortality in elderly patients with thermoregulatory failure, *Arch Intern Med* 149:1521, 1989.

Lach H et al: Disaster planning: Are gerontological nurses prepared? *J Gerontol Nurs* 31(11):21-28, 2005.

Mason C: Using technology to improve delivery of care, *Generations* 29(5):70-72, 2005.

Morimoto T, Itoh T: Thermoregulation and body fluid osmolality, *J Basic Clin Physiol Pharmacol* 9(1):51, 1998.

National Association of Triads, Inc. *NATI resources: Frauds, scams, and the senior citizen* (website): *www. nationaltriad.org/tools/ NATI_Resource_Frauds_and_Scams.pdf*. Accessed July 10, 2006.

Pittiglio L: Use of reminiscence therapy in patients with Alzheimer's disease, *Lippincott's Case Manag* 5(6):216, 2000.

Schwartz B et al: Global environmental change: what can health care providers and the environmental health community do about it now? *Environ Health Perspect* 114(12):1807-1812, 2006.

Sweeney M, Chiriboga D: Evaluating the effectiveness of a multimedia program on home safety, *Gerontologist* 43(3):325-334, 2003.

Sykes K: A healthy environment for older adults: the aging initiative of the Environmental Protection Agency, *Generations* 29(2):65-69, 2005.

Tanner E: Assessing home safety in homebound older adults, *Geriatr Nurs* 24(4):250-255, 2003.

Warner M: *The complete guide to Alzheimer's proofing your home*, Layafette, Ind, 2000, Purdue University Press.

Wongsurawat N et al: Thermoregulatory failure in the elderly, *J Am Geriatr Soc* 38:899, 1990.

CHAPTER 17

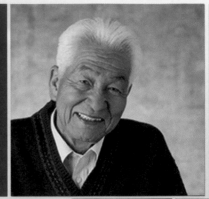

Economic, Residential, and Legal Issues

Kathleen Jett

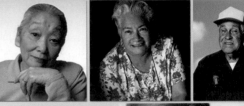

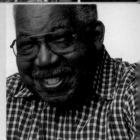

AN ELDER SPEAKS

When I was growing up, life was hard. We were so poor we couldn't do much but to hold on tight. When I was lucky I could get work plowing a field for $1 an acre. You work hard and you make do. There were not such things as going to a doctor or hospital; you did the best you could and pray you don't get sick. . . . Then when I turned 65 I got a little check from the government and a red, white, and blue insurance card [Medicare card]. The check isn't much, about $521 a month [SSI], but you know I consider myself blessed and much better off than ever before. And now I don't worry about my health; I will be taken care of, praise the Lord.

Aida at 74 in 1994

LEARNING OBJECTIVES

On completion of this chapter, the reader will be able to:

1. Explain the basic mechanisms used to finance health care in the United States.
2. Briefly explain the history of Social Security and some of the anticipated challenges.
3. Specifically explain legal issues of concern to elders.
4. Define the characteristics of a managed care organization.
5. List several types of long-term care and the various means of financing.
6. Discuss several types of housing for elders.
7. Describe the role of the nurse-advocate in relation to legal, health, and economic issues of concern to the older adult.

Economics, health care, and the law interact intimately with the organization of American health care and the needs of the aging population (Box 17-1). The health care system is huge in size and in its consumption of money. More than $1 trillion is spent on health care each year. This amount is equal to the entire budget of Italy and just behind France (Sultz and Young, 2001). Yet over 44 million people are uninsured and persons from racial and ethnic minority groups are disproportionately affected (Burnette, 2006). For adults with limited capacity to understand or consent to care or manage their own finances, the problems are significantly exacerbated.

Health care encompasses a wide variety of services, providers, products, and institutions. Each has its own interest groups, patterns of work, method of financing, and set of laws and regulations. Services, providers, products, and institutions all interact with each other and are therefore influenced by each other and the laws that govern them. Complex federal and state laws affect health care in many areas, many of which are common to all participating in the health care system and some of which are specific to older adults and persons with long-term disabilities. Moreover, health care and its systems are undergoing profound change. The changes include the increasing number of managed care organizations, changes in the roles of health care providers, and more recently, the creation of the Medicare Part D program.

Complicating much of the functioning of the health care system is the fact that the issues affecting the legal environment are unsettled. Fundamental policy questions remain unresolved. The regulation versus competition issues and the tension surrounding the locus of health care decision making—whether centralized in either professional or governmental hands or devolved authority to consumers and their agents—remain undetermined.

Economic factors are always a consideration in the delivery of health care, regardless of who pays for it. In the United

Special thanks to Alice G. Rini, the previous edition contributor, for her content contributions to this chapter.

428

BOX 17-1 Legal and Economic Needs of Older Adults

- Health and personal care planning
- Residents' rights in long-term care
- Housing issues
- Litigation and administrative advocacy
- Fiduciary representation
- Retirement planning
- Legal capacity
- Income, estate, and gift taxes
- Public benefits
- Insurance matters

From National Elder Law Foundation: *Becoming a certified elder law attorney* (website). Available at *www.nelf.org*.

States, the system of health care providers, payers, insurers, and beneficiaries is complex. The federal government purchases or provides the majority of care through its insurance plans (Medicare, Railroad Medicare, Medicaid, and TRI-CARE) and directly through the Veterans Administration. State governments are also significantly involved through the shared Medicaid plan and in public and mental health services.

Economic conflict exists in several areas: (1) between generations—younger workers, who pay Social Security and Medicare taxes, and disabled and retired persons, who use the greatest amount of health care dollars toward the end of their lives; (2) between providers, who find that reimbursement for care has decreased significantly, and regulators, who are struggling with cost containment; and (3) between Medicare beneficiaries, who are constrained by rules limiting the care for which Medicare will pay, and legislators, who understand the power of the older voter.

As reviewed in Chapter 1 and several other previous chapters, the proportion of persons older than 65 years is steadily increasing and growth of this age cohort is anticipated to be dramatic as more of the "baby-boomers" age. This has implications for ensuring incomes and ultimately providing care to the most frail.

Gerontological nurses are and will be faced with not only knowing how best to provide care but also understanding the economic and legal aspects of late life and health care. This chapter is intended to explain and clarify the legal, political, and economic issues that nurses in all gerontological practice situations need to know to be effective in providing care, education, guidance, and referrals to appropriate resources. Included is a review of the residential options available to persons as they age.

FINANCE IN LATE LIFE

Before the industrial revolution of the late 1800s, persons in most countries and cultures worked until they were no longer physically able to do so. In many cases the "work" of the individual changed with time and as capabilities diminished and did not cease until shortly before death. Care, when necessary, was provided by family members and the community (see Chapter 20) (Bohm, 2001).

It was not until the rigors of industrial work that opportunities disappeared for those with declining abilities. The term "retire" was defined as "withdraw from service" but changed to mean "no longer fit for service" between the mid-1800s and the early 1900s (Achenbaum, 1978). Care became less available as whole families joined the urban workforce. Congregate living, including nursing homes, and Social Security as a form of ongoing income for eligible workers were created as a result of the social changes of the time.

In the early 1900s, almshouses and poor houses emerged to provide care for frail indigent persons who did not have family available or able to care for them. Most of these facilities were supported by charitable organizations. Later, the government became involved, and when the primary population in almshouses was the elderly, many essentially became public nursing institutions. In some places the law supported the use of public monies for a formerly private purpose—the care of the elderly—and local governments were authorized to purchase land and erect facilities for the care of the elderly and could tax its citizens to maintain them (*Mason County Infirmary v. Smith's Comm.*, 1901). In the early 1900s it was determined that the care of indigent elderly could be construed to be a public responsibility (*Maydwell v. Louisville*, 1903). Because the concept of personal responsibility continued to exist, poor persons who were admitted to care facilities were required to contribute any property they owned that could be used to help pay for the care and maintenance provided (Nacev and Rettig, 2002, p. 142, fn. 26).

Social Security

Considered by many to be one of the most successful federal programs, Social Security was established in 1935, in the depths of the Great Depression. The primary function of the program was to provide monetary benefits to older former workers and was viewed as a means to prevent or minimize the dependency of older members on younger members of society (Weinberger, 1996).

Social security and a number of programs that followed were set up as "age-entitlement" programs. This meant that an individual could receive the benefits simply because of their age and regardless of their need. In other words, the monetary support is available to those persons at a certain age regardless of their personal resources. They were and are, however, limited to American citizens and legal residents older than a certain age or totally and permanently disabled who have paid into the system through payroll taxes for at least 10 years or are married to someone who has worked the required years. The amount of benefit is calculated in part on the person's average salary during 35 of his or her working years. If fewer than 35 years were worked, the years are counted as zero income and still used in the calculation (Hooyman and Kiyak, 2005). This has been most beneficial to white men, who are more likely to have worked the most consistently and at higher salaries than all other groups of workers. The amount of benefit increases each year on January 1st as a cost-of-living adjustment (COLA). In 2007 the average Social Security benefit was $1044 for the 49 million recipients.

The program has been managed on what is called a *pay-as-you-go system*. Payroll taxes on the first $97,500 of income are collected from employees and employers and are immediately distributed to beneficiaries (retirees and the disabled or eligible spouses). Social Security funds, although individually deposited by employers and employees, are not reserved for any one individual. No one has an account set aside in his or her name. All funds that are not immediately paid out to beneficiaries are "borrowed" by the federal government for regular operating expenses. The government converts the borrowed funds into government bonds, reflecting the debt of the government to Social Security, and places these in a "trust fund" watched over by the trustees of the fund. However, no funds are specifically identified to pay back those monies borrowed from the Social Security Trust Fund (Weinberger, 1996).

At the time of its inception, the system was constructed to transfer funds from those believed to be relatively well off (workers) to those believed to be relatively and uniformly poor (retirees). As long as the amount of contributions from workers exceeds that paid to beneficiaries, the program, as designed, can exist, or remain solvent. The combination of the increasing number of beneficiaries, the decreasing number of workers (in proportion to the beneficiaries), and the intangible nature of the "trust fund" has resulted in concern that the program will cease to exist in the near future—a potential threat to the future incomes of retirees who have spent their lives paying into a system that may not be available to them in their later years.

The trustees of the Social Security Trust Fund have for many years reported that the fiscal integrity of the fund is in jeopardy and that reform is needed (Friedman, 1999). The 1994 trustees' report expressed concern that if reform and change were not instituted quickly, the magnitude of the changes needed would be great and would threaten the existence of the program (Social Security and Medicare Board of Trustees, 1994). In 2006 the prediction was revised to anticipate the insolvency of Medicare reserves as early as 2018 followed by the insolvency of the Social Security funds by 2040 when the income into the fund will finance only 74% of benefits required (Trustees, 2006). Details of the changing status of Social Security (and Medicare) are provided to the public annually and may be accessed at *www.ssa.gov/OACT/TR/index.html.*

Despite deep concern, a solution has not been found and the George W. Bush Administration suggestion to privatize the Social Security systems has not been completely accepted. Although such a plan might work well for persons who have the resources and skills to plan far ahead, it may be a significant, if not insurmountable, problem for those on very limited incomes or without financial acumen in their working years. One attempt to delay the problem has been implemented by raising the age of "retirement." The age at which one becomes eligible for Social Security benefits is increasing slowly and will transition to 67 years old for those born in 1960 or after.

Supplemental Security Income. Not all older persons living in the United States have Social Security benefits adequate to provide even the most basic necessities of life. This has been true especially for persons who have spent their lives employed in the agriculture industry or as domestic workers and paid very low wages, often on a cash basis. Supplemental Security Income (SSI) was established in 1965 by Title XIX of the Social Security Act. SSI provides for a minimum level of economic support to persons regardless of their earning power in early life or when capable of working. SSI either provides total support or supplements a low Social Security benefit. In 2006 the SSI benefit for approximately 7 million people was a maximum of $603 month for a single person and $904 for a couple, although some states supplement this amount to some extent (Social Security Administration [SSA], 2006).

Other Late Life Income

Finally, financing late life may include private retirement or pension plans. Individuals may pay into the plans themselves (e.g., IRAs) or through their employers (e.g., 401K accounts). Either the private retirement, pension funds, or a combination of these are invested in private sector financial instruments (e.g., stocks, bonds, or real estate holdings) or perhaps in government treasury notes. Those funds are held for the beneficiary and may become part of his or her estate if the beneficiary dies before collecting the pension. Some private retirement annuities provide for several choices for receipt of funds after retirement. The retiree could elect to take his or her pension based on his or her own life only or based on the retiree's and a spouse's life. In other words, a person may set up a plan so that he or she receives all or most of the benefit during his or her lifetime rather than providing for any survivor benefit. Notification of the potential survivor of such a choice is not always required (Hooyman and Kiyak, 2005). The amount received is actuarially determined based on the life expectancy of one or two beneficiaries and whether a guaranteed minimum number of years is selected.

FINANCING HEALTH CARE

In many countries across the globe, health care is a universal entitlement. That is, some level of health care is available to all persons either living in or working in the country, and health care is considered a right. In these settings, health care providers are considered workers alongside of others in the service sector. The universal services are supported to a large extent by payroll taxes, which can be significant. The insurance risk is shared among all citizens. Although these plans have significant benefits, challenges have also been encountered, such as long waits for elective or non-urgent procedures and rationing of other types of services. As the population in a particular country prospers, a "second tier" of care has developed, that which can be purchased. That is, some of the services that are more limited in the country's plan can be purchased if one can afford to do so in what is called a "fee-for-service" model. This results in considerable ethical and moral dilemmas.

In the United States, health care has always been a purchsed service—not a right. Health care is purchased either directly in a fee-for-service model, such as the one just noted, or indirectly through capitated insurance plans. The cost of the plan is directly proportional to the benefits provided. The three main types of purchased plans are (1) fee-for-service, (2) purchased (Original Medicare, private insurance, some prospective payment plans [PPOs]), and (3) Medicare Advantage Plans (managed care plans [MCPs] and health maintenance organizations [HMOs]) (Box 17-2).

With the fee-for-service model, payments are made only after a charge has been incurred and are made at the rate charged. In these plans there is usually little or no restriction on which services are "purchased" or at what cost. The participant pays a monthly premium to Medicare. As of January 1, 2007, this premium is based on income as reported to the Internal Revenue Service. In the Original Medicare and most other purchased plans, the patient is responsible for paying premiums to the insurer and is required to make a co-pay and pay the co-insurance when services are received; in this way, the patient is sharing the cost. In the Medicare Advantage Plans, the patient is assigned to specific providers and vendors who have entered into a prior (prospective) agreement with the insurer about services provided and patient co-pays. These plans were created in an attempt to control the skyrocketing costs associated with the fee-for-service model. With the Medicare Advantage Plans, a provider or health care system receives a flat capitated rate from Medicare for each potential recipient of care. Within pre-established guidelines, all medically necessary services must be provided by that provider or health care system.

Persons without insurance purchase all health care in an "out-of-pocket" manner. They are expected to pay whatever the charge is for a received service. Although the number of uninsured persons is expected to increase each year, most elders fall under one of the safety nets of Medicare, Medicaid or both. These services are described in the following sections.

BOX 17-2 Terms Related to Financing Health Care

Managed care organization (MCO): A for-profit or not-for-profit company that manages a system of health care delivery in which patients agree to use health care providers from a panel of physicians, nurse practitioners, therapists, hospitals, pharmacies, and home care agencies, among others designated by the MCO. The MCO monitors the cost of care provided to patients to control the cost of care.

Integrated delivery systems: A group of individual entities such as a hospital and physicians that join together into a single entity to provide integrated health care services to contracted clients/patients.

Payers: In the health care context, payers are the entities who pay for health care on behalf of persons who have paid premiums or fees to the payer or, in the case of some government programs, on behalf of persons who are unable to pay themselves.

Provider: One who provides something; a generic term referring to all persons and agencies that provide health care.

Insurer: An individual or organization that underwrites an insurance risk and that agrees to pay compensation or benefits to the insured according to a contract. The insured is the person covered by the insurance contract; with a health insurance contract, the insured is the patient.

Beneficiary: A person who derives a benefit from something; in health care, the person who is a subscriber to an MCO or HMO or who is receiving benefits through Medicare is said to be a beneficiary of those organizations since the person receives medical benefits from his/her association with the organizations.

Preferred provider organization (PPO): A health care delivery system through which providers contract to offer medical services to benefit plan enrollees on a fee-for-service basis at various reimbursement levels in return for more patients and/or timely payment. Enrollees may use any provider in the PPO or outside the PPO, but they have a financial incentive (e.g., lower coinsurance payments) to use providers within the PPO.

Health maintenance organization (HMO): A health insurance company to which subscribers (patients) pay a predetermined co-pay in return for a range of medical services from physicians and other health care providers who are approved by the organization. Premiums are usually paid by Medicare through a capitated system.

Medicare Modernization Act: A legal ruling that changed several aspects of the traditional Medicare insurance plans. Among the changes were coverage for several preventive services, a one time "welcome to Medicare" physical, and the implementation of a public-private partnership to offer partial drug coverage under the new Medicare Part D, which supplements the existing Medicare Parts A, B, and C.

Prescription drug plans (PDPs): Insurance plans for prescription drug coverage that are individually managed and owned by either private or corporate organizations. Most are "for-profit." If deemed "credible," they are considered an option for purchasing under the Medicare Part D plan.

Medicare

History. In 1934 President Franklin D. Roosevelt appointed the Committee on Economic Security (CES) to craft a Social Security bill. The original report included a health insurance plan, but because of much opposition to it, Roosevelt deferred the health insurance part of the bill to avoid losing Social Security (see earlier discussion) (Corning, 1969). The American Medical Association opposed any national program of health insurance, believing it to be "socialized medicine," and made efforts to prevent its implementation (Goodman, 1980). *Fortune* magazine polled the American public in 1942 and found that 76% of those polled opposed government-financed medical care (Cantril, 1951).

In the early 1960s President Johnson recognized that the numbers of older persons, those with serious disabilities, and poor children were increasing significantly and too often persons from these vulnerable groups were without access to needed health services. Although opposition continued, Johnson proposed amendments (Title XVIII and Title XIX) to the Social Security Act to address these social problems. In Senate and House hearings, some legislators described the amendments as steps that would continue to destroy independence and self-reliance and would tax the poor and middle class to subsidize the health care of the wealthy (Twight, 1997).

Nonetheless, legislation was passed in 1965 and 1966 to expand the Social Security system by establishing Medicare, Railroad Medicare (for retired railroad workers), and Medicaid. These were set up as entitlement programs; if the person met set criteria, he or she could receive the services. For Medicare, one's own resources were not included in the criteria for eligibility and became a version of "universal health care" for most persons ages 65 years and older. Medicaid's criteria included income and asset restrictions. Initially, all three plans were set up as fee-for-service plans. In a short time after the implementation of these plans, millions more persons could receive health care and the costs for the services escalated rapidly.

Medicare Part A was created as an entitlement insurance to cover the costs of hospital and limited nursing home care for eligible beneficiaries (Box 17-3). Medicare Part B was created as a purchasable and affordable voluntary insurance plan that covered outpatient and health care provider services (see Box 17-3). Prescription drug coverage in the form known as *Medicare Part D* was not

---

BOX 17-3 Fundamentals of Original Medicare Parts A and B*

MEDICARE PART A

Medicare Part A is designed primarily to partially cover the costs of inpatient hospital care and other specialized care as listed below:

- Acute hospitalization coverage, through a prospective payment system, includes costs of semiprivate rooms, meals, nursing services, operating and recovery room, intensive care, drugs, laboratory and radiology fees, blood products, and other necessary medical services and supplies. There is a deductible for days 1-60. This is repeated anytime the person is rehospitalized after 60 days. After 60 days, there is a daily co-pay that increases over time. There is no coverage after 150 days. Deductibles and co-pays increase every year. The deductibles and co-pays are either paid out-of-pocket or by Medicaid or Medigap policies.
- Nursing home care is covered by Medicare only if the person had been in an acute care setting for 3 days before the admission and only as long as a skilled service is needed and for a maximum of 100 days. While the facility is paid on a prospective payment system similar to the acute care setting, for the patients, the first 20 days are covered at 100%, and for days 21-100 a substantial daily co-pay is required. There is no coverage if skilled care is not continuously needed.
- Home health care may be covered by Medicare (also prospective payment) on an intermittent and/or part-time basis for skilled nursing care, physical therapy, and rehabilitative services. The person must be ill enough to be considered homebound. Custodial care is not covered. Medicare pays 80% of the approved amount for durable medical equipment and supplies.
- Hospice care is provided for terminally ill persons expected to live less than 6 months who elect to forgo traditional medical treatment for the terminal illness. Medicare pays for all but limited co-pays for outpatient drugs and inpatient care. Hospice Medicare replaces Medicare Parts A and B for all costs associated with the terminal condition.
- Inpatient psychiatric care is a limited number of days in a lifetime; partial payment; other limitations apply.

MEDICARE PART B

Medicare Part B is designed to cover some of the costs associated with outpatient or ambulatory services. Deductibles and co-pays are required in most cases:

- Physician and nurse practitioner services, including some prescribed supplies and diagnostic tests
- Physical, occupational, and speech therapy for the purpose of rehabilitation
- Limited durable medical equipment
- Clinical laboratory services fully covered if deemed medically necessary after a deductible
- Outpatient hospital treatment, blood, and ambulatory surgical services
- Limited preventive services
- Diabetic supplies (excluding insulin and other medications)

*See *www.cms.gov* for the latest information about covered services and associated costs. These are all subject to change.

added until U.S. President George W. Bush's administration in 2006.

Like Social Security, Medicare Part A was designed as a pay-as-you-go system; that is, taxes collected from employers and employees are used for payment of current Medicare beneficiaries and are not placed in a fund earmarked for taxpayers' future medical expenses. Of the costs of Medicare Part B and Part D, 75% comes from the general revenue of the federal government. The remainder comes primarily from the beneficiaries themselves in the form of premiums and co-pays. In 2006, the first year of Medicare Part D, 12% of the costs was paid for by state governments in exchange for support of persons previously covered under Medicaid (Trustees, 2006).

Medicare is administered by the Centers for Medicare and Medicaid Services (CMS) and is a part of the Department of Health and Human Services, a special entity created to improve the administration of the programs. In 2006 nearly 47 million persons older than 65 years, blind, disabled, or with end-stage renal disease were covered by some part of Medicare (Jett, 2006). Expenses related to Medicare made up 2.7% of the gross domestic product (GDP) in 2005 (Trustees, 2006).

Medicare Part A. A person automatically receives a Medicare card (red, white, and blue) indicating Medicare Part A coverage when he or she turns 65 years and has paid Medicare taxes for at least 30 quarters (10 years). In 2007, if a person has not worked before the age of 65 years, he or she may be eligible to purchase Part A coverage for a monthly fee of up to $410 per month (Centers for Medicare and Medicaid Services [CMS], 2006). Medicare Part A is a hospital insurance plan covering acute care and acute and short-term rehabilitative care and some costs associated with hospice care and home health care under certain circumstances. The coverage and co-payments vary by setting under the original fee-for-service plans. When acute care is needed, the co-payments can be quite high, including co-pay of $992 (as of 2007) for days 1 to 60, $248 for days 61 to 90, and $496 for days 91 to 150. After 150 days in an acute care setting, each beneficiary has a 60-day lifetime reserve at the co-pay cost of $496 per day. After the 60-day reserve is used, the acute stay of over 150 days is not covered (CMS, 2007).

Rehabilitative care, usually provided in skilled nursing facilities, is paid for only if it occurs within 3 days of a hospital discharge and as long as the patient requires what is called *skilled care* (only that which is provided by a licensed nurse or physical or occupational therapist). Medicare Part A will pay 100% of the first 20 days of a nursing home stay, with a co-pay of up to $124 per day for days 21 to 100 and no coverage after that (CMS, 2006). At any time the person no longer needs skilled care, Medicare coverage stops. Medicare does not cover additional charges that may be incurred during a long-term care stay, such as incontinence supplies and laundry.

When the assistance needed is limited to personal care or medication supervision, it is not covered by Medicare at all. Similarly, for home health care, for the costs to be paid by Medicare the care must be provided at the written direction of a physician. Ongoing supervision can be provided by either a physician or a nurse practitioner. It must be through a certified agency and for the purposes of active rehabilitation as seen in the nursing home setting. There are no co-payments for home health care and limited co-pays for hospice care.

Medicare Part B. In the 7 months surrounding a person's 65th birthday (from 3 months before), all persons who are eligible for Medicare Part A must select and apply for Part B through the local Social Security Administration offices (*www.socialsecurity.gov*). Medicare Part B covers the costs associated with the services provided by physicians; nurse practitioners; outpatient services (e.g., laboratory services); qualified physical, speech, and occupational therapists; and some home health care providers.

The Original Medicare Plan is based on a traditional fee-for-service arrangement. The advantages of the Original Medicare Plan include choice and access. Participants can seek the services of any provider they choose and without a referral. Providers all over the United States accept Medicare, and participants can change providers as often as desired. When a patient receives medically necessary services from a provider, a bill for the cost of the care is sent to Medicare or to the patient, who can submit the claims; the provider or the patient is then reimbursed. Charges incurred are paid by Medicare at a rate based on an "allowable charge." If a provider "accepts assignment," there is no additional charge to the patient other than the allowable charge. A provider who does not accept assignment may charge the patient up to 15% above the allowable charge. With the Original Medicare Plan, the patient is responsible for an annual deductible, co-pays, coinsurance charges, and

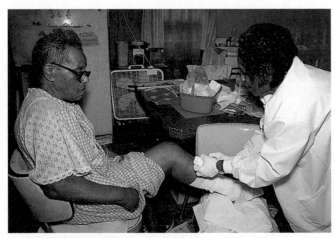

Wound care is usually a "covered service" under Medicare A when provided by a registered nurse in a person's home and all other requirements are met. (From Lewis SM et al: *Medical-surgical nursing: assessment and management of clinical problems,* ed 7, St Louis, 2007, Mosby.)

a monthly premium based on income and marital status. Unless the patient has a Medigap policy (described on p. 435) all of these fees are paid for "out-of-pocket." The premium is usually deducted directly from the monthly Social Security check. All costs are adjusted on a yearly basis (CMS, 2005).

Preferred Provider Organization (PPO) plans work like the Original Medicare Plan except that only specific providers (those in the network) can be used. In most cases a referral from a selected or assigned primary care provider is required to see a specialist. The additional services, fees, and co-pays vary by plan. A patient may choose to be seen by a provider outside the PPO network for an additional charge.

Medicare Advantage Plans (sometimes called Medicare C) are prospective payment models. Medicare pays a predetermined fee to the health care organization or provider on a regular basis in what is known as a capitated payment plan. All costs of care are expected to be paid for by this capitated amount. HMOs that have been granted Medicare per capita waivers cannot refuse applicants based on preexisting health conditions. All traditional services covered by Medicare Part A and Part B must be provided, and additional services, co-pays, and deductibles are predetermined. Not all Medicare Advantage Plans are offered at all locations in the United States.

Medicare Advantage Plans may provide a cost savings to the member as well as extra benefits. In most cases a member of the plan pays no premium. However, special rules must be followed, and the member may be charged extra co-pays for additional services. The member is also restricted to certain providers and hospitals. There are fewer out-of-pocket costs unless an individual decides to see a provider or to seek a service without a referral or outside the system to which he or she has subscribed; such services are usually not covered at all. Referrals are required for all services other than that of the primary health care provider. The negative aspects of HMOs and managed care plans are the access barriers to specialists and high-tech procedures and treatments.

The best of these plans are complete health care systems with highly trained physicians, nurse practitioners, and nurses working out of single or regional and completely equipped medical centers. Medicare Advantage Plans and other managed care plans differ from other plans in that they are expected to emphasize preventive medicine, comprehensive care, periodic physical examinations, and immunizations. Some HMOs provide extensive health education services, support groups, and telephone support services to homebound patients. The supplemental services offered may save the participant a considerable amount in the costs of medications, assistive devices, and professional consultation charges.

Capitation or set limits for reimbursement are imposed on managed care plans by Medicare. Capitated plans are further limited in that the plan is paid a certain fixed amount each day for each enrollee regardless of the amount of care given. All necessary care must be provided from this amount. This model has created abuses and horror stories in which elders were denied needed treatments to save money for the corporate providers. Patient protection laws now allow consumers to lodge complaints and initiate legal action against these abuses. The Center for Patient Advocacy supported a much-needed bill that became law in October 1999. This law allows appeals when an managed care plan denies care, guarantees access to specialists when needed, ensures that health-related decisions are made by health care providers rather than bureaucrats, and holds managed care plans legally accountable for medical decisions that cause harm.

Medicare Part D. In 2003 the Medicare Modernization Act established a prescription drug benefit for eligible recipients of Medicare, known as *Medicare Part D;* the plan was implemented January 1, 2006. It is an elective prescription drug plan (PDP) with associated out-of-pocket premiums and co-payments. All persons with either Medicare Part A or Medicare Part B are eligible to voluntarily purchase a Medicare Part D PDP.

Help with the costs associated with Medicare Part D is available for persons with low incomes (below 150% of the poverty level) and those who receive Medicaid (Box 17-4). For persons with both Medicare and Medicaid (called *"dual eligibles"*), the new plan is not voluntary and replaced the former drug benefit under Medicaid. Dually eligible persons who did not choose a plan in the fall of 2005 were arbitrarily assigned to a PDP (Resnick and Jett, 2005). However, it is unclear whether this method of enrollment will continue.

The PDPs established under Medicare Part D are all commercial plans that have contractual arrangements with

---

BOX 17-4   **Low Income Eligibility for Assistance with the Costs of Medicare Part D**

INCOME (AS OF 2005)

Must be no greater than 150% of the federal poverty level
- $1197/month for individual (higher for Alaska and Hawaii)
- $1604/month for married couple (higher for Alaska and Hawaii)
- Adjusted for family size

RESOURCES (AS OF 2007)

Value of assets* limited to:
- $11,710 for individual
- $23,410 for married couple (includes $1500/personal burial plans)

Data from McClellan M: Medicare D prescription coverage, *Geriatrics* 60(10), 7-9, 2005; Social Security Administration: *Help with Medicare drug plan costs* (website): *www.ssa.gov.* Website expires May 31, 2008.
*Does not include the home the person lives in.

CMS. To be included as an option, the company must agree to follow the rules set forth by CMS and change as directed. With the agreement to provide the minimum level of benefits established by the Medicare Part D regulations, the plan is deemed "credible" by CMS and becomes accepted as equivalent (Stefanacci, 2006a).

The initial enrollment period for the realization of full benefits was November 15, 2005, to December 31, 2005. All persons who had completed the application process by the close of the initial enrollment were to begin receiving benefits on January 1, 2006. The second period of enrollment began January 1, 2006, and continued until May 15, 2006.

With few exceptions, the costs for those who enroll after May 15, 2006 are assessed a 1% per month penalty fee, and most persons with existing Medicare coverage can enroll only from November 15th to December 31st of each year (the "open enrollment" period). As persons become newly eligible for Medicare, they can enroll for all three plans at the same time or within 60 days at the prices in effect at that time (Wortz, 2006).

Once enrolled in either Medicare Part D or another credible PDP, a person cannot change a plan until the next open enrollment period except under special circumstances. These circumstances include those who are admitted to, reside in, or discharged from a skilled nursing facility and persons with dual-eligibility.

Of the 47 million persons potentially eligible for PDPs, as many as 27 million have coverage through an employer or pension-sponsored "credible" plan or through a government plan such as the Veterans Administration or Indian Health Services. In the first 6 months of 2006, 1 million previously uncovered people voluntarily enrolled in a managed care plan that included drug benefits and 9 million enrolled in one of the plans made possible the new Medicare Part D. Finally, 5.9 million "dual-eligibles" either selected a plan or were arbitrarily enrolled in one. An estimated 6 million Medicare beneficiaries had not enrolled as of May 15, 2006 (Stefanacci, 2006b).

Most PDPs are set up in a similar way. The standard Medicare Part D drug benefit premium in 2006 was about $37 a month and could be deducted from the beneficiary's Social Security check or paid directly to the plan. The annual deductible was $250. After the person had spent $250, the PDP covered 75% of the cost of the approved drugs up to $2000 with a 25% co-pay (Medicare paid $1500, the person paid $500). The next $2850 in costs was paid directly by the individual (called the "*donut hole*"). When the total costs for approved drugs reached $5100 ($3600 out of pocket), the PDP paid 95% (5% co-pay) of all drug costs for the rest of the year. The premiums and co-pay amounts are expected to change annually and vary greatly from plan to plan. The deductible and donut-hole are repeated yearly. Although most PDPs have donut holes, a person may elect a plan with lower co-pays or broader drug coverage for a higher monthly premium. No plan approved as a Medicare Part D plan can have lower benefits (McClellan, 2005; CMS, 2007).

Nurses, nurse practitioners, physicians, pharmacists, and community volunteers have spent and continue to spend hours helping beneficiaries enroll at appropriate times and select the plan that best meets their needs. This sometimes onerous task can be instrumental in promoting healthy aging.

Supplemental or Medigap Insurance Policies

Because of the potentially high co-payments associated with Medicare, persons who are able to do so often purchase supplemental insurance plans known as *Medigap policies*. Medigap policies feature standardized benefits, and generally several different policies are available from which to select in each state. Persons searching for an appropriate Medigap plan can be referred to the Medicare website for their state or request a print copy of the standard plans (available at *www.medicare.gov*). Standard plans are designated A through J, and all include the basic benefits of Medicare Part A coinsurance, the cost of an extra 365 days of hospital care after the Medicare Part A benefit ends, Medicare Part B coinsurance or co-payment, and the first three pints of blood each year. Plans A through J cover increasing benefits and therefore have increasing costs as the number of benefits increases. In some areas, beneficiaries may choose a "Medigap Select" policy, which restricts enrollees to certain physicians, hospitals, and other providers. Medigap Select policies tend to be less costly.

Medigap insurance policies cover only the deductibles and part of the coinsurance amounts based on Medicare-approved amounts contracted with providers. Physicians and nurse practitioners who agree to accept the Medicare assignment amount cannot charge a patient with both Medicare and a Medigap policy any uncovered charges. Providers who do not accept Medicare assignment can charge the difference between the plans and the actual charge.

Care for Veterans

Nearly 7 million World War II veterans and 3 million Korean War veterans are now older than 65 years. Medical program expenses for the veterans of our wars have become a major fiscal responsibility, from approximately $16.9 billion in 1997 to well over $100 billion as a result of the Gulf War and the wars in Iraq and Afghanistan (Kennedy School, 2007). The Veterans Health Administration (VA) system has long held a leadership position in gerontological research, medical care, and extended care. In fact, a great deal of the research that guided gerontologists in earlier years was generated through the VA system, as were innovations in care. In addition, the majority of geriatric fellowships have been provided through the VA hospitals. The VA system has been a forerunner of the various continua of care providers now in place. Early on, this system provided VA-run nursing homes, home care and community-based programs, respite care, blindness rehabilitation, mental health, and numerous other services in addition to acute medical/surgical provisions.

Persons and their dependents who have been part of the uniformed services may be eligible for health care services through veterans hospital networks. At one time, veterans hospitals and services were available on an as-needed basis for anyone who had served at any time. It was not necessary for individuals to use their Medicare benefits. However, this system is undergoing a process of significant change. One of the first changes that veterans noted was restrictions placed on the use of veterans hospitals and services. Instead of coverage of any health problems, priorities were set for those problems that were in some way deemed "service connected"; in other words, the health care problem had to be linked to the time the person was on active duty.

Veterans older than 65 years are now expected to obtain and use Medicare for their non–service-connected health problems, with the responsibilities for co-pays and deductibles the same as for other beneficiaries. An outcry among veterans and veteran groups resulted in the development of a free Medigap policy known as TRICARE for Life (TFL).

TRICARE for Life. TRICARE is the health care insurance program provided by the Department of Defense for eligible beneficiaries. The TFL is for Medicare-eligible beneficiaries ages 65 years and older and their dependents or widows or widowers older than 65 years. This plan requires that the person enroll in both Medicare Part A and Part B and pay the premiums for Part B. As a Medigap policy, TFL covers those expenses not covered by Medicare, such as co-pays and prescription medicines. Dependent parents or parents-in-law may be eligible for pharmacy benefits if they turned age 65 years on or after April 1, 2001, and are enrolled in Medicare Part B. For more information about this, see *www.tricare.osd.mil.*

Medicaid

Medicaid is a health insurance program jointly funded by federal and state governments using tax dollars collected into the general funds of each. It provides health services for low-income children, pregnant women, those who are permanently disabled, and persons older than 65 years. For elders with low incomes, Medicaid offsets the high Medicare co-pays and deductibles and provides additional health benefits.

Medicaid was created in 1965 as part of Title XIX of the Social Security Act at the same time as Medicare. It makes payments for health care provided to Medicaid recipients directly to health care providers. Because it is a joint program, CMS administers the program at the federal level, and a state agency administers at each state level (Nacev and Rettig, 2002). Eligibility for Medicaid is determined by the state and is based on income and assets, categorical need, and lack of ability to afford, even with Medicare, the medical care required.

Federal law requires states to provide a certain minimum level of service, and states may add other coverage such as

prescription drugs (now replaced by Medicare Part D), vision care, dentures, prostheses, case management, and other medical or rehabilitative care provided by a licensed health care practitioner. In most cases, Medicaid covers more services than Medicare, including custodial care in nursing homes and preventive care with no co-pays or deductibles; however, this is highly variable by state and by the year and depends on the state's fiscal health and political priorities.

If institutional long-term care is needed, a single adult without a dependent child but with a low income (less than approximately $1200 a month and few assets) is required to contribute all but $35 dollars of his or her monthly income to partially cover the actual costs of care. The difference between the person's contribution and Medicaid's allowable charge is paid by a combination of state and federal revenues. This ensures that the neediest disabled adults are cared for. Persons with incomes above the limit set by the state are not eligible for assistance with health care expenses.

If a person who requires the financial support of Medicaid for a nursing home stay has a spouse who is able to remain in the community, the spouse is permitted to keep a percentage of the couple's income and cash as well as the family home, a car of any value, and personal property.

Because some people who believed they would soon need nursing home care transferred funds to become eligible for Medicaid and avoid using their own funds for that care, laws have been enacted to preclude ineligible persons from defrauding government programs. Some transfers are permitted, such as to a spouse or a disabled, dependent child. Any other transfer, to another person or to a trust, is considered an improper transfer and will be invalid for the purpose of qualifying for Medicaid. When a person applies for Medicaid, a "look-back period" determines if funds have been transferred that would normally be available to the applicant. Transfers to recipients other than a trust have a look-back period of 36 months; transfers to a trust have a look-back period of 60 months. If transfers were made, Medicaid support will not begin until the costs incurred and paid equal the amount of the transfer. For example, a person who transfers $100,000 and is in a nursing home where the monthly rate is $4000 would be ineligible for Medicaid for 25 months ($4000 × 25 months = $100,000). This is known as "spend-down." These regulations attempt to ensure that individuals pay what they can for the care they need but still provides a safety net when funds are exhausted.

In 2004 Medicaid provided health care insurance to 4.5 million persons 65 years of age or older (10% of all Medicaid beneficiaries) at a cost of over $11,345 per person, and for 7.5 million disabled persons at $10,040 per person. State Medicaid programs paid for 41% of all of the U.S. nursing home and home health care. This included $37.2 billion ($21,898 per beneficiary) for 1.7 million of the people in nursing homes and $3.5 billion ($3475 per person) for one million at home (CMS, 2006).

The majority of the Medicaid funds are used to provide long-term nursing home care for older and disabled adults. The federal government has attempted to slow the flow of

Medicaid monies to pay for nursing home and other care for the non-poor by a series of laws enacted to require people to pay as much as they can from their own funds. Examples include the following (Teske, 2000):

- The 1993 Omnibus Budget Reconciliation Act (OBRA) permitted states to recover the costs of nursing home care from a deceased person's estate.
- The 1996 Health Insurance Portability and Accountability Act (HIPAA) reduced the allowable methods of hiding or transferring monies before needing or entering long-term care.
- The 1997 Balanced Budget Act targeted lawyers and other estate planners, holding them responsible for attempting to circumvent laws that required persons to pay for their own long-term care.

Long-Term Care Insurance

Some persons are electing to purchase additional insurance (long-term care insurance [LTCI]) for their potential long-term care needs. Ideally, these policies would cover the expenses related to co-pays for long-term care and coverage for what is called *custodial care* or help with day-to-day needs (as opposed to skilled care). Traditionally, these policies were limited to care in long-term care facilities and provided a flat-rate reimbursement to residents for their costs. However, these policies are becoming more creative and innovative and may cover home care costs instead or in addition to under some circumstances. Many plans are being marketed. Even the American Nurses Association (ANA) has a plan available to ANA members that is underwritten by American Express.

LTCI plans are not for everyone. Because they do not receive any governmental funding support, the costs can be prohibitive, especially as one ages. At the age of 50 years, a LTCI policy can cost approximately $850 a year. This number would increase to $1800 a year at the age of 65 years and $5500 a year for those who purchase a plan at the age of 85 years (American Health Care Association [AHCA], 2005). The purchaser must be cautioned to read the policy carefully and understand all the details, limitations, and exclusions. Particular concerns are related to Alzheimer's disease because many policies exclude these individuals from home benefits and include very limited institutional benefits. The best LTCI packages are those that have been negotiated by a large employer or state organization or association. It is also advisable to have the elder or family member check consumer reports of the particular insurance company and its reliability before applying for a policy.

RESIDENTIAL OPTIONS IN LATE LIFE

Although the expenses related to long-term care in general and residing in a nursing home in particular are significant, older adults live in the community the majority of the time. Of the millions of households headed by older persons, the majority reside in their own homes and the majority of these homes are paid for. Whereas most persons want to

TABLE 17-1

Comparison of Numbers of Licensed Facilities in the United States, 2007

Type of Facility	Number of Facilities
Assisted living facility	39,500
Senior housing	21,203
Nursing home	16,100
Continuing care community	2240

Data from American Association of Homes and Services for the Aging: *Aging services: the facts* (website): *www.aahsa.org.* Accessed June 26, 2007.

TABLE 17-2

Comparison of Occupancy by Type of Residential Setting, 2007

Type of Residential Setting	Number of Residents
Nursing home	1.4 million
Assisted living facility	900,000
Continuing care community	745,000

Data from American Association of Homes and Services for the Aging: *Aging services: the facts* (website): *www.aahsa.org.* Accessed June 26, 2007.

TABLE 17-3

Comparison of Average Residential/Care Costs Across the Continuum, 2007

Type of Facility	Cost
Nursing home (private room)	$6234/mo $76,806/yr
Assisted living facility	$2714/mo $32,572/yr
Life care community (non-profit)	Entry fee: $60,000-$120,000 $2672/mo $32,064/yr

Data from American Association of Homes and Services for the Aging: *Aging services: the facts* (website): *www.aahsa.org.* Accessed June 26, 2007.

remain in their homes for economic and personal reasons, some seniors, by choice or by need, move from one type of residence to another. A number of options exist, especially for those with the financial resources that allow them to have a choice (Tables 17-1, 17-2, and 17-3). Residential options range along a continuum from remaining in one's own home; to senior retirement communities; to shared housing with family members, friends or others; to residential care communities such as assisted living settings; to, for those with the most needs, nursing facilities (Figure 17-1). A growing number of older adults are also able to move to

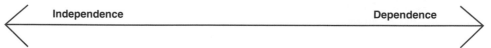

Independence

Home ownership
Single-room occupation (SRO)
Condominium ownership
Apartment dwelling
Shared housing
Congregate lifestyles

Independent to partial dependence

Retirement communities
Public housing complexes
Residence with family
Foster homes
Board and care
Residential homes
Continuing care retirement
  communities (CCRCs)

Partial dependence to complete dependence

Nursing facilities
Skilled nursing facilities
Acute care facilities
Inpatient hospice care facilities

Independence ⟷ Dependence

FIGURE 17-1 Continuum of residential options based on level of assistance needed.

a comprehensive life care community or continuing care retirement community (CCRC).

Senior Retirement Communities

Communities designed for elders are proliferating. Numerous combinations of single family homes, apartments, activities, optional services, meals in the home, cafeterias, restaurants, housekeeping, golf, tennis, and security are available. In some cases, emergency services and health clinics are adjacent. These are all designed to make independent living feasible with the least effort on the part of the elder. Some senior communities are luxurious and have a wide range of physical and cultural amenities; others are simpler, providing only the basic necessities. Prices are consistent with the level of luxury provided and the range of services available.

Although the costs of the majority of senior communities are borne by the consumers, for elders with limited incomes, federally subsidized rental options are available in some areas of the country. Older adults benefiting from this option are assisted through rental housing subsidized by the U.S. Department of Housing and Urban Development (HUD). Although not all HUD housing is designated for senior living, Section 202 of the Housing Act, U.S. Department of Housing and Urban Development, approved the construction of low-rent housing units especially for elders. These units may also have provisions for health care, recreation, and transportation. More than 91% of these apartment units have waiting lists of eight or more applicants for each vacancy that occurs. Under Section 8 of the Housing Act of 1983, tenants locate their own unit. Usually the tenant pays 30% of his or her adjusted gross income toward the rent and HUD assists with supplementary vouchers ranging from 30% to 120% of the tenant's contribution to meet the fair market value of the rental.

An ideal public housing complex for low-income older adults will provide modern facilities, security, accessible services, privacy, and some entertainment and activities. An important consideration in planning low-cost housing units

for older adults is the potential for evolution of services. Residents rarely move out, and as they age, their ability and independence are likely to decrease.

Shared Housing

Shared housing has become a choice for many because of either cultural preferences or need. The sharing may relieve the economic burdens of maintaining a home after widowhood or retirement on a fixed income. It also has the potential to relieve the emotional burden that some experience in living alone.

Mutigenerational Shared Housing. The factors most likely to result in shared housing among adult relatives and elders are widowhood, a small support network, and low economic status. However, strong cultural influences predict the frequency of multigenerational residences as well. Among elders from Asia and South America and among African-Americans, it is often an expectation, although increasing industrialization in any country changes these traditional patterns. Shared housing has many variations, but the important issue is for social policy and supports to provide choices for the individual and the family.

A variation of multigenerational housing has long existed in what has become known as "granny flats." These may be apartments added to existing homes or the construction of small housing units on family property with privacy as well as sharing of time and resources. Such arrangements allow families to be close enough to be of assistance if needed but to remain separate. They are practical and economical, and their production has continually expanded in Australia in particular. In the United States, use of this model is minimal but existing "mother-in-law" cottages and apartments have served a similar purpose for many families for years. Another popular model in certain areas is the use of mobile homes. These may in fact be mobile and moved onto family property or may in reality be quite immobile and set in established mobile home parks that cater to older adults and their needs.

Co-habitation or Group Homes. A third model of shared housing is that of opening homes to others. Older people often live in houses with ample space geared to family life, purchased in their young adult years. It is estimated that one half of the space is underused. Sharing a house can be easily implemented by locating, screening, and matching older people looking for houses to share with those who have them. The National Shared Housing Resource Center (NSHRC) has established subgroups nationally to assist individuals interested in home sharing. Those who have done so report feeling safer and less lonely. Studies on home sharing focus on the effects on well-being, finances, health, social life, and daily satisfaction. Most successful is the intergenerational model, in which an elder with a home locates a younger person to share the home (Bergman, 1994). In each situation the individuals must consider the following:

- Will men and women live together?
- Will the house include older peers only or people of all ages?
- Will there be equal or reciprocal exchange?
- Will the house provide temporary or permanent residence?
- Will residents sign an agreement form?
- Will residents respect privacy?
- What is the motivation for moving into a shared house: financial need, companionship, or services and assistance?

Small groups of older adults living under the same roof are a growing trend. The following are characteristics of successful group homes:

- They usually have a nonprofit sponsor.
- Services include housekeeping, cooking, maintenance, and social services.
- Spontaneity and interaction are encouraged but not forced.

Residential Care Facilities

Residential care facility is the broad term for a range of non-medical, community-based residential settings that house two or more unrelated adults and provide services such as meals, medication supervision or reminders, activities, transportation, or assistance with activities of daily living (ADLs). These kinds of facilities are for elders who need more care than is available in shared housing or for whom shared housing is not an option when nursing home care is not needed. Residential care facilities are known by more than 30 different names across the country, including *adult congregate living facilities, foster care homes, personal care homes, homes for the elderly, domiciliary care homes, board and care homes, rest homes, family care homes, retirement homes,* and *assisted living facilities* (Hawes, 1999).

Residential care facilities are the fastest growing housing option available for older adults in the United States. This kind of facility is viewed as more cost-effective than nursing homes while providing more privacy and a homelike environment. Medicare does not cover the cost of care in these types of facilities. In some cases, costs may be covered by private and long-term care insurance and some other types of assistance programs. The trend is growing for states to establish waiver programs to extend Medicaid services to this type of housing, but most residents of these types of facilities pay privately for their care. The rates charged and what services those rates include vary considerably as do regulations and licensing.

Foster Care. Adult foster care is meant to provide assistance and supervision in a homelike setting that will enhance function and the quality of life and allow the elder to remain in a community-based setting. The operational definition of adult foster care is that which offers a community-based living arrangement to adults who are unable to live independently because of physical or mental impairment or disabilities and are in need of supervision or personal care.

Homes providing adult foster care offer 24-hour supervision, protection, and personal care in addition to room and board. They may also provide additional services. Adult foster care serves a designated small number of individuals (generally from one to six) in a homelike and family-like environment; one of the primary caregivers often resides in the home (Folkemer et al., 1996). A growing number of homes are under corporate ownership, and in these situations the homelike atmosphere can be lost. However, with state-regulated, outcome-oriented quality assurance strategies focused on achieving maximum function, autonomy, and social integration, adult foster care may fill a real need.

Assisted Living. A popular type of residential care can be found in assisted living facilities (ALFs), also called *board and care homes* or *adult congregate living facilities (ACLFs).* In 2006 approximately 36,000 facilities provided housing to approximately 1 million persons (National Center for Assisted Living [NCAL], 2006). An ALF is defined as a "special combination of housing, personalized supportive services, and health care designed to meet the needs, both scheduled and unscheduled, of those who need help with activities of daily living" (Munroe, 2003, p. 100). Assisted living is a residential long-term care choice for seniors who need more than an independent living environment can offer but do not need the 24 hr/day skilled nursing care and the constant monitoring of a skilled nursing facility. The mean age of ALF residents is 85 years, and most are women (Box 17-5). Assisted living settings may be a shared room or a single-occupancy unit with a private bath, kitchenette, and communal meals, but all provide some support services (Munroe, 2003). Assisted living provides security with independence and privacy, and it supports physical and social well-being with the health care supervision it provides.

Assisted living is more expensive than independent living and less costly than skilled nursing home care, but it is not inexpensive. Many facilities are part of large nationwide for-profit chains. Costs vary by geographical region, size of a unit, and relative luxury and can range from a low of $1200 per month to well over $5000 per month with an

BOX 17-5 Profile of the Resident of an Assisted Living Facility

- 85 years old
- Female (76%)
- Needs help with at least two activities of daily living (ADLs)
  - Bathing: 68%
  - Dressing: 47%
  - Toileting: 34%
  - Transferring: 25%
  - Eating: 22%
- Needs help with instrumental activities of daily living (IADLs)
  - Housework: 91%
  - Medications: 86%
- Length of stay: 27 months
  - 34% move to a nursing facility
  - 30% die while a resident

Data from National Center for Assisted Living: *Assisted living resident profile*, 2006. (website): *www.ncal.org*.

average cost of $2627 a month (NCAL, 2006). Most ALFs offer two or three meals each day, light weekly housekeeping, and laundry services, as well as optional social activities at various times of the day. Each added service increases the cost of the setting but also allows for persons with resources to remain in the setting longer as functional abilities decline. Some states provide Medicaid reimbursement for a limited number of low-income seniors who live in modest ALFs, but generally the cost is borne by the consumer.

Many seniors and their families prefer ALFs to nursing homes because they cost less, are more homelike, and offer more opportunities for control, independence, and privacy. However, many residents of ALFs have chronic care needs and over time may require more care than the facility is able to provide. Services (e.g., home health, hospice, homemakers) can be brought into the facility, but some question whether this replaces the need for 24-hour supervision by registered nurses (RNs). Not every ALF has an RN or licensed practical/vocational nurse (LPN/LVN), and in most states, any skilled nursing provided by the staff other than nurse-delegated assistance with self-administered medications is prohibited. Wallace (2003) noted that litigation involving ALFs is increasing related to understaffing, inability to meet resident needs, inadequate staff training, inappropriate administration of medications, lack of monitoring and medical supervision, and lack of communication with family about changes in resident status.

The Joint Commission and the Commission for Accreditation of Rehabilitation Facilities have published standards for accreditation of ALFs, but many persons are advocating for more comprehensive federal and state standards and regulations. Advanced-practice gerontological nurses are well suited to the role of primary care provider in ALFs, and many have assumed this role.

Continuing Care Retirement Communities

Persons with at least moderate financial resources may elect to join life care communities (CCRCs), which provide the full range of residential options, from single family homes to skilled nursing facilities all in one location. Most of these communities provide access to these levels of care for a community member's entire remaining lifetime, and for the right price, the range of services may be guaranteed. Having all levels of care in one location allows community members to make the transition between levels without life-disrupting moves. For married couples in which one spouse needs more care than the other, life care communities allow them to live nearby in a different part of the same community. This industry is maturing. In 2006 more than 2000 CCRCs were in the United States, providing homes for 150,000 older adults (American Association of Homes and Services for the Aging [AAHSA], 2006). Most CCRCs are non-profit. They usually charge an entrance fee, which can range from $75,000 to more than $400,000, that covers and reflects the cost of the residence in which the member will live, the possible future care needed, and the quality and quantity of the community services. More information about life care communities is available from the American Association of Homes and Services for the Aging (AAHSA) (*www.ahasa.org*).

Population-Specific Communities

As the number of senior communities expands, older adults have more options of moving somewhere that they find especially welcoming. These options include communities that emphasize a particular sport, like tennis or golf. Or groups of people come together to form intentional communities, buying a cluster of home tracks and building in such a way to support their particular lifestyles or needs or personalities. Still others provide unique additional services, such as those in communities that specialize in providing residences for persons with, for example, a mental illness, alcoholism, mental retardation, or a developmental disability.

Gay, lesbian, bisexual, and transgendered (GLBT) seniors face several problems in housing in their older years. They often have little family support and may face discrimination in housing options. A survey of New York gay persons revealed that two thirds of them lived alone, a much higher number than heterosexual persons of the same age, and were at greater risk for isolation. The need for assisted living may be higher for this population than for others, but many GLBT seniors say that they do not feel welcome at such residences. Those who wish to live together are discouraged from doing so by some organizations. Nurses should be aware of this heretofore invisible group of aging persons who need access to welcoming resources.

Nursing Homes

Nursing homes are the settings for the delivery of around-the-clock care for those needing specialized care that cannot be provided elsewhere. When used appropriately, nursing homes fill an important need for families and elders. In 2006 there were 18,000 licensed nursing homes; the majority of these are for-profit, and Medicaid provides most of the funding followed by the resident in an out-of-pocket arrangement (AAHSA, 2006).

The settings called *nursing homes* most often include up to two levels of care: a *skilled nursing care* (also called *subacute care*) facility requires licensed professionals with a focus on rehabilitation or the management of complex medical needs; and a *chronic care* facility requires 24-hour personal assistance that is supervised and augmented by licensed nurses. The settings that provide chronic care *(nursing facilities)* may include dementia-specific units and palliative care units. For many elders, the nursing home becomes their final home.

Resident Characteristics. Approximately 1.6 million individuals in the United States are nursing home residents, and this number is expected to rise dramatically in the next 30 years as the population ages, especially those older than 85 years (see Chapter 1). Clearly this calls for increased education and recruitment of gerontological nurses to this setting as well as creation of new models of care.

Residents of nursing homes are predominantly women, 80 years or older, Caucasian, widowed, and dependent in ADLs and instrumental activities of daily living (IADLs). More than 60% are cognitively impaired. Nursing home residents represent the most frail of the older adult population. In many cases, their needs for 24-hour care could not be met in the home or residential care setting or their needs may have exceeded the family's ability to provide required care.

Costs of Care. Costs for nursing homes vary significantly with the location but average $74,095 a year (see Table 17-3). Costs vary by geographical location, ownership, and amenities. The purchase of long-term care insurance is becoming a popular option for many Americans. Estimates are that this trend will continue, and by the year 2020, financing of long-term care by private insurance will increase to 6.6% (Lueckenotte, 2000).

The majority of the costs of care in nursing homes is borne by the individuals themselves and the state-federal Medicaid programs. Medicare covers only the first 20 days of service that qualifies as skilled and rehabilitative. It requires a significant co-pay for the next 80 days if the needs continue. Medicare does not cover the cost of care in nursing facilities or on nursing units (compared with "skilled" units); however, for eligible persons, Medicaid does provide coverage for all levels in a nursing home. For many older people, the costs are excessive. Concern is growing nationwide related to the financing of long-term care and the ability of states and the federal government to continue to support costs through the Medicaid programs. Reimbursement levels now do not cover actual costs, and there is fear that if further cuts are made, the often precarious quality of care in these settings will be further compromised.

Regulations and Quality of Care. Nursing homes are one of the most highly regulated industries in the United States. Although nursing homes recognize the need to enact

legislation to ensure quality, the lack of additional funding for legislated initiatives has left many nursing homes struggling to maintain quality and meet standards with few resources. Criteria and standards often create a bureaucratic structure and a punitive environment that challenges those caring for nursing home residents. The Omnibus Budget Reconciliation Act (OBRA) of 1987 and the frequent revisions and updates are designed to improve the quality of resident care and have had a positive impact. Some of the requirements of OBRA and subsequent legislation include the following: comprehensive resident assessments, increased training requirements for nursing assistants, elimination of the use of medications and restraints for discipline or convenience, higher staffing requirements for nursing, social work staff, standards for nursing home administrators, and quality assurance activities.

Regulations have also been created to preserve the rights of the residents of nursing homes. Residents in these long-term care facilities have rights under both federal and state law. The staff of the facility must inform residents of these rights and protect and promote their rights. The rights to which residents in long-term care are entitled should be conspicuously posted in the facility (Box 17-6). Also, the *Long-Term Care Ombudsman Program* is a nationwide effort to support the rights of both the residents and the facilities. In most states the program provides trained volunteers to investigate rights and quality complaints or conflicts. Each facility is required to post the name and contact information of the ombudsman assigned to the facility.

BOX 17-6 Bill of Rights for Long-Term Care Residents

- The right to voice grievances and have them remedied
- The right to information about health conditions and treatments and to participate in one's own care to the extent possible
- The right to choose one's own health care providers and to speak privately with one's health care providers
- The right to consent to or refuse all aspects of care and treatments
- The right to manage one's own finances if capable, or choose one's own financial advisor
- The right to be transferred or discharged only for appropriate reasons
- The right to be free from all forms of abuse
- The right to be free from all forms of restraint to the extent compatible with safety
- The right to privacy and confidentiality concerning one's person, personal information, and medical information
- The right to be treated with dignity, consideration, and respect in keeping with one's individuality
- The right to immediate visitation and access at any time for family, health care providers, and legal advisors; the right to reasonable visitation and access for others

NOTE: This list of rights is a sampling of federal and several states' lists of rights of residents or participants in long-term care. Nurses should check the rules of their own state for specific rights in law for that state.

LEGAL ISSUES IN GERONTOLOGICAL NURSING

The gerontological nurse is the ideal person to formally advocate for older adults as an ombudsman or in a less formal way by involvement in ensuring the delivery of quality care. At the same time, especially in the days after the implementation of HIPAA regulations, it is imperative for the nurse to be cognizant of several keys legal issues frequently encountered in the work of gerontological nursing.

Advocacy

An advocate is one who maintains or promotes a cause; defends, pleads, or acts on behalf of a cause for another; fights for someone who cannot fight; and often gets involved in getting someone to do something he or she would not otherwise do.

Topics for advocacy can include protection of specific rights, such as promoting the least restrictive residential alternative for another, finding the best nursing home, or telling court personnel one's opinion of a proposed conservator. Other areas include the rights of medical patients, the right to have in-home supportive services, and maintenance of government benefits, such as veterans' benefits, Medicare, Social Security (SS) and Supplemental Security Income (SSI), and food stamps. Advocates function in various arenas: with their own and other disciplines within their own agencies, with other agencies, with physicians, with families, with neighbors and community representatives, with legislators, and with courts.

In a health care situation, advocacy is acting for or on behalf of another in terms of pleading for and supporting the best interests of that other person with respect to choice, provision, and refusal of health care. Nurses act as advocates of their clients when they support the person as a free agent who has autonomy in the health care situation (Rini, 1998). However, situations occur in the care of older adults when the elder is either not strong enough or does not have the mental capacity to exert measures to protect his or her own interests. When this occurs, the extent of an individual's capacity may be determined.

Capacity (Competence)

The evaluation of a patient's cognitive capacity and judgment is at the core of most legal dilemmas that health care personnel face, whether an issue of consent, involuntary placement in an institution, or civil or criminal law. *Competency* and *capacity* are legal terms that have precise meanings related to an individual's ability to understand the consequences of his or her actions and decisions (Goldstein, 2002). A patient has capacity unless the courts have declared otherwise (Springhouse, 2002). Capacity is also task specific—the patient must be able to handle finances/daily business and make medical decisions. He or she may be declared to have no or limited capacity for one but not the other.

Consent is a concept that arises from the idea of human self-determination and autonomy. In the health care situation, consent is related to accepting or refusing care and treatments and is expressed in the legal doctrine of informed consent. Decisional capacity and ability to consent are presumed of all adults regardless of age unless there is a reason to believe the person cannot understand the provided information or is unable to make an informed decision. Informed consent requires the disclosure of information about a proposed treatment that might be material to a client's decision about consenting to the treatment. State law generally specifies the extent of information to be disclosed. Most courts have upheld providing information that a reasonable health care provider would disclose in the same or similar circumstances or that which a reasonable client would consider material to his or her decision.

Consent for treatment is based on one's decision-making capacity. Such capacity is determined by the provider(s) proposing the care or treatment and intending to carry it out in day-to-day nursing practice. Informed consent means that the person is able to understand the nature and purpose of the procedure or that which is proposed and is able to appreciate its possible risks and benefits. Consent for research participation is a more detailed and extensive process, because treatments provided in such circumstances may not necessarily directly benefit the client.

When the capacity of an individual is impaired, legal options protect the person and ensure that decision making, as needed, can be done in a manner in which the person would want if the person were able. These options include powers of attorney, conservatorship, and guardianship. It is important that the nurse understand the differences among the options and the meaning of each.

Powers of Attorney. A power of attorney (POA) is a legal document and device in which one person designates another person (e.g., family member, friend) to act on his or her behalf. The two types are a regular or general POA and

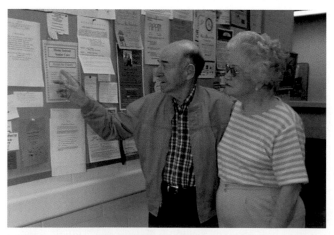

Information about legal and other resources is available at many public settings such as libraries and community centers. (From Lewis SM et al: *Medical-surgical nursing: assessment and management of clinical problems,* ed 7, St Louis, 2007, Mosby; courtesy Rick Brady, Riva, MD.)

a durable POA. The appointed person becomes known as the *attorney-in-fact*. The attorney-in-fact named in a general POA usually has the right, for example, to make financial decisions and pay bills but not to make decisions related to health care.

The attorney-in-fact appointed in a durable POA usually has additional rights and responsibilities to make health-related decisions for persons when they are unable to make them for themselves. The appointed person is also known as the *health care surrogate*. A health care surrogate is expected to use "substituted judgment" in making decisions; that is, the decision is expected to be that which the person would have made for herself or himself if able to do so and not what the surrogate would make for herself or himself in the same situation. Therefore it is always advisable that the choice of the surrogate is someone who is willing to uphold the wishes of the persons or holds similar values. Whether the health care surrogate is allowed to make end-of-life decisions is determined by state statutes.

Powers of attorney are in effect only at the specific request of the elder or, in the case of the durable power of attorney, in the event that he or she is unable to act on his or her own behalf. As soon as the person regains abilities, the POA is no longer in force unless the individual requests it to continue. The elder retains all of the rights and responsibilities afforded by usual law. This is the least restrictive form of assistance with decision making for persons with impaired capacity. An important aspect of the power of attorney is that persons who are given decision-making rights are those who are have been chosen by the elder rather than a court.

Guardians and Conservators. Guardians and conservators are individuals, agencies, or corporations who have been appointed by the court to have care, custody, and control of a disabled person and manage his or her personal or financial affairs (or both). Disabled in this sense means legally disabled, not medically disabled, meaning the person is unable to manage personal and financial business. Such a disability includes an inability to make informed decisions about personal matters and lack of capacity to provide for one's physical health and safety, including, but not limited to, health care, food, shelter, and personal hygiene.

Whereas a *conservator* is the person appointed to control the finances of the ward, the person appointed to be responsible for the person is usually called the *guardian*. The conservator or guardian continues in that role until the court rescinds the order and in no other way. Each state is slightly different in how this is handled. In many, the ward, as a person without any legal standing, is unable to petition the courts to have his or her rights restored.

In some states, limits are set according to the degree of protection needed. Total dependency means the person cannot meet basic needs for survival and is unable to manage the environment in any self-sustaining way. Some dependency means the person may be able to manage certain challenges of life; health or judgment may interfere with management of other needs. In the latter situation, a limited

guardian may be appointed to protect the person in very specific ways.

The appointments of a guardian or conservator are made at court hearings in which someone demonstrates the incapacity of the elder. Often the elder is not present. The elder is declared *incapacitated* (formerly called *incompetent*). The elder is then considered a ward, and all legal rights are lost. All decision making is the legal right and responsibility of the conservator or guardian. As with an attorney-in-fact, substituted judgment is expected to form the basis of decision making.

The guardian, who replaces the attorney-in-fact if present, must take custody of the ward, establish safe shelter, provide for care and maintenance, provide appropriate consent for medical or other professional care, manage financial resources carefully, protect and ensure the rights of the ward, and file an annual report with the appointing court (Nacev and Rettig, 2002). Whether the guardian can make end-of-life decisions depends on the structure of the guardianship and state law.

A guiding principle in guardianships is to accomplish the care and protection needed in the least restrictive way; this is not so different from the care nurses provide in long-term care and home care situations. The law supports the idea that a person has a right to as much autonomy as he or she can manage without sacrificing safety.

There are considerable pros and cons in the use of conservatorships and guardianships, including high risk for exploitation by the conservator. These should be considered only in extreme cases. Nurses working with older adults and their families can encourage the use of advanced planning, including the appointments of health care surrogates and powers of attorney as alternatives that are less restrictive, noting that the definitions and rules vary from state to state.

▲ PROMOTING HEALTHY AGING: IMPLICATIONS FOR GERONTOLOGICAL NURSING

Gerontological nurses are frequently called upon to advocate for older adults and interpret legal situations in their daily practice. This is especially true for elders who appear to have diminished capacity, regardless of legal status. Nurses are expected to provide safety and security to the persons under their care, to the extent possible. This includes helping facilitate residential options that are the most appropriate to the individual's needs and personal preferences. It also may mean wrestling with difficult and problematic legal and ethical issues in the provision of care. Two of the more common issues in nursing care of frail older adults are refusal of treatment and release of information.

As just noted, unless otherwise adjudicated (declared by the courts), each individual has presumed capacity to control his or her life, including what happens to his or her body. This has received a significant amount of legal support through the passage of the Patient Self-Determination Act of the 1980s (see Chapter 26) and HIPAA of 1997. The dilemma occurs when it appears clear to the nurse that the patient does not understand the consequences of his or her decisions. It is always necessary to determine whether the appearance of incapacity is truly one of impairment or whether it is inconsistent with the preferences, expectations, or values of the nurse, caregiver, or potential health care surrogate.

The nurse is expected to work toward preserving the individual's integrity, independence, dignity, and assets to the extent possible. In some situations this results in conflict. While working in a nursing facility, one of the authors (K.J.) regularly heard from previously distant or uninvolved relatives of somewhat impaired elders; these relatives would declare that they were the "power of attorney" and therefore had the right to override an individual's apparent decisions or choices or would insist on access to the person's medical and health information. In such a situation, several nursing actions are recommended. First, the nurse should clarify the issues at hand and the conflicts that may be presented. Second, the nurse can work with other professionals to conduct an assessment of gross measures of the elder's capacity, including knowledge of and confidence in the person making the POA claim while realizing that these are clinical judgments and do not replace court decisions or legal action. Third, if, in the clinical judgment of the health care team, it is in the person's best interest to have help with decision making, the nurse must clarify the type of POA that is held (if it is regular or durable) and if applicable, respond accordingly. This would include obtaining a copy of the document for the patient's record and having it reviewed by an attorney for authenticity

Human Needs and Wellness Diagnoses

Self-Actualization and Transcendence
(Seeking, Expanding, Spirituality, Fulfillment)
Develop interests and fulfillments beyond the
constraints of imposed restrictions
Seeks spiritual development and transcendence
Upholds values, ethics, and legalities

Self-Esteem and Self-Efficacy
(Image, Identity, Control, Capability)
Exerts reasoned choices and takes responsibility for decisions
Asks for assurance of competence and quality from service providers and advisors
Plans for various contingencies that may occur
Seeks professional guidance when needed
Develops awareness of resources to obtain services as needed
Seeks knowledge of rights and privileges

Belonging and Attachment
(Love, Empathy, Affiliation)
Develops appropriate and gratifying
interactions with providers
Maintains significant relationships regardless
of restricted income or health care
Discusses specific plans with loved ones for
when incapacity or death occurs

Safety and Security
(Caution, Planning, Protections, Sensory Acuity)
Knows how to access needed assistance for
legal, economic, and health needs
Seeks sources of economic viability
Plans for death (i.e., living wills, power of attorney for health care,
end-of-life care, burial methods)
Recognizes impact of legalities on options

Biological and Physiological Integrity
(Air, Fluids, Comfort, Activity, Nutrition, Elimination, Skin Integrity)
Recognizes and seeks assistance when needed to
maintain basic needs

These are not all the possible wellness diagnoses that may be identified. The above
are examples of nursing diagnoses that should be considered when planning care
for the older adult.

and specificity. Health information can be released only to persons approved by the patient, through permission or the written permission such as that implied by the POA.

On the other hand, if the nurse is presented with proof that the patient has been adjudicated to have limited or no capacity, the guardian indeed is the decision maker and sole representative of the patient or resident. The guardian is then the person who will decide who has access to the patient's information. The facility in which the person resides will need to have its own legal consultation in determining the authority of the documents and in guiding the health care team in any specific directions in any legal documents. However, as an advocate, the nurse still has a responsibility to protect the patient from neglect or exploitation from all sources, including guardians (see Chapter 18).

Although nursing has long recognized the need for gerontological specialization, the law and lawyers have not always done so, with the exception of a few categories. It is interesting to note that the National Elder Law Foundation (NELF) is one of the few specialty organizations that certifies lawyers who have demonstrated knowledge pertinent to the needs of older adults in several categories. These needs are outlined in Box 17-1.

These categories of need relate to both legal and economic concerns of older adults and differ little from those with which nurses have been dealing for years as they care for their elderly clients. Gerontological nursing as a specialty has been evolving and has become more important as the population of older adults has increased and their health care and other needs have been identified, acknowledged, and codified. Nurses who are consulted by clients about legal issues should not attempt to provide legal advice but, instead, should refer their clients to an attorney,

preferably one who is certified by NELF. The state or local bar association is able to assist nurses and their clients with this information.

KEY CONCEPTS

- Health care and its systems are undergoing profound changes, including the increase in the number of managed care organizations and changes in the roles of health care providers. All of these changes affect the care of the older adult.
- The fiscal integrity of the Social Security Trust Fund is in jeopardy, and reform is needed for it to remain solvent.
- Between Medicare, Medicaid, and Veterans Benefits, most U.S. citizens and legal residents ages 65 years and older have some type of health insurance.
- The costs of Medicare increase each year in proportion to the cost-of-living adjustment (COLA) through Social Security.
- Supplemental Security Income (SSI) provides a minimal level of support for all eligible persons; however, this support is extremely low. The majority of older adults who rely on SSI as their major form of income are persons from minority groups and never-married women.
- The residential options available to persons as they age are most limited by the individual person's economic resources.
- The majority of persons older than 65 years will spend some time in a nursing home at some time in their life.
- Protective measures are available for persons with limited or absent capacity through power-of-attorney, guardians, and conservators.
- The nurse has a responsibility to ensure the safety and security of those persons to whom care is provided. This responsibility does not change with the change in the persons' legal status or capacity.

CASE STUDY: Potential Abuse and Neglect

Mr. and Mrs. J.

Mr. and Mrs. J, ages 62 and 60, respectively, have been married for 35 years. Mr. J. was a midlevel executive with a flourishing company. With company stock options and an attractive pension plan, their future looked bright. They owned their home, a split-level, four-bedroom house in a lovely suburban community located on the bay. Their small cabin cruiser gave them a great deal of pleasure, and they also frequently took commercial cruises. Their lifestyle was geared to their upper-middle-class income, as were their friends. When Mr. J. was 58 years old, the company was sold to a multinational corporation based outside the United States, and Mr. J. no longer had a position with the new company. The stock dropped in price, the pension plan was inadequate if drawn on early, and there was a penalty for drawing on tax-deferred funds before age 59½ years. It appeared the pension funds were poorly invested and would not bring the expected returns. Though their health is good, they are concerned about the future of Medicare, managed care, and whether to buy long-term care insurance. Mrs. J. had never worked outside the home and has no salable skills. What they had thought to be a very comfortable retirement became one of serious concern. They had saved a considerable amount in their middle years, but it was soon depleted as it was used for general expenses. Now Mr. J. has begun to draw on his Social Security at a reduced benefit rate, and Mrs. J. is collecting Social Security based on her husband's benefits. Combined, their retirement income is about $2800 per month. This is insufficient to maintain the style of living to which they are accustomed. They are able to get by, but their income will not be adequate for maintaining and repairing their 35-year-old house, maintaining their boat, or their present social life. In addition, taxes keep going up as property values continue to rise. Mrs. J. says, "We really don't know what to do to ensure that we will have sufficient income for our needs 20 years from now. I'm really frightened about our future."

Jake

Jake had retired after 20 years as a sergeant in the U.S. Army. For several years he did odd jobs, often as a mechanic in a nonunion shop or helping friends with home and mechanical repairs. He simply never found his niche after leaving the service. Some thought his war experiences had created serious psychological problems for him. His wife, a successful nursing faculty member, had a good retirement plan. When his wife realized she was dying of cancer, she selected spousal survivor benefits in her retirement and insurance policies. After her death, Jake was financially secure though grief stricken because he had depended on his wife's practical and emotional support. Two years later, Jake met Jane and soon realized he wished to marry her but found that his spousal retirement and Social Security benefits would be terminated if he married. Jake contacted a friend of his deceased wife to discuss his feelings and thoughts with her. He said, "I will not be content unless I marry Jane, but without the benefits I now receive I won't be able to manage. I wonder what I should do."

Based on one of the case studies, develop a nursing care plan using the following procedure*:
- List comments of the client that provide subjective data.
- List information that provides objective data.
- From these data, identify and state, using accepted format, two nursing diagnoses you determine are most significant to this client at this time. List two client strengths that you have identified from data.
- Determine and state outcome criteria for each diagnosis. These must reflect some alleviation of the problem identified in the nursing diagnosis and must be stated in concrete and measurable terms.
- Plan and state one or more interventions for each diagnosed problem. Provide specific documentation of the source used to determine the appropriate intervention. Plan at least one intervention that incorporates the client's existing strengths.
- Evaluate the success of the intervention. Interventions must correlate directly with the stated outcome criteria to measure the outcome success.

Critical Thinking Questions

1. What would be the focus of your first interaction with Mr. and Mrs. J.?
2. Discuss various options that may provide them more economic security. Compare the benefits they might obtain from a reverse annuity mortgage with the benefits of selling the home and entering a life-care community. Discuss the pros and cons. How would you initiate such a discussion?
3. Discuss the limitations of Medicare and the out-of-pocket costs that elders experience.
4. How common is a situation such as that of Mr. and Mrs. J?
5. What major economic and legal issues are concerns of yours as you contemplate your old age?
6. Discuss the pros and cons of managed health care.
7. Do you believe it is acceptable to spend the majority of our health dollars on the very old when several million children have no health care?
8. Is age a valid criterion for denial of certain medical services?
9. Discuss the meanings and the thoughts triggered by the elder's viewpoint expressed at the beginning of the chapter. How do these vary from your own experience?
10. Discuss Social Security with an older relative and its effectiveness for him or her.
11. Consider Jake's dilemma and propose various solutions, remembering his personal history and cohort.
12. How have your parents' expenditure patterns changed as they age?
13. What do you believe the "baby boomers" should do about their future economic situation and health care?

* Students are advised to refer to their nursing diagnosis text and identify possible or potential problems.

RESEARCH QUESTIONS

What do elders find most helpful about Medicare? Least helpful?

How would elders like to see Medicare changed?

What are elders' thoughts and attitudes about managed care?

Who do elders most frequently contact when they need legal and economic advice?

How many elders feel secure about their economic future?

What are the current average out-of-pocket costs for elder health care?

How do elders feel about the rationing of health care based on age or survivability?

Are the poverty-inducing effects of widowhood and retirement different in specific ways in various ethnic groups?

What are the prevalent attitudes of the elderly persons with whom you are acquainted regarding their economic future?

REFERENCES

Achenbaum WA: *Old age in a new land*, Baltimore, 1978, Johns Hopkins Press.

American Association of Homes and Services for the Aging (AAHSA): *Aging services: the facts*, 7/26/06. (website): *www.aahsa.org*. Accessed June 26, 2007.

American Health Care Association (AHCA): *Paying for long term care*, 2005. (website): *www.ahca.org*. Accessed October 17, 2006.

Bergman G: Shared housing—not only for rent, *Aging Today* 15(1):1, 1994.

Bohm D: Striving for quality in American nursing homes, *DePaul J Health Care Law* 4:317, 2001.

Burnette M: Closing the health insurance gap: what nurses can do to help uninsured and underinsured minority patients get the care and coverage they need, *Minority Nurse* Summer: 28-31, 2006.

Cantril H: *Public opinion 1935-1946*, Princeton, NJ, 1951, Princeton University Press.

Centers for Medicare and Medicaid Services (CMS): *Medicare and you, 2007*, Baltimore, 2006, The Centers.

Centers for Medicare and Medicaid Services (CMS): *Technical summary: overview of Medicaid*, 2006. (website): *www.cms.gov*. Accessed October 16, 2006.

Corning P: *The evolution of Medicare: from idea to law*, research report No 29, Washington, DC, 1969, U.S. Department of Health, Education and Welfare, Social Security Administration, Office of Research and Statistics, U.S. Government Printing Office.

Folkemer D et al: *Adult foster care for the older adult: a review of state regulatory and funding strategies*, Washington, DC, 1996, American Association of Retired Persons.

Friedman M: *Speaking the truth about Social Security reform*, Cato briefing paper No 46, April 12, 1999. (website): *www.socialsecurity.org/pubs/articles/bp-046es.html*.

Goldstein MK: Ethics. In Ham RJ et al, editors: *Primary care geriatrics*, St Louis, 2002, Mosby.

Goodman JC: *The regulation of medical care: is the price too high?* Cato public policy research monograph No 3, San Francisco, 1980, Cato Institute.

Hawes C: A key piece of the integration puzzle: managing the chronic care needs of the frail elderly in residential care facilities, *Generations* 23(2):51-55, 1999.

Hooyman NR, Kiyak HA: *Social gerontology: a multidisciplinary perspective*, ed 7, New York, 2005, Pearson.

Jett KF: Medicare D: a new drug benefit in its first year, *ADVANCE for Nurses*, 26(8):19-23, 2006.

Kennedy School: *Linda Bilmes testifies before the House Subcommittee on Veteran's Health Care Costs* (website): *www.ksg.harvard.edu*. Accessed March 13, 2007.

Lueckenotte A: *Gerontological nursing*, ed 2, St Louis, 2000, Mosby.

Mason County Infirmary v Smith's Comm, 1901 KY Lexis 234 (KY 1901).

Maydwell v Louisville, 76 S.W. 1091, 92 (KY 1903).

McClellan M: Medicare D prescription coverage, *Geriatrics* 60(10):7-9, 2005.

Munroe D: Assisted living issues for nursing practice, *Geriatr Nurs* 24(2):99-105, 2003.

Nacev AN, Rettig J: A survey of key issues in Kentucky elder law, *North KY Law Rev* 29(1):139, 2002.

National Center for Assisted Living (NCAL): *Assisted living: facilities profile*, 2006. (website): *www.ncal.org*. Accessed October 17, 2006.

Resnick B, Jett K: *The Medicare Modernization and Improvement Act: the Medicare Part D drug benefit: tips for nurses*. Published by the John A Hartford Foundation Institute for Geriatric Nursing, 2005. (website): *www.hartfordign.org*.

Rini AG: Legal and ethical issues, section VIII. In Luggen AS et al: *NGNA core curriculum for gerontological advanced practice nurses*, Thousand Oaks, Calif, 1998, Sage.

Social Security Administration (SSA): *SSI fact sheet*, 2006. (website): *www.ssa.gov*.

Social Security and Medicare Board of Trustees: *Annual Report*, 1994. Available at www.socialsecurity.gov.

Springhouse: *Better elder care*, Springhouse, Pa, 2002, Springhouse.

Stefanacci R: How to help your patients choose the right prescription drug plan, *Ann Long-Term Care* 14(4):17-18, 2006a.

Stefanacci R: Clarifying Medicare part D enrollment numbers, *Ann Long-Term Care* 14(6):13-17, 2006b.

Sultz HA, Young KM: *Health care USA: understanding its organization and delivery*, Gaithersburg, Md, 2001, Aspen.

Teske R: *How to cope with the coming crisis in long-term care*, Heritage Lecture #658, April 2000. (website): *www.heritage.org/Research/HealthCare/h1658.cfm*.

Trustees: *OASDI Trustees report*, 2006. (website): *www.ssa.gov/OACT/TR/TR02/index.html*. Accessed October 15, 2006.

Twight C: Medicare's origin: the economics and politics of dependency, *Cato J* 16(3):1997.

Wallace M: Is there a nurse in the house? The role of nurses in assisted living, *Geriatr Nurs* 24(4):218-235, 2003.

Weinberger M: *Social Security: facing the facts*, Washington, DC, 1996, Cato Project on Social Security privatization (website): *www.socialsecurity.org/pubs/ssps/ssp3.html*.

Wortz C: Seeing through the political spin, *Ann Long-Term Care* 14(6):16-18, 2006.

CHAPTER 18

Frailty, Vulnerability, and Elder Mistreatment

Kathleen Jett

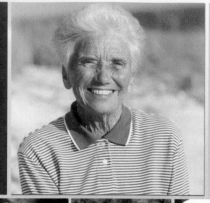
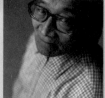
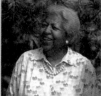

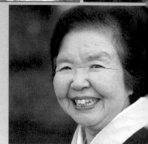

AN ELDER SPEAKS

I used to walk the ½ mile to the mail box every day, but it seems now my get-up-and-go has gone-up-and-went. Some days I feel that I ain't good for nuthin!

Mary, living alone at 84

LEARNING OBJECTIVES

On completion of this chapter, the reader will be able to:

1. Explain the concepts of frailty and vulnerability.
2. Identify the types of frailty commonly seen.
3. Discuss the relationship of frailty to independent functioning.
4. Propose strategies the nurse can use to promote healthy living for those who have been identified as frail or vulnerable.
5. Differentiate the types of elder mistreatment.
6. Identify persons at risk for abuse or neglect.

7. Describe strategies that may be used to minimize the risk for elder mistreatment.
8. Identify the nurse's legal responsibility in his or her own home state when neglect or abuse is suspected.

In every society, one of the hallmarks of maturity is the increasing capacity of the individual to meet self-care needs, that is, those tasks associated with personal care (activities of daily living [ADLs]) and home maintenance (instrumental activities of daily living [IADLs]). The adult is always expected to be able to meet his or her most basic needs independently. During most of one's life, if illness or injury occurs, temporary dependence of some type may occur, but it is expected that it is fleeting and full capacity will return.

Some very old individuals maintain their capacities because of being genetically, physically, functionally, emotionally, and spiritually sturdy. However, for many, the combination of an accumulation of years and chronic illness leads to the diminution of maximum self-care capacity and a lessened ability to rebound from acute health problems. For those older than 70 years, up to 60% require assistance in at least one ADL (Wendel and Durso, 2006). The diminution of independent ability can be the result of limitations in either physical or cognitive functioning, but the ultimate effect is the same and that which can be described as *frailty*.

Frailty results in vulnerability or susceptibility in a number of ways. A frail elder is more likely to become ill, to experience an accidental injury such as a fall, or to have symptoms of cognitive impairment (delirium) from seemingly minor alterations in health or in the environment. Unfortunately, the frail elder is also significantly more likely to become a victim of abuse or neglect.

In this chapter, the concepts of frailty and vulnerability in aging are explored and abuse and neglect are discussed in some depth. We close with specific strategies the gerontological nurse can use to promote healthy aging even among the most frail and to assume a leadership role in identifying and preventing abuse and neglect.

FRAILTY

Gerontologists have long been attempting to define and measure frailty in older adults. Quantitatively, frailty is usually measured in terms of one's ability to perform ADLs or IADLs (see Chapter 6). The qualitative meaning of frailty is more elusive. An elder may appear frail to one person (or

Special thanks to Priscilla Ebersole, the previous edition contributor, for her content contributions to this chapter.

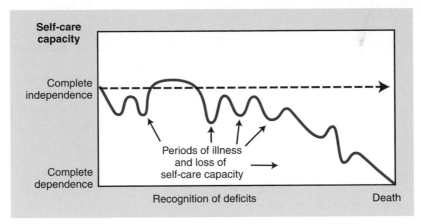

FIGURE 18-1 The frailty trajectory. (Courtesy Kathleen Jett.)

nurse) and rather robust to another. Various adjectives have been applied to persons considered frail, such as *fragile, delicate, brittle,* or even *"easily disturbed."* It is more often described as something that you know when you see it. But still, the view is highly subjective in nature.

Frailty can also be viewed on a trajectory, beginning with the point when the limitations in one's self-care capacity are no longer temporary (Figure 18-1). The frailty trajectory begins with the loss of complete self-care independence, progresses to complete dependence, and ends in death. At first the person may be only minimally dependent, such as needing someone to provide transportation or help with another IADL. As the frailty progresses, the needs for assistance increase, first with IADLs and later with ADLs. While on the frailty trajectory, the elder who experiences an acute illness or injury or exacerbation of a chronic condition may lose capacity more quickly or may never return to the previous level of independence or dependence. Individuals may be mentally or physically frail.

Mental Frailty

Mental frailty may be the first sign of physical frailty. Mental frailty can be conceptualized as the narrowing of the sense of self as the trappings of identity are eroded by loss, changing appearance, and insufficient physiological reserve to support the lifestyle that has formed an individual's persona. Wolanin (1996) conceptualizes mental frailty as the increasing difficulty in the later years in maintaining the "continuity of self" that characterizes a person's identity and capacity for personal integration. Changes may require more residual energy than an individual can muster in a particularly challenging situation. Anxiety, confusion, and paranoia may be signals that indicate the inability to adapt to the changing demands.

Splinting is an important concept in the consideration of frailty and life on the frailty trajectory. Splinting was identified by Wolanin and further developed conceptually by Virginia Burggraf and Pricilla Ebersole (2001). When an elder has exceeded adaptive ability and is psychologically distressed, the presence of a trusted person and routine activities help support (splint) the individual until he or she re-

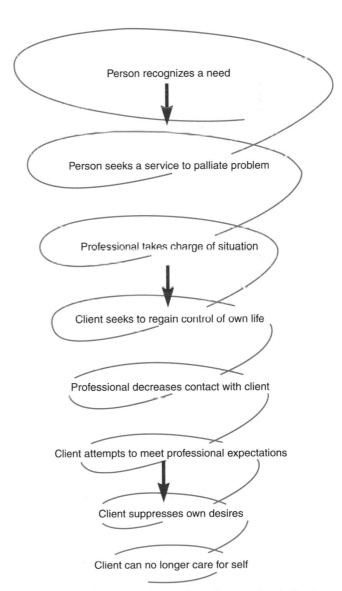

FIGURE 18-2 Spiral of dependency. (Courtesy Patricia Hess.)

gains psychic balance. Couples often function in a splinting manner as they lean on each other for stability but cannot function adequately without each other.

Physical Frailty

Physical frailty is thought to begin physiologically with sarcopenia and the biological markers of increased homocysteine and cytokines (Morley, 2002). Anorexia and malnutrition may be significant findings as well. Physical frailty is evidenced by increased susceptibility to disease and accident, diminished physiological function, and compromised host-defense mechanisms. Sometimes this has been seen in what gerontological nurses have called *failure to thrive (FTT)*. FTT has been described as present when a person has unexplained weight loss, nutritional deficits, decline in physical and cognitive function, and depressive symptoms such as remaining in bed, isolating self, giving up, and feeling helpless (Kimball and Williams-Burgess, 1995). Gaffney (1995) suggests that FTT is the result of a "downward spiral" similar to that conceptualized by Hess in 1985 (Figure 18-2). As a catch-all phrase, FTT is used less often now in nursing and is no longer an acceptable term in medical diagnostics or billing.

VULNERABILITY

Frailty is most important to gerontological nurses because of its relationship to vulnerability. Frailty and vulnerability are inextricably linked. As early as 1988, Buchner and Wagner described frailty as "a state of reduced physiologic reserve associated with increased susceptibility to disability" (p. 1).

Vulnerability is a difficult concept to define clearly because all humans are vulnerable at some time. In addressing the vulnerability of elders, we are particularly concerned about their susceptibility to abuse, fraud, illness, accident, and debilitation. Not only are frail elders vulnerable to physiological disturbance but also they are socially vulnerable to various abuses, mentally vulnerable to stressors, and spiritually vulnerable to reduced opportunities for self-actualization. Recognition of this vulnerability and proactive interventions are the keys to longer periods of healthy survival and shorter periods of disability before death, that is, more stabilization of self-care capacity on the frailty trajectory (see Figure 18-1). The most important issue in facilitating shortened morbidity is to be aware of the vulnerability of the very old and to strengthen their support systems and enhance their adaptive capacities.

Physical Vulnerability

Physical vulnerability affects all elders to some degree. However, for those on the frailty trajectory, energy wanes; sensory, immune, and environmental competence decrease; and falls and infectious processes become more common. Several co-morbid conditions cause particular difficulty for frail elders.

Bone and Joint Problems. Problems with osteoarthritis are almost universal by the eightieth birthday. Mobility is greatly decreased in the oldest-old, largely because of degenerative joint disease (osteoarthritis) and osteoporosis (see Chapter 15 for further discussion). These conditions may be accompanied by severe discomfort and require special attention to achieve comfort (see Chapter 11). Because osteoarthritis affects weight-bearing joints and the spine, it is a key factor in instability and falls. Of women older than 75 years, 90% have some degree of osteoporosis. Fractures, falls, pain, and restricted mobility result. A fall may presage immobility, decline, and death.

Visual and Hearing Problems. One half of the oldest-old report having trouble with their vision, even with glasses. Approximately 21% have much trouble seeing, and 12% report blindness in one or both eyes. Most very old elders have hearing loss that has not been adequately assessed. Sensory appraisal and augmentation, when possible, are critical to maximizing function and preventing accidents (see Chapter 14).

Cognitive Impairment. In the oldest-old, especially those older than 85 years, a minimal level of cognitive impairment is common. Statistics vary, but several sources agree that approximately 35% of people 85 years and older who are living in the community are cognitively impaired and 40% of these are severely impaired (see Chapter 23).

Spiritual Vulnerability

Toward the end of life, individuals may become preoccupied with the meanings, significance, and consequences of the events of life. Some people are burdened with great sorrow and desire to redo events or make restitution. These feelings are discussed more fully in Chapters 26 and 27. Nurses need to be aware that intense preoccupation with spiritual issues and the gravity of unresolved disappointments may sap the energy of an individual, especially when little time or energy is left to make amends.

ELDER MISTREATMENT

Unfortunately, a person in need of the assistance of others is vulnerable for abuse and neglect; that is, the person is at risk for harm and injury at the hands of a frustrated, angry, fraudulent, careless, or disturbed caregiver. Mistreatment of older frail and vulnerable adults is found in all socioeconomic, racial, and ethnic groups in the United States. It is one of our most unrecognized and underreported social problems today. Elder mistreatment may be intentional but may also be accidental.

Mistreatment includes several types of abuse and neglect; however, the definitions of exactly what constitutes any of these vary somewhat by state. It can be seen in any configuration of family and in every setting. The abuse tends to be episodic and recurrent rather than isolated.

In recognition of the escalating problem of elder mistreatment across the globe, countries are busy defining the problem and establishing plans for prevention. Federal definitions of elder abuse, neglect, and exploitation appeared for the first time in the 1987 Amendments to the Older Americans Act. These definitions were provided in the law only as guidelines for identifying the problems and not for enforcement purposes. The specific definitions of elder abuse or mistreatment are now defined by state law and vary considerably from one jurisdiction to another. In 1992 the U.S. Congress passed the Family Violence Prevention and Services Act mandating an analysis of the problem and the Vulnerable Elder Rights Protection Act, which established the National Ombudsman Program (see Chapter 17). In December 2001, the first National Summit on Elder Abuse in the United States was held to identify future directions in the protection of abused elders. The National Center for Elder Abuse (NCEA) provides detailed information on the state of elder abuse and related laws (see *www.elderabusecenter.org*).

In more contemporary times, defining mistreatment is becoming more difficult as our countries become more diverse. Cultural differences are numerous in the identification and definition of abuse (Malley-Morrison et al., 2006). Given our diverse society, this must be considered. For example, Moon (2001) examined the attitudes toward elder abuse, the tolerance of abuse, and the tendency to blame the victims in a group of first-generation Chinese, Japanese, Korean, and Taiwanese Americans. None of the respondents were in favor of reporting suspected or known abuse or of outside intervention, and their tolerance for abuse was associated with victim blaming. The Korean Americans were significantly more tolerant of financial exploitation than the other groups and were more likely to blame the victim.

Just how much mistreatment is occurring is almost impossible to ascertain; estimates of abuse range from 4% to 6% of elders from several countries (Wang et al., 2006). In the United States, the number of older adults experiencing mistreatment is estimated at more than 2 million (Lantz, 2006). However, up to 80% of actual mistreatment may be unreported, or one in five cases (Lantz, 2006; Meiner, 2006).

In a recent cross-sectional study of abuse among community-dwelling women older than 55 years, nearly half reported having experienced some type of abuse and many of them reported repeated abuse (Fisher and Regan, 2006). Usually victims are unwilling or afraid to report the problem because of shame, embarrassment, intimidation, or fear of retaliation. The abuser may be the only caregiver available to the elder, and reporting or complaining could leave the elder without care at all (Box 18-1).

Most abuse occurs in the home setting, where the majority of caregiving occurs. Most abusers are spouses or adult children. The majority (84%) of the documented cases are among white elders (Meiner, 2006). The incidence of elder abuse is expected to increase with the increase in numbers of persons in need of care, the increased conflicting demands on the caregiver's time, and the increased pressure to report suspicions of abuse.

The most common types of mistreatment are financial exploitation and physical, psychological, and sexual abuse. Medical abuse is also seen, wherein the person is subjected to unwanted treatments or procedures; or medical neglect occurs, in which desired treatment is withheld. A particular problem in the elderly is pain under-treatment, a form of medical neglect (Lewis, 2006). Caregiver neglect implies that the caregiver has not met his or her obligation to the elder for whom he or she is recognized as responsible and includes abandonment (Fulmer, 2002). Self-neglect means that a person is not caring for herself or himself in the manner in which most peers would. In all cases, the vulnerable person is harmed.

Abuse

Abuse is intentional and may be physical, psychological, or sexual and always violates a person's rights (Box 18-2). When the abuser or neglectful person is a caretaker (e.g., a nurse), the caretaker is subject to tort litigation; that is, he or she can be sued for the injuries to the elderly person and

---

BOX 18-1   Women and Abuse

A study conducted by Bonnie Fisher and Saundra Regan examined the types of abuse, repeated abuse and the experiences of multiple abuse by women over 60. Eight hundred forty-two women living in the community responded to a telephone survey. Almost one half of the women have experienced some type of abuse since the age of 55; many of these reported repeated abuse. The abused women were more likely than the non-abused women to complain of health problems, including bone and joint problems, digestive problems, depression or anxiety, chronic pain, high blood pressure, or heart problems.

Data from Fisher BS, Regan SL: The extent and frequency of abuse in the lives of older women and their relationship with health outcomes, *Gerontologist* 46(2):200-209, 2006.

BOX 18-2   Types of Elder Mistreatment*

Physical abuse: The use of physical force that may result in bodily injury, physical pain, or impairment.

Sexual abuse: Nonconsensual sexual contact of any kind with an elderly person, including with those persons unable to give consent.

Emotional or psychological abuse: The infliction of anguish, pain, or distress through verbal or nonverbal acts, including intimidation or enforced social isolation.

Medical abuse: Subjecting a person to unwanted medial treatments or procedures; medical neglect occurs when a medically necessary and desired treatment is withheld.

Financial or material abuse or exploitation: The illegal or improper use of an elder's funds, property, or assets.

Neglect: The refusal or failure to fulfill any part of a person's previously agreed obligation or duties to an elder dependent on the person for care or assistance.

Abandonment: The desertion of an elder by an individual who had assumed the responsibility of providing care or assistance.

Elder mistreatment implies that the recipient of the mistreatment is in a situation or condition in which the ability to protect oneself is limited in some way. Otherwise the actions are more accurately described as *domestic violence, sexual assault,* or *fraud.*

may have to pay monetary damages. If the abuse or neglect is of such a nature that it rises to a criminal act or if the abuse has to do with theft or conversion of property or money, the caretaker is subject to criminal prosecution. Many states have reporting statutes that require certain persons, including nurses, who become aware of abuse, neglect, or exploitation to report it to appropriate authorities. Who that authority is can be found in state laws (National Center on Elder Abuse [NCEA], 2006).

Physical Abuse. Physical abuse is the use of physical force that may result in bodily injury, physical pain, or impairment. It includes but is not limited to acts of violence such as striking (with or without an object), hitting, beating, pushing, shoving, shaking, slapping, kicking, pinching, and burning. The inappropriate use of chemical and physical restraints, force-feeding, and physical punishment of any kind also are examples of physical abuse (NCEA, 2006). Any unexpected injury, bruise, or change in behavior of the elderly person may be a sign that requires further investigation (see the discussion that follows).

Psychological Abuse. Emotional or psychological abuse includes but is not limited to verbal assaults, insults, threats, intimidation, humiliation, and harassment. Psychological abuse is the infliction of anguish, pain, or distress through verbal or nonverbal acts (Meiner, 2006). Treating an older person like a child; isolating an elderly person from his or her family, friends, or regular activities; and enforced social isolation are examples of psychological abuse (NCEA, 2006). This type of abuse may be a deliberate effort to dehumanize the person, sometimes to mitigate the guilt of providing poor care or abusing the person emotionally.

Sexual Abuse. Sexual abuse is nonconsensual sexual contact of any kind with another person, regardless of age. Sexual contact with a person incapable of giving consent is also considered sexual abuse. It includes but is not limited to unwanted touching and all types of sexual assault or battery, such as rape, sodomy, coerced nudity, and sexually explicit photographing (NCEA, 2006). Nurses and other health care providers may observe injuries from rough or forceful sexual activity; however, sometimes injury may not be present but certain behaviors may be revealing. Fear of certain persons, resistance to necessary touch in the genital area, or reports of sexual contact cannot be ignored.

Financial or Material Exploitation

Financial or material exploitation is the illegal or improper use of another's funds, property, or assets. Exploitation may be accomplished by force, such as demanding that the person sign checks or other documents with the threat of withholding care. It can also be done with stealth through deceit, misrepresentation, or fraud, such as cashing an elderly person's checks without authorization or permission, forging a signature, or misusing or stealing an older person's money or possessions. Also, conservatorship, guardianship,

or power of attorney can be improperly used (see Chapter 17). Whereas other forms of abuse have external signs, it is often difficult to detect financial exploitation. Care is costly, and much of the elderly person's assets may be gone before it is noted that far more has been used than seems to be needed. Changes in banking practices, failure to pay medical or other care bills, unexpected changes in a will, and finding personal valuable items missing are all evidence of possible financial exploitation and should be reported to proper authorities.

Undue Influence. Undue influence is often used as a means of achieving financial or material exploitation. As described by Quinn (2002, p. 11):

> Undue influence is the substitution of one person's will for the true desires of another...Undue influence takes place when one person uses his or her role and power to exploit the trust, dependency or fear of another to gain psychological control over the weaker person's decision-making, usually for financial gain.

Undue influence may occur in an insidious way because the victim is often isolated from friends and family and convinced that the only one who cares is the caretaker; or a younger person attempts to defraud a lonely widow or widower of assets through romance and marriage. In these cases, intervention is difficult because the victim has developed trust and reliance on the abuser and has usually entered into the relationship voluntarily. Undue influence may be exerted on the elder, and a companion or home care provider will manage to convince the elder to transfer assets and even the deed to the home. These situations are being examined more carefully in the courts, and some states are activating legal protections against undue influence (Quinn, 2002; Quinn and Tomita, 2003). Quinn has developed guidelines for nurses attempting to identify signs of undue influence (Box 18-3).

Neglect

Neglect is the most common form of elder mistreatment and may be at the hands of a caregiver or oneself. Neglect of self and neglect by caretakers are often difficult to define because they are intertwined with energy, lifestyle, and resources. Nurses must be cautious in setting specific boundaries around neglect. However, when basic needs go unmet, intervention may be required. Physical neglect is the most common and obvious occurrence and may be indicated by a person's failure to thrive, untreated medical conditions (medical neglect), badly neglected grooming, malnutrition, and dehydration (NCEA, 1999).

Caregiver Neglect. Neglect is passive abuse not characterized by physical violence. Caregiver neglect is seen as an act of omission or withholding needed goods and services such as food, medication, medical treatment, and personal care necessary for the well-being of the frail elder. It also includes behavior that ignores the person's obvious needs even though the caretaker is present.

BOX 18-3 Signs and Symptoms of Undue Influence

- Elder takes actions inconsistent with his or her life history. Actions run counter to the person's previous long-time values and beliefs.
- Elder makes sudden changes with regard to financial management. Examples include cashing in insurance policies or changing titles on bank accounts or real property.
- Elder changes his or her will and previous disposition of assets.
- Elder is taken to practitioners different from those he or she has always trusted. Examples include bankers, stockbrokers, attorneys, physicians, and realtor.
- Elder is systematically isolated from or is continually monitored with others who care about him or her.
- Someone suddenly moves into the person's home or the elder is moved into someone's home under the guise of providing better care.
- Someone attempts to get income checks directed differently from the usual arrangement.
- Documents are suddenly signed frequently as the elder nears death.
- A history of mistrust exists in the elder's family, especially with financial affairs, and the elder places unusual trust in newfound acquaintances.

- Someone promises to provide lifelong care in exchange for property on the elder's death.
- Statements of the elder and the alleged abuser vary concerning the elder's affairs or disposition of assets.
- A power imbalance exists between the parties in matters of finances or health.
- Someone shows unfairness to the weaker party in a transaction. The stronger person unduly benefits by the transaction.
- The elder is never left alone with anyone. No one is allowed to speak to the elder without the alleged abuser having a way of finding out about it.
- Unusual patterns arise in the elder's finances. For instance, numerous checks are written out to "cash," always in round numbers, and often in large amounts.
- The elder reports meeting a "wonderful new friend who makes me feel young again." The elder then becomes suspicious of family and begins to avoid family gatherings.
- The elder is pressed into a transaction without being given time to reflect or contact trusted advisors.

From Quinn M: Undue influence and elder abuse: recognition and intervention strategies, *Geriatr Nurs* 23(1):11-16, 2002.

Neglect by a caregiver may occur for many reasons. Sometimes it is the result of caregiver stress, the result of feeling overwhelmed by the responsibilities of caregiving. Or it can be active neglect that is deliberate and malicious (Quinn and Tomita, 2003). However, some acts of neglect occur because of incompetence, unawareness of importance of the neglected care, no legal requirement to give such care, unavailability of resources, or exhaustion. The caregivers' own frailty and advanced age are often mitigating factors. Passive neglect—simply ignoring or not attending to needs—is most prevalent.

Self-Neglect. Elder self-neglect is a behavior of the individual person. It is usually a function of a person's diminished physical or mental capacity that threatens his or her own health or safety. Self-neglect generally manifests itself in an older person as a refusal or failure to provide himself or herself with adequate safety, food, water, clothing, shelter, personal hygiene, or health care. Self-neglect may be associated with increasing severity of physical or mental impairments but may also reflect a lifestyle of alcoholism and drug abuse (Quinn and Tomita, 2003). However, in some situations, a mentally competent person who understands the consequences of his or her decisions makes a conscious and voluntary decision to engage in acts that threaten his or her health or safety as a matter of personal choice. It is an ethical and legal question as to how much health care professionals should intervene in these situations unless it can definitely be determined that the person lacks capacity or competence.

Risk Factors

Dyer and colleagues (2000) and other investigators have found that individuals older than 75 years who are diagnosed with depression or dementia are the most likely to be mistreated. Victims are most likely to be female and living in a household with family members.

Elder abuse requires an abuser, an elder, and the context of caregiving (Burke and Laramie, 2004). There are multiple risk factors for one to be or become an abuser or abused (Box 18-4). Persons who are abusing alcohol or other substances, have emotional or mental illnesses, or have a history of abusing or being abused are more likely to be abusers, as are caregivers who are exhausted and frustrated (see Box 18-4). Wang and colleagues (2006) found that in Taiwan, abusers were most likely to be younger women with higher levels of education and higher levels of burden.

The abuser is usually the caregiver but may also be the care recipient. Caregivers, be they informal (e.g., spouses) or formal (e.g., nursing assistants), may be subjected to verbal and physical abuse by the person for whom they are caring. This may be a lifelong pattern that intensifies in the current situation.

Although any older person who is frail and therefore vulnerable can be abused, women are at particular risk. The typical abused elder is a white, 75-year-old woman who lives alone and is frail, confused, or depressed (Lantz, 2006). The risk for abuse is intensified if the person has been abused in the past or if his or her behavior is considered aggressive, combative, or provocative; that is, the person is viewed as overly demanding or unappreciative (Harrell et al., 2002).

BOX 18-4 Profiles of Abused and Abusers

ABUSED ELDERS

Woman age 80 years or older
Lives alone or with abuser
Has mental or physical disability
Is dependent on abuser

ABUSERS

Middle-aged male sibling or offspring
Has mental health and substance abuse problems
Is financially dependent on abused
Has history of abuse and being abused

Adapted from Utley R: Screening and intervention in elder abuse, *Home Care Provid* 4(5):198, 1999.

The level of dependency is also a factor; the more dependent the elder, the more vulnerable he or she is to being abused. Men or women who had abused the caregiver earlier in life may be at risk for retaliation. Because both the majority of caregiving and the majority of abuse occur within the family, this is the context. Caregiver/care recipient relationships that were conflicted earlier in life will continue to be so.

Abuse and exploitation can also occur in the situation of a hired caregiver. When a number of providers are giving care, monitoring becomes especially difficult. Situations of potential formal caregiver abuse include those in which there is inadequate supervision of patient care, poor coordination of services, inadequate staff training, theft and fraud, drug and alcohol abuse by staff, tardiness and absenteeism, unprofessional and criminal conduct, and inadequate record keeping. The nurse should pay particular attention to the caregiver who is alone, with no support from others and no opportunities for respite. The abuse may be a lifelong pattern in which the victim has always felt somewhat at fault and will remain in the situation.

▲ PROMOTING HEALTHY AGING: IMPLICATIONS FOR GERONTOLOGICAL NURSING

Frailty in late life presents a significant challenge to both the persons experiencing it and those who provide care. How does one adjust to diminished self-care capacity without a loss of self-esteem? How does one continue to find meaning in life when one's abilities change? How can personal integrity stand the test of time? How does one provide assistance to others without promoting dependence? How does one help maximize the quality of life and health of those on a frailty trajectory while spontaneously addressing issues of multiple co-morbid conditions (see Chapter 1), recurrent stress (see Chapter 24), polypharmacy (see Chapter 12), soaring health care costs (see Chapter 17), and problems with access to health care (see Chapters 15, 21, and 22)? And finally, how does the gerontological nurse protect vulnerable elders in a respectful and life-affirming manner?

BOX 18-5 Signs of and Responses to Elder Mistreatment

SIGNS AND SIGNALS

Obvious physical signs of violence
Feeling of the victim that he or she has done something wrong
Isolation from others outside the relationship
Restriction of elder's contact with others
Perpetrator easily irritated or agitated and demonstrates poor control of anger
Verbalized threats toward elder or caregiver

ACTIONS TO BE TAKEN

Assess the presence of physical danger
Identify appropriate options:
- Seek legal advice
- Get a protective order
- Have the abuser arrested
- Support victim's decision to leave or stay
- Develop a workable safety plan

Reestablish contact with family and friends
Identify emergency actions that will assist the victim:
- Give specific information on places of sanctuary

Modified from Davey P, Davey D: Domestic violence: a clinical view, *Home Health Focus* 2(10):78-79, 1996.

Assessment

Good nursing care always begins with assessment. Frail elders benefit the most from comprehensive assessments. Several tools that are of particular usefulness are described in Chapter 6, including the original OARS (Pfeiffer, 1975) and the more limited but contemporary SPICES (Wallace and Fulmer, 2002). Models of both assessment and planning that are in use and refinement are part of the NICHE (Nurses Improving Care for Health Systems Elders) and ACE (Acute Care of the Elderly) initiatives (Wendel and Durso, 2006). An ACE unit is specifically designed and staffed to meet the needs of frail elders. This begins with a thorough interdisciplinary assessment and sophisticated care planning to support the elder and his or her family after discharge.

When working with frail elders, nurses must always be vigilant in their sensitivity to the potential for abuse, observing for signs and symptoms in all their interactions with vulnerable elders. In addition to the obvious physical signs (Box 18-5), the nurse looks for more subtle signals. Is there an unusual delay between the beginning of a health problem and when help is sought? Are appointments often missed without reasonable explanations? Are the histories given by the elder and the caregiver inconsistent? Also, behavioral indications may suggest an abusive situation. Does the caregiver do all of the talking in a situation, even though the elder is capable? Does the caregiver appear angry, frustrated, or indifferent while the elder appears hesitant or frightened? Is the caregiver or the care recipient aggressive toward one another or the nurse?

If abuse is suspected, a full and specialized assessment should be done, including a determination of the safety of the victim and the desires of the victim if competent. Assessment of mistreatment involves several components. Terry Fulmer at the John A. Hartford Foundation presents a detailed assessment that is considered one of the best practice protocols. Her tool can be found in Figure 18-3. Because of the sensitive nature of such an assessment, specialized training is recommended for all gerontological nurses (Fulmer et al., 2004).

Interventions

In response to the findings of the assessment, the gerontological nurse intervenes to maximize health and self-care capacity and to protect vulnerable elders. The PACE model, such as On Lok, is one effective approach that provides an alternative to nursing home placement. Instead, the strengths identified in the assessment are enhanced and strategies are formulated to limit the effect of the weakness. For example, the elder whose cognitive abilities are threatened by isolation may be involved in the day activities of a social senior center, with transportation to and from the center provided. For the physically fragile, a home health aide may be available to assist with personal care, not because the person is completely incapacitated but to preserve energy for more life-affirming interactions. Both of these strategies may support the person on the frailty trajectory in a way that may slow decline or minimize exacerbations of dependence during times of stress. On Lok is considered a best-practice model for geriatric interdisciplinary care (Kornblatt, 2002). Unfortunately, under the current health care system in the United States, motivation or fiscal support is limited for such life-affirming interventions if rehabilitation or restoration to complete independence is not a clear possibility. Too often, value-added programs are limited to those who can afford them.

Although responses to frailty may be restricted or selective to resources that are available, the nurse's response to potential abuse or neglect of the vulnerable may be mandated. In most jurisdictions in the United States, nurses have a legal responsibility to protect the vulnerable, be they children, persons with disabilities, or elders with limited physical of cognitive capacity. The gerontological nurse is in an ideal position not only to detect potential elder mistreatment but also to plan an active role in its prevention. However, here more than in any other situation is it imperative for the nurse to have at least a working knowledge of the laws that protect vulnerable elders.

Mandatory Reporting. In most states and U.S. jurisdictions, licensed nurses are "mandatory reporters," that is, persons who are required to report suspicions of abuse to the state, usually to a group called *Adult Protective Services* or *APS*. Failure to report suspicions may result in civil and/or criminal penalties (Meiner, 2006). The standard for reporting is one of reasonable belief; that is, the nurse

must have a reasonable belief that a vulnerable person either has been or is likely to be abused, neglected, or exploited. Actual knowledge is not required (Guido, 2006). Usually these reports are anonymous. If the nurse believes the elder to be in immediate danger, the police should be notified. How the nurse accomplishes this varies with the work setting. In hospitals and nursing homes, this is often reported first internally to the facility social worker. In the home care setting, the report is made to the nursing supervisor. It would be very unusual for the nurse not to go through his or her employer. However, the nurse who is a neighbor, friend, or privately paid caregiver may be under obligation to make the report. In the nursing home or licensed assisted living facility, the nurse has the additional resource of calling the state long-term care ombudsman for help.

In each state, ombudsmen are either volunteers or paid staff members who are responsible for acting as advocates for vulnerable elders in institutions. All reports, either to the state ombudsman or to adult protective services, will be investigated. A unique aspect of elder abuse compared with child abuse is that the physically frail but mentally competent adult can refuse assessment and intervention and often does. Abused but competent elders cannot be removed from harmful situations without their permission, much to the frustration of the nurse and other health care providers.

Prevention of Abuse. In the ideal situation, gerontological nurses are alert to potential mistreatment of vulnerable elders and take steps to prevent the occurrence of abuse or neglect. In some situations, the abuse may be preventable, and in others, it is less likely to be preventable. If the abuse is the result of psychopathological conditions, especially if the situation is long-standing, the nurse probably cannot prevent the abuse. However, nurses can make sure that the potential victims know how to get help if it is needed and the resources that are available to them, and nurses can provide support and encouragement that it is possible to leave the situation. The nurse can also work with the elder, caregiver, and community supports to increase the exposure of the elders to others.

If the abusive behavior is learned or a response to stress, the situation may be subject to change. Learned abuse, theoretically, can be unlearned and may respond to a close working relationship with a mentoring professional who can demonstrate positive problem solving and new ways of managing difficult situations.

If the abuse is based in the stress of the caregiving situation, nurses can be very proactive and help all involved take action to lessen the stress. This may include finding respite services, changing the situation entirely (giving permission to the caregiver to give up the role), referring to support groups for expression of frustrations and peer support, teaching people how to use crisis hotlines, professional consultation, victim support groups, victim volunteer companions, and, above all, thoughtful and compassionate care for the

1. General Assessment	Very Good	Good	Poor	Very Poor	Unable to Assess
a. Clothing					
b. Hygiene					
c. Nutrition					
d. Skin integrity					

Additional Comments:

2. Possible Abuse Indicators	No Evidence	Possible Evidence	Probable Evidence	Definite Evidence	Unable to Assess
a. Bruising					
b. Lacerations					
c. Fractures					
d. Various stages of healing of any bruises or fractures					
e. Evidence of sexual abuse					
f. Statement by elder re: abuse					

Additional Comments:

3. Possible Neglect Indicators	No Evidence	Possible Evidence	Probable Evidence	Definite Evidence	Unable to Assess
a. Contractures					
b. Decubiti					
c. Dehydration					
d. Diarrhea					
e. Depression					
f. Impaction					
g. Malnutrition					
h. Urine burns					
i. Poor hygiene					
j. Failure to respond to warning of obvious disease					
k. Inappropriate medications (under/over)					
l. Repetitive hospital admissions due to probable failure of health care surveillance					
m. Statement by elder re: neglect					

Additional Comments:

4. Possible Exploitation Indicators	No Evidence	Possible Evidence	Probable Evidence	Definite Evidence	Unable to Assess
a. Misuse of money					
b. Evidence					
c. Reports of demands for goods in exchange for services					
d. Inability to account for money/property					
e. Statement by elder re: exploitation					

Additional Comments:

5. Possible Abandonment Indicators	No Evidence	Possible Evidence	Probable Evidence	Definite Evidence	Unable to Assess
a. Evidence that a caretaker has withdrawn care precipitously without alternate arrangements					
b. Evidence that elder is left alone in an unsafe environment for extended periods without adequate support					
c. Statement by elder re: abandonment					

Additional Comments:

6. Summary	No Evidence	Possible Evidence	Probable Evidence	Definite Evidence	Unable to Assess
a. Evidence of abuse					
b. Evidence of neglect					
c. Evidence of exploitation					
d. Evidence of abandonment					

Additional Comments:

FIGURE 18-3 Abuse and neglect assessment. (From Fulmer T: *Elder abuse and neglect assessment. Try This: best practices in nursing care to older adults,* Hartford Institute for Geriatric Nursing, #15, May 2002.)

victim and the perpetrator (Quinn and Tomita, 2003; Reis and Nahmiash, 1995; Pillemer and Wolf, 1986). See Box 18-6 for tips for the prevention of elder mistreatment.

Finally, for elders who become mentally incompetent, legal protection may be necessary. Gerontological nurses can become familiar with the laws that specifically affect older adults in their state. This can be done by speaking with an elder law attorney or selecting continuing education programs to update knowledge in the field of client legal protections. Once informed of the laws affecting frail elders, nurses are in a position to assist elders and family members in seeking legal representation when necessary and in selecting the approach that will solve the problems in the least restrictive manner possible. Although initiating these interventions is usually the responsibility of the social worker and enacted by

---

BOX 18-6   Tips for the Prevention of Elder Mistreatment

- Make professionals aware of potentially abusive situations.
- Educate the public about normal aging processes.
- Help families develop and nurture informal support systems.
- Link families with support groups.
- Teach families stress management techniques.
- Arrange comprehensive care resources.
- Provide counseling for troubled families.
- Encourage the use of respite care and day care.
- Obtain necessary home health care services.
- Inform families of resources for meals and transportation.
- Encourage caregivers to pursue their individual interests.

Human Needs and Wellness Diagnoses

Self-Actualization and Transcendence
(Seeking, Expanding, Spirituality, Fulfillment)
Seeks meaning in vulnerability
Rises above physical frailty
Seeks spiritual enlightenment
Enjoys life

Self-Esteem and Self-Efficacy
(Image, Identity, Control, Capability)
Asserts self to obtain sufficient material resources
Maintains dignity and self-assurance
Maintains grooming
Maintains balance in lifestyle demands and rewards

Belonging and Attachment
(Love, Empathy, Affiliation)
Maintains healthy affiliations
Accepts assistance from others when needed
Maintains important ties with family and friends
Demonstrates appropriate compassion for others
Is aware of others' needs as well as his or her own

Safety and Security
(Caution, Planning, Protections, Sensory Acuity)
Reports needs and vulnerabilities to appropriate authorities
Knows how and when to obtain protective assistance
Plans in advance for avoiding threatening situations
Avoids situations of potential risk
Is free from fear

Biological and Physiological Integrity
(Air, Fluids, Comfort, Activity, Nutrition, Elimination, Skin Integrity)
Has basic needs adequately met
Sustains appropriate weight and hydration
Is free of bruises, contusions, lesions, and fractures
Is free from pain

These are not all the possible wellness diagnoses that may be identified. The above are examples of nursing diagnoses that should be considered when planning care for the older adult.

lawyers and judges, the nurse should understand the basic concepts and the types of legal protection for elders and other incapacitated persons (see Chapter 17).

KEY CONCEPTS

- Many elders have diminishing abilities to perform independent ADLs or IADLs because of chronic disease superimposed on the normal changes with aging. This is called *frailty*.
- Frailty can be visualized on a trajectory from initial loss of total independence to death. Vulnerable elders are easily influenced and subject to catastrophic responses to changes or demands of their environment.
- Frail elders are vulnerable to discomfort and prolonged recovery from injury or illness.
- Frail elders must have basic needs met and supportive networks available to maintain physical and psychological function.
- Failure to thrive (FTT) in elderly people is poorly understood but is likely a deprivation of caring individuals and the downward spiral of dependency.
- *Elder mistreatment* is an umbrella term that covers abuse, neglect, exploitation, and abandonment.
- The nurse has a legal responsibility in most states to report suspected mistreatment of frail or disabled elders.
- Availability of comprehensive resources and coordinated care can keep frail and vulnerable elders safe, functional, and independent longer.

RESEARCH QUESTIONS

Discuss your concept of frailty in late life, and propose a clear definition of the concept.

What are the physiological principles that best explain the concept of frailty in aging?

Discuss various legal mechanisms for protecting the frail elderly.

What is the distinction between frailty and vulnerability?

Refer to the chapter on relationships (see Chapter 20), and describe factors in a spousal or partnered relationship that may be functional or detrimental to the frail elderly.

What are your responsibilities in reporting elder abuse in your state?

How do health care agencies define frail elderly?

Which agencies offer services specifically designed for the elderly, and what are these services?

What proportion of individuals older than 80 years are considered frail, and based on what criteria?

Is the increasing population (older than 85 years) shifting toward more durability or increasing frailty in recent decades?

Are shelters available to frail elders who are attempting to escape from abuse?

CASE STUDY: Elder Abuse

Mrs. Henry, 87 years old, was admitted to the medical/surgical floor of a community hospital with a fractured right orbit and ruptured eye globe. Her husband attends to her with care and concern, trying to anticipate her needs. He is active and appears much younger than his stated age of 85. The emergency department report states the cause of the injury as "fall at home." Although Mrs. Henry is alert and oriented, she appears very thin, frail, and withdrawn. Her husband also voices concern that she seems confused at times. When the gerontological clinical nurse specialist arrives to do a basic intake, she reports to the nurses that she is concerned that Mrs. Henry has been abused. Her husband answers all the questions posed to his wife, and as he does so, Mrs. Henry seems to withdraw even further from both him and the staff. Mr. Henry does not leave his wife's side for hours. Finally he leaves for a quick cup of coffee, and the nurse who had been providing care quickly goes into the room and asks Mrs. Henry what happened. She begins to cry and says that her husband hit her. She is immediately offered shelter and protection. She declines, saying that she has no where else to go but back home and that she will be okay. The husband returns to find the nurse talking to his wife privately and immediately gathers up her things and they leave the hospital against medical advice.

Based on the case study, develop a nursing care plan using the following procedure*:

- List Mrs. Henry's comments that provide subjective data.
- List information that provides objective data.

- From these data, identify and state, using accepted format, two nursing diagnoses you determine are most significant to Mrs. Henry at this time. List two of Mrs. Henry's strengths that you have identified from the data.
- Determine and state outcome criteria for each diagnosis. These must reflect some alleviation of the problem identified in the nursing diagnosis and must be stated in concrete and measurable terms.
- Plan and state one or more interventions for each diagnosed problem. Provide specific documentation of the source used to determine the appropriate intervention. Plan at least one intervention that incorporates Mrs. Henry's existing strengths.
- Evaluate the success of the intervention. Interventions must correlate directly with the stated outcome criteria to measure the outcome success.

Critical Thinking Questions

1. Identify the risk factors for elder abuse in this situation.
2. Provide the subjective data suggesting abuse.
3. Provide the objective data suggesting abuse in this situation.
4. Describe the nurse's legal responsibility to Mrs. Henry at this time.
5. Why might Mrs. Henry believe she has no options?
6. Describe the next step the nurse will take on the departure of this patient.

---

* Students are advised to refer to their nursing diagnosis text and identify possible or potential problems.

REFERENCES

Buchner D, Wagner E: Preventing frail health, *Clin Geriatr Med* 8(1):1, 1988.

Burggraf V, Ebersole P: *Elderly couples splinting*, Personal communication, 2001.

Burke MM, Laramie JA: *Primary care of the older adult: a multidisciplinary approach*, ed 2, St Louis, 2004, Mosby.

Dyer CB et al: The high prevalence of depression and dementia in elder abuse and neglect, *J Am Geriatr Soc* 48(2):205, 2000.

Fisher BS, Regan SL: The extent and frequency of abuse in the lives of older women and their relationships with health outcomes, *Gerontologist* 46(2):200-209, 2006.

Fulmer T: *Elder abuse and neglect assessment. Try this: best practices in nursing care to older adults*, Hartford Institute for Geriatric Nursing, #15, May 2002.

Fulmer T et al: Progress in elder abuse screening and assessment instruments, *J Am Geriatr Soc* 52(2):297-304, 2004.

Gaffney D: Commentary on failure to thrive: the silent epidemic of the elderly, *APNSCAN* 6:10, August, 1995.

Guido GW: *Legal and ethical issues in nursing*, ed 4, Upper Saddle River, NJ, 2006, Prentice-Hall.

Harrell R et al: How geriatricians identify elder abuse and neglect, *Am J Med Sci* 323(1):34, 2002.

Hess P: Crisis, stress, depression and control. In Ebersole P, Hess P, editors: *Toward healthy aging: human needs and nursing response*, ed 2, St Louis, 1985, Mosby.

Kimball MJ, Williams Burgess C: Failure to thrive: the silent epidemic of the elderly, *Arch Psychiatr Nurs* 9(2):99, 1995.

Kornblatt S: Best practice: the On Lok model of geriatric interdisciplinary team care, *J Gerontol Social Work* 40(1/2):15-22, 2002.

Lantz MS: Elder abuse and neglect: help starts with recognizing the problem, *Clin Geriatrics* 14(9):10-13, 2006.

Lewis M: Pain. In Meiner S, Lueckenotte A, editors: *Gerontologic nursing*, ed 3, St Louis, 2006, Mosby.

Malley-Morrison K et al: International perspectives on elder abuse: five case studies, *Educ Gerontol* 32(1):1-11, 2006.

Meiner S: Legal and ethical issues. In Meiner S, Lueckenotte A, editors: *Gerontologic nursing*, ed 3, St Louis, 2006, Mosby.

Moon A: Elder mistreatment among four Asian American groups: an exploratory study on tolerance, victim blaming, and attitudes toward their party intervention. *J Gerontol Social Work*, 36(1/2): 153-169, 2001.

Morley JE: Frailty, *Aging Successfully* 12(1):5, 12-13, 17, 2002.

National Center on Elder Abuse (NCEA): *Types of elder abuse in domestic settings*, Elder abuse series information #1, 1999. (website): *www.elderabusecenter.org*. Accessed November 10, 2006.

National Center on Elder Abuse (NCEA): *International and cultural perspectives—an update of the literature*, 2006. (website): *www.elderabusecenter.org*. Accessed November 10, 2006.

Pfeiffer E: *Multidimensional functional assessment, the OARS method: a Duke manual*, Center for the Study of Aging and Development, 1975.

Pillemer KA, Wolf RS: *Elder abuse: conflict in the family*, Dover, Me, 1986, Auburn House.

Quinn M: Undue influence and elder abuse: recognition and intervention strategies, *Geriatr Nurs* 23(1):11, 2002.

Quinn M, Tomita SK: *Elder abuse and neglect: causes, diagnoses and intervention strategies*, ed 3, New York, 2003, Springer Series on Social Work.

Reis M, Nahmiash D: When seniors are abused: an intervention model, *Gerontologist* 35(5):666, 1995.

Wallace M, Fulmer T: *SPICES: an overall assessment tool for older adults. Try This Series* from the Hartford Institute for Geriatric Nursing, 2002. (website): *www.hartfordign.org*. Accessed November 20, 2006.

Wang J-J et al: Psychologically abusive behavior by those caring for the elderly in domestic context, *Geriatr Nurs* 27(5):284-291, 2006.

Wendel VI, Durso SC: A case study: challenges and issues caring for the older adult across the spectrum of settings, *J Nurse Practitioners* 2(9):600-606, 2006.

Wolanin MO. *Mental frailty*, Personal communication, February 20, 1996.

CHAPTER 19

Intimacy and Sexuality in Late Life

Theris A. Touhy

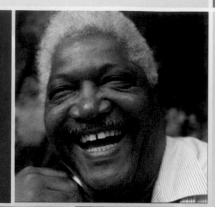
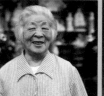
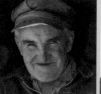

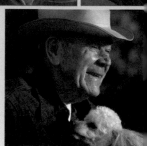

AN ELDER SPEAKS

These early morning hours are terribly lonely ... that's when I have such a longing for someone who loves me to be there just to touch and hold me ... and to talk to.

Sister Marilyn Schwab (From Schwab M: *A gift freely given: the personal journal of Sister Marilyn Schwab,* Mt Angel, Ore, 1986, Benedictine Sisters.)

LEARNING OBJECTIVES

On completion of this chapter, the reader will be able to:

1. Discuss touch and intimacy as integral components of sexuality.
2. Discuss the therapeutic benefits of touch for older people.
3. Discuss the physiological, social, and psychological factors that affect the older adult's sexual function.
4. Describe the various approaches to sexuality assessment that may reduce nurse-client anxiety in discussing a sensitive area.
5. Identify the risks to sexual integrity.
6. Formulate and validate appropriate nursing diagnoses.
7. Discuss interventions that foster sexual integrity.

TOUCH

Touch affects almost anything we do. It is the oldest, most important, and most neglected of our senses. Touch is 10 times stronger than verbal or emotional contact. All other senses have an organ on which to focus, but touch is everywhere. Touch is unique because it frequently combines with other senses. An individual can survive without one or more of the other senses, but no one can survive and live in any degree of comfort without touch. In the absence of touching or being touched, people of all ages can become sick and become touch starved (Ackerman, 1995). According to Kim and Buschmann (2004, p. 35):

> Touch is experienced physically as sensation as well as affectively as emotion and behavior. The interaction of touch affects the autonomic, reticular, and limbic systems, and thus profoundly affects the emotional drives.

The human yearning for physical contact is embedded in our language in such figurative terms as "keep in touch," "handle with care," and "rubbed the wrong way" (Huss, 1977). We will focus on touch as an overt expression of closeness, intimacy, and sexuality. We believe an individual must recog-

nize the power of touch and its intimacy to fully comprehend sexuality. Touch and intimacy are integral parts of sexuality, just as sexuality is expressed through intimacy and touch. Together, touch and intimacy can offer the older adult a sense of well being. Touch is the first sensory system to become functional. Throughout life, touch provides emotional and sensual knowledge about other individuals—an unending source of information, pleasure, and pain.

We love and are loved by virtue of our skin sensation and appearance. How our skin is arranged affects others' willingness to touch us. Even though beauty is said to be only skin deep, skin is significant. The wrinkled skin of the old person shows the beautiful lines of hard work and experience. Old hands and old faces tell much of the bearer's capacity for intimacy. Sensations of old skin, clean, dry, and powdered or cologned, linger in the remote memories of many individuals who were held by a grandmother or grandfather. These features provide our foundation for intimacy with the old.

Response to Touch

The Touch model proposed by Hollinger and Buschmann (1993) proposes that attitudes toward touch and acceptance

Special thanks to Patricia Hess, the previous edition contributor, for her content contributions to this chapter.

of touch affect the behaviors of both caregivers and patients. Two types of touch occur during the nurse-patient relationship: procedural and non-procedural. Procedural touch (*task-oriented* or *instrumental touch*) is physical contact that occurs when a particular task is being performed. Non-procedural touch (*expressive physical touch*) does not require a task but is affective and supportive in nature, such as holding a patient's hand (Kim and Buschmann, 2004).

Nurses should recognize the influence of their own personality, cultural expectations, and early exposure to touching. Everyone has definite feelings and opinions about touch based on his or her own life experience. "Individuals learn the boundaries of tactual communication culturally" (Kim and Buschmann, 2004, p. 37). Touch only if it is comfortable. Individuals quickly discern the discomfort of another if touch is not an integral part of behavior. It is important to remember is that the comfort of touching depends on the location of touch, the situation, social status, culture, and age.

A test of the person's readiness to be touched is to initiate a hand clasp or handshake. The person can feel the tension or the welcoming relaxation that occurs. Some people respond warmly to a firm touch and others to a light or casual touch. Useful information may be obtained through a handshake. Does the individual grasp firmly or hesitate? Does he or she relinquish quickly or hold on? Are the fingers intertwined or held together? Is the hand limp, passive, or responsive, or is it tremulous, sweaty, or cold?

Fear of Touching

Often a nurse will touch in a condescending way (a pat on the head or a tweak of the toe) or in a circumscribed nursing treatment. Of all health care professionals, nurses have the most frequent opportunities to provide gentle, reassuring, renewing touch. The intimacy of the nurse-patient contacts may influence a nurse to be overly circumspect. However, the use of touch involves risk and may be misinterpreted by the nurse or patient. Stirring sexual feelings, if that is a response to gentle touching, is a human response and need not frighten. Older men and women have stated they miss the touching and holding of their earlier lives. These older adults may seek such comfort by sexually provocative behaviors. Nurses need not encourage such overt behavior but must be cognizant of the underlying needs of intimacy.

Nurses sometimes respond negatively to a breach in the "status" of touch. A status system of touch exists that is significant to health care. A person of higher status may touch an individual of an inferior status, but the reverse is discouraged. Similarly, name familiarity may be used by an individual in a superior position but is greatly resented if the lower-ranking person presumes the same liberty. Because this notion is embedded in many hierarchical structures, treating everyone with respect regarding their name and propensity for touch is prudent. Instant familiarity is seldom useful. It should not be surprising when a patient reciprocates with the same level of intimacy as the nurse initiates. Therapeutic, caring touch by the nurse is a potent healing intervention. It is important that touching be done with respect regarding the person's comfort and with the nurse's intention of providing a comforting and healing modality within the nurse-patient relationship.

Touch Zones

Hall (1969) identifies different categories of touching—expanding or contracting zones around which every individual extends the sensory experience of touching, smelling, hearing, and seeing. Entering the zone of intimacy, which is identified as being in an area within an arm's length of the individual's body and is the space used for comforting, protecting, and lovemaking, is part of the nurse's function (Figure 19-1). Illness, confinement, and dependency seen in institutionalization are stresses on the intimate zone of touch. Just as caregivers enter a room without knocking, so they often intrude into the intimate circle of touch without asking. A person's need for privacy and personal space is

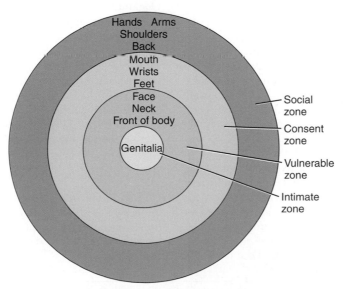

FIGURE 19-1 Zones of intimacy or sexuality.

strongly related to acceptance and response to touch (Buschmann et al., 1999). If the need for privacy and distance is great, touch should be used judiciously. The parameters of the intimate zone of touch are examined in this chapter to emphasize the importance of understanding behavior that might occur when the nurse enters this arena.

The social zone includes the areas of the body that are the least sensitive or embarrassing to be touched and that do not necessarily require permission to be handled. The consent zone requires the nurse to seek out or ask permission to touch or initiate procedures to these areas. The vulnerable zone is highly sexually charged and will be protected. The most intimate area, the genitalia, is the most personally protected area of the body and causes the most stress and anxiety when approached, touched, and viewed by the caregiver.

Touch Deprivation

Montagu (1986) noted that "tactile hunger" becomes more powerful in old age when other sensuous experiences are diminished and direct sexual expression is often no longer possible or available. Furthermore, Montagu believes the cause of illness may be greatly influenced by the quality of tactile support received. Do older people suffer touch deprivation? Many elders do if they are separated from caring others. Older men, in particular, may find it hard to reach out to others for comforting and caring touch. The previous lifestyles of these men often discouraged touch, except in the intimacy of sexual contact, which may no longer be available to them (Montagu, 1986). Older women are allowed

considerably more freedom to touch, although they may lack the opportunity.

In the cases of the isolated or institutionalized older person, higher death rates are more related to the quality of human relationships than they are to the degree of cleanliness, nutrition, and physical disabilities on which we focus. Sansone and Schmitt (2000) noted that older people in nursing homes experience touch every day as they are bathed, dressed, toileted, fed, and positioned. The type of touch they desire is not task-oriented touch but "gentle, patient, conscious touch of another person that says to them, 'I'm here, I care, you are important to me.' It's the kind of touch that goes beyond routine and bonds one human being with another" (p. 304).

Adaptation to Touch Deprivation. People can survive extreme sensory deprivation as long as the sensory experiences of the skin are maintained. An outstanding feature of touch according to Ackerman (1995) is that it does not have to be performed by a person or other living thing. Some sustenance or peace for the old may be gained from the self-contained stimulation of a rocking chair or slowly stroking an animal's fur or wearing something that provides sensory stimulation. Thayer (1982) describes these activities as *self-adapters*.

Music, perceived through the skin as well as the ears, may be another source of touch stimulation that is self-induced. Skin touched by the vibrations of music is enveloped and caressed. Music and dancing seem to be two important mechanisms of enjoyment of older people. In later years,

---

BOX 19-1	**Evidence-Based Practice:** Pilot Study to Test the Effectiveness of Healing Touch on Agitation in People with Dementia

PURPOSE

The purpose of this pilot study was to assess the effectiveness of Healing Touch (HT) in lowering agitation levels of residents with dementia.

SAMPLE/SETTING

A Dementia Special Care Unit, an 18-bed secured unit, at the Veterans Affairs Medical Center in Prescott, Arizona, was the site for the study. Fourteen male residents with similar average scores on the Cohen-Mansfield Agitation Inventory were placed in either a control group (8) (receiving usual care) or a treatment group (6) (receiving HT).

METHOD

A Healing Touch Practitioner used 2 HT techniques (unruffling and modified mind clearance) for 10 minutes daily for 4 weeks with the treatment group. Mean agitation scores using the Cohen-Mansfield Agitation Inventory and t tests were used for data analysis. Qualitative results were obtained from a data sheet which the Healing Touch Practitioner used to record her observations and comments from the participants. Data on use of psychotropic medication use were also obtained.

RESULTS

HT significantly lowered the frequency of agitation behaviors in male dementia residents exhibiting higher agitation scores. Qualitative comments from the participants included feelings of relaxation, enjoyment. Five of six residents in the treatment group who were receiving psychotropic medications had dose reductions during the intervention, and two of the six had dose increases within the first 2 weeks after the HT interventions were stopped. The small sample size limits the inferences from the study and the placebo effect is also to be considered since the participants received extra attention as a result of the HT treatment. Another limiting variable is that all participants were men and the HT practitioner was a woman.

IMPLICATIONS

HT may be an effective intervention to reduce agitation levels in persons with dementia. Further study is indicated and should include larger and more gender diverse sample sizes, longer time periods, and comparison to other types of placebo treatments.

Data from Wang K, Hermann C: Pilot study to test the effectiveness of Healing Touch on agitation in people with dementia, *Geriatr Nurs* 27(1):34-40, 2006.

older adults often return to dancing after decades of ignoring the pleasurable activity. Perhaps this desire is a response to the need for more touch.

Therapeutic Touch

Touch is a powerful healer and a therapeutic tool that nurses can use to satisfy "touch hunger" of older people. Nursing has recognized the importance of touch and has the social sanctions to touch the body in the intimate and personal care of a person, an opportunity too often not fully used for the betterment of the older person's adaptation to environment and location in time and space. Touch can serve as a means of providing sensory stimulation, reducing anxiety, relieving physical and psychological pain, and comforting the dying, as well as sexual expression.

Kreiger's experiments with therapeutic touch (1975) demonstrate physiological and psychological improvement in patients who are exposed to consistent "doses" of touch. "Hands-on healing and energy based interventions have been found in cultures throughout history, dating back at least 5000 years" (Wang and Hermann, 2006, p. 34). "Laying on of the hands" and the power of touch to heal had largely disappeared with the scientific revolution. The phenomenon has reemerged as healing touch and therapeutic touch movements. A growing body of research supports the healing power of touch, and *Energy Field, Disturbed* is an approved nursing diagnosis (Wang and Hermann, 2006, p. 34). Many nurses have learned how to perform therapeutic and healing touch and use these modalities in their practice with people of all ages. Positive outcomes of interventions utilizing touch in nursing homes, particularly with people with dementia and agitated behaviors, have been reported (Kim and Buschmann, 2004; Kolcaba et al., 2006; Remington, 2002; Sansone and Schmitt, 2000; Snyder and Burns, 1995; Wang and Hermann, 2006; Woods et al., 2005) (Box 19-1).

Research has demonstrated the positive effects of massage with acutely ill and dying patients, as well as patients in rehabilitation settings (Holland and Pokorny, 2001; Sansone and Schmitt, 2000). Massage stimulates circulation, dilates blood vessels, relaxes tense muscles, and cleans toxins out of the body through the flow of lymph. Pain relief, improved sleeping patterns, lower blood pressure, reduced stress hormone levels, and increased appetite have also been associated with massage (Roberson, 2003). "The psychosocial benefits of massage include mental and tactile stimulation, unconditional one-on-one attention, nurturing, companionship and pleasure" (Sansone and Schmitt, 2000, p. 304). Further research on the use of touch with older people is needed. Touch is a powerful tool to promote comfort and well-being when working with elders.

INTIMACY

Although intimacy is often thought of in the context of sexual performance, it encompasses more than sexuality and includes five major relational components: commitment, affective intimacy, cognitive intimacy, physical intimacy, and interdependence (Blieszner and deVries, 2001; Troll, 2001; Youngkin, 2004). "Intimacy is from a Greek work meaning 'closest to; inner lining of blood vessels'" (Steinke, 2005, p. 40). It is a warm, meaningful feeling of joy. Intimacy includes the need for close friendships; relationships with family, friends, and formal caregivers; spiritual connections, knowing that one matters in someone else's life, and the ability to form satisfying social relationships with others (Blieszner and deVries, 2001; Piercy, 2001; Ramsey, 2001; Steinke, 2005).

Youngkin (2004) points out that older people may be concerned about changes in sexual intimacy but (p. 46):

> …social relationships with people important in their lives, the ability to interact intellectually with people who share similar interests, the supportive love that grows between human beings (whether romantic or platonic), and physical nonsexual intimacy are equally—and in many instances more—important than the physical intimacy of direct sexual relations. All of these facets of intimate life are integrally woven into the fabric of aging, along with other influences that can make life rewarding.

Intimacy needs change over time with others, but the need for intimacy and satisfying social relationships is an important component of successful aging (Steinke, 2005).

SEXUALITY

As a major aspect of intimacy, sexuality includes the physical act of intercourse, as well as many other types of intimate activity. It includes components such as sexual desire, activity, attitudes, body image, and gender-role activity (Zeiss and Kasl-Godley, 2001). Sexuality provides the opportunity to express passion, affection, admiration, and loyalty. It can also enhance personal growth and communication. Sexuality also allows a general affirmation of life (especially joy) and a continuing opportunity to search for new growth and experience (Butler and Lewis, 2002; Lewis, 1995).

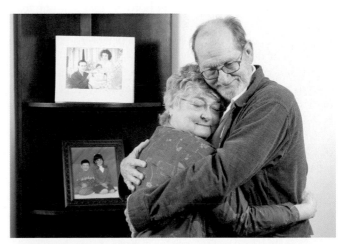

Love and affection are important to older persons. (From Sorrentino SA, Gorek B: *Mosby's textbook for long-term care assistants,* ed 5, St Louis, 2007, Mosby.)

NURSE CREDENTIALLING PROGRAMS
HEALTH SCIENCES DIVISION

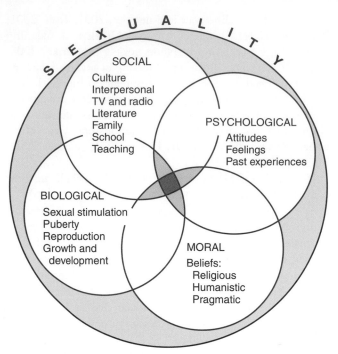

FIGURE 19-2 Interrelationship of dimensions of sexuality.

Sexuality, similar to food and water, is a basic human need, yet it goes beyond the biological realm to include psychological, social, and moral dimensions. The constant interaction among these spheres of sexuality work to produce harmony. The linkage of the four dimensions composes the holistic quality of an individual's sexuality.

The social sphere of sexuality is the sum of cultural factors that influence the individual's thoughts and actions related to interpersonal relationships, as well as sexuality related to ideas and learned behavior. Television, radio, literature, and the more traditional sources of family, school, and religious teachings combine to influence social sexuality. The belief of that which constitutes masculine and feminine is deeply rooted in the individual's exposure to cultural factors.

The psychological domain of sexuality reflects a person's attitudes, feelings toward self and others, and learning from experiences. Beginning with birth, the individual is bombarded with cues and signals of how a person should act and think about the use of "dirty words" or body parts. Conversation is self-censored in the presence of or in discussion with certain people. The moral aspect of sexuality, the "I should" or "I shouldn't," makes a difference that is based in religious beliefs or in a pragmatic or humanistic outlook.

The final dimension, biological sexuality, is reflected in physiological responses to sexual stimulation, reproduction, puberty, and growth and development. Because of the interrelatedness, these dimensions affect each other directly or indirectly whenever an aspect of sexuality is out of harmony. Figure 19-2 illustrates the interrelationship of the sexuality dimensions.

Sexuality is a vital aspect to consider in the care of the older person regardless of the setting. Sexuality exists throughout life in one form or another in everyone. All older people have a need to express sexual feelings, whether the individuals are healthy and active or frail. Sexuality is linked with the person's personality and identity and has a significant role in promoting better life adaptation (Billhorn, 1994; Butler and Lewis, 2002; Wiley and Bortz, 1996). Sexuality can be envisioned as part of Maslow's Hierarchy of Needs, with physical reproduction the lowest level and a progression to the higher levels with increased communication, trust, sharing, and pleasure with or without a physical action. Figure 19-3 focuses on the hierarchy of sexuality.

Acceptance and Companionship

Sexuality validates the lifelong need to share intimacy and have that offering appreciated. Sexuality is love, warmth, sharing, and touching between people, not just the physical act of coitus. Margot Benary-Isbert in her book "The Vintage Years" (1968) expresses the essence of sexuality most eloquently (p. 200):

> Let us not forget old married couples who once shared healthy and happy days as they now share the unavoidable limitations of old age and grow even closer together in love and patience. When they exchange a smile, a glance, one can guess that they still think each other beautiful and loveable.

Benary-Isbert continues "...as long as we live with our companion all these seem worthwhile because each one desires to make life as easy as possible for the other" (Benary-Isbert, 1968, pp. 201-202). The Hite report (Hite, 1977) identified touching at night, listening to the breathing and the heart beat, and open talking that occur in bed as important features of sexuality expressed by older women; a study by Nay (1992) confirms this contention. Berlin concludes: "Sexuality can mean anything which gives sexual or emotional pleasure, excitement, or comfort" (1978, p. 2).

Femininity and Masculinity

Males and females possess characteristic behavioral traits, which Jung refers to as the *anima* (female) and *animus* (male). Past social pressures did not often allow the appearance of sensitivity, gentleness, and sentimentality in most men. Men were expected to be strong, to be in control of situations, and to handle their emotions. On the other hand, women were not viewed as aggressive or the major decision makers.

Often seen and perpetuated among older adults are socially accepted standards characteristic of masculine and feminine behavior, which reflect male and female role models dominant in their formative years. Jung's work has shown this view to be so, indicating that strong attitude types (male and female) and roles and functions associated with these attitudes are developed as adaptations of the person to the demands of the environment.

Man believed that repressing his feminine traits was virtuous; and woman, until recently, repressed her animus. Both men and women, however, are not consciously aware that they possess the opposite sexual identity. Goldblatt (1972) contends that neither gonads nor chromosomal sex is a determinant of sexual behavior. Money and Tucker

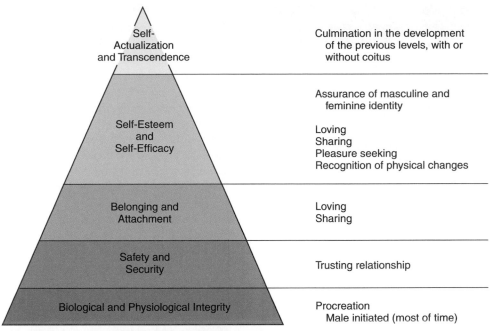

FIGURE 19-3 Progression of sexual emphasis through life.

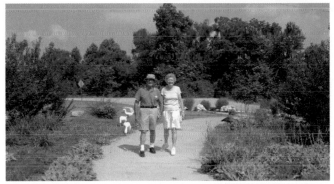

Older couples enjoy love and companionship. (From Monahan F et al: *Phipps' medical-surgical nursing: health and illness perspectives,* ed 8, St Louis, 2006, Mosby.)

(1975) in their work "Sexual Signatures" believe that social stimulation provides gender identity and limits the individual's concept of self. In essence, society expects men to be men and women to be women.

In the later part of life, self-knowledge deepens. People tend to discover traits in their nature that were previously suppressed or heretofore remained in the unconscious. At this time, the emergence of the anima (in men) and animus (in women) may be seen. Jung identified this experience as the expression of the psyche that in the first half of life was turned inward. In late life, directed outward, this expression becomes indicative of the capacity for fuller living. Men become more comfortable with tenderness, "more dependent on the marriage for their sense of well-being, and more willing to accommodate for the sake of preserving peace" (Huyck, 2001, p. 11). Women become more assertive and self-confident. The person's ability to accord his or her other nature its due recognition will enhance sexuality.

SEXUAL HEALTH

The World Health Organization defines sexual health as "the integration of somatic, emotional, intellectual, and social aspects of sexual being, in ways that are positively enriching and that enhance personality, communication, and love" (Woods, 1979, p. 75). According to Maddocks (1975) and Denny and Quadango (1992), sexual health is a realistic phenomenon that includes four components: personal and social behaviors in agreement with individual gender identity, comfort with a range of sexual role behaviors and engagement in effective interpersonal relations with both sexes in a love or long-term commitment, response to erotic stimulation that produces positive and pleasurable sexual activity, and the ability to make mature judgments about sexual behavior congruent with one's beliefs and values.

These interpretations speak of the multifaceted nature of the biological, psychosocial, cultural, and spiritual components of sexuality and imply that sexual behavior is the capacity to enhance self and others. Sexual health is individually defined and wholesome if it leads to intimacy (not necessarily coitus) and enriches the involved parties.

Expectations

A large number of cultural, biological, psychosocial, and environmental factors influence the sexual behavior of older adults. The older person may be confronted with barriers to the expression of their sexuality by reflected attitudes, health, culture, economics, opportunity, and historic trends (Butler and Lewis, 2002).

Factors affecting a person's attitudes on intimacy and sexuality include family dynamics and upbringing and cultural and religious beliefs (Youngkin, 2004). Older people often internalize the broad cultural proscriptions of sexual

BOX 19-2   Sexuality and Aging Women: Common Myths
• Masturbation is an immature activity of youngsters and adolescents, not older women.   • Sexual prowess and desire wane during the climacteric, and menopause is the death of a woman's sexuality.   • Hysterectomy creates a physical disability that results in the inability to function sexually.   • Sex has no role in the lives of the elderly, except as perversion or remembrance of times past.   • Sexual expression in old age is taboo.   • The elderly are too old and frail to engage in sex.   • The young are considered lusty and virile; the elderly are considered lecherous.   • Sex is unimportant or over.   • Elderly women do not wish to discuss their sexuality with professionals.

Adapted from Morrison-Beedy D, Robbins L: Sexual assessment and the aging female, *Nurs Pract* 14(12):35, 1989.

behavior in late life that hinder the continuance of sexual expression. Much sexual behavior stems from incorporating other people's reactions. Jarvik and Small (1988) and Butler and Lewis (1990) indicate that older people do not feel old until they are faced with the fact that others around them consider them old. Similarly, older adults do not feel asexual until they are continually treated as such. American society continues to struggle with open acceptance of sexual expression for the young but continues to remain hostile to the attempts of older people to do the same. Sexual interest and activity in the elderly are sometimes regarded as deviant behavior and described in such terms as "dirty old man," "lecher," and "old biddy." The same activity attempted by a younger person would be viewed as appropriate. An often quoted statement by Alex Comfort (1974) sums it up nicely: "In our experiences, old folks stop having sex for the same reasons they stop riding a bicycle—general infirmity, thinking it looks ridiculous, no bicycle." Box 19-2 presents some of the myths about sexuality in older people that may be held by older people themselves and by society in general.

Redefinitions

Sexuality in the older person shifts its focus from procreation to an emphasis on companionship, physical nearness, intimate communication, and a pleasure-seeking physical relationship. Some researchers have coined the phrase "from procreation to recreation," which refers to this change in sexual emphasis. This redefinition of sexuality within Maslow's hierarchical framework simply means the most basic level of function might be male-initiated sex for the purpose of reproduction, and the more complex levels involve a relationship of greater communication, trust, love, sharing, and the giving of pleasure with or without coitus.

Activity Levels

For both heterosexual and homosexual individuals, research supports that (Zeiss and Kasl-Godfrey, 2001, p. 20):

> ...liberal and positive attitudes toward sexuality, greater sexual knowledge, satisfaction with a long-term relationship or a current intimate relationship, good social networks, psychological well-being, and a sense of self-worth are associated with greater sexual interest, activity and satisfaction.

Both early studies of sexual behavior in older adults and more recent ones indicate that men and women remain sexually active and find their sexual lives satisfying. The National Council on Aging (NCOA) publication "Sex After 60: A Natural Part Of Life" says "an active sex life may be as normal a part of aging as having grandchildren." According to the NCOA survey of 1300 older Americans, almost half of older people surveyed are sexually active (having intercourse at least once a month) and find sex equal to or more satisfying than it was in their 40s. Men were more than twice as likely as women to report wanting sex more often, and this was true in all age segments, even in men ages 80 years and older. Men are more sexually active than women, most likely because women live longer and may not have a partner (National Council on Aging [NCOA], 2006).

Even though many older women retain a strong drive, the population imbalance of the sexes limits opportunity to be sexually active. Older women outnumber older men and thus have fewer opportunities. Statistics show that by the age of 85 years, there are 83 men for every 100 women in the United States (Butler and Lewis, 2002). Older women may feel that having a new relationship (inside or outside of marriage) is unacceptable after being widowed or divorced or that it is abnormal to have a continued interest in sexual activity (Zeiss and Kasl-Godley, 2001). Also, older women have been viewed by themselves and society (Burke and Knowlton, 1992; Nay, 1992) as sexually unattractive.

Although her sample of older women was a small segment of the total study, Hite (1977) helps emphasize that sexuality and the capacity to experience sexual pleasure are lifetime attributes for women. A septuagenarian commented, "At my age and without responsibility I do not want matrimony but I have a continuing sex drive which keeps me looking 15 to 20 years younger than my chronological age" (p. 509).

Cohort and Cultural Influences

The era in which a person was born influences attitudes about sexuality (Youngkin, 2004). Women in their 80s today may have been strongly influenced by the prudish, Victorian atmosphere of their youth and may have experienced difficult marital adjustments and serious sexual problems early in their marriages. Sexuality was not openly expressed or discussed. The next generation of older people ("baby boomers") has experienced other influences, including more liberal attitudes toward sexuality, the women's movement, a higher number of divorced adults, the human immunodeficiency virus (HIV) epidemic, and increased numbers of gay and lesbian couples, that will affect their views and attitudes as they age. The boomers and beyond, as they find themselves experiencing sexuality beyond the age they had assigned to their elders, may alter current perceptions.

Most of what is known about sexuality in aging has been gained through research with well-educated, healthy, white older adults. Further research is needed among culturally, socially, and ethnically diverse older people, those with chronic illness, and gay, lesbian, and bisexual older people (Zeiss and Kasl-Godley, 2001). It is important to come to know and understand the older person within his or her social and cultural background and not make judgments based on one's own belief system.

Alternative Sexual Lifestyles: Lesbian, Gay, Bisexual, and Transgender

Estimates suggest that between 1 and 3 million gay and lesbian individuals older than 60 years are in the United States (Agronin, 2004). Gay and lesbian older people face the "double stigma" of being both old and homosexual, with lesbians facing the triple threat of being women, elderly, and having a different sexual orientation (Agronin, 2004; Deevey, 1990). Whereas discrimination in health and social systems affects gays and lesbians of all ages, gay and lesbian elders may be even more at risk for discrimination as a result of life-long experiences with marginalization and oppression. They are "less likely to seek out health services or identify themselves as gay or lesbian to health care providers" (Brotman et al., 2003, p. 172).

Knowledge is lacking about aging lesbian, gay, bisexual, and transgender (LGBT) individuals. Reasons for this include difficulties in studying the LGBT population because of problems with definition, differences in self-identification, societal attitudes, and a lack of support for research with this population (Blando, 2001). Research has been conducted primarily with middle-class white gay men and lesbians in urban areas (Blando, 2001). As a result of invisibility and discrimination, the needs of gay and lesbian elders and their families receive limited recognition in health and social services (Brotman et al., 2003). Even less is known about bisexual and transgender older people.

Older gay men and lesbians are as diverse as the remainder of the heterosexual elder population. Many gay men and lesbians age successfully, are healthy, and are active with satisfied lives. Some gay and lesbian people are coupled, have children, and are open about their sexual orientation, and some are not. Some of these individuals have only recently "come out"; others have been "out" most of their lives; and some find themselves isolated in the larger society. Older gays and lesbians are more likely to have kept their relationships hidden than those who grew up in the modern day gay liberation movement (Brotman et al., 2003). In the limited research available, a considerable proportion of gay men and lesbians are in long-term relationships, countering the stereotype they are alone and lonely (Blando, 2001). Information about the older homosexual continues to be limited except for the major works by Berger, "Gay and

Gray: The Older Homosexual Man," (1995) and Kehoe's study of lesbians (1988), which provides major insight into the lifestyles of gay males and lesbians.

Older lesbians have been labeled the "invisible minority" (Hooyman and Kiyak, 2005, p. 268). These women tend to keep a very low profile, although conservative estimates are that over 2 million now reside in the United States, preferring rural settings, whereas gay men prefer urban areas. An interesting note is that approximately one third of the lesbians "come out" after the age of 50 years. Most lesbians married, raised children, divorced, and lead double lives (Butler and Lewis, 2002).

An intensive study of 100 lesbians between 60 and 86 years of age found that most lived alone, were retired from helping professions, and had college or advanced degrees. Eighty-four percent felt positive about being lesbian, and almost one half had, at one time, been married. The majority desired special senior centers or retirement communities for lesbians (Kehoe, 1988). More recent studies reported that lesbians are comfortable with their sexual orientation and have a positive self-image and feelings about being identified as a lesbian (Hooyman and Kiyak, 2005; Jones and Nystrom, 2002; Martin and Lyon, 2001; Wojciechowski, 1998). According to Hooyman and Kiyak (2005, p. 269):

> Most lesbians remain sexually active, although sexual frequency generally declines. The extent to which sexual activity is considered to be an integral part of a lesbian relationship varies, although sexuality in a broader sense continues to play an important role in their lives. For some, lesbianism is a wider female interdependence and sense of positive self-identity rather than a sexual relationship as such.

Younger gay men have been found to have had multiple liaisons, but the number of gay men with partners does increase with age, peaking among those 46 to 55 years old. However, with the impact of acquired immunodeficiency syndrome (AIDS) on this population, a decrease in multiple liaisons has become evident. "Older gay men are more likely to be in long-term relationships (average length 10 years) or none at all rather than in short-term relationships" (Hooyman and Kiyak, 2005, p. 269). After age 60 years, the percent of gay men in relationships decreases. The situation has been attributed to several factors, for example, the death of a loved one and rejection of the idea of a single lifelong partner.

Health care providers lack sufficient information and sensitivity when caring for older LGBTs. This sensitivity is of utmost importance when attempting to obtain a health history. Using open-ended questions such as "Who is most important to you?" or "Do you have a significant other?" is much better than asking "Are you married?" This form of the question allows the nurse to look beyond the rigid category of family. Euphemisms are frequently used for a life partner (roommate, close friend). Asking individuals if they consider themselves as primarily heterosexual, homosexual, or bisexual is also better. This question conveys recognition of sexual variety. An older lesbian woman in a health care situation may refer to herself indirectly by saying "people like us." Nurses need to become more aware of these nuances and try to understand the fear of discovery that is apparent in the older gay man and lesbian woman. These elders are of a generation in which they were and may still be closeted because of the homophobic experiences they had through their younger years.

Better support and care services for gays and lesbians by care providers should include working through homophobic attitudes and discomfort discussing sexuality, learning about special issues facing older gay men and lesbians, and becoming aware of the gay and lesbian resources in the community. LGBT elders living in metropolitan areas may find organizations particularly designed for them, such as Senior Action in a Gay Environment (SAGE), (SAGE-Net is now in nine states and Ontario, Canada); New Leaf Outreach to Elders (formerly GLOE, San Francisco); Rainbow Project (Los Ange-

les); Gay and Lesbians Older and Wiser (GLOW, Ann Arbor, Mich.); and the Lesbian and Gay Aging Issues Network (LGAIN). Other resources are listed in the Resources section at the end of this chapter. Finally, facilities or agencies already in the community need to be assessed from the perspective of the client, patient, or resident who may be gay or lesbian. Programs to increase awareness of the needs of LGBT elders and reduce discrimination are necessary (Brotman et al, 2003).

Research regarding the subject of LGBTs among older adults is needed because so little is known about these elders. The Gerontological Society of America has established a research interest group, Rainbow Research, devoted to issues of older LGBT individuals. The American Society on Aging Lesbian and Gay Issues Network also addresses concerns of LBGT elders (see the Resources section at the end of this chapter). Chapter 20 also provides further discussion of relationship and family issues of elder LGBT individuals.

TABLE 19-1
Physical Changes in Sexual Responses in Old Age

Female	Male
EXCITATION PHASE	
Diminished or delayed lubrication (1-3 min may be required for adequate amounts to appear)	Less intense and slower erection (but can be maintained longer without ejaculation)
Diminished flattening and separation of labia majora	Increased difficulty regaining an erection if lost
Disappearance of elevation of labia majora	Less vasocongestion of scrotal sac
Decreased vasocongestion of labia minora	Less pronounced elevation and congestion of testicles
Decreased elastic expansion of vagina (depth and breadth)	
Breasts not as engorged	
Sex flush absent	
PLATEAU PHASE	
Slower and less prominent uterine elevation or tenting	Decreased muscle tension
Nipple erection and sexual flush less often	No color change at coronal edge of penis
Decreased capacity for vasocongestion	Slower penile erection pattern
Decreased areolar engorgement	Delayed or diminished erectal and testicular elevation
Labial color change less evident	
Less intense swelling or orgasmic platform	
Less sexual flush	
Decreased secretions of Bartholin glands	
ORGASMIC PHASE	
Fewer number and less intense orgasmic contractions	Decreased or absent secretory activity (lubrication) by Cowper gland before ejaculation
Rectal sphincter contraction with severe tension only	Fewer penile contractions
	Fewer rectal sphincter contractions
	Decreased force of ejaculation (approximately 50%) with decreased amount of semen (if ejaculation is long, seepage of semen occurs)
RESOLUTION PHASE	
Observably slower loss of nipple erection	Vasocongestion of nipples and scrotum slowly subsides
Vasocongestion of clitoris and orgasmic platform	Very rapid loss of erection and descent of testicles shortly after ejaculation
	Refractory time extended (time required before another erection ranges from several to 24 hours, occasionally longer)

Data compiled from Miller CA: *Nursing care of older adults,* Glenview, Ill, 1990, Scott Foresman/Little Brown, Higher Education; Saxon SV, Etten MJ: *Physical changes and aging,* ed 3, New York, 1994, Tiresias Press; Shippee-Rice R: Sexuality and aging. In Fogel C, Lauver D, editors: *Sexual health promotion,* Philadelphia, 1990, Saunders.

Biological Changes with Age

Acknowledgement and understanding of the age changes that influence coitus may partially explain alteration in sexual behavior to accommodate these changes and facilitate continued pleasurable sex (see Chapter 4). Characteristic physiological changes during the sexual response cycle do occur with aging, but these vary from individual to individual depending on general health factors. The "use it or lose it" phenomenon also applies here: the more sexually active the person is, the fewer changes he or she is likely to experience in the pattern of sexual response. Illnesses and medications also affect sexual response. Physical alteration is one variable in the total picture of sexuality and is therefore included as one of the main factors that influence the act of intercourse. Many texts explain biological changes in depth. Table 19-1 summarizes physical changes in the sexual response cycle.

Older people who do not understand the physical changes that affect sexual activity become concerned that their sex life is approaching its natural conclusion with the onset of menopause or, for men, when they discover a change in the firmness of their erection or the decreased need for ejaculation with each orgasm or when the refractory period is extended between episodes of intercourse. A major nursing role is to provide information about these changes, as well as appropriate assessment and counseling within the context of the individual's needs. Assessment and interventions are discussed on p. 476.

SEXUAL DYSFUNCTION

Sexual dysfunction, which occurs in both men and women, has a physiological or psychological base or a combination of both. Psychological dysfunction is more common than physical impairment (Butler and Lewis, 2002; Ham, 2002). A major problem confronting older men is the fear of or the actual occurrence of impotence, now called *erectile dysfunction (ED)*. What men generally call *impotence* is diminished potency and frequency of sexual activity. Impotence, according to Ham (2002), is a psychogenic or organic pathological condition that has its origins in excessive use of alcohol, preoccupation with work problems, monotony in the relationship, anger, fatigue, or neurological or vascular conditions. Sexual dysfunction in women has not been accorded the same intensive research as has dysfunction in men even though it is as much a quality-of-life issue as it is in men.

Male Dysfunction

Impotence (ED) is defined as the inability to achieve and sustain an erection sufficient for satisfactory sexual intercourse in at least 50% or more attempts. ED has become recognized as a common problem among men older than 50 years (Butler and Lewis, 2000; Moon, 2000). Until recently, ED had been a neglected area of health that is fraught with myths and superstition. ED transiently occurs to men of all ages at least once in their life; however, the prevalence of ED

BOX 19-3   Causes of Erectile Dysfunction

- Vascular problems
- Endocrine problems
- Neurological problems
- Structural abnormalities of the penis
- Depression
- Zinc deficiency
- Alcoholism
- Diabetes mellitus
- Medications
- Psychological problems

Compiled from Buczny B: Impotence: the problem men don't talk about, *J Gerontol Nurs* 18(5):25, 1992; Butler R, Lewis M: *The new love and sex after 60,* New York, 2002, Ballantine Books; Gerchafsky M: Impotence in older men: a newly recognized problem, *Adv Nurse Pract* 3(3):13, 1995.

---

increases with age, with estimates that 50% of men ages 40 to 70 years and nearly 70% of those ages 70 years and older experience ED (Agronin, 2004).

For most older men, ED is caused by an underlying medical diagnosis. Nearly one third of ED is a complication of diabetes. Alcoholism, medications, depression, and prostate cancer and treatment are also causes of ED in older men. An erection is governed by the interaction among the hormonal, vascular, and nervous systems. A problem in any of these systems can cause ED. Of course, multiple causes exist for this problem in older men (Box 19-3). Various medications that affect the sympathetic and parasympathetic nervous system interfere with the man's capacity to have an erection or to ejaculate. Adrenergic agents block impulses that affect contractility of the prostate gland and seminal vesicles and depress or interfere with ejaculation. The anticholinergic preparations affect penis erection by vasocongestion in the venous channels. The ganglionic blocking agents possess properties of both the adrenergic and anticholinergic preparations and affect both penis erection and ejaculation (Butler and Lewis, 2002). A few medications have been found to increase sexual desire. The phenothiazines and testosterone increase the libido in the older woman, and L-dopa heightens sexual desire in the older man (Butler and Lewis, 2002).

Because of professional discomfort discussing sexuality or lack of knowledge about sexuality in older people, medications are often prescribed to both older men and women without attention to the sexual side effects. If medications that affect sexual function are necessary, adjustment of doses, use of alternative agents, and prescription of antidotes to reverse the sexual side effects are important (Agronin, 2004). Table 19-2 lists some medications that alter sexual function.

Most men who undergo surgical procedures such as transurethral resection and other types of prostatectomies, Y-V–plasty of the bladder neck, resection of the colon for cancer, or a sympathectomy may experience ED or have retrograde ejaculations caused by interference with autonomic innervation in the pelvis (Butler and Lewis, 2002).

TABLE 19-2
Drugs Adversely Affecting Sexuality

Drug Class	Example	Drug Effect on Sexuality
Dopamine agonists	Levodopa Requip Mirapex	Increased desire
Diuretics	Lasix Bumex Aldactone	Incontinence
Anticholinergics*	Detrol Reglan Benadryl Lasix	Impaired ejaculation
Antipsychotics	Risperdal Zyprexa	Inhibit erection Inhibit ability to ejaculate, even when the capacity for erection remains
Sedatives-hypnotics	Ambien Restoril	Depress sexual arousal
Antidepressants	Paxil Prozac	Inhibit sexual desire Lack of orgasm
Antihypertensives	HCTZ Aldactone Atenolol Clonidine Lisinopril Cardizem	Erectile dysfunction Incontinence Inhibition of orgasm
Alcohol		Erectile dysfunction Women's sexual function
Anxiolytics/Benzodiazepines	Ativan Xanax	Decreased sexual desire Inhibition of orgasm
Anticonvulsants	Dilantin Tegretol	Decreased desire Erectile dysfunction

From Meiner SE, Lueckenotte A: *Gerontologic nursing,* ed 3, St Louis, 2006, Mosby. Data from Messinger-Rapport B et al: Sex and sexuality: is it over after 60? *Clin Geriatr* 11(10):45-53, 2003; Nusbaum M et al: Chronic illness and sexual functioning, *Am Fam Phys* 67:347, 2003; Butler R, Lewis M: Sexuality. In Beers MH, Berkow R, editors: *The Merck manual of geriatrics,* ed 3, Whitehouse Station, NJ, 2000, Merck Research Laboratories.
*Many drugs have anticholinergic properties.

Particularly after a prostatectomy, a space remains where the enlarged prostate had been. The principle that fluid travels the path of least resistance applies here. At the point of ejaculation, the semen moves backward into the bladder rather than forward through increased resistance, which produces a retrograde, or dry, ejaculation. A lack of knowledge regarding this physiological change further convinces men that their sexual activity is over when, in fact, it is not. Erection can be attained and orgasmic pleasure achieved. Any surgery that involves the male perineum has a high risk of causing ED resulting from potential nerve damage in that area. Newer surgical procedures that spare the nerves may result in less effect on sexual functioning.

The use of phosphodiesterase inhibitors such as sildenafil (Viagra), vardenafil (Levitra), and tadalafil (Cialis) has revolutionized treatment for ED regardless of cause (Agro-

nin, 2004). Use of these medications to treat female arousal disorders has been inconclusive to date but they may be helpful for select women. Further research is needed and may lead to the development of better drug therapies for women (Mayer et al., 2005). Contraindications to the use of these medications include nitrate therapy, heart failure with low blood pressure, certain antihypertensive regimens, and other medications and cardiovascular conditions. See Chapter 12 for further discussion of contraindications and side effects. Before the availability of these medications, intracavernosal injections with the drugs *papaverine* and *phentolamine,* vasoactive agents that reduce resistance of arteriolar and cavernosal smooth muscle tissue of the penis, were used. Penile implants of the semirigid, adjustable-malleable, or hinged and inflatable types are available when impotence does not respond to other treatments or is irreversible. The hinged and inflatable types, which are inserted in the testicular area, are the most popular. Still evolving is penile revascularization surgery (the shifting of blood vessels to restore normal blood circulation to the penis). Candidates for this type of surgery are those with arteriosclerosis and other peripheral vascular conditions and those who have experienced trauma to the penis and surrounding area. This type of surgery requires extraordinary surgical skill and is only for men who meet the criteria of localized, identifiable lesions (Beers, 1995; Butler and Lewis, 2002).

Female Dysfunction

Female dysfunction is considered "persistent impediment to a person's normal pattern of sexual interest, response, or both" (Kaiser, 2000, p. 1174). Female sexual function can be influenced by factors such as culture, ethnicity, emotional state, age, and previous sexual experiences, as well as changes in sexual response with normal aging. For heterosexual women, frequency of intercourse depends more on the age, health, and sexual function of the partner or the availability of a partner rather than on their own sexual capacity. Dyspareunia occurs in one third of women older than 65 years, resulting from inadequate lubrication, irritation, dryness, atrophic vaginitis, and altered anatomical structure, as well as intromission (the altered angle of intercourse penetration). In many instances, using water-soluble lubricants such as K-Y, Astroglide, Slip, and HR lubricating jelly can resolve the difficulty. Vaginismus (a problem related to dyspareunia) is the involuntary, forceful, and painful spasms of the lower vaginal muscles caused by vaginal infection, vaginal mucosal irritation, and fear of losing control or being hurt during intercourse (Barnes, 2000; Butler and Lewis, 2002; Kaiser, 2000).

Women can experience arousal disorders resulting from drugs such as anticholinergics, antidepressants, and chemotherapeutic agents and from lack of lubrication from radiation, surgery, and stress. Orgasmic disorders also may result from drugs used to treat depression. Radiation to the pelvis is another factor in orgasmic dysfunction as is anorgasmia resulting from decreased libido. Unlike ED, studies of vascular insufficiency are less clear in women with sexual dysfunction. Prolapse of the uterus, rectoceles, and cystoceles can be surgically repaired to facilitate continued sexual activity. Urinary incontinence (UI) is another condition that may affect sexual activity for both men and women. Appropriate assessment and treatment are important because many causes of UI are treatable. (See Chapter 7 for a discussion of UI.)

INTIMACY AND CHRONIC ILLNESS

Chronic illnesses and their related treatments may bring many challenges to intimacy and sexual activity. Steinke (2005), in an excellent article discussing intimacy needs and chronic illness, suggests that although some research has been done on the effects of myocardial infarction on sexual function, less information is available for patients with heart failure, implantable cardioverter-defibrillators (ICDs), hypertension, arthritis, chronic pain, or chronic obstructive pulmonary disease (COPD).

Often, patients and their partners are given little or no information about the effect of illnesses on sexual activity or strategies to continue sexual activity within functional limitations. Timing of intercourse (mornings or when energy level is highest), oral or anal sex, masturbation, appropriate pain relief, and different sexual positions are all strategies that may assist in continued sexual activity (Table 19-3).

TABLE 19-3
Chronic Illness and Sexual Function: Effects and Interventions

Condition	Effects/Problems	Interventions
Arthritis	Pain, fatigue, limited motion Steroid therapy may decrease sexual interest or desire	Advise patient to perform sexual activity at time of day when less fatigued and most relaxed Suggest use of analgesics and other pain-relief methods before sexual activity Encourage use of relaxation techniques before sexual activity such as a warm bath or shower, application of hot packs to affected joints Advise patient to maintain optimum health through a balance of good nutrition, proper rest, and activity Suggest that he or she experiment with different positions, use pillows for comfort and support Recommend use of a vibrator if massage ability is limited Suggest use of water-soluble jelly for vaginal lubrication

Continued

TABLE 19-3

Chronic Illness and Sexual Function: Effects and Interventions—cont'd

Condition	Effects/Problems	Interventions
Cardiovascular disease	Most men have no change in physical effects on sexual function; one fourth may not return to pre–heart attack function; one fourth may not resume sexual activity Women do not experience sexual dysfunction after heart attack Fear of another heart attack or death during sex Shortness of breath	Encourage counseling on realistic restrictions that may be necessary Instruct patient and spouse on alternative positions to avoid strain Suggest that patient avoid large meals several hours before sex Advise patient to relax; plan medications for effectiveness during sex
Cerebrovascular accident (stroke)	Depression May or may not have sexual activity changes Often erectile disorders occur; decrease in frequency of intercourse and sexual relations Change in role and function of partners Decreased physical endurance, fatigue Mobility and sensory deficits Perceptual and visual deficits Communication deficit Cognitive and behavioral deficits Fear of relapse or sudden death	Encourage counseling Instruct patient to use alternative positions Suggest use of a vibrator if massage ability is limited Suggest use of pillows for positioning and support Suggest use of water-soluble jelly for lubrication Instruct patient to use alternative forms of sexual expression
Chronic obstructive pulmonary disease (COPD)	No direct impairment of sexual activity although affected by coughing, exertional dyspnea, positions, and activity intolerance Medications may lead to erectile difficulties	Encourage patient to plan sexual activity when energy is highest Instruct patient to use alternative positions Advise patient to plan sexual activity at time medications are most effective Suggest use of oxygen before, during, or after sex, depending on when it provides the most benefit
Diabetes	Sexual desire and interest unaffected Neuropathy and/or vascular damage may interfere with erectile ability. About 50% to 75% of men have erectile disorders; a small portion have retrograde ejaculation Some men regain function if diagnosis of diabetes is well accepted, if diabetes is well controlled, or both Women have less sexual desire and vaginal lubrication Decrease in orgasms/absence of orgasm can occur; less frequent sexual activity; local genital infections	Recommend possible candidates for penile prosthesis Instruct patient to use alternative forms of sexual expression Recommend immediate treatment of genital infections
Cancers		
Breast	No direct physical affect. There is a strong psychological effect: Loss of sexual desire Body-image change Depression Reaction of partner	Encourage individual or group counseling
Most other cancers	Men and women may lose sexual desire temporarily Men may have erectile dysfunction; dry ejaculation; retrograde ejaculation Women may have vaginal dryness, dyspareunia Both men and women may experience anxiety, depression, pain, nausea from chemotherapy, radiation, pelvic surgery, hormone therapy, nerve damage from pelvic surgery	

For individuals with cardiac conditions, manual stimulation (masturbation) may be an alternative that can be used early in the recovery period to maintain sexual function if the practice is not objectionable to the patient. Studies show that masturbation is less taxing on the heart and makes less oxygen demand. Although self-stimulation is steeped in myth and fear, masturbation is a common and healthy practice in late life. Individuals without partners or those whose spouses are ill or incapacitated find that masturbation is helpful. As children, today's older population was discouraged from practicing this pleasurable activity with stories of the evils of fondling a person's own genitals. Masturbation provides an avenue for resolution of sexual tensions, keeps sexual desire alive, maintains lubrication and muscle tone of the vagina, provides mild physical exercise, and preserves sexual function in individuals who have no other outlet for sexual activity and gratification of their sexual need (Butler and Lewis, 2002).

One couple who had long sustained a satisfactory sexual relationship was unable to imagine engaging in the alternative modes of sexual expression (cunnilingus, mutual masturbation, and repositioning) suggested when the wife developed severe osteoarthritis. The old gentleman brought the worn and dog-eared illustrative pamphlet back to the nurse in the health clinic. "She just won't go for it, nurse!" In such cases, the most well-meant advice may not be useful. To resolve such incompatible needs, the nurse may best counsel the most sexually active and liberal partner in ways to achieve orgasm while still remaining sexually comforting for the other partner.

Tabloski (2006) provides age-appropriate illustrations of coital positions for older people with cardiovascular disease that can be used in teaching. Steinke (2005) also provides specific suggestions and teaching plans that will be very useful for nurses working with older people for sexual counseling after myocardial infarction and for older people with CHF, COPD, ICDs, and hypertension.

FACTORS AFFECTING INTIMACY AND SEXUALITY IN LONG-TERM CARE FACILITIES

Environmental Factors

Environmental barriers result predominantly from the lack of privacy available to the older individual. Lack of privacy can occur when the older person lives with adult children. If a parent has a suitor in to visit, they may not have a place to go without other family members around. If the older person is in a nursing home, further barriers may be present including lack of privacy, absence of a suitable partner, and family and staff attitudes about the appropriateness of sexual activity. Research is needed on sexuality in nursing homes, but surveys suggest that a significant number of older people residing in nursing homes might choose to be sexually active if they would have privacy and an available partner (Messinger-Rapport et al., 2003). Intimacy and sexuality among nursing home residents include the opportunity to have not only coitus but also other forms of intimate expressions such as hugging, kissing, hand holding, and masturbation.

Nursing homes are required by federal regulation to allow married spouses to share a room if they desire, but no other requirements related to sexual activity in nursing homes exist (Messinger-Rapport et al., 2003). However, what about unmarried individuals in intimate relationships or gay and lesbian partners? In research with older gays and lesbians and their families (Brotman et al., 2003), participants reported being terrified of going into care facilities and having to hide their relationships or lose their partners and friends. One lesbian couple who had been living together for several decades were separated by health care professionals and family members who were not aware of the nature of their partnership. Another partner in a lesbian relationship changed her last name to her partner's so that they would be taken for sisters and put in the same room.

Wallace (2003a) noted the following:

> Addressing the continuing sexual needs of older residents of long-term care facilities is a highly needed and yet very difficult task to accomplish...despite the perceived difficulty among all involved, the sexual needs of older adults must be addressed with the same priority as nutrition, hydration, and other well-accepted needs.

The institutionalized older person has the same rights as noninstitutionalized elders have to engage in or abstain from sexual activity.

Privacy is a major issue in nursing homes that can prevent fulfillment of intimacy and sexual needs. Bauer (1999) in a study exploring nursing home caregivers' experiences of residents' sexuality reported that caregivers had an understanding of the right for privacy but varied considerably regarding this practice. Suggestions for providing privacy and an atmosphere accepting of sexual activity include the availability of a private room, not interrupting when doors are closed and sexual activity is taking place, allowing residents to have sexually explicit materials in their room, and providing adaptive equipment such as siderails or trapezes and double beds (Wallace, 2003a; Zeiss and Kasl-Godley, 2001). For safety, Wallace (2003a) suggests that a trusted staff member should be informed about the sexual activity and the call light should be within reach. In one facility where one of the authors (T.T.) worked, the staff would assist one of the female residents to be freshly showered, perfumed, and in a lovely nightgown when she and her partner wanted to have sexual relations.

Bauer (1999) also points out that privacy can be violated by sharing intimate information about the resident's life and activities with other caregivers or, worse, by laughing, joking, or teasing about the activity. Unless the information is essential to providing care to the resident, Bauer suggests that this is "mere gossip" (p. 40) and should be avoided. Staff education about sexuality (see the following discussion) may assist in promoting more comfort and respect.

Caregiver and Family Attitudes

Attitudes about intimacy and sexuality among nursing home staff and, often, family members may reflect general societal attitudes that older people do not have sexual needs or that sexual activity is inappropriate. Wallace (2003a) suggests that families may have difficulty understanding that their older relative may want to have a new relationship. Caregivers often view residents' sexual acts as problems rather than expressions of the need for love and intimacy. Reactions may include disapproval, discomfort, and embarrassment, and caregivers may explicitly or implicitly discourage or deny intimacy needs. A lack of knowledge about intimacy and sexuality in late life and a lack of knowledge in handling related issues are major reasons for staff reactions (Low et al., 2005; Zeiss and Kasl-Godley, 2001).

Staff, family, and resident education programs to promote awareness, provide education on sexuality and intimacy in late life, and discuss interventions to respond to residents' needs are important in long-term care settings. Education should include the opportunity to discuss personal feelings about sexuality, normal changes of aging, and the impact of diseases and medications on sexual function, as well as role playing and skill training in sexual assessment and intervention (Bauer, 1999; Low et al., 2005; Lyder, 1994; Skinner, 2000; Steinke, 2005; Wallace, 2003a; Zeiss and Kasl-Godley, 2001). The Hebrew Home for the Aged in Riverdale, New York, initiated model sexual policies in 1995 that have been used to develop a guide for long-term care facilities in developing sexual policies (*www.fhs.mcmaster.ca/mcah/cgec/toolkit.pdf*). Additional resources listed at the end of this chapter may also be helpful in education programs.

INTIMACY, SEXUALITY, AND DEMENTIA

Intimacy and sexuality remain important in the lives of persons with dementia and their partners throughout the illness. Intimacy and sexuality may "serve as a nonverbal form of communication and intimacy when other cognitive skills and functions have declined" (Agronin, 2004, p. 13). As dementia progresses, particularly in persons living in long-term care facilities, intimacy and sexuality issues may present challenges, especially regarding the impaired person's ability to consent to sexual activity (Agronin, 2004; Messinger-Rapport et al., 2003; Wallace, 2003a) and requires accurate assessment and documentation.

Determination of a cognitively impaired person's ability to consent to participation in a sexual activity involves concepts of voluntary participation, mental competence, and the understanding of the risks and benefits (Messinger-Rapport et al., 2003). It is important for the person to understand the potential physical risks but also the "psychological risks including risk of loss through transfer, death, or discharge of his or her partner" (Messinger-Rapport et al., 2003, p. 52). Resources and guidelines for determination of competent decision making for sexual activity in persons with cognitive impairment can be found in Davies et al. (1998);

Gordon and Sokolowski, 2004; Gwyther and Willer (2004); and Lichtenberg and Strzepek (1990); and at *www.fhs. mcmaster.ca/mcah/cgec/toolkit.pdf*.

Inappropriate sexual behavior such as exposing oneself, masturbating in public, or making inappropriate sexual advances or sexual comments may also occur in the nursing home setting and is most distressing to staff. Messinger-Rapport et al. (2003) suggest that these behaviors may be triggered by unmet intimacy needs. Encouraging family and friends to touch, hug, kiss, and hold hands when visiting may help to meet touch and intimacy needs and decrease inappropriate sexual behavior. Also, allowing the person to stroke a pet or hold a stuffed animal may be helpful. When sexually inappropriate behavior does occur, it should be assessed like any other behavior as to cause, precipitating factors, and response to interventions. Aggressive or violent behavior may require limit setting, working with the resident and family, providing for sexual expression in a nonharmful manner, and pharmacological treatment if indicated (Messinger-Rapport et al., 2003). Staff will need opportunities for discussion and assistance with interventions.

AIDS AND THE ELDERLY

Individuals ages 50 years and older account for 12% to 15% of AIDS cases in the United States. The number of AIDS cases in this age-group has increased 22% since 1991 (Older Americans and HIV, 2001). After leveling off in the late 1990s after the introduction of the highly active antiretroviral treatment (HAART), the number of individuals older than 50 years diagnosed with HIV/AIDS is rising again, particularly among the African-American and Latino populations. In the context of reporting HIV statistics, the Centers for Disease Control and Prevention (CDC) considers an *older adult* to be older than 50 years rather than the commonly used 65 years (Uphold et al., 2004). AIDS is rising faster among the older population than it is in those ages 24 years and younger. Women older than 60 years make up one of the fastest growing risk groups (Goodroad, 2003). The incidence of HIV in older people is expected to continue to increase "as more individuals become infected later in life and as those who were infected in early adulthood live longer" (Uphold et al., 2004, p. 16).

The compromised immune system of an older individual makes him or her even more susceptible to HIV or AIDS than a younger person. AIDS is not exclusively a young person's disease, but it is frequently underreported in the elderly because the symptoms of fatigue, weakness, weight loss, and anorexia are common to other elder disease conditions or may be attributed to "normal aging." In addition, the idea that elders are not sexually active limits physicians' and other care providers' objectivity to recognize HIV-AIDS as a possible diagnosis.

Contrary to popular belief, HIV-AIDS in the elderly population is not the result of blood transfusions alone nor is it confined to the homosexual population. Research shows that elders are sexually active and thus at risk for HIV-AIDS. In the state of Florida, 25% of all HIV cases occur in older heterosexuals (Older Americans and HIV, 2001). People older than 50 years were one-sixth as likely to use condoms during sex and one-fifth as likely to have been tested for HIV. Because procreation is not an issue with elders, they are least likely to use condoms. Responsible sexual behavior is a leading health indicator in *Healthy People 2010* and applies to young as well as older individuals. Lack of awareness about HIV in older people often results in late diagnosis and treatment. This is especially problematic for older people since HIV tends to progress faster in older persons (Older Americans and HIV, 2001).

Older women who are sexually active are at high risk for HIV-AIDS (and other sexually transmitted infections) from an infected partner, resulting in part from normal age changes of the vaginal tissue—a thinner, drier, friable vaginal lining. Older men may frequent prostitutes (a potentially high-risk group for HIV-AIDS). Gay men may increase their risk of HIV exposure after the death of a long-term mate by turning to a more available younger partner, who may have HIV. In general, elders lack adequate knowledge about HIV-AIDS and believe that HIV-AIDS "just does not happen in my generation." This view places elders at high risk for HIV and AIDS. Further, older people may have limited access to HIV tests and age-appropriate information.

Physicians do not usually ask sexually active elders about their sexual activity and health. Studies indicate that 40% of primary care physicians do not assess HIV risk in people older than 60 years (Older Americans and HIV, 2001). The U.S. Preventive Services Task Force (USPSTF) advises that all adults at high risk for HIV be screened. Box 19-4 presents high-risk factors for HIV. A study at the University of California, San Francisco, of 3200 predominantly heterosexual Americans older than 50 years found that approximately 10% had at least one risk factor for HIV infection. Assessment and screening for other sexually transmitted infections (gonorrhea, chlamydia, syphilis, trichomonas, human papillomavirus [HPV]) should also be a part of primary care for sexually active elders. If symptoms of another disease such as herpes arise, testing should occur as well.

AIDS in older adults has been called the "Great Imitator." In addition to the vague signs mentioned earlier, symptoms include dementia with increased neurological abnormalities and unexplained diffuse encephalopathy that is demonstrated in progressive and chronic dementia. Elders may be misdiagnosed as having Alzheimer's disease (AD) (Schuerman, 1994; Whipple and Scura, 1996) instead of AIDS—the actual problem. AIDS dementia is rapid in onset, as opposed to the slow, progressive decline associated with AD. Confusion and other cognitive difficulties may wax and wane. Aphasia, which is seen in AD, is usually absent in AIDS dementia. Extrapyramidal symptoms suggestive of parkinsonism may occur but without the tremors and ataxia. Leg tremors, peripheral neuropathy with progressive weakness, and a positive Babinski reflex may also be seen when diagnosing AIDS.

Other AIDS problems that the elder might exhibit include opportunistic infections, malignancies, *Pneumocystis carinii* pneumonia (PCP), tuberculosis, esophageal or recurrent genital candidiasis, toxoplasmosis, non-Hodgkin's lymphoma, Kaposi's sarcoma, or herpes zoster. Women may develop candidiasis or HPV infections as a first sign of AIDS (Butler and Lewis, 2002; Goodroad, 2003; Schuerman, 1994; Whipple and Scura, 1996). It should be remembered that conditions that persist or reoccur should be suspect for HIV-AIDS and that the elder should be tested given that the incubation period for AIDS may be as long as 10 years.

Elders need to understand that they are at high risk for HIV-AIDS. As of 1999, 78,000 people older than 50 years developed AIDS. This number is ten times that of the decade before. Educational materials and programs need to be developed that include information about what HIV-AIDS is and how it is and is not transmitted, the need to use condoms for protection when engaging in sexual activity, symptoms of which to be aware, and the treatments that are available. Physicians, nurse practitioners, and other health professionals need to become comfortable taking a complete sexual history and talking about sex with the elderly. In addition, the myth that elders do not engage in sexual activity must be put to rest. An innovative program in Broward County, Florida, the *Seniors HIV Intervention Project (SHIP)*, educates seniors as educators and peer counselors to deliver educational workshops on HIV/AIDS in churches, condominiums, and other community sites. Websites with specific information about HIV and older people that can be used in prevention and education can be found in the Resources section at the end of this chapter.

BOX 19-4 HIV: High-Risk Behaviors

- Men who have had sex with men after 1975
- Men and women reporting unprotected sex with multiple partners
- Past or present injection drug users
- Persons being treated for sexually transmitted infections
- Persons with a history of blood transfusions between 1978 and 1985

NOTE:

- A person is considered high-risk if he/she reports at least one risk factor or lives in a high-prevalence area.
- Individuals who ask for testing without reporting any risk factors may also be considered at higher risk for HIV.

From *Screening for human immunodeficiency virus infection,* U.S. Preventive Services Task Force, July 2005.
HIV, Human immunodeficiency virus.

▲ PROMOTING HEALTHY AGING: IMPLICATIONS FOR GERONTOLOGICAL NURSING

Nurses have multiple roles in the area of sexuality and older people. The nurse is a facilitator of a milieu that is conducive to the older person asking questions and expressing his or her sexuality. The nurse has the responsibility to help maintain the sexuality of older people by offering opportunity for discussion. Nusbaum et al. (2005) reported that older women had a similar number of sexual concerns as younger women but were less likely to be asked about sexual health during health care visits. Older women wanted health care providers to ask about their sexual functioning although participants reported some discomfort discussing the topic with younger physicians.

To assist and support older people in their sexual needs, nurses should be aware of their own feelings about sexuality and their attitudes towards intimacy and sexuality in older people (single, married, and homosexual). Only after confronting one's own attitudes, values, and beliefs can the nurse provide support without being judgmental. Rarely are sex histories elicited from the elderly patient. Physical examinations often do not include the reproductive system unless it is directly involved in the present illness. However, when questions about sexual issues are asked or when the elderly are examined, the nurse needs to be particularly cognizant of the era and culture in which the individual has lived to understand the factors affecting conduct.

The nurse should be an educator and provide information and guidance to older people who need it. Older persons should be asked about their sexual satisfaction, because they may not mention it voluntarily. Anticipation of problems in older individuals' sexual experiences can ward off anxiety, misconceptions, and an arbitrary cessation of sexual pleasure. Validation of the normalcy of sexual activity or a discussion of the physiological changes that occur with age or the effect of illness and treatment that may interfere with sexual activity by altering the routine or interfering with physical performance may be needed. Counseling may also be needed for the older person to adapt to natural physiological changes and image-altering surgical procedures. The nurse may also be a consultant and counselor to others who give care to older people.

Assessment

Discussion of sexuality and sexuality problems may be uncomfortable for both nurse and elder. Nonetheless, learning the significance of sexual function to the elder and the perception of sexual function the elder has without bringing the nurse's own biases into the interaction is important. The PLISSIT model (Annon, 1976) is a helpful guide for discussion of sexuality (Box 19-5). Youngkin (2004) provides suggestions for use of the PLISSIT model with older people:

- **Permission:** Obtain permission from the client to initiate sexual discussion (Wallace, 2003b). Allow the person to discuss concerns related to sexual issues, and

---

BOX 19-5   PLISSIT Model

P Permission from the client to initiate sexual discussion
LI Providing the Limited Information needed to function sexually
SS Giving Specific Suggestions for the individual to proceed with sexual relations
IT Providing Intensive Therapy surrounding the issues of sexuality for the clients (may mean referral to specialist)

Compiled from Annon J: The PLISSIT model: a proposed conceptual theme for behavioral treatment of sexual problems, *J Sex Educ Ther* 2(2):1-15, 1976; Wallace M: Best practices in nursing care to older adults: sexuality, *Dermatol Nurs* 15(6):570-571, 2003; Youngkin E: The myths and truths of mature intimacy: mature guidance for nurse practitioners, *Adv Nurse Pract* 12(9):45-48, 2004.

gather information about what might have changed in the person's life to affect sexual needs and response. Questions such as "What concerns or questions do you have about fulfilling your sexual needs?" (Wallace, 2003b) or "In this era of HIV and other sexually transmitted infections, I ask all my patients about sexual practices and concerns. Are there any questions I can answer for you?" (Nusbaum et al., 2005).

- **Limited Information:** Provide the limited information to function sexually (Wallace, 2003b). Offer teaching about the normal age-associated changes that affect sexual performance or how illness may affect sexuality. Encourage the person to learn more about the concern from books and other sources.
- **Specific Suggestions:** Offer suggestions for dealing with problems such as lubricants for atrophic vaginitis; use of condoms to prevent sexually transmitted infections; proper use of ED medications; how to communicate sexual and other needs; ways to increase comfort with coitus or ways to be intimate without coital relations.
- **Intensive Therapy:** Refer as appropriate for complex problems that require specialist intervention.

Box 19-6 provides other suggestions for assessment. Additional suggestions for sexuality assessment can be found at the John A. Hartford Foundation Institute for Geriatric Nursing website (*www.hartfordign.org*).

Interventions

Interventions will vary depending on the needs identified from the assessment data. A variety of suggested interventions for maintaining sexual function for older people with chronic conditions was presented in Table 19-3, and ED was discussed with available options of treatment. Perhaps one of the most important interventions is education regarding normal age changes related to sexual function and the dimensions of sexuality that provide pleasure.

Counseling and Advocacy. Although older people do seek counseling on sexuality and sexual concerns, we do not always hear them and many of us are not well enough prepared to help them. Successful and continuing sexual activ-

BOX 19-6   Guidelines for Health Care Providers in Talking to Older Adults about Sexual Health

Health care providers should spend time with older adults.
- Be available to discuss the subject.
- Give us your full attention.
- Allow time to ask questions.
- Take time to answer questions.

Health care providers should use clear and easy-to-understand words.
- Use plain, everyday language.
- Explain medical terms in plain English.
- Give explanations or answers to questions in simple terms.

Health care providers should help older adults feel comfortable talking about sex.
- Help us to break the ice.
- Make us feel comfortable in asking questions.
- Offer permission to express feelings and needs.
- Do not be afraid or embarrassed to discuss sexuality problems.

Health care providers should be open-minded and talk openly.
- Do not assume there are no concerns.
- Be open.
- Ask direct questions about sexual activity and attitudes.
- Discuss sexual concerns freely.
- Answer questions honestly.
- Just talk about it.
- Do not evade sexual concerns.
- Be willing to discuss sexual problems.
- Probe sexual concerns if elder wishes.

Health care providers should listen.
- Be prepared to listen.
- Listen so we feel you are interested in our problems.
- Let us talk.

Health care providers should treat older adults with a respectful and nonjudgmental attitude.
- See us as individuals with sexual needs.
- Accept us for what we are: gay, straight, bisexual.
- Be nonjudgmental.
- Show genuine concern and respect.

Health care providers should encourage discussion.
- Make opportunities for one-to-one discussion.
- Provide privacy.
- Promote candid discussion.
- Provide discussion groups to ask questions.
- Develop support groups.

Health care providers can give advice or suggestions.
- Provide information.
- Offer to find solutions and alternatives to given situations.
- Provide explicit pamphlets; explain sexual positions, lubrication.
- Discuss old taboos.
- Give suggestions of ways to help solve sexual problems.

Health care providers need to understand that sex is not just for the young.
- Try to eliminate the idea that sex and love are just for younger people.
- Acknowledge that sexual impulses are healthy and do not disappear as individuals age.
- Treat older adults as normal sexual beings and not as asexual elderly people.
- Recognize that sex can improve—can become even better when one is older.

From Johnson B: Older adults' suggestions for health care providers regarding discussions of sex, *Geriatr Nurs* 18(2):65-66, 1997.

ity is but one sign of healthy aging. Some nurses have extensive education in sexuality and can provide intensive therapy for people with sexual problems. Although the nurse in the acute or long-term care facility may not be well prepared to engage in sex therapy, being knowledgeable about sexual changes that occur in aging or with illness, providing information about sexual issues in anticipation of questions or in response to questions asked, treating expressions of sexuality as normal, and referring individuals with complex problems to specialists are important nursing responses.

Evaluation

Elders whose sexuality needs are fulfilled will consider their sexual life with satisfaction. This attitude will be apparent through verbal and nonverbal expression, the individual's self-image, and involvement and concern about others.

In summary, the nurse has a variety of roles in ensuring the sexuality of older people: facilitator, educator, consul-

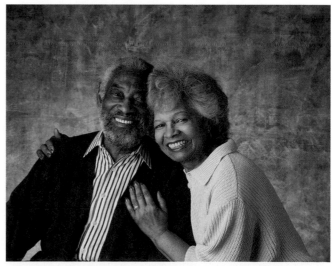

Sexuality is an important need in late life and affects pleasure, adaptation, and a general feeling of well-being. (Copyright © Getty Images.)

Human Needs and Wellness Diagnoses

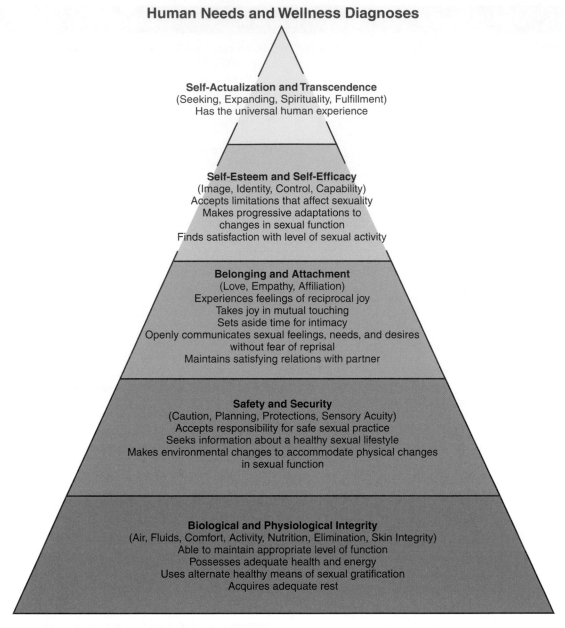

Self-Actualization and Transcendence
(Seeking, Expanding, Spirituality, Fulfillment)
Has the universal human experience

Self-Esteem and Self-Efficacy
(Image, Identity, Control, Capability)
Accepts limitations that affect sexuality
Makes progressive adaptations to
changes in sexual function
Finds satisfaction with level of sexual activity

Belonging and Attachment
(Love, Empathy, Affiliation)
Experiences feelings of reciprocal joy
Takes joy in mutual touching
Sets aside time for intimacy
Openly communicates sexual feelings, needs, and desires
without fear of reprisal
Maintains satisfying relations with partner

Safety and Security
(Caution, Planning, Protections, Sensory Acuity)
Accepts responsibility for safe sexual practice
Seeks information about a healthy sexual lifestyle
Makes environmental changes to accommodate physical changes
in sexual function

Biological and Physiological Integrity
(Air, Fluids, Comfort, Activity, Nutrition, Elimination, Skin Integrity)
Able to maintain appropriate level of function
Possesses adequate health and energy
Uses alternate healthy means of sexual gratification
Acquires adequate rest

These are not all the possible wellness diagnoses that may be identified. The above
are examples of nursing diagnoses that should be considered when planning care
for the older adult.

tant, counselor, and advocate. Sexuality is an amalgamation of biological, psychological, and social moral elements that affect pleasure, adaptation, and a general feeling of well-being in older people.

KEY CONCEPTS

- Touch provides sensory stimulation, reduces anxiety, and provides pain relief, comfort, and sexual expression.
- The absence of touch, a powerful sense, threatens survival.
- Sexuality is love, sharing, trust, and warmth, as well as physical acts. Sexuality provides an individual with self-identity and affirmation of life.
- Sexual activity continues in old age, though adaptations are needed for the age-related changes of the male and female genital systems.

- Generally speaking, medications, ill health, and lack of a partner affect sexual activity.
- Further research is needed to promote knowledge and understanding of the sexual health of older adults with alternative lifestyles, such as gay men, lesbians, and bisexual and transgender individuals.
- AIDS awareness and the practice of safe sex among older adults are still lacking. Health professionals, too, do not consider older adults at risk for AIDS, even though the incidence of AIDS in the older population is rapidly increasing. Finding appropriate services for the older adult with AIDS may prove difficult.
- The major role of the nurse in older adult sexuality in the community or long-term care settings is education and counseling about sexual function, adaptations for age-related changes and chronic conditions, and the maintenance of sexuality for the older adult's health and pleasure.

CASE STUDY: Sexuality in Late Life

George was a 70-year-old man who had been widowed for 6 years. He lived alone in a lovely home in the hills of San Francisco. His many friends tried to introduce him to a lady who would be attractive to him, but they were unaware of his real concerns. Although George was attracted to young, energetic women, often barely older than his daughters, he was justifiably cautious regarding their sincere attraction to him because he had a considerable estate. In addition, his sexual desire was waning and his capacity for sexual performance was unpredictable. One thing George expressed fairly frequently was, "I don't like demands made on me." To further complicate the picture, George had begun to take medication to reduce his benign prostatic hypertrophy (BPH) that had become increasingly troublesome. The medication further reduced his sexual desire. In addition, George's sleep pattern was disturbed by the need to arise three or four times each night to void. George came to the clinic for follow-up evaluation of his BPH, and while talking with the nurse, he began crying uncontrollably, much to his embarrassment and the nurse's surprise because George had always seemed a rather stolid and stoic fellow, reluctant to discuss feelings.

Based on the case study, develop a nursing care plan using the following procedure*:

- List George's comments that provide subjective data.
- List information that provides objective data.
- From these data, identify and state, using accepted format, two nursing diagnoses you determine are most significant to George at this time. List two of George's strengths that you have identified from the data.
- Determine and state outcome criteria for each diagnosis. These criteria must reflect some alleviation of the problem identified in the nursing diagnosis and must be stated in concrete and measurable terms.
- Plan and state one or more interventions for each diagnosed problem. Provide specific documentation of the sources used to determine the appropriate intervention. Plan at least one intervention that incorporates George's existing strengths.
- Evaluate the success of the intervention. Interventions must correlate directly with the stated outcome criteria to measure the outcome success.

Critical Thinking Questions

1. How would you begin discussing sexuality with George?
2. What are the factors that may be underlying George's sexual distress?
3. Discuss BPH and its prevalence and usual effects.
4. With a partner, role play and demonstrate your interpersonal interaction with George in this situation.
5. What resources or recommendations would you suggest for George?

* Students are advised to refer to their nursing diagnosis text and identify possible or potential problems.

RESEARCH QUESTIONS

What do women find are the most troubling changes in their sexuality as they grow older?

What do men find are the most troubling changes in their sexuality as they grow older?

What are the differences in sexual feelings and expression in the 60-year-old, the 70-year-old, the 80-year-old, and the 90-year-old individual?

What are the chronic disorders that most affect sexual performance of men and women, and how are they affected?

How many individuals older than 60 years have ever been given the opportunity to provide a thorough sexual history?

What community and health resources are available to meet the needs of LGBT older adults?

What is the knowledge level of people older than 65 years about HIV/AIDS?

RESOURCES

AIDS Action
1706 Sunderland Place NW
Washington, DC 20036
(202) 530-8031
www.aidsaction.org

American Psychological Association
Aging and human sexuality resource guide
www.apa.org/pi/aging/sexuality.html

Gay and Lesbian Carers Network
U.K. organization for lesbian women and gay men caring for a partner, relative, or friend with dementia
www.alzheimer's org.uk/Gay_Carers/gaycarers.htm

Gay and Lesbian Elder Housing
www.gleh.org

Gerontological Society of America
Rainbow Research Group
Contact Karen Friedriksen-Goldsen at fredrikk

Intimacy, sexuality and sexual behavior in dementia: how to develop practice guidelines and policy for long term care facilities
www.fhs.mcmaster.ca/mcah/cgec/toolkit.pdf

LGBT Aging Project
www.lgbtagingproject.org

National Association on HIV Over Fifty (HIV and Older Adults Tip Sheet)
http://hivoverfifty.org

National Center for Lesbian Rights
www.nclrights.org

National Council on Aging
Love and life: a healthy approach to sex for older adults (brochures, training materials, video)
www.ncoa.org

National Institute on Aging, Age Page, Sexuality in Later Life
http://niapublications.org/agepages/sexuality.asp

SeniorSex.org
Older adult sexuality reference

Survivor Project
www.survivorproject.org

Films on Sexuality
A Thousand Tomorrows: Intimacy, Sexuality and Alzheimer's
Forever Young
Freedom of Sexual Expression: Dementia and Resident Rights in
Long Term Care Facilities
Sexuality in Later Life
The Forgotten Tenth (HIV and Older Adults)
All Available from Terra Nova Films
9848 S. Winchester Ave.
Chicago, IL 60643
www.terranova.org

Eager for Your Kisses
www.newday.com

Rose by Any Other Name
Addresses issues of sexuality in nursing homes
www.keller.com/tricepts/rose.html

Sexuality and Aging
www.gpn.unl.edu or www.mediarights.org

REFERENCES

Ackerman D: *A natural history of the senses*, New York, 1995, Vantage Books.
Annon J: The PLISSIT model: a proposed conceptual scheme for behavioral treatment of sexual problems, *J Sex Educ Ther* 2(2):1-15, 1976.
Agronin M: Sexuality and aging: an introduction, *CNS Long-Term Care*, Summer:12-13, 2004.
Barnes MM: Female genital disorders. In Beers MH, Berkow R, editors: *The Merck manual of geriatrics*, ed 3, Whitehouse Station, NJ, 2000, Merck Research Laboratories.
Bauer M: Their only privacy is between their sheets, *J Gerontol Nurs* 25(80:37-41, 1999.
Beers MH: Male hypogonadism and impotence. In Abrams WB et al, editors: *The Merck manual of geriatrics*, ed 2, Whitehouse Station, NJ, 1995, Merck Research Laboratories.
Benary-Isbert M: *The vintage years*, New York, 1968, Abingdon Press.
Berger R: *Gay and gray: the older homosexual man*, Binghamton, NY, 1995, Hawthorn Press.
Berlin H: Your doctor discusses: sexuality in mature/late life, *Planning for Health* 21:2, 1978.
Billhorn DR: Sexuality and the chronically ill older adult, *Geriatr Nurs* 15(2):106, 1994.
Blando J: Twice hidden: older gay and lesbian couples, friends and intimacy, *Generations* xxv(2):87-89, 2001.
Blieszner R, deVries B: Perspectives on intimacy, *Generations* xxv(2):7-8, 2001.
Brotman S et al: The health and social service needs of gay and lesbian elders and their families in Canada, *Gerontologist* 43(2):172-202, 2003.
Burke MA, Knowlton CN: Sexuality. In Burke MM, Walsh MB, editors: *Gerontological nursing*, St Louis, 1992, Mosby.
Buschmann MBT et al: Implementation of expressive physical touch in depressed elders, *J Clin Geropsychol* 5(4):291-300, 1999.

Butler R, Lewis M: Sexuality. In Abrams WB, Berkow R, editors: *Merck manual of geriatrics*, Rahway, NJ, 1990, Merck Sharpe and Dohme Research Laboratories.
Butler R, Lewis M: Sexuality. In Beers MH, Berkow R, editors: *The Merck manual of geriatrics*, ed 3, Whitehouse Station, NJ, 2000, Merck Research Laboratories.
Butler R, Lewis M: *The new love and sex after 60*, New York, 2002, Ballantine Books.
Comfort A: Sexuality in old age, *J Am Geriatr Soc* 22(10):440-442, 1974.
Davies HD et al: Sexuality and intimacy in Alzheimer's patients and their partners, *Sex Disabil* 16(3):173-203, 1998.
Deevey S: Older lesbian women: an invisible minority, *J Gerontol Nurs* 16(5):35, 1990.
Denny NW, Quadango D: *Human sexuality*, St Louis, 1992, Mosby.
Goldblatt R: Factors influencing sexual behavior, *J Am Geriatr Soc* 20(2):49, 1972.
Goodroad BK: HIV and AIDS in people older than 50, *J Gerontol Nurs* 29(4):18, 2003.
Gordon M, Sokolowski M: Sexuality in long-term care: ethics and action, *Ann Long-Term Care* 12(9):45-48, 2004.
Gwyther L, Willer L: Ask the expert: how do we assess and determine the mental capacity of our patients with Alzheimer's disease and dementia for consent to conjugal visits with their spouse? *Ann Long-Term Care* 12(4):27-28, 2004.
Hall ET: *The hidden dimensions*, Garden City, NY, 1969, Doubleday.
Ham RJ: Sexuality. In Ham RJ, Sloane PD, editors: *Primary care geriatrics*, ed 4, St Louis, 2002, Mosby.
Hite S: *The Hite report*, New York, 1977, Dell.
Holland B, Pokorny M: Slow stroke back massage: its effect on patients in a rehabilitation setting, *Rehabil Nurs* 26(5):182-186, 2001.
Hollinger, LM, Buschmann MT: Factors influencing the perception of touch by elderly nursing home residents and their health caregivers, *J Gerontol Nurs* 21(1):37-47, 1993.
Hooyman N, Kiyak HA: *Social gerontology: a multidisciplinary perspective*, ed 7, 2005, Boston, Pearson.
Huss AJ: Touch with care or a caring touch, *Am J Occup Ther* 31:12, 1977.
Huyck M: Romantic relationships in later life, *Generations* xxv(2):9-17, 2001.
Jarvick L, Small G: *The psychology of CJ Jung*, New York, 1988, Crown.
Jones T, Nystrom N: Looking back . . . (looking forward: addressing the lives of lesbians, *J Women Aging* 14:59-73, 2002.
Kaiser FE: Sexual dysfunction in men; sexual dysfunction in women. In Beers MH, Berkow R, editors: *The Merck manual of geriatrics*, ed 3, Whitehouse Station, NJ, 2000.
Kehoe M: Have you ever seen a lesbian over 60? *Aging Connection* 4(4):4, 1988.
Kim EJ, Buschmann MBT: Touch-stress model and Alzheimer's disease: using touch intervention to alleviate patients' stress, *J Gerontol Nurs* 30(12):33-39, 2004.
Kolcaba K et al: Effects of hand massage on comfort of nursing home residents, *Geriatr Nurs* 27(3):85-91, 2006.
Kreiger D: Therapeutic touch: the imprimatur of nursing, *Am J Nurs* 75:784, 1975.
Lewis MI: Sexuality. In Abrams WB et al, editors: *Merck manual of geriatrics*, ed 2, Whitehouse Station, NJ, 1995, Merck Research Laboratories.

Lichtenberg PA, Strzepek DM: Assessment of institutionalized dementia patients' competencies to participate in intimate relationships, *Gerontologist* 30(1):119-120, 1990.

Low L et al: Promoting awareness of sexuality of older people in residential care, *Elec J Hum Sex* 8, August 24, 2005. (website): *www.ejhs.org/volume8/sexuality_of_older_people.htm*.

Lyder CH: The role of the nurse practitioner in promoting sexuality in the institutionalized elderly, *J Am Acad Nurse Pract* 6(2):61-63, 1994.

Maddocks J: Sexual health and health care, *Postgrad Med* 58:52, 1975.

Martin D, Lyon P: Positively gay: new approaches to gay and lesbian life. In Berzon B, editor: *Positively gay: new approaches to gay and lesbian life*, Berkeley Calif, 2001, Celestial Arts.

Mayer M et al: Phosphodiesterase inhibitors in female sexual dysfunction, *World J Urol* 23(6):393-397, 2005.

Messinger-Rapport B et al: Sex and sexuality: is it over after 60? *Clin Geriatr* 11(10):45-53, 2003.

Money J, Tucker P: *Sexual signatures: being a man or woman*, Boston, 1975, Little, Brown.

Montagu A: *Touching: the human significance of the skin*, ed 3, New York, 1986, Harper & Row.

Moon TD: Male genital disorders. In Beers MH, Berkow R, editors: *The Merck manual of geriatrics*, ed 3, Whitehouse Station, NJ, 2000, Merck Research Laboratories.

National Council on Aging: Sex after 60: a natural part of life. (website): *www.ncoa.org/content.cfm?sectionID=109&detail=134*. Accessed August 30, 2006.

Nay R: Sexuality and the aged women in nursing homes, *Geriatr Nurs* 13(6):312, 1992.

Nusbaum M et al: Sexual health in aging men and women: addressing the physiological and psychological sexual changes that occur with age, *Geriatrics* 60(9):18-21, 2005.

Older Americans and HIV, 2001. (website): *http://aidsaction.org*. Accessed August 8, 2006.

Piercy K: We couldn't do without them: the value of close relationships between older adults and their nonfamily caregivers, *Generations* xxv(2):41-47, 2001.

Ramsey J: Spiritual intimacy in later life: implications for clinical practice, *Generations* xxv(2):59-63, 2001.

Remington R: Calming music and hand massage with agitated elderly, *Nurs Res* 51(5):319-323, 2002.

Roberson L: The importance of touch for the patient with dementia, *Home Healthc Nurse* 21(1):16-17, 2003.

Sansone P, Schmitt L: Providing tender touch massage to elderly nursing home residents: a demonstration project, *Geriatr Nurs* 21(6):303-308, 2000.

Schuerman DA: Clinical concerns: AIDS in the elderly, *J Gerontol Nurs* 20(7):11, 1994.

Skinner KD: Creating a game for sexuality and aging: the sexual dysfunction trivia game, *J Contin Educ Nurs* 31(4):185-189, 2000.

Snyder M, Burns K: Efficacy of hand massage in decreasing agitation behaviors associated with care activities in persons with dementia, *Geriatr Nurs* 16(3):60-63, 1995.

Steinke E: Intimacy needs and chronic illness, *J Gerontol Nurs* 31(5):40-50, 2005.

Tabloski P: *Gerontological nursing*, Boston, 2006, Pearson Prentice Hall.

Thayer S: Social touching. In Schiff W, Foulke E, editors: *Tactile perception: a source book*, Cambridge, 1982, Cambridge University Press.

Troll L: When the world narrows: intimacy with the dead? *Generations* xxv(2):55-58, 2001.

Uphold CR et al: HIV and older adults, *J Gerontol Nurs* 30(7):16-24, 2004.

Wallace M: Sexuality and aging in long-term care, *Ann Long-Term Care* 11(2):53-59, 2003a. (website): *www.annalsoflongtermcare.com/article/315*. Accessed August 8, 2006.

Wallace M: Best practices in nursing care to older adults: sexuality, *Dermatol Nurs* 15(6):570-571, 2003b.

Wang K, Hermann C: Pilot study to test the effectiveness of healing touch on agitation in people with dementia, *Geriatr Nurs* 27(1):34-40, 2006.

Whipple B, Scura KW: The overlooked epidemic: HIV in older adults, *Am J Nurs* 96(2):23, 1996.

Wiley D, Bortz II WM: Sexuality and aging: usual and successful, *J Gerontol A Biol Sci Med Sci* 51a(3):M142, 1996.

Wojciechowski C: Issues in caring for older lesbians, *J Gerontol Nurs* 24:28-33, 1998.

Woods DL et al: The effect of therapeutic touch on behavioral symptoms of persons with dementia, *Altern Ther Health Med* 11(1):66-74, 2005.

Woods NF: Sexuality and aging. In Reinhardt AN, Quinn MD, editors: *Current practice in gerontological nursing*, vol 1, St Louis, 1979, Mosby.

Youngkin E: The myths and truths of mature intimacy, *Adv Nurse Pract* September:45-48, 2004.

Zeiss A, Kasl-Godley J: Sexuality in older adults' relationships, *Generations* xxv(2):18-25, 2001.

CHAPTER 20

Relationships, Roles, and Transitions

Theris A. Touhy

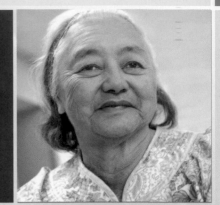

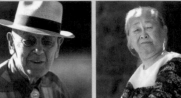

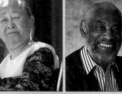

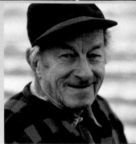

A YOUTH SPEAKS

I'm really worried about retirement! That is ridiculous at my age, but I keep reading and hearing about Social Security and Medicare running out of money for the baby boom generation. Those are my parents! What about me?

Joseph, age 30

AN ELDER SPEAKS

I thought when my children left home that my most important job was done. But they came home again and again, and then my mother-in-law came to live with us. Finally, the kids were really on their own and married, so now I take care of the grandchildren while they both work to make ends meet. I just pray daily that my husband will remain healthy. I don't think I could deal with one more thing.

Esther, age 64

LEARNING OBJECTIVES

On completion of this chapter, the reader will be able to:

1. Identify several important roles that elder members of society usually fulfill.
2. Discuss changes in family structure and functions that are occurring.
3. Describe the various roles of grandparents.
4. Enumerate several caregiver concerns and current societal supports.
5. Relate some of the factors that must be considered in the decision to retire.
6. Explain the issues in adapting to a major role change such as retirement or widowhood.
7. Discuss the development of a volunteer role in late life.
8. Discuss nursing responses with older adults experiencing caregiver roles or other transitions.

This chapter examines the various relationships, roles, and transitions that are characteristic in late life. Important relationships include that of spouse, partner, parent, grandparent, great-grandparent, sibling, and friend. The role functions of these relationships shift as societal norms and economics change. Biomedical technology, political agendas, social expectations, and worldwide economic fluctuations are continually changing the face of aging. Even more changes are expected among singles, families, and retirees as the first wave of "baby boomers" enters young-old age. The major concerns of this group are adequate health care coverage, the preservation of Social Security, and caregiving demands (American Association of Retired Persons [AARP],

2002a, 2002b). This major change in the aging landscape is only one of many massive social changes that have altered the patterns of work, family, and kinship structures in recent decades. The chief concerns in this chapter are the impact of these numerous changes on the quality of life and the range of possibilities for elders in their most important affiliations. Individuals live longer, families are smaller, more women work, and caregiving has become an expectable concern. Thus social change and individual need continue to change the nature of the life course and affiliative inclinations.

Role transitions likely to occur in late life include working to retirement and volunteering, grandparenthood, wid-

Special thanks to Priscilla Ebersole, the previous edition contributor, for her content contributions to this chapter.

owhood, divorce, and becoming a caregiver and service recipient. These transitions may occur predictably or by unanticipated events. Retirement is an example of a predictable event that can and should be planned long in advance. Divorce, widowhood, and widowerhood may occur unexpectedly and create emotional chaos in the transitional phase. Transitions that are signaled by experiences of family and friends or anticipatory events alert a person to the impending shift and sometimes define the passage through ritualized activities. Most difficult are the transitions that incorporate losses rather than gains in status, influence, and opportunity. The move from independence to dependence and becoming a care recipient is particularly difficult. Conditions that influence the outcome of transitions include personal meanings, expectations, level of knowledge, preplanning, and emotional and physical reserves. The ideal outcome is when gains in satisfaction and new roles offset losses.

RELATIONSHIPS

The classic study of Lowenthal and Haven (1968) has been reviewed in detail and elaborated many times since its inception. The importance of caring relationships and the presence of a confidante as a buffer against "age-linked social losses" is demonstrated in the study. Maintaining a stable intimate relationship was more closely associated with good mental health and high morale than was a high level of activity or elevated role status. Individuals seem able to manage stresses if some relationships are close and sustaining. Increasingly evident is that a caring person may be a significant survival resource. Frequently nurses become the caring other in an older person's life, especially among elders living in nursing homes (Touhy, 2001). Social bonding increases health status through as yet undetermined physiological pathways, though studies in psychoneuroimmunology are giving us clues.

This segment of the chapter familiarizes the reader with relationships as experienced in old age within generations and between generations. A network of kin, friends, and acquaintances can sustain the older adult and give life meaning. We might use the analogy of a tree that withstands storms and drought through an extensive root system, which provides stability and nourishment that may be helpful; such is old age. The ground around the tree must be tended to keep it thriving. We may find ourselves best caring for older people by caring for those who are important to them.

Primary relationships are intimate associations that provide a strong sense of sharing and belonging; these are the deep roots of our tree analogy. Relationships that are more formal, impersonal, superficial, and circumstantial are often time limited, sometimes intense but with a tendency to dissipate. These relationships are the surface network of roots that extend outward in many directions and are sustained by their profusion but wither with neglect or insignificance. Thus the primary network may need professional strengthening to bear the increasing demands.

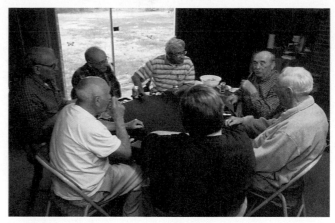

Friends play an important role in the lives of older adults. (From Lewis SM et al: *Medical-surgical nursing: assessment and management of clinical problems,* ed 6, St Louis, 2004, Mosby; courtesy Rick Brady, Riva, MD.)

Friendships

Friends are often a significant source of support in late life. Lifelong friendships are often sustaining in the face of overwhelming circumstances. They provide the critical elements of satisfactory living that families may not, providing commitment and affection without judgment. Personality characteristics between friends are compatible because the relationships are chosen and caring is shared without obligation. Bleiszner (2001) found that 88% of individuals between 65 and 85 years of age maintained contact with friends and neighbors, and these contacts, in many cases, were as meaningful as those with family. Trust, demonstrations of caring, and mutual problem solving were important aspects of the friendships.

Friends may share a lifelong perspective or may bring a totally new intergenerational viewpoint into one's life. Late-life friendships often develop out of changing situations, such as shared tenancies, widowhood, moves, and involvement in volunteer pursuits. As desires and pursuits change, some friendships evolve that the person never would have considered in his or her youth. Friends function in many ways: (1) act as surrogate kin, (2) ease the loneliness of widowhood or widowerhood, and (3) validate one's generational viewpoint. Considering the obvious importance of friendship, it seems to be a neglected area of exploration and a seldom considered resource for professionals working with older people. Because close friendships have such influence on the sense of well-being of elders, anything done to sustain them will be helpful. Nurses may include in their assessment questions about older individuals' friendships and their importance and availability.

Mentoring Relationships

Professionals and, in some other situations, older adults may develop intense reciprocal relationships with younger adults, and vice versa. These relationships often have an intimacy that is similar to that of parent and offspring (Fingerman, 2001a). In the case of the elder, a relationship may fill a need for offspring who were never produced. In some cases, these relationships may be more satisfactory because the inherent generational expectations are attenuated by the absence of obligation. Elder retired academics often become involved with young neophyte students and professionals, the elder benefiting from fresh ideas and the younger from the wisdom of the elder. When the relationship is not one of mentoring, it may be a replacement of the idealized parent or grandparent who is no longer or was never available. "Catherine was the great-grandmother I never knew." "Priscilla was a model of gracious aging." "Mary Opal was a mentor and a surrogate mother."

FAMILIES

The idea of family evokes strong impressions of whatever an individual believes the typical family should be. Because everyone comes from a family, these impressions have powerful symbolic meanings. However, in today's world, the definition of family is in a state of flux. As recently as 100 years ago, the norm was the extended family made up of parents, their grown children, and the children's children, often living together and sharing resources, strengths, and challenges. As cities grew and adult children moved in pursuit of work, parents did not always come along and the nuclear family evolved. The norm in the United States became two parents and their two children, or at least that was the norm in what has been considered mainstream America. This pattern was not as common, nor is it yet, in many families of color, especially living in what are called "ethnic neighborhoods," where the extended family is still the norm.

Other variations on the idea of family have developed. Approximately 42% of today's families are married couples without children. The high divorce and remarriage rate results in households of blended families of children from previous marriages and the new marriage. Single-parent families, blended families, childless families, and fewer families altogether are common. Four- and five-generation families are also becoming common (Kutza, 2001).

Still other families are composed of same-gender couples, which may or may not include children. Others without biological families either by choice or circumstance have created their own "families" through communal living with siblings, friends, or others. Indeed, it is not unusual for childless persons residing in long-term care facilities to refer to the staff as their new "family."

Family members form the nucleus of relationships and are the primary source of social support for older people. Nearly 94% of elders have living family members. Most older adults possess a large intergenerational web of significant people, including sons, daughters, stepchildren, in-laws, nieces, nephews, grandchildren, and great-grandchildren, as well as partners and former partners of their offspring. All these people may play an important part in maintaining late life satisfactions.

In coming to know the older adult, the gerontological nurse comes to know the family as well, learning of their

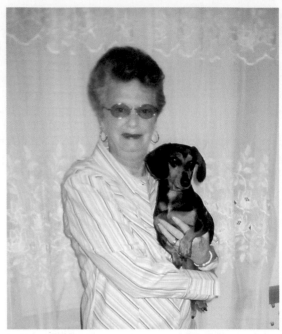

Pets are a part of the family and are particularly beneficial to older adults. They provide companionship, comfort, and caring. (From Monahan F et al: *Phipps' medical-surgical nursing: health and illness perspectives*, ed 8, St Louis, 2006, Mosby.)

special gifts and their life challenges. The nurse works with the elder within the unique culture of his or her family of origin, present family, and support networks, including friends.

Roles and Relationships

As families change, the roles of the members or expectations of one another may change as well. Grandparents may assume parental roles for their grandchildren if their children are unable to care for them; or grandparents and older aunts and uncles may assume temporary caregiving roles while the children, nieces, and nephews work. Adult children of any age may provide limited or extensive caregiving to their own parents or aging relatives who become ill or impaired. A spouse or a sibling may become a caregiver as well. This caregiving may be temporary or long term.

Close-knit families are more aware of the needs of their members and work to resolve problems and find ways to meet the needs of members, even if they are not always successful. Emotionally distant families are less available in times of need and have greater potential for conflict. If the family has never been close and supportive, it will not magically become so when members grow older. Resentments long buried may crop up and produce friction or psychological pain. Long-submerged conflicts and feelings may return if the needs of one family member exceed those of the others.

Traditional Couples

The traditional couple in the United States is husband and wife. Although this relationship is often the most binding if it extends into late life, the chance of a couple going through old age together is exceedingly slim. Approximately 40% of men and 80% of women older than 75 years have no spouse (U.S. Administration on Aging, 2000). Men who survive their spouse into old age ordinarily have multiple opportunities to remarry if they wish. A woman is less likely to have an opportunity for remarriage in late life. Couple relationships are becoming more diverse, involving varying degrees of habit, culture, intimacy, shared backgrounds, and instrumental and emotional support (Connidis, 2001).

In late marriages or remarriage, developing an intimate, sharing relationship between individuals who have had 75 or 80 years of separate experiences often brings conflicting ideologies into the new relationship and can be an enormous challenge. Older people who remarry usually choose someone they have previously known and with whom they share similar backgrounds and interests. Often, older couples live together but do not marry because of economic and inheritance reasons (Hooyman and Kiyak, 2005).

The needs, tasks, and expectations of couples in late life differ from those in earlier years. Some couples have been married more than 60 or 70 years. These years together may have been filled with love and companionship or abuse and resentment or anything in between. However, in general, marital status (or the presence of a long-time partner) is positively related to health, life satisfaction, and well-being. For all couples, the normal physical and sociological circumstances in late life present challenges. Some of the issues that strain many of these relationships include (1) the deteriorating health of one or both partners, (2) limitations in income, (3) conflicts with children or other relatives, (4) incompatible sexual needs, and (5) mismatched needs for activity and socialization.

Nontraditional Couples

As the variations in families grow, so do the types of coupled relationships. Among the types of couples we see today are lesbian, gay, bisexual, and transgender (LGBT) couples. Although the number of LGBT people of any age has remained elusive, an estimated 3 million LGBT people are in the United States. The number is projected to increase to as many as 4 million by 2030 (deVries, 2005-2006). Although these couples are less often seen in the aging population, they are still there but may not be obvious because of long-standing discrimination and fear. Many older LGBT individuals have been part of a live-in couple at some time during their life (Hooyman and Kiyak, 2005). Some research has suggested that older lesbian women and gay men may adapt more successfully to old age as a result of coping over a lifetime with discrimination and prejudice (deVries, 2005-2006; Jones and Nystrom, 2002; Wojciechowski, 1998). However, the experience of discrimination and prejudice may also deter older lesbian women and gay men from accessing health care services. As society becomes more willing to accept persons in these relationships, they may be more willing to share with us who they are. The majority of research has involved lesbian and gay couples and much less is known about bisexual and transgender relationships.

Although the issue of same-gender couples marrying is before the courts, it is not legal in most states to do so. In some cases the couples enter into marriage-type commitments and, where possible, legally register as "domestic partners." Lesbian women and gay men in long-term committed relationships often share homes, resources, and professional interests. Their families may include children (biological and adoptive), parents, siblings, and friends. In some cases the couples may be estranged from families of origin and come to late life with a network of close friends who make up their "family." These nonrelatives become surrogate family and take on the instrumental and affection attributes of family. Because these family members are not relatives in the traditional sense, they may not be recognized by the health care system, leading to considerable stress to all involved.

Other issues such as Social Security and pension benefits, health insurance, and access to appropriate housing and services for future care needs have been identified as concerns by both older lesbian women and gay men (deVries, 2005-2006). In a study of lesbian women 55 years of age and older, Jones and Nystrom (2002) reported the most common concerns related to aging included "housing, financial security, illness, the impact of losing the support of partners and friends through death, and how to ensure that they and their partners would continue to have control over their own lives" (p. 72). Interest in and availability of retirement and long-term care communities designed to meet the needs of lesbian and gay older men and women have increased (deVries, 2005-2006).

If a same-gender relationship was unknown to the public, the grief surrounding the loss of the partner becomes difficult because the loss may be unrecognized by others and may pass without ritual or social sanctions. This type of grief has been defined as "disenfranchised grief," which can be particularly difficult to resolve (Doka, 2002). Much more knowledge of cohort, cultural, and generational differences among age-groups is needed to understand the recent, dramatic changes in the lives of lesbians and gays in family lifestyles. Issues of concern to society and the LGBT that need further investigation are the impact of homophobia on late-life health, retirement and leisure issues, and the hidden incidence of abuse and neglect (Claes and Moore, 2000). Chapter 19 discusses the sexual health needs of older LGBT individuals.

Elders and Their Adult Children

In adulthood, relationships between the generations become increasingly important for most people. Older parents enjoy being told about the various activities and successes of their offspring, and these adult children begin to see aspects of themselves that are and have developed from their parents. At times, the relationships may become strained because the younger adults are more concerned with their own spouses, partners, and children. The parents are no longer central to their lives, though offspring may be central to the lives of their parents (Fingerman, 2001a). The most difficult situations occur when the elder parents are openly critical or judgmental about the lives of their offspring. In the best of situations, adult children shift to the role of friend, companion, and confidant to the elder, a concept known as *filial maturity*.

Contrary to popular opinion, older people are not neglected by families and most older people see their children on a regular basis, with approximately 80% reporting weekly contact with at least one of their children (Hooyman and Kiyak, 2005). Even children who do not live close to their older parents maintain their close connections, and "intimacy at a distance" can occur (Hooyman and Kiyak, 2005; Silverstein and Angelli, 1998). By and large, elders and their children have relationships that are reciprocal in nature and characterized by affection and mutual support. These relationships are both the most important and potentially the most conflicted. Family resources are shared from birth and usually in some way until and after death. These resources may be tangible, such as money, belongings, and housing. Intangible resources may include advice, support, guidance, and day-to-day assistance with life. Elders provide a family history perspective, models for growing old, assistance with grandchildren, a sense of continuity, and a philosophy of aging. The older family members often serve as kin-keepers. *Kin-keeper* is a term used to denote a family member who arranges get-togethers, develops the family history and rituals, and in other ways promotes solidarity and unity among the kin.

Consider the example of Grandma Daisy, who always merited a special visit from any of the kin in her vast northwestern network. A pioneer settler in her small community, she knew the names, ages, and whereabouts of the children and spouses and the grandchildren and spouses of all of her eight children. They seldom saw one another but always felt a connecting link through Grandma Daisy. When she died at age 94, a great portion of the family history and sense of solidarity died with her. She was a true kin-keeper.

Grandparenting

About 80% of elders older than 65 years have three or more grandchildren, and nearly 50% are great-grandparents. Only about 13% of adults older than 65 years have no grandchildren (Hooyman and Kiyak, 2005; National Council on the Aging [NCOA], 2002). As the term implies, the "grands" are a step beyond parents in their concerns, exposure, and responsibility. The age, vitality, and proximity of both grandchild and grandparent produce a kaleidoscope of possible activities and interactions as both progress through their aging processes. Historically, the emphasis has been on the progressive aging of the grandparent as it affects the affinity, but little is said about the effects of the growth and maturation of the grandchild as these affect the relationship.

Although grandchildren are most affectionate and involved with grandparents from ages 3 to 13 years, with many stages and activities in between, the relationship matures as the grandchild does and becomes more affiliative and appreciative. With grandparent, adolescents can be both childish and playful or discuss adult issues, but they do not need

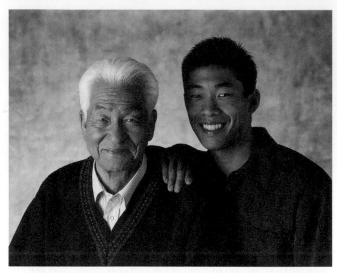

Grandparenting is an important role for elders. (Copyright © Getty Images.)

to swing wildly between dependence and independence as they do with parents. As adolescents approach adulthood and become absorbed with their own lives, the grandparental relationship is less intense or involved, other than with those who are primary caregivers in the child's daily life. Young adults are often given economic assistance as their material needs grow and those of the grandparents diminish. In addition, mileposts of achievement are particularly important to recognize. One of the authors (P.E.) writes:

> My older grandchildren are as proud of me and my accomplishments as I am of theirs. The most meaningful time has been taking a planned vacation to someplace of the grandchild's choice on the child's ninth birthday; just one grandchild and I having exclusive time together. I have been fortunate enough to be able both energetically and economically to do this with each of the eight grandchildren. A latecomer, 12 years younger than the others, has been an unexpected great joy.

Box 20-1 provides a set of guidelines for grandparents.

Gender and lineage are greatly influential in the meaning of grandparenthood (Somary and Stricker, 1998). Chan and Elder (2000) note a great matrilineal advantage in grandparenting relationships, but the role of grandfathers is also significant in the lives of many children. This area needs further study. The majority of grandchildren "perceive their grandparents as having active and influential roles in their lives" (Roberto and Skoglund, 1996, p. 107). The views of a grandmother as seen by an 8-year-old child are presented in Box 20-2.

Great-Grandparenting

Great-grandparenthood rarely has been studied, although 40% to 50% of older people in the United States will live long enough to become great-grandparents (U.S. Administration on Aging, 2000). Stereotypically, great-grandparents have been consigned to a rocking chair and shawl. Today, for a man or woman 65 years of age, still young and vital, being

BOX 20-1 Guidelines for Grandparenting

- Grandchildren need your attention and interest in their activities.
- Celebrating special times creates memories and continues traditions.
- Grandchildren need help exploring their world while they are young.
- Offering assistance without interference is recommended.
- Rule-making is not a grandparent's task.
- Do not give advice about child rearing.
- Give the child undivided attention during projects, games, and reading.
- Be a link with the past; tell grandchildren about their parents and about you when you were a child.
- Support the parents in their decisions; never undermine.
- Offer the gift of your time: nature walks, baking cookies, and so on.

LONG-DISTANCE GRANDPARENTING

- Brief and frequent cards and letters are useful; send clippings, cartoons, and riddles; use colorful stickers and stamps.
- Audiotapes and videotapes that you produce are appreciated; storytelling, reading, or singing.
- Celebrate special days and firsts (lost tooth, first day of school, mastery of a new situation).
- Telephone frequently.
- Visit as often as you can.

From Good grandparenting, *Mayo Clin Health Lett* 11(1):6, 1993.

BOX 20-2 A Grandmother as Seen by an 8-Year-Old Child

"A grandmother is a woman who has no children of her own. That is why she loves other people's children."

"Grandmothers have nothing to do. They are just there: when they take us for a walk they go slowly, like caterpillars along beautiful leaves. They never say, 'Come on, faster, hurry up!'"

"Everyone should try to have a grandmother, especially those who don't have a TV."

From *Ageing in Focus,* March 2006.

a great grandparent is not unusual; there are also many great-great-grandparents. This trend is expected to continue with the increase in the number of older people who are predicted to age in better health than current cohorts of elderly (Hooyman and Kiyak, 2005).

In most cases, the great-grandparental role is modeled after the role as grandparent. The middle generation's attitudes and involvement with their parents and grandparents largely determine the quality of the relationship. For most people, the intensity of the relationship is diminished compared with that of grandparenting. As more and more older adults become great-grandparents, we will learn more about the significance of the role. An area ripe for investi-

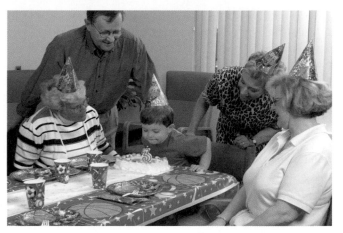

Grandparents take part in family activities. (From Sorrentino SA, Gorek B: *Mosby's textbook for long-term care assistants,* ed 5, St Louis, 2007, Mosby.)

gation is that of the increasing number of grandparents who have virtually raised a grandchild and then see the progeny of that child more as a grandchild than they do a great-grandchild.

Siblings

Late-life sibling relationships are poorly understood and have been neglected by researchers. As individuals age, they often have more contact with siblings than they did in the years when family and work demands were more pressing. About 80% of older people have at least one sibling. For many elders, these relationships became increasingly important because they have a long history of memories and are of the same generation, similar backgrounds, and often ambivalent early relationships (Bedford and Avioli, 2001). Sibling relationships become particularly important when they are part of the support system, especially among single or widowed elders living alone. The strongest of sibling bonds is thought to be the relationship between sisters. When blessed with survival, these relationships remain important into late old age (Scott, 1996). In some remarkable cases, such as the Delaney sisters, the two personalities complement each other and function well together in coping with the demands of independent living at great old age. Bessie, age 101 years, was feisty and abrupt, whereas Sadie (age 103 years) did what was needed with quiet determination (Delaney and Delaney, 1993). Of course, much has to do with age differences, place in the family, and personality. Service providers should inquire about sibling relationships of past and present significance. Consider the following:

> I remember the days when I detested Buddy, especially in our adolescence, but he is the only one still alive who has been a part of my entire life. Now, when we reflect on our divergent paths it is with a mixture of pleasure and poignancy. When our parents, other siblings, and mates died, we held each other together. Others call him Joe, but he will always be my Buddy.

The loss of siblings has a profound effect in terms of awareness of one's own mortality, particularly when those of the same gender die. When an elder reaches the age of the sibling who died, the reaction can be quite disruptive. Not only is grieving activated, but also rehearsal for one's own death may occur. In some cases in which an elder sibling survives younger ones, there may be not only a deep grief but also pangs of guilt: "Why them and not me?"

Other Kin

Interaction with collateral kin (cousins, aunts, uncles, nieces, nephews) generally depends on proximity, preference, and the general availability of primary kin. The quality of relationships varies but is still a potential source of joy, support, assistance, or conflict. Maternal kin (related through female bloodlines) may be emotionally closer than those in one's paternal line (Jett, 2002). These relatives may provide a reservoir of kin from which to find replacements for missing or lost intimate relationships for singles or childless people as they grow older.

Surrogate Family Forms: Fictive Kin

Fictive kin are non–blood kin who serve as "genuine fake families," as expressed by Virginia Satir. These non-relatives become surrogate family and take on some of the instrumental and affectional attributes of family. Fictive kin are important in the lives of many elders, especially those with no close or satisfying family relationships and those living alone or in institutions. Fictive kin includes both friends and, often, paid caregivers. Primary care providers such as nursing assistants, nurses, or case managers often become fictive kin. Professionals who work with older people need to recognize the instrumental and emotional support, as well as the mutually satisfying relationships, that occur between friends, neighbors, and other fictive kin who assist dependent older adults.

CAREGIVING ROLES

Mary Lund (2005, p. 152), quoting Rosalyn Carter, offers the following reflection on caregiving:

> There are four kinds of people in the world: those who have been caregivers, those who are currently caregivers, those who will be caregivers, and those who will need caregivers.

Lund (2005) suggests that assuming a caregiving role:

> …is a time of transition that requires a restructuring of one's goals, behaviors, and responsibilities. It requires taking on something new but it is also about loss—of what was and what could have been. Caregiving responsibilities often create conflicts with obligations to work or family. There is the emotional pain of seeing a parent or spouse become physically or cognitively incapacitated. Caregivers experience the whole range of human emotions: guilt, anger, frustration, exhaustion, anxiety, fear, grief, sadness, love, and the not-to-be underestimated satisfaction of having done a good job (p. 152).

Gerontological nurses are most likely to encounter elders with their family and friends in situations relating to caregiving of some kind. Family members provide 80% of care for older adults in the United States (Curry et al., 2006). The

majority of caregiving takes place in the home of the elder or that of the caregiver. In 2004, a study by the National Alliance for Caregiving (NAC) and the American Association of Retired People (AARP) estimated that there were 44.4 million caregivers in 22.9 million homes. The face of informal caregiving has changed and may include family, friends, and paid and unpaid workers, as well as volunteers in the home. "Researchers estimate that family caregiving for older adults in 2000 had an economic value of $257 billion. Without the involvement of informal caregivers caring for older relatives, the cost of providing care would stagger the health care system" (Schumacher et al., 2006, p. 42). Even though generally considered a women's issue, in more and more cases, male caregivers, including those other than spouses (e.g., brothers, nephews, sons), are assuming a full range of caregiving roles (Houde et al., 2001). Thirty-nine percent of caregivers are men (Lund, 2005; National Alliance for Caregiving [NAC] and AARP, 2004). Family caregiving has become a normative experience (similar to marriage, working, or retirement) for many of America's families and cuts across racial, ethnic, and social class distinctions (Lund, 2005). In 17% percent of white households and 15% of African-American households, at least one person is providing care to an adult 50 years of age or older (Schumacher et al., 2006).

Earlier studies have suggested that caregiver burden may be less in African-Americans and that ethnic minority caregivers rely less on formal support than do whites. Results of a meta-analysis of ethnic differences in stressors, resources, and psychological outcomes of family caregiving (Pinquart and Sorensen, 2005) raise questions about assumptions that ethnic minority caregivers rely less on formal support or that they experience less caregiver burden or depression. This study points out the need for further research into ethnic differences in caregiving, an area of particular need in light of the increasing number of ethnically and racially diverse elders (Box 20-3).

Although caregiving is a means to "give back" to a loved one and can be a source of joy in the giving, it is also stressful and can be physically and emotionally demanding, leading to increased medical illnesses and a greater risk of mortality (Zarit, 2006). Caregivers are considered to be "the hidden patient" (Schulz and Beach, 1999, p. 2216). Caregivers frequently experience depression and physical and emotional exhaustion (Box 20-4). Whereas not all caregivers experience consequential stress, the circumstances that are more likely to cause problems with caregiving include competing role responsibilities (e.g., work, home), advanced age of the caregiver, high-intensity caregiving needs, insufficient resources, dementia of the care recipient, and prior relational conflicts between the caregiver and care recipient (Navaie-Waliser et al., 2002). In addition, appraisal, coping responses, and social support have been reported to be significant predictors of stress in the caregiving role (McCarty, 1996). Box 20-5 presents caregiver needs.

The positive benefits of caregiving have been given more attention in recent years, but further research is needed to

---

BOX 20-3 Evidence-Based Practice: Ethnic Differences in Stressors, Resources, and Psychological Outcomes of Family Caregiving: A Meta-Analysis

PURPOSE

This study examines ethnic differences in caregiver background variables, objective stressors, filial obligations, beliefs, psychological and social resources, coping processes, and psychological and physical health.

SAMPLE/SETTING

A conceptual model of ethnic differences was used to guide an analysis of 116 articles describing research on White, non-Hispanic, African-American, Hispanic, Asian-American, and Native American caregivers from English language sources.

METHOD

Meta-analysis of research on caregiving with statistical analysis of ethnic differences reported. The following hypotheses were examined:

- Compared with White caregivers, ethnic minority caregivers would be younger, more likely to be female, adult children, and employed, and more likely to have lower socioeconomic status.
- Minority caregivers would face higher levels of care receiver impairments, use more informal and less formal support, and report higher levels of filial obligation beliefs, cognitive coping, uplifts, and positive well-being than White caregivers.
- Low levels of service use and stronger impairments of psychological and physical health will be found in Hispanic and Asian-American caregivers than in African-Americans.

RESULTS

Ethnic minority caregivers provided more hours of care; had fewer financial resources and less education but used more informal support and cognitive and emotion-focused coping than Whites. African-American caregivers reported better psychological health, whereas results were inconsistent for Hispanic. Asian-American caregivers exhibited poorer psychological health than Whites. Most ethnic differences were small and should not be overinterpreted. Elevated levels of stressors were found for the minority groups, but African-Americans were less burdened and depressed while Hispanic and Asian-American caregivers were more depressed than White caregivers. Again, most differences were small. Advantages and disadvantages for caregivers are not identical across ethnic groups. Ethnic caregivers received more informal and less formal support than Whites. However, only Asian-American caregivers used significantly less formal support than Whites and this may be related to language barriers. Hispanic and Asian caregivers reported lower levels of relational quality with the care recipient than Whites.

IMPLICATIONS

Future research should focus on the similarities and differences between ethnic groups such as language-related barriers of service use, different types of acculturation, and differences between ethnic subgroups (e.g., Mexican-American and Cuban-Americans). Studies comparing motivation for care provision, coping processes, and emotional strengths of different ethnic groups are needed to explain caregiver outcome differences. Differences between groups were small and ethnicity explained only 1.5% to 5% of the observed variance in caregiver burden and depression. There was no evidence that minority caregivers rely less on formal support than do Whites as a result of differences in value systems. Caregiver interventions with African-Americans need to focus on improving the physical health of caregivers, and improving the quality of relationship between caregiver and care receiver may be especially useful for Hispanics and Asian-American caregivers. Interventions with White caregivers may benefit from knowledge gained from studies of ethnic minority caregivers who report more positive benefits from caregiving. The benefits that African-Americans have in using positive appraisal to cope with high stress levels may be useful additions to all caregiver interventions. Further research comparing more homogeneous ethnic groups to Whites or to each other is needed, and we should be cautious accepting untested ad hoc explanations such as African-Americans do not need formal services because they use more informal support.

Data from Pinquart M, Sorensen S: Ethnic differences in stressors, resources, and psychological outcomes of family caregiving: a meta-analysis, *Gerontologist* 45(1):90-106, 2005.

---

help understand what factors influence how caregivers perceive the experience. Positive benefits of caregiving may include enhanced self-esteem and well-being, personal growth and satisfaction, and finding or making meaning through caregiving (Chappel and Reid, 2002; Hunt, 2003; Pinquart and Sorensen, 2005). "Giving and receiving care among family members involves complex interactions that can be stressful, with potentially positive and negative consequences for each member of the dyad" (Sebern, 2005, p. 170). Most attention in caregiving research has been given to the caregiver and less to the care recipient or the relationship between the caregiver and care recipient.

Patricia Archbold and her colleagues have studied caregiving as a role, examining how the relationships between the caregiver and care recipient (mutuality) and the preparation of the caregiver (preparedness) influence reactions to caregiving (Archbold et al., 1990). Mutuality is defined as "an enduring quality of a relationship with four components: shared values, love, shared activities, and reciprocity (Sebern, 2005, p. 175). Caregivers who have a positive relationship with the care recipient experience less stress and find caregiving more meaningful. Nursing interventions to assist in preparing the caregiver for the caregiving role, particularly at the time of discharge from the hospital, also seem to prevent or reduce role strain. Nurses working with older people and their caregivers need to assess both the quality of the caregiver–care recipient relationship and how prepared the caregiver is for assuming the role (Archbold et al., 1990). Sebern (2005) suggests the construct of shared care as a framework for understanding both the caregiving and

BOX 20-4 Suggestions to Reduce Caregiver Stress

To reduce caregiver stress, nurses are advised to use all means and resources at their disposal to do the following:

- Restore a sense of control and effectiveness in the situation.
- Reinforce any social supports that are available to the caregiver.
- Find opportunities for group participation with other caregivers.
- Advise routine times of respite, and assist caregiver in finding respite sources.

Schmall et al.* suggest the following:

- Tailor programs and services to the unique situation of caregiver and care recipient.
- Urge the caregiver to take care of self.
- Encourage caregiver to maintain activities important to his or her well-being.
- Allow the caregiver to express negative and angry feelings they may have about the care recipient and the caregiving experience.
- Encourage the caregiver's efforts to use all available resources and assistance.
- Include all directly involved parties in decisions about care.
- Praise whatever is being done well, and encourage letting go of things that have not gone well.

*Schmall VL, Stiehl R: *Coping with caregiving: How to manage stress when caring for older relatives,* Corvallis, OR, 2003, Pacific Northwest Extension. Available at *http://extension.oregonstate.edu/catalog/PDF/PNW/PNW315.pdf.*

BOX 20-5 Caregiver Needs

- Finding time for myself
- Keeping the person I care for safe
- Balancing work and family responsibilities
- Managing emotional and physical stress
- Finding easy and satisfying activities to do with the care recipient
- Learning how to talk to physicians
- Making end-of-life decisions
- Moving or lifting the care recipient; bathing and dressing
- Managing the challenging behaviors of the care recipient
- Negotiating health care and home and community-based services
- Managing complex medication schedules or high-tech medical equipment
- Choosing a home health agency, assisted living or skilled nursing facility
- Managing incontinence or toileting problems
- Finding non-English educational material

From Curry L et al: Educational needs of employed family caregivers of older adults: evaluation of a workplace project, *Geriatr Nurs* 27(3):166-173, 2006; Family Caregiver Alliance: Caregiver assessment: principles, guidelines and strategies for change, Report from a National Consensus Development Conference (vol 1), San Francisco, 2006, The Alliance.

BOX 20-6 Suggestions for Caregivers

- Educate yourself about the disease or medical condition
- Find a health care professional who understands the disease
- Consult with other experts to help plan for the future (legal, financial)
- Tap your social resources for assistance
- Find a confidante
- Take time for relaxation and exercise
- Use community resources
- Maintain your sense of humor
- Explore religious beliefs and spiritual values
- Set realistic goals

From U.S. Department of Health and Human Services Administration on Aging, National Family Caregiver Support Program Resources: Taking Care of Yourself. (website): *www.aoa.gov.* Accessed June 28, 2007.

receiving relationship and individualizing interventions to assist in enhancing the relationship to promote positive outcomes. Further research is needed to understand the complexities of the caregiving and care receiving role and provide a theory base for nursing interventions. Box 20-6 presents some suggestions for caregivers.

With the increase in the older adult population, declining household size, and a shortage of direct health care workers, projections are that there will be fewer caregivers for older people in the future. A new American Association of Retired Persons (AARP) Public Policy Institute Report (2006), *Who's Caring for the Caregivers?*, found that "the use of paid, formal care by older persons with disabilities in the community has been decreasing, while their sole reliance on family caregivers has been increasing." (Accessed August 13, 2006 from *www.aarp.org/research/press-center/presscurrentnews/caring_for_caregivers.html.*)

Caregiving is considered in some depth here because it is one of the most crucial phenomena today. Caregiving for older people with Alzheimer's disease and other dementias presents some unique challenges and is discussed in Chapter 23.

Caring for Parents

The role of elders with adult children is usually studied as a caregiving issue. Adult children are sometimes said to reverse roles with parents when the parents become old and dependent. This scenario has a demeaning connotation, as if the elder becomes a child again. In illness and deterioration of the elder, the adult child may at times feel parental, but the inner child always remains in need of the protective and guiding parent. No matter how mature a person becomes, the parent symbolizes security and acceptance, regardless of the reality or facts. These dynamics often make the caregiving role very complex and difficult.

A 2004 study by the NAC and AARP found that 61% of caregivers were women with an average age of 46 years, although 13% were 65 years of age or older, and in most cases, adult daughters were providing care for their older mothers.

Middle-aged caregivers, "the sandwich generation," often struggle to balance the demands of work and parenting with caregiving for an older relative. Fingerman (2001b) provides research-based findings of the positive and negative emotions that occur between older mothers and their adult daughters, one of the most frequently encountered caregiving relationships.

Filial obligation is associated with a sense of duty toward one's parents that is inherent in the relationship. In some cultures and in many ethnic groups, this sense of duty is strong. As a result, it is expected that children will set aside their own needs to meet those of the parent. If the children have active lives and demanding careers or face multiple needs of their own children, conflicts with the needs of the parents are fairly certain. Many children find ways to overcome the conflicts and provide a substantial amount of elder care as just noted. The major concerns arise when the child caregiver is not available or willing to assume these responsibilities if he or she is needed.

Spousal Caregiving

Among older adults receiving care in the community, 23.4% received this from spouses (Burton et al., 2003). Elderly spouses caring for disabled partners have special needs and may face many role changes. "An older woman may need to learn to drive, manage money, or make decisions by herself. Male caregivers may need to take on unfamiliar household chores such as cooking or laundry, or helping their partner with personal hygiene" (Lund, 2005, p. 152). The spouse may have significant health problems that are neglected in deference to the greater needs of the incapacitated partner. The disabled spouse may need physical care that is beyond the capabilities of the spouse/caregiver.

The nurse should be alert to situations in which health care personnel may be able to provide supports and resources that make it possible for an individual to assume new responsibilities without being totally overwhelmed. When a spouse is ill and the mate needs to take over functions for both, someone must be available to give reinforcement, encouragement, and relief. An adult day program, routine visits from a community health nurse, or periodic assistance from a home health aide or a housekeeper may make it possible for the couple to continue to live together. One important consideration is counseling the couple to maintain as much independent function as possible for both people.

Aging Parents Caring for Developmentally Disabled Children

Although we tend to think of caregivers as middle-aged adults caring for elders, an unknown number of elders are caring for their middle-aged children who are physically and mentally disabled. Earlier in the past century these developmentally disabled children usually died before reaching adulthood; now, with improved care, they are surviving. An estimated 4.3 million people in the United States with developmental disabilities live at home, and a quarter of them are being cared for by a family member who is at least 60 years old (Ansberry, 2004). Often this has been a burden carried by parents for their entire adult life and will end only with the death of the parent or the adult child. The phenomenon of an aging parent caring for an aging child is beginning to receive attention by both organizations for aging and organizations for developmentally disabled individuals (Ansberry, 2004). The Planned Lifetime Assistance Network (PLAN), available in some states through the National Alliance for the Mentally Ill, provides lifetime assistance to individuals with disabilities whose parents or other family members are deceased or can no longer provide for their care (Hooyman and Kiyak, 2005; www.nami.org).

Grandparents Raising Grandchildren

In recent years, more grandparents have become, by default, the primary caregivers of grandchildren because the parents are unable to provide the care needed as a result of child abuse, teen pregnancy, imprisonment, joblessness, military deployment, drug and alcohol addictions, illness, death, and other social problems (AARP, 2005; Butler and Zakari, 2005). In the United States, an estimated 400,000 to 600,000 grandparents have assumed parental roles for their grandchildren (6.3% of all children younger than 18 years in the United States) (AARP, 2005; NAC, 2004). Grandparents raising grandchildren is a global phenomenon as well. The AARP report *Intergenerational Relationships: Grandparents Raising Grandchildren* states that although the number of children being raised by grandparents in the United States is significantly high, it is much less than the millions of children in Africa and other developing countries who are being raised by grandparents or other relatives. Grandparents in these developing countries face great challenges in providing basic subsistence for their grandchildren, and often for themselves. The *Grandmother Project* (*www.aarp.org/research/family/grandparenting/may_06_gubser_grandmother.html*) is a U.S. nonprofit organization working to strengthen the leadership role of grandmothers in improving health for women and children in Laos, Senegal, Mali, Uzbekistan, and Albania. Outcomes of the project include greater confidence among grandmothers, increased community respect for elder women, and improvements in advice to young women on pregnancy, infant feeding, and neonatal health.

In the United States, the number of grandparents raising grandchildren has increased by more than 30% since 1990 and continues to grow. The most recent U.S. Census showed that more than one fourth of grandparents ages 65 years and older who reported living with grandchildren 18 years of age and younger have primary responsibility for them (Butler and Zakari, 2005; U.S. Census Bureau, 2004).

Of grandparents caring for grandchildren, 20% were older than 65 years and 50% of the children were younger than 6 years (Troope, 2000). Unmarried older women and African-American grandparents are more likely to assume a primary caregiver role with their grandchildren although the phenomenon is increasingly prevalent in all races, ethnic groups,

BOX 20-7   Suggested Nursing Interventions with Grandparent Caregivers

- Early identification of at-risk grandparents
- Comprehensive assessment of physical, psychosocial, and environmental factors affecting those in the caregiving role for grandchildren
- Anticipatory guidance and counseling about child growth and development and other child-raising issues
- Referral to resources for support and counseling
- Advocacy for policies supportive of grandparents who have assumed a caregiving role for grandchildren

Data from Butler F, Zakari N: Grandparents parenting grandchildren: assessing health status, *J Gerontol Nurs* 31(3):43-54, 2005.

and social classes around the world. Thirteen percent of African-American children, 8% of Hispanic children, and 4% of Asian and Caucasian children are being raised by grandparents. A large proportion of Native American children are also being raised by grandparents, with estimates that in some Indian tribes, up to 60% of children are in this situation (AARP, 2005). AARP (2003) reports on research related to African-American, Hispanic, and Native American caregiving grandparents *(www.aarp.org/research/family/grandparenting/aresearch-import-483.html)*.

Research is lacking related to the physical and mental health consequences of grandparents raising grandchildren, and no clear data are available on the effect of grandparent caregiving on health status (Butler and Zakari, 2005; Grinstead et al., 2003). As with other types of caregiving, there are both blessing and burdens (Davidhizar et al., 2000). Grandparents who are caregivers report that it provides a sense of purpose that keeps them going, and in some cases, children raised solely by grandparents fare better than those in single-parent families (Roe and Minkler, 1998-1999).

For many grandparents, however, economic, health, and social challenges associated with caregiving may include limited income and financial support through the welfare system, lack of informal support systems, loss of leisure and social activities in retirement, and shame or guilt related to their children's inability to parent (Butler and Zakari, 2005; Grinstead et al., 2003; Hooyman and Kiyak, 2005). Too often, both the children and their grandparents are in need of help. As expected, many of these children have multiple loss and grief issues and need mental health services (Brown-Standridge and Floyd, 2000). Box 20-7 provides research-based suggestions for nursing interventions with older adults who are providing primary care to their grandchildren.

The U.S. government has recognized that increasing numbers of older adults are raising grandchildren, great-grandchildren, and other younger relatives. However, there is a continued need to develop services that support grandparents as sole caregivers. Some of the funds distributed through the Older Americans Act have been earmarked to support this group. Nurses can refer the grandparents to their local area agency on aging to inquire about available re-

sources. The AARP also provides resources for grandparents (see the Resources section at the end of this chapter).

Long-Distance Caregiving

Because of the increasing mobility of today's society, more children move away from home for education or employment and do not return home. When the parent needs help, it must be provided "long distance." In 2004 the NAC estimated that more than 7 million caregivers lived more than 1 hour away from the care recipient. Of these caregivers, 70% were employed full time and most lost work hours regularly because of their added responsibilities. This is perhaps one of the most difficult situations, and it presents unique challenges. The usual impulse is to move the elder into the family's home or to a more accessible location for the family, but this may not be best for an elder who has lived a long time in one community and has many supports there. Box 20-8 presents factors to consider when planning to add an older person to the household. Plans and alternatives should be discussed before emergency events and may prevent the need for hasty decisions. Conferring with a geriatric care manager in advance of any evidence of problems may forestall the need to move the parent into the adult child's home. Issues that need to be considered include identifying a local person who will be available quickly in emergency situations; identifying reliable individuals or services that will provide daily monitoring if necessary; identifying acceptable facilities for assisted living if that becomes necessary; determining which family member is most likely to be free to travel to the elder if needed; and being sure that legalities regarding advance directives, a will, and power of attorney (for health care and financial) have been established.

A profession and industry have emerged to assist the geographically distant family member to ensure that an elderly relative will be cared for; this profession is made up of geriatric care managers, some of whom are nurses or social workers. A care manager can be hired to do everything a family member would do if able, from being available in an emergency, to helping with estate planning, to making arrangements for a move to a nursing home. Often care managers know of resources that can assist the elder to remain independent and yet assure the family that safety and other needs are being met. These services are available primarily to those who are able to pay for them since they are not covered by private insurance, Medicare, or any public agencies. Although these services are expensive, they are far less expensive than alternative living arrangements or institutional placement.

Similar services may be available for persons with very low incomes by asking the local area agency on aging about the local "Community Care for the Elderly" programs. Some states also have *nursing home diversion projects* to provide home support to those who would otherwise qualify for Medicaid coverage for nursing home care. When incomes are too high to qualify for Medicaid and too low to pay for private care managers, the persons and their families must

---

BOX 20-8   Planning to Add an Older Person to the Household

Questions you need to ask:
- What are the needs of the new member and of the family?
- Where will space be allotted for the new member?
- How will this new member be included in existing family patterns?
- How will responsibilities be shared?
- What resources in the community will assist in the adjustment phase?
- Is the environment safe for this new member?
- How will family life change with the added member, and how does the family feel about it?
- What are the differences in socialization and sleeping patterns?
- What are the older person's strong needs and expectations?
- What are the older person's skills and talents?

Modifications you need to make:
- Arrange semiprivate living quarters if possible.
- Regularly schedule visits to other relatives to give each family times of respite and privacy.
- Arrange adult day health programs and senior activities for the older person to help keep contact with members of his or her own generation. Consider how the older person will feel about giving up familiar surroundings and friends.

Discuss potential areas of conflict:
- Space: especially if someone has given up his or her space to the older relative.

- Possessions: older people may want to move possessions into house; others may not find them attractive or may insist on replacing them with new things.
- Entertaining: times when old and young feel the need or desire to exclude the other from social events.
- Responsibilities and chores: the older person may feel useless if he or she does nothing and may feel in the way if he or she does something; young may feel that their position is usurped or may be angry if they wait on parent.
- Expenses: increased cost of home maintenance, food, clothing, and recreation may not be shared appropriately.
- Vacations: whether to go together or alone; the young may feel uneasy not taking older person out and resentful if they must.
- Child rearing: disagreement over child-rearing policies.
- Child care: grandparental babysitting may be welcomed by family and resented by older person, or if not allowed, older person feels lack of trust in capability.

Decrease areas of conflict by the following:
- Respecting privacy.
- Discussing space allocations.
- Discussing elderly person's furnishings before move.
- Making it clear in advance when social events include everyone or exclude someone.
- Clearing decisions about household tasks—all should have responsibility geared to ability.
- Paying a share of expenses and maintaining a separate phone reduce strain and increase feelings of independence.

---

do the best they can. Long-distance care then depends on the goodness of neighbors, local friends, and apartment managers and frequent trips by the long-distance caregiver to the elder.

Role of Nonfamily Caregivers

Close relationships often develop between older adults and their nonfamily caregivers. Over 50% of family caregivers use nurses, homemakers, and other personal care providers to assist in the care of their elder dependents (Piercy, 2001). These providers may include friends and hired or volunteer caregivers from a church or agency. Piercy (2001) found that only 40% of the care recipients actually had living relatives. The caregivers not only provide substantial physical care but also are involved with the elder, when possible, in social activities such as dining, concerts, and church events. Conditions that foster closeness include continuity of caregiver, social isolation of the elder, homogeneity of the client-caregiver, and the caregiver performing extra tasks and small personal attentions. The client will sometimes describe a paid caregiver as "my family." Elders and their caregivers in nursing homes often describe their relationship "like family" as well (Touhy et al., 2005). A caveat should be added that is explained in Chapter 18—dependent and lonely elders with assets may be vic-

timized by apparently doting caregivers who may exert undue influence.

▲ Promoting Healthy Aging: Implications for Gerontological Nursing

Nurses are often the primary care providers and case managers for elders and their families both in the home and in the institutional setting. The nurse monitors progress and manages chronic disorders of the elder within the context of the family. Support for families in the caregiving role is an important nursing intervention and one that needs continued attention by policymakers.

Family Assessment. A comprehensive assessment of the elder includes assessment of the family: who are the members; what is the family history; and what are their usual roles and their strengths, contributions, and deterrents to the function of the family unit. Assessing the family's needs and strengths, as well as its sources of stress, particular methods of coping, meaning of caregiving, cultural values, support system, and family dynamics, will help the nurse know the family and design responses that may strengthen the family unit.

Often, nurses see families in times of crisis when an older family member needs care. It is important to encourage the expression of feelings from all involved family members, as

BOX 20-9 Family Support System Assessment*

Size	Number in extended family who are accessible
	Number of daughters who are accessible
	Number of sons who are accessible
	Number of grandchildren, nephews, nieces, confidants, siblings
Ability	Economic status of each:
	Poverty
	Lower middle
	Middle
	Upper middle
	Wealthy
Willingness	Frequency of involvement:
	Monthly
	Weekly
	Daily
	Constant
Functions	Contributions to elderly member:
	Money
	Chores
	Transportation
	Listening and psychological support
	Functional assistance
Deterrents	Other demands:
	Work
	Travel
	Adolescent children
Recent stresses	Poor health
	Job change
	Moves
	Deaths

*The strengths of the family or possible dysfunctional aspects can be assessed in a superficial but helpful manner by using the Family APGAR (Smilkstein G: Validity and reliability of the family APGAR as a test of family function, *J Fam Pract* 15[2]:303-311, 1982).

BOX 20-10 Nursing Actions to Create and Sustain a Partnership with Caregivers

- Surveillance and ongoing monitoring
- Coaching: helping caregivers apply knowledge and develop skills
- Teaching: providing information and instruction
- Fostering partnerships: fostering communication and collaboration between the caregiver and the care recipient and between them and the nurse
- Providing psychosocial support: attending to psychosocial well-being
- Rescuing: providing a safety net by stepping in to provide direct care and making clinical decisions
- Coordinating: orchestrating the work of other health care team members and the activities of the caregiver

Data from Eilers J et al: Independent nursing actions in cooperative care, *Oncol Nurs Forum* 32(4):849-855, 2005; Schumacher K et al: Family caregivers: caring for older adults working with their families, *Am J Nurs* 106(8):40-49, 2006.

Caregiver Assessment. Family members who assume the caregiving role, as just discussed, experience both stressors and benefits. The stresses, expectations of future needs and problems, and the positive aspects of the caregiving situation should be explored. Caregiver assessment includes how the family member can help the care recipient and how the health care team can help the person providing care. In light of the physical and emotional stressors often associated with the caregiving role, nurses need to monitor the physical and emotional health of both the caregiver and the care recipient and provide support as necessary. A partnership model, combining the "nurse's professional expertise with the caregiver's knowledge of the family member, is recommended" (Schumacher et al., 2006, p. 47). Box 20-10 presents a research-based model to guide nursing interventions with caregivers.

The Family Caregiver Alliance (2006) principles to guide caregiver assessment include the following: (1) caregiver assessment should include the needs and preferences of both the care recipient and the family caregiver; (2) caregiver assessment should reflect culturally competent practice; (3) caregiver assessment should be multidimensional and conducted with a multidisciplinary approach; and (4) caregiver assessment should result in a plan of care developed collaboratively with the caregiver that specifies the provision of services and intended measurable outcomes. Box 20-11 presents the components of caregiving assessment.

Several validated caregiver assessment instruments are available, including the Preparedness for Caregiving Scale and the Mutuality Scale (Archbold et al., 1992) (website: *www.geronurseonline.org*) and the Caregiver Strain Index developed by Robinson (1983) (Figure 20-1).

Caregiver Interventions. The New York University (NYU) Spouse Caregiver Intervention Study reported by Mittleman (2002) found the most useful of the interventions studied included a few sessions of counseling with the care-

well as the older person, and maintain a nonjudgmental attitude. It is important for the nurse to be aware of his or her vision of what a "family" should be and what a "family" should do. Our values should not enter into assessment and intervention with clients. Meiner and Lueckenotte (2006, p. 137) remind us that we should not "label families as 'dysfunctional' but rather build upon the strengths within each family and provide support and resources for limitations." Thus the nurse's role is to teach, monitor, and strengthen the family system so as to maintain health and wellness of the entire family structure.

A mutually constructed, written assessment of a family's needs and coping capacities can be both comprehensive and specific and becomes a document of the family's strengths in times of stress. Including the family in the discussion of the outcome of the assessment is recommended for all settings, especially in long-term care facilities and home care. Box 20-9 presents a family assessment.

BOX 20-11 Recommended Domains and Constructs of Caregiver Assessment

DOMAINS	CONSTRUCTS
Context	Caregiver relationship to care recipient Physical environment (home, facility) Household status (e.g., number in home) Financial status Quality of family relationships Duration of caregiving Employment status (work/home/volunteer)
Caregiver's perception of health and functional status of recipient	Activities of daily living (ADLs) (e.g., bathing, dressing) Instrumental activities of daily living (IADLs) (e.g., managing finances, using the telephone) Psychosocial needs Cognitive impairment Behavioral problems Medical tests and procedures
Caregiver values and preferences	Caregiver/care recipient willingness to assume/accept care Perceived filial obligation to provide care Culturally based norms Preferences for scheduling and delivering care and services
Well-being of the caregiver	Self-rated health Health conditions and symptoms Depression or other emotional distress (e.g., anxiety) Life satisfaction/quality of life

Consequences of caregiving	Perceived challenges:
	   Social isolation
	   Work strain
	   Emotional and physical health
	   Financial strain
	   Family relationship strain
	Perceived benefits:
	   Satisfaction of helping family member
	   Developing new skills and competencies
	   Improved family relationships

Skills/abilities/knowledge to provide recipient with needed care	Caregiving confidence and competencies Appropriate knowledge of medical care tasks (e.g., wound care)
Potential resources that caregiver could choose to use	Formal and informal helping network and perceived quality of social support Existing or potential strengths (e.g., what is presently going well) Coping strategies Financial resources (health care and service benefits, entitlements such as Veteran's Affairs, Medicare) Community resources and services (caregiver support programs, religious organizations, volunteer agencies)

From Recommended Domains and Constructs, p. 16, Family Caregiver Alliance, 2006: *Caregiver assessment: principles, guidelines and strategies for change,* Report from a National Consensus Development Conference (vol 1), San Francisco, The Alliance. *www.caregiver.org.*

giver and other involved family members and a support group for primary caregivers, as well as ongoing telephone support. These interventions, when available, can alleviate much of the stress of caregiving (Box 20-12 and Table 20-1).

With many caregivers trying to balance caregiving responsibilities while still working, educational programs offered in the workplace can be beneficial for both the caregiver and the employer (Curry et al., 2006). Box 20-13 presents suggested topics for programs. Several caregiver education and support programs are also available on-line (see the Resources section at the end of this chapter).

Respite Care. Respite is the provision of temporary relief to the caregiver and is perhaps the most significant intervention with families. Respite may be in many forms, including the temporary stay of the elder in a care facility,

I am going to read a list of things that other people have found to be difficult. Would you tell me if any of these apply to you? (Give examples.)

	Yes = 1	No = 0
Sleep is disturbed (e.g., because is in and out of bed; wanders around at night)		
It is inconvenient (e.g., because helping takes so much time; it's a long drive over to help)		
It is a physical strain (e.g., because of lifting in and out of a chair; effort or concentration is required)		
It is confining (e.g., helping restricts free time; cannot go visiting)		
There have been family adjustments (e.g., because helping has disrupted routine; there has been no privacy)		
There have been changes in personal plans (e.g., had to turn down a job; could not go on vacation)		
There have been other demands on my time (e.g., from other family members)		
There have been emotional adjustments (e.g., because of severe arguments)		
Some behavior is upsetting (e.g., because of incontinence; has trouble remembering things; accuses people of taking things)		
It is upsetting to find _____ has changed so much from his/her former self (e.g., he/she is a different person than he/she used to be)		
There have been work adjustments (e.g., because of having to take time off)		
It is a financial strain		
Feeling completely overwhelmed (e.g., because of worry about _____; concerns about how to manage)		
TOTAL SCORE (Count yes responses. Any positive answer may indicate a need for intervention in that area. A score of 7 or higher indicates a high level of stress.)		

FIGURE 20-1 Caregiver strain index. (From Robinson B. *J Gerontol* 38:344, 1983. Copyright © The Gerontological Society of America. Reproduced by permission of the publisher. Available at *www.hartfordign.org*.)

participation in an adult day program, or in-home relief by a relief informal or formal caregiver. Adult day services are a valuable resource for community-dwelling elders and can also provide needed respite for caregivers. The types of adult day services include the following: adult day social care, which provides social activities, meals, recreation, and some health-related services; adult day health care, which offers more intensive therapeutic, health, and social services for elders with severe medical problems and for those at risk for nursing home placement; and Alzheimer's-specific day programs, which provide social and health services to persons with Alzheimer's and related dementias. Participants can attend these programs for several hours a day or full days, and some also provide services on Satur-days. Adult day programs have grown in the last 20 years, with approximately 4000 centers nationwide. The average cost of services is around $56/day, but some provide services with a sliding-scale fee. Fees are not covered under Medicare, but Medicaid does cover costs if the elder qualifies financially. Private medical insurance policies and long-term care insurance may also pay for adult day services depending on the policy (National Adult Day Services Association, 2007). Local Area Agencies on Aging can provide information on adult day services and other forms of respite care. Respite care is also offered by many long-term care facilities. Nurses need to encourage caregivers to use this resource to provide needed relief from caregiving and to restore their energy and well-being.

TABLE 20-1

Positive Outcomes Reported by the Clients and Caregivers

Outcomes	Caregivers' Comments	Clients' Comments
Social enjoyment		It was an outing. An excuse to go out and talk to people!
Increased knowledge	I am more aware now. I know what things to look for.	I enjoyed the assessment. I learned from it.
Reduced stress	The support was very good. There was tremendous amount of guilt going on…Assessment helped us to deal with these things.	I was reassured that this was part of an illness. I had an explanation why this was happening.
Enhanced skills and feelings of competence	It proved very useful for our learning process in terms of her management (referring to client) and my own coping.	I learned how to cope better with my disability. I'm more positive as a result of it.
Better family communication and collaboration	They helped with communication with family. Our children now better understand how to support me.	
Improved decision-making	I don't know what we would have done without the geriatric services…It helped us to make decisions.	
Greater access to services	Everything came out of that assessment: the diagnosis, home services, day program.	
Positive health outcomes	If it wasn't for the assessment, she wouldn't be here today. She may have died in her apartment.	

From Aminzadeh F et al: Comprehensive geriatric assessment: exploring clients' and caregivers' perceptions of the assessment process and outcomes, *J Gerontol Nurs* 28(6):9, 2002.

BOX 20-12   Goals of Family Support Groups

- Learn to accept the elder as he or she is now, let go of the past.
- Learn the balance between protectiveness and smothering.
- Recognize one's own needs as fundamental to caring for others.
- Learn to share and cope with disappointment.
- Discuss resurgence of feelings of loss during holidays and anniversaries.
- Share knowledge of how to deal with family and community.
- Develop a caring and sharing network within the group.
- Deal with feelings of guilt, helplessness, and hopelessness.
- Identify realistic ways to assist in the care of the elder.

Modified from Richards M: Family support groups, *Generations* 10(4):68, 1986.

BOX 20-13   Topics For Workplace Caregiver Assistance Programs

- Normal and healthy aging
- Communicating effectively with older adults
- Medication use
- Caring for the caregiver
- Specific health information
- Community resources
- Supplemental services
- Housing and long-term care options
- Medicare, Medigap, and other insurance (e.g., long-term care)
- Support groups
- End-of-life and legal information (e.g., advance directives)

From Curry L et al: Educational needs of employed family caregivers of older adults: evaluation of a workplace project, *Geriatr Nurs* 27(3):166-173, 2006.

An innovative intervention that may help caregivers obtain some relief from care is video respite. The care recipient in the home or institution can view videotapes of music, memories, and pictures that were developed by researchers at the Gerontology Center at the University of Utah for persons with dementia (Lund et al., 1995; Meiner and Lueckenotte, 2006). The researchers report that persons with Alzheimer's disease watch and participate with the tapes, and nursing home staff report that the tapes have a calming effect on the residents (see the Resources section at the end of this chapter). Families can also make their own videos or DVDs with family memories or messages from loved ones that can be played for care recipients.

Interventions with caregivers must always consider the great variability in family structures, resources, traditions, and history. The range of adaptations is enormous, and the goal is always to restore the balance of the system to the greatest extent possible and support caregivers in their caring. The family can be visualized as a mobile with many parts, and when one is touched, each part shifts to regain the balance. The intrusion of professionals in a family system will temporarily unbalance the system and may provide an opportunity to restore the balance in a healthier manner, sometimes by adding an element or increasing the weight of one or decreasing the weight of another. When the nurse works with a family from a different culture and who may have rituals and routines unfamiliar to him or her, the nurse needs to be particularly careful to respect these differences. The nurse can work with the family to make the best use of their strengths, whatever they may be. Each family member can be valued for what he or she brings to the situation. According to Schumacher et al (2006, p. 48):

> Family members must not be allowed to 'fail' while providing care; a nurse should be available to step in when demands of the situation exceed family members' capabilities. And the nurse should be prepared to step back when the family's support is what's needed.

Box 20-10 presents suggested nursing interventions for working with caregivers.

TRANSITIONS

Numerous minor role changes occur in the aging process, but the transitions expected by most elders are related to the work role and the role of spouse or partner. Transitions require letting go of certain habits and structures and developing new ones. Some feelings of loss and bewilderment are nearly always present, and new roles and opportunities often are anticipated. Age-related transitions are socially created, shared, and recognized. A transition is socially recognized and entails a reorientation of perceptions and expectations of and by the individual. Transitions that make use of past skills and adaptations are less stressful than those that are entirely unfamiliar. Some shifts, such as those from functional independence to functional dependence, cut across many aspects of life and require major changes in lifestyle.

To the degree that an event is perceived as expected and occurring at the right time, a role transition may be comfortable and even welcomed. Those persons who must retire "too early" or are widowed "too soon" will have more difficulty adapting than those who are of an age when these events are expected. The speed and intensity of a major change may make the difference between a transitional crisis and a gradual and comfortable adaptation. Role changes that produce crises are usually abrupt losses of familiar functions at a time when meaningful substitute functions are not available. Anticipatory planning, awareness of potential problems, positive or negative attitudes, and a sense of control (by far the most important) make role transitions easier.

The most common roles of older people are retiree, parent, grandparent, great-grandparent, spouse, homemaker, widow, kin, friend, citizen, volunteer, church member, acquaintance, patient, and service recipient. In cases of role accumulation, such as that of grandparent, some previous development will be applicable, with modification, to the new role. Likewise, the shifts in parent-child relationships are gradual and do not require complete role deletion or role reversal. Those transitions that make use of past skills and adaptations may be least stressful. Cohort, cultural, and gender differences are inherent in all of life's major transitions.

Retirement

Retirement is no longer just a few years of rest from the rigors of work before death. It is a developmental stage that may occupy 30 years of one's life and involve many stages. The transitions are blurring because numerous pursuits and opportunities may occur after one has "retired." Tafford (2002) addressed this relatively new segment of adult life. She examines the unprecedented aging in the life cycle and contends that people know as little about it as they did about adolescence at the turn of the century (Age Beat On Line, 2002). The numerous patterns and styles of retiring have produced more varied experiences in retirement. More older people are working longer or changing careers after formal retirement. Some do so because of economic need, whereas others have a desire to remain involved and productive.

Older people who did not expect retirement at the time when they left the workforce may suffer detrimental effects and be in need of counseling or assistance. They may experience job separation as a crisis and a traumatic role transition triggered by an unplanned job termination; this could be the result of illness or company downsizing, a euphemism for cutting out jobs.

Others, given the opportunity to work past retirement age, must weigh the benefits. Part-time work during retirement is viewed by the working public of all ages as a desirable option. Employers seek older workers because they are reliable and dependable. Seniors older than 65 years can now earn any amount without endangering Social Security benefits. Obviously, health status and financial status affect decisions and abilities to work or engage in new work opportunities (Figures 20-2 and 20-3).

Labor Force Participation. Just as Social Security was initially seen as a mechanism for resolving unemployment, early retirement is a means of regulating the labor supply. Employers encourage early retirement of older, more expensive workers by offering attractive incentives. Early retirement packages may be so attractive that individuals retire earlier than they had planned or expected and without sufficient preparatory time.

Clearly, the goals of government and industry are in conflict related to the older workforce. Government cannot afford a large body of nonworking individuals, and industry cannot afford to keep these individuals in top-salaried positions. With recent events that have seriously threatened pension security and portability, more workers are remaining in the workforce. "The long-term trend toward ever-earlier retirement has halted" (Ekerdt and Dennis, 2002, p. 1). The work scene continually changes and becomes more complex as government policies, technology, and world economics continually destroy jobs and create new ones. The balance between downsizing and creating new jobs is variable across regions and industries.

Retirement Planning. Decisions to retire are often based on financial resources, attitude toward work, chronological age, health, and self-perceptions of ability to adjust to retirement (Box 20-14). Retirement planning is advisable during early adulthood and essential in middle age. However, people differ in their focus on the past, present, and future and their realistic ability to "put away something" for

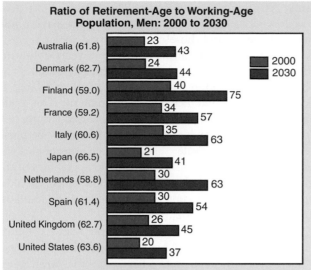

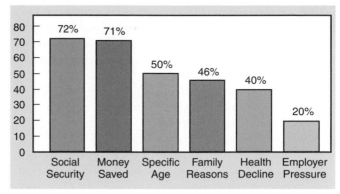

FIGURE 20-3 Reasons for retiring. (From National Council on the Aging [NCOA]: *American perceptions of aging in the 21st century,* Washington, DC, 2002. [website]: *www.ncoa.org.*)

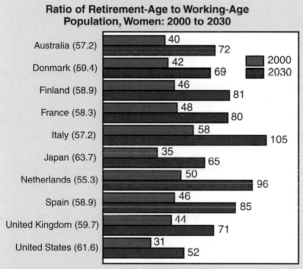

Note: Ratios represent the number of persons at or above average retirement age per 100 persons between age 20 and the average retirement age in 1995. Each national average is shown in parentheses.

FIGURE 20-2 Ratio of retirement-age to working-age population, male and female workers, selected countries, 2000 to 2030. (From Organization for Economic Cooperation and Development, 1998; and US Census Bureau, 2000.)

future needs. Retirement preparation programs are usually aimed at employees with high levels of education and occupational status, those with private pension coverage, and government employees. Thus the people most in need of planning assistance may be least likely to have any available or the resources for an adequate retirement. Individuals who are retiring in poor health, minority persons, and those in lower socioeconomic levels may experience greater concerns in retirement and may need specialized counseling. These groups are often neglected in retirement planning programs.

BOX 20-14   Issues in Retirement Potential

1. Financial need versus resources
2. Employability
3. Rewards derived from employment:
   - Wages sufficient for needs and morale
   - Satisfaction level, possibility for resolution of job frustrations
   - Meaning of job, contact with friends, source of prestige
4. Psychosocial characteristics—attitudes toward retirement:
   - Attitudes of significant others (advising? directing?)
   - Strength of work ethic
   - Effect of retirement on prestige
5. Personality factors:
   - Time orientation (past, present, future)
   - Active versus passive in planning
   - Rationalism versus fatalism as life stance
   - Type-A versus type-B personality (hard-driving, easy-going)
   - Inner-directed versus other-directed (enjoyment of self or need for high level of external motivation)
6. Level of information about retirement:
   - Planning programs on job, adult education, or community programs
   - Awareness of friends and family who have retired and how influenced by them
7. Pressures to retire:
   - Compulsory, age discriminatory
   - Unemployment (how long?)
   - Job retrogression (being moved down the ladder)
   - Skill obsolescence (opportunities for developing other skills?)
   - Peer pressure (organized or informal)
   - Employer pressure (reduced incentives to continue work, increased incentives to retire)
   - Family pressure (spouse's working status)
   - Health, discomfort, or disability interfering with job performance and dependability

Working couples must plan together for retirement. Decisions will depend on their career goals, shared future interests, and the quality of their interpersonal relationship. The following are some questions one must weigh when deciding to retire or continue working:

- What do I want to do?
- Who needs me, and what are my best opportunities?
- What am I best able to do?
- What is the meaning of my life?
- What should my life accomplish or contribute?
- Am I financially independent for the rest of my life if I live 30 or more years?
- Can I afford to completely retire from paid work?

Retirement education plans are supplied through group lectures, individual counseling, booklets, DVDs, and computerized modules. However, at this juncture and in light of the many hazards experienced by pre-retirees, planning is often insufficient. Dennis (2002) notes that many individuals have very high expectations for the final third of their lives. Although federal laws encourage increased participation in company-sponsored 401(k) plans, many of these plans are unreliable. The proposals for the privatization of Social Security also contribute to uncertainty about retirement benefits. When considering retirement, Dennis notes areas for consideration include the adequacy of (1) company-provided retirement benefits; (2) Social Security and Medicare benefits; (3) company-provided postretirement health care; and (4) financial planning. Thoughtful financial planning must include distribution options and tax consequences (LaRock, 2001).

The adequacy of retirement income depends not only on work history but also on marital history. The poverty rates of older women are excessively high. Couples who had previous marriages and divorces may have significantly lower available economic resources than those in first marriages. Child support, divorce settlements, and pension apportionment to ex-spouses may have diminished retirement income. This problem is an ever-increasing impediment to retirement because, among couples presently approaching retirement age, fewer than half are in a first marriage (U.S. Divorce Statistics, 2002). Policies have been based on the traditional lifelong marriage, and this is no longer appropriate.

Dennis (2002) notes that retirement planning is really life planning and that the process is best accomplished when, early on, individuals determine their goals, values, and motivations in life. This assessment requires personal reflection and thought about the choices in everyday life that provide satisfaction and that the individual will wish to continue in late life (Shagrin, 2002). Retirement planning has become a highly specialized professional field. For people who can afford it, engaging a retirement planner in early adulthood is wise. Nurses need to be familiar with these sources of information and discuss the need for retirement planning with their clients.

Special Considerations in Retirement. Retirement security depends on the "three-legged stool" of Social Security pensions, savings, and investments (Stanford and Usita, 2002). Older people with disabilities, those who have lacked access to education or held low-paying jobs with no benefits, and those not eligible for Social Security are at economic risk during retirement years. Minority older persons, women, immigrants, and gay and lesbian men and women often face greater challenges related to adequate income and benefits in retirement. The traditional idea of retirement as a time of increased leisure, new interests, and relaxation and enjoyment may not be possible for many older people. "Future retirement policies will need to consider the rapidly changing demographics of the aging population and the special barriers faced by older people of color, women, immigrants, and gays and lesbians" (Stanford and Usita, 2002, p. 47).

Inadequate coverage for women in retirement is common because their work histories have been sporadic and diverse. Women are often called on to retire earlier than anticipated because of family needs. Whereas most men have always worked outside the home, it has been only within the past 30 years that this has been the expectation of women. Therefore large cohort differences exist.

Traditionally, the variability of women's work histories, interrupted careers, the residuals of sexist pension policies, Social Security inequities, and low-paying jobs created hazards for adequacy of income in retirement. The scene is gradually changing in many respects, but the gender bias remains. Basing retirement calculations on gender and projected survival statistics is now illegal, though until the early 1980s, women were allotted less pension income based purely on their expected longevity compared with men. Although this is no longer true, women who retired 20 or 25 years ago remain penalized because of gender.

Older women are likely to have several years of no earnings calculated in the averages that determine the amount of their Social Security benefits. Some women find that they will receive more if their Social Security benefits are calculated on their husband's earnings; this may be true even though widowed or divorced. The Social Security Administration must be contacted regarding these matters because many variables may be used.

The complexity of the issues includes differences between retirement patterns of single and married women and men. Single and married women differ in the degree of dependency on their own benefits and work history. Pension coverage and health are useful predictors of retirement for men but not as much for women. For single women, recent income is an important factor in the decision to retire. For women and men, the most significant factors in adaptation to retirement are health, income, and social involvement.

Barriers to equal treatment for LGBT couples include job discrimination, unequal treatment under Social Security, pension plans, and 401(k) plans (Cahill and South, 2002). LGBT couples are not eligible for Social Security survivor benefits, and unmarried partners cannot claim pension plan rights after the death of the pension plan participant. These policies definitely place LGBT elders at a disadvantage in retirement planning.

Nurse's Role in Assisting in Retirement Preparation. Successful retirement adjustment depends on socialization needs, energy levels, health, adequate income, variety of interests, amount of self-esteem derived from work, presence of intimate relationships, social support, and general adaptability. Nurses may have the opportunity to work with people in different phases of retirement or participate in retirement education and counseling programs (Box 20-15). Talking with clients older than 50 years about retirement plans, providing anticipatory guidance about the transition to retirement, identifying those who may be at risk for lowered income and health concerns, and referring to appropriate resources for retirement planning and support are important nursing interventions.

It is important to build on the strengths of older adults' life experiences and coping skills and to provide appropriate counseling and support to assist older people to continue to grow and develop in meaningful ways during the transition from the work role. In ideal situations, retirement offers the opportunity to pursue interests that may have been neglected while fulfilling obligations. However, for too many older people, retirement presents challenges that affect both health and well-being and nurses need to be advocates for policies and conditions that allow all older people to maintain quality of life in retirement.

Volunteer Role. Retirement is often thought of as a time to develop secondary interests and challenges. Many older people volunteer and contribute to filling gaps in services that might otherwise be unmet. Some of the formal volunteer programs for older people include the National Network on Aging (Nursing Home Ombudsman Program, National Nutrition Program), Senior Corps (Foster Grandparents [FGP], Retired Senior Volunteer Program [RSVP]), Volunteers in Service to America (VISTA), Senior Companion, Peace Corps, Legal Service Corporation, SCORE (Small Business Administration), Department of Veterans Affairs, and National Volunteer School Program (teacher aides). Many of these volunteers are paid or given other inducements to supplement low incomes. Numerous other volunteer opportunities are available in local communities including community agencies, hospitals, and other health care facilities. Some of the many ways volunteers may be involved are seen in Box 20-16.

Volunteer Training. Training programs, supervision, and ongoing support are critical to the success of volunteer programs. The following considerations guide the development of successful volunteer programs:

- Administrative support of volunteers
- Clearly determined goals for the program
- A specific orientation program with printed support materials to give volunteers
- Buddy systems to orient and reinforce the volunteer role and expectations
- Periodic evaluations and modifications as needs are indicated by volunteer participants
- Determination of specific awards and rewards to sustain interest and involvement

Individuals should be encouraged to begin minimal participations in volunteer programs before discontinuing the work role. This can serve as a bridge of continuity. Certain steps are identified in the full development of a role as a volunteer. These can be seen in Box 20-17. Group involvement and group meetings will solidify and strengthen the identification with the volunteer role. One of the most predominant reasons for joining volunteer groups is the social contact with other volunteers. Many volunteer activities involve working with people who are in need of special attention. These situations provide opportunities for expressing altruistic motives. Investment of self and contact with others seem to result in an enriching experience. Some, such as the Foster Grandparents Program, are particularly fulfilling.

Today's elders are perhaps the only ones who have, in large numbers, the health, vitality, education, affluence, and opportunity to make retirement the most creatively produc-

---

BOX 20-15   Phases of Retirement

Remote: Future anticipation with little real planning
Near: Preparation and fantasizing regarding retirement
Honeymoon: Euphoria and testing of the fantasies
Disenchantment: Letdown, boredom, sometimes depression
Reorientation: Developing a realistic and satisfactory lifestyle
Stability: Personal investment in meaningful activities
Termination: Loss of role resulting from illness or return to work

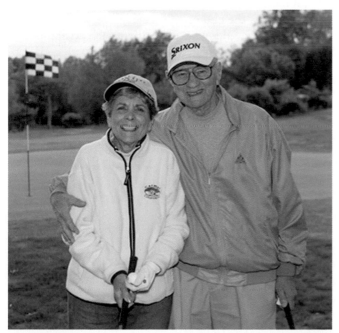

A retired couple enjoys golf as a leisure-time activity. (From Sorrentino SA, Gorek B: *Mosby's textbook for long-term care assistants,* ed 5, St Louis, 2007, Mosby.)

BOX 20-16   Volunteer Community Services

- Perform in a choral group in nursing homes.
- Sew for institutionalized children.
- Help deprived persons obtain entitlements.
- Provide widow-to-widow help.
- Perform American Cancer Society clerical work.
- Assist at nutrition programs.
- Make dolls for hospitalized children.
- Assist children in school remedial reading programs.
- Organize food co-op, sell to elders at discount prices.
- Raise money with bazaars, white elephant sales for nutrition programs.
- Serve as musicians for senior dances.
- Teach language classes in senior centers.
- Become "fix it" men.
- Prepare kits for Red Cross Blood Mobile.
- Telephone the homebound.
- Present puppet shows to schoolchildren, bringing history alive.
- Serve coffee and act as language interpreters at gerontological centers.
- Help residents settle into new living arrangements, nursing or retirement homes.
- Assist with shopping, walking around.
- Teach remedial math to schoolchildren.
- Present slide shows in churches and senior centers as museum volunteers.
- Assist in childcare shelters.
- Work with developmentally disabled—teach swimming, cooking, and activities of daily living.
- Alert isolated elderly to services and Supplemental Security Income (SSI).

BOX 20-17   Steps in Development of Volunteer Role

1. Volunteer role uses skills from previous work or community experience. A gain in status, prestige, and community sanction is experienced.
2. Volunteer role improves interest in self and others. Dependence is reduced, and interdependence is created.
3. Feedback is gained from recipients of services. Self-view is improved, and resourcefulness is recognized.
4. Social and psychological stimulation is found in volunteer settings. Personal growth and development occur as skills are refined.
5. Community rewards and recognition are awarded. New roles of social significance are internalized.

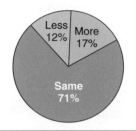
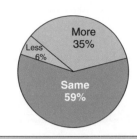

Widowed Persons' Interests

Survey Question: Compared to when your spouse was alive, do YOU have more interest, less interest, or about the same amount of interest in having contact with relatives and friends?

Friends' & Relatives' Interests

Survey Question: Do your relatives and friends show more interest, less interest, or about the same amount of interest in having contact with you?

FIGURE 20-4 Effect of widowhood on social participation. (From Utz RL et al. *Gerontologist* 42[4]:522, 2002. Copyright © The Gerontological Society of America. Reproduced by permission of the publisher.)

---

tive and gratifying stage of life. Retirement can be the time when the individual is free to pursue a lifelong avid interest. For the fortunate individuals, retirement years can indeed be the best years of their life and the most gratifying.

Widows and Widowers

Losing a partner after a long close and satisfying relationship is the most difficult adjustment one can face, aside from the loss of a child. The loss of a spouse is a stage in the life course that can be anticipated but seldom is. Nearly 50% of all women and 12% of all men ages 65 years and older are widowed (deVries, 2001).

The death of a life partner is essentially losing one's self and one's core. The mourning is as much for self as for the individual who has died. Part of oneself has died with the partner, and even with satisfactory grief resolution, that self will never return. Even those widows and widowers who reorganize their lives and invest in family, friends, and activities often find that many years later they still miss their "other half" profoundly (Figure 20-4).

With the loss of the intimate partner, several changes occur simultaneously that involve social status, economics, and self-image. Individuals who have been self-confident and competent seem to fare best. The transitional phase of

grief, if handled appropriately, leads to the confirmation of a new identity, the end of one stage of life, and the beginning of another. Seldom in life is there such an abrupt and distinct breach that creates intense pain but offers the opportunity for the emergence of a new identity. Patterns of adjustment can be seen in Box 20-18. Knowing the stages of the transition to a new role as a widow or widower may be useful, although each individual is unique in this respect. Individuals respond to losses in ways that reflect the nature and meaning of the relationships as well as the unique characteristics of the bereaved (deVries, 2001). Gender differences are found in the literature on widowhood. Bereaved husbands may be more socially and emotionally vulnerable. Many studies have found that widowers adapt more slowly than widows to the loss of a spouse and often remarry quickly. Common bereavement reactions of widowers are listed in Box 20-19 and should be discussed with male clients.

Nurse's Role with Widows and Widowers. Nurses working with the bereaved will need to review Lindemann's classic grief studies to understand the initial somatic responses of the bereaved (Lindemann, 1944). Feelings of the bereaved one are not orderly or progressive; they are con-

---

BOX 20-18   Patterns of Adjustment to Widowhood

STAGE ONE: REACTIONARY

(First Few Weeks)

Early responses of disbelief, anger, indecision, detachment, and inability to communicate in a logical, sustained manner are common. Searching for the mate, visions, hallucinations, and depersonalization may be experienced.

Intervention: Support, validate, be available, listen to talk about mate, reduce expectations.

STAGE TWO: WITHDRAWAL

(First Few Months)

Depression, apathy, physiological vulnerability occur; movement and cognition are slowed; insomnia, unpredictable waves of grief, sighing, and anorexia occur.

Intervention: Protect against suicide, and involve in support groups.

STAGE THREE: RECUPERATION

(Second 6 Months)

Periods of depression are interspersed with characteristic capability. Feelings of personal control begin to return.

Intervention: Support accustomed lifestyle patterns that sustain and assist person to explore new possibilities.

STAGE FOUR: EXPLORATION

(Second Year)

Individual begins new ventures, testing suitability of new roles; anniversaries or holidays, birthdays, and date of death may be especially difficult.

Intervention: Prepare individual for unexpected reactions during anniversaries. Encourage and support new trial roles.

STAGE FIVE: INTEGRATION

(Fifth Year)

Individual will feel fully integrated into new and satisfying roles if grief has been resolved in a healthy manner.

Intervention: Assist individual to recognize and share own pattern of growth through the trauma of loss.

BOX 20-19   Common Widower Bereavement Reactions

- The search for the lost mate
- The neglect of self
- The inability to share grief
- The loss of social contacts
- The struggle to view women as other than wife
- The erosion of self-confidence and sexuality
- The protracted grief period

---

flicted, ambivalent, suicidal, full of rage, and often suspicious. Widows and widowers may exhibit personality disorganization that would be considered mentally aberrant or frankly psychotic under other circumstances. Some people handle grief with less apparent decompensation. Grief reactions must be accepted as personally valid and useful evidences of healing. deVries (2001) discusses the ongoing bonds and connections (dreaming of the deceased, ongoing daily communication, "checking in") with the deceased that persist long after death and counsels professionals to reexamine the idea that there is a timetable for "resolution" of grief. Rather, according to deVries, "Grief reflects the intimacy of relationships that need not end with the physical absence of individuals" (p. 79).

With adequate support, reintegration can be expected in 2 to 4 years. People with few familial or social supports may need professional help to get through the early months of grief in a way that will facilitate recovery. Supporting the grieving person requires an extension of self to reconnect the severed person with a world of warmth and caring. No one nurse or one family member can accomplish this task alone. Hundreds of small, caring gestures build strength and confidence in the grieving person's ability and willingness to survive. Additional information about dying, death, and grief can be found in Chapter 26.

Divorce and the Elderly

In the past, divorce was considered a stigmatizing event; however, today it is so common that a person is inclined to forget the ostracizing effects of divorce from 60 years ago. There are large generational and individual differences in expectations from marriage, but older couples are becoming less likely to stay in an unsatisfactory marriage (Lanza, 1996). Health care professionals need to avoid assumptions and be alert to the possibility of marriage dissatisfaction in old age. Nurses need to ask, "How would you describe your marriage?"

At age 65 years and older, 11.5% of women and 9.2% of men are divorced (U.S. Census Bureau, 2001). People who divorce in late life have been largely neglected in research and support services. The number of people who seek divorce after that age is unknown, but divorce, as well as marriage and remarriage, must often be considered within the context of economics. In the past few years, the number of divorced elders has increased much more rapidly than the increase in the elderly population. This statistic may be largely a cohort effect. As divorces increase in couples of all ages, many more enter the ranks of older people. Today, 50% of all first marriages and 60% of remarriages end in divorce (U.S. Divorce Statistics, 2002).

Long-term relationships are varied and complex, with many factors forming the glue that holds them together. Lanza (1996) studied the divorces of older women and found them attributed to their husbands' infidelity, retirement, or simply growing apart. Wives often tended to blame themselves, believing that they were in some way deficient and that otherwise the divorce would not have occurred. Lanza concluded that marital breakdown is more devastating in old age because it is often unanticipated and may occur concurrent with other significant losses.

Health care workers must be concerned with supporting a client's decision to seek a divorce and with assisting him or her in seeking counseling in the transition. A nurse should alert the client that a divorce will bring on a grieving process similar to the death of a spouse and that a severe disruption in coping capacity may occur until the client adjusts to a new life. The grief may be more difficult to cope with because no socially sanctioned patterns have been established, as is the case with widowhood. In addition, tax and fiscal policies favor married couples and many divorced elderly women are at a serious economic disadvantage in retirement.

Transition from Health to Illness

Recognition of and adaptation to chronic disorders and disabilities (see Chapter 10) are transitions that many elders will face. For example, the move from being a "healthy" elder to an elderly "diabetic" requires changes in lifestyle,

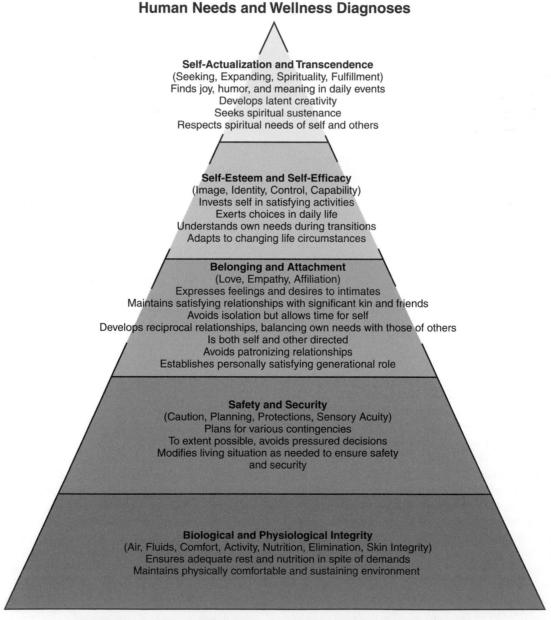

Human Needs and Wellness Diagnoses

Self-Actualization and Transcendence
(Seeking, Expanding, Spirituality, Fulfillment)
Finds joy, humor, and meaning in daily events
Develops latent creativity
Seeks spiritual sustenance
Respects spiritual needs of self and others

Self-Esteem and Self-Efficacy
(Image, Identity, Control, Capability)
Invests self in satisfying activities
Exerts choices in daily life
Understands own needs during transitions
Adapts to changing life circumstances

Belonging and Attachment
(Love, Empathy, Affiliation)
Expresses feelings and desires to intimates
Maintains satisfying relationships with significant kin and friends
Avoids isolation but allows time for self
Develops reciprocal relationships, balancing own needs with those of others
Is both self and other directed
Avoids patronizing relationships
Establishes personally satisfying generational role

Safety and Security
(Caution, Planning, Protections, Sensory Acuity)
Plans for various contingencies
To extent possible, avoids pressured decisions
Modifies living situation as needed to ensure safety
and security

Biological and Physiological Integrity
(Air, Fluids, Comfort, Activity, Nutrition, Elimination, Skin Integrity)
Ensures adequate rest and nutrition in spite of demands
Maintains physically comfortable and sustaining environment

These are not all the possible wellness diagnoses that may be identified. The above
are examples of nursing diagnoses that should be considered when planning care
for the older adult.

self-concept, and relationships. The transitions that occur in facing the end of life are discussed in Chapter 26.

▲ Promoting Healthy Aging: Implications for Gerontological Nursing

Role transitions and losses often characterize the aging experience. For some older adults, these can be devastating and will require support from nurses and other health professionals. Nurses can provide anticipatory guidance to assist older people in preparing for these transitions. It is important to build upon the strengths of older adults' life experiences and coping skills and to provide appropriate counseling and support to assist older people continue to grow and develop in meaningful ways. During the transition from familiar roles to new ones, an individual needs the freedom to try various possibilities in an accepting atmosphere that encourages success, tolerates failure, and recognizes that progress is not accomplished by slow, even steps. In reality, progress follows a more wayward, uneven course. One is easily distracted and often falls back to the familiar. The nurse is most helpful in providing an accepting milieu that encourages independence and exploration, as well as the awareness that transitions all create some anxiety. Useful nursing interventions will assist the older adult in maintaining self-esteem and developing new and satisfying roles.

Future generations of older adults will redefine what we now consider "norms" for aging and roles for older people. Research is needed to provide the foundation for nursing interventions with family caregivers, particularly among racially and ethnically diverse families and nontraditional families. Our goal as gerontological nurses is to create opportunities for each older adult to thrive, not merely survive, in late life.

KEY CONCEPTS

- Roles define individual and societal expectations of function.
- In a rapidly changing society, roles quickly become anachronistic.
- Transitions are akin to shedding of skin as a new one is generated.
- Ability to successfully negotiate transitions and develop new and gratifying roles depends on personal and environmental supports, timing, clarity of expectations, personality, and degree of change required.
- Elders may perceive more losses than gains in the transitions of aging.
- Caring family or pseudo-family relationships are critical to an elder's adaptation to the transition in aging.
- Caregiving activities occupy much of an elder's time, either as the caregiver or the recipient of care.
- Grandparents are increasingly assuming primary caregiving roles with grandchildren.
- Mid-life individuals are often caring for individuals from generations before and after them.
- A major transitional issue for an elder is moving from health to illness and redefining the individual in terms of a chronic disorder. Nurses must ensure that this new definition does not become the identity of the individual.

- The work role transition is the major change for men and is increasingly becoming so for women, though women often continue their homemaker-caregiver role without interruption.
- Numerous patterns of retirement exist, and therefore retirement per se cannot be viewed categorically.
- Pre-retirement planning and post-retirement follow-up significantly affect positive adaptation to the transition.
- Definite gender differences exist in the roles and transitions common to the aging process.
- Volunteerism is becoming increasingly attractive to elders who feel the need to express their altruistic motives; some opportunities also supplement retirement income.
- Loss of spouse is the role change that has the greatest potential for life disruption, and nursing support can make a significant positive difference in the transition.
- Widowers are a neglected group in the literature and in the service arena. These men are particularly vulnerable to maladaptive behaviors and deterioration.

RESEARCH QUESTIONS

What are the resources for older LGBT couples in your community?

What are the roles and activities of great-grandparents with great-grandchildren?

What are the differences between grandparenting and great-grandparenting?

What are the reactions of elders to the care given by their offspring?

How many elders had been with one company for the majority of their working life?

How does retirement affect these individuals?

What are the patterns of adaptation of widowers? How do the patterns differ for young-old and old-old?

Who divorces in late life and for what reasons?

RESOURCES

AARP: Lean on Me
Support and minority outreach for grandparents raising grandchildren
www.aarp.org/research/family/grandparenting/aresearch-import-483. html

A Prescription for Caregivers
Video
Contact Wendy Lustbader at (425) 462-5722

AARP Grandparent Information Center
www.aarp.org/families/grandparents/gic/a2004-01-16-grandparentsin-focenter.html

Caregiver.com
www.caregiver.com/

Children of Aging Parents
www.caps4caregivers.org/index.htm

Educated Caregiver Video Series
Available from Life View Resources
(800) 395-5433

CASE STUDY: Retirement

Sandy was a professor at a small, private college in a metropolitan area. Although she had taught nursing for 25 years and loved her work, it had been a demanding year and she was very tired. A rumor had recently circulated that the college was in trouble financially. Some of the most affluent alumni could no longer be counted on for gifts and endowments because the football coach had not produced a winning team for several years. Because the tuition was becoming exorbitant, the college had recently lost some students to one of the three state college campuses within driving distance of the city. The trustees of the college, in a move to cut expenses, offered an incentive to professors who were willing to retire early; an extra year of service credit was presented for every 6 years worked. Sandy was only 55 years old but thought that the 4 years of extra credit would bring her near the minimum retirement age for Social Security (an error, of course, because her age did not change with her service credit). Rather impulsively, Sandy decided to accept the offer after telling colleagues, "Well, you know how I love to travel. Why wait until I'm too old to enjoy retirement? Why don't you think about the offer, too? This is a once-in-a-lifetime opportunity." Near the end of the academic year, the celebrations began: recognition, plaques, expressions of gratitude from students, and envy from her associates. The send-off was wonderful. In the summer, Sandy withdrew her savings and booked a cruise to the Greek islands. The journey was lovely, and she enjoyed every moment. Sandy began to feel depressed when she got off the ship but knew it was only because the elegant cruise was over. However, as fall came around, Sandy began to feel more depressed. Most of her friends were teachers, and they were all back at work. Sandy briefly thought of going to Pittsburgh to visit her sister but decided against the idea because she and her sister had really never been very compatible. Then Sandy was hit with some of the realities of early retirement: she was unable to withdraw any of her considerable tax-deferred savings before she was 59½ years of age without significant penalty, her health insurance coverage was considerably less comprehensive after retirement, her colleagues were all busy, and she was very bored. Then the real blow fell. The college, in desperation, had dipped into the retirement funds to remain solvent, and the retirees' pensions were now at risk. Sandy's sister, who was a nurse, called to announce that she wanted to come and stay a few days while she attended a conference in the city. When she arrived, Sandy overwhelmed her with the litany of woes. If you were Sandy's sister, what would you do?

Based on the case study, develop a nursing care plan using the following procedure*:

- List Sandy's comments that provide subjective data.
- List information that provides objective data.
- From these data, identify and state, using accepted format, two nursing diagnoses you determine are most significant to Sandy at this time. List two of Sandy's strengths that you have identified from the data.
- Determine and state outcome criteria for each diagnosis. These criteria must reflect some alleviation of the problem identified in the nursing diagnosis and must be stated in concrete and measurable terms.
- Plan and state one or more interventions for each diagnosed problem. Provide specific documentation of the source used to determine the appropriate intervention. Plan at least one intervention that incorporates Sandy's existing strengths.
- Evaluate the success of the intervention. Interventions must correlate directly with the stated outcome criteria to measure the outcome success.

Critical Thinking Questions

1. Identify several important family and social roles that elder members of your family fulfill.
2. What are the factors to consider in role transitions, and how can transitions be made smoother?
3. What factors must be considered in the decision to retire?
4. Discuss the differences you would expect in adaptation to retirement between an individual who retired because of ill health and one who retired because he or she desired to do so.
5. How do you think retirement differs for men and women?
6. Describe what you think would be an ideal retirement.
7. Plan specific ways in which you would present a retirement seminar to workers in a computer microchip factory.
8. Explain the major issues in adaptation to a major role change such as retirement and widowhood.
9. Discuss how you think an individual can prepare for widowhood.
10. Discuss the meanings and the thoughts triggered by the young person's and elder's viewpoints expressed at the beginning of the chapter. How do these vary from your own experience?

* Students are advised to refer to their nursing diagnosis text and identify possible or potential problems.

Eldercare Online
www.ec-online.net/Community/Activists/can.htm

Ethnic Elders Care Network
www.ethniceldercare.com

Family Caregiver Alliance, National Center on Caregiving
www.caregiver.org

Family Caregiver Support Network
www.caregiversupportnetwork.org

Foster Grandparents Program and Retired Senior Volunteer
Program
www.seniorcorps.gov/about/programs/fg.asp

Generations United
http://ipath.gu.org

Grandmother Project
www.aarp.org/research/family/grandparenting/may_06_gubser_grand-mother.html

National Adult Day Services Association
www.nadsa.org

National Center on Grandparents Raising Grandchildren
http://chhs.gsu.edu/nationalcenter/

Prescription for Caregivers: Take Care of Yourself
Terra Nova Films
www.terranova.org

Service Corps of Retired Executives (SCORE)
http://www.score.org/

U.S. HHS Administration on Aging
National family caregiver support program
www.aoa.gov

Video Respite Series by Innovative Caregiving Resources
(800) 249-5600

Video Respite Series
www.alzstore.com

Well Spouse Foundation
www.wellspouse.org

REFERENCES

Age Beat Online: The Newsletter of the Journalists Exchange on Aging, 2(15), July 2002. Available at www.asaging.org.

American Association of Retired Persons (AARP) Public Policy Institute: *Characteristics of uninsured 50-64-year-olds in 2000*, Washington, DC, 2002a, The Association. (website): *www.aarp.org/ppi.*

American Association of Retired Persons (AARP) Public Policy Institute: *Health care coverage among 50-64 year-olds in 2000*, Washington, DC, 2002b, The Association. (website): *www.aarp.org/ppi.*

American Association of Retired Persons (AARP) Public Policy Institute: *Lean on me: support and minority outreach for grandparents raising grandchildren*, Washington, DC, 2003, The Association. (website): *www.aarp.org.*

American Association of Retired Persons (AARP) Public Policy Institute: *Intergenerational relationships: grandparents raising grandchildren*, Washington, DC, 2005, The Association. (website): *www.aarp.org.*

American Association of Retired Persons (AARP) Public Policy Institute: *Who's caring for the caregivers?* Washington, DC, 2006, The Association. (website): *www.aarp.org.*

Ansberry C: Parents devoted to a disabled child confront old age, *Wall Street Journal On Line*, January 7, 2004. (website): *www.online.wsj.com.*

Archbold PG et al: Mutuality and preparedness as predictors of caregiver role strain, *Res Nurs Health* 13:375-384, 1990.

Archbold PG et al: Clinical assessment of mutuality and preparedness in family caregivers to frail older people. In Funk SG et al, editors: *Key aspects of elder care: managing falls, incontinence, and cognitive impairment*, New York, 1992, Springer.

Bedford VH, Avioli PS: Variations on sibling intimacy in old age, *Generations* 25(2):34, 2001.

Bleiszner R: "She'll be on my heart": intimacy among friends, *Generations* 25(2):48, 2001.

Brown-Standridge MD, Floyd CW: Healing bittersweet legacies: revisiting contextual family therapy for grandparents raising grandchildren in crisis, *J Marital Fam Ther* 26(2):185, 2000.

Burton L et al: Transitions in spousal caregiving, *Gerontologist* 43(2):230-241, 2003.

Butler FR, Zakari N: Grandparents parenting grandchildren: assessing health status, *J Gerontol Nurs* 31(3):43-54, 2005.

Cahill S, South K: Policy issues affecting lesbian, gay, bisexual, and transgender people in retirement, *Generations* 26(11):49, 2002.

Chan CG, Elder GH: Matrilinear advantage in grandchild-grandparent relations, *Gerontologist* 40(2):189, 2000.

Chappell N, Reid R: Burden and well-being among caregivers: examining the distinction, *Gerontologist* 42(6):772-780, 2002.

Claes JA, Moore W: *J HHS Admin* 23(2):181, Fall 2000.

Connidis I: *Family ties and aging*, Thousand Oaks, Calif, 2001, Sage.

Curry L et al: Educational needs of employed family caregivers of older adults: evaluation of a workplace project, *Geriatr Nurs* 27(3):166-173, 2006.

Davidhizar R et al: The changing role of grandparenthood, *J Gerontol Nurs* 25(1):24-29, 2000.

Delaney S, Delaney E: *Having our say: the Delaney sisters' first 100 years*, New York, 1993, Kodansha International.

Dennis H: The current state of retirement planning, *Generations* 13(2):38, 2002.

deVries B: Grief: intimacy's reflection, *Generations* 25(2):75-79, 2001.

deVries B: Home at the end of the rainbow, *Generations* 29(4):64-68, 2005-2006.

Doka KJ: Disenfranchised grief: lessons for those serving older clients, *Aging Today* 23(4):13, 2002.

Ekerdt D, Dennis H: Introduction to retirement: new chapters in American life, *Generations* 26(11):entire issue, 2002.

Family Caregiver Alliance: *Caregiver assessment: principles, guidelines and strategies for change*, Report from a National Consensus Development Conference (vol 1), San Francisco, 2006, The Alliance.

Fingerman KL: A distant closeness: intimacy between parents and their children in later life, *Generations* 25(2):26, 2001a.

Fingerman KL: *Aging mothers and their adult daughters: a study in mixed emotions*, New York, 2001b, Springer.

Grinstead L et al: Review of research on the health of caregiving grandparents, *J Adv Nurs* 44(3):318-326, 2003.

Hooyman N, Kiyak H: *Social gerontology*, Boston, 2005, Pearson.

Houde SC et al: Men providing care to older adults in the home, *J Gerontol Nurs* 27(8):13, 2001.

Hunt C: Concepts in caregiver research, *J Nurs Scholarsh* 35(1):27-32, 2003.

Jett KF: Making the connection: seeking and receiving help by elderly African Americans, *J Qualitative Health Res* 12(3):373-387, 2002.

Jones T, Nystrom M: Looking back . . . looking forward: addressing the lives of lesbians 55 and older, *J Women Aging* 14(3/4):59-76, 2002.

Kutza EA: Living longer, living better: policy presumptions and new family structures, *Pub Pol Aging Rep* 11(3):12, 2001.

Lanza ML: Divorce experienced as an older woman, *Geriatr Nurs* 17(4):166, 1996.

LaRock S: Key components, topics of successful preretirement counseling program, *Employee Benefit Plan Rev*, November 2001.

Lindemann E: Symptomatology and management of acute grief, *Am J Psychiatry* 101(2):141-148, 1944.

Lowenthal MF, Haven C: Interaction and adaptation: intimacy as a critical variable, *Am Sociol Rev* 33:20, 1968.

Lund DA et al: Video respite: an innovative resource for family, professional caregivers, and persons with dementia, *Gerontologist* 35(5):683-687, 1995.

Lund M: Caregiver, take care, *Geriatr Nurs* 26(3):152-153, 2005.

McCarty E: Caring for a parent with Alzheimer's disease: process of daughter caregiver stress, *J Adv Nurs* 23(4):792-803, 1996.

Meiner S, Lueckenotte A: *Gerontological nursing*, St Louis, 2006, Mosby.

Mittleman MS: Family caregiving for people with Alzheimer's disease: results of the NYU spouse caregiver intervention study, *Generations* 26(1):104, 2002.

National Adult Day Services Association: *Adult day services: the facts* (website): www.nadsa.org. Accessed May 13, 2007.

National Alliance for Caregiving (NAC) and AARP: *Caregiving in the U.S.*, 2004. (website): *www.caregiving.org.*

National Council on the Aging (NCOA): American perceptions of aging in the 21st century, Washington, DC, 2002, The Council. (website): *www.ncoa.org.*

Navaie-Waliser M et al: When the caregiver needs care: the plight of vulnerable caregivers, *Am J Public Health* 92(3):409, 2002.

Piercy KW: We couldn't do without them: the value of close relationships between older adults and their nonfamily caregivers, *Generations* 25(2):41, 2001.

Pinquart M, Sorensen S: Ethnic differences in stressors, resources, and psychological outcomes of family caregiving: a meta-analysis, *Gerontologist* 45(1):90-106, 2005.

Roberto KA, Skoglund RR: Interactions with grandparents and great-grandparents: a comparison of activities, influences, and relationships, *Int J Aging Hum Dev* 43(2):107, 1996.

Robinson B: Validation of a caregiver strain index, *J Gerontol* 38:344, 1983.

Roe KM, Minkler M: Grandparents raising grandchildren: challenges and responses, *Generations* 22(4):25, 1998-1999.

Schulz R, Beach SR: Caregiving as a risk factor for mortality: the caregiver health effects study, *JAMA* 262:2215, 1999.

Schumacher K et al: Family caregivers: caring for older adults, working with their families, *Am J Nurs* 106(8):40-49, 2006.

Scott JP: Sisters in later life: changes in contact and availability. In Roberto K, editor: *Relationships between women in later life*, New York, 1996, Haworth Press.

Sebern M: Shared care, elder and family member skills used to manage burden, *J Adv Nurs* 52(2):170-179, 2005.

Shagrin SS: Retirement saving and financial planning, *Generations* 26(11):40, 2002.

Silverstein M, Angelli J: Older parents' expectations of moving closer to their children, *J Gerontol* 53B:S153-163, 1998.

Somary K, Stricker G: Becoming a grandparent: a longitudinal study of expectations and early experiences as a function of sex and lineage, *Generations* 38(1):53, 1998.

Stanford P, Usita P: Retirement: who is at risk? *Generations* 26(11):45-48, 2002.

Tafford A: *The bonus decades*, New York, 2002, Basic Books.

Touhy T: Nurturing hope and spirituality in nursing homes, *Holist Nurs Pract* 15(4):45-56, 2001.

Touhy T et al: Expressions of caring as lived by nursing home staff, families and residents, *Int J Human Caring* 9(3):31-37, 2005.

Troope M: *Grandparents and other relatives raising children*, Washington, DC, 2000, Generations United.

U.S. Administration on Aging: *Facts about older Americans*, 2000. (website): *www.aoa.gov.*

U.S. Census Bureau: *Statistical abstract of the United States: 2002*, ed 122, Washington, DC, 2001, U.S. Government Printing Office.

U.S. Census Bureau: *Facts for features*, 2004. (website): *www.census.gov/Press-Release/www/2001/cb01fff12..html.*

U.S. Divorce Statistics: *DivorceMagazine.com*, December 2002. (website): *www.divorcemag.com/statistics/statsUS.shtml.*

Wojciechowski C: Issues in caring for older lesbians, *J Gerontol Nurs* 24(7):28-33, 1998.

Zarit SH: Assessment of family caregivers: a research perspective. In Family Caregiver Alliance, *Caregiver assessment: voices and views from the field*, Report from a National Consensus Development Conference (vol II), San Francisco, 2006, Author.

CHAPTER 21

Culture, Gender, and Aging

Kathleen Jett

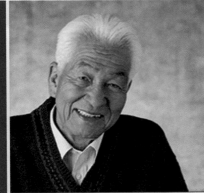

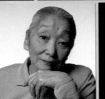

A YOUTH SPEAKS

The old ones, in their seventies or eighties, with long memories of hardships faced and perhaps only partially (if at all) surmounted, deprived of education, made to feel hopelessly inarticulate, and obviously out of "the American mainstream," they are nevertheless men and women who seem to have held stubbornly to a peculiar notion: that they are eminently valuable and important human beings, utterly worth the respect, even admiration, not to mention the love, of their children and grandchildren.

Description of the Chicanos of New Mexico in Coles R: *The old ones,* Albuquerque, 1973, University of New Mexico Press.

LEARNING OBJECTIVES

On completion of this chapter, the reader will be able to:

1. Recognize the current knowledge related to health disparities and their potential impact on older adults of color and women.
2. Relate major historical events that have affected each cohort of elders.
3. Compare several different ethnically based approaches to health care.
4. Describe several of the unique circumstances related to gender and aging.
5. Identify personal factors contributing to ethnic and cultural sensitivity.
6. Discuss approaches that facilitate an appreciation of diverse cultural and ethnic experiences.
7. Accurately identify situations in which expert interpretation is necessary.
8. Understand key points of working with interpreters.
9. Formulate a care plan incorporating ethnically sensitive interventions.
10. Develop gerontological nursing interventions geared toward reducing health disparities.

Interest in and attention to culture and gender issues in health care are increasing. Entire programs of study related to gender and those of culture and aging exist; however, the combination of gender, aging, and culture is rare. In the care of older adults, the term *ethnogeriatrics* refers to the nexus of culture, aging, and health, whereas the term *transcultural nursing* refers to provision of nursing care across cultures.

In the field of gerontology, this interest is stimulated to a great extent by two major issues: the realization of a demographic imperative and the recognition of the significant health disparities in the Unites States. The *demographic imperative* refers to the significant increases in both the total numbers of older adults and the relative proportion of older adults in most countries across the globe (see Chapter 1).

These numbers also reflect a "gerontological explosion" of older adults from ethnically distinct groups. *Health disparities* refer to the differences both in the state of health and in health outcomes among groups of persons. Those found to be especially vulnerable to health disparities include older women, men and women from ethnically distinct groups, and the poor. Among older poor adults, women of all races and ethnicities predominate.

Today's nurse is expected to provide competent care to persons with different life experiences, cultural perspectives, values, and styles of communication. The nurse may need to effectively communicate with persons regardless of the languages spoken. In doing so, the nurse may depend on limited verbal exchanges and attend more to facial and body expres-

Special thanks to Patricia Hess, the previous edition contributor, for her content contributions to this chapter.

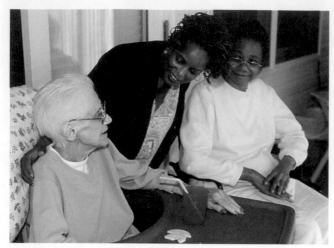

Nurses are caring for more elders from multiple ethnicities. (From Lewis SM et al: *Medical-surgical nursing: assessment and management of clinical problems,* ed 6, St Louis, 2004, Mosby.)

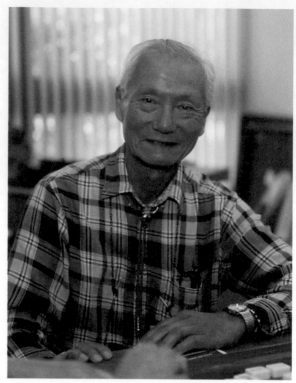

The number of older Asian Americans is increasing. (From Lewis SM et al: *Medical-surgical nursing: assessment and management of clinical problems,* ed 7, St Louis, 2007, Mosby.)

sions, postures, gestures, and touching. However, these forms of communication are heavily influenced by culture and ethnicity and may be easily misunderstood. To be able to skillfully assess and intervene, nurses must first develop cultural sensitivity through awareness of their own ethnocentricities. Effective nurses develop cultural competence through new cultural knowledge about ethnicity, culture, language, and health belief systems and develop the skills needed to optimize intercultural communication.

This chapter provides an overview of culture, gender, and aging, as well as strategies gerontological nurses can use to best respond to the changing face of elders and, in doing so, help reduce health disparities. These strategies include increasing cultural sensitivity, knowledge, and skills in working with diverse groups of older adults.

THE GERONTOLOGICAL EXPLOSION

The need to address culture, gender, and aging co-exists with the demographic imperative (see Chapter 1). Worldwide, the number of older adults has increased significantly; at the same time, in the United States the percentage of persons of ethnic groups other than white of European descent has increased. It is projected that by 2050 those persons from groups that have long been counted as statistical minorities will assume membership in what can be called the *emerging majority* (Table 21-1).

Although older adults of color will still be outnumbered by their white counterparts for years to come, tremendous growth is anticipated. It would not be unusual for nurses working in states with the greatest number of refugee or immigrant elders (California, Nevada, Florida, Texas, New Jersey, Illinois) to care for persons from a variety of backgrounds in the same day (Gelfand, 2003) (Figures 21-1 through 21-4). The largest growth in the older adult population is occurring among persons who consider themselves Hispanic—from less than 5% of the total older adult

TABLE 21-1

Growth of Minority Groups as a Proportion of the U.S. Population

Year	Percentage of U.S. Population
1970	16%
1998	27%
2050	50%

From Administration on Aging (AOA): *Achieving cultural competence,* 2001.

population in 2000 to 16.4% by 2050. The number of older African-Americans will grow from 8% of those older than 65 years to 12.2%. The percentage of older Asian or Pacific Islanders is projected to increase from 2.4% to 6.5% and Native Americans and Alaskans from 0.4% to 0.5% (Administration on Aging, 2004) (Figures 21-5 and 21-6). It must be noted, however, that these and many of the figures available today are drawn from the U.S. census in which persons of color are often underrepresented and those who reside illegally are not included at all. In reality, the numbers of ethnic elders in the United States may be or become substantially higher.

Even within the broad census racial and ethnic categories, there is considerable diversity. The broad terms are useful statistically but are considerably less useful for the gerontological nurse caring for an ethnic elder. One who identifies as a "Native American" is a member of one of over 500 tribal

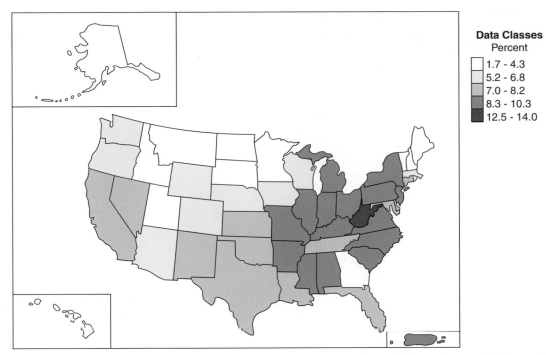

FIGURE 21-1 Percent of persons ages 65 years and older (black or African-Americans alone). (From U.S. Census Bureau, 2000.)

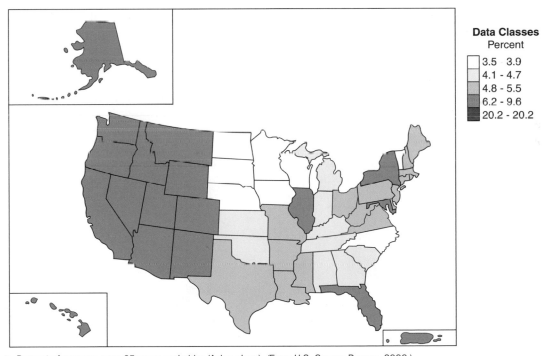

FIGURE 21-2 Percent of persons ages 65 years and older (Asian alone). (From U.S. Census Bureau, 2000.)

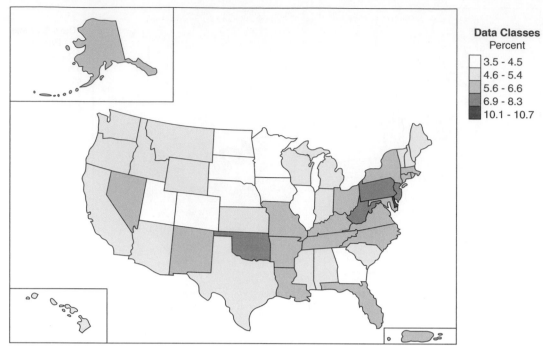

FIGURE 21-3 Percent of persons ages 65 years and older (American Indian or Alaskan native alone). (From U.S. Census Bureau, 2000.)

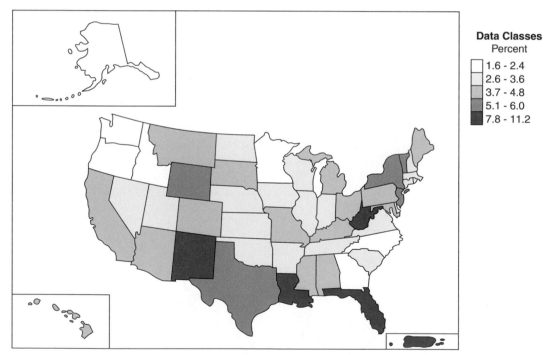

FIGURE 21-4 Percent of persons ages 65 years and older (Hispanic or Latino, any race). (From U.S. Census Bureau, 2000.)

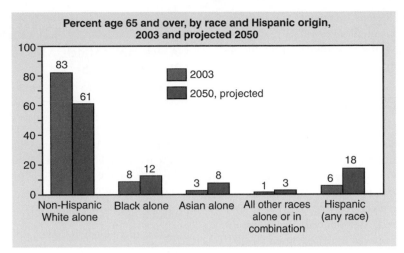

FIGURE 21-5 Population ages 65 years and older, by race and Hispanic origin, 2003 and projected. (From U.S. Census Bureau, Population Estimates and Projections, 2004.)

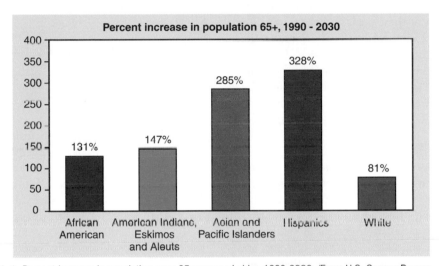

FIGURE 21-6 Percent increase in population ages 65 years and older, 1990-2030. (From U.S. Census Bureau, January 2000.)

groups, each with both common and unique cultural features. An elder identified as Asian/Pacific Islander is from one of over a dozen countries that rim the Pacific Ocean and speaks one (or more) of over 1000 languages or dialects. Persons classified as black Americans are usually assumed to identify themselves as African-American, although an increasing number are from any one of the Caribbean Islands, each with a distinct culture and, in some cases, language.

Adding to the diversity in the United States is the number of persons emigrating from an increasing number of countries. The immigrant population is growing at a faster rate than that of the native born. In 2003 Gelfand reported that the median age of those born elsewhere was 52 years—persons who will soon be the recipients of gerontological nursing. Although access to the United States varies with global politics, older adults are continually being reunited with their adult offspring, where they assist with homemaking and care for younger children in the family as they are cared for themselves. It is becoming increasingly common for communities to provide and support senior centers with activities and meals reflective of their diverse participants.

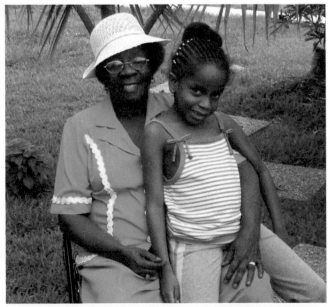

Older Haitian-American grandmothers often care for their grandchildren while the parents work. (Courtesy M. Tamara Adonis-Rizo.)

The diversity of values, beliefs, languages, and historic life experiences of elders today challenges nurses to gain new awareness, knowledge, and skills to provide culturally and linguistically appropriate care.

HEALTH DISPARITIES AND OLDER ADULTS

In 1979 the first national goals for health were published in the United States and included (1) increasing the healthy life span, (2) increasing access to health care, and (3) decreasing health disparities. Objectives for each goal were created and monitored whenever possible. Although some objectives were accomplished, the majority were not. In 2000 both the goals and objectives were redefined for 2010 to focus on (1) increasing the quality of life lived and (2) reducing health disparities, with the emphasis on the latter (U.S. Department of Health and Human Services [USDHHS], 2000). Both of these goals and their associated objectives have significant implications for the consideration of culture, gender, and aging and for the practice of gerontological nursing. This entire text is directed toward meeting these goals, with specific strategies found throughout, especially relating to the first goal. This chapter specifically addresses the second, that of decreasing health disparities.

Types of Health Disparities

Health disparities have been defined in a number of different ways; however, their commonality is the statistical appreciation of differences in the incidence, prevalence, mortality, and burden of diseases and other adverse health conditions that exist among specific population groups in the United States. As noted earlier, the elderly, persons of color, and women are all among the specific populations that experience more of a disparity burden than white men.

In 2003 the Institute of Medicine (IOM) prepared an analysis of the state of the science on the health disparities. It began with the acknowledgement that persons of color had difficulty accessing the same care as their white counterparts. The researchers were to determine the state of care while controlling for access issues.

The result of the study was that, even when controlling for unequal access, health care treatment in and of itself was unequal (Smedley et al., 2002) (Box 21-1). The barriers to quality care were found to be wide, ranging from those related to geographical location to age, gender, race, ethnicity, and sexual orientation. Disparities were consistently found across a wide range of disease areas and clinical services. Among the findings were the following:

- Disparities are found even when clinical factors, such as stage of disease presentation, co-morbidities, age, and severity of disease, are taken into account.
- Disparities are found across a range of clinical settings, including public and private hospitals and teaching and non-teaching hospitals.
- Disparities in care are associated with higher mortality among minorities.

BOX 21-1   Examples of Health Disparities

AFRICAN-AMERICANS (COMPARED WITH WHITES)

50% more likely to have a stroke
50% more likely to die of the stroke
20% more likely to die of heart disease
1.5 times more likely to have HTN
2.5 times more likely to have diabetes
30% more likely to have DM-related amputations
African-American with a TIA: 62% fewer get anticoagulation

MEXICAN AMERICANS

2 times more likely to have DM
Get 36% fewer prescriptions post-MI

NATIVE HAWAIIANS

5.7 times more likely to have DM than whites living in Hawaii

Data from Office of Minority Health (OMH) Report: *The black population*, 2002; Institute of Medicine (IOM): *Unequal treatment, 2003*.
HTN, Hypertension; *DM*, diabetes mellitus; *TIA*, transient ischemic attack; *MI*, myocardial infarction.

One of the most upsetting conclusions of the study was that the color of one's skin or presumed ethnic group was enough to negatively influence the health care one would and did receive in the United States.

Older adults of color have been described as facing "double jeopardy" for health disparities because of two risk factors (age and ethnicity) for vulnerability. For women, the risk becomes "triple jeopardy," and poverty adds a fourth factor. Many of the specific examples of disparities for older adults and women were presented in Chapter 10 in the discussions related to differences in life expectancy and incidence and prevalence of various chronic diseases. Others can be found in any of the publications of the Agency for Healthcare Research and Quality (*www.ahrq.gov*) or the Office for Minority Health (*www.omhrc.gov*).

Reducing Health Disparities

The IOM study also provided a number of recommendations for reducing health disparities. However, before change can occur, all health care providers must become more culturally competent. The end point is not just to become competent but to become culturally proficient, that is, able to move smoothly between the world of the nurse and the world of the patient (in this case, the world of the elder). Moving toward culturally proficient gerontological nursing care is one of the major strategies to reduce the existing and seemingly persistent health disparities. This requires cultural awareness and sensitivity, knowledge, and skills.

Nurses should become aware of and understand the considerable problems that many older women in general and men and women from ethnically distinct groups encounter in the pursuit and receipt of health care and the considerable disparities in health outcomes. Through this awareness, more compassionate and relevant care can be provided.

By increasing awareness, nurses learn of their personal biases, prejudices, attitudes, and behaviors toward persons different from themselves in age, gender, sexual orientation, social class, economic situations, and many other factors. Through increased knowledge, nurses can better assess the strengths and challenges of the older adult and know when and how to effectively intervene to support rather than hinder cultural strengths. Skills in cultural competence include putting cultural knowledge to use in assessment, communication, negotiation, and intervention.

Cultural Awareness. The development of competence begins with increased awareness of our own beliefs and attitudes and those commonly seen in the community at large and in the community of health care (Box 21-2). Increased awareness requires openness and self-reflection. Consider the following:

> A gerontological nurse responded to a call from an older patient's room. For some unknown reason, he repeatedly and without comment dropped his watch on the floor while talking to the nurse. She calmly picked it up, handed it back to him, and continued talking. During one of the droppings, an aide walked in the room, picked up the watch, and attempted to hand it back to him. The patient immediately started yelling and cursing at the aide for attempting to steal his watch. When telling this story, the nurse thought the whole situation odd, but not too remarkable. It was not until she was learning about subtle racism in health care settings, that she realized the more harmful, racist behavior of the man—he was white, and so was she; the aide was black.

If the nurse is white, it is realizing that whiteness alone often means special privilege and freedoms. Older adults of color may not have had the same advantages or experiences as the nurse (McIntosh, 1989). Cultural awareness means recognizing the presence of the "ism's" (e.g., racism, social classism, ageism) and how these have the potential to impact not only health care but also the quality of life for older adults (Smedley et al., 2002). Awareness includes considering how the nurse feels about gender. For example, is sexuality accepted in the same way in older men as in older women?

An awareness of one's thoughts and feelings about others who are culturally different from oneself is necessary. These thoughts and feelings can be hidden from oneself but may be evident to clients. To be aware of these thoughts and feelings about others, one can begin to share or write down personal memories of those first experiences of cultural differences. Questions such as "How did it happen? How did I feel? How did they react?" are a good starting point for the process of cultural self-discovery.

Cultural awareness has several levels. The first is the self-level, requiring self-understanding of one's experiences and values. The second level involves the ability to work with and build relationships with a member from another cultural group. The third level is the recognition of factors beyond

---

BOX 21-2   Steps to Cultural Sensitivity and Competence

- Know yourself: examine your own values, attitudes, beliefs, and prejudices and your cultural heritage and identity.
- Confront biases and stereotypes.
- Do not judge: do not measure others' behavior against your beliefs and values.
- Keep an open mind: attempt to look at the world through other cultures' perspectives.
- Respect differences among people: each group has strengths and weaknesses.
- Appreciate inherent worth of diverse cultures, value them equally, and do not consider them inferior to one's own.
- Listen! Develop the ability to hear things that transcend language, and foster understanding of the client and his or her cultural heritage and the resilience that supports family and community that comes from within the culture.
- Be willing to learn: this requires interest in people's beliefs, values, and practices.
- Travel, read, and attend local ethnic and cultural events in the community.
- Develop an awareness and understanding for the complexities of the health care delivery system—its philosophy, problems, biases, and stereotypes—and become keenly aware of the socialization process that brings the care provider into this complex system.
- Be resourceful and creative: there are many ways to accomplish the same thing.
- Adapt your nursing interventions to suit different cultures and individuals.

Data from Grossman D: Enhancing your cultural competence, *Am J Nurs* 94(7):58, 1994; Spector RF: *Cultural diversity in health and illness,* ed 4, East Norwalk, Conn, 1996, Appleton & Lange.

---

culture, such as health, safety, and poverty, that affect members of a cultural group. On the fourth level, it is important to understand how one's own community history affects how others are viewed. On the last level, one must be able to step outside of cultural bias and accept that other cultures have different ways of perceiving the world that are equal to our own.

Cultural Knowledge. Cross-cultural knowledge can minimize frustration and cultural conflict among older adult clients, nurses, and other health care providers. It will allow the nurse to more appropriately and effectively improve client health outcomes.

Cultural knowledge is both what the nurse brings to the caring situation and what the nurse learns about older adults, their families, their communities, their behaviors, and their expectations. Essential knowledge includes the elder's way of life (ways of thinking, believing, and acting). This knowledge is obtained formally or informally through the professional experience of nursing and caring. Over time, the nurse builds up a reservoir of information about the beliefs of his or her clients and how they behave.

Some nurses prefer to use what can be called an "encyclo-pedic" approach to details of a particular culture or ethnic group, such as proper name usage, greeting, eye contact, gender roles, foods, and beliefs about relevant topics (e.g., the meaning of aging, the appropriate expression of pains, death practices, caregiving). This information is available in many well-done compendiums of cross-cultural information (see the Resources section at the end of the chapter for suggestions). This chapter discusses concepts that have more global application to nursing care and the ethnic elder rather than specific details about any one culture group.

Definitions of Terms. Cultural knowledge includes the appropriate use of terms, especially race, culture, and ethnicity. Often used interchangeably, each actually has a separate meaning. *Race* is usually defined in terms of hereditary make-up as expressed in traits, such as eye color, facial structure, hair texture, and especially skin tones. The four major racial groups worldwide are Caucasoid, Mongoloid, Negroid, and Australoid, usually referred to in terms of underlying skin tones of white, red, black, and yellow respectively. However, the relative importance of race is diminishing because of widespread mixing of the gene pool, making it increasingly uncommon for any one person to be genetically homoge-neous (Gelfand, 2003). Acknowledgement of this heteroge-neity was demonstrated when a new racial category of "mixed" was finally added to the 2000 census.

Culture is the shared and learned beliefs, expectations, and behaviors of a group of people. Style of dress, food pref-erences, language, and social behavior are reflections of culture. Beliefs about aging may be relatively consistent within one culture group (Jett, 2003). Culture guides think-ing, decision making, and action. Cultural beliefs about ag-ing are often portrayed in the media, both in print and on the screen. For example, the 2005 movie "In Her Shoes" portrays a number of stereotypes about aging, both positive and negative. A particular characteristic of culture is that it is transmitted from one member to another through the process called *enculturation*. Culture provides directions for individuals as they interact with family and friends within the same group. Culture allows members of the group to predict each other's behavior and respond in ways that are considered appropriate (Spector, 2004).

Acculturation is the process by which a person from a mi-nority or marginalized culture adopts that of the dominant or majority culture in which they find themselves. There has been much concern about aging immigrants and how culture facilitates or hinders the adjustments needed in late life in the United States. Pierce and colleagues (1978-1979) and Spector (2004) wrote that various types of acculturation were more critical to functional adaptation than others. For example, outward adaptation that incorporates language, dress, and behavior was seen as superficially important. On a deeper level, traditional personal value orientations, includ-ing concepts of time, person to nature, and relationships, were more likely to remain in the original cultural context.

These have been a source of conflict between parents and children when caregiving is needed. The parents may expect the children to provide all the care that is needed. The more acculturated children may feel significant conflict as their "American" lives do not reflect or support their filial duties.

Ethnicity is a complex phenomenon. It is a social differen-tiation based on cultural criteria. Most important, it is a shared identity. Persons from a specific ethnic group may share common geographical origins, migratory status, race, language or dialect, or religion. Traditions, symbols, litera-ture, folklore, food preferences, and dress are often expres-sions of ethnicity (Jett, 2006). These persons may or may not share a common race. For example, persons who consider themselves Hispanic (the largest ethnic group in the United States) may be from any race and from any one of a number of countries. However, most persons who consider them-selves Hispanic share the Catholic religion and the Spanish language. It is more accurate to ask an elder to self-identify ethnicity rather than make assumptions.

Beliefs About Health, Illness, and Treatment. Fun-damental cultural knowledge is that of beliefs about health, illness, and treatment. The individual's beliefs are influenced by others within the family and culture. Older adults have lifelong experiences with illness of self, family, and others within their ethnic groups. The significance they attach to illness symptoms and their reactions to these are related to the outcomes they have experienced or observed in the past. The diversity of the population has brought the strong po-tential for a clash of health belief systems, language, and at-titudes about health and illness between the care provider and the client. Many of the beliefs and practices do not fit into the traditional format of health care as most care pro-viders know it. This set of beliefs can be loosely divided into three theoretical categories: magico-religious, naturalistic/holistic, and biomedical.

Biomedical. The biomedical, scientific, or Western med-ical belief system espouses that disease is the result of abnor-malities in structure and function of body organs and sys-tems. It is still a dominant belief that permeates the thinking of those educated in Western health care. The objective term *disease* is used by care providers, and *illness* is a subjec-tive term to describe symptoms of discomfort or sickness. A personal state of illness has distinct social dimensions. As-sessment and diagnosis are directed at identifying the patho-gen or process causing the abnormality and removing or destroying the cause or at least repairing or modifying the problem through treatment. Clinicians use the scientific method, as well as laboratory and other procedures, to treat the disease or disease process. Prevention in this belief sys-tem is to avoid pathogens, chemicals, activities, and dietary agents known to cause malfunction.

Magico-Religious. In the magico-religious theory of ill-ness and disease causation, both are caused by the actions of a higher power, e.g., God, gods, or supernatural forces or agents such as ghosts, ancestors, or evil spirits (Gerdner et al., 2006). Health is viewed as a blessing or reward of God and illness as a punishment for a breach of rules, breaking a taboo, or displeasing or failing to please the source of power. Beliefs about illness and disease causation attributed to the wrath of God are prevalent among members of the Holiness, Pentecostal, and Fundamentalist Baptist churches. Examples of magical causes of illness are voodoo, especially among persons from the Caribbean; root work among southern African-Americans; hexing among Mexican Americans and African-Americans; and Gaba among Filipino Americans. Treatments may consist of or include religious practices such as praying, meditating, fasting, wearing amulets, burning candles, and establishing family altars. Such practices may be used both curatively and preventively. Another preventive strategy is to ensure that one maintains good relationships with others.

Significant conflict with nurses may result when a patient refuses biomedical treatments because to do so may be viewed as a sign of disrespect for God, as challenging God's will. Although this approach is more common in certain groups, most of us believe in this approach to some extent. How many nurses and their older patients have prayed to a higher power that health be restored or maintained? This belief system can be traced back to the ancient Egyptians, thousands of years ago, and persists in whole or in part in many groups. Current practices included in this group are "laying of the hands" and prayer circles. It is not uncommon to hear an older adult pray for a cure or to lament "What did I do to cause this?"

Naturalistic or Holistic. The naturalistic or holistic health belief system is based on the concept of balance and stems from the ancient civilizations of China, India, and Greece (Jackson, 1993). Many people throughout the world view health as a sign of balance—of the right amount of exercise, food, sleep, evacuation, interpersonal relationships, or geophysic and metaphysical forces in the universe, such as chi. Disturbances in this balance result in disharmony and subsequent illness. Diagnosis requires the determination of the type of imbalance. A common manifestation of this theoretical approach is in the yin/yang of ancient China and in the hot/cold theory common throughout the world.

The yin/yang theory is an ancient Chinese theory that has been used continuously for the past 5000 years. Health is viewed as a state of perfect balance between the yin and the yang, dark and light, male and female. When one is in balance, a feeling of inner and outer peace is experienced. Illness represents an imbalance of yin and yang. Balance may be restored by herbs, acupuncture (insertion of the needles into points along the body's meridians), acupressure (application of pressure or massage to the same meridian points), or controlled deep-breathing exercises.

Naturalistic or holistic health beliefs are used throughout Asia and are gaining acceptance in the United States. Older adults who were raised in one of the countries on the Pacific Rim (especially Asia and the Pacific Islands) or in a traditional Native American community frequently rely on these beliefs. The naturalistic system practiced in India and some of its neighboring countries is known as *ayurvedic medicine*. It is often applied along with practices of Western medicine.

Another variation of naturalistic beliefs is the hot/cold theory. Illness is classified as either hot or cold and believed to be the result of an excess of heat or cold that has entered the body and caused an imbalance. Hot and cold are generally metaphorical, although at times temperature is an aspect. Various foods, medicines, environmental conditions, emotions, and body conditions, such as menstruation and pregnancy, may possess the characteristics of either hot or cold (Spector, 2004). Diagnosis is concerned with identifying the type of disease as either hot or cold. Remedies are similarly divided into hot and cold. Treatment then is focused on using the opposite element; if the disease is the result of excess hot, treatment will be with something that has cold properties, and vice versa. The treatments may take the form of herbs, food, dietary restrictions, or medications from Western medicine that have hot and cold properties, such as antibiotics, massage, poultices, and other therapies.

Orientation to Time. The concept and use of time is culturally constructed and has significant implications in the use of health care. Time orientation has long been theoretically recognized but often overlooked as a factor influencing the use of health care, especially preventive practices (Lukwago et al., 2001). Older adults are more likely to use the orientation of their culture of origin, which may contrast significantly with that of the health care system in the United States.

A future time orientation is consistent with that of Western medicine. Prevention today is important because of its effect on future health. One who is ill today can make an appointment for the "next available" opening; in other words, the health problem can "wait" until an office appointment with a health care provider tomorrow—the problem will still be there and the delay will not necessarily affect the outcome. This also means that health screenings today are believed to be valuable in that they may detect a potential problem today for treatment or prevention for future development at a later time—days, weeks, or years ahead. The strength and acceptance of this orientation is seen in the influence of the document *Healthy People 2010* (USDHHS, 2000) as the national agenda for health care.

Quite different from a future orientation are those of the past or present orientation. Persons oriented to the present experience a problem now, and treatment is believed to be needed at the time of the problem and may not be needed in the future. The outcome is seen as current and not future. Preventive actions are not consistent with this approach.

Persons oriented to the past view the health of the present dependent on the actions of the past, either from a past life, earlier in this life, or events or circumstances of one's ancestors. Dishonoring ancestors by failure to perform certain rituals may result in illness. Illness today may be a punishment for past deeds.

Conflicts between the future-oriented Westernized world of the nurse and those with past or present orientations are not hard to imagine. Such elders are likely to be labeled as *noncompliant* for failure to keep appointments or for failure to participate in preventive measures, such as a turning schedule for a bed-bound patient or immunizations. Members of present-oriented groups are often accused in the media of overusing hospital emergency departments, when in fact it may be the only option available for today's treatment of today's problems.

The nurse can, however, listen closely to the elder and find out which orientation has the most value to him or her and find ways to work with it rather than expect (often unsuccessfully) the person to conform. In this way we are reaching out beyond our ethnocentrism to improve the quality of the gerontological nursing care.

Orientation to Family and Self. Another useful concept in caring for ethnic elders is orientation to family and self (Hofstede and Pedersen, 2002). White Americans of European descent tend to highly value autonomy and individuality, with identity bound first to oneself. In a large, classic study by Rathbone-McCune (1982), she found that European American elders would go to great lengths and live with significant discomfort rather than ask for help. To seek or receive help was considered a sign of weakness and dependence, to be avoided at all costs. The reliance on the individual is institutionalized in the passing of the Patient Self-Determination Act of 1990. In it, the rights and responsibilities of the individual to participate in all decisions regarding his or her health are articulated.

This orientation is in sharp contrast to that of a collectivist, or the belief in familism (Lukwago et al., 2001). The identity of a member of a collectivist culture is drawn from family (broadly defined) ties rather than individual accomplishments. The "family" is more important than the individual, and decisions are made by a group and for the benefit of the group rather than the individual. On the surface, the Health Insurance Portability and Accountability Act (HIPAA) rules established to protect the privacy of the individual are in direct conflict with this cultural pattern. Within family groups, the exchange of help and resources is both expected and commonplace. This orientation applies to most groups other than European Americans. Jett (2002) found that help-seeking and help-giving among frail, elderly African-American women were common experiences. The receipt of help was considered a sign of the love of others, a reflection of the status of the elder. The greater the affection of others, the higher the level of help received, and that "...good things will come to you" (Jett, 2002, p. 384).

When a European American nurse who values individuality provides care for an elder who has a collectivist perspective or visa versa, the potential for cultural conflict exists, illustrated by the following scenario:

> An older Filipino woman is seen in her home by a Euro-American public health nurse and found to have a blood pressure of 210/100 mm Hg and a blood sugar of 380 mg/dL. The nurse insists on calling the client's physician and arranging immediate transportation to the health facility of the physician's choice. The older Filipino woman insists that she must wait until her son-in-law and daughter get out of work to tell them of her condition. The daughter and her husband must decide where and when the client will go for treatment. She is concerned about the welfare of the family and wants to ensure that income is not lost by leaving work early. The family also jointly decides if they can afford a physician's visit and a possible hospitalization, since the client does not have health insurance. The nurse's main concern is the health of the individual elder, and the elder's concern is her family. The nurse is operating from the value that says an individual is independent and responsible for personal health care decisions.

Intensity of Relationships. Another concept that has implications for working with elders in cross-cultural situations is "context," which refers to the characteristics of relationships and behaviors toward others (Hall, 1977, 1990). The context is loosely divided into high and low and refers to the intensity of the interactions, with expressions of emotion and inclusion of family and a relationship with the nurse. When caring for the *high-context* elder, he or she will inquire of the nurse's health, family, or work. In return, the caring nurse first is expected to inquire about family members and appear friendly and genuinely interested in the person, and, second, be concerned with what might be called nursing tasks. Body language is more important than spoken words; it conveys the intended message. The quality of the relationship between the nurse and the person is more important than, perhaps, the needs of the person. The majority of cultures across the globe are high context in nature.

In sharp contrast are those whose relationships and behaviors are low context, such as the culture of Western medicine and nursing. This is common among persons from northern Europe, especially from the United Kingdom and Germany. *Low-context* health care encounters are tasks-oriented and only secondarily concerned about the relationship between the nurse and the older adult. Individual identity is not as important. For example, Mrs. Gomez is not the 82-year-old immigrant from Mexico, mother of seven and grandmother of 30; instead, she is the "fractured hip in 203." For the person who is low context, small talk may be considered a waste of time. A direct approach is expected, with a literal message such as "Just tell me what is wrong with me!" Nonverbal communication is infrequent, and verbal communication is used only when necessary.

The culturally competent nurse is skilled enough to assess the patterns of those cared for and to move between the contexts to provide the highest quality of caring.

Cohort Experiences. One approach to knowledge about any group of elders is from the perspective of cohort experiences and concept of cohort effect. A cohort is a group of people born within the same time span, usually a decade. These rigid boundaries fit nicely with statistical and actuarial tables but not so well with people. However, it is useful to consider the cohort experiences of major national and world events. Groups of people, usually born within the same time period, may share a common historical context. The term *cohort* is usually applied to such a group. For example, men born between 1920 and 1930 were very likely to have been active participants in World War II and the Korean War. In comparison, men born between 1940 and 1950 were likely to have been involved in the Vietnam conflict, an entirely different experience. It is not surprising that these two groups of men have different world perspectives and different health problems. Likewise, most women born between 1920 and 1930 were raised with what are known as *traditional values and roles* and may have either never worked outside the home or been limited to lower-paying "women's work," such as domestic services, teaching, and nursing. In contrast, women born between 1930 and 1940 had pressure to work outside the home and also had considerably more opportunities, partially as a result of the feminist revolution of the 1960s. For some ethnic elders it may be more appropriate to think in terms of existential time; before and after the Jim Crow Era for African-American elders in the rural south, or before and after the Mariel Boatlift of 1980 for Cuban Americans.

Obstacles to Cultural Knowledge. Gerontological nurses providing culturally competent care help reduce health disparities through awareness of and sensitivity to both overt and covert barriers to caring. Among these barriers are ethnocentrism, stereotyping, and other "ism's." As a result of any of these, we may see cultural conflict in the nursing situation. Cultural conflict can occur any time a person interacts with another whose beliefs, values, customs, languages, and behavior patterns differ from their own. For example, an immigrant Korean nurse is instructed to ambulate an 80-year-old African-American client. The patient says that he is tired and wants to remain in bed. The nurse does not insist. The European American nurse manager reprimands the immigrant Korean nurse for not ambulating the patient as ordered. The immigrant Korean nurse says to another Korean nurse: "Those Americans do not respect their elders; they talk to them as if they were children."

In the traditional Korean culture, men are the decision makers and older adults are revered. The European American nurse complains to a colleague that "those Asian nurses allow men to run all over them." Those from the culture known as *mainstream American* or *European American* do not necessarily consider age or gender in these circumstances. In the responses of both nurses, each denigrated the other's culturally prescribed behavior to underscore that his or her own cultural response was "correct."

Ethnocentrism. Ethnocentrism is a belief that one's own ethnic group is superior to that of another's and is exemplified in the nursing situation just described. In nursing, we have a unique culture and usually expect our clients to adapt to us. We expect them to be on time for appointments, to follow our instructions, and to listen to what we say. If we are caring for elders in an institutional setting, we expect them to agree with, for example, the frequency of prescribed bathing, eating (and timing of this), and sleep and rest cycles. The better acculturated an elder is to the culture of the institution and nurse, the less the potential for conflict. She will eat the meals provided even if the food does not look or taste like what she has always eaten. A non–English-speaking resident will accommodate the staff with or without an interpreter.

Stereotyping. Although cultural knowledge is helpful and essential, it should be applied cautiously. Stereotyping is the application of limited knowledge about one person with specific characteristics to other persons with the same general characteristics and limits the recognition of the heterogeneity of any group. Relying on knowledge of a positive stereotype can be useful as a starting point in understanding but can also be used to limit understanding of the uniqueness of the individual and impose unrealistic expectations. For example, a common stereotype of older African-Americans may be that the church is a source of support. If the nurse simply assumes this to be true, it could have a negative outcome, such as fewer referrals for other forms of support (e.g., home-delivered meals). On the other hand, this stereotype can be used to shortcut the assessment. In discussing discharge plans with an African-American elder, the nurse may say, "Is your church one of the resources you will be able to depend on when you return home?"

The "Ism's." The "ism's" refer to the use of personal and/or social characteristics to label people, which in turn can affect not only their self-esteem but also their life experience. "Ism's" assume negative beliefs, attitudes, or behavior toward a person or groups of persons based on a particular characteristic. The "ism's" usually result in differential treatment and discrimination that are directed at a specific ethnic or minority group. Elders in the United States are frequently exposed to ageism, in the presumption of incapacity based solely on chronological age; women face sexism based on their gender; persons of color face racism based on their skin color; and the poor face classism based on their socioeconomic status. All of these serve to perpetuate health disparities, and all are amenable to change by the sensitive and knowledgeable gerontological nurse.

Cultural Skills. Promoting healthy aging and providing the highest quality of care for ethnic elders requires not only awareness and knowledge but also the ability to apply both with a new or refined set of skills. In doing so, the self-esteem of the elder is enhanced. The appropriate use of communication and language is a foundational skill and intimately tied to the concept of the self. The self is continuously constructed and inextricably bound up with the linguistic categories available in a given culture (Berman, 1991). Communication is an issue not only of language but also of idiom, style, jargon, voice tone, inflection, and body language. We can conceive of ourselves only within the language we know. To make each contact with the elderly fully meaningful, shared communication is essential.

Communication also means listening carefully to the person, especially for his or her perception of the situation, and attending not just to the words but also to the nonverbal communication and the meaning behind the stories. Listen to the elder's perception of the situation, desired goals, and ideas for treatment. Cultural skills include nurses' ability to explain their perceptions clearly and without judgment, acknowledging that both similarities and differences exist between their perceptions and goals and those of the elder.

Unspoken Communication. Communication begins long before a word is spoken. In many cultures the unspoken message may be as or more important than what is heard. For persons with dementia, from any culture, this is especially true.

The Handshake. A handshake is the customary and expected greeting in what is called "mainstream America." A firm handshake is thought to be a sign of good character and strength. Yet this is not always the case. To an elder Native American, a firm or vigorous handshake may be interpreted as a sign of aggression. Their handshake may instead be more of a passing of the hand with light touch as a sign of respect rather than of weakness. To Soviet older adult immigrants, a handshake may be interpreted as insolent and frivolous (Tripp-Reimer and Lauer, 1987). In the Muslim culture, cross-gender physical contact (including handshakes) may be considered highly inappropriate or even forbidden. Before the nurse makes physical contact with an elder of any culture, he or she should ask the elder's permission.

Eye Contact. Making eye contact during verbal communication is another highly valued behavior in the mainstream American culture. Direct eye contact is taught to be a sign of being honest, trustworthy, and straightforward. Nursing students are taught to establish and to maintain eye contact when interacting with clients, but this behavior may be misinterpreted by older adults of different ethnic groups.

The less-acculturated ethnic elder may avoid eye contact, not as a sign of deceit but as a sign of respect. A more traditional Native American elder may not allow the nurse to make eye contact, moving his or her eyes slowly from the floor to the ceiling and around the room. Direct eye contact is considered disrespectful in most Asian cultures. Looking one directly into the eyes implies equality. Older adults may avoid eye contact with physicians and nurses because the health professionals are viewed as authority figures. In some cultures, direct eye contact between genders is considered a sexual advance. The gerontological nurse can follow the lead of the elder by being open to eye contact but not forcing this type of contact in any way.

The Use of Silence. The value, use, and interpretation of silence also vary markedly from one culture to another. In general, Eastern cultures value silence over the use of words;

in Western cultures, the opposite is true. For older adults of many Eastern cultural groups, especially those in which the Confucian philosophy is embraced, silence is a sign of respect for the wisdom and expertise of the speaker. Silence is expected by young family members and by family members who have less authority. In traditional Japanese and Chinese families, silence during a conversation may indicate the speaker is giving the listener time to ponder what has been said before moving on to another idea. In Native American cultures, it is believed that one learns self-control, courage, patience, and dignity from remaining silent. Silence during a conversation may signify that the listener is reflecting on what the speaker has just verbalized. French, Spanish, and Soviet older adult immigrants may interpret silence as a sign of agreement (Tripp-Reimer and Lauer, 1987; Purnell and Paulanka, 2003).

Spoken Communication. Unspoken communication is usually accompanied by a spoken component. If both the nurse and the elder speak the same language, communication is facilitated although attentions to cross-cultural factors are not precluded. However, when different languages are spoken, interpretation and sometimes translation are needed for optimal care. Translation is the exchange of one written language for another, such as in the translation of patient education materials. Interpretation, on the other hand, is the processing of language from one spoken language to another in a manner that preserves the meaning and tone of the original language without adding or deleting anything. The job of the interpreter is to work with two different linguistic codes in a way that will produce equivalent messages (Haffner, 1992). The interpreter tells the elder what the nurse has said and the nurse what the elder has said without adding meaning or opinion.

An interpreter is needed any time the nurse and the elder speak different languages, when the elder has limited English proficiency, or when cultural tradition prevents the elder from speaking directly to the nurse. The more complex the decision making, the more important are the interpreter and his or her skills, such as when determining the elder's wishes regarding life-prolonging measures.

It is ideal to engage interpreters who are trained in medical interpretation and who are the same gender, social status, and, in some cases, age of the elder. Unfortunately, too often children or even grandchildren are called upon to act as interpreters. When they are not available, secretaries or housekeepers are asked to fill this role. When doing so, the nurse must realize that either the interpreter or the elder may "edit" his or her comments because of cultural restrictions about the content, that is, what is or is not appropriate to speak about to parent, child, or stranger.

When working with an interpreter, the nurse first introduces herself or himself to the client and the interpreter and sets down guidelines for the interview. Sentences should be short, employing the active tense, and metaphors should be avoided because they may be impossible to convert from one language to another. The nurse asks the interpreter to say

BOX 21-3   Hints for Working with Interpreters

- Before an interview or session with a client, meet with the interpreter to explain the purpose of the session.
- Encourage the interpreter to meet with the client before the session to identify the educational level and attitudes toward health and health care and to determine the depth and type of information and explanation needed.
- Look and speak directly to the client, not the interpreter.
- Be patient. Interpreted interviews take more time because long, explanatory phrases often are needed.
- Use short units of speech. Long, involved sentences or complex discussions create confusion.
- Use simple language. Avoid technical terms, professional jargon, slang, abbreviations, abstractions, metaphors, or idiomatic expressions.
- Encourage interpretation of the client's own words rather than paraphrased professional jargon to get a better sense of the client's ideas and emotional state.
- Encourage the interpreter to avoid inserting his or her own ideas and to avoid omitting information.
- Listen to the client and watch nonverbal communication (facial expression, voice intonation, body movement) to learn about emotions regarding a specific topic.
- Clarify the client's understanding and the accuracy of the interpretation by asking the client to tell you in his or her own words what he or she understands, facilitated by the interpreter.

Modified from Lipson JG et al, editors: *Culture and nursing care: a pocket guide,* San Francisco, 1996, UCSF School of Nursing Press.

exactly what is being said, use the first person, and direct all conversation to the client.

For more information on working with interpreters, see Box 21-3 and refer to the detailed guidelines and protocols available from Enslein and colleagues at the University of Iowa (Enslein et al., 2001, 2002).

GENDER

Gender, which refers to the personal, cultural meaning of biological differences, is fundamental to personal identity and is the primary way in which experiences are organized. Gender incorporates those and other less-measurable characteristics that are the result of a coalescence of cohort, culture, and genetics. Environmental influences, social expectations, and early socialization, as well as innate capacities, all seem to fall within the purview of these three categories. As a matter of interest, the previous editions of this textbook did not have a category related to gender alone because little was available related to gender and aging.

Consideration of aging from a cultural perspective provides rich context for providing the highest quality gerontological care. When adding knowledge about gender issues, our perspectives can broaden and our sensitivities deepen. Gender studies in general have become increasingly popular.

The goals of a gender-focused research center include such aims as the following:
- Basic and clinical research related to gender-specific needs and characteristics
- Developing and testing gender-specific therapeutic strategies
- Providing gender-appropriate health recommendations
- Disseminating research findings that promote understanding of gender-specific issues

However, to identify the relevance of gender is exceedingly difficult and requires a breadth of perspective. In the past two decades we have moved from simply describing biological differences to emphasizing the shaping of gender roles by socialization patterns, and we are now in a phase of describing gender in terms of social structure and cultural patterns (Hooyman and Kiyak, 2006). Unfortunately, few studies have been done in the sub-area of gender and aging.

From a demographic perspective, gender differences can be quite remarkable, from life expectancy to social support. Women usually live longer than men and are much more likely to live alone after widowhood. Men who survive their wives often remarry and live alone significantly less often than women. However, women usually have larger social networks outside the work environment than do men, which could potentially reduce social isolation after the death of a spouse or companion (Hooyman and Kiyak, 2006). And gender-related health problems emerge: women increasingly confront osteoporosis and breast and uterine cancer, whereas men are vulnerable to prostate enlargement and prostatic cancer. Heart disease is the number-one cause of death for both men and women, yet women are treated less aggressively than are men.

Older Women

Older women are the fastest growing segment of the population, especially among those older than 85 years. At least 55% of those ages 65 to 74 years and 71% of those older than 85 years are women (Hooyman and Kiyak, 2006). Older women are also more likely than men to be widowed or divorced, live alone, live in a nursing home or assisted living facility, live longer (Figures 21-7 and 21-8), and provide 24-hour care to spouses or family members at some time in their later lives (Figure 21-9). They are also more likely to live in significant poverty, especially after becoming widowed or divorced, be or become victims of abuse, and face ageist discrimination and societal devaluing (see "double jeopardy" and "triple jeopardy" discussion on p. 514).

Social Status. The social status of women varies by culture and is quite different from that of their male counterparts. The variations have implications for the gerontological nurse that might be overlooked. Women who live alone are more likely to be white, never married, never had children or who have outlived their children, or have outlived

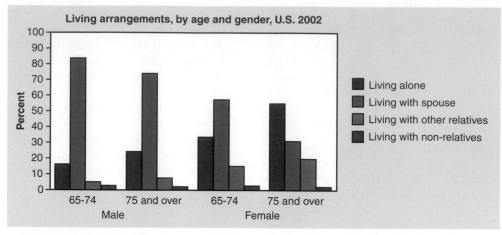

FIGURE 21-7 Living arrangements, by age and gender, United States, 2002. (From U.S. Census Bureau.)

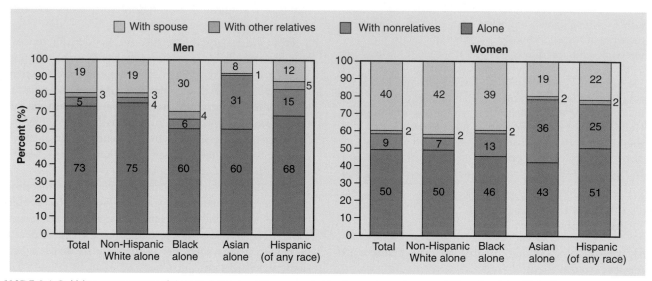

FIGURE 21-8 Living arrangements of the population age 65 years and older, by gender and race and Hispanic origin, 2003. (From U.S. Census Bureau, Current Population Survey, Annual Social and Economic Supplement.)

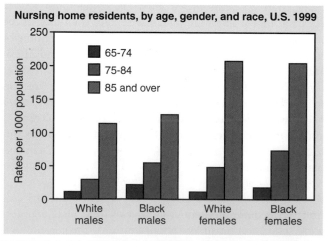

FIGURE 21-9 Nursing home residents, by age, gender, and race, United States, 1999. (From The National Nursing Home Survey.)

their husbands, especially women of color (Hooyman and Kiyak, 2006). Older women are highly unlikely to re-marry, both by personal choice and by an inadequate number of potential partners (Figure 21-10). If they live with others, it probably will be, first, a spouse or partner and, second, a daughter. Only rarely do white women live with other relatives, but this is much more common for women of color. Whereas most women in European American groups hold a lower status compared with men, older women of color often hold elevated social status, respected for both their age and their contributions to the family, community, and church. Women, in sharp contrast to men, often have an extended social support network made up of not only family but also friends and neighbors. This may be especially strong among lesbian women who, over a life-time, have created a tight fictive-kin group to replace their estranged family (when this is the situation).

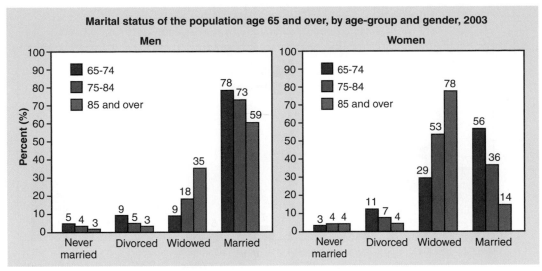

FIGURE 21-1O Marital status of the population age 65 years and older, by age-group and gender, 2003. (From U.S. Census Bureau, Current Population Survey, Annual Social and Economic Supplement.)

Economic Status. Overall, older women are at a significant economic disadvantage. This has implications in many ways, from the ability to purchase transportation to see health care providers, to the ability to pay for health care, to the opportunities to live in safe and well-maintained "healthy" homes. Of those who are older than 65 years and considered poor, 75% are women—the older a woman is, the more likely she is to be poor (this is called the "feminization of poverty"). Income and marital status are connected, with most widowed and never-married women having the lowest incomes of all.

At retirement, one's Social Security income is calculated looking back on the past 30 years of employment. Non–income-producing years are counted as zero income and are still included in the calculation. For women, this is usually particularly relevant because of discontinuous employment as a result of interruptions with childbirth and other caregiving responsibilities. The continuing low wages for women (compared with men) exacerbate the problem. Women, on average, continue to earn approximately 75% of that of men in the same positions and professions, which again is ultimately reflected in their Social Security income.

Another structural problem facing women is pension laws. Although no longer allowed in large organizations, smaller companies are still permitted to have their pension "survivor benefit" optional without survivor consent. This means that the wage earner may opt to receive higher pension payments while living with no or little continuation to his or her survivor. And for the small companies, notification is not required. This means that the survivor benefit can be declined without informing the potential survivor.

While the author worked as a hospice nurse, she cared for a couple during the husband's very long and difficult death. There was concern about the wife's health as a 24-hour caregiver with no children and no nearby relatives. Their income was very limited, but she thought it was adequate to pay their bills and maintain their small home in a rural, isolated community, although her husband "handled all of those things." After his death, she found that he had opted for a "no survivor benefit" pension. She was almost immediately profoundly impoverished and in danger of becoming homeless with few options.

Health Status. Women are more likely to have multiple chronic diseases rather than an acute illness that is the cause of death for many men (Figure 21-11). Rather than cause death, these health conditions are more likely to lead to problems with everyday activities and functioning (those things one needs to do to get through the day). Because of the number of illnesses, women take more prescription medications, which they may not be able to pay for. If poor, women—especially women of color—are more likely to receive a lower quality of care or do not get care because of costs.

Many areas of health specific to women (e.g., breast health, menopause) and as they affect women (e.g., osteoporosis, heart disease) are slowly receiving more attention (Helzner et al., 2005; O'Dell and McGee, 2006; Watson et al., 2006). Before the 1990s, almost all research that was later applied to women (e.g., the safety of synthetic estrogen) was actually conducted on men. The study called "The Woman's Health Initiative" (in progress) is the first major wide-range project using women to study women's health issues. This study has already revolutionized what we thought we knew about the effect and safety of hormone replacement therapy (HRT).

Yet the quality and receipt of health care depend largely on the access through health insurance. If an older woman (especially divorced or widowed) is not yet 65 years of age (when she may qualify for Medicare), does not have insur-

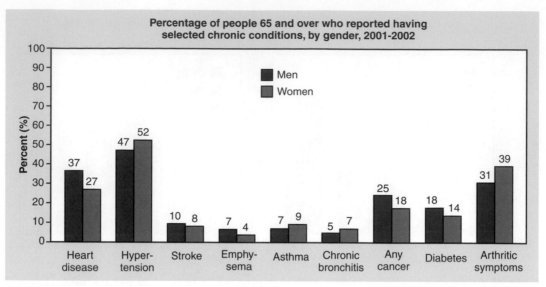

FIGURE 21-11 Percent of persons age 65 years and older who reported having select chronic conditions, by gender, 2001-2002. (From Centers for Disease Control and Prevention [CDC], National Center for Health Statistics, National Health Interview Survey.)

ance, and becomes ill, she is in serious trouble. Women are more likely to be working for employers who do not provide health benefits, for example, many nursing homes, domestic services, and small businesses. If insurance is available, she may not earn enough to purchase the plan but her income may be too high to qualify for Medicaid. Helping women (and men) who lose insurance through divorce has been attempted. "Conversion" laws require that one's former spouse (either deceased or divorced) continue to provide access to insurance for up to 3 years after the death or divorce—although the premium may be prohibitive.

A small percentage of elders experience multiple serious and/or disabling conditions that leave them unable to care for themselves. Whereas the family provides most of this care, about 5% seek this care in institutions, usually nursing homes. Women outnumber men two to one among those considered to be frail. Women who had been living alone go to nursing homes more than anyone else.

Despite the difficulties of aging for women, maturity brings new opportunities for many. They may find caregiving responsibilities rewarding. Or, with children grown, they have free time for the first time in their lives and go back to school, develop new interests, or become master athletes or gardeners or mentors to others.

Older Men

When considering men and aging, there is an interesting paradox. Until the past 10 to 15 years, the majority of research was done with groups composed entirely or primarily of men. Yet most of the aging literature, when gender specific, is about older women, since they make up the majority of the population 65 years of age and older.

Inferences about social and economic status can be easily made about older men when learning about their contrast with older women as noted earlier. The differences in

health status, especially when combined with racial and ethnic differences, bear closer examination and will become more interesting in the coming years. For example, men used to predominate in those with lung cancer, greatly influenced by occupation exposure to toxins and smoking. Now lung cancer is the leading type of cancer death for both men and women. The number of women with chronic obstructive pulmonary disease (COPD) is also increasing because of increased cigarette smoking. Men die younger than women, with black men having the shortest life span of all. Yet our understanding of all of these phenomena is still limited.

The primary focus on older men has been in specific health issues that are theirs alone (Philpot and Morley, 2000). Benign prostatic hypertrophy is now recognized as affecting most men at some time in their lives. Erectile dysfunction (ED) may be receiving the most attention because of the increase in pharmacological interventions now possible and the openness of ED discussion in the media. Prostate cancer is now recognized as particularly important to African-American men because of its higher prevalence and death rate when compared with all other men (USDHHS, 2000). And finally, men have joined women in their fight against the aging process, with the rising popularity of hair implants, hair color "designed for men," and other cosmetic surgery and treatments.

A number of questions arise when discussing gender issues related to aging, including the following:

- Why, if older women have so many disadvantages, do they survive longer and seemingly maintain morale, in spite of being old, poor, and alone?
- Why is it so difficult for men to seek medical help before life-threatening conditions occur?
- What effect will the baby boomers have on gender parity or disparity?

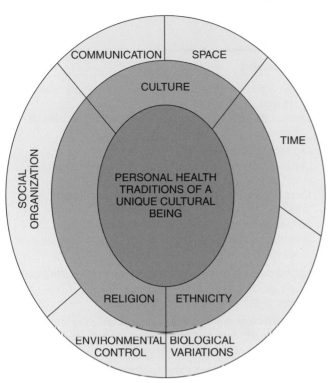

FIGURE 21-12 Personal health traditions of a unique cultural being. (From Spector RE: *Cultural diversity in health and illness*, ed 5, Upper Saddle River, NJ, 2000, Pearson Education.)

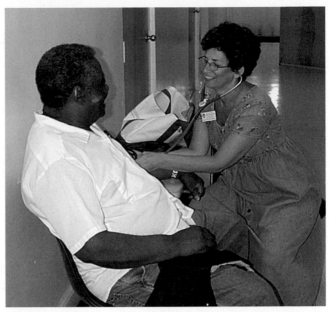

Nurses provide care in a number of settings. (Courtesy Kathleen Jett.)

▲ PROMOTING HEALTHY AGING: IMPLICATIONS FOR GERONTOLOGICAL NURSING

To fully understand another culture or gender, one must enter into an unknown conceptual world in which time, space, religion, tradition, and wellness are expressed through a unique language that conveys these formulations about the nature of the world and humanity. Heritage consistency is a component of many features: communications, space, time, socialization, environment, and biology (Figure 21-12). These in turn affect culture, religion, and ethnicity. Collectively, the personal uniqueness is established.

Assessment

The contact between elders and gerontological nurses often begins with assessment. During that time, the nurse and the elder have an opportunity to come to know each other. Listening is the key to the assessment as the nurse tries to understand the situation and the person. A thorough assessment includes a cultural assessment. A comprehensive cultural assessment takes time. It is clear that not all situations allow for this, but even if it must be done bit by bit over time, it will give the caregiver a better understanding of how to work with and within the culture of the client. One must also remember that great generational cohort and cultural differences may exist between practitioner and client.

Several tools or instruments can help the nurse elicit the elder's health care beliefs while identifying his or her own perceptions of the beliefs. The explanatory models developed by Kleinman and associates (1978) and Pfeifferling (1981) have helped nurses and other health care professionals obtain needed information in a culturally sensitive manner. An adaptation of these models for use in obtaining a meaningful cultural health assessment appears in Box 6-1. Another framework for a meaningful and more detailed cultural assessment, as well as interventions, was offered by Evans and Cunningham (1996) and is presented in Table 21-2.

Key information in the assessment is the determination of the health beliefs as discussed earlier. Most people (nurses and patients alike) ascribe to more than one belief system, combining Western biomedical approaches with those that may be considered more traditional. People choose from among the beliefs or include several of them in their attempt to make sense of health, illness, and treatments. To optimize the healthy aging of the person who depends on the nurse for intervention and caring, the nurse should learn to be sensitive to the possibility that the person may hold one or more of these beliefs. Significant conflict with nurses may result when a patient refuses biomedical treatments because the patient believes that accepting the treatment is a sign of disrespect for God (as challenging God's will) or because he or she does not believe the treatment will restore balance. Learning more about the person's beliefs regarding disease causation and effective treatment will allow the nurse to work between the cultures of medicine and the person to promote better health.

However, information about beliefs alone is inadequate; the gerontological nurse should incorporate cultural assessment into a holistic assessment as described in Chapter 6. Nursing concerns must focus on overall health care for persons by assisting them to gain access to needed services

TABLE 21-2

Nursing Care for the Ethnic Elder

	Assessment	Interventions
Ethnicity	Number of years living in United States Age at immigration (immigrant vs refugee) Degree of affiliation with ethnic group or assimilation to U.S. culture	Be sensitive to historical events that influence elders' perception of self and authority of health care providers. Demonstrate respect for elder by using surname and providing care in a manner sensitive to cultural norms.
Communication	English as primary or secondary language Level of fluency Barriers to communication such as sensory deficits, lack of privacy, distractions, or cultural taboos Meaning of nonverbal gestures	Use translator for exchange of health information. Document system for communicating basic needs between patient and staff. Provide patient access to sensory aids (glasses, hearing aids, pocket talkers). Eliminate background noise, and provide optimum lighting. Offer gestures of assistance with basic needs (warm blanket, glass of water).
Health perception	Perception of health problem, causes, and prognosis Response to pain, illness, and death	Educate patient/family about disease process and medical treatments. Identify and document reasons for behavior. Develop system for identifying and rating pain.
Folk practices	Use of cultural healers, herbal medicines, alternative health practices and beliefs	Obtain order for use of folk remedies as indicated. Educate patient regarding contraindications for folk remedy, and discourage use if dangerous.
Health care system	Previous hospitalization experiences Current hospitalization planned or emergency?	Encourage patient to express fears regarding hospitalization and treatments. Keep patient/family informed of patient's progress as appropriate.
Religion	Spiritual practices and beliefs Level of incorporation of spiritual practices into healing/dying process	Allow privacy and space for religious articles and practices. Arrange for visit from spiritual leader as requested. Refer patients to hospital chaplain. Document beliefs about death and burial and healing.
Food	Beliefs regarding food and healing Use of hot/cold paradigm Specific food preferences	Obtain consultation with dietitian. Incorporate food preferences into menu selection. Ask family to supply familiar foods. Document use of hot/cold practices as they relate to nursing care.
Social support	Current living situation Support of family or community (or both)	Encourage family participation in care if desired. Encourage visits or phone calls with peers.
Decision making	Primary decision maker for health care How does the patient make decisions? Who is needed for decisions?	Involve family when providing patient with health care information. Arrange for family conference if disparity exists between goals of patient, family, or health care team.
Discharge planning	Expectations for care after hospitalization and during future years of aging Financial status that affects discharge planning and both short-term and long-term health status Ability of patient/family to support discharge needs	Involve family in discharge planning. Obtain consult for social services. Refer patient to community resources for legal advice, transportation, meals, shopping, and emotional support.

From Evans CA, Cunningham BA: Caring for the ethnic elder, *Geriatr Nurs* 17(3):105, 1996.

through ascertaining affordability, efficacy, accessibility and availability of information, client satisfaction, respect for clients' health beliefs, illness perspective, and informal support systems.

Designing Interventions

Finally, promoting healthy aging in cross-cultural situations includes the ability to develop a plan of action that considers the perspective of both the elder/family and the nurse/health care system and to negotiate an outcome that is mutually acceptable. Skillful cross-cultural nursing means de-

veloping a sense of mutual respect between the nurse and the elder. It is working "with" the client rather than "on" the client.

The LEARN Model. The LEARN Model (Berlin and Fowkes, 1983) uses the perspective shown in the explanatory model and expands it to the person: nurse interaction. The LEARN Model is a useful tool in guiding the nurse in the clinical setting while interacting with elders of any ethnicity. Through it, the nurse will increase his or her cultural sensitivity and in doing so will be instrumental in providing more culturally competent care, thus helping reduce health disparities.

L Listen carefully to what the elder is saying. Attend to not just the words but to the non-verbal communication and the meaning behind the stories. Listen to the elder's perception of the situation, the desired goals and ideas for treatment.

E Explain your perception of the situation and the problems.

A Acknowledge and discuss both the similarities and the differences between your perceptions and goals and those of the elder.

R Recommend a plan of action that take both perspectives into account.

N Negotiate a plan that is mutually acceptable.

Given the necessary data, the nurse can use this information to negotiate a clear understanding of problems and solutions with the client or the identified support figure in the person's life. Once an understanding is reached, the nurse may need to include consultation or collaboration with traditional or alternative healers if the client believes they are important. Locate priests, monks, rabbis, ministers, or indigenous healers if they are who are desired or believed to be helpful. When alternative healing methods are used, respect them as judiciously as those you may be implementing. A sense of caring is conveyed in these gestures of personal recognition. Unbiased caring can surmount cultural differences.

Models of Cross-Cultural Care. Ethnic elders can also be found in senior centers, especially those that have introduced culturally appropriate food and activities. The impact of cultural relativism in a senior center was described by Ochoco and Shimamoto as far back as 1987. They found that many of the participants who were ethnically distinct had been passive, dependent, and depressed during the "usual" center activities. Two thirds of the participants were widowed women who had originally emigrated from Japan and depended highly on their children. By introducing ethnic-related activities at a senior center in Hawaii, they were able to increase patient self-esteem, independence, and satisfaction. The community health nurse who activated the group wished to strengthen the sense of self in group members through a focus on cultural heritage. In addition to health-teaching sessions and education about the aging process, the nurse used reminiscence and construction of a collective oral history to stimulate interaction and the sense of accomplishment. This model has been adapted in many community and institutional settings. In providing culturally relevant care, the uniqueness of the person is honored.

The On Lok Project in San Francisco is the ultimate model of the provision of long-term care services to diverse elders. Originally designed to meet the home care needs of Chinese and Italian immigrants, it now has the capacity to provide every level of short- and long-term care, as well as residential options, to all persons. Services are provided in the language of the elder and in the manner that optimizes each person's cultural heritage (Bodenheimer, 1999;

Kornblatt et al., 2002, 2003). Nurses can learn from the work of On Lok and other programs to enhance the care and encourage the health of ethnic elders.

Modifications of existing long-term care services to enhance the well-being of ethnic elders may include the following:

1. Ensuring that the resident has access to professional interpreter services if needed
2. Developing programs that reflect the diversity of the residents and the staff
3. Considering monocultural facilities or units where population demographics warrant
4. Employing staff who reflect the diversity of residents or clients

INTEGRATING CONCEPTS

Promoting healthy aging in the care of ethnic elders frequently provides the gerontological nurse with new challenges and necessitates a slightly different conceptualization of Maslow's Hierarchy. Unfortunately, poverty is very common in many households of persons of color or of women living alone, and meeting basic needs, especially food and health care, may be difficult. Older immigrants who have never worked in the United States will not qualify for Medicare and may not qualify for Medicaid. The nurse must be sensitive to this possibility without making assumptions or stereotyping. The nurse can assess the components of biological integrity and, if necessary, facilitate the elder or family obtaining whatever supports (e.g., food stamps, home-delivered meals) that are possible and appropriate.

Whereas some ethnic elders have been in the United States most of their lives or their move to the United States was not traumatic, many others have experienced horrific events in their home country or during their immigration process and may hold a unique regard for safety and security. The staff of a Jewish nursing home complained that it was particularly difficult getting some of the residents with dementia to shower. It was some time before they realized that a number of their residents were Holocaust survivors. As the residents' dementia progressed, they were no longer able to distinguish the difference between a shower for hygiene and the fear of "going to the showers" (i.e., to the gas chamber) in the concentration camps of their youths (G. Weissman, personal communication, April 21, 2003).

A sense of belonging for the ethnic elder may be closely tied to self-esteem. Cultural and sexual identity may be one of the major elements of self-concept and a key to self-esteem, and increasingly so as a person becomes more mentally or physically frail. Often ethnic elders are closely tied to family and community and, in some cases, religious communities. Estrangement from their country of origin may be ameliorated if they live in homogeneous communities and may be exacerbated if they live in social isolation or away from persons with similar backgrounds. The ethnic community (e.g., barrios, Nihonmachi, Chinatown) serves as a buffer and a means of strengthening cohesiveness for elders and

Human Needs and Wellness Diagnoses

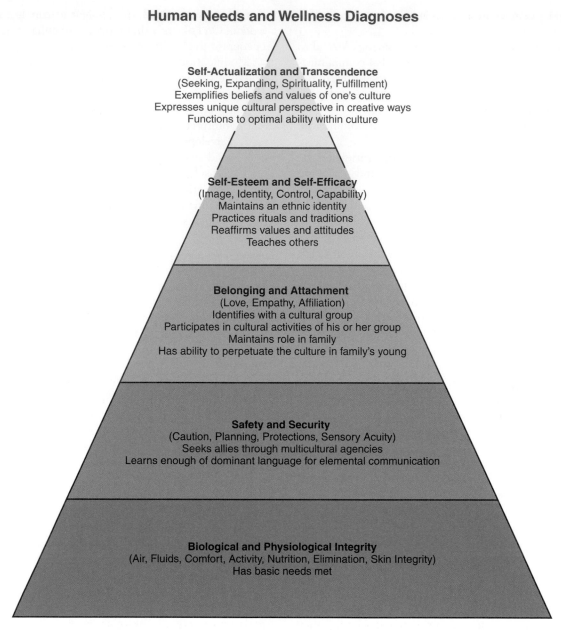

Self-Actualization and Transcendence
(Seeking, Expanding, Spirituality, Fulfillment)
Exemplifies beliefs and values of one's culture
Expresses unique cultural perspective in creative ways
Functions to optimal ability within culture

Self-Esteem and Self-Efficacy
(Image, Identity, Control, Capability)
Maintains an ethnic identity
Practices rituals and traditions
Reaffirms values and attitudes
Teaches others

Belonging and Attachment
(Love, Empathy, Affiliation)
Identifies with a cultural group
Participates in cultural activities of his or her group
Maintains role in family
Has ability to perpetuate the culture in family's young

Safety and Security
(Caution, Planning, Protections, Sensory Acuity)
Seeks allies through multicultural agencies
Learns enough of dominant language for elemental communication

Biological and Physiological Integrity
(Air, Fluids, Comfort, Activity, Nutrition, Elimination, Skin Integrity)
Has basic needs met

These are not all the possible wellness diagnoses that may be identified. The above
are examples of nursing diagnoses that should be considered when planning care
for the older adult

others of various cultural groups. Within the community, members are protected from discrimination and the strange language and customs of the society outside.

Family, religion, community, and history are important reference points for self-worth and identity for any individual or ethnic group. Familial supports are variable among groups, social classes, and subcultures, yet the nuclear or extended family is the chief avenue of transmitting cultural values, beliefs, customs, and practices. The family provides orientation, stability, and sanctuary. In a simplistic sense we may say that Asians value familial piety; Hispanics, the extended family (*compadres* translates to co-parents); blacks, extended or fictive-kin supports; and Native Americans, a system of kinship and line of descent.

Church or religiosity plays a major role in defining many cultures. Religion may function as a consistent experience that affords psychic support in the individual's life. In many black communities, religion is a pervasive force and the place to instill self-determination toward change (Hooyman and Kiyak, 2006; Moriwaki and Kobata, 1983; Walls, 1992). The Issei seek religious tradition in the face of aging and death (Kitano, 1969). Padilla and Ruiz (1976) note that Hispanics tend to seek Spanish-speaking clergy rather than mental health professionals when they have emotional problems.

Changes are threatening the historical role of the elder and the traditional family. Economic independence and mobility of the younger members of the family are chipping away at the insulation afforded by the community. Intergenerational discontinuities of assimilation create a communication gap between the young and the old. Often the elderly are not proficient in the language of the dominant culture, and the younger members may not retain the language of their parents. This may cause isolation and estrangement between the oldest and youngest generations. Members of ethnic minorities are extremely vulnerable in old age. They experience double jeopardy because they may be devalued because of age and ethnicity. Attitudes and economic inequality also contribute to their problems.

Throughout this chapter older adults are viewed, individually and collectively, as they have been defined and developed by the influence of their time and place in history,

their gender, and distinctive group practices and beliefs that have served as the foundation for the self-system.

The study of the uniqueness and individuality of each surviving elder is one of the most complex and intriguing opportunities of our day. Realistically, it will be almost impossible to become familiar with the whole range of clinically relevant cultural differences of older adults one may encounter, but to attempt to serve them holistically and sensitively is the most challenging opportunity.

KEY CONCEPTS

- Population diversity is rapidly increasing and will continue to do so for many years. This suggests that nurses will be caring for a greater number of minority elders than they have in the past.

CASE STUDY: Where Do I Belong? Who Am I?

Georgia thought she was a misfit. She had always thought this. She felt that she was born in the wrong time and most of the time was in the wrong place. She was born in China in 1920, the child of missionary parents. Her parents had built and managed a school for orphaned children in Shanghai. There were many problems and uprisings in China, and when she was 15, the political situation and threat of war were so intense that her parents were asked to leave the school and return to the United States. They were then sent to an Appalachian mining village to manage a small school and clinic. Having grown to adolescence in China, she felt more Chinese than Anglo. She had a difficult adjustment in the poverty-stricken rural mining village in Appalachia, so unlike where she had been. In a few years, her parents sent her to a private religious college, attended mainly by the children of the affluent elders of the church. She married a young army officer, and they were immediately sent to France. Her life from then on seemed to consist of nothing but moves as she followed her husband about. She was grateful that she had never had children; as she said, "My life has always seemed so unsettled, I don't think I could have provided any stability for children." As she aged, she developed crippling arthritis and her husband provided much of her care. When she was widowed at 80, she almost immediately entered a nursing home. There she found that most of the staff were Filipino and talked among themselves in Tagalog. Again, she felt out of step with the prevailing culture in which she found herself. She became very difficult to get along with, and the staff were at their wits end trying to please her. You recently went to work as director of nursing in the facility where Georgia is. How will you help her and the staff maximize their life satisfactions?

Based on the case study, develop a nursing care plan using the following procedure*:

- List Georgia's comments that provide subjective data.
- List information that provides objective data.
- From these data, identify and state, using accepted format, two nursing diagnoses you determine are most significant to Georgia at this time. List two of Georgia's strengths that you have identified from data.
- Determine and state outcome criteria for each diagnosis. These must reflect some alleviation of the problem iden-

tified in the nursing diagnosis and must be stated in concrete and measurable terms.
- Plan and state one or more culturally relevant interventions for each diagnosed problem. Provide specific documentation of the source used to determine the appropriate intervention. Plan at least one intervention that incorporates Georgia's existing strengths.
- Evaluate the success of the intervention. Interventions must correlate directly with the stated outcome criteria to measure the outcome success.

Critical Thinking Questions

1. Define the terms *culture, ethnicity, ethnocentricity, cultural sensitivity,* and *cultural competence*.
2. Identify several personal values or beliefs that are derived from your ethnic and cultural roots.
3. Relate major historical events that have affected your birth cohort, and explain in what way your cohort has been affected.
4. Discuss several different ethnically based approaches to health care.
5. Describe characteristics that you believe are specific to your gender.
6. Construct a cultural genogram, and discuss your roots.
7. Discuss ways in which you have learned to appreciate cultural and ethnic differences.
8. Privately list your stereotypes and "ethnocentrisms" for various ethnic groups, and explore the basis of these beliefs (taught, fear, experience, lack of knowledge). Then consider what can be done to be more culturally sensitive and competent.
9. Select a food or particular behavior and examine differences in custom that arise from ethnic/cultural interpretations.
10. Describe the advocacy role of nurses who care for ethnic elderly.
11. Formulate a care plan incorporating ethnically sensitive interventions.
12. Plan strategies to provide care that is culturally sensitive and acceptable to Georgia without losing a focus on the individual's own aging experience.

---

* Students are advised to refer to their nursing diagnosis text and identify possible or potential problems.

- Recent research has revealed significant and persistent disparities in the outcomes of health for persons from minority groups, with the members of these groups bearing the burden of morbidity and mortality in most areas.
- One of the major goals of *Healthy People 2010* is to reduce health disparities in the nation.
- Nurses can contribute to the reduction of health disparities through increasing their own cultural awareness, knowledge, and skills.
- Cultural competency and sensitivity require awareness of issues related to culture, race, gender, sexual orientation, social class, and economic situations.
- Ethnicity is a complex phenomenon encompassing language, traditions, symbols, and folklore expressed as identity.
- Culture is a complex concept reflecting the interrelationship of many components. It includes shared beliefs, expectations, and behaviors.
- Stereotyping negates the fact that significant heterogeneity exists within cultural groups.
- Health beliefs of various groups emerge from three general belief systems: biomedical, magico-religious, and naturalistic. Elders may adhere to one or more of these systems.
- Gender affects values, perceptions, and the approach to health care assessment and treatment.
- Two cultural patterns that have great potential for conflict between the elder and the health care system are orientation to time and orientation to family and self.
- Effective cross-cultural care to elders includes skills related to language, both verbal and nonverbal.
- The more complex the decision making, the more important the quality of communication; for those with limited English proficiency, expert interpretation is needed whenever serious decisions are needed, for example, end-of-life care or treatment changes.
- The use of family, children, or support staff as interpreters is not recommended and may result in censored interpretation because of rules of cultural etiquette unknown to the nurse.
- The LEARN Model provides a useful framework for working with ethnic elders.

RESEARCH QUESTIONS

What are the chief difficulties in providing nursing care for individuals from an entirely different background from one's own?

Which personality types thrive best in a homogeneous environment, and which thrive best in a heterogeneous environment?

What are the factors that identify a group as an ethnic minority?

What are the enduring cohort differences that are unlikely to change throughout life?

How is cultural sensitivity incorporated into a curriculum?

What are the outcomes of an integrated cultural approach versus a separate-course approach in a curriculum?

Why, if older women have so many disadvantages, do they survive longer and seemingly maintain morale in spite of being old, poor, and alone?

Why is it so difficult for men to seek medical help before life-threatening conditions occur?

What effect will the baby boomers have on gender parity or disparity?

REFERENCES

Administration on Aging: *Addressing diversity*, 2004. (website): *www.aoa.gov*. Accessed September 1, 2006.

Berlin E, Fowkes W: A teaching framework for cross-cultural health care: application in family practice, *West J Med* 139(6):934-993, 1983.

Berman HJ: From the pages of my life, *Generations* 15(2):33, 1991.

Bodenheimer T: Long-term care for frail elderly people: the On Lok model, *N Engl J Med* 341(17):1324-1328, 1999.

Enslein J et al: *Evidence-based protocol: interpreter facilitation for persons with limited English proficiency*. Research dissemination core product, 2001. Available for the University of Iowa Gerontological Nursing Interventions Research Center.

Enslein J et al: Evidence-based protocol: interpreter facilitation for individuals with limited English proficiency, *J Gerontol Nurs* 28(7):5-13, 2002.

Evans CA, Cunningham BA: Caring for the ethnic elder, *Geriatr Nurs* 17(3):105, 1996.

Gelfand D: *Aging and ethnicity: knowledge and service*, ed 2, New York, 2003, Springer.

Gerdner LA et al: Chronic confusion and memory impairment among elders: honoring differing cultural beliefs in America, *J Gerontol Nurs* 32(3):23-31, 2006.

Haffner L: Translation is not enough: interpreting in a medical setting, *West J Med* 157(3):255-259, 1992.

Hall ET: *Beyond culture*, Garden City, NY, 1977, Anchor Press.

Hall ET: *Understanding cultural differences*, Yarmouth, Me, 1990, Intercultural Press.

Helzner EP et al: Race and sex differences in age-related hearing loss: the health, aging and body composition study, *J Am Geriatr Soc* 53(12):2119-2127, 2005.

Hofstede G, Pedersen P: *Exploring culture: exercises, stories and synthetic culture*. Yarmouth, Me, 2002, Intercultural Press.

Hooyman N, Kiyak HA: *Social gerontology*, ed 7, Boston, 2006, Allyn & Bacon.

Jackson LE: Understanding, eliciting, and negotiating clients' multicultural health beliefs, *Nurse Pract* 18(4):30, 1993.

Jett KF: Making the connection: seeking and receiving help by elderly African Americans, *Qual Health Res* 12(3):373-387, 2002.

Jett KF: The meaning of aging and the celebration of years among rural African American women, *Geriatr Nurs* 24(5):290-293, 2003.

Jett KF: Cultural influences. In Meiner S, Lueckenotte AG, editors: *Gerontologic nursing*, ed 3, St Louis, 2006, Mosby.

Kitano H: *Japanese Americans*, Englewood Cliffs, NJ, 1969, Prentice-Hall.

Kleinman A et al: Culture, illness, and care: clinical lessons from anthropologic and cross-cultural research, *Ann Intern Med* 88:251-258, 1978.

Kornblatt S et al: Best practices: the On-Lok model of geriatric interdisciplinary team care, 2002. Available from On Lok SeniorHealth at *www.onlok.org*.

Kornblatt S et al: Cultural awareness in health and social services: the experience of On Lok, *Generations* 26(3):46-53, 2003.

Lukwago S et al: Development and validation of brief scales to measure collectivism, religiosity, racial pride, and time orientation in urban African American women, *Fam Community Health* 24(3):63-71, 2001.

McIntosh P: *White privilege: unpacking the invisible knapsack.* Working paper #189. Wellesley College Center for Research on Women, 1989. (website): *www.utoronto.ca/acc/events/peggy1. htm.*

Moriwaki S, Kobata F: Ethnic minority aging. In Woodruff R, Birren J, editors: *Aging,* ed 2, Monterey, Calif, 1983, Brooks/Cole.

Ochoco L, Shimamoto Y: Group work with the frail ethnic elderly, *Geriatr Nurs* 8:185, 1987.

O'Dell KK, McGee S: Acupuncture for urgency in women over 50: what is the evidence? *Urol Nurs* 26(1):23-30, 2006.

Padilla A, Ruiz R: Prejudice and discrimination. In Hernandez CA et al, editors: *Chicanos: social and psychological perspectives,* ed 2, St Louis, 1976, Mosby.

Pfeifferling JH: A cultural prescription for mediocentrism. In Eisenberg L, Kleinman A, editors: *The relevance of social science for medicine,* Boston, 1981, Reidel.

Philpot CD, Morley JE: Health issues unique to the aging man, *Geriatr Nurs* 21(5):234-239, 2000.

Pierce R et al: Generation and ethnic identity: a typological analysis, *Int J Aging Hum Dev* 9:19, 1978-1979.

Purnell LD, Paulanka BJ: *Transcultural health care,* Philadelphia, 2003, Davis.

Rathbone-McCune E: *Isolated elders: health and social intervention,* Rockville, Md, 1982, Aspen.

Smedley B et al, editors: *Unequal treatment: confronting racial and ethnic disparities in health care,* Institute of Medicine, National Academy Press, 2002. Special report.

Spector RE: *Cultural diversity in health and illness,* ed 6, Upper Saddle River, NJ, 2004, Prentice Hall Health.

Tripp-Reimer T, Lauer GM: Ethnicity and families with chronic illness. In Wright LM, Leahy M, editors: *Families and chronic illness,* Springhouse, Pa, 1987, Springhouse.

U.S. Department of Health and Human Services (USDHHS): *Healthy People 2010,* ed 2, (2 vols), Washington, DC, November 2000, U.S. Government Printing Office.

Walls CT: The role of the church and family support in the lives of older African Americans, *Generations* 17(3):33, 1992.

Watson J et al: Serum antioxidants, inflammation and total mortality in women, *Am J Epidemiol* 163(1):18-26, 2006.

Weissman G: Personal communication, April 21, 2003.

CHAPTER 22

Nursing and Aging in Rural and Frontier Settings

Kathleen Jett

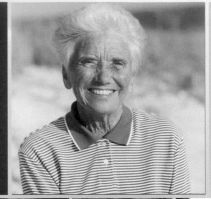
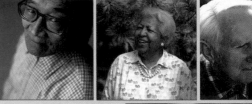
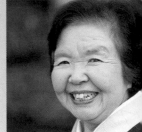

AN ELDER SPEAKS

Where we live, if you even think you are going to have a heart attack you had better call the rescue wagon, because it is going to take them at least 20-30 minutes or more to get to you— if they ever do!

Chuck, age 75

LEARNING OBJECTIVES

On completion of this chapter, the reader will be able to:

1. Differentiate urban, rural, and frontier settings, and suggest differences that may influence aging and nursing.
2. Develop an understanding of the multiple complex issues facing rural older adults.
3. Describe the common personal and cultural characteristics of the older adult in the rural setting.
4. Identify potential challenges to accessing and receiving health care in rural and frontier settings.

5. Discuss strategies to facilitate nursing care and healthy aging in rural settings.
6. Compare features of rural and urban nursing practice.

Older adults living in rural and frontier settings are different from their urban counterparts, and these differences have both advantages and disadvantages. This chapter gives the reader an awareness of the life ways and culture of older rural Americans and what it is like to practice nursing in a rural community. The information is drawn from the gerontological, sociological, and nursing literature. Relevant historical perspectives are highlighted, along with rural concepts, characteristics, health status, and health care features. It is important for the reader to understand the difficulty in generalizing research information across rural settings because great regional diversity exists in the social, cultural, ethnic, and economic structures of rural communities across the United States and other nations.

The roles of rural nurses are distinct from those of their urban peers. Gerontological nursing in the rural setting presents unique challenges. Rural nurses provide care to sparse populations living in large, often isolated geographical areas that have limited resources. They are challenged to become

expert generalists, to be nonjudgmental, and to develop the characteristics of resiliency, creativity, and resourcefulness in themselves and in those to whom they provide care. They often have little or no separation between their professional and personal lives. On the other hand, they are respected, hold public visibility, and have a great deal of autonomy and flexibility in delivering care (Bushy, 2000). See Table 22-1 for a comparison of rural and urban nursing practice.

AGING IN RURAL AMERICA

The lives of older persons in the rural setting are often portrayed in a romanticized stereotype of leading peaceful, healthy, independent existences with strong families and environments to support them in their aging years. As more data become available, this stereotype is disappearing and more dependable information is emerging about the day-to-day realities of older rural men and women and their families.

Special thanks to JoAnn G.G. Congdon, the previous edition contributor, for her content contributions to this chapter.

TABLE 22-1

Comparison of Rural and Urban Nursing Practice on Select Characteristics*

Feature	Rural	Urban
Clients	Of all ages and across the life span Personally acquainted with many of them Sense of connectedness to the community despite geographic distances	More likely to focus on one or two age-groups Usually not personally acquainted
Scope of practice	Expected to wear many hats Interface with other disciplines Greater opportunity for expanded roles	More precise job description for each discipline
Roles	Generalist role Role overlaps with other disciplines	More opportunities to specialize Disciplines have more clearly delineated roles
Resources (materials, other professionals, technology, fiscal, and other)	Sometimes fewer formal services Greater flexibility in planning and delivering nursing care Informal networking facilitates continuum of caregiving	Usually have more (there always are some limitations) Greater structure in planning and delivering nursing care within an institution
Patient/client health conditions and diagnosis	Exposure to clients with wide range of health conditions and diagnoses Opportunities to become an "expert generalist"	Specialize; work with fewer types of conditions and diagnoses
Degree of autonomy	Greater Fewer peers with whom to consult	More limited Better access to peers and other professionals
Pace	Generally slower	Usually more intense; hurried
Public visibility	High public visibility—known by many locals Difficult to remain anonymous	Less visibility Easier to maintain anonymity
Discharge planning and client follow-up	Familiarity with clients means increased opportunities for nurse-client interaction outside of facility; continues informally after discharge (in community settings) Creativity encouraged to prevent fragmentation of care	Formal referrals to other agencies and providers
Coordination of a continuum of care for clients	Extended family and familiarity among community residents facilitate integration of informal services with formal services Flexibility in planning continuum of care with family system	Reduced access to informal networks Greater reliance on formal services
Status in community	Nursing viewed as an occupation of status, usually highly esteemed Few nurses means high public visibility Acknowledged as a community health resource Well thought of by community (individual variations)	Denser population means less public visibility More nurses and other health professionals—recognition is dispersed among them
Community involvement (informal health education; local policy development)	Multiple roles in home and community social systems (church, school, civic groups, etc.) Plays many roles in health care facility that extend into community roles Little differentiation (less clear boundaries between work, home, and community)	Community activities/roles shared by more people having a particular interest in that activity
Confidentiality	Can be problematic due to familiarity among residents and the visibility of their actions to others	Less problematic because of less familiarity and public visibility but must always be a concern
Quality-of-life issues	Small-town atmosphere Family, recreation, and lifestyle opportunities differ from those of highly populated settings Regional variations—vary from community to community	Regional variations—vary from community to community

From Bushy A: *Orientation to nursing in the rural community*, Thousand Oaks, Calif, 2000, Sage.
***Note:** There are wide variations among and between rural and urban communities and individuals. Therefore these characteristics are experienced in varying degrees by individual residents in both settings.

Since the 1980s and 1990s, sociologists Krout and Coward, nurses Magilvy and Congdon, and others have been prolific researchers of rural aging. In 1998, Krout and Coward explained that the increased interest in rural aging within the field of gerontology was related to a number of factors, including the following:

- A growing exposure of the aging population in research journals and scholarly publications
- An increase of federal and foundation funding for research related to the aging population
- The farm crisis of the early 1980s, which heightened national and academic awareness of rural issues
- The national awareness of the changing demographics of Americans, particularly the rapid aging of the overall population
- The growing interest of gerontologists to better understand the diversity of older Americans and the importance that residence plays as a variable that adds to this diversity

RURAL CONCEPTS

Definitions

Rural areas have several prominent features, including low population size and density, small communities, physical remoteness, distance from urban resources, and relative dominance of natural ecology. A newer term "frontier" refers to a subset of areas that are even more sparsely populated, geographically isolated, and less accessible. "Rural" is now defined by one of exclusion, that is, areas that are not considered metropolitan statistical areas (MSAs) or their surrounding communities. MSAs are areas that include a city of 50,000 or more or an urbanized area with at least 50,000 inhabitants and a total MSA population of 100,000 or more (Rural Information Center Health Service, 2001). Rurality is determined by considering a combination of three factors: population density, raw population size, and residence outside of a town of 2500 or more. On the other hand, frontier rural areas are defined more simply in terms of

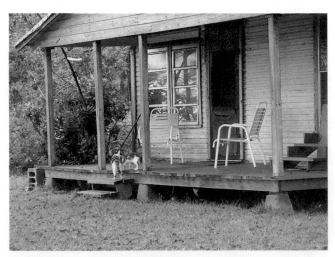

Rural north Florida. (Courtesy Kathleen Jett.)

population density that is less than 7 persons per square mile. Frontier areas have been measured by percentage of any one state, with the range from 0.02% of Michigan and 0.2% of Florida and Louisiana to 52.3% of Alaska, 54.1% of Montana, and 73.9% of Wyoming (Zelarney and Ciarlo, 2000). However, the use of these national definitions for rural does not accurately describe the differences among rural regions, farms, non-farms, villages, towns, and urban satellite areas. A well-known prominent characteristic of rural America is its diversity. Rural America varies not only by region, community size, and type but also, most distinctly, by its social and economic diversity (Havens et al., 2001).

For the purposes of this chapter, a discussion of the complexities of the finer distinctions between urban and rural differences is not necessary; therefore *rural* is defined as "a generic term referring to the end of the residential continuum that includes towns and open country with small or widely dispersed populations remote from large metropolitan cities" (National Institute of Nursing Research [NINR], 1995, p. 26).

Characteristics of Rural Older Adults

Approximately one in four persons age 65 years and older in the United States lives in a rural community; that is, 25% of the 36.5 million Americans 65 years and older. This rate is similar to those living in inner city cores. This number is projected to increase to 71.5 million by the year 2030. Even though rural residence is sometimes equated with farm life, most rural older adults live in or near small towns.

Age, Gender, and Race Composition. An exodus of the younger generation from rural communities to urban areas has depopulated many rural communities. Younger persons and professionals are attracted to metropolitan areas for better economic security and more lucrative employment opportunities. The availability of both skilled and semiskilled jobs is decreasing in rural America with plant closings or transfers to Mexico and off-shore sites (Leight, 2003). In rural areas, as compared with urban, the percentage of individuals ages 19 to 54 years is lower and the percentage of those older than 55 years is higher. An interesting phenomenon accompanying this rural-urban age difference is the high age-dependency ratio. This ratio is calculated by the number of elders and children (those older than 64 years and younger than 18 years) divided by the number of working-age persons (19 to 64 years of age). The result indicates the extent to which working-age persons are available to support those who are more dependent—mainly children and the elderly. The rural age distributions indicate that the nonmetropolitan areas have the smallest number of working-age persons and thus a potentially smaller base of support for the very young and the elderly. Many rural areas have been "aging" (1) through the loss of young adults who move to more urban areas for economic and job-related purposes and (2) from an influx of retirees. Older persons who remain in the rural areas and retirees become an ever-increasing proportion of the total population (Reeder, 1998).

Because women have a longer life expectancy than men have in general, their overall number compared with men is greater in all settings. In rural settings in the age-group of 65 to 74 years, women make up 51.8% of the population, with this number increasing to 65.9% of those 85 years old and older. These figures are comparable in non-metropolitan and metropolitan settings with a slight decrease in the rural setting for women in the age-group 65 to 74 years. However, in the age-group of 65 to 84 years and living on farms, the number of men exceeds the number of women (U.S. Department of Agriculture [USDA], 2005). The difficulty of living alone on a farm and the trend of older farm widows to move into small towns may account for these figures. Among those ages 85 years and older, the sex ratios are lower but the pattern is similar (McLaughlin and Jensen, 1998).

The older rural population is less racially and ethnically diverse than those younger than 65 years, but the diversity is increasing, especially among aging farm workers and other immigrants (Averill, 2005). The extent of racial and ethnic diversity varies from region to region of the country. For example, rural African-American elders have greater concentrations in the southern states, American Indians are concentrated more in the Southwest and northern plains, and Hispanics in the Southwest (Ham et al., 2003). Although the number of whites is greater in both rural and urban areas, the predominance of whites is much more pronounced in many of the rural and frontier areas. Overall in the non-metropolitan areas in the United States, 92% of persons older than 65 years are white; 6.2% black; 2.6% Hispanic; and fewer than 1% each Native American and Asian. Although the relative number of Native Americans, Native Alaskans, and Aleuts is small, of their population over 50% reside in non-metropolitan areas (McLaughlin and Jensen, 1998).

Marital Status, Housing, and Family Conditions.

Marital status and living arrangements of older persons have significant influence on overall well-being, social support, poverty status, and health. Older adults who live alone are much more likely to lack social support and are more likely to experience health problems, poverty, and a lower quality of life. Older adults in rural areas are slightly more likely to be married than are urban elders, yet widowhood increases with age for all, regardless of setting. In the non-metropolitan setting, 17.2% of those 65 to 74 years old are widowed, with the number increasing to 65.1% of those 85 years old and older. Widowed women significantly outnumber men (6.7% vs. 26.9% ages 65 to 74 years old, and 36.9% vs. 79.7% 85 years old and older [USDA, 2005]).

Home ownership can be a valuable asset, and most older persons in all areas own their own homes. However, rural elders are more likely to own their own homes and to be free of mortgage payments than their urban counterparts (Goldsmith et al., 2000). The advantage seems to stop there because rural elders tend to have older homes that are lower in value and in need of more repairs, as measured by incomplete plumbing, deficient kitchen facilities, electrical de-

fects, and insufficient heating and maintenance (Rogers, 1999).

The out-migration pattern of rural young generations noted earlier has contributed to some erosion of traditional family structures and networks. On one hand, as this migration pattern continues, healthy older persons have the potential of becoming an important source of human capital for rural communities and are in-migrating (Dorfman, 1998). On the other hand, as the remaining and growing older population become an increasing proportion of the rural population, the demand for more health and social services and long-term care in these rural communities increases concomitantly (Averill, 2005).

Education, Income, and Poverty.

Educational level is often a proxy measure for economic security; that is, the higher the education, the greater are one's economic opportunities. In both education and income there are notable rural-urban differences, especially for the oldest-old. Among those 85 years old and older in rural settings, approximately 45% never finished high school compared with approximately 30% of those in urban settings (USDA, 2005). This low educational level has contributed to lifelong limited employment opportunities, lesser incomes, lower retirement incomes, higher poverty rates, and decreased health status.

Changes in both educational attainment and economic security have already been seen between the oldest-old and the younger-old in the rural settings (USDA, 2005). Higher-educated older persons will be better informed and have the skills to take advantage of community programs and services designed to benefit them. Analogous with the higher educational levels will come higher expectations and demands for an increase in the quality and number of health care services for older rural persons (Rogers, 1999).

Poverty is a major problem for rural elders, especially widows (USDA, 2005). Women living alone in rural areas have the highest rate of poverty or near-poverty, nearly double the number of urban men in the same situation (Brown and May, 2005). McCulloch (1998) attributed several explanations for this representation of rural older women: lower levels of education, lower earnings, scarce employment opportunities, competition for jobs that fall within a narrower range of occupations, less prospects for promotion, more part-time employment or employment without benefits, lower pensions, and the high likelihood that rural older women will be living alone as they age.

The United States Department of Agriculture (USDA) defines persistent poverty counties as counties in which 20% or more of the population live below the poverty line; they are the most heavily concentrated in the Southeast, in Appalachia, in the Southwest, and on Native American reservations. In some areas of rural Appalachia, the unemployment rates can reach 37% to 50% (Brown and May, 2005). These are families who have members who are employed, but they cannot afford to buy health insurance nor do they qualify for public assistance because their income level is above the poverty line. The families that do have some coverage struggle with medical and prescription co-payments and deductibles. Bushy (2000) reported that persistent poverty counties have decreased over the past three decades.

Health Status

Aging in the rural setting has been considered "triple jeopardy" (Coward et al., 1996). In addition to coping with the problems of aging, rural elders face increased vulnerability because of their residence in sparsely populated and remote locales and contending with a greater prevalence of certain conditions that negatively affect health just by living in rural America. This vulnerability translates to increased risk for premature morbidity and mortality, decreased functional status, and decreased quality of life (Leight, 2003). Poor economic conditions and stress-producing rural occupations such as farming, fishing, mining, and forestry may exacerbate common chronic conditions.

Rural-dwelling older adults are also at increased risk for disease and disability because of their multiple complex health problems, lower socioeconomic status, cultural issues, and barriers to accessible health services (Averill, 2005; Congdon and Magilvy, 1996).

At the same time, researchers caution that the epidemiological findings in one geographical region do not necessarily generalize to others because of the heterogeneity of rural populations and regions (Wallace and Wallace, 1998). Although rural-urban differences are seen, they are not universal across all settings, or in all indicators of health; therefore not all rural elders are at a disadvantage (Coward et al., 1994).

Chronic Conditions. As persons age, regardless of residential, economic, environmental, or social variables, their number of major chronic health conditions increases. Chronic diseases are the major causes of morbidity and mortality among people ages 65 years and older in the United States (Hennessy et al., 2001). However, there are some overall variations in urban/rural rates of chronic health conditions. Rural residents have higher rates of the following: arthritis and associated functional limitations and disability, cataracts, hearing impairments, loss of extremities, deformities or orthopedic impairments, ulcers, diabetes, bladder and kidney problems, hypertension, and emphysema (Wallace and Wallace, 1998).

Older adults living in rural or frontier settings also have higher rates of heart disease, diabetes, depression, and injuries (Averill, 2005). Isolated farmers are particularly vulnerable to depression and work- and stress-related illnesses. Elderly rural residents older than 60 years also evaluated their health as only fair or poor—6% more often than their urban counterparts (Ham et al., 2003).

Acute Conditions. Older rural residents experience a greater number of acute conditions such as infections, parasitic diseases, acute bronchitis, pneumonia, digestive system conditions, total injuries, sprains and strains, open wounds, lacerations, and non-migraine headaches; also, the number of older rural residents injured per year is higher than that of their urban counterparts (Wallace and Wallace, 1998). New research is also indicating an increased rate in falls and falls with injuries among rural elders (Quandt et al., 2006). Many of the injuries encountered in rural areas are the result of farm-related occupations along with operating dangerous machinery and working in risky weather conditions.

Migration to and from Rural Communities

In recent years there has been migration both into and out of rural communities. The majority of out-migration has been of young adults who move to metropolitan areas to seek employment and changes in lifestyle. There they remain and raise their children, returning to rural communities only to visit family members who have remained. Another group of persons who have migrated out are elders who, after a decline in health, a decline in functional ability, or the death of a spouse move from their homes to join younger family members in the urbanized areas of the country (Longino and Smith, 1998).

The older adults who have remained in their rural or frontier towns and farms are being joined by new retirees. The older persons who are migrating into rural communities tend to be younger, in good health, married, white, and relatively stable economically (Gale, 2002). They often have preestablished links with the rural community through vacationing, visiting relatives or friends, or following associates who migrated earlier (Fuguitt et al., 2002). Some communities that have been struggling to survive are actively recruiting both tourists and retirees; however, this is not without controversy and concern regarding the loss of the "small-town cohesiveness" (LaCaille, 2005). The reasons for rural migration vary greatly and include a desire to return to rural roots, the fatigue of crowded and hurried conditions in the cities, a search for tranquility and beauty of the country, and the belief that life is simpler, less stressful, and less costly in rural areas. For many there is an expectation of the ability to increase their quality of life (Longino and Smith, 1998).

Significant and uneven rural population shifts occurred throughout the 1990s, with much of the rural population growth concentrated in about 40% of rural counties (Health and Human Services Rural Task Force, 2002). The inward migration dynamics of elderly persons and the substantial continued out-migration of young people tends to complicate the age, social, economic, and net migration structures of some rural counties. In the short run, this migration pattern appears to benefit the rural areas economically, but more research is needed to fully understand the long-term impact of elderly migration on rural communities.

CULTURAL CHARACTERISTICS

The concept of culture is used most often with reference to different societies or national origins, but it can also mean the differences by geographical regions or other subgroups within a nation. Culture is usually defined as a pattern of learned behaviors, values, and beliefs (see Chapter 21). Cultural characteristics become especially important when considering the changing needs of elders over time and their influence on help-seeking.

Rural life can be considered a culture and characterized by a propensity to be self-reliant and independent, use a high level of self-care activities, seek help through an informal health care system, value privacy, and expect reciprocity in relationships (see *exchange theory* in Chapter 2). They are also known for their loyalties to their communities and neighbors (Averill, 2005; Higuchi et al., 2006; Sanford and Townsend-Rocchiccioli, 2004; WK Kellogg Foundation, 2002). Leight (2003) and Brown and May (2005) add hardiness and ruggedness to the characteristics.

Independence

Although, theoretically, the high value placed on independence could serve as the impetus to allow an individual to accept assistance, it usually leads to a pattern of resisting and neither seeking nor accepting help (Longino and Smith, 1994; Weinert and Long, 1990; Winstead-Fry et al., 1992). Longino and Smith (1994) found that "dependence, even on medical authority, is not considered a virtue among many rural elders" (p. 237). In a study of rural caregivers, a dependence on self, family, friends, and clergy sometimes precluded the use of formal services, even when they would have been beneficial (Sanford and Townsend-Rocchiccioli, 2004).

Others have described rural residents as having a "greater suspicion of governmental and agency assistance, and greater investment in the maintenance of self and family independence" (McCulloch, 1995, p. 331). Magilvy and colleagues (1994) reported that some elderly persons refused home care services because they viewed the government paperwork to qualify for these services as infringing on their privacy.

Rabiner and colleagues (1997) studied the relationship between metropolitan and non-metropolitan residential location and self-report related to one's ability to perform basic, mobility, and instrumental activities of daily living; they also assessed the degree to which the levels and types of functional limitations affect metropolitan versus non-metropolitan older adults' performance of self-care activities. They found many insignificant differences between the rural and urban participants in their abilities to perform functional tasks, but older adults from non-metropolitan areas were more likely to report performing self-care activities both in the presence and absence of disability. The researchers concluded that non-metropolitan older adults may discount the significance of declining functional status, thus normalizing the trajectory of aging in a different way than do their metropolitan counterparts. This may be influenced by the tendency to define health in functional terms, including the ability to continue to work (Brown et al., 2004; Leight, 2003).

Magilvy and Congdon (1994) described rural older persons who tolerated significant health problems so they could remain in their own homes. They further explained that financial, social, and geographical constraints may lead some rural older adults to lowered health expectations that prevents them from seeking advanced health care services (Congdon and Magilvy, 1998b). Still others have suggested that older people who grew up in rural environments are more likely to have limited expectations and a more developed sense of fatalism (Foner, 1986). Rabiner and colleagues (1997) also proposed that rural older adults may compare their current situation with that of their peers and consider their health to be better than the health of those in their peer group.

Spirituality and Faith

In a series of ethnographic studies on the health of rural older adults, Congdon and Magilvy (1998a; Magilvy and Congdon, 2000) reported that churches and religions were vital forces in the communities they studied and that many family and social activities were centered in the rural churches. The faith community assumed a responsibility to minister to the body as well as to the spirit and soul. Older adults, their families, caregivers, and ministers of faith believed that health care and faith were important in achieving healing and positive health outcomes. A strong integration of faith, spirituality, and health existed in the lives of rural older adults. Many rural residents believed that the church held the community together and that religion and spirituality were important for physical and mental well-being.

Martinez's (1999) work in southern Colorado supports the notion that spirituality is integral to rural life and health; she found that as rural older adults aged, their emphasis on spiritual health intensified. Older residents often described health as a balance of the spiritual, emotional, and physical aspects of the self. Health was achieved and maintained when one's actions were in harmony with one's values of faith, spirituality, and religion. For the rural Hispanic elders in her study, life's joys and sufferings provided opportunities to serve God, family, and community in the spirit of their faith.

In a discussion of rural health promotion programs, Mochenhaupt and Muchow (1994) reported that rural churches are appropriate and available sites for the delivery of health promotion and disease prevention services. Churches are trusted in rural areas, whereas outsiders (persons outside the community) may be viewed with suspicion and doubt. Rural church-based health promotion was most successful when it occurred within congregations and was incorporated into the healing mission and leadership of the church. Unfortunately, because of the long distance, some of the benefits of a faith community may not be accessible to frontier families and elders or to those with transportation challenges (Averill, 2005).

Care delivery approaches in rural settings that are culturally congruent and compatible with people's values are the most likely to succeed. Parish nursing has been suggested as an example of a health delivery program that is highly likely to succeed in rural locations (Brown et al., 1996). The concept of parish nursing is culturally well suited to many rural settings in that it places care in a trusted community institution and can provide improved access to and comprehensiveness of care.

HEALTH SERVICES IN RURAL SETTINGS

The provision of health services of any kind in the rural setting presents unique challenges ranging from the cultural resistance just noted, to health care shortages at every level, to the seemingly insurmountable transportation barriers.

Transportation

In any setting, health care services are accessed through various forms of transportation, which is an almost universal problem for older adults at some point. In the urban setting, some of the transportation challenges can be overcome by the use of public transportation, enlisting friends and family, hiring drivers, or moving to a location near the needed services. For home-delivered services, the transportation and time costs in the urban setting are minimal, especially in densely populated areas (Jett et al., 2005).

Transportation and access to services are increasingly serious problems in rural settings. In most locations, only limited public or nonprofit transport systems are available and, if available, are underutilized. Additional transportation barriers include long distances to health care services, poor and inadequate road conditions, and lack of dependable vehicles (Bushy, 1998). Approximately one third of rural residents travel 20 to 30 miles to the nearest health care providers, with 5% driving over 30 miles (Sanford and Townsend-Rocchiccioli, 2004). At the same time the number of home health agencies has significantly decreased in the past several years (Sanford and Townsend-Rocchiccioli, 2004).

If rural residents are to maintain access to goods and services and any quality of life, they must typically rely on their own private vehicles. It is not uncommon for older rural residents to continue to drive despite considerable problems with vision, hearing, reflexes, and mobility (Magilvy and Congdon, 1994). Researchers report hearing numerous stories from rural health care providers and family members about even the oldest-old making incredible efforts and taking risks to drive despite their tremendous physical and mental handicaps. For older drivers of any setting, the loss of driving privileges is synonymous with the loss of independence (Jett et al., 2005).

Barriers to Care

Although a variety of health care facilities serve the health needs of people living in rural settings, usually fewer and a narrower range of services are available to and used by rural older adults and the barriers to health care are significant. The barriers include inadequate access, difficulty navigating the managed care system, transportation limitations, and the cultural beliefs noted earlier (Averill, 2005; Brown et al., 2004; Higuchi et al., 2006). Research has consistently found that rural elders have lower levels of service awareness and tend to distrust the service bureaucracy (Krout, 1998; San-

ford and Townsend-Rocchiccioli, 2004). Other rural elders have been found to depend highly on informal care, including the use of traditional self-care strategies, their own assessments of their health problems, and dependence on family and friends rather than formal service providers (Brown et al., 2004). For health care providers, challenges exist in their blurred roles of neighbor, friend, and formal service provider. For the immigrant populations, language barriers may exacerbate the problems of access to health care (Averill, 2005).

Primary Care. Primary care services in rural settings are scarce, and specialty care is even less available. Even in the presence of the considerable number of chronic and debilitating conditions in the older rural population, they see health care providers less often and later in their illness. Referrals to specialists and services including radiology, dentistry, pharmacy, and dietetics may be impossible, especially in frontier communities. Instead, hospitalizations are more frequent and stays are shorter. Yet out-of-pocket costs for rural elders are about 23% of their income compared with 18% in the urban setting. Twice as many elders (10%) have no insurance coverage other than Medicare (Ham et al., 2003).

Part of the problem with access to care in rural settings is the limited number of health care providers. Although 25% of the population are in rural areas, only 9% of the physicians are available. The expanding role and utilization of nurse practitioners and physician assistants may eventually lessen the problems.

Many of the providers work in rural health systems. These include ambulatory practices that are part of a hospital, rural community health care centers, nurse-managed centers associated with regional schools of nursing, and Indian Health Services. Still other providers reach out to rural residents through videoconferencing and Internet and telemedicine. In some cases, collaborations of interdisciplinary caregivers have been successful (National Rural Health Association, 2005).

Unfortunately, the problems of provision of rural primary care are daunting. Problems of sustainability include low reimbursement rates and the burden of multiple licensing requirements when providing care in multiple states (e.g., through telemedicine).

Rural Hospitals. America's rural hospitals are commonly an integral and major component of the rural community. They have long-standing relationships with their communities and are interwoven into rural life. They are sources of community identity, worth, self-respect, and pride and are a major employer and purchaser in the local economy (Schlenker and Shaughnessy, 1996).

Most rural hospitals are nonprofit, but some are owned by state and local governments and corporations. In 1996 there were 2226 rural hospitals in the United States. Most of these were and are small, fewer than 100 beds, and depend heavily on Medicare revenues (Rural Information Center Health

Service, 2001). Compared with urban settings, rural hospitals are modest institutions in terms of beds, employees, and revenues; are usually housed in older physical plants; and provide a narrower range of medical services. In the 1980s the United States experienced a crisis in health care costs and dramatic national cost-containment efforts took place. Rural hospitals did not fare well from the increased external regulations and cost-cutting changes; consequently, closures accelerated. Between the early 1980s and 2000, more than 400 rural hospitals closed or changed the type of service offered (Center for Rural Health, 2002).

In some rural communities where full-service hospitals have closed, limited-service hospitals are being used as a means of maintaining some level of health care. These hospitals provide emergency and low-intensity services (services that do not require intensive or critical care units) and are allowed flexibility in staffing and licensing requirements (Shreffler et al., 1999). Evaluation studies have indicated that these limited-service institutions are a cost-effective solution for maintaining access to acute care services for sparsely populated, remote rural communities that cannot maintain a fully licensed hospital (Shreffler et al., 1999).

Duncan (1994) suggested that rural hospitals, like rural residents, experience a kind of multiple jeopardy. He explained that elderly patients who have the greatest need for local hospital services may also be the least economically desirable, because Medicare reimbursement rates are below costs for rural hospitals. Survival of rural hospitals depends, in part, on providing services for patients who pay at rates that provide a reasonable margin of profit. These patients are the privately insured or Medicare patients with generous Medigap coverage. Schlenker and Shaughnessy (1996) attributed some rural hospital survival to increased diversification of services, such as swing beds (see the next paragraph) and long-term care. The long-term care services include home health and skilled nursing care. Rural hospitals are more involved in long-term care than are their urban counterparts, and this pattern of involvement is increasing.

A unique example of long-term care use by rural hospitals was the advent of swing beds. Swing beds are acute care hospital beds that are used to provide nursing home care on an as-needed basis. The term *swing bed* refers to a change in the level of nursing and medical care without the patient being moved from the facility or, frequently, even from the bed (Palumbo, 1992). The Omnibus Budget Reconciliation Act of 1980 allowed eligible rural hospitals with fewer than 50 beds to be certified by Medicare and Medicaid to provide swing bed care. The assumption was that it would be more cost effective to provide long-term care in low-occupancy hospitals in rural areas than to build new nursing homes. Swing beds allow rural hospitals to fill beds, provide post–acute care for patients, provide a bed for a patient until one becomes available in a nursing home, or provide beds for patients who would have to travel long distances to obtain skilled nursing care (Rowles, 1996). This swing bed program may make the difference between survival and closure for some rural hospitals. In addition to the swing bed program, in recent years many rural hospitals have added their own long-term care units, which are part of or adjacent to the hospital. However, the recent changes in the reimbursement model to prospective payment for both home and skilled care may further challenge the existence of these services.

Community Nursing Homes. In rural areas, frail elders who are isolated from family and friends as a result of out-migration are more likely to reside in nursing homes than are their urban counterparts. More nursing home beds are available and more are likely to be used for custodial care as well as skilled care because of a near-absence of intermediate care facilities such as the board and care homes and assisted living facilities seen elsewhere (see Chapter 17) (Ham et al., 2003).

In a study conducted in rural Colorado, Magilvy and colleagues found that nursing homes were viewed with mixed feelings by rural older adults and their family members (Magilvy et al., 2000). Caring for one's aging parents was a tradition in the rural communities studied, but frequently, health care providers believed that families kept their older members in the home beyond a reasonable period. Hispanic family members especially struggled to meet family obligations of "caring for our own." A religious leader in the Hispanic community supported the view that some families waited too long to seek assistance with caregiving, as evidenced by caregivers becoming exhausted and care deteriorating. Although family remains an important and treasured aspect of the Hispanic culture, societal, economic, and family changes have altered the ability of families to provide support to Hispanic elders. Responsibilities for caregiving are beginning to fall to non-family care providers such as home care nurses, case managers, personal care providers, homemakers, and nursing home staff.

On the other hand, many older adults and their family caregivers were relieved and thankful for the available nursing homes because they would not have been able to provide care without them. The nursing homes contributed to the wholeness of the community and to the health and well-being of the residents. They served as an extension of the home and were considered a rich part of the community. Some older adults felt relieved that they were not burdening their families, and for some, making the decision to move to a nursing home enabled them to maintain a sense of independence and autonomy within the family system (Magilvy et al., 2000).

Rural nursing homes have evolved into an important health care resource because often they are the only long-term care option available. Because of this, rural nursing homes have developed in a different way than their urban counterparts. Glover (2001) pointed out that moving to a local nursing home enables long-time rural residents to continue to be part of the community. The residents are well known by the nursing home staff and vice versa.

However, transitions to nursing homes were often problematic and of a crisis nature. Most admissions occurred after hospitalizations, and decisions were made quickly with little or no planning (Congdon and Magilvy, 2001; Jett et al., 1996; Magilvy et al., 2000). Families had often not considered care beyond the hospital. For some older persons and their families, accessing any type of assistance was intimidating and they dreaded dealing with institutional bureaucracy, filling out endless forms, and gaining certification of eligibility for services. The presence of an ill or frail spouse or limited family resources could also complicate the transition. After hospitalization for an acute illness or during a period of extreme family or individual stress, the nursing home was sometimes the only choice.

Home Care. Home care has been shown to enhance quality of life and promote a holistic, family-centered approach to the care of rural older adults with acute, post-acute, rehabilitative, chronic, and end-of-life conditions (Congdon and Magilvy, 1998b). Home care focuses on a variety of needs and services that include both medical services and social services (see Chapter 17).

In rural America, the types of home care services and availability of services may differ by region and, in part, are limited by the availability of staff. The number and availability of providers and agencies are inconsistent across the country. In urban areas, the home health industry is highly competitive with a preponderance of for-profit agencies. In the entire state of predominantly rural Alabama, only 31 agencies provide care to 4000 patients, down from the 8000 cared for before the Balanced Budget Act of 1997 (Sanford and Townsend-Rocchiccioli, 2004). Magilvy (1994) reported that geographical conditions, economic variables such as funding and reimbursement mechanisms, and local adaptations in the provision of home care that are consistent with local preferences and culture all contribute to the diverse patterns of care. Home care is delivered in a number of settings and by an array of professionals, paraprofessionals, and agencies. It can be delivered in the person's own home, in the home of a relative, in assisted living facilities, or in foster or group care. However, the majority of long-term rural home care is provided by informal sources such as family caregivers or friends in the community or by freestanding clinics or agencies affiliated with hospitals (Brown and May, 2005).

Congdon and Magilvy (1998b) observed that home care as an integral part of long-term care can be both a socially and culturally acceptable form of holistic health care for an older rural population that fiercely values independence and freedom from institutional restraints. In a series of ethnographic studies, they reported that care at home facilitates independence, self-care activities, and the management of complex health needs over time (Congdon and Magilvy, 1998b; Magilvy and Congdon, 2000; Congdon and Magilvy, 2001). Rural lifestyles and culture challenged persons to use their informal resources and to live with and tolerate significant health problems. Combined with the

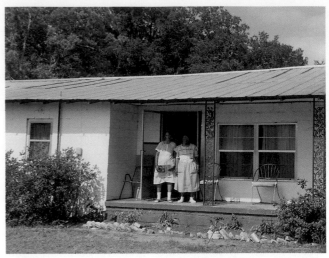

Co-habitation for the purposes of survival and caregiving is a common occurrence in some rural communities. (Courtesy Kathleen Jett.)

informal support of family and neighbors, home care surfaced as a major strength in health care delivery and transitions for rural older adults and their families. The commitment and resourceful strategizing of rural nurses were central to accessing both informal and formal home care services for older persons and to the successful delivery of the services.

Informal Care. Family members and circles of informal care are the primary sources of assistance for both healthy and frail older adults living in rural community settings (Sanford and Townsend-Rocchiccioli, 2004). Spouses, adult children, extended relatives, friends, and neighbors provide unpaid services that include assistance with meals, household tasks, shopping, personal care, health-related care, errands, transportation, and companionship. Congruent with rural culture, health care providers such as nurses and health care aides as members of the community are also integral parts of the formal as well as the informal system. Nurses and other health care providers live, shop, work, and worship in the rural communities and are neighbors and friends of elders needing care. For example, a public health nurse's brief trip to the grocery store might entail an extended conversation with a neighbor about a health problem or a commitment to drop off health care supplies to a homebound person on her way home from work (Magilvy and Congdon, 1994).

Community churches, religious organizations, caring ministries, senior centers, home-delivered meals, and local meal sites are also part of the informal but essential network that assists frail older adults to remain independent in their own homes. Some senior centers have posted lists of programs that offer volunteers who are willing to clean, cook, chop wood, or do other chores to assist elderly persons in need (Magilvy and Congdon, 1994).

The informal care systems are strong and highly developed in rural settings. Weinert and Long (1990) contended that these informal systems are the core of rural health care and that the formal health services and providers frequently support the informal system. To understand this strong informal care system, it helps to place it in the context of rural culture and life. Important characteristics such as dignity, independence, a need for privacy, the importance of reciprocity, and hardiness are embedded in rural culture. For example, Craig (1994) described the significance of reciprocal relationships that emerged among older residents and their community members. The need to reciprocate for the help one received was critical for the older adults in her study. This reciprocity was not only beneficial for the integrity of the older adults but also enhanced the health of the entire community. Magilvy and Congdon (1994) summarized their findings of the informal care system by extending a word of caution. Although research supports the view that the informal circle of care is a substantial strength of the rural health care system (p. 32):

> Policy makers and health care providers cannot relinquish responsibility for care to the informal network. Critical examination of whose needs are being met at whose expense must be constantly assessed if meaningful and ethical services are to be provided.

RURAL NURSING PRACTICE

Rural nursing is defined as "the provision of health care by professional nurses to persons living in sparsely populated areas" (Long and Weinert, 1998, p. 4). Organized efforts for rural nursing service were initiated early in the twentieth century by frontier nurses such as Lillian Wald and Mary Breckinridge. In 1912 Lillian Wald was instrumental in establishing the *Rural Nursing Service*, which was renamed a year later the *Town and Country Nursing Service*. Mary Breckinridge began the *Frontier Nursing Service* in 1925 in rural Appalachia and greatly expanded the nursing role in primary health care (Weinert and Long, 1991). High standards for nurses were strictly maintained in the early education and experience of rural nurses. Because Wald believed that rural work was diverse, demanding, and independent, she recruited only the most capable and dedicated women for rural nursing. Breckenridge, disturbed with the limited preparation and education of the lay midwives who were practicing in rural regions of the Appalachians, replaced them with frontier nurses who were prepared in general nursing, public health, and midwifery. The context and framework for nursing in rural environments that were established by Wald and Breckenridge are still relevant in today's nursing world (Bushy, 2000).

Scharff (1998, p. 21) described rural nursing practice as follows:

> Being rural means being a long way from anywhere and pretty close to nowhere. Being rural means being independent or perhaps being alone. Being a rural nurse means that when a nurse saves a life, everyone in town recognizes that she or he was there, and when a nurse loses a life, everyone in town recognizes that she or he was there. Being rural means turning inward for answers, because there may be nobody to turn to outward. Being rural means that when a nurse walks into the emergency room, it may be her or his spouse or child who needs a nurse and at that moment, being a nurse takes priority over being anyone else. Being a rural nurse means being able to deal with what she or he has got, where she or he is, and being able to live with the consequences.

Key Concepts of Rural Nursing

In their ongoing work to develop a theory base for rural nursing, Long and Weinert (1998) noted a pattern of certain concepts and relational statements appearing repeatedly in their data collected in rural Montana. These concepts and perceptions included the notion of "outsiders" and "insiders" and the potential of significant isolation of the rural providers, including nurses.

Rural nurses feel a sense of isolation from their peers, have a lack of privacy about their personal lives, have difficultly separating their roles in the community from their roles of professional caregiver, and are expected to perform a variety of diverse and unrelated tasks while working. Although the demand of the nurse is one of generalist, the need for specialty knowledge related to care of the older adult is increasing with the aging of the community members. On a single shift, a hospital nurse may work in the delivery room, in the emergency room, and on a medical-surgical unit. During the weekend or an evening shift, the nurse may be expected to carry out the tasks reserved for a pharmacist or dietitian. The lack of anonymity also extends to rural clients and their families. Persons living in a rural setting understand that there are very few secrets in a rural community. Everyone seems to know everything (Glover, 2001). For example, rural persons may be reluctant to access mental health services, knowing that others may recognize their car outside the clinic and know they are there. This lack of anonymity leads to the reduced use of rural mental health services. Home care nursing may include visits via helicopters or stays away from home as nurses travel throughout the state.

Glover (2001) added that rural nurses must learn to be aware of the unspoken community rules or they will risk being considered untrustworthy or outsiders. Scharff (1998), in her study of rural nurses in western Montana, northern Idaho, and eastern Washington, described the *newcomer* and the *old-timer*, terms that are commonly used in rural areas in relation to nursing staff tenure and group acceptance. Nurses who move to rural communities to work cannot expect to be accepted immediately. It generally takes time to make the transition from a newcomer to an old-timer. No particular time limit is identified when a nurse finally makes this transition and no clear way to arrive at a level of acceptance. Scharff estimated that it generally takes 3 to 5 years in combination with a certain amount of competence and common sense to be fully accepted. Scharff summarized her thoughts on rural nursing by stating that "the newcomer practices nursing in a rural setting, unlike the old-timer who practices rural nursing" (p. 38). Long and Weinert (1998) suggested that involvement in community activities may facilitate being known in the community and thus assist with acceptance. They caution that nurses who choose to maintain a separate professional and personal life may have a more difficult time adjusting to rural culture and environment. Glover (2001, p. 333) added that "health care providers who separate themselves and don't identify with the community may be viewed with suspicion and their judgments challenged."

Current Changes in Rural Nursing

Workforce Differences. Rural nurses are older than their urban counterparts, partly because of their longevity in the rural communities and rural health care institutions. As rural communities lose population and rural hospitals close, the percentage of nurses working in rural hospitals also declines. With the aging of the rural population and the increasing numbers of older persons, rural nurses are needed to provide acute, chronic, and long-term care to growing numbers of elderly persons. The increasing use of biotechnology such as telemetry and telehealth systems allows rural health care providers to consult quickly and efficiently with urban-based experts. Because of these changes, hospital and home care nurses need acute care skills to manage the increased complexity of care in rural areas (Bushy, 2000).

Workforce estimates project that the demand for rural nurses with baccalaureate degrees will increase with the extension of managed care organizations in rural communities (Bushy, 2000). As in urban areas, there is a shift from hospital acute care to community-based care. The greatest nursing needs will be in public health, home care facilities, ambulatory care, and nursing education programs. The question is whether rural facilities will be able to compete economically for nurses with higher educational levels. Rural registered nurses with baccalaureate degrees make lower salaries than their urban counterparts, have lower raises as experience and longevity on the job increase, and receive lower bonuses for earning advanced practice preparation (Bushy, 2000). On the other hand, some authors argue that the cost of living is lower and the quality of life higher in rural settings; thus nurses must assess all the variables when considering the advantages and disadvantages of rural nursing.

Strategies to educate, recruit, and retain rural nurses and other health care providers are underway across the country. Innovative educational programs using computer and interactive technologies are being delivered to rural outreach sites. In many cases, nursing school loan repayment is possible with commitments to work in rural settings through the National Health Services Corp. Many schools of nursing are offering and encouraging clinical rotations in rural sites, using local providers in collaboration with academic faculty as preceptors. Introducing rural high school students to the profession of nursing, exposing nursing students to rural environments, recruiting students with rural backgrounds to nursing schools, and increasing

the use of advanced practice nurses in underserved rural areas are examples of the wide variety of strategies nationwide to recruit and retain nurses and other health care providers in rural areas.

Changes in the Nature of Nursing. Historically, through a variety of practices, rural nurses have been committed to providing care to those most in need and to improving the health of their communities. Rural nurses are noted for their resilience, flexibility, ingenuity, and adaptability and for their connectedness to their communities. They are part of the rural system that values taking care of one's own. However, the past two decades of national health care turbulence and economic challenges have directly affected the roles of rural nurses. Congdon and Magilvy (1995) studied home care nursing in eight rural Colorado counties. One of their key findings was the theme of the changing spirit of rural nursing. Rural nurses perceived overwhelming documentation requirements as impeding rural practice, decreasing the quality of nursing care, and changing the spirit of rural community nursing from an emphasis on caring and community service to a focus on reimbursement. One nurse, in a comment that was heard repeatedly throughout the study, said, "The back of public health nursing is being broken because of the priority on generating revenue. Preventive care that emphasizes teaching and self care is being replaced by a system obsessed with only cost-containment" (Congdon and Magilvy, 1995, p. 20).

Customarily, rural nurses will spend extra time and effort to provide care because they feel linked to the community with strong ties and relationships. Most of their patients are not strangers. Rural nurses take pride in their self-directedness and independence in practice, and they are not unlike their rural patients in their dislike for too many government regulations and policies. Care is usually not refused just because a person cannot afford it. "Freebies," or free care, was observed, but nurses said the practice is not as prevalent as in the past, in part because of the "paperwork" demands in practice today and the need to maximize the number of patients seen rather than the quality of service delivery—to assume maximum reimbursement.

In Congdon and Magilvy's study (1995), the majority of the nurses who provided direct care in the home were prepared at less than the baccalaureate level and had little or no formal education for public health or home care roles. Some of them discussed openly their desire for skills to work more effectively within the changing health care system. However, one of the successful strategies that the rural nurses used to deal with the frustrating and seemingly ever-changing reimbursement regulations was to collaborate and network with other nurses in adjacent geographical areas. The nurses creatively pooled their resources, worked to ensure that home care staff kept current with the changes, and learned coping and management techniques from each other. Taking this opportunity to optimize their collective strength and working together to problem solve led to increased job satisfaction for the home care nurses and helped rekindle the spirit of rural nursing.

▲ PROMOTING HEALTHY AGING: IMPLICATIONS FOR GERONTOLOGICAL NURSING

The basis of rural nursing practice has been built by the pioneering work of such leaders in rural nursing as JoAnn Congdon (who wrote an earlier version of this chapter) and her colleague Joan Magilvy. Since then, Centers on Rural Aging have been established in key universities and include interdisciplinary teams of researchers and health care professionals. The challenges of aging in rural settings and the estab-

lished national recommendations present some unique opportunities for nurse to play an active role in the promotion of health.

In 2004 the West Virginia University Center on Aging presented conclusions and recommendations on policies on global rural aging from which nursing actions can be drawn (Hermanova and Richardson, 2004). The emphasis was on the promotion of healthy and active aging. These conclusions and implications for gerontological nursing include the following:

- Work within the determinants of healthy and active aging while considering a multiplicity of factors. This begins with a thorough assessment of the situation, one that includes components that have less meaning

Human Needs and Wellness Diagnoses

Self-actualization and Transcendence
(Seeking, Expanding, Spirituality, Fulfillment)
Seeks spiritual fulfillment in natural environment
Finds transcendence in isolation
Develops creative self-expressions
Seeks knowledge of self and rural culture

Self-Esteem and Self-Efficacy
(Image, Identity, Control, Capability)
Maintains independence to extent possible
Avoids stereotypical judgments of rurality
Makes wise choices within limits of capability and accessibility

Belonging and Attachment
(Love, Empathy, Affiliation)
Develops and maintains reciprocally
sustaining relationships
Recognizes vulnerability of isolation and
makes plans to avoid excess
Maintains non-rural affiliations
Expands generational contacts

Safety and Security
(Caution, Planning, Protections, Sensory Acuity)
Develops transportation options for necessary goods and services
Modifies dwelling to accommodate changes of aging
Exerts appropriate caution in all activities
Plans ahead for possible emergencies

Biological and Physiological Integrity
(Air, Fluids, Comfort, Activity, Nutrition, Elimination, Skin Integrity)
Develops appropriate methods of sustaining basic needs with
particular attention to adequate shelter, warmth, and nutrition
Respects need for routine health monitoring
and health maintenance

These are not all the possible wellness diagnoses that may be identified. The above
are examples of nursing diagnoses that should be considered when planning care
for the older adult.

in urban settings, such as how food is obtained and services are accessed and if basic utilities are consistently available.

- The importance of adequate nutrition, safe drinking water, and a healthful environment. Nurses can be involved in planning and program development in their communities. They can make sure to include these aspects of a holistic assessment in any care setting—acute, long-term, or home care.

- The necessity of educating elders and their families about normal changes of aging, risk factors for health problems, and early warning signs of impending health deterioration. The earlier the signs are noted, the more likely the person can overcome the common access issues in the rural and especially the frontier setting (see quote at the beginning of the chapter). All education must be culturally appropriate and must consider the participants' level of literacy. All programs should be geared toward empowerment rather than dependence.

- Recognition of the importance of the informal network of care providers. The rural gerontological nurse works within the preexisting patterns of care and behavior to create a patchwork of care, optimizing the strength of all available resources.

- The need to emphasize the highest level of wellness and independence possible. This includes working with existing self-care practices to maximize their effectiveness and attempting to de-stigmatize such health issues as mental health problems to ensure adequate care and intervention. The gerontological nurse in the rural setting works with all three levels of prevention/promotion simultaneously (prevention, early detection, and rehabilitation).

- Professionals working in the rural setting must understand and work within the existing culture, concerns, and needs as presented by the elders and their families. For example, because work is of major importance to rural residents, health care clinics, programs, and appointments must fit with rural work schedules. Health promotion education and programs should be related to work issues and the prevention of long-term disabilities that may prevent persons from carrying out their work or usual activities. These features will be more meaningful to rural residents than preventive measures that emphasize a more comfortable way of living.

- The characteristic of rural residents to be self-reliant may influence rural persons to delay seeking health care until they are seriously ill or debilitated. Nurses must learn to be nonjudgmental about this feature and to stress appropriate preventive health strategies or behav-iors. With appropriately delivered information, rural residents can learn to make health-promoting decisions regarding the delicate balance of relying solely on self-care behaviors and seeking professional care.

KEY CONCEPTS

- Great regional diversity exists in the social, cultural, ethnic, and economic structures of rural communities across the United States.

- Approximately 25% of persons ages 65 years and older live in rural communities.

- The older rural population is less racially and ethnically diverse than those younger than 65 years or persons of any age in urban settings.

- Younger persons and professionals are leaving rural areas for increased economic opportunities in urban areas.

- Retirees are leaving urban areas for rural retreats.

- Rural older adults are at risk for disease and disability because of their multiple complex health problems, low socioeconomic status, and barriers to appropriate health care services.

- Health risk factors of rural older adults include obesity, physical inactivity, smoking, moderate drinking, poverty, inadequate or lack of health insurance, chronic diseases, poor dental health, higher death rates, and serious injuries from motor vehicle accidents.

- Rural older adults have a propensity to be self-reliant, are independent, engage in a high level of self-care activities, seek health assistance through an informal system of care, value "insider care," and demonstrate an expectation of reciprocity.

- Older rural persons have a tendency to underreport health problems and to tolerate significant health problems to remain independent in their own homes.

- Financial, social, geographical, and cultural constraints may lead some older rural persons to have lowered health expectations and prevents them from seeking advanced health care services.

- A strong integration of the value of independence, faith, spirituality, and health exists in the lives of rural older adults.

- Family members and the informal system of care are the primary sources of assistance for community-dwelling rural older adults.

- Rural older adults define health in terms of being able to work or carry out their usual daily activities.

- Rural health care providers must cope with a certain amount of professional isolation, a lack of anonymity, and a sense of role diffusion.

- Rural nurses are not unlike their rural patients in their dislike for too many government regulations and policies.

- Successful rural nurses are expert generalists and increasingly expert specialists, especially in care of the older adult as their communities "gray" around them.

CASE STUDY: Community and Conflict

Maude, an 85-year-old widow and retired schoolteacher, developed breast cancer with metastases. She lived alone and was active in her community. She developed pain and swelling of her right leg and was hospitalized. She was diagnosed with deep venous thrombophlebitis. Maude was discharged to home with treatment, but she soon realized that she could not live independently, even with substantial help from her church and friends. She chose to move into a nursing home that was right down the street, where her friends could continue to visit. Many of the staff at the nursing home had been friends of her daughter, and she had watched many of them grow up. At the time of admission to the nursing home, Maude was of sound mind. She completed a medical power of attorney form and named her only child, Sarah, as her medical power of attorney representative. Sarah had moved away years ago, and the two were not close. Maude was always trying to find ways to improve their relationship. Over time, Maude became confused and forgetful. The physicians said that she had less than 6 months to live and recommended a comfort care plan. Maude had continuous problems with pain in her right leg. She began to vomit blood. Sarah was contacted, and she insisted that her mother be hospitalized to get the bleeding stopped. She did not want her mother to bleed to death. She disagreed with the physician about the comfort care plan and demanded that everything be done for her mother, including hospitalization for tests and cardiopulmonary resuscitation (CPR) if necessary. The staff in the nursing home was upset with the decisions of the daughter. Sarah had never come to visit her mother, and she had never asked Maude what her wishes were regarding end-of-life care. The staff, by contrast, had a rich sense of what Maude would want, based on numerous conversations with her as she faced her own illness and death, and through conversations with her about other friends and family members. They had watched her gradual decline, and they wanted to make sure that she remained comfortable. They believed Sarah's decisions were based on guilt and not based on any actual knowledge of her mother's wishes or experience of her mother's care. (Modified from *Journal of Rural Health* 17(4):333, 2001.)

Based on the case study, develop a nursing care plan using the following procedure*:

- List Maude's comments that provide subjective data.
- List information that provides objective data.
- From these data, identify and state, using accepted format, two nursing diagnoses you determine are the most significant to the client at this time. List two of Maude's strengths that you have identified from data.

- Determine and state outcome criteria for each diagnosis. These must reflect some alleviation of the problem identified in the nursing diagnosis and must be stated in concrete and measurable terms.
- Plan and state one or more interventions for each diagnosed problem. Provide specific documentation of the source used to determine the appropriate intervention. Plan at least one intervention that incorporates the client's existing strengths.
- Evaluate the success of the intervention. The intervention must correlate directly with the stated outcome criteria to measure the outcome success.

Critical Thinking Questions

1. Although this case could also happen in an urban setting ("the daughter from out of town" is a familiar scenario), what specific features of the case are characteristic of a rural setting?
2. Why do you think Maude chose to move into this particular nursing home?
3. Why do you think the nursing home staff feels a strong ethical responsibility to intervene in Maude's behalf? Taking into account what you have learned about the rural health care system, what is at stake for the nursing home staff?
4. What are your thoughts on confidentiality? Do you think it is an issue in this rural case study?
5. How do informal systems operate in rural communities?
6. What are the critical aspects that facilitate continuity between the informal and formal health care systems in a rural community?
7. What is the relationship between spirituality and rural health behaviors, quality of life, and the management of chronic illness?
8. What is the impact of a community-based parish nursing program on the health and quality of life of rural older adults?
9. How can rural nurses facilitate smooth transitions among levels of health care for rural older adults and their families?
10. How do rural bioethical issues of the older adult differ from urban ones?
11. How can health care providers balance the ethical obligation of confidentiality and maintain the trust of the rural community?

* Students are advised to refer to their nursing diagnosis text and identify possible or potential problems.

REFERENCES

Averill JB: Studies of rural elderly individuals: merging critical ethnography with community-based action research, *J Gerontol Nurs* 31(12):11-18, 2005.

Brown EJ et al: Rural Floridians' perceptions of health, health values, and health behaviors, *South Online J Nurs Res* 3(5), 2004.

Brown JW, May BA: Rural older Appalachian women's formal patterns of care, *South Online J Nurs Res* 2(6), 2005.

Brown NJ et al: An approach to care management for rural older adults: parish nursing, *New Horiz* 5:7, 1996.

Bushy A: Health issues of women in rural environments, *J Am Med Womens Assoc* 53(2):53, 1998.

Bushy A: *Orientation to nursing in the rural community*, Thousand Oaks, Calif, 2000, Sage.

Center for Rural Health: *North Dakota Medicare Rural Flexibility Program: working with critical access hospitals to stabilize the rural health delivery system*, 2002. University of North Dakota, School of Medicine (website): *www.med.und.edu*. Accessed May 23, 2007.

Congdon JG, Magilvy JK: The changing spirit of rural community nursing: documentation burden, *Public Health Nurs* 12(1):18, 1995.

Congdon JG, Magilvy JK: Health status of rural older adults, *New Horiz* 5(24):4, 1996.

Congdon JG, Magilvy JK: Rural nursing homes: a housing option for older adults, *Geriatr Nurs* 19(3):157, 1998a.

Congdon JG, Magilvy JK: Home health care: supporting vitality for rural elders, *J Long Term Home Health Care* 17(4):9, 1998b.

Congdon JG, Magilvy JK: Themes of rural health and aging: a program of research, *Geriatr Nurs* 22(5):234, 2001.

Coward RT et al: An overview of health and aging in rural America. In Coward RT et al, editors: *Health services for rural elders*, New York, 1994, Springer.

Coward RT et al: Obstacles to creating high quality long-term care services for rural elders. In Rowles G et al, editors: *Long-term care for the rural elderly*, New York, 1996, Springer.

Craig C: Community determinants of health for rural elderly, *Public Health Nurs* 11(4):242, 1994.

Dorfman LT: Economic status, work, and retirement among the rural elderly. In Coward RT, Krout JA, editors: *Aging in rural settings*, New York, 1998, Springer.

Duncan RP: Rural hospitals and rural elders. In Coward RT et al, editors: *Health services for rural elders*, New York, 1994, Springer.

Foner A: *Aging and old age: new perspectives*, Englewood Cliffs, NJ, 1986, Prentice Hall.

Fuguitt G et al: Recent trends in older population changes and migration from non-metropolitan areas 1970-2000, *Rural American* 17(3):11-19, 2002.

Gale F: The graying farm sector: Legacy of off-farm migration, *Rural American* 17(3):1-2, 2002.

Glover JJ: Rural bioethical issues of the elderly: how do they differ from urban ones? *J Rural Health* 18(1):332, 2001.

Goldsmith H et al: *Low density counties with different types of sociodemographic, economic and health/mental health characteristics*, Letter to the field No. 18, 2000. (website): *www.wiche.edu/MentalHealth/Frontier/letter18.html*. Accessed December 15, 2006.

Ham R et al: *Best practices in service delivery to the rural elderly*, West Virginia Center on Aging Report to Congress, 2003. (website): http:/dpaweb.hss.state.ak.us. Accessed December 15, 2006.

Havens B et al: Finding and using rural aging data: an international perspective, *J Rural Health* 17(4):350, 2001.

Health and Human Services Rural Task Force Report to the Secretary: *One department serving rural America*, 2002, U.S. Department of Health and Human Services.

Hennessy CH et al: The public health perspective in health promotion and disability prevention for older adults: the role of the Centers for Disease Control and Prevention, *J Rural Health* 17(4):364, 2001.

Hermanova HM, Richardson SK: *Conclusions and recommendation for policies on rural aging in the first decades of the 21st century.* Report to the International Conference on Aging, West Virginia University Center on Aging, International Rural Aging Project 1997-2004, 2004.

Higuchi KA et al: A new role for advanced practice nurses in Canada: bridging the gap in health services for rural older adults, *J Gerontol Nurs* 32(7):49-55, 2006.

Jett KF et al: The influence of community context on the decision to enter a nursing home, *J Aging Stud* 10(3):237-254, 1996.

Jett KF et al: Imposed vs. involved: different strategies to bring about driving cessation in cognitively impaired older adults, *Geriatr Nurs* 26(2):111-116, 2005.

Krout JA, Coward RT: Aging in rural environments. In Coward RT, Krout JA, editors: *Aging in rural settings*, New York, 1998, Springer.

LaCaille JP: Retirement communities in rural America, 2005. (website): *www.nal.usda.gov*. Accessed December 15, 2006.

Leight SB: The application of a vulnerable populations conceptual model to rural health, *Public Health Nurs* 20(6):440-448, 2003.

Long KA, Weinert C: Rural nursing: developing the theory base. In Lee HJ, editor: *Conceptual basis for rural nursing*, New York, 1998, Springer.

Longino CF, Smith MH: Epilogue: reflections on health services for rural elders. In Coward CN et al, editors: *Health services for rural elders*, New York, 1994, Springer.

Longino CF Jr, Smith MH: The impact of elderly migration on rural communities. In Coward RT, Krout JA, editors: *Aging in rural settings*, New York, 1998, Springer.

Magilvy JK, Congdon JG: Circles of care: rural home care for older adults, *Rural Clinician Q* 4(2):3, 1994.

Magilvy JK, Congdon JG: The crisis nature of health care transitions for rural older adults, *Public Health Nurs* 17(5):336, 2000.

Magilvy JK et al: Circles of care: home and community support for rural older adults, *Adv Nurs Sci* 16(3):22, 1994.

Magilvy JK et al: Caring for our own: health care experiences of rural Hispanic elders, *J Aging Stud* 14(2):17, 2000.

Martinez RJ: Close friends of God: an ethnographic study of health of older Hispanic adults, *J Multicultl Nurs Health* 5(1):40, 1999.

McCulloch BJ: Aging and kinship in rural context. In Blieszner R, Bedfor VH, editors: *Handbook of aging and the family*, Westport, Conn, 1995, Greenwood Press.

McCulloch BJ: *Old, female, and rural*, New York, 1998, Haworth Press.

McLaughlin DK, Jensen L: The rural elderly: a demographic portrait. In Coward RT, Krout JA, editors: *Aging in rural settings*, New York, 1998, Springer.

Mochenhaupt RE, Muchow JA: Disease and disability prevention and health promotion for rural elders. In Krout JA, editor: *Providing community-based services to the rural elderly*, Newbury Park, Calif, 1994, Sage.

National Institute of Nursing Research (NINR): *Community-based health care: nursing strategies, report of the NINR Priority Expert Panel*, NIH Pub No 95, Bethesda, Md, 1995, National Institutes of Health.

National Rural Health Association: *Collaboration: modern relationships between rural community health centers and hospitals*, 2005. (website): *www.nrharural.org*. Accessed December 10, 2006.

Palumbo MV: Swing beds: providing extended care in rural acute-care hospitals. In Winstead-Fry P et al, editors: *Rural health nursing*, New York, 1992, National League for Nursing Press.

Quandt S et al: Predictors of falls in a multiethnic population of rural adults with diabetes, *J Gerontol Biol Sci Med Sci* 61A(4):394-398, 2006.

Rabiner DJ et al: Metropolitan versus nonmetropolitan differences in functional status and self-care practice: findings from a national sample of community dwelling older adults, *J Rural Health* 13(1):14, 1997.

Reeder R: *Retiree-attraction policies for rural development*, AIB-741, Economic Research Service, Washington, DC, 1998, U.S. Department of Agriculture.

Rogers CC: *Changes in the older population and implications for rural areas*, Rural development research report No 90, Food and Rural Economics Division, Economic Research Service, Washington, DC, 1999, US Department of Agriculture.

Rowles GD: Nursing homes in the rural long-term care continuum. In Rowles GD et al, editors: *Long-term care for the rural elderly*, New York, 1996, Springer.

Rural Information Center Health Service (RICHS): *Rural health statistics*, Beltsville, Md, 2001. (website): *www.nal.usda.gov/ric/richs/stats.htm*.

Sanford JT, Townsend-Rocchiccioli JT: The perceived health of rural caregivers, *Geriatr Nurs* 25(3):145-148, 2004.

Scharff JE: The distinctive nature and scope of rural nursing practice: philosophical bases. In Lee HJ, editor: *Conceptual basis for rural nursing*, New York, 1998, Springer.

Schlenker RE, Shaughnessy PW: The role of the rural hospital in long-term care. In Rowles GD et al, editors: *Long-term care for the rural elderly*, New York, 1996, Springer.

Shreffler MJ et al: Community decision-making about critical access hospitals: lessons learned from Montana's medical assistance facility program, *J Rural Health* 15(2):180, 1999.

U.S. Department of Agriculture (USDA): *Rural population and migration: rural older population*, 2005. (website): *www.ers.usda.gov/briefing/population/older*. Accessed November 29, 2006.

WK Kellogg Foundation: *Perceptions of rural America*, Battle Creek, Mich, 2002. (website): *www.wkkf.org*. Accessed December 20, 2006.

Wallace RE, Wallace RB: Rural-urban contrasts in elder health status: methodologic issues and findings. In Coward RT, Krout JA, editors: *Aging in rural settings*, New York, 1998, Springer.

Weinert C, Long KA: Rural families and health care: refining the knowledge base, *J Marriage Fam Rev* 15(1/2):57, 1990.

Weinert C, Long KA: The theory and research base for rural nursing practice. In Bushy A, editor: *Rural nursing*, vol 1, Newbury Park, Calif, 1991, Sage.

Winstead-Fry P et al: *Rural health nursing*, New York, 1992, National League for Nursing Press.

Zelarney P, Ciarlo J: *Defining and describing frontier areas in the U.S: an update*. Letter #22. 2000. (website): *www.wiche.edu*. Accessed December 1, 2004.

CHAPTER 23

Cognition and Caring for Persons with Cognitive Impairment

Theris A. Touhy

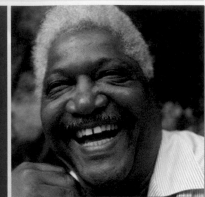
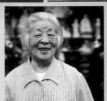

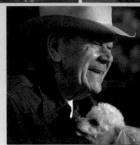

A STUDENT SPECULATES

I imagine I am in my late eighties and my husband and I live with our daughter. I am experiencing an unpleasant physical change; I am losing my memory. I can sharply remember all details about events that happened a long time ago but often fail to recall what happened 2 hours ago. Although this situation scares me and I wonder what will happen if my family gets tired of my forgetfulness, I remind myself that I live with the people who love and care for me very much and will not desert me when I need them the most.

Tatyana, age 30

AN ELDER SPEAKS

It has been quite a relief to be in this retirement home…everyone here forgets names and words, and I don't feel alone when I'm forgetful.

Liz, age 78

LEARNING OBJECTIVES
On completion of this chapter, the reader will be able to:

1. Discuss concepts related to cognition, memory, and learning in late life.
2. Differentiate between delirium, dementia, and depression.
3. Describe the parameters and methods used in a comprehensive assessment of cognitive function.
4. Describe nursing models of care for persons with dementia.
5. Discuss common concerns in care of persons with dementia and nursing responses.
6. Identify effective communication strategies that nurture personhood in elders with dementia.
7. Develop a nursing care plan for an individual with delirium.
8. Develop a nursing care plan for an individual with dementia.

COGNITIVE FUNCTION

This chapter addresses normal cognition of the older adult and the various situations, disorders, and diseases that influence cognitive processes and at times produce temporary or permanent cognitive decline. We remain oriented to the healthy aging model while we examine each of the states of mentation in late life as having the potential for comfort and pleasures. All elders are deserving of active nursing intervention to maintain the highest practicable level of function and satisfaction.

We have artificially separated cognitive function from mental health, though they are in most ways interdependent. The mind is in some ways limited by the capacities of the brain, yet just as in medicine, there is a danger of evaluating the person by the measured and tested efficiency of cells and organs. Nowhere is this more important than in examining the cognition of older people. Citing John Morris, professor of neurology at Washington University in St. Louis, Crowley (1996) says that if brain function becomes impaired in old age, it is a result of disease, not aging.

Special thanks to Ann Schmidt Luggen, the previous edition contributor, for her content contributions to this chapter.

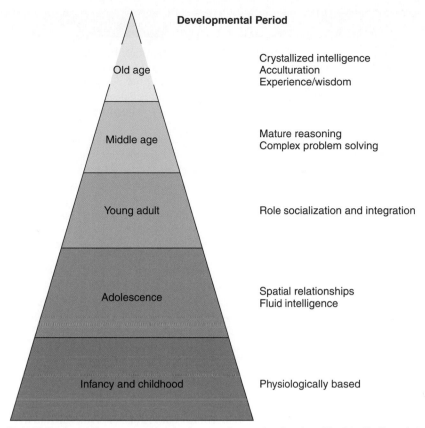

Developmental Period

Old age — Crystallized intelligence
Acculturation
Experience/wisdom

Middle age — Mature reasoning
Complex problem solving

Young adult — Role socialization and integration

Adolescence — Spatial relationships
Fluid intelligence

Infancy and childhood — Physiologically based

FIGURE 23-1 Life span cognitive developmental strengths. (Developed by Priscilla Ebersole.)

Adult Cognition

Cognition is the process of acquiring, storing, sharing, and using information (Bunton, 2001). Cognitive function includes the following 12 categories: attention span, concentration, intelligence, judgment, learning ability, memory, orientation, perception, problem solving, psychomotor ability, reaction time, and social intactness (McDougall et al., 2003). Cognitive development of older people is often measured against the norms of young or middle-aged people, which may not be appropriate to the distinctive characteristics of elders. Most tests of cognitive abilities were designed to test children or young adults and do not address cultural or ethnic differences. Therefore these tests may have little relevance for daily function of older people. Intelligence in old age is dynamic, and certain abilities change and even improve with age (Figure 23-1). More and more theorists are speculating about the possibility of unique cognitive powers of old age, as did Plato. Reflective regression (intense reliving and reviewing of old memories) and life review seem to be forms of cognitive development characteristic of late life. Individuals focus more on memories and meaning.

The determination of intellectual capacity and performance has been the focus of a major portion of gerontological research. In general, cognitive functions may remain stable or decline with increasing age (Beers and Berkow, 2000). The cognitive functions that remain stable include attention span, language skills, communication skills, comprehension of discourse, and visual perception. The cogni-

tive skills that decline are verbal fluency, logical analysis, selective attention, object naming, and complex visuospatial skills (Beers and Berkow, 2000). Fluid intelligence (often called *native intelligence*) is skills that are biologically determined, independent of experience or learning. Measures of fluid intelligence include spatial orientation, abstract reasoning, word fluency, and inductive reasoning. Crystallized intelligence is knowledge and abilities that the person acquires through education and life. Measures of crystallized intelligence include verbal meaning, word association, social judgment, and number skills. Older people perform more poorly on performance scales (fluid intelligence), but scores on verbal scales (crystallized intelligence) remain stable. This is known as the *classic aging pattern* (Hooyman and Kiyak, 2005). Interrelationships between intelligence quotient (IQ) and mental and physical health are exceptionally strong. However, in general, intellectual abilities appear to plateau in the 50s and 60s and begin to decline in the 70s, with declines in fluid intelligence beginning earlier than in crystallized intelligence.

Late adulthood is no longer seen as a period of growth cessation and arrested cognitive development; rather it is seen as a life stage programmed for plasticity and the development of unique capacities. Education, pulmonary health, general health, and activity levels all influence cognitive ability in late life. Other reasons have been advanced for the variations of intellectual performance of the older adult being tested (Box 23-1). Elderly people do maintain their abil-

---

BOX 23-1 Complexities of Accurately Assessing Intellect in Old Age

- The old are most frequently compared with college students, whose chief occupation is proving their intellectual capacity.
- Young adults are in the habit of being tested and have developed test wisdom, a skill never developed by the elderly or one that has grown rusty with disuse.
- Test material may not be relevant to the world of older adults, especially those of different cultures.
- The ability to concentrate is inversely related to anxiety.
- Intellectual function declines differentially. The old are assumed deficient in encoding during learning, storing information for retention, and/or speed of retrieving stored information.
- Adrenal or stress hormones may be responsible for some of the gradual changes in the brain during aging.
- Older people always perform more slowly than younger people in tasks involving neuromuscular learning because of slower reaction time and an increase in cautious behavior.
- Older people often perform poorly on test items because they are less likely to guess and more likely not to answer any items that seem ambiguous to them.

- Cautiousness has often been described as the reason older adults do not perform as well as younger people in memory tasks. Other personality traits, such as greater activity levels, less impulsiveness, and greater emotional stability, also seem to influence how well older people perform on memory tests.
- Older people may have difficulty focusing attention and ignoring irrelevant stimuli.
- Subject attrition in longitudinal studies of older adults shows evidence of the survival of the intellectually superior.
- No evidence suggests general slowing of central nervous system activity in old age as had been commonly presumed and reported by researchers.
- Intellectual performance relying on verbal functions shows little or no decline with age, but speeded tests using nonverbal psychomotor functions show a great decline.
- Social cognition and social context are related in terms of elder function. The elderly who maintain the best cognitive function are also those with a high social interactional level.

---

ity to understand situations and learn from new experiences. These findings are significant to satisfaction in old age because the capacity for effective lifestyle management and cognitive resources contributes to adaptation and enjoyment in old age.

The Aging Brain

It has been generally assumed that cognitive function declines in old age because of a decreased number of neurons, decreased brain size, and diminished brain weight. Although these losses are features of aging, they are not consistent with deteriorating mental function nor do they interfere with everyday routines (Sugarman, 2002). Neuron loss occurs mainly in the brain and spinal cord and is most pronounced in the cerebral cortex. The neuronal dendrites atrophy with aging, resulting in impairment of the synapses and changes in transmission of the chemical neurotransmitters dopamine, serotonin, and acetylcholine. This causes a slowing of many neural processes. However, overall cognitive abilities remain intact. We now understand that continued development requires appropriate levels of challenge and stimulation throughout life. Untapped potential exists for patterning and learning through stimulating brain cells to expand function. This is shown most remarkably in the retraining of speech and other functions after a stroke. When working with the older adult to maintain and improve cognitive functions, there must be regular input and "exercise" of the brain around ideas that are significant and interesting to the older person. The phrase "use it or lose it" applies to cognitive as well as physical function. Maintenance and improvement of brain health is a concept that is receiving much attention in gerontology.

Memory Retrieval. Memory is defined as the ability to retain or store information and retrieve it when needed. Memory is a complex set of processes and storage systems. Three components characterize memory: immediate recall; short-term memory (which may range from minutes to days); and remote or long-term memory (Gallo et al., 2003). Biological, functional, environmental, and psychosocial influences affect memory development throughout adulthood. Recall of newly encountered information seems to decrease with age, and memory declines are noted for complex tasks and strategies. Even though some older adults show decrements in processing information, reaction time, perception, and attentional tasks, the majority of functioning remains intact and sufficient. Familiarity, previous learning, and life experience compensate for the minor loss of efficiency in the basic neurological processes. In unfamiliar, stressful, or demanding situations, these changes may be more marked.

Age-associated decline in memory is a major focus of research in aging and dementia. Normal older adults may complain of memory problems, but their symptoms do not meet the criteria for dementia. The term *age-associated memory impairment (AAMI)* has been used to describe memory loss that is considered normal in light of the person's age and educational level. *Mild cognitive impairment (MCI)* is considered to be present when the individual has greater levels of memory impairment than other individuals of the same age with other aspects of cognitive functioning remaining intact (Butler et al., 2004; Gallo et al., 2003; Peterson, 2004). Some research indicates that about 50% of people with MCI will develop dementia within 3 years of diagnosis but it is unclear whether MCI is a "transitional state to dementia or a separate condition entirely" (Butler et al., 2004, p. 119). AAMI and MCI refer only to memory loss, whereas dementia is defined as cognitive impairment severe enough to affect daily functioning. Many medical or psychiatric difficulties (depression, anxiety) also influence memory abilities, and it is important for older adults with memory complaints to have a comprehensive evaluation. In many cases, memory impairment is related to reversible and treatable conditions. If an irreversible dementia is detected, it is important to accurately diagnose the type of dementia and provide appropriate treatment. Clearly, the knowledge about memory and changes related to aging is still developing.

Scientists are finding that nerve cell regeneration does occur in the hippocampus of the brain, where memory formation occurs (National Institutes of Health, 2002). They have found that stress decreases the capacity for generation of new nerve cells. Still other research on the "plasticity" of the brain is based on physical changes that occur in the brain that result from new memories and the addition of new neurons. Higher participation in mentally stimulating activities, social interaction, and physical exercise appears to be associated with a lower risk of Alzheimer's disease (Butler et al., 2004). This is good evidence for us to continue to learn and grow and experience the world around us even into very old age.

Cognitive stimulation and memory training utilizing techniques such as mnemonics (strategies to enhance coding, storage, and recall), internal and external aids, cognitive games (e.g., scrabble, chess, crossword puzzles), spaced retrieval techniques, and Montessori-based activities (discussed on p. 570) may be helpful for cognitively intact elders, as well as for those with cognitive impairment (Camp and Skrajner, 2004; Knapp et al., 2006). Many games and aids are available that may be useful to enhance memory and stimulate cognitive function. One of the health maintenance organizations (HMOs) (Humana) in Florida is offering a free brain fitness computer CD to its members (*www.positscience.com*). Ruth Tappen and colleagues at Florida Atlantic University are studying the effect of several therapeutic interventions, including cognitive games and memory training techniques, on the function of older people with mild to moderate memory impairment. All older adults should remain active and engaged in stimulating activities for the mind as well as for the body.

Learning in Late Life

Basic intelligence remains unchanged with increasing years. Spatial awareness and intuitive, creative thought may decline (Batchelor, 2001). Verbal abilities do not change. However, elderly people may have many barriers to learning. These include memory impairment, vision and hearing impairment, cultural and cohort variations, education levels, and low literacy skills. Adults ages 60 years and older are a heterogeneous group in their characteristics and in their literacy skills. A 2004 report by the Institute of Medicine (IOM) titled "Health Literacy: A Prescription to End Confusion" revealed that nearly one half of adults nationwide have problems understanding and using the health information they receive (*www.iom.edu/?id=19750*). Individuals residing in urban settings, those with poor education or low income, minorities, older people, and people for whom English is a second language are more likely to perform at lower levels of literacy (Wilson et al., 2003). Limited literacy skills influence learning, as well as understanding of health-related information such as prescription directions, consent documents, and health education materials. "Limited literacy is, in fact, an occult, silent disability and a secret that most people do not share even with members of their own family" (Dreger and Tremback, 2002, p. 282).

The older adult demands that teaching situations are relevant; new learning must relate to what the elder already knows. The elder is in control of what and how much is learned and the degree of participation in a learning situation, and the elder will monitor his or her own progress and pace. Many elders still have special learning needs based on education deprivation in their early years and consequent anxiety about formalized learning. Box 23-2 summarizes some ways to enhance the learning of older people.

Nurses must discover the preferred learning mode and setting appropriate to the needs and desires of the elder (Figure 23-2). Also, the nurse should provide the elder with information about media resources that may make knowledge readily available and easier to understand. Increasingly, elders are taking charge of their own health learning and scanning the Internet for information about health and lifestyles. Approximately 15% of older people are on-line, and those numbers will continue to grow as the "baby boomers" bring their computers with them into senior citizenship (Clark, 2002). Innovations such as a user-friendly talking computer touch screen are being used with good outcomes to assist low-literacy elders in health and disease prevention initiatives (Hahn et al., 2004). Many reliable Internet resources related to health and aging are available. The National Institute of Aging website (*www.nia.nih.gov/health/*) provides excellent resources for health-related topics. The "Age Page" series is especially helpful and includes a variety of one-page informational sheets for consumers and health professionals. Nurses are beginning to recognize the necessity of revising the traditional teaching/learning strategies, which often are limited to giving information in the form of brochures and mini-lectures with return demonstration. In addition, attention to literacy skills and cultural variations is important to enhance learning and usefulness. Figure 23-3 presents a nutrition guide developed by one of the authors in collaboration with elders of Afro-Caribbean descent to adapt traditional foods for healthy nutrition.

Numerous opportunities exist for older learners within the established educational institutions or in special programs. Many universities have "senior scholar" or lifelong learning programs designed especially for elders. The Elderhostel program is an example of a program designed for elders to participate in continued learning combined with travel. Other resources are listed in the Resources section at the end of this chapter. Nursing approaches to enhance learning for older

BOX 23-2   Guiding Older Adult Learners

- Make sure the client is ready to learn before trying to teach. Watch for clues that would indicate that the client is preoccupied or too anxious to comprehend the material.
- Sit facing the client so that he or she can watch your lip movements and facial expressions.
- Speak slowly.
- Keep your tone of voice low; elderly persons can hear low sounds better than high-frequency sounds.
- Present one idea at a time.
- Use extra voice and media amplification.
- Emphasize concrete rather than abstract material—make learning practical.
- Encourage the learner to develop various mediators or mnemonic devices (visual images, rhymes, acronyms, self-designed coding schemes).
- Use high contrast on visuals and handout material (e.g., larger-font black print on white paper).
- Pay attention to reading ability; use techniques other than printed material, such as drawings, pictures, and discussion.
- Provide enough time to respond, because older adults' reaction times may be longer than those of younger persons.

- Focus on a single topic to help the client concentrate.
- Keep environmental distractions to a minimum.
- Take appropriate breaks and defer teaching if the client becomes distracted or tired or cannot concentrate for other reasons.
- Invite another member of the household to join the discussion.
- Use audio, visual, and tactile cues to enhance learning and help the client remember information.
- Provide regular feedback.
- Use past experience; connect new learning to that already learned.
- Ask for feedback to ensure that the information has been understood.
- Compensate for physical discomfort and sensory decrements.
- Support a positive self-image in the learner.
- Use creative teaching strategies.
- Respond to identified interests of learners.
- Emphasize and integrate emotional and personal values in the acquisition of skills and ideas.

Modified from *Bridging principles of older adult learning: reconnaissance phase final report,* Washington, DC, 1999, SPRY Foundation.

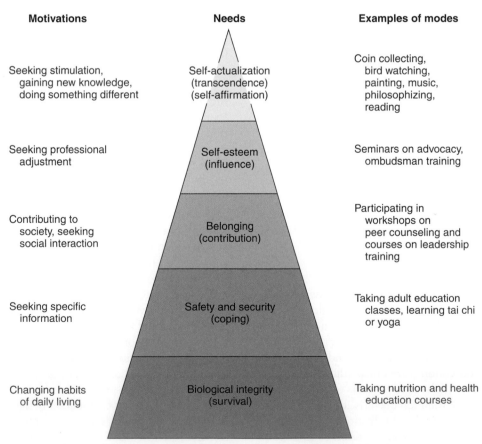

Motivations	Needs	Examples of modes
Seeking stimulation, gaining new knowledge, doing something different	Self-actualization (transcendence) (self-affirmation)	Coin collecting, bird watching, painting, music, philosophizing, reading
Seeking professional adjustment	Self-esteem (influence)	Seminars on advocacy, ombudsman training
Contributing to society, seeking social interaction	Belonging (contribution)	Participating in workshops on peer counseling and courses on leadership training
Seeking specific information	Safety and security (coping)	Taking adult education classes, learning tai chi or yoga
Changing habits of daily living	Biological integrity (survival)	Taking nutrition and health education courses

FIGURE 23-2   Learning and growing in late life. (Developed by Priscilla Ebersole.)

Healthy Eating
Caribbean Style

Say 'YES' to GREEN, Say 'NO' to RED, Say 'SOMETIMES' to YELLOW

GREEN	YELLOW	RED
Eat or use any of these every day in limited amounts.	Do not eat more that 1-3 times a month.	Do not eat or use at all.

Dairy

Low Fat Milk 1% Sugar Free Ice Cream Evaporated milk	Canola Oil Olive Oil Vegetable oil	
Coconut Milk Whole Milk	Coconut Oil Peanut Oil Palm Oil Butter Lard	

Oils

Sweets & Snacks

Crackers (Low fat)
Cookies (Nonsweetned, low fat)
Fruits

Peanuts (1 handful)
Peanut butter

Cane Syrups
Burnt Sugar
White Sugar

Proteins 4-5 ounces a day (one handful)

POULTRY	SEAFOOD		Patty	Chicken & Beef Liver
Chicken Hen	Conch Crabs Cod Fish Fresh Fish Boiled Fish Baked Fish	Snapper Smoked Herring Salmon Smoked Fish Lobster	Pork Chops Goat broiled Lamb Salted Cod Fish Eggs (3 per week) Lean Meatballs	Stewed Chicken Feet Fried Beef Fritters Meat fat drippings Meat prepared in gravy/sauce Stewed Cow Foot Pig Feet Pies Tripe Bacon
MEAT Lean Stew Beef				

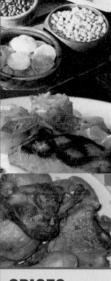

SPICES

Salt, small amt
Pepper
Scotch Bonnet
Vinegar
Ginger
Garlic
Peppers
Thyme
Sage
Cinnamon
Cloves
Mint
Nutmeg
Lemon Grass
Peppermint

Starches 9-11 servings (4-5 oups) per day

Grits Oatmeal Porridge Yellow Rice Brown Rice	Macaroni Whole Wheat Breads Banana Bread Crackers Oatmeal	Sweet Potatoes White Potatoes Corn Cassava Yucca Yam	

Beans

Black Eye Peas
Red Beans
Lima Beans
Pigeon Beans
Black Beans

SAUCES

Lo-fat Red Sauce

Fruits & Vegetables 9 servings (4 cups) per day

Spinach Tomatoes Fresh Okra Eggplant Leeks Onions Mushrooms Pumpkin Avocado Beet	Calabaza Scallion Shallot Malanga Tamarind Watercress Heart of Palm Breadfruit Cabbage	Apricot Banana Any Fresh Fruit Bananas Sour apple Tamarind Custard Apple Raisins Watermelon	Papaya Canteloupe Guava Sour Orange Pineapple Strawberries Peaches Plums Mango	Oranges Tangerines Grapefruit Lemons Limes Guava

BEVERAGES

Gingerale
Punch
Milo Malt Drink

FIGURE 23-3 Healthy eating. (Copyright © 2006 M.T. Adonis-Rizzo and K.F. Jett.)

people include the use of teaching learning strategies that are relevant to older learners and appropriately adapted based on an assessment of the person's needs including cognitive status, sensory impairments, culture, education, and literacy. Also, nurses should provide suggestions for resources available to the elder and encourage continued learning, self-development, and growth. Learning and self-actualization activities are further discussed in Chapter 27.

COGNITIVE IMPAIRMENT

Cognitive impairment (CI) is a term that describes a range of disturbances in cognitive functioning, including disturbances in memory, orientation, attention, and concentration (Warner and Butler, 2001). Other disturbances of cognition may affect intelligence, judgment, learning ability, perception, problem solving, psychomotor ability, reaction time, and social intactness.

Cognitive Assessment

The evaluation of cognition requires a formal focused assessment (Box 23-3). Casual informal interviews with those who are socially adept or highly educated may not uncover a cognitive deficit that is present. Solomon and Murphy (2006) noted that fewer than one half of patients with Alzheimer's disease are currently diagnosed and an estimated 95% of cases of mild dementia are not detected by clinicians. An older person with a change in cognitive function needs a thorough assessment to rule out reversible causes and to accurately diagnose the type of dementia that may be present. In addition to objective evaluations, McDougall et al. (2003) also recommend a subjective or self-report evaluation of memory self-efficacy such as the Memory Efficacy (ME) screen.

A complete assessment, including laboratory workup, should be performed to rule out any medical causes of cognitive impairment. Screening for depression using instruments such as the Geriatric Depression Scale (GDS) should be conducted. Formal cognitive testing, neuropsychological examination, interview (family and patient), observation, and functional assessment are additional components of a comprehensive assessment. Computerized tomography (CT), magnetic resonance imaging (MRI), and an electroencephalogram (EEG) may be indicated in the diagnostic process. Several evidence-based guidelines are available for assessment of changes in mental status and diagnosis of dementia, including assessing cognitive function (Foreman et al., 2003); assessment, treatment, and care (American Medical Directors Association [AMDA], 2005); and diagnosis of dementia (American Geriatrics Society, 2001; Knopman et al., 2001; Lyketsos et al., 2006). All these guidelines are available at *www.guidelines.gov*. Chapter 6 presents a discussion of instruments to assess cognitive function.

The Three D's of Cognitive Impairment

Dementia, delirium, and depression have been called the *three D's of cognitive impairment* because they occur frequently in older adults. These conditions are not a normal conse-

quence of aging, although incidence increases as one grows older. Older people, particularly those with dementia and acute illnesses and stressors, are especially prone to delirium. Because cognitive and behavioral changes characterize all three D's, it can be difficult to diagnose delirium superimposed on dementia or depression. Inability to concentrate, with resulting memory impairment and other cognitive dysfunction, is common in late-life depression. The term *pseudodementia* has been used to describe the cognitive impairment that may accompany depression in older adults (depression is discussed in Chapter 25). Knowledge about cognitive function in aging and appropriate assessment and evaluation are keys to differentiating these three syndromes. Table 23-1 presents the clinical features and the differences in cognitive and behavioral characteristics in delirium, dementia, and depression. An evidence-based guideline, "Caregiving Strategies for Older Adults with Delirium, Dementia, and Depression," developed by the Registered Nurses Association of Ontario (RNAO) (2004), is available at *www.guidelines.gov*.

Delirium

Delirium is usually a complication of a medical illness, a drug or substance effect on the brain, or a surgical procedure involving general anesthesia. Environmental factors such as noise, relocation, and the use of invasive devices and restraints influence the development and escalation of delirium. The condition usually occurs as a result of complex interactions among multiple causes and is more common in older people. Factors predisposing older adults to delirium include normal age-related changes in the brain and nervous system, diminished eyesight and hearing, greater use of medications, and diseases that injure the brain and predispose to delirium such as dementia. Delirium is given many labels: *acute confusional state, acute brain syndrome, confusion, reversible dementia, metabolic encephalopathy,* and *toxic psychosis.*

The accepted definition of delirium from the American Psychiatric Association's Diagnostic and Statistical Manual of Mental Disorders (DSM-IV) is as follows (Rapp et al., 2001):

- Delirium is a disturbance of consciousness with reduced ability to focus, sustain, or shift attention; a change in cognition; or the development of a perceptual disturbance that occurs over a short period of time and tends to fluctuate over the course of a day.

- Associated features of delirium may include sleep-wake cycle disturbances, altered psychomotor behavior (e.g., restlessness, agitation, inattention, somnolence), behavioral manifestations such as attempts to escape one's environment, disruptive vocalizations (e.g., screaming, calling out, cursing, moaning), removal of medical equipment, and aggressive behavior such as striking out.

The exact pathophysiological mechanisms involved in the development and progression of delirium remain uncertain, and further research is needed to understand the neuropathogenesis of delirium. Delirium is thought to be related to disturbances in the neurotransmitters in the brain that

BOX 23-3   Overview of Cognitive Assessment

A. Concepts and categories
1. Definition: cognitive function: the processes by which an individual perceives, registers, stores, retrieves, and uses information
2. Categories of cognitive change/decline
   a. The dementias (e.g., Alzheimer's, vascular) are chronic, progressive, insidious, and permanent states of cognitive impairment
   b. Delirium/acute confusion: an acute and sudden impairment of cognition that is considered temporary, generally an identifiable, biophysical cause
   c. Impairment in thought processes
B. Assessment
1. Methods of assessment
   a. Formal—cognitive testing using standardized instruments
      i. Advantages: standardized; enables comparison across individuals and nurses
      ii. Disadvantages: individual performance influenced by pain, education, fatigue, cultural background, and perceptual and physical abilities
   b. Informal—through structured observations of nurse-individual interactions
      i. Advantages: may have greater meaning about individual's actual cognitive ability-performance
      ii. Disadvantages: difficult to make judgments regarding change in individual condition; variability in interpretation
2. Other considerations for assessment
   a. Characteristics of the environment for assessment
      i. Physical environment
         —Comfortable ambient temperature
         —Adequate lighting but not glaring
         —Free of distractions (e.g., should be conducted in the absence of others and other activities)
         —Position self to maximize individual's sensory abilities
      ii. Interpersonal environment
         —Use individual's self-paced rate for assessment
         —Emotionally nonthreatening
   b. Timing considerations
      i. Timing should reflect the actual cognitive abilities of the individual and not extraneous factors
      ii. Times of the day to generally avoid
         —Immediately on awakening from sleep, wait at least 30 minutes
         —Immediately before or after meals
         —Immediately before or after medical diagnostic or therapeutic procedures
         —When patient has pain or discomfort
3. Parameters of assessment
   a. Alertness/level of consciousness: the most rudimentary cognitive function and level of arousal, or responsiveness to stimuli determined by interaction with individual and determination of level made on the basis of the individual's best eye, verbal, and motor response to stimuli
      i. Alertness—able to interact in a meaningful way with the examiner
      ii. Lethargy or somnolence—not fully alert; individual tends to drift to sleep when not stimulated, diminished spontaneous physical movement, loses train of thought, ideas wander
      iii. Obtundation—transitional stage between lethargy and stupor; difficult to arouse, meaningful testing futile, requires constant stimulation to elicit response
      iv. Stupor or semicoma—individual mumbles/groans in response to persistent and vigorous physical stimulation
      v. Coma—completely unable to be aroused, no behavioral response to stimuli
   b. Attention: ability to attend/concentrate on stimuli: can follow through with directions, especially a three-stage command; is easily distracted
   c. Memory: ability to register, retain, and recall information both new and old. Does individual remember your name? Is individual able to learn and remember new information?
   d. Orientation: to time, place, and person
   e. Thinking: ability to organize and communicate ideas; thoughts should be organized, coherent, and appropriate perception: presence/absence of illusions, delusions, or visual or auditory hallucinations
   f. Psychomotor behavior: ability to comprehend and perform simple motor skills; execution ability: ask the individual to perform certain ADLs/IADLs, or to perform a three-step command, and to copy a figure
   g. Insight: ability to understand oneself and the situation in which one finds oneself
   h. Judgment: ability to evaluate a situation (real or hypothetical) and determine an appropriate action
C. Outcomes of assessment
1. Individual
   a. Detection of deviations will be prompt and early with appropriate care and treatment instituted in a timely manner
   b. Plans of care will appropriately address corrective and supportive cognitive function
2. Health care provider
   a. Assessment and documentation of cognitive function
   b. Appropriate strategies to address any deviation in cognitive function
   c. Competence in cognitive assessment
   d. Evidence of ability to differentiate among the different types of cognitive change/decline
3. Institution
   a. Documentation of cognitive function will increase
   b. Referral to appropriate advanced practitioners (e.g., geriatrician, geriatric/gerontologic or psychiatric clinical nurse specialist or nurse practitioner, consultation-liaison service) will increase

From Foreman MD et al. *Geriatr Nurs* 17(5):228, 1996.
ADLs, Activities of daily living; *IADLs,* instrumental activities of daily living.

TABLE 23-1

Differentiating Delirium, Depression, and Dementia

Characteristic	Delirium	Depression	Dementia
Onset	Sudden, abrupt	Recent, may relate to life change	Insidious, slow, over years and often unrecognized until deficits obvious
Course over 24 hr	Fluctuating, often worse at night	Fairly stable, may be worse in the morning	Fairly stable, may see changes with stress
Consciousness	Reduced	Clear	Clear
Alertness	Increased, decreased, or variable	Normal	Generally normal
Psychomotor activity	Increased, decreased, or mixed Sometimes increased, other times decreased	Variable, agitation or retardation	Normal, may have apraxia or agnosia
Duration	Hours to weeks	Variable and may be chronic	Years
Attention	Disordered, fluctuates	Little impairment	Generally normal but may have trouble focusing
Orientation	Usually impaired, fluctuates	Usually normal, may answer "I don't know" to questions or may not try to answer	Often impaired, may make up answers or answer close to the right thing or may confabulate but tries to answer
Speech	Often incoherent, slow or rapid, may call out repeatedly or repeat the same phrase	May be slow	Difficulty finding word, perseveration
Affect	Variable but may look disturbed, frightened	Flat	Slowed response, may be labile

Adapted from Rapp CG et al: Acute confusion/delirium protocol, *J Gerontol Nurse* 27(4):21-33, 2001. Reprinted with permission from SLACK, Inc., Thorofare, NJ.

modulate the control of cognitive function, behavior, and mood. Irving and Foreman (2006) note that "there is growing evidence of cholinergic failure as a common pathway in delirium" (p. 122). Poor cerebral blood flow is also a factor in the development of delirium (Flaherty and Morley, 2004). The causes of delirium are potentially reversible; therefore accurate assessment and diagnosis are critical.

Incidence. Delirium is a prevalent and serious disorder estimated to affect 14% to 80% of all older adults hospitalized for treatment of an acute physical illness; and it may develop in more than 8 of 10 patients in the intensive care unit (ICU) (Ely et al., 2001; Foreman et al., 2001). As many as one fourth of all older patients in the hospital experience delirium, and the rates are even higher among those in ICU, those who have undergone surgery, and those with dementia (Fick et al., 2005). The prevalence of delirium after general surgery is 5% to 10% and is as high as 65% after orthopedic surgery, particularly hip fracture repair (Rigney, 2006).

In the acute care setting, delirium often is not recognized by health care providers. Studies indicate that delirium is unrecognized in 66% to 84% of patients (Hustey and Meldon, 2002; Sanders, 2002). Sixty-five percent of physicians and 43% of nurses failed to recognize delirium in hospitalized older adults, and even when specifically asked to document cases of delirium, nurses identified fewer than 50% of those who were moderately to severely delirious (Foreman et al., 2001; Inouye et al., 2001; Rigney, 2006).

Older people with dementia are especially vulnerable to the development of delirium. Acute changes in mental status in persons with dementia are often attributed to the underlying dementia or "sundowning." Delirium is thought to occur 4 to 5 times more often in persons with dementia and is less likely to be recognized and treated than is delirium without dementia (Fick and Mion, 2005). Yet, only a few studies have investigated the prevalence of delirium superimposed on dementia (DSD) in either the community or hospital settings. A study investigating DSD in community-dwelling older adults showed a prevalence rate of 13% and significant associated health care costs and utilization (Fick et al., 2005). The authors of this study note that "despite over 20 years of research on delirium, we still do not know the natural history of and effective treatment strategies for persons with dementia who develop delirium" (Fick et al., 2005, p. 752).

Consequences. Delirium during hospitalization is associated with high morbidity and mortality, functional decline, increased length of hospital stay and hospital readmissions, increased services after discharge, and high rates of institutionalization (Flaherty and Morley, 2004; Kalisvaart et al., 2005; Rigney, 2006). Delirium also accounts for more than $4 billion of Medicare expenditures (Rigney, 2006). At the time of discharge from the hospital, approximately 30% to 90% of patients who experienced delirium continue to manifest symptoms. In a study of older patients admitted to a home care agency after hospital discharge, 46% were delirious upon admission. Of even greater significance, 50% of that group lived alone.

A study of older people admitted to skilled care facilities found that delirium affects functional outcomes and the longer the episode of delirium, the greater the effect (Marcantonio et al., 2003). Several studies reported that patients with delirium continue to manifest symptoms up to 6 months after discharge, with persistent memory deficits of particular significance (Foreman et al., 2001). Although delirium is considered a reversible cause of altered mental status, a significant number of older adults with delirium never return to their baseline cognitive status, especially in the presence of preexisting dementia (Marcantonio et al., 2003; McCusker et al., 2001; Rigney, 2006).

Confusion: What Does It Really Mean? Contributing to the problem of diagnosis of delirium is our lack of knowledge and understanding about cognition and behavioral changes that may occur in older adults. Cognitive changes in older people are often labeled *confusion* by nurses and physicians, are frequently accepted as part of normal aging, and are rarely questioned. In a landmark book entitled *Confusion: Prevention and Care*, Wolanin and Phillips were some of the first gerontological nurses to describe this phenomenon (1981, p. 2):

> The term *confusion* is used to describe a constellation of behaviors that caregivers recognize as being deviant from those expected from the person in a certain place or at a certain time...Confusion in the young is a temporary phenomenon. In the middle aged it is a reversible event that has a definite etiology. When the cause is removed, the confusional state clears. Historically, the confusional state of the elderly is linked to...hopeless and permanent dementia.

More recently, in a report on the occurrence of delirium in elderly patients with hip fracture, Millisen et al. (2002, p. 27) stated that "confusion is used as a descriptive term or symptom (e.g., dementia is characterized by severe confusion), or as a diagnosis (e.g., the patient is confused)." A variety of signs and symptoms are used by physicians and nurses when labeling a person confused. These include disorientation, inability to concentrate, memory loss, anxiety, restlessness, sleep disturbances, or psychotic symptoms such as delusions or hallucinations. Clarity and agreement are lacking regarding the definition of confusion, and for many, confusion implies an irreversible, untreatable condition. Nurses may report clients' behavioral manifestations within their own framework, seldom exploring the meaning to the individuals. It is essential to recognize and diagnose delirium rather than label all acute changes in mental status with the

---

BOX 23-4   Clinical Subtypes of Delirium

HYPOACTIVE DELIRIUM

"Quiet or pleasantly confused"
Reduced activity
Lack of facial expression
Passive demeanor
Lethargy
Inactivity
Withdrawn and sluggish state
Limited, slow, and wavering vocalizations

HYPERACTIVE DELIRIUM

Excessive alertness
Easy distractibility
Increased psychomotor activity
Hallucinations, delusions
Agitation and aggressive actions
Fast or loud speech
Wandering, nonpurposeful repetitive movement
Verbal behaviors (yelling, calling out)
Removing tubes
Attempting to get out of bed

MIXED

Unpredictable fluctuations between hypoactivity and hyperactivity

---

general term *confusion*. Confusion is not a consequence of normal aging, and any change in the mental status of an older person needs thorough assessment. Failure to recognize delirium by assuming confusion to be normal contributes to the morbidity and mortality associated with this condition.

Clinical Subtypes of Delirium. Delirium is categorized according to the level of alertness and psychomotor activity. The clinical subtypes are hyperactive, hypoactive, and mixed. Box 23-4 presents the characteristics of each of these clinical subtypes. In non–ICU settings, approximately 30% of delirium is hyperactive, 24% hypoactive, and 46% mixed. Because of the increased severity of illness and use of psychoactive medications, hypoactive delirium may be more prevalent in the ICU. Although the negative consequences of hyperactive delirium are serious, the hypoactive subtype may be missed more often and associated with a worse prognosis because of the development of complications such as aspiration, pulmonary embolism, pressure ulcers, and pneumonia. Increased hospital stays, longer duration of delirium, and higher mortality have been associated with hypoactive delirium (Truman and Ely, 2003). A recent study found that nurses reported delirium only when it was hyperactive (Speciale et al., 2005). A website (*www. icudelirium.org*) sponsored by The ICU Delirium and Cognitive Impairment Study Group from Vanderbilt University Medical Center and the Veterans Affairs TN Valley Geriatric Research Education and Clinical Center

---

BOX 23-5 Diseases and Disorders Placing Older People at Risk for Delirium

- Pharmacological agents, especially anticholinergics, hypnotics, anxiolytics, antipsychotics, nonsteroidal antiinflammatory drugs (NSAIDs), antidepressants
- Hypoxemia and metabolic disturbances
- Infection, especially respiratory and urinary tract
- Dehydration, with and without electrolyte disturbances
- Electrolyte imbalances
- Withdrawal syndromes (alcohol and sedative-hypnotic agents)
- Major medical and surgical treatments (especially hip fracture)
- Nutritional deficiencies
- Dementia
- Circulatory disturbances (congestive heart failure [CHF], myocardial infarction [MI], cerebrovascular accident [CVA])

- Anemia
- Pain (either unrelieved or inadequately treated)
- Sensory deficits
- Social isolation, lack of family contact
- Retention of urine and feces
- Emergency admission or admission from a long-term care facility
- Use of invasive equipment
- Restraint use
- Abrupt loss of significant person
- Multiple losses in short span of time
- Move to radically different environment (hospitalization, nursing home)

(GRECC) provides information and resources related to brain dysfunction in critically ill patients.

Delirium Risk Factors. Identification of risk factors, prompt and appropriate assessment, and continued surveillance are the cornerstones of delirium prevention. More than 35 potential risk factors have been identified for delirium. Acute illness, infections, metabolic disturbances, alcohol or drug abuse, sensory impairments, surgery, hip fracture, and cognitive impairment are common risk factors for delirium (Box 23-5). Unrelieved or inadequately treated pain significantly increases the risk of delirium (Irving and Foreman, 2006; Milisen et al., 2002; Morrison et al., 2003). Medications account for 22% to 39% of all deliriums, and all medications, particularly those with anticholinergic effects and any new medications, should be suspect. Invasive equipment such as nasogastric tubes, intravenous lines, catheters, and restraints also contribute to delirium by interfering with normal feedback mechanisms of the body. The "Acute Confusion/Delirium Protocol" developed by Rapp et al. (2001) provides a screening and surveillance form identifying risk factors that can be used on hospital admission and during the course of the hospital stay.

Assessment. Several instruments can be used to assess the presence and severity of delirium. To detect changes, it is very important to determine the person's usual mental status. If the person cannot tell you this, family or other caregivers who are with the patient can be asked to provide this information. If the patient is alone, the responsible party or the institution transferring the patient can provide this information by phone. Do not assume the person's current mental status represents his or her usual state, and do not attribute altered mental status to age alone or assume that dementia is present. All patients, regardless of their current cognitive function, should have formal assessment to identify possible delirium, especially delirium superimposed on dementia. Strategies to assist in assessing and managing delirium in

persons with dementia can be found at *www.hartfordign.org/publications/trythis/AssesMangeDeleriumWDementia.pdf.*

The Mini-Mental State Examination (MMSE) (Folstein et al., 1975) is considered a general test of cognitive status that helps identify mental status impairment. Although the MMSE alone is not adequate for diagnosing delirium, it represents a brief, standardized method to assess mental status and can provide a baseline from which to track changes. The MMSE is discussed in Chapter 6. Several delirium-specific assessment instruments are available, such as the Confusion Assessment Method (CAM) (Inouye et al., 1990) and the NEECHAM Confusion Scale (Neelon et al., 1996). The CAM-ICU is another instrument specifically designed to assess delirium in an intensive care population and has recently been validated for use in critically ill, nonverbal patients who are on mechanical ventilation (Ely et al., 2001; Rigney, 2006). The CAM instrument is available at *www.hartfordign.org/publications/trythis/issue13.pdf.*

Assessment using the MMSE, CAM, and NEECHAM should be conducted on admission to the hospital, throughout the hospitalization for all patients identified at risk for delirium, and for all patients who exhibit signs and symptoms of delirium or develop additional risk factors. Documenting specific objective indicators of alterations in mental status rather than using the global nonspecific term *confusion* will lead to more appropriate prevention, detection, and management of delirium and its negative consequences.

Prevention and Treatment. An awareness and identification of the risk factors for delirium and a formal assessment of mental status are the first-line interventions for prevention. Many nursing interventions, in addition to treatment of underlying physical causes, can assist in the prevention of delirium. Nurses play a pivotal role in identification of delirium, and it is imperative that they accurately report patients' mental status to the medical team (Irving and Foreman, 2006). Multidisciplinary approaches, including education, to delirium prevention seem to show the most

---

BOX 23-6   Suggested Interventions to Prevent Delirium

- Know baseline mental status, functional abilities, living conditions, medications taken, alcohol use.
- Assess mental status using Mini-Mental State Exam (MMSE), Confusion Assessment Method (CAM), or NEECHAM Confusion Scale, and document.
- Correct underlying physiological alterations.
- Compensate for sensory deficits (hearing aids, glasses, dentures).
- Encourage fluid intake (make sure fluids are accessible).
- Avoid long periods of giving nothing orally.
- Explain all actions with clear and consistent communication.
- Avoid multiple medications, and avoid problematic medications.
- Be vigilant for drug reactions or interactions; consider onset of new symptoms as an adverse reaction to medications.
- Avoid use of sleeping medications—use music, warm milk, noncaffeinated herbal tea to alleviate discomfort.
- Attempt to find out why behavior is occurring rather than simply medicating for it (e.g., need to toilet, pain, fear, hunger, thirst).
- Avoid excessive bed rest; institute early mobilization.

- Encourage participation in care for activities of daily living (ADLs).
- Minimize the use of catheters, restraints, or immobilizing devices.
- Use least restrictive devices (mitts instead of wrist restraints, reclining geri-chairs with tray instead of vest restraints).
- Hide tubes (stockinette over intravenous [IV] line), or use intermittent fluid administration.
- Activate bed and chair alarms.
- Place the patient near the nursing station for close observation.
- Assess and treat pain.
- Pay attention to environmental noise.
- Normalize the environment (provide familiar items, routines, clocks, calendars).
- Minimize the number of room changes and interfacility transfers.
- Do not place a delirious patient in the room with another delirious patient.
- Have family, volunteer, or paid caregiver stay with the patient.

---

promising results, but continued research is needed to evaluate what type of approach has the most beneficial effect in specific clinical settings. An innovative approach, borrowing the concept of a "doula" from maternity care and creating a delirium doula, is mentioned in the literature (Balas et al., 2004; Irving and Foreman, 2006). Of interest, this concept was designed by student nurses who had completed a maternity placement where doulas were utilized. The proposed role of the delirium doula would include providing support, adjusting the environment to meet the patient's behavior or needs, and assisting the patient to get help when required. Flaherty et al. (2003) reported a 40% reduction in delirium development among high-risk patients using a specialized delirium unit that utilized a multidisciplinary team approach, behavioral interventions as first-line treatment, and higher nurse-patient staffing ratios.

A well-researched multidisciplinary program of delirium prevention in the acute care setting, the Elder Life Program (Bradley et al., 2005; Inouye et al., 1999; Rubin et al., 2006), focuses on managing six risk factors for delirium: cognitive impairment, sleep deprivation, immobility, visual impairments, hearing impairments, and dehydration. Patient outcomes with the use of this model include a 40% reduction in the incidence of delirium and a decrease in the number of days and episodes of delirium. Most of the interventions can be considered quite simple and part of good nursing care. Examples include the following: offering herbal tea or warm milk instead of sleeping medications, keeping the ward quiet at night by using vibrating beepers instead of paging systems, using silent pill crushers, removing catheters and other devices that hamper movement as soon as possible, encour-

aging mobilization, assessing and managing pain, and correcting hearing and vision deficits. Fall risk reduction interventions such as bed and chair alarms, low beds, reclining chairs, volunteers to sit with restless patients, and keeping routines as normal as possible with consistent caregivers are other examples of interventions. Box 23-6 presents other nursing interventions. Further information on the Elder Life Program can be found at *http://elderlife.med.yale.edu/public/public-main.php*.

Pharmacological interventions to treat the symptoms of delirium may be necessary if patients are in danger of harming themselves or others or if non-pharmacological interventions are not effective. However, pharmacological interventions should not replace thoughtful and careful evaluation and management of the underlying causes of delirium. Pharmacological treatment should be one approach in a multicomponent program of prevention and treatment. Research on the pharmacological management of delirium is limited, but with "improved understanding of the neuropathogenesis of delirium, it is conceivable that drug therapy could become primary to the treatment of delirium" (Irving and Foreman, 2006, p. 122). In a recent study, low-dose haloperidol prophylactic treatment reduced the severity and duration of postoperative delirium in high-risk elderly patients who had hip surgery but had no effect on reducing the incidence of delirium. The study protocol also included consultation by experienced geriatric nurses and geriatricians and a comprehensive delirium protocol that included many of the non-pharmacological interventions discussed previously. Short-acting benzodiazepines are often used to control agitation but may worsen mental status. Psychoactive medications

---

BOX 23-7 Communicating with a Person Experiencing Delirium

- Know the person's past patterns.
- Look at nonverbal signs, such as tone of voice, facial expressions, gestures.
- Speak slowly.
- Be calm and patient.
- Face the person and keep eye contact—get to the level of the person rather than standing over him or her.
- Explain all actions.
- Smile.
- Use simple, familiar words.
- Allow adequate time for response.
- Repeat if needed.
- Tell the person what you want him or her to do rather than what you don't want him or her to do.
- Give one-step directions; use gestures and demonstration to augment words.
- Reassure of safety.
- Keep caregivers consistent.
- Assume that communication and behavior are meaningful and an attempt to tell us something or express needs.
- Do not assume the person is unable to understand or is demented.

---

should be given at the lowest effective dose, monitored closely, and reduced or eliminated as soon as possible so that recovery can be assessed (Rigney, 2006).

Caring for patients with delirium can be a challenging experience. Patients with delirium can be difficult to communicate with, and disturbing behaviors such as pulling out intravenous (IV) lines or attempting to get out of bed disrupt medical treatment and compromise safety. It is important for nurses to realize that behavior is an attempt to communicate something and express needs. The patient with delirium feels frightened and out of control. The more calm and reassuring the nurse is, the safer the patient will feel. Box 23-7 presents some communication strategies that are helpful in caring for people experiencing delirium.

Dementia

Features of Dementia. In contrast to delirium, which is usually a reflection of an acute physiological disturbance or severe depression, dementia is an irreversible state that progresses over years in the decline of intellectual function. Dementia is considered a syndrome, not a diagnosis. Dementia has more than 70 causes, and any persons with symptoms of dementia should have a thorough workup to determine the etiology. Ham (2002) defines dementia as:

> ...a clinical state in which a persistent change in cognitive function occurs, with memory loss, and at least one other type of cognitive deficit. These losses are severe enough to impair social and occupational function and to be a clear change from a prior level of function, not occurring during the course of a delirium (p. 253).

Other clinical features of the syndrome of dementia include at least one of the following:
- Aphasia—loss of ability to speak with relevance and fluency
- Apraxia—inability to carry out purposeful movements although motor and sensory abilities are intact
- Agnosia—inability to recognize common objects or faces of familiar people despite intact sensory abilities
- Disturbances in executive functioning (planning, organizing, sequencing, abstracting) (Figure 23-4)

Types of Dementia. Dementia can be categorized as primary or secondary. Primary dementias are progressive disorders caused by pathological conditions of the brain (e.g., Alzheimer's disease [AD]; secondary dementias produce pathological conditions of the brain as a result of other conditions (e.g., dementia related to the effects of alcohol). Many dementias in old age can be described as mixed dementia, produced by a number of primary and secondary causes. For example, dementia can be caused by a combination of AD, vascular brain changes, and prior alcoholism (two primary causes and one secondary cause). Box 23-8 presents the primary dementias and common secondary dementias.

Although dementia has approximately 70 causes, dementia of the AD type is the most common, accounting for 50% to 60% of all dementias. AD affects more than 5 million individuals older than 65 years in the United States and more than 16 million individuals worldwide. The prevalence, incidence, and cumulative risk of AD appear to be much higher in African-Americans than in non-Hispanic whites. Higher rates of vascular dementia are also found among African-Americans, most likely related to the higher incidence of hypertension and diabetes (Alzheimer's Association, 2006, *www.alz.org*).

The actual proportion of people with pure AD is probably smaller, and recent studies indicate that half of all people with AD have concomitant vascular disease or cortical Lewy bodies (Bhidayasiri, 2006). The prevalence of AD increases with age, doubling approximately every 5 years in individuals between the ages of 60 and 95 years. An estimated 50% of individuals older than 85 years have AD. If current trends continue, by the year, 2050, the prevalence of AD is expected to more than triple and one in four individuals will either have AD or be caring for someone who does. It is the fourth leading cause of death in the United States and carries an annual cost of $110 billion (Ham, 2002; Solomon and Murphy, 2006).

Dementia has a number of other causes. These include vascular dementia (VaD) (about 10% of dementias); diffuse Lewy body dementia (DLBD) (about 15% to 25% of dementias); and mixed dementias (usually AD and vascular). Other less commonly occurring dementias are frontotemporal dementia (FTD); Creutzfeldt-Jakob disease (CJD) (subacute spongiform encephalopathy); and human immunodeficiency virus (HIV)–related dementia. Normal pressure hydrocephalus (NPH) causes a dementia characterized

Functional Dementia Scale

Circle one rating for each item:
1 None or little of the time
2 Some of the time
3 Good part of the time
4 Most or all of the time

Patient _____

Observer _____

Position or relation to patient _____

Facility _____

1	2	3	4	(01)	Has difficulty in completing simple tasks on own, e.g., dressing, bathing, doing arithmetic.
1	2	3	4	(02)	Spends time either sitting or in apparently purposeless activity.
1	2	3	4	(03)	Wanders at night or needs to be restrained to prevent wandering.
1	2	3	4	(04)	Hears things that are not there.
1	2	3	4	(05)	Requires supervision or assistance in eating.
1	2	3	4	(06)	Loses things.
1	2	3	4	(07)	Appearance is disorderly if left to own devices.
1	2	3	4	(08)	Moans.
1	2	3	4	(09)	Cannot control bowel function.
1	2	3	4	(10)	Threatens to harm others.
1	2	3	4	(11)	Cannot control bladder function.
1	2	3	4	(12)	Needs to be watched so doesn't injure self, e.g., by careless smoking, leaving the stove on, falling.
1	2	3	4	(13)	Destructive of materials around him, e.g., breaks furniture, throws food trays, tears up magazines.
1	2	3	4	(14)	Shouts or yells.
1	2	3	4	(15)	Accuses others of doing him bodily harm or stealing his possessions—when you are sure the accusations are not true.
1	2	3	4	(16)	Is unaware of limitations imposed by illness.
1	2	3	4	(17)	Becomes confused and does not know where he/she is.
1	2	3	4	(18)	Has trouble remembering.
1	2	3	4	(19)	Has sudden changes of mood, e.g., gets upset, angered, or cries easily.
1	2	3	4	(20)	If left alone, wanders aimlessly during the day or needs to be restrained to prevent wandering.

FIGURE 23-4 Functional Dementia Scale. (From Moore JT et al: A functional dementia scale, *J Fam Pract* 16:498, 1983.)

by ataxic gait, incontinence, and memory impairment. This disease is reversible and treated with a shunt that diverts cerebrospinal fluid away from the brain. Many dementias present with symptoms of cognitive impairment, but associated features, as well as age of onset, vary among the different types of dementing syndromes (Box 23-9). It is important for people with symptoms of cognitive impairment to receive a comprehensive evaluation by professionals expert in the diagnosis of dementia. Accurate diagnosis is important, since treatment and prognosis vary. Advances in technology and knowledge about dementia-type disorders have resulted in better diagnosis of the different types of dementia.

Alzheimer's Disease. AD was first described by Dr. Alois Alzheimer in 1906 and is a cerebral degenerative disorder of unknown origin. AD destroys proteins of nerve cells of the cerebral cortex by diffuse infiltration with nonfunctional tissue called *neurofibrillary tangles* and *plaques*. The tangles and plaques represent the death of nerve cells throughout the brain. The brain shrinks to about one third

---

BOX 23-8 Primary and Secondary Dementias

PRIMARY, PROGRESSIVE DEMENTIAS

Alzheimer's disease (dementia of the Alzheimer's type [DAT])
Diffuse Lewy body dementia
Vascular dementia (includes Binswanger's disease, multiinfarct dementia)
Frontotemporal dementia (includes Pick's disease)
Huntington's disease
Creutzfeldt-Jakob disease

COMMON SECONDARY DEMENTIAS

Alcohol-associated dementia
Parkinson's-associated dementia (subcortical)
Human immunodeficiency virus/acquired immunodeficiency syndrome–associated dementia
Postanoxic encephalopathy
Poststroke dementia
Progressive supranuclear palsy

BOX 23-9   Classification of Dementing Disorders

DEMENTING DISORDER	SUGGESTIVE FEATURES
Vascular dementia (VaD)	Stepwise deterioration (<50%) Focal neurological signs Neuroimaging evidence of cerebrovascular insufficiency
Dementia with Lewy bodies (DLB)	Fluctuations in performance Visual hallucinations, delusions Bilateral symmetric parkinsonism Neuroleptic hypersensitivity
Frontotemporal lobe dementia (FTD) (Pick's disease)	Early personality changes Early age of onset (before 60) Cortical atrophy selective to frontal and temporal lobes Early language dysfunction Relatively preserved memory and visuospatial function
Parkinson disease dementia (PDD)	Asymmetric parkinsonian features Later onset of dementia, at least 1 year after onset of parkinsonian features Subcortical dementia with impairment of frontal-executive functions
Creutzfeldt-Jakob disease (CJD) and vCJD (transmissible spongiform encephalopathy)	CJD: Rare form dementia characterized by tiny holes that give the brain a "spongy" appearance under microscope May be hereditary, occur sporadically, or through transmission from infected individuals Symptoms occur about age 60 90% of patients die within 1 year Failing memory, behavioral changes, lack of coordination, visual disturbances vCJD (bovine spongiform encephalopathy/mad cow disease) Occurs in younger patients and may be caused by contaminated feed

Data from National Institute of Neurological Disorders and Stroke, 2006. (website): *www.ninds.nih.gov/disorders*; Bhidayasiri R: When it's not AD: atypical dementing illnesses, Part 1: *CNS Senior Care* 5(2):17, 2006.

of its normal weight. The tangles consist of a protein called *tau* that "clogs" the insides of brain cells and their connections. Deposits of beta amyloid accumulate abnormally in the brains of patients with AD. The disease is progressive and is accompanied by increasing memory loss, inability to concentrate, personality deterioration, and impaired judgment. The course of AD ranges from 1 to 15 years; typical life expectancy is 8 to 9 years after symptom onset, with death usually occurring as a result of pulmonary infections, urinary tract infections, pressure ulcers, or iatrogenic disorders. Risk factors include increasing age, family history and genetics, Down's syndrome, female gender, environmental toxins, low formal education and occupational attainment, previous head trauma, and cerebrovascular disease. Diabetes also seems to increase the risk of AD.

The cause of the disorder is still unknown, and research is ongoing. Current research focuses on many aspects of AD: anatomy, biochemistry, diagnosis, genetics, language, memory, nutrition, perception, pharmacology, physiology, psychosocial issues, and virology. Some research indicates that flaws in processes governing production, accumulation, or disposal of beta amyloid are the primary causes of AD (Alzheimer's Association, 2006, *www.alz.org*). Other clinical research trials have begun looking at homocyste-

ine, which is linked to an increased risk of developing AD over time. This amino acid is known to be linked to an increase in heart disease risk, and higher homocysteine levels may increase the risk for AD. The well-known Nun Study conducted by Dr. David Snowden at University of Kentucky has brought new speculation about AD. From 1991 to 1993, 675 Catholic sisters joined this study and donated their brains at death. It was found that the presence of tiny strokes or transient ischemic attacks (TIAs) in combination with the plaques and tangles significantly increased the clinical manifestations of AD. This study also found that cognitive ability in youth is linked to development of AD in late life. The women who had poor scores on measures of cognitive ability as young adults were found to be at higher risk for AD and low cognitive function in late life.

The two recognized forms of AD are familial and sporadic. Familial AD is quite rare and usually occurs before the age of 60 years. In familial AD, the person has inherited an abnormal variation (mutation) in one of three genes that are known causes of the disease: PS1, PS2, and APP. The gene mutations influence the production of beta amyloid. Sporadic AD is not inherited in any direct pattern, but genetic variations may influence susceptibility to AD. Gene research

BOX 23-10   DSM-IV-TR Criteria for Dementia of the Alzheimer's Type

1. Multiple cognitive deficits manifested by the following:
   a. Memory impairment
   b. Aphasia, apraxia, or executive function disturbance
2. Significant impairment of social and work-related function caused by deficits in cognition in 1a and 1b and is a decline from previous functioning.
3. There is a gradual onset of deficits and progressive cognitive decline.
4. The cognitive deficits in 1a and 1b are not caused by the following:
   a. Central nervous system disturbances that cause progressive memory deficits, such as Parkinson's disease, cerebrovascular disorders, subdural hematoma, brain tumor
   b. Conditions known to cause dementia, such as hypothyroidism, pernicious anemia, folic acid deficiency, neurosyphilis, hyperparathyroid disease with hypercalcemia
   c. Substances, drugs
5. The deficits are not caused by delirium.
6. The deficits are not accounted for by major depression or schizophrenia.

Reprinted with permission from American Psychiatric Association: *Diagnostic and statistical manual of mental disorders*, DSM-IV-TR, Washington, DC, 2000, The Association.

is an area of active investigation. For more information on current research, see *www.alz.org*.

Diagnosis of Alzheimer's Disease. The only confirmatory method of diagnosing AD is to perform a brain biopsy or autopsy. AD is diagnosed most thoroughly based on the history from the family and testing to rule out other disorders that may mimic the disease. Probable AD can be clinically diagnosed if the onset is typically insidious with progression and if no other systemic or brain diseases could account for the progressive cognitive deficits. Symptoms are usually present several years before a diagnosis is made. Symptoms of apathy and depression may be the first and earliest signs of AD, occurring up to 3 years before the disease is diagnosed (*Apathy may be harbinger of early cognitive decline*, 2006). The history given by the family is another important part of assessing and diagnosing probable AD. A recent survey by the Alzheimer's Foundation of America (2006) found that the stigma associated with Alzheimer's disease among patients and families can delay the diagnosis for up to 6 years after symptoms first appear. A delayed diagnosis means that patients and families are without critical support, resources, and treatment (*www.alzfdn.org*). The components of a comprehensive assessment were presented on p. 554 and in Box 23-3. Box 23-10 presents the DSM-IV-TR criteria for dementia of the Alzheimer's type.

Cultural Differences. Research is limited regarding the influence of culture and ethnicity on the recognition and interpretation of cognitive changes and the assessment, diagnosis, and treatment of AD and other dementias. Further

research is needed to understand how individuals from racially and culturally diverse groups view dementia and how cultural beliefs about disease etiology and symptoms influence diagnosis, treatment, and help-seeking behaviors (Hargrave, 2006; Neary and Mahoney, 2005). Studies (Hargrave, 2006) have shown that African-Americans may view dementia as a:

> …normal consequence of aging, a form of mental illness, or manifestation of culture-specific physical syndromes (e.g., "worriation" or "spells"). These health beliefs may lead to normalizing or minimizing symptoms, promote denial, and delay help-seeking behaviors (p. 37).

Hispanics may attribute the etiology of dementia to a "lack of balance in one's lifestyle, punishment for bad behavior, or mental illness (locos) or a temporary state of nervous, or nervousness" (Neary and Mahoney, 2005, p. 169). However, recent studies suggest that limited knowledge about dementia is a more significant deterrent to recognizing its symptoms and seeking assessment and treatment (Neary and Mahoney, 2005; Hargrave, 2006). Development of culturally and linguistically appropriate sources of information about dementia is important (Neary and Mahoney, 2005). The Diversity Toolbox, prepared by the Alzheimer's Association, is an important resource for nurses and other health professionals working with culturally and racially diverse older adults. Other resources about dementia for ethnically and culturally diverse individuals are found in the Resource section at the end of this chapter.

Drug Treatment. Drug therapy with cholinesterase inhibitors (CIs) has transformed the treatment of AD, offering hope for enhanced function and reduction of the speed of decline. CIs approved to treat AD include donepezil (Aricept), rivastigmine (Exelon), and galantamine (Reminyl). The most recently approved drug, memantine (Namenda), is a new class of medication (N-methyl-D-aspartate [NMDA] antagonist) indicated for the treatment of moderate to severe AD. Unlike the CIs, which increase the amount of acetylcholine in the brain, memantine blocks the effect of abnormal glutamate activity that may lead to neuronal cell death and cognitive dysfunction. Memantine may be used alone or in combination with the CIs. These medications may also positively affect the behavioral manifestations of AD.

Current treatment guidelines recommend CI therapy as first-line treatment in patients with mild to moderate AD. Duration of therapy should be long-term, even if the patient shows slight decline, provided that function is better than it would have been without treatment (Doody et al., 2001; Ham et al., 2002). Side effects are generally mild and include gastrointestinal disturbances, sleep disturbances, and sedation. Starting at a low dose with slow titration is recommended to minimize side effects. Rivastigmine (Exelon) is now available in a patch that may be more convenient to use, have fewer side effects, and provide a consistent day-long dose. Medication therapy is directed toward the symptoms of AD and does not affect the neuronal decline that will eventually produce severe disability. However, medications are likely to produce a plateau of brain function and functional abilities and delay the progression of AD. Positive effects on the behavioral manifestations of AD have also been shown with drug therapy. A recent study reported that the use of CIs was associated with a decreased risk of rapid cognitive deterioration, institutionalization, and weight loss (Gillette-Guyonnet et al., 2006).

Vascular Dementia. Vascular dementia refers to a group of heterogeneous disorders arising from cerebrovascular insufficiency or ischemic or hemorrhagic brain damage. VaD is the second most prevalent type of dementia in the United States. VaD often co-exists with AD, is more common among African-Americans and Japanese Americans, and is associated with advancing age, male gender, and stroke (Bhidayasiri, 2006; Fladd, 2005). The ratio of VaD to AD is generally 1:5, and dementia after stroke is thought to occur in one quarter to one third of stroke cases. Hypertension, cardiac disease, diabetes, smoking, alcoholism, and hyperlipidemia are additional risk factors for VaD (Box 23-11).

The major subtypes of VaD include single strategic stroke, multiple infarcts, and subcortical small vessel disease. Subcortical small vessel disease is thought to be responsible for approximately two thirds of VaD cases and is more likely to lead to progressive dementia. Binswanger's disease is a type or subcortical dementia associated with hypertension. Onset is usually in the sixth or seventh decade with symptoms of reduced speed of information processing, decreased spontaneity, apathy, emotional blunting, and falls (Bhidayasiri, 2006). Symptoms of VaD vary depending on the size, location, and type of damage. Focal neurological signs are commonly present and include hemiparesis, visual field deficits, hemisensory loss, and pseudobulbar palsy. Differentiating VaD from AD is difficult, and the two diseases often exist together (mixed dementia) (Bhidayasiri, 2006). Difficulties with balance and movement are seen earlier with VaD, and this may also help in differential diagnosis. Disorders of balance and movement are not commonly seen in AD until late in the disease. Fladd (2005) suggests that the main feature that differentiates subcortical VaD from other dementias is psychomotor slowness. According to Bhidayasir (2006, p. 17):

> On neuroimaging, white matter lesions consisting of ill-defined regions with altered signal around the frontal and occipital horns of the anterior ventricles, often extending into the centrum semiovale, are seen. However, more than 60% of patients with AD present with incomplete white matter infarction as well. Increasing evidence shows that brain lesions associated with the two disorders occur together and interact in important ways to increase the likelihood of cognitive decline.

Diagnostic criteria for VaD include the DSM-IV criteria, the Hachinski Ischemic Score, and the National Institute of Neurological Disorders and Stroke-Association Internationale pour la Recherche et l'Enseignement en Neurosciences (NINDS-AIREN) (Bhidayasiri, 2006).

Management of hypertension, diabetes, and hyperlipidemia is important in the primary prevention of VaD. Secondary prevention includes treatments to prevent the recurrence of a vascular accident (use of antihypertensive and antiplatelet medications) or minimize further cognitive damage (use of CIs). The use of acetylcholinesterase inhibitors is also recommended for the symptomatic treatment of VaD (Fladd, 2005).

BOX 23-11   Vascular Brain Disease

Vascular brain disease may result from any of the following:
- Arteriosclerotic plaques blocking circulation to cerebral cells
- Blood dyscrasias interfering with platelet and clot formation
- Cardiac decompensation resulting in insufficient perfusion to the brain
- Cerebrovascular hemorrhage (strokes) of small or large magnitude
- Diabetic deterioration of blood vessels
- Primary hypertension causing deterioration of capillary walls because of sustained pressure (Cerebral cells dependent on the deteriorated capillaries no longer function. Over time, hypertensive persons show greater decrements in cognitive performance than persons with normal blood pressure.)
- Rupture of cerebrovascular or aortic aneurysms
- Sustained severe anemia
- Systemic emboli lodging in cerebrovascular pathway
- Transient ischemic attacks (TIAs) lasting up to 24 hours, resulting from spasms of blood vessels in certain segments of the brain, which produce temporary disturbances in sensation, cognition, and motor activity and are often a warning sign of impending stroke

---

Developmentally Disabled Elders

The number of developmentally disabled elders (DDEs) is rapidly increasing, primarily because of medical advances and healthier living conditions that have extended life expectancy. Individuals with Down's syndrome (trisomy 21) who survive until old age develop the pathogenic hallmarks of AD (Beers and Berkow, 2000). Functional limitations in the biological, social, and psychological spheres may be a major cause of frailty in the DDE. Those elders particularly depend on their environment for stimulation, and in its absence, behaviors suggestive of dementia may emerge.

Many aspects of the aging process apparently are prematurely experienced by the developmentally disabled. Their average age of death is younger than healthy persons—death in women/men is 79/73 in healthy adults but 67/63 in elders who are developmentally disabled (Brown, 2002). Thus they may experience musculoskeletal changes, sensory decline, problems from medication use over long periods, and certain disease states earlier. It is important to look for behavioral changes in those who have communication problems because these may indicate an underlying health disorder. Age-related hearing loss and vision loss are two of the problems that affect DDEs just as they affect healthy adults, but these problems may be discovered only by observing and acting on behavioral changes (Bagley, 2002; Flax, 2002). Retirement needs and responses to relocation present special considerations. Caregiving concerns for elders who are developmentally disabled are discussed in Chapter 20.

▲ PROMOTING HEALTHY AGING: IMPLICATIONS FOR GERONTOLOGICAL NURSING

Person-Centered Care

Irreversible dementia such as Alzheimer's disease has no cure, and although new medications offer hope for improved function, the most important treatment for the disease is competent and compassionate person-centered care. "Since Alzheimer's affects mind and personality, as well as physical function, there is a great danger that the person can become obscured by the disease, defined by symptoms rather than by her or his unique spirit and continuing sense of self" (Sifton, 2001, p. iv). Person-centered care looks beyond the disease and the tasks we must perform to the person within and our relationship with them. The focus is not on what we need to "do to the person" but rather on the person himself or herself and how to enhance well-being and quality of life. Gerontological nurses know that the person, not the disease, is always the focus of care, and they practice from a belief that the person with dementia is still a whole person, someone who can think, feel, learn, grow, and be in a relationship (Touhy, 2004). "The person with dementia is not an object, not a vegetable, not an empty body, not a child, but an adult, who, given support, might exercise choices and respond to a respectful approach" (Woods, 1999, p. 35). Person-centered care fosters abilities, supports limitations, ensures safety, enhances quality of life, prevents excess disability, and offers hope. Care for persons with dementia is more than keeping their bodies alive, safe, and clean; performing tasks; and managing behavior—the care must also nourish their souls (Touhy, 2004). Person-centered care is care that establishes connections and a sense of security; respects and appreciates the person; and supports the person's need to love and be loved, to be known and accepted, to give and to share, and to be productive and successful (Bell and Troxel, 2001).

The current view of Alzheimer's disease in the popular and professional press is negative, hopeless, and frightening. We hear people with Alzheimer's described as victims, empty shells (Moore and Hollett, 2003), ex-people (Pulsford, 1997), and bodies from which the personhood has been removed (Keane, 1994). Nursing students used the terms *afraid, frustrated, sad,* and *nervous* to describe their feelings when caring for a person with dementia (Beck, 1996). The actions of people with dementia are often described as aggressive, agitated, inappropriate, and burdensome (Fazio, 2001; Talerico and Evans, 2000). Despite a growing body of evidence on the importance of person-centered care, therapeutic communication techniques, and therapeutic work with people with dementia, the emphasis in the literature and in practice continues to be on the care of the body (bathing, feeding) and

the management of aggressive and problematic behavior. Discussions of how to prevent catastrophic reactions and handle aggressive behavior are far more common than discussions of how to nurture personhood and quality of life. The emphasis on the decline associated with the disease, the catastrophic behaviors, and the loss of humanness promotes despair, hopelessness, and fear for professional caregivers, patients, and families (Touhy, 2004).

Nursing Models of Care for Persons with Dementia

Gerontological nurses often provide direct care for people with dementia in the community, hospitals, and long-term care facilities. They also work with families and staff, teaching best practice approaches to care and providing education and support. Much of the care of people with dementia takes place in the home and is provided by a spouse or other family member or in a nursing home where it is provided by nursing assistants. Gerontological nurses will be most effective when they assist caregivers in all settings to understand the nature of dementia and the interventions likely to be most effective. Overall, interventions must match expectancies with capacities, incorporate earlier life skills and interests, and provide a calm, caring, and structured environment. Several nursing models of care are useful in guiding practice and assisting families and staff in providing care to people with dementia.

PLST Model. The progressively lowered stress threshold (PLST) model (Hall and Buckwalter, 1987; Hall, 1994) was one of the first models used to plan and evaluate care for people with dementia in every setting. The PLST model categorizes symptoms of dementia into four groups: (1) cognitive or intellectual losses, (2) affective or personality changes, (3) conative or planning losses that cause a decline in functional abilities, and (4) loss of the stress threshold causing behaviors such as agitation or catastrophic reactions. Symptoms such as agitation are a result of a progressive loss of the person's ability to cope with demands and stimuli when the person's stress threshold is exceeded. Five common stressors that may trigger these symptoms are fatigue; change of environment, routine, or caregiver; misleading stimuli or inappropriate stimulus levels; internal or external demands to perform beyond abilities; and physical stressors such as pain, discomfort, acute illness, and depression.

Using this model, care is structured to decrease the stressors and provide a safe and predictable environment. Outcomes reported when the model was used on an Alzheimer's special care unit included increased hours of sleep; decreased nighttime awakening; decreased sedative and tranquilizer use; increased food intake and weight; increased socialization; decreased episodes of anxious, agitated, combative behaviors; increased caregiver satisfaction with care; and increased functional level (Hall and Buckwalter, 1997). Hall (1994) offers many suggestions for both institutional caregivers and families caring for a person with dementia at home. Using principles of the PLST model, DeYoung et al.

(2003) designed a behavior management unit in a long-term care facility. Reported outcomes included a decrease in aggressive, agitated, and disruptive behaviors. Staff training was an important part of this program and included an emphasis on knowing the patient well and modifying the environment. McCloskey (2004) offers practical suggestions based on the PLST model in the acute care environment when caring for patients with dementia. Box 23-12 presents the principles of care derived from the PLST model.

Need-Driven, Dementia-Compromised Behavior Model.

The need-driven, dementia-compromised behavior (NDB) model (Algase et al., 2003; Kolanowski, 1999; Rich-

---

BOX 23-12   Principles of Care Derived from PLST Model

1. Maximize functional abilities by supporting all losses in a prosthetic manner.
2. Establish caring relationship, and provide person with unconditional positive regard.
3. Use behaviors indicating anxiety and avoidance to determine appropriate limits of activity and stimuli.
4. Teach caregivers to try to find out causes of behavior and to observe and evaluate verbal and nonverbal responses.
5. Identify triggers related to discomfort or stress reactions (factors in the environment, caregiver communication).
6. Modify the environment to support losses and promote safe function.
7. Evaluate care routines and responses on a 24-hour basis, and adjust plan of care accordingly.
8. Provide as much control as possible—encourage self-care, offer choices, explain all actions, do not push or force the person to do something.
9. Keep environment stable and predictable.
10. Provide ongoing education, support, care, and problem solving for caregivers.

Adapted from Hall GR, Buckwalter KC: Progressively lowered stress threshold: a conceptual model for care of adults with Alzheimer's disease, *Arch Psychiatr Nurs* 1(6):399-406, 1987.

---

ards et al., 2000) is a framework for the study and understanding of behavioral symptoms of dementia. All behaviors have meaning and are a form of communication, particularly as verbal communication becomes more limited (Ortigara, 2000). The NDB model proposes that the behavior of persons with dementia carries a message of need that can be addressed appropriately if the person's history and habits, physiological status, and physical and social environment are carefully evaluated (Kolanowski, 1999). Rather than behavior being viewed as disruptive, it is viewed as having meaning and expressing needs. Behavior reflects the interaction of background factors (cognitive changes as a result of dementia, gender, ethnicity, culture, education, personality, responses to stress) and proximal factors (physiological needs such as hunger or pain, mood, physical environment [e.g., light, noise]) with social environment (e.g., staff stability and mix, presence of others) (Richards et al., 2000). Optimal care is provided by manipulating the proximal factors that precipitate behavior and by maximizing strengths and minimizing the limitations of the background factors. For instance, sleep disruptions are common in people with dementia. If the person is not getting adequate sleep at night, agitated or aggressive behavior during the day may signal the need for more rest. Interventions to modify proximal factors interfering with sleep, such as noise, frequent awakenings during the night, and daytime boredom, can help meet the need for rest and sleep and decrease agitation or aggression.

Cohen-Mansfield's treatment routes for exploring agitation (TREA) model (2000) is another useful framework for detecting the needs of the person with dementia. The decision-making algorithms for understanding and responding to behaviors such as verbal agitation and physical aggression presented as part of this model help design interventions. Table 23-2 presents some reasons for unmet needs in people with dementia using Maslow's framework.

Other authors have discussed the importance of viewing all behavior as meaningful rather than disruptive or problematic and encourage nurses to avoid labeling the behavior of persons with dementia as *aggressive* (Cohen-Mansfield, 2000; Smith and Buckwalter, 2005; Talerico and Evans,

---

TABLE 23-2

Reason for Unmet Needs in Persons with Dementia

Maslow's Hierarchical Needs	Internal and External Conditions Affecting Need Fulfillment
Physiological—rest, fluids and nutrition, elimination, pain and comfort	Unable to communicate needs, unaware of needs of self, lack of availability to caregiver, caregiver unresponsiveness or inability to understand and respond to needs
Safety, protection from injury, feeling secure	Unaware of needs, safety risks, limitations; unable to use prior coping mechanisms
Love and belonging, acceptance, need for social contacts	Unable to obtain the means for meeting needs, unable to communicate easily, environment not supportive of establishing connections, limited interaction and stimulation
Self-esteem, respect, control	Does not receive positive feedback, environment does not provide support, often viewed as "nonperson"
Self-actualization, finds meaning in life and death	No meaningful activities offered, communication limited, no opportunities to meet spiritual needs, may be seen as "empty shell" with no higher-level needs

Adapted from Cohen-Mansfield J. *Alzheimer Care Q* 1(4):23, 2000.

2000; Volicer and Mahoney, 2002). Terms such as *disruptive* and *aggressive* focus on the caregiver's negative response (disturbed, disrupted) rather than on the perspective of the person with dementia (fearful, protective)) (Talerico and Evans, 2000). Behavioral symptoms usually occur during personal care activities and are associated with higher levels of disability and communication deficits. Fear, pain, discomfort, unfamiliar surroundings and people, illness, fatigue, depression, need for autonomy and control, caregiver approaches, and environmental stressors are frequent precipitants of behavioral symptoms (Box 23-13).

BOX 23-13 Conditions Precipitating Behavioral Symptoms in Persons with Dementia

- Communication deficits
- Pain or discomfort
- Acute medical problems
- Sleep disturbances
- Perceptual deficits
- Depression
- Need for social contact
- Hunger, thirst, need to toilet
- Loss of control
- Misinterpretation of the situation or environment
- Crowded conditions
- Changes in environment or people
- Noise, disruption
- Being forced to do something
- Fear
- Loneliness
- Psychotic symptoms
- Fatigue
- Environmental overstimulation or understimulation
- Depersonalized, rushed care
- Restraints
- Psychoactive drugs

Adapted from Talerico K, Evans L. *Alzheimer Care Q* 1(2):78, 2000.

Nurses must use appropriate assessment to understand the meaning of behavior and determine what interventions would be most helpful to meet the needs being expressed. Yet behaviors are frequently treated without appropriate assessment. Putting yourself in the place of the person with dementia and trying to see the world from his or her eyes will help understand behavior. Questions of What, Where, Why, When, Who, and What Now are important components of assessment of behavior. Box 23-14 presents a framework for asking questions about the possible meanings and messages behind observed behavior.

Kovach et al. (2006a) proposed the consequences of NDB (C-NDB) as an extension of the NDB model. The C-NDB theory suggests that failure to recognize behaviors as symptoms leads to undertreatment of many needs, worsening behaviors, and new behaviors and needs. "Expressing needs behaviorally can set off a series of cascading effects that may lead to negative outcomes for the individual with dementia, the caregiver, and the environment" (p. 14). Findings of a recent study of the effectiveness of an innovative nursing assessment and treatment intervention, the serial trial intervention (STI), an approach to behaviors associated with advanced dementia, suggest the positive effects of the STI on patient discomfort and short-term resolution of behaviors (Kovach et al., 2006a, b). The STI is further discussed in Chapter 11.

The overuse of the atypical antipsychotic medications to treat behavioral responses is of concern in light of the side effects of such medications. None of these medications are approved for use in treatment of behavioral responses in dementia. In a recent study, Schneider and colleagues (2006) reported that the benefits of such medications are uncertain and adverse effects offset any advantages. Chapter 12 discusses the appropriate use and monitoring of psychoactive medications. A careful understanding of behavior and adaptation of responses and the environment offer a more therapeutic approach to the behavioral responses in dementia.

BOX 23-14 Framework for Asking Questions About the Meaning of Behavior

WHAT?

What is being sought? What is happening? Does the behavior have a physical or emotional component or both? What are the person's responses? What would be done if the person was 20 years old instead of 80? What is the behavior saying? What is the emotion being expressed?

WHERE?

Where is the behavior occurring? Environmental triggers?

WHEN?

When does the behavior most frequently occur? After what (e.g., activities of daily living [ADLs], family visits, mealtimes)?

WHO?

Who is involved? Other residents, caregivers, family?

WHY?

What happened before? Poor communication? Tasks too complicated? Physical or medical problem? Person being rushed or forced to do something? Has this happened before and why?

WHAT NOW?

Approaches and interventions (physical, psychosocial)? Changes needed and by whom? Who else might know something about the person or the behavior or approaches? Communicate to all and include in plan of care.

Adapted from Hellen C: *Alzheimer's disease: activity focused care*, Boston, 1998, Butterworth-Heinemann; Ortigara A. *Alzheimer Care Q* 1(4):91, 2000.

Teri et al. (2003) and Livingston et al. (2005) provide other resources on non-pharmacological approaches for behavioral responses including exercise training, behavioral management techniques, and psychological interventions. Non-pharmacological interventions and nursing responses derived from the use of frameworks just described place the focus of care on understanding the person with the disease. Gerontological nurses with this focus create environments and relationships that value and respect older adults with dementia rather than ones that punish or control.

Communicating with Persons with Dementia

The experience of losing cognitive and expressive abilities is both frightening and frustrating. Memory impairments and communication disorders such as aphasia, apraxia, and agnosia can mean that people experiencing cognitive impairment have difficulty expressing their personhood in ways easily understood by others. However, the need to communicate and the need to be treated as a person remain despite memory and communication impairments. No group of patients is more in need of supportive relationships with skilled, caring health care providers. People with cognitive and communication impairments "depend on their relationship with and trust of others to provide emotional support, solve problems, and coordinate complex activities" (Buckwalter et al., 1995, p. 15). Communication with the person experiencing cognitive impairment requires special skills and patience.

Communication is a complex process and consists of reciprocal exchanges between a listener and a speaker. Communication has both receptive and expressive components. Nonverbal communication (gestures, facial expressions) and behavior are important methods of communication. Receptive components include listening and comprehending what is said; expressive components include formulating and generating ideas into logical expression (Hendryx-Bedalov, 2000). Dementia affects both expressive and receptive communication components and alters the way people speak, the words they use, and their understanding. Early in the disease, word finding is difficult and remembering the exact facts of a conversation is also challenging. The following illustrates (Snyder, 2001, pp. 8, 11, 16):

> I'm aware that I'm losing larger and larger chunks of memory…I lose one word and then I can't come up with the rest of the sentence. I just stop talking and people think something is really wrong with me. For awhile, I'll search for a word and I can see it walking away from me. It gets littler and littler. It always comes back, but at the wrong time. You just can't be spontaneous.

People with dementia often use nonsensical or "made-up" words such as calling an electric razor a "whisker grinder." Automatic language skills (e.g., hello) are retained for the longest time. The person may wander from the topic of the conversation and bring up seemingly unrelated topics. As the disease progresses, verbal output may become less frequent although the grammar and sounds of the language being spoken remain relatively intact. The person with dementia may fail to pick up humor or sarcasm or abstract ideas in conversation. Nonverbal and behavioral responses become especially important as a way of communication as verbal skills become more limited.

Apraxia and agnosia occur with dementia and become progressively more severe as the disease progresses. Apraxia (inability to perform purposeful actions including speech) affects the ability to perform activities of daily living (ADLs), as well as communication, for persons with dementia. Difficulties arise because they cannot always coordinate the idea of the action they want to take with the motor response or coordination needed to carry out the action (Snyder, 2001). Agnosia (inability to recognize objects and people, even with good vision) can also affect communication. If you would serve a tray of food to persons with dementia, hand them a fork, and ask them to start eating, they may not recognize the fork as an eating utensil or identify the food and therefore would not respond. Caregivers may think that the person is not capable of feeding himself or herself and needs assisted feeding. An understanding of agnosia and the use of cues, gestures, and demonstration, coupled with serving one food at a time with one utensil, would have promoted self-feeding.

Much of the literature on communication with persons experiencing dementia describes a person's attempts at speech in the later stages as nonsensical and devoid of meaning or insight, contributing to the impression of a diminishing self and inability to enter into therapeutic and meaningful communication and relationships. If nurses practice from this framework, custodial and task-oriented care is all that can be offered and there is little purpose in initiating conversation to understand the individual. A growing body of literature on the experiences of people with dementia and recent research suggests that the person with dementia maintains an awareness of self and the ability to express emotions and feelings and to enter into meaningful relationships with others even into the later stages of the disease.

To effectively communicate with a person experiencing dementia, it is essential to believe that the person is trying to communicate something; it is as essential for the nurse to believe that what the person is trying to communicate is important enough to make the effort to understand. Nurses must understand and appreciate that every time they communicate with someone they affect the relationship with that person in either positive or negative ways depending on their attitude and skills (Buckwalter et al., 1995). Kitwood (1999) provided a simple way to learn techniques that enhance communication with the person with dementia (Box 23-15). The best thing we can do is to treat everything the person says, however jumbled it may seem, as important and an attempt to tell us something. It is our responsibility as professionals to know how to understand and respond. The person with dementia cannot change his or communication; we must change ours.

Evidence-Based Communication Strategies. Research conducted by Ruth Tappen of Florida Atlantic University and her colleagues provided insight into communica-

BOX 23-15   Communicating Effectively with Persons with Dementia

Envision a tennis game: the caregiver is like the tennis coach, and whenever the coach plays the ball, he or she seems to be able to put the ball where the person on the other side of the net can return it. The coach also returns the ball in such a way as to keep the rally going; he or she does not return it to score a point or win the match but, rather, returns the ball so that the other player is able to reach it and, with encouragement, is able to hit it back over the net again. Similarly, in our communication with people with dementia, our conversation and words must be put into play in a way that the person can respond effectively and share thoughts and feelings.

tion strategies that were helpful in creating and maintaining a therapeutic relationship with people in the moderate to later stages of dementia. The research challenged some of the commonly held beliefs about communication with persons with cognitive impairment, such as avoiding the use of open-ended questions, keeping communication focused only on simple and task-oriented topics and questions that can be answered with yes or no, and avoiding discussion of feelings. In the Tappen et al. studies (1997, 1999), conversations between 23 participants in the middle and late stages of Alzheimer's disease and advanced practice nurses were analyzed to clarify what type of communication techniques were helpful in creating and maintaining a therapeutic relationship. Interviewers were told "to avoid frequent correction of the individual, encourage the individual to engage in conversation, attempt to make the conversation as meaningful as possible, and to assume that any attempt at communication had some meaning to it, however difficult it was to ascertain that meaning" (Tappen et al., 1997, p. 250). Findings were compared with recommendations in the literature, and specific communication strategies were developed (Williams-Burgess and Tappen, 1999). More than 80% of the participants' responses were relevant in the context of the conversation.

General principles of communication with person with dementia include the following:

- Treat the individual as an adult.
- Assume they do understand you.
- Notice emotion expressed in nonverbal behavior.
- Augment conversation with gestures, touch.
- Allow time to respond.
- Communication strategies differ depending on the purpose of communication (e.g., performing ADLs, encouraging expression of feelings).
- Remember that there is a person behind the disease.
- Come to know the person—his or her past and present likes, dislikes, patterns, uniqueness.

Box 23-16 presents further suggestions for communication.

In the past, structured programs of reality orientation (RO) (orienting the person to the day, date, time, year, weather, upcoming holidays) were often used in long-term care and chronic psychiatric units as a way to stimulate interaction and offer hopeful interventions. This intervention is still often noted as being of benefit for persons with dementia. However, it has been found that structured RO may place unrealistic expectations on persons with middle- to late-stage dementia and may be distressing when they cannot remember these things. An often-told story in gerontological nursing is about a researcher who was going into the nursing home daily administering the MMSE to residents with dementia as part of her study. One morning, one of the residents hurried to the nursing station quite agitated and frantically kept asking, "What day is it today?" The nurse asked her why she was so upset about the day and she responded, "It's not me but there is a young woman who comes in every day asking that question and I want to help her out."

This is not to say that we should not orient the person to daily activities, time of day, and other important events, but it should be offered without the expectation that they will remember. Caregivers can provide orienting information as a part of general conversation (e.g., It's quite warm for December 10 but it will be a beautiful day for our lunch date). Rather than structured reality orientation, a better approach is going to where the persons are in their world rather than trying to bring them to yours. Identifying with elements of the individuals' past and helping them and their caregivers appreciate the connections and the feelings are more therapeutic approaches. Validation therapy, developed by Naomi Feil in the 1980s, involves following the patient's lead and responding to feelings expressed and issues of importance to the person rather than interrupting to supply factual data.

Deborah Hoffman, in her wonderful film "Complaints of a Dutiful Daughter" chronicles her mother's journey through Alzheimer's disease and humorously describes her frustration with trying to keep her mother oriented and in the present. When her mother thought Deborah was one of her sorority sisters from college and talked to her about all the good times they had, she would correct her mother and tell her "I'm your daughter; I didn't go to college with you." After many such conversations and corrections, she finally realized that it was okay if her mother thought she was one of the sorority girls—it made her mother happy to talk about good times and they could laugh and reminisce together.

Therapeutic Activities

Meaningful and enjoyable activities for persons with dementia provide cognitive stimulation and opportunities for interaction with others. Participation in therapeutic activities enhances feelings of self-worth, promotes a sense of belonging and accomplishment, and encourages expression of feelings and thoughts. "Activities for persons with dementia should be considered rehabilitative if they can increase or prevent further decline in adaptation and functional levels" (Camp and Skrajner, 2004, p. 426). It is important for caregivers in the home, as well as those in assisted-living and nursing homes, to provide meaningful and therapeutic activities for persons with dementia. Such activities are of benefit in enhancing communication and enjoyable interac-

BOX 23-16 Four Useful Strategies for Communicating with Individuals Experiencing Cognitive Impairment

SIMPLIFICATION STRATEGIES (USEFUL WITH ADLs)

- Give one-step directions.
- Speak slowly.
- Allow time for response.
- Reduce distractions.
- Interact with one person at a time.
- Give clues and cues as to what you want the person to do. Use gestures or pantomime to demonstrate what it is you want the person to do—for example, put the chair in front of the person, point to it, pat the seat, and say "Sit here."

FACILITATION STRATEGIES (USEFUL IN ENCOURAGING EXPRESSION OF THOUGHTS AND FEELINGS)

- Establish commonalities.
- Share self.
- Allow the person to choose subjects to discuss.
- Speak as if to an equal.
- Use broad openings, such as "How are you today?"
- Employ appropriate use of humor.
- Follow the person's lead.

COMPREHENSION STRATEGIES (USEFUL IN ASSISTING IN UNDERSTANDING OF COMMUNICATION)

- Identify time confusion (in what time frame is the person operating at the moment?).
- Find the theme (what connection is there between apparently disparate topics?). Recognize an important theme, such as fear, loss, happiness.
- Recognize the hidden meanings (what did the person mean to say?).

SUPPORTIVE STRATEGIES (USEFUL IN ENCOURAGING CONTINUED COMMUNICATION AND SUPPORTING PERSONHOOD)

- Introduce yourself, and explain why you are there. Reach out to shake hands, and note the response to touch.
- If the person does not want to talk, go away and return later. Do not push or force.
- Sit closely, and face the person at eye level.
- Limit corrections.
- Assume meaningfulness.
- Use multiple ways of communicating (gestures, touch).
- Search for meaning.
- Know the person's past life history as well as daily life experiences and events.
- Recognize feelings, and respond.
- Treat with respect and dignity.
- Show interest through body posture, facial expression, nodding, and eye contact. Assume a pleasant, relaxed attitude.
- Attend to vision and hearing losses.
- Do not try to bring the person to the present or use reality orientation. Go to where the person is, and enjoy the conversation.
- When leaving, thank the person for his or her time and attention as well as information.
- Remember that the quality, not the content or quantity, of the interaction is basic to therapeutic communication.

ADLs, Activities of daily living.

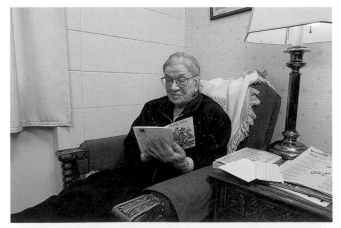

Meaningful activities provide cognitive stimulation. (From Sorrentino SA, Gorek B: *Mosby's textbook for long-term care assistants,* ed 5, St Louis, 2007, Mosby.)

tion for both the caregiver and the person with dementia. Buettner and Kolanowski (2003) provide guidelines for recreation therapy in the care of persons with dementia.

Research has shown that activities for persons with dementia that involve "external memory aids and procedural learning assist in increasing engagement with the environment and more positive affect than standard activities programming" (Camp and Skrajner, 2004, p. 426). Cameron Camp and colleagues have created Montessori-based activities based on the work of Maria Montessori, an Italian educator who developed an educational method for children. The Montessori method utilizes task breakdown, guided repetition, progressions from simple to complex and concrete to abstract, extensive use of external cues, and reliance on procedural memory rather than explicit memory. These techniques are part of the principles that have been found useful in interventions for cognitive stimulation and therapeutic work with persons with dementia. Activities are structured to the person's functional and cognitive level and can be modified to accommodate a wide range of cognitive abilities. A recent study investigated training persons with early-stage dementia to function as leaders for Montessori-based activities for people with more advanced dementia (Camp and Skrajner, 2004). Camp has authored two training manuals to guide the implementation of Montessori-based activities (Camp, 1999, 2001).

Group work, such as reminiscence and storytelling, is another therapeutic approach to encouraging communication, providing opportunities for enjoying memories and conversation, and promoting interaction that enhances self-esteem. Chapter 25 discusses group work in more detail. Bastings (2003, 2006) has described a storytelling modality designed for individuals with cognitive impairment called *Time Slips* (www.timeslips.org). Group members, looking at a picture, are encouraged to create a story about the picture. The pictures can be fantastical and funny, such as from greeting cards, or more nostalgic, such as Norman Rockwell paintings. All contributions are encouraged and welcomed, there are no right or wrong answers, and everything that the individuals say is included in the story and written down by the scribe. Stories are read back to the participants during the session, using their names to identify their contributions. At the beginning of each session, the story from the last session is read to the participants. Care is taken to compliment each member for his or her contribution to the wonderful story. The stories created are full of humor and creativity and often include discussions of memories and reminiscing. John Killick (1999, p. 49), writer in residence at a nursing home in Scotland, stated:

> Having their words written down is empowering for people with dementia. It affirms their dignity and gives an assurance that their words still have value…One woman said, "Anything you can tell people about how things are for me is important. It's a rum do, this growing ancient … The brilliance of my brain has slipped away when I wasn't looking."

One of the authors (TT) has used the storytelling modality extensively with mild to moderately impaired older people with great success as part of a research study on the effect of therapeutic activities for persons with memory loss. Potential outcomes include increased verbalization and communication, socialization, alleviation of depression, and enhanced quality of life. Qualitative responses from group participants and families indicate their enjoyment with the process. At the end of the 16-week group, the stories are bound into a book and given to the participants with a picture of the group with each member's name listed. Many of the participants and their families have commented on pride they feel at their "book" and have even shared them with grandchildren. In Bastings' work (Bastings, 2003), some of the stories were presented as a play. Although further research is indicated in relation to the outcomes of this intervention, it seems to have poten-

tial as a beneficial and cost-effective therapeutic intervention in many settings.

Despite the inability of the person with dementia to always express his or her thoughts and feelings in ways to which we are accustomed, people with dementia still have higher-order needs such as those for belonging, self-esteem, and meaningful relationships. The care relationship and the environment need to support the meeting of all of their needs. According to Buckwalter et al. (1995, p. 15):

> Gerontological nurses who are sensitive to communication and interaction patterns can assist both formal and informal caregivers in using more personal verbal and nonverbal communication strategies which are humanizing and show respect for the person. Similarly, they can monitor and try to change object-oriented communication approaches, which are not only insensitive and dehumanizing, but also often lead to diminished self-image and angry, agitated responses on the part of the patient with cognitive impairment.

Assessment and evaluation of interactions and communication patterns, use of therapeutic communication techniques, and teaching others effective communication are important roles for gerontological nurses. The story in Figure 23-5 describes a nursing situation that one nurse experienced in caring for a patient with dementia who was being admitted to a nursing home. Written from the perspective of the nurse and his knowing the patient, the story provides insight into important nursing responses, such as person-centered care, therapeutic communication, and establishing meaningful relationships.

Common Care Concerns

Nutrition, ADLs, maintenance of health and function, safety, and caregiver needs and support are the major care concerns for patients, families, and staff who care for people with dementia. Mary Opal Wolanin, a gerontological nursing pioneer, suggested that nurses are not as interested in the neurofibrillary tangles in the brain as they are in trying to smooth out the environmental and relational tangles. The overriding goals in caring for older adults with dementia are to maintain function and prevent excess disability, structure the environment and relationships to maintain stability, compensate for the losses associated with the disease, and create a therapeutic milieu that nurtures the personhood of the individual and maintains quality of life. Two common care concerns are discussed in the remainder of this chapter—ADL care and wandering. Nutrition is discussed in Chapter 9 and caregiver needs and support in Chapter 20.

Providing Care for Activities of Daily Living. The losses associated with dementia interfere with the person's communication patterns and ability to understand and express thoughts and feelings. Perceptual disturbances and misinterpretations of reality contribute to fear and misunderstanding. People with dementia often struggle to understand the world and to make their needs known. Often, bathing and the provision of other ADL care such as dress-

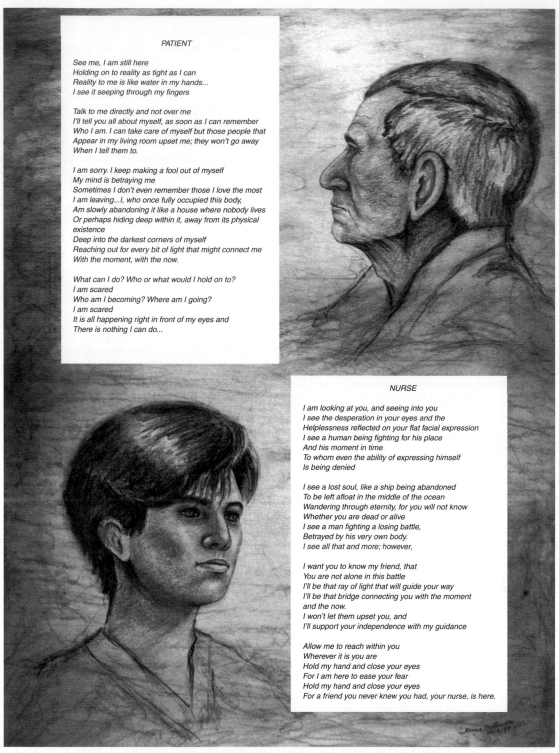

PATIENT

See me, I am still here
Holding on to reality as tight as I can
Reality to me is like water in my hands...
I see it seeping through my fingers

Talk to me directly and not over me
I'll tell you all about myself, as soon as I can remember
Who I am. I can take care of myself but those people that
Appear in my living room upset me; they won't go away
When I tell them to.

I am sorry. I keep making a fool out of myself
My mind is betraying me
Sometimes I don't even remember those I love the most
I am leaving...I, who once fully occupied this body,
Am slowly abandoning it like a house where nobody lives
Or perhaps hiding deep within it, away from its physical
existence
Deep into the darkest corners of myself
Reaching out for every bit of light that might connect me
With the moment, with the now.

What can I do? Who or what would I hold on to?
I am scared
Who am I becoming? Where am I going?
I am scared
It is all happening right in front of my eyes and
There is nothing I can do...

NURSE

I am looking at you, and seeing into you
I see the desperation in your eyes and the
Helplessness reflected on your flat facial expression
I see a human being fighting for his place
And his moment in time
To whom even the ability of expressing himself
Is being denied

I see a lost soul, like a ship being abandoned
To be left afloat in the middle of the ocean
Wandering through eternity, for you will not know
Whether you are dead or alive
I see a man fighting a losing battle,
Betrayed by his very own body.
I see all that and more; however,

I want you to know my friend, that
You are not alone in this battle
I'll be that ray of light that will guide your way
I'll be that bridge connecting you with the moment
and the now.
I won't let them upset you, and
I'll support your independence with my guidance

Allow me to reach within you
Wherever it is you are
Hold my hand and close your eyes
For I am here to ease your fear
Hold my hand and close your eyes
For a friend you never knew you had, your nurse, is here.

FIGURE 23-5 Nurse and person. (Copyright © 1998 by Jaime Castaneda, Lake Worth, Fla.)

ing, grooming, and toileting are the cause of much distress for both the person with dementia and the caregiver. Bathing and care for ADLs, particularly in nursing homes, can be perceived as an attack by persons with dementia who may respond by screaming or striking out. A rigid focus on tasks or institutional care routines, such as a shower three mornings each week, can contribute to the distress and precipitate distressing behaviors. Being touched or bathed against one's will violates the trust in caregiver relationships and can be considered a major affront (Rader and Barrick, 2000). The behaviors that may be exhibited by the person with dementia are not deliberate attacks on caregivers by a violent person. The message is, in the words of Rader and Barrick (2000, p. 49), "Please find another way to keep me clean, because the way you are doing it now is intolerable." To care effectively for older adults with dementia, nurses and other caregivers need to try to put themselves in the place of the person with dementia and try to see the world from his or her eyes. The following paragraph will illustrate:

> You are asleep in the chair at home when suddenly you are awakened by a person you have never seen before trying to undress you. Then he or she puts you naked into a hard, cold chair and wheels you down a hallway. Suddenly cold water hits you in the face and the person is touching your private areas. You don't understand why the person is trying to do this to you. You are embarrassed, frightened, cold, angry. You hit and scream at this person and try to get away.

It is very important to remember that behavior is an expression of needs, and as such, the focus needs to be on understanding what the person is trying to communicate through behavior. Family members and nurses caring for people with dementia must understand that they are the ones who must change their behavior, reactions, and approaches because the person with dementia cannot do this. In research in nursing homes, Rader and Barrick (2000) have provided comprehensive guidelines for bathing people with dementia in ways that are pleasurable and decrease distress. Asking the question "What is the easiest, most comfortable, least frightening way for me to clean the person right now?" guides the choice of interventions (Radder and Barrick, 2000, p. 42). Knowing the person's lifetime bathing routines and preferences; providing care only when the person is receptive; respecting refusals to participate in care; explaining all actions; realizing that a bath is not an essential intervention; encouraging self-care to the extent possible; making bathrooms and shower areas warm, comfortable, and safe; being attentive to pain and discomfort; and using alternative bathing methods such as a towel bath or sponge bath are some suggested responses. Box 23-17 presents a summary of some of these guidelines that both nurses and family caregivers may find helpful.

Wandering. Wandering is one of the most difficult management problems encountered in home and institutional settings. Wandering has been defined as purposeless walking that involves random movement and frequent changes in direction, pacing, or doing laps (Rowe, 2003). Wandering can lead to falls, elopement (leaving the home or facility), disturbances in care routines such as eating, and interference with the privacy of others (Algase et al., 2003). Wandering behavior may also result in people with dementia going outside and getting lost, a phenomenon studied by Rowe (2003). The Alzheimer's Association estimates that 60% of people with dementia will wander and become lost in the community at some point. Conclusions from Rowe's (2003) research, a retrospective review of records of Safe Return (a nationwide federally funded identification program of the Alzheimer's Association), advised that all people with dementia should be considered capable of becoming lost. Caregivers need to prevent people with dementia from leaving homes or care facilities unaccompanied, register the person in the Safe Return program, and have a plan of action in case the person does become lost.

Rowe also suggests that police must respond rapidly to requests for searches and the general public should be informed about how to recognize and assist people with dementia who may be lost (2003). Box 23-18 presents specific recommendations from this study.

The stimulus for wandering arises from many internal and external sources. Wandering can be considered a rhythm, intrinsically and extrinsically driven. People with dementia who wander may have more visual-spatial impairments, anxiety and depression, and a history of a prior active lifestyle. Agenda behaviors were identified and studied by Rader et al. (1985) and are defined as "the verbal and nonverbal planning actions that cognitively impaired persons use in an effort to fulfill their social, emotional, and physical needs (p. 196). Rader and colleagues proposed three factors that may contribute to wandering: fear caused by separation from people and environments with which the person was previously most connected and comfortable; frustration that develops when the agenda is thwarted by caregivers with a different agenda; and the need to be needed. The following excerpts about wandering from an article by Laurenhue (2001) provide a great deal of insight into this concern from the person's perspective:

> Wandering and restlessness is one of the by-products of Alzheimer's disease...When the darkness and emptiness fills my mind, it is totally terrifying...Thoughts increasingly haunt me. The only way I can break the cycle is to move (Davis, 1989, p. 96).
>
> Very often, I wander around looking for something which I know is very pertinent, but then after awhile I forget all about what it was I was looking for. When I'm wandering around, I'm trying to touch base with—anything, actually. If anything appeared I'd probably enjoy it, or look at it or examine it and wonder how it got there. I feel very foolish when I'm wandering around not knowing what I'm doing and I'm not always quite sure how to do any better. It's not easy to figure out what the heck I'm looking for (Henderson, 1998, p. 24).

Algase et al. (2003) described how the NDB model can be used to research, understand, and design interventions related to wandering. With this framework, predisposing background factors and proximal factors all play a role in wandering behavior. Wandering behaviors can be predicted through careful observation and knowing the person's patterns. For example, if the person with dementia starts wandering or trying to leave the home around dinnertime everyday, meaningful activities such as music, exercise, and refreshments can be provided at this time. Research suggests that wandering may be less likely to occur when the person is involved in social interaction. Environmental interventions such as camouflaging doorways, providing enclosed outdoor gardens and paths for walking, and electronic bracelets that activate alarms at exits are some examples. Box 23-19 presents suggestions for additional interventions. A guideline for approaches to prevent and manage wandering in the hospitalized older adult can be found at *www.hartfordign.org*. An evidence-based protocol

BOX 23-17 Guidelines for Bathing Persons with Dementia

- Speak calmly, slowly, facing the person, and using his or her name.
- Tell the person what you are doing at all times, and avoid surprises.
- Praise and reassure.
- Bathe the person before he or she is dressed for the day.
- Wash the most sensitive area (as defined by the person being bathed) last.
- Keep covered and warm.
- Minimize the number of moves during the bath or shower.
- Pat dry rather than rub to decrease discomfort.
- Medicate for pain before bathing if indicated.
- Keep room and water temperatures comfortable. Install an extra heater in the tub room so the air and water temperatures are not as disparate.
- Avoid background noises and conversations. Hang beach towels in the bathing room if there is a lot of "echo" from sounds.
- Wash hair last, be sure patient is well covered and warm, wet head with washcloths, use small amount of baby shampoo, and rinse using small amounts of water from a small pitcher or bowl, deflecting water from face and ears.
- Give the person a tub bath, shower, bed bath, sponge bath at sink, or towel bath, depending on preference of the resident. Assess the best time of day for the person's bath—usually when the resident is the most calm and does not have other activities or appointments challenging his or her stress threshold. Follow accustomed patterns for bathing (method, frequency, time of day).
- If the person is very resistive, postpone the bath, return when more receptive. Do not push or force. Bathing is rarely an emergency situation.
- Transfer residents with sufficient staff, proper techniques, and proper equipment. Do not use a shower chair to transfer the person to the bathing room. Replace tubs with hydraulic chair lifts with ones that use an easy-access side panel.
- Undress the person in the bathing room. As the person is undressed, cover each unclothed area with a bath blanket. If comforting, put the person in the tub with bath blankets or towels that cover the person and are raised only in the area needed to allow a hand and washcloth to do the washing.
- Run the water into the tub before the person enters the bathing room. Running water before bringing the person to the tub room not only keeps the tub room warm but

also controls unwanted noise and distraction. It also allows the caregiver and person to engage in conversation. Some people can tolerate 1 inch of water, and some are not bothered by 5 inches. Keep this and other likes and dislikes in the care plan.
- Have all equipment, linens, and clothing ready and organized before the person enters the bathing room to facilitate an organized and consistent bathing process.
- Allow the resident to feel the water before getting into the tub. Use reassuring phrases such as "This is nice" or "This feels good."
- Try some aromatherapy. Give the resident a choice between two. For example, allow the resident to smell the bath oils and ask, "Do you like the rose or herb scent?"
- Use a calm, unhurried approach. Have one consistent caregiver give the bath, explaining what will be done and asking the person if he or she is comfortable. Use reassuring words, especially when the person seems confused or fearful.
- Keep stimulation as singular and focused as possible. For example, two people should not bathe different parts of the body. If water is running, decrease or stop tactile stimulation.
- Encourage the resident to participate in the bath when possible. If the person has difficulty, try putting your hand over the person's hand while washing.
- Give the person a washcloth or shampoo bottle to hold during the bath, and encourage self-care to the extent possible.
- Placing a sock or pillowcase over the shower head decreases the force of the spray. Use only a hand-held shower to provide focused and controlled spraying.
- Use music to redirect and relax. Songs with which the caregiver and person can sing along can be helpful in giving the person control of the bath.
- Decorate the tub room in a homelike fashion. The tub room should look like a bathroom, not a laboratory. Encourage the staff to bring their personalities into the bathing routine. Pictures of children, pets, and familiar landscapes and objects are helpful for supporting engaging behaviors.
- "Seize the moment." If an accidental food spill soils the clothes, it may be the perfect time to change clothes in the tub room and suggest a bath. "As long as we're changing your clothes, let's freshen up, wash your face and hands, and soak your feet a while."

From Ebersole P et al: *Gerontological nursing and healthy aging*, ed 2, St Louis, 2005, Mosby. From Kovach CR, Meyer-Arnold EA. *Geriatr Nurs* 18(3):107-111, 1997; Rader J. *Alzheimer Care Q* 1(4):35-49, 2000.

for wandering (Futrell and Mellilo, 2002) can be found at *www.guidelines.gov*.

Environmental Alterations. Both home and institutional settings can be modified to be more supportive for people with dementia. Many nursing homes resemble little hospitals and can be cold, impersonal, and confusing places for people with dementia. The culture change movement to humanize and make nursing home environments more

person-centered and homelike is a welcome change to the more commonly found environments. Many facilities have established special care units (SCUs), designed for the needs of people with dementia. In nursing homes, space can be designed to be a more homelike environment with smaller areas more like rooms in a house. Family rooms, small-group dining rooms, kitchens on the unit where residents can participate in meal preparation and eat together, private spaces, natural light, elimination of noises such as overhead paging

BOX 23-18 Recommendations to Avoid People with Dementia Getting Lost

- Do not leave the person with dementia alone in the home.
- Secure the environment so that the person cannot leave by himself or herself while the caregiver is asleep or busy.
- If the person lives in a nursing facility, keep in supervised area; do frequent checks; use bed, chair, and door alarms and Wanderguard bracelets; identify potential wanderers by special arm bands; and disguise doorways.
- Place locks out of reach, hide keys, and lock windows.
- Consider motion detectors or home security systems that alert when doors are opened.
- Register the person in the Safe Return program of the Alzheimer's Association, and ensure that the person wears the Safe Return jewelry or clothing tags at all times.
- Let neighbors know that a person with dementia lives in the neighborhood.
- Prepare a search and rescue plan in case the person becomes lost.
- Keep copies of up-to-date photos ready for distribution to searchers, police, hospital, and the media.
- Conduct a search immediately if the person becomes lost.
- Call the local law enforcement agency and the Safe Return program to report the missing person.
- If the person is not found within 6 to 12 hours (or sooner depending on weather conditions), search any wooded areas or fields near where the person was last seen. People with dementia may not seek help or respond to calls and may try to hide from searchers; search in an organized manner with as many searchers as possible.

Adapted from Rowe M: People with dementia who become lost, *Am J Nurs* 103(7): 32-39, 2003.

BOX 23-19 Interventions for Wandering or Exiting Behaviors

- Face the person, and make direct eye contact (unless this is interpreted as threatening).
- Gently touch the person's arm, shoulders, back, or waist if he or she does not move away.
- Call the person by his or her formal name (e.g., Mr. Jones).
- Listen to what the person is communicating verbally and nonverbally; listen to the feelings being expressed.
- Identify the agenda, plan of action, and the emotional needs the agenda is expressing.
- Respond to the feelings expressed, staying calm.
- Repeat specific words or phrases, or state the need or emotion (e.g., "You need to go home, you're worried about your husband.").
- If such repetition fails to distract the person, accompany him or her and continue talking calmly, repeating phrases and the emotion you identify.
- Provide orienting information only if it calms the person. If it increases distress, stop talking about the present situations. Do not "correct" the person or belittle his or her agenda.
- At intervals, redirect the person toward the facility or the home by suggesting, "Let's walk this way now" or "I'm so tired, let's turn around."
- If orientation and redirection fail, continue to walk, allowing the person control but ensuring safety.
- Make sure you have a backup person, but he or she should stay out of eyesight of the person.
- Have someone call for help if you are unable to redirect. Usually the behavior is time limited because of the person's attention span and the security and trust between you and the person.

Adapted from Rader J et al: How to decrease wandering, a form of agenda behavior, *Geriatr Nurs* 6(4):196-199, 1985.

systems, spa-like bathrooms, and outdoor walking and sitting areas are some examples. There are many other ideas and descriptions of more appropriate designs for institutions (Eastman, 2001; Lindstrom, 2004). Hurley et al. (2004) developed a home/safety injury model that may help teach caregivers how to create safer homes. Resources to assist caregivers in both institutional and home settings in making environmental modifications to maintain function and ensure safety are listed in the Resources section at the end of this chapter and in Chapters 15 and 16.

Caregiving for Persons with Dementia

In the United States, more than 5 million households are providing care for someone with dementia. Predictions are that the prevalence of persons with dementia will increase 27% by 2020, 70% by 2030, and 300% by 2050. Of persons with dementia, 85% to 90% are cared for at home, and this care is particularly demanding (Robinson et al., 2005). The financial costs of caring for people with dementia is estimated to cost the nation $80 to $90 billion a year in both direct expenditures as well as indirect costs, such as lost productivity of the patients and family members (Dibartolo, 2002). Unless a cure is found, more people will become caregivers to persons

with dementia. These caregivers experience more adverse consequences than caregivers of those with other chronic illnesses and are more likely to experience depression and health problems than other caregivers (McCarty and Drebing, 2003; Robinson et al., 2005). Spousal caregivers comprise approximately 50% of all primary family caregivers. They are at most risk for adverse effects related to their own advanced age and the long duration of the illness (Dibartolo, 2002).

According to a recent Harris Poll conducted by the Alzheimer's Foundation of America (2006), 97% of the caregivers agreed that Alzheimer's disease is a life-changing event for the family, with 75% feeling overwhelmed by the pressures of caregiving. Factors that influence the stress of caregiving include grief over the multiple losses that occur, the physical demands and duration of caregiving (up to 20 years), and resource availability (Dibartolo, 2002). Behavioral symptoms, difficulties in providing ADL care, and communication problems have been found to be the best predictors of caregiver distress and care-receiver institutionalization (Farran et al, 2004).

Peterson (2006) suggests that grief is a major dimension of caregiving for persons with dementia, beginning on the day of diagnosis and continuing long after the death of the person. "Losses come in smaller steps such as the day the doctor told her that her husband should not drive, the moment when he asked her his daughter's name, and the most excruciating, his placement in residential care" (Peterson, 2006, p. 15). Often, caregivers do not recognize grief and do not seek help. Marwit and Meuser (2002) reported on the development of an inventory to assess grief in caregivers of persons with Alzheimer's disease, and it may be useful in both practice and research.

Most research has focused on caregiving in the late stages of dementia and on the "burden" of caregiving. Few studies have addressed the experience of caregiving in early-stage dementia; this is increasingly important as more people are being diagnosed early in the disease process. Many authors suggest that the "concept of burden alone does not adequately explain the complexities of caregiving for an older person with dementia" (Suwa, 2002, p. 5). Warmth, pleasure, comfort, spiritual growth, self-transcendence, and other positive dimensions of caregiving have also emerged in qualitative studies (Acton, 2002; Farran et al, 2004). In the study by the Alzheimer's Foundation of America (2006), 77% of survey participants reported that they have become stronger than they thought; 64% believed that they have become more compassionate as a result of caregiving; and 59% said they feel closer to the patient since they began caring for them. Further research is needed to help us understand how we can extend caring to both the caregiver and the person with dementia in ways that maintain person-

Human Needs and Wellness Diagnoses

Self-Actualization and Transcendence
(Seeking, Expanding, Spirituality, Fulfillment)
Seeks mind and spirit expansion
Recognizes limits of paranormal understanding
Seeks intellectual stimulation
Develops wisdom from experience

Self-Esteem and Self-Efficacy
(Image, Identity, Control, Capability)
Has feelings of pride and self-worth
Actively seeks to increase knowledge
Maintains strong sense of identity

Belonging and Attachment
(Love, Empathy, Affiliation)
Recognizes own personality idiosyncrasies
Accepts personality foibles in others
Conveys affection to intimates
Assumes appropriate role in relationships

Safety and Security
(Caution, Planning, Protections, Sensory Acuity)
Consciously exercises memory
Incorporates memory cues in life patterns as needed
Avoids situations that cause cognitive insecurity
Relies less on automatic behaviors and monitors actions for safety

Biological and Physiological Integrity
(Air, Fluids, Comfort, Activity, Nutrition, Elimination, Skin Integrity)
Attends to basic needs
Understands importance of these in maintaining cognitive function,
particularly aeration, extra activity, nutrition, and comfort

These are not all the possible wellness diagnoses that may be identified. The above are examples of nursing diagnoses that should be considered when planning care for the older adult.

hood, enhance relationships, promote quality of life, and balance the stresses with the joys (Haak, 2000). Additional information on caregiving is found in Chapter 20.

Nursing Roles in the Care of Persons with Dementia

Many of the interventions to prevent delirium and to care for people with cognitive impairment are achieved by applying the principles of good gerontological nursing care. An understanding of these principles and how to adapt responses and the environment to people with cognitive impairment will ensure the meeting of basic needs and enhance quality of care and quality of life. Some may seem like basic nursing, but they are often not practiced, leading to iatrogenesis, distress, and excess disability. Often these consequences are more problematic than the illnesses themselves. Our care, however well intentioned, must not increase disability. It must be based on knowledge and research to be considered best practice. We also have a responsibility to teach others about best practices.

The four roles of a successful caregiver for someone with dementia presented by Rader and Tornquist (1995) provide a framework for competent and compassionate care and promotion of healthy aging for older adults with cognitive impairment:

Magician role: To understand what the person is trying to communicate both verbally and nonverbally, we must be a magician who can use our magical abilities to see the world through the eyes, ears, and feelings of the person. We know how to use tricks to turn an individual's behavior around or prevent it from occurring and causing distress.

Detective role: The detective looks for clues and cues about what might be causing distress and how it might be changed. We have to investigate and know as much about the person as possible to be a good detective.

Carpenter role: By having a wide variety of tools and selecting the right tools for the job, we build individualized plans of care for each person.

CASE STUDY: Cognitive Impairment

William was 69 years old and had been a successful builder until his retirement from business 4 years ago. His wife, Caroline, of 30 years was a high school teacher. Their marriage had been minimally gratifying, but both enjoyed their work and had felt they led a full and satisfying life. They had no children but had developed a large social network over the years; most were friends who were in some way work related. Six months ago William began to seem restless; he was easily angered and embarrassed himself and his wife several times by being verbally abusive during a social function with their friends. William was also less careful about his grooming; because he had always been most meticulous about his appearance, his wife was quite alarmed that he seemed not to notice or care. After returning from one particularly exhausting vacation trip, William became enraged when he thought someone had stolen his wallet. He ignored his wife's efforts to calm him and became even angrier. Later his wife found his wallet in an inner suit jacket pocket. He ordinarily kept his wallet in the back pocket of his trousers. His wife began to feel anxious and frightened of him, though he had never physically abused her. She urged him to see the physician for a "general checkup" but was not surprised that he refused. She went to the physician for tranquilizers to quell her anxiety. He gave her a prescription for Prozac and sent her on her way. Her nurse-neighbor dropped by one day and found her in tears saying, "I just can't stand it anymore. William is not like himself. We used to have such fun and now he is angry all the time." As the nurse-neighbor, how would you help Caroline and William?

Based on the case study, develop a nursing care plan using the following procedure*:

- List William's comments that provide subjective data.
- List information that provides objective data.

- From these data, identify and state, using accepted format, two nursing diagnoses you determine are most significant to William at this time. List two of William's strengths that you have identified from data.
- Determine and state outcome criteria for each diagnosis. These must reflect some alleviation of the problem identified in the nursing diagnosis and must be stated in concrete and measurable terms.
- Plan and state one or more interventions for each diagnosed problem. Provide specific documentation of the source used to determine the appropriate intervention. Plan at least one intervention that incorporates William's existing strengths.
- Evaluate the success of the intervention. Interventions must correlate directly with the stated outcome criteria to measure the outcome success.

Critical Thinking Questions

1. Is there any evidence that cerebral cells may regenerate?
2. What memory aids might you suggest for a person who is complaining of memory problems?
3. What are some of the differences between delirium, dementia, and depression?
4. What nursing interventions will assist in preventing delirium in the hospitalized elder?
5. Identify several signs of early dementia.
6. How can Alzheimer's disease be diagnosed accurately?
7. Discuss some specific interventions to promote comfort during bathing for persons with dementia?
8. What type of communication techniques would be helpful in assisting with ADL activities for a person with dementia?
9. Discuss evidences of intact cognition or signs of dementia in elders you have known who are between ages 85 and 90 years.

---

* Students are advised to refer to their nursing diagnosis text and identify possible or potential problems.

Jester role: Many people with dementia retain their sense of humor and respond well to the appropriate use of humor. This does not mean making fun of but rather sharing laughter and fun. "Those who love their work and do it well employ good doses of humor as part of the care of others as well as for self-care" (Rader and Barrick, 2000, p. 42). The jester spreads joy, is creative, energizes, and lightens the burdens (Laurenhue, 2001; Rader and Barrick, 2000).

KEY CONCEPTS

- It has long been assumed that cognitive decline is a necessary concomitant of aging, but recent studies demonstrate the potential of the aging brain for regeneration.
- The distinctive cognitive capacities of older adults have hardly been investigated and are poorly understood.
- Age-associated memory impairment (AAMI) refers to memory loss that is considered normal in light of the person's age and educational level. Mild cognitive impairment (MCI) describes memory impairment beyond that which is believed to constitute normal aging but other aspects of cognitive functioning remain intact. MCI may be a precursor to Alzheimer's disease.
- Nurses need to advocate for thorough assessment of any elder who appears to be experiencing genuine cognitive decline and inability to function in important aspects of life.
- Delirium, sometimes referred to as an *acute confusional state,* is the result of physiological imbalances and may be caused by a variety of biological disturbances. Delirium is characterized by fluctuating levels of consciousness, sometimes in a diurnal pattern, and frequent misperceptions and illusions. It is often unrecognized and attributed to age or dementia. People with dementia are more susceptible to delirium. Knowledge of risk factors, preventive measures, and treatment of underlying medical problems is essential to prevent serious consequences.
- Medications and pain are frequently the causes of delirious states in older people.
- Irreversible dementias follow a pattern of inevitable decline accompanied by decreased intellectual function, personality changes, and impaired judgment. The most common of these is Alzheimer's disease.
- Alzheimer's disease has been the subject of enormous research in attempts to understand the causes. Genes, latent viruses, enzyme and neurotransmitter deficiencies, environmental toxins, and psychosocial stressors have all been implicated to some degree. Research is continuing in attempts to discover ways to protect against or halt the progress of the disease. There is no known cure although some medications seem to slow the progress of the dementia for a time.
- *Vascular dementia* refers to a group of heterogeneous disorders arising from cerebrovascular insufficiency or ischemic or hemorrhagic brain damage. VaD is the second most prevalent type of dementia in the United States and often co-exists with AD. The major subtypes of VaD include single strategic stroke, multiple infarcts, and subcortical small vessel disease. Subcortical small vessel disease is thought to be responsible for approximately two thirds of VaD cases and is more likely to lead to progressive dementia. Hypertension, cardiac disease, diabetes, smoking, alcoholism, and hyperlipidemia are additional risk factors for VaD. Prevention and treatment of risk factors are important.
- Assessment of cognitive impairment is complex. Nurses may do a cursory assessment with any number of brief mental status examinations and need to request more thorough assessment when there is an indication of dementia.
- Individuals with cognitive impairment respond best to calmness and patience, adaptations of communication techniques, and environments and relationships that enhance function, support limitations, ensure safety, and provide opportunities for a meaningful quality of life. Because cognitively impaired persons may be unable to express their feelings and needs in ways that are easily understood, the gerontological nurse must always try to understand the world from their perspective.

RESOURCES

Learning in Late Life
AARP's Directory of Centers for Older Learners
www.aarp.org

Elderhostel
www.elderhostel.org

Lifetime Education and Renewal Network (LEARN)
www.asaging.org/networks/learn/about.cfm

Cognitive Impairment
Websites
Accelerate Cure/Treatments for Alzheimer's Disease
www.act-ad.org

Alzheimer's Association
225 N. Michigan Ave., Floor 17
Chicago, IL 60601
(800) 272-3900
www.alz.org

Alzheimer's Caregiver Support Online
www.alzonline.net

Alzheimer's Disease Education and Referral Center
PO Box 8250
Silver Spring, MD 20907
(800) 438-4380
www.alzheimers.org

Alzheimer's Foundation
http:alzfnd.org

Alzheimer's Solutions
3122 Knorr St.
Philadelphia, PA 19149
(212) 624-2098
www.caregiving-solutions.com

*Films and Videos**
Alzheimer's disease: a multi-cultural perspective
Terra Nova Films
www.terranova.org

Alzheimer's disease: inside looking out
www.terranova.org

Bathing without a battle: personal care of individuals with dementia
www.bathingwithoutabattle.unc.edu

Beloved strangers: caring for a loved one with Alzheimer's disease
www.bathingwithoutabattle.unc.edu

Best friends
Discusses the innovative best friends approach to caring for older people with Alzheimer's disease and related dementias
Health Professions Press
www.healthpropress.com

Breakfast Club: enhancing the communication ability of Alzheimer's patients
Alzheimer's Association
www.alz.org

Communicating in Alzheimer's disease
Caregivers describe their challenges and solutions for communicating with the person with the disease
Alzheimer's Association
www.alz.org

Hoffman D: *Complaints of a dutiful daughter*, 1994
www.wmm.com

Interacting with Alzheimer's patients: tips for family and friends
Alzheimer's disease do's and dont's
Video Press
University of Maryland, School of Medicine, Baltimore
Also, Alzheimer's Association
www.alz.org

Recognizing and responding to emotion in persons with dementia
Alzheimer's Association
www.alz.org

Feature Films
Iris, 2001
The Notebook, 2004
Away from Her, 2007

---

*Many other films are available—see Alzheimer's Association website resources at *www.alz.org*.

REFERENCES

Acton G: Self-transcendent views and behaviors: exploring growth in caregivers of adults with dementia, *J Gerontol Nurs* 28(12):22-30, 2002.

Algase D et al: Wandering in long-term care, *Ann Long-Term Care* 11(1):33-29, 2003.

Alzheimer's Association: *African-Americans and Alzheimer's disease: The silent epidemic*, 2006 (website): *www.alz.org*. Accessed January 20, 2007.

Alzheimer's Association: *Fact sheet: Experimental Alzheimer's drugs targeting beta-amyloid and the "amyloid hypothesis,"* 2006 (website): *www.alz.org*. Accessed January 20, 2007.

Alzheimer's Foundation of America: *I CAN: Investigating caregivers' attitudes and needs*, 2006 (website): *www.alzfdn.org*. Accessed January 20, 2007.

American Geriatrics Society: Guidelines abstracted from the American Academy of Neurology's dementia guidelines for early detection, diagnosis, and management of dementia, 2001 (website): *www.americangeriatrics.org/products/positionpapers/aan_dementia.shtml*. Accessed January 20, 2007.

American Medical Directors Association (AMDA): *Dementia*, 2005 (website): *www.guidelines.gov*.

American Psychiatric Association: *Diagnostic and statistical manual of mental disorders*, DSM-IV-TR, Washington, DC, 2000, The Association.

Apathy may be harbinger of early cognitive decline, *CNS Senior Care* 5(2):1, 2006.

Bagley M: *Hearing changes in aging people with mental retardation*, 2002. (website): *www.thearc.org/faqs/hearinginaging*.

Balas M et al: Delirium doulas: an innovative approach to enhance care for critically ill older adults, *Crit Care Nurse* 24:34-46, 2004.

Bastings A: Reading the story behind the story: context and content in stories by people with dementia, *Generations* 27:25-29, 2003.

Bastings A: Arts in dementia care: "This is not the end...it's the end of this chapter," *Generations* 30(1):16-20, 2006.

Batchelor N: Normal aging changes. In Luggen AS, Meiner S, editors: *NGNA core curriculum for gerontological nurses*, ed 2, St Louis, 2001, Mosby.

Beck CT: Nursing students' experience caring for cognitively impaired elderly people, *J Adv Nurs* 23(5):992-998, 1996.

Beers MH, Berkow R: *Merck manual of geriatrics*, ed 3, Whitehouse Station, NJ, 2000, Merck Research Laboratories.

Bell V, Troxel D: Spirituality and the person with dementia: a view from the field, *Alzheimer's Care Q* 2(2):31-45, 2001.

Bhidayasiri R: When it's not AD: atypical dementing illnesses, Part 1: *CNS Senior Care* 5(2):1, 17, 2006.

Bradley E et al: After adoption: sustaining the innovation: a case study of disseminating the Hospital Elder Life Program, *J Am Geriatr Soc* 53(9):1455-1461, 2005.

Brown A: Aging with developmental disability, *Women's Health Issues*, 2002. (website): *www.thearc.org/faws/whealth*.

Buckwalter K et al: Shining through: the humor and individuality of persons with Alzheimer's disease, *J Gerontol Nurs* 21(11):11-16, 1995.

Buettner L, Kolanowski A: Practice guidelines for recreation therapy in the care of persons with dementia, *Geriatr Nurs* 24(1):18-25, 2003.

Bunton D: Normal changes with aging. In Maas ML et al, editors: *Nursing care of older adults: diagnoses, outcomes, and interventions*, St Louis, 2001, Mosby.

Butler R et al: Maintaining cognitive health in an ageing society, *J Royal Soc Prom Health* 124(3):119-121, 2004.

Camp C: *Montessori-based activities for persons with dementia*, Baltimore, Md, 1999, Health Professions Press.

Camp C: *Montessori-based activities for persons with dementia*, Baltimore, Md, 2001, Health Professions Press.

Camp C, Skrajner J: Resident-assisted Montessori programming (RAMP): training persons with dementia to serve as activity group leaders, *Gerontologist* 44(3):426-431, 2004.

Clark DJ: Older adults living through and with their computers, *Comput Inform Nurs* 20(3):117-124, 2002.

Cohen-Mansfield J: Nonpharmacological management of behavioral problems in persons with dementia: the TREA model, *Alzheimer Care Q* 1(4):22-34, 2000.

Crowley SL: Aging brain's staying power, *AARP Bulletin* 37(4):1, 1996.

Davis R: *My journey into Alzheimer's disease*, Wheaton, Ill, 1989, Tyndale House Publishers.

DeYoung S et al: Decreasing aggressive, agitated, or disruptive behavior participation in a behavior management unit, *J Gerontol Nurs* 28(6):22-30, 2003.

Dibartolo M: Exploring self-efficacy and hardiness in spousal caregivers of individuals with dementia, *J Gerontol Nurs* 28(4):24-33, 2002.

Doody RS et al: Practice parameter (an evidence based review): report of the quality standards subcommittee of the American Academy of Neurology, *Neurology* 56(9):1154-1166, 2001.

Dreger V, Tremback T: Optimize patient health by treating health literacy and language barriers, *AORN J* 75(2):280-285, 2002.

Eastman P: Environmental therapy aids Alzheimer's patients, *Caring for the Ages* 2(9):1, 18, 2001.

Ely EW et al: Evaluation of delirium in critically ill patients: validation of the Confusion Assessment Method for the intensive care unit (CAM-ICU), *Crit Care Med* 29(7):1370-1379, 2001.

Farran C et al: Caring for self while caring for others: the two-track life of coping with Alzheimer's disease, *J Gerontol Nurs* 30(5):38-46, 2004.

Fazio S: Person-centered language is an essential part of person-centered care, *Alzheimer Care Q* 2(2):87-90, 2001.

Fick D et al: Delirium superimposed on dementia in a community-dwelling managed care population: a 3-year retrospective study of occurrence, costs, and utilization, *J Gerontol A Biol Sci Med Sci* 60A(6):748-753, 2005.

Fick D, Mion L (2005). *Assessing delirium in persons with dementia*, Geriatric Nursing Hartford Foundation Try This Dementia Series, 2005. (website): *www.hartfordign.org/resources/education/tryThis.html.*

Fladd D: Subcortical vascular dementia, *Geriatr Nurs* 26(2):117-121, 2005.

Flaherty JH, Morley JE: A call to improve current standards of care, *J Am Geriatr Soc* 51(7):341-343, 2004.

Flaherty JH et al: A model for managing delirious older inpatients, *J Am Geriatr Soc* 51(7):1031-1035, 2003.

Flax M: *Aging with developmental disabilities: changes in vision*, 2002. (website): *www.thearc.org/faqs/visfact.*

Folstein MF et al: *Mini-mental state: a practical method for grading the cognitive status of patients for the clinician*, Oxford, 1975, Pergamon.

Foreman M et al: Assessing cognitive function. In Mezey M et al, editors: *Geriatric nursing protocols for best practice*, New York, 2003, Springer.

Foreman MD et al: Delirium in elderly patients: an overview of the state of the science, *J Gerontol Nurs* 27(4):12-20, 2001.

Futrell M, Mellilo KD: *An evidence based protocol for wandering*, 2002. (website): *www.guidelines.gov.*

Gallo JJ et al: *Handbook of geriatric assessment*, ed 3, Boston, 2003, Jones & Bartlett.

Gillette-Guyonnet S et al: Outcome of Alzheimer's disease: potential impact of cholinesterase inhibitors, *J Gerontol A Biol Sci Med Sci* 61A(5):516-520, 2006.

Haak N: One joy will scatter a hundred griefs, *Alzheimer Care Q* 1(4):1-3, 2000.

Hahn EA et al: The talking touchscreen: a new approach to outcomes assessment in low literacy, *Psychooncology* 13(2):86-95, 2004.

Hall GR: Caring for people with Alzheimer's disease using the conceptual model of progressively lowered stress threshold in the clinical setting, *Nurs Clin North Am* 29(1):129-141, 1994.

Hall GR, Buckwalter KC: Progressively lowered stress threshold: a conceptual model for care of adults with Alzheimer's disease, *Arch Psychiatr Nurs* 1(6):399-406, 1987.

Ham RJ: Dementias (and Delirium). In Ham RJ et al, editors: *Primary care geriatrics*, St Louis, 2002, Mosby.

Hargrave R: Caregivers of African-American elderly with dementia: a review and analysis, *Ann Long-Term Care* 14(10):36-40, 2006.

Henderson C: *Partial view: an Alzheimer's journal*, Dallas, 1998, Southern Methodist Press.

Hendryx-Bedalov P: Alzheimer's dementia: coping with communication decline, *J Gerontol Nurs* 26(8):151-155, 2000.

Hooyman N, Kiyak H: *Social gerontology*, ed 7, Boston, 2005, Pearson.

Hurley A et al: Promoting safer home environments for persons with Alzheimer's disease, *J Gerontol Nurs* 30(6):43-51, 2004.

Hustey F, Meldon S: The prevalence and documentation of impaired mental status in elderly emergency department patients, *Ann Intern Med* 39:248-253, 2002.

Inouye SK et al: Clarifying confusion: the confusion assessment: a new method for detection of delirium, *Ann Intern Med* 113(12):941-948, 1990.

Inouye SK et al: A multicomponent intervention to prevent delirium in hospitalized older patients, *N Engl J Med* 340(9):669-676, 1999.

Inouye SK et al: Nurses' recognition of delirium and its symptoms: comparison of nurse and researchers ratings, *Arch Intern Med* 161(20):2467-2473, 2001.

Irving K, Foreman M: Delirium, nursing practice and the future, *Int J Older People Nurs* 1:121-127, 2006.

Kalisvaart K et al: Haloperidol prophylaxis for elderly hip-surgery patients at risk for delirium: a randomized placebo-controlled study, *J Am Geriatr Soc* 53(10):1658-1666, 2005.

Keane WL: The patient's perspective: the Alzheimer's Association, *Alzheimer Dis Assoc Disord* 8(suppl 3):151-155, 1994.

Killick J: "What are we like here?" Eliciting experiences of people with dementia, *Generations* 13(3):46-49, 1999.

Kitwood T: *Dementia reconsidered: the person comes first*, Bristol, Pa, 1999, Open University Press.

Knapp M et al: Cognitive stimulation therapy for people with dementia: cost-effectiveness analysis, *Br J Psychiatry* 188:574-580, 2006.

Knopman DS et al: Practice parameter: diagnosis of dementia (an evidence-based review): report of the Quality Standards Subcommittee on the American Academy of Neurology, *Neurology* 56(9):1143-1153, 2001.

Kolanowski AM: An overview of the Need-Driven Dementia-Compromised Behavior Model, *J Gerontol Nurs* 25(9):7-9, 1999.

Kovach C et al: Behaviors of nursing home residents with dementia: examining nurse responses, *J Gerontol Nurs* 32(6):13-21, 2006a.

Kovach C et al: Effects of the serial trial intervention on discomfort and behavior of nursing home residents with dementia, *Am J Alzheimers Dis Other Demen* 21(5):147-155, 2006b.

Laurenhue K: Each person's journey is unique, *Alzheimer Care Q* 2(2):79-83, 2001.

Lindstrom A: Designer's challenge, *Caring for the Ages* 5(4):1, 16, 18, 27, 2004.

Livingston G et al: Systematic review of psychological approaches to the management of neuropsychiatric symptoms of dementia, *Am J Psychiatry* 162:1996-2021, 2005.

Lyketsos C et al: Position statement of the American Association Geriatric Psychiatry regarding care for persons with dementia resulting from Alzheimer's disease, *Am J Geriatr Psychiatry* 14:561-573, 2006.

Marcantonio ER et al: Delirium symptoms in post-acute care: prevalent, persistent, and associated with poor functional recovery, *J Am Geriatr Soc* 51:523-532, 2003.

Marwit S, Meuser T: Development and initial validation of an inventory to assess grief in caregivers of persons with Alzheimer's disease, *Gerontologist* 42(6):751-765, 2002.

McCarty E, Drebing C: Exploring professional caregivers' perceptions: balancing self-care with care for patients with Alzheimer's disease, *J Gerontol Nurs* 29(9):42-48, 2003.

McCloskey R: Caring for patients with dementia in an acute care environment, *Geriatr Nurs* 25(3):139-144, 2004.

McCusker J et al: Delirium in older medical inpatients and subsequent cognitive and functional status: a prospective study, *Can Med Assoc J* 165:575-583, 2001.

McDougall G et al: Aging memory self-efficacy: elders share their thoughts and experience, *Geriatr Nurs* 24(3):162-168, 2003.

Millisen K et al: Documentation of delirium in elderly patients with hip fracture, *J Gerontol Nurs* 28(11):23-29, 2002.

Moore T, Hollett J: Giving voice to persons living with dementia: the researcher's opportunities and challenges, *Nurs Sci Q* 16:164-167, 2003.

Morrison R et al: Relationship between pain and opioid analgesics on the development of delirium following hip fracture, *J Gerontol A Biol Sci Med Sci* 58:M76-81, 2003.

National Institutes of Health: *Memory loss,* 2002. (website): *www.nlm.nih.gov/medlineplus/ency/article/003257.htm.*

Neary S, Mahoney D: Dementia caregiving: the experiences of Hispanic/Latino caregivers, *J Transcult Nurs* 16(2):163-170, 2005.

Neelon VJ et al: The NEECHAM confusion scale: construction, validation and clinical testing, *Nurs Res* 45(6):324-330, 1996.

Ortigara A: Understanding the language of behaviors, *Alzheimer Care Q* 1(4):89-92, 2000.

Peterson D. Grief and dementia, *Aging Today,* May-June, 5,13, 2006.

Peterson R: MCI as a useful clinical concept, *Geriatric Times* 5(1), 2004. (website): *www.geriatrictimes.com/g040215.html.*

Pulsford D: Therapeutic activities for people with dementia—what, why (and why not)? *J Adv Nurs* 26(4):704-709, 1997.

Rader J, Barrick A: Ways that work: bathing without a battle, *Alzheimer Care Q* 1(4):35-49, 2000.

Rader J, Tornquist E: *Individualized dementia care,* New York, 1995, Springer.

Rader J et al: How to decrease wandering, a form of agenda behavior, *Geriatr Nurs* 6(4):196-199, 1985.

Rapp C et al: Acute confusion/delirium protocol, *J Gerontol Nurs* 27(4):21-33, 2001.

Registered Nurses Association of Ontario (RNAO): *Caregiving strategies for older adults with delirium, dementia and depression,* Toronto (ON), 2004. (website): *www.guidelines.gov.*

Richards K et al: Deriving interventions for challenging behaviors from the need-driven dementia-compromised behavior model, *Alzheimer Care Q* 1(4):62-76, 2000.

Rigney T: Delirium in the hospitalized elder and recommendations for practice, *Geriatr Nurs* 27(3):151-157, 2006.

Robinson K et al: Response by Robinson, Buckwalter, and Reed, *West J Nurs Res* 27(20):145-147, 2005.

Rowe MA: People with dementia who become lost, *Am J Nurs* 103(7):32-39, 2003.

Rubin FH et al: Replicating the Hospital Elder Life Program in a community hospital and demonstrating effectiveness using quality improvement methodology, *J Am Geriatr Soc* 54(6):969-974, 2006.

Sanders AB: Missed delirium in older emergency department patients: a quality-of-care problem, *Ann Emerg Med* 39(3):338-341, 2002.

Schneider LS et al: Effectiveness of atypical antipsychotic drugs in patients with Alzheimer's disease, *N Engl J Med* 355(15):1525-1538, 2006.

Sifton C: Life is what happens while we are making plans, *Alzheimer Care Q* 2(2):iv-vii, 2001.

Smith M, Buckwalter K: Behaviors associated with dementia, *Am J Nurs* 105(7):40-52, 2005.

Snyder L: The lived experience of Alzheimer's—understanding the feelings and subjective accounts of persons with the disease, *Alzheimer Care Q* 2(2):8-22, 2001.

Solomon P, Murphy C: Should we screen for Alzheimer's disease? A review of the evidence for and against screening for Alzheimer's disease in primary care practice, *Geriatrics* 60(11):26-29, 2006.

Speciale A et al: Staff training and use of specific protocols for delirium management, *J Am Geriatr Soc* 53(8):1445-1446, 2005.

Sugarman RA: Structure and function of the neurologic system. In McCance KL, Huether SE, editors: *Pathophysiology: the biologic basis for disease in adults and children,* ed 4, St Louis, 2002, Mosby.

Suwa S: Assessment scale for caregiver experience with dementia, *J Gerontol Nurs* 28(12):5-12, 2002.

Talerico K, Evans L: Making sense of aggressive/protective behaviors in persons with dementia, *Alzheimer Care Q* 1(4):77-88, 2000.

Tappen RM et al: Communicating with individuals with Alzheimer's disease: examination of recommended strategies, *Arch Psychiatr Nurs* 11(5):249-256, 1997.

Tappen RM et al: Persistence of self in advanced Alzheimer's disease, *Image J Nurs Sch* 31(2):121-125, 1999.

Teri L et al: Exercise plus behavioral management in patients with Alzheimer's disease, *JAMA* 290(15):2015-2022, 2003.

Touhy T: Dementia, personhood and nursing: learning from a nursing situation, *Nurs Sci Q* 17(1):43-49, 2004.

Truman B, Ely EW: Monitoring delirium in critically ill patients: using the Confusion Assessment Method for the intensive care unit, *Crit Care Nurs* 23(2):25-36, 2003.

Volicer L, Mahoney D: Are nursing home residents with dementia aggressive? *Gerontologist* 42:875-876, 2002.

Warner J, Butler R: *Alzheimer's disease: clinical evidence number 6,* London, 2001, BMJ Publishers.

Williams-Burgess C, Tappen R: Can we create a therapeutic relationship with nursing home residents in later stages of AD? *J Psychosoc Nurs* 37(3): 28-35, 1999.

Wilson F et al: Literacy, readability and cultural barriers: critical factors to consider when educating older African Americans about anticoagulant therapy, *J Clin Nurs* 12(2):275-282, 2003.

Wolanin MO, Phillips LR: *Confusion: prevention and care,* St Louis, 1981, Mosby.

Woods B: Dementia challenges assumptions about what it means to be a person, *Generations* 13(3): 39, 1999.

CHAPTER 24

Stress, Crises, and Health in Aging

Theris A. Touhy

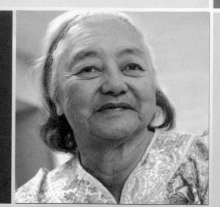

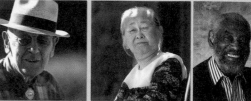

A STUDENT SPEAKS

My grandmother told me that every day should be an adventure. It isn't enough I have to worry about school, gang fights, gaining weight, and everything else. Now I have to worry about something happening to her! She travels all the time.

Ashley, age 15

AN ELDER SPEAKS

You know, I'm 83 years old! I've seen so many changes in my lifetime but the world seems such a dangerous place now. I worry so about my grandchildren and the things they must deal with in the future.

Sarah, age 83

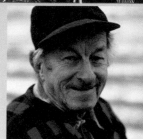

LEARNING OBJECTIVES

On completion of this chapter, the reader will be able to:

1. Identify several aspects of stress.
2. Relate several stressors that are likely to occur in late life.
3. Recognize physiological responses to stress.
4. Discuss common reactions to crises.
5. Discuss coping styles and methods of resolving stress and crises.
6. Describe several methods of restoring a sense of control.
7. Discuss strategies for crisis intervention that gerontological nurses can use with older adults.
8. Explain the healthful aspects of resolving stress and crisis.

STRESS

Stress is a given in any complex society. Stress is any event or situation that brings about bodily or mental tension. Without stress there would likely be little motivation in living other than filling most basic needs. Perhaps many of the stressors we subject ourselves to are unnecessary, but these are highly individual matters. Some people thrive on high levels of stress; others are depleted by it. This chapter discusses the ability of individuals to cope with stress and crises and the mechanisms that translate these into illness or healthy adaptations. The focus is on stress and crises and the events that are probable in the process of growing old and that may create disruptions in daily life that drain one's inner resources or require the development of new and unfamiliar coping strategies. Post-traumatic stress disorder, a more intense response to major life stressors, is discussed in

Chapter 25. As a society, we are experiencing nonspecific stressors that are unpredictable and uncontrollable and produce a constant level of anxiety and insecurity. However, it is more intense for some individuals than others (depending to a large extent on their earlier life experiences). Becoming alert to evidences of decompensation and helping individuals regain equilibrium on a healthier level are the goals of this chapter.

Types of Stressors

Acute Stress. Acute stress is seldom productive in that it is an internal state perceived as a threat to self. A stress response exists whenever there is a discrepancy between what the individual expects and that which requires change or recognition of uncertainty. Healthy stress levels motivate one toward growth, whereas a stress overload diminishes one's ability to cope effectively. Stress may arise from exter-

Special thanks to Priscilla Ebersole, the previous edition contributor, for her content contributions to this chapter.

nal events and situations or inner dictates. Most people recognize visible manifestations of acute stress such as increased body movement or excessive talking, irritability, sweaty or clammy hands, insomnia, and accelerated heart rate. Manifestations of acute stress may be more subtle in frail elders (e.g., wringing of the hands, picking at bed linens, behavior disturbances, memory impairment).

Proximal Stressors. Proximal stressors are those that are in the present and that require prompt action and inner resources to avert crises. Proximal stressors are often acutely uncomfortable, are pronounced, and require immediate adaptive energy daily for a brief time. The effects of these are mitigated by personality, available resources, environmental situation, contextual issues, and presence of chronic stressors. The number and frequency of stressors experienced in a given period must be considered.

Distal Stressors. Distal stressors have "gone underground," and the individual may be unaware of their presence. They are usually chronic and sometimes imbedded in personality. These are likely to be attenuated as current demands fluctuate as some taxing situations are resolved.

Chronic Stressors. Chronic stressors tend to be those categorized as constant or remote events and are contextual, such as a nongratifying marriage, childhood scars, or inability to carry out desired activities. For elders, contextual issues often involve a living situation that produces constant discomfort and dismay, functional disabilities, enduring chronic illnesses and pain, abusive caregivers, generally poor health, and internalized ageism. Inability to manage activities of daily living (ADLs) is a major and ongoing stress factor for older persons. Anxiety responses and chronic disorders may erupt during an increase in stressful or worrisome events.

Chronic stress is likely to activate depression, and this creates physiological changes that can result in illness and further exacerbate stress. This cyclic process may be the source of numerous illnesses. Perhaps some of the aging process itself is a result of a lifetime of numerous stresses and adaptive demands; essentially, the body runs out of energy.

Hassles. Hassles are the small daily events—everyday stressors that are seldom given much thought. Hassles are generally minor harassments. These include everyday irritants in daily life involving home maintenance, transportation, balancing checkbooks, finances, waiting in lines for goods or services, or waiting on hold during phone calls. An overload of daily hassles may adversely affect well-being and health status even more than major life disruptions. Home maintenance and environmental and social hassles are particularly onerous for older people who have depleted energies.

In combination with major stressful life events, hassles create psychological and sometimes physiological problems.

Gerontologists seriously consider the impact of hassles on stress levels, coping energy, and style of coping. It may be useful to keep a diary of daily events because many individuals are unaware of small hassles; the diary may help identify irritating problems and patterns that are readily subject to solution. Stetson (1997) uses diaries to assist individuals to identify self-healing activities in which they select one hassle they wish to modify and then develop a concrete plan to accomplish that with weekly, measurable goals.

Worry. In a comparison of worries between younger and older adults, results indicated that no significant differences in overall worry existed between the groups. However, older people worried more about health, family concerns, and world issues than did younger adults in the sample. Fakouri and Lyon (2005) reported similar results in a study of the relationship between worry and perceived health and life satisfaction in a group of community-dwelling older people. In this sample, reports of worry were relatively low, with the 85- to 89-year-old participants reporting the least amount of worry. The authors hypothesize that "worry may actually diminish with advancing age because of a decrease in future extension" (p. 22). Worry was associated with lower life satisfaction and negative emotions in this study. Asking older people about their worries and how they affect well-being may be an important part of nursing assessment. Powers and colleagues (1992) developed a worry scale that may assist the elderly more specifically appraise their worries (Figure 24-1).

Stressors Experienced in the Process of Aging. Some stressors that are common to older people are listed in Box 24-1. The narrowing range of biopsychosocial homeostatic resilience and changing environmental needs as one ages may produce a stress overload that can occur unexpectedly. Among older adults, stress may appear as a cognitive impairment that will be alleviated as the stress is reduced to the parameters of the individual's adaptability.

Stress tolerance is variable and based on current and ongoing stressors. For example, if an elder has lost a significant person in the previous year, the grief may be manageable. If he or she has lost a significant person and developed painful, chronic health problems, the consequences may be quite different and can be highly stressful.

Assessment of Stress Levels

Assessing stress level is a complex issue with many variables, both personal and environmental. The confluence of daily hassles; distal, chronic, and proximal stressors; worries; and functional capacities all create a stress load. Though many life event stress evaluation scales have been developed, none that exist today can measure age variances as well as these other factors. These scales can be used as tools to focus discussion of the various events and to suggest other factors that may be creating stress. Adolph Meyer's seminal concept (1951) of evaluating numerous strands in a lifeline perspective is likely to be useful. A discussion of the clustering of

Instructions: Below is a list of problems that often concern many Americans. Please read each one carefully. After you have done so, please fill in one of the spaces to the right with a check that describes how much that problem worries you. Make only one check mark for each item.

THINGS THAT WORRY ME...

	Never	Rarely (1-2 times per month)	Sometimes (1-2 times per week)	Often (1-2 times a day)	Much of the time (more than 2 times a day)

Finances

1. that I'll lose my home
2. that I won't be able to pay for the necessities of life (such as food, clothing, or medicine)
3. that I won't be able to support myself independently
4. that I won't be able to enjoy the "good things" in life (such as travel, recreation, entertainment)
5. that I won't be able to help my children financially

Health

6. that my eyesight or hearing will get worse
7. that I'll lose control of my bladder or kidneys
8. that I won't be able to remember important things
9. that I won't be able to get around by myself
10. that I won't be able to enjoy my food
11. that I'll have to be taken care of by my family
12. that I'll have to be taken care of by strangers
13. that I won't be able to take care of my spouse
14. that I'll have to go to a nursing home or hospital
15. that I won't be able to sleep at night
16. that I may have a serious illness or accident
17. that my spouse or a close family member may have a serious illness or accident
18. that I won't be able to enjoy sex
19. that my reflexes will slow down
20. that I won't be able to make decisions
21. that I won't be able to drive a car
22. that I'll have to use a mechanical aid (such as a hearing aid, bifocals, a cane)

Social conditions

23. that I'll look "old"
24. that people will think of me as unattractive
25. that no one will want to be around me
26. that no one will love me anymore
27. that I'll be a burden to my loved ones
28. that I won't be able to visit my family and friends
29. that I may be attacked by muggers or robbers on the streets
30. that my home may be broken into and vandalized
31. that no one will come to my aid if I need it
32. that my friends and family won't visit me
33. that my friends and family will die
34. that I'll get depressed
35. that I'll have serious psychological problems

Other worries

FIGURE 24-1 The Worry Scale. (From Powers CB et al: Age differences and correlates of worrying in young and elderly adults, *Gerontologist* 32[1]:82, 1992. Copyright © The Gerontological Society of America. Reproduced by permission of the publisher.)

events and situations at various times can be very revealing. Figure 24-2 can be used as a model.

Stress Management

The effects of stress on aging and adaptation have been researched extensively in the past 25 years. Researchers concerned with the effects of stress on the lives of elders have examined many moderating variables and have concluded that cognitive style, coping strategies, social skills, personal efficacy, support systems, and personality are all significant to stress management. Factors that influence one's ability to manage stress are presented in Box 24-2.

CRISES

Crises constitute a major temporary disruption in coping capacity, whereas stress involves ineffectual or effectual coping and may be sustained over long periods. The term *crisis* was first introduced by Erich Lindemann (1944) after the Cocoanut Grove fire. It is defined as the lack of defense or coping mechanisms to deal with sudden and unexpected intrusions into a life situation that was previously experienced as satisfactory. A distinction between crisis and stress is related to time. Crises occur abruptly, are time limited, and are always resolved as an individual initiates some action and reestablishes equilibrium on a higher or lower level of personal organization.

Any stressors that occur in the lives of older people may actually be experienced as a crisis if the event occurs abruptly, is unanticipated, or requires skills or resources the

---

BOX 24-1   Stressors in Late Life

- Incompetency proceedings
- Inheritance conflicts
- Abandonment: fear of dying alone/not being found/ painful death
- Hospitalization
- Institutionalization
- Separation from personal physician
- Sensory changes (vision and hearing)
- Housing and home maintenance
- Lack of protection when frail and vulnerable
- Limited mobility and lack of transportation
- Unnamed concerns about the future
- Functional impairment, inability to be independent in activities of daily living (ADLs)
- Fear of dementia
- Social losses, loss of driver's license
- Acute and chronic pain
- Medications
- Abuse and neglect
- Loss of pet
- Rent increases or increases in other living expenses
- Caregiving of a partner with dementia
- Illness
- Relocation
- Loss of children
- Loss of cohorts
- Loss of siblings
- Loss of friends
- Dispersal of significant belongings

BOX 24-2   Factors Influencing Ability to Manage Stress

- Health and fitness
- A sense of control over events
- Awareness of self and others
- Patience and tolerance
- Resilience
- Hardiness
- Social support
- Personal stability zones or a strong sense of self
- Beliefs and values

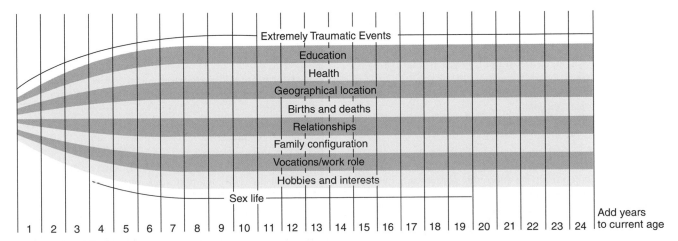

FIGURE 24-2 Life chart.

elder does not possess. Some individuals have developed, through a lifetime of coping with stress, a tremendous stress tolerance, whereas others will be thrown into crisis by changes in their life with which they feel unable to cope. The critical factor is the personal perception of the event.

Long ago, Robert Butler (1967), the first director of the Institute on Aging, identified four factors that significantly affect individual perception of crisis events in old age:

1. **Extrinsic factors.** The social or personal impact of losses and the degree of lifestyle reorganization required to adapt are significant in crisis resolution.
2. **Intrinsic factors.** Personality traits such as a pessimistic or optimistic outlook on life affect interpretation of events.
3. **Reserve capacity.** Depletion as a result of physical disabilities, chronic illness or stress, and brain damage may predispose one to experience small irritations as crises.
4. **Past history.** Capacity for surviving, adapting, and maintaining a positive self-view throughout life will influence ability to tolerate crises and stress in old age.

These factors are still relevant in identifying the various influences on crisis impact for older people. Important to remember is the great individual variability in definition of a crisis event. For some, the loss of a pet canary is a crisis; others accept the loss of a good friend with grief but without personal disorganization.

The disequilibrium of crises usually does not remain for more than a few weeks, thought to be about 6 weeks, but this is not necessarily true of older persons; this is an area that deserves investigation. Ultimately, crises are expressed in higher levels of coping or deterioration in efficacy and feelings of failure. A crisis event for one person may be perceived only as a stressor by another.

Major crises events for elders have always been the death of children, spouse, and siblings. Now the undercurrent of terrorizing events made boldly evident to the entire population has resulted in amplified reactions to all other crises and sometimes intense reactivation of early traumatic life experiences. Crises common to older people are listed in Box 24-3.

BOX 24-3   Crises Common in Late Life

- Abrupt internal and external body changes and illnesses
- Other-oriented concerns: children, grandchildren, spouse, or partner
- Loss of significant people
- Acute discomfort and pain
- Breach in significant relationships
- Fires, thefts
- Injuries, falls
- Aphasia, abrupt loss after stroke
- Major unexpected drain on economic resources; for example, house repair, illness
- Abrupt changes in living arrangements, especially without warning, to a new location, home, apartment, room, or institution
- Death of roommates in institutions

Relocation

One of the major stressors, and often a crisis for both the older person and his or her family, is relocation. In light of the strong instinctual nature of territorial needs, it is not surprising that much attention has been given to the crisis of relocation. Regardless of the type of move and its desirability or undesirability, some degree of stress will be experienced. Relocation to a long-term care facility is identified as one of the most stressful and one that many older people fear. With each move, if the adaptation is to be satisfying, one must begin to claim personal space by somehow placing one's stamp of individuality on the new surroundings. Because the older adult is particularly likely to move or be moved, the subject of relocation is significant. Nurses in hospitals, the community, and long-term care institutions frequently care for elders who have experienced relocation.

The first issue to address in any move is whether it is necessary and whether it will provide the least restrictive lifestyle appropriate for the individual. Questions that must be asked to assess the impact on the individual after a move are presented in Box 24-4.

Nurses' concerns are with assessing the impact of relocation and determining methods to mitigate any negative reactions. The growing numbers of persons who will spend some of their later years in institutions have made this an urgent issue.

Relocation Stress Syndrome. *Relocation Stress Syndrome* is a nursing diagnosis describing the confusion resulting from a move to a new environment. Characteristics of

---

BOX 24-4   Assessment of Relocation

- Are significant persons as accessible in the new location as they were before the move?
- Is the individual developing new and reciprocal relationships in the new setting?
- Is the individual functioning as well, better, or not as well in the new location? This determination cannot be made immediately but must be assessed at least 6 weeks after the move.
- Was the individual given options before the move?
- Was the individual given the opportunity to assess the new environment before making a decision to move?
- Has the individual been able to move important items of furniture and memorabilia to the new setting?
- Has a particular individual who is familiar with the environment been available to assist with orientation?
- Was the decision to move made hastily or with inadequate information?
- Does the new situation provide adequately for basic needs (food, shelter, physical maintenance)?
- Are individual idiosyncratic needs recognized, and is there an opportunity to actualize them?
- Does the new situation decrease the possibility of privacy and autonomy?
- Is the new living situation an improvement over the previous situation, similar, or worse?

relocation stress syndrome include anxiety, insecurity, altered mental status, depression, insecurity, loss of control, and physical problems (Iwasiw et al., 2003). An abrupt and poorly prepared transfer actually increases illness and disorientation. An individual who has functioned quite well before a major move may show previously unrecognized signs of dementia when in an unfamiliar environment. An accurate assessment of mental status before the move must be obtained from family or significant others. If this is not possible, it must be temporarily assumed that the changes in cognitive functioning are a transient response. An elder who has been transferred to an institution from a residence in which considerable autonomy was possible may react more intensely than one whose change in lifestyle has not been so severe. Some, of course, move to a much more comfortable and supportive situation and adapt well.

To avoid some of the effects of relocation stress syndrome, the individual must have some control over the environment, preparation regarding the new situation, and maintenance of familiar situations to the greatest degree possible. Nurses must carefully assess and monitor older people for relocation stress syndrome effects. Working with families to help them plan relocations, understanding the effects of relocation, and implementing effective approaches are also necessary. It is important that some familiar and some treasured items accompany the transfer. Too often, elders arrive at long-term care institutions via ambulance stretcher from the hospital with nothing but a hospital gown. Everything familiar and necessary in their lives remains at the home they have left when they became ill. Even more distressing is when families or responsible parties sell the home to finance long-term care stays without the input of the elder. It is no wonder so many residents with dementia in nursing homes wander the hallways looking for home and for something familiar and comforting. Family members will need considerable support when an elder is moved into an institution. No matter what the circumstances, the family invariably feels that they have in some way failed the elder. These issues are discussed in more depth in Chapter 20. A summary of relocation stress syndrome and nursing actions to prevent relocation stress are presented in Box 24-5.

BOX 24-5 Relocation Stress Syndrome

Relocation stress syndrome is a physiological and/or psychosocial disturbance as a result of transfer from one environment to another.

DEFINING CHARACTERISTICS

Major
Change in environment or location
Anxiety
Apprehension
Increased confusion
Depression
Loneliness

Minor
Verbalization of unwillingness to relocate
Sleep disturbance
Change in eating habits
Dependency
Gastrointestinal disturbances
Increased verbalization of needs
Insecurity
Lack of trust
Restlessness
Sad affect
Unfavorable comparison of posttransfer and pretransfer staff
Verbalization of being concerned or upset about transfer
Vigilance
Weight change
Withdrawal

RELATED FACTORS

Past, concurrent, and recent losses
Losses involved with the decision to move
Feeling of powerlessness
Lack of adequate support system
Little or no preparation for the impending move
Moderate to high degree of environmental change
History and types of previous transfers
Impaired psychosocial health status
Decreased physical health status

SAMPLE DIAGNOSTIC STATEMENT

Relocation stress syndrome related to admission to long-term care setting as evidenced by anxiety, insecurity, and disorientation

EXPECTED OUTCOMES

1. The resident will socialize with family members, staff, and/or other residents.
2. Preadmission weight, appetite, and sleep patterns will remain stable. If previous patterns were dysfunctional, more appropriate health patterns will develop.
3. The resident will verbalize feelings, expectations, and disappointments openly with members of the staff and/or family.
4. Inappropriate behaviors (e.g., "acting out," refusing to take medicines) will not occur.

Expected Short-Term Goals
1. The resident will become independent in moving to and from areas within the facility during the next 3 months.
2. The resident will react in a positive manner to staff effort to assist in adjusting to nursing home placement in the next 3 months.
3. The resident will express his or her thoughts or concerns about placement when encouraged to do so during individual contacts in the next 3 months.

Continued

BOX 24-5   Relocation Stress Syndrome—cont'd

EXPECTED OUTCOMES—cont'd

Expected Short-Term Goals—cont'd

4. During the next 3 months, the resident will not develop physical or psychosocial disturbances indicative of translocation syndrome as a result of the change in living environment.

Expected Long-Term Goals

1. The resident will verbalize acceptance of nursing home placement within the next 6 months.
2. The resident will indicate acceptance of nursing home placement through positive body language within the next 6 months.

SPECIFIC NURSING INTERVENTIONS

1. Identify previous coping patterns during admission assessment. Clearly document these, and share the information with other staff members.
2. Include the resident in assessing problems and developing the care plan on admission.
3. Adjust for limitations in sensory/perceptual disturbances when planning care for residents. Visual disturbances need special intervention to assist residents in finding their way around.
4. Staff members will introduce themselves when entering the resident's room, indicating the nature of their relationship with the resident. Example: "Hello, Mr. S. My name is Nancy. I'll be your nurse attendant today, helping you with your meals and your bath."

5. Each staff member providing care for the resident should make it a point to spend at least 5 minutes each day with new admissions to "just visit."
6. Allow the resident as many opportunities to make independent choices as possible.
7. Identify previous routines for activities of daily living (ADLs). Try to maintain as much continuity with the resident's previous schedule as possible. Example: If Mr. S. has taken a bath before bed all of his life, adjust his schedule to continue that practice.
8. Familiarize the resident with unit schedules.
9. Encourage family participation through frequent visits, phone calls, and activity sessions. Be sure to let the family know schedules.
10. Establish familiar landmarks for the resident when leaving his or her room so that he or she can recognize areas more quickly.
11. Encourage family members to bring familiar belongings from home for the resident's room decorations.
12. Provide reorientation cues frequently. Example: "You are in the dining room. Your room is down the hall three doors just past the window."
13. Encourage the resident to talk about expectations, anger, and/or disappointments and the recent life changes that he or she has experienced.
14. Review the patient's medication list with the physician to verify the need for medications that might promote disorientation.
15. Provide for constructive activities. Initiate activity therapy consultation.

BOX 24-6   Guidelines for Assessment of Crises

Stage 0—No crisis but rather a request for information.

Stage 1—Mild crisis with ability to mobilize own resources after ventilating concern.

Stage 2—Emerging crisis; client insightful but desiring specific help.

Stage 3—Emergent crisis, second grade. Client recognizes need for assistance but uncertain what, where, or how to obtain. Counseling and referral necessary. Future crisis likely but client open and willing to use help when necessary.

Stage 4—Moderate crisis. Decompensation impending, behaviors mostly ineffective but client making attempts to resolve problem. Assistance can be deferred for a short time.

Stage 5—Moderately severe crisis. Client agitated, disoriented, severely depressed.

Stage 6—Severe crisis. Client presents likelihood of a life-threatening situation; client pleading for help, praying, trying ineffectively to escape the situation.

Stage 7—Very severe crisis. Client in an immediate life-threatening situation; unable to focus on present situation; often engaged in irrelevant activities, for example, looking for makeup or comb when the house is on fire.

Crisis Assessment

Crisis assessment must consider the recency of the event, the effectual or ineffectual efforts to cope, and the available supports. Guidelines for determining the seriousness of crises are presented in Box 24-6.

The elderly themselves and their families need more education in recognizing the early warnings of an impending crisis. Any of the reactions identified in stages 3 through 7 (see Box 24-6) need immediate attention. Referrals may come from family members, a nonrelative, or a professional. Rarely does the older person seek crisis assistance. Therefore the first action is to assess the degree of crisis and respond to the appropriate level of disorganization.

Crisis Intervention

Once an event has been identified as being of crisis proportions, the following actions must be taken:

- Immediately support the individual and communicate concern.
- Ensure that a responsive person is available at any time the individual needs support.
- Identify to the individual any positive adaptive efforts.
- Identify and establish some patterns of coping.

BOX 24-7 Crisis Intervention with Older People

- Crises are often not as clearly delineated as in younger people and are more likely to be overlapping.
- Older people may be unaware of their crisis state; professional assessment of symptoms is often necessary, especially in case of cognitive impairment, depression, paranoia.
- Older people may be reluctant to seek help because of pride of independence, stoic acceptance of difficulty, unawareness of resources, fear of "being put away."
- Change is stressful; therefore intervention should impose as few changes as possible.
- Older people who are resilient deal with stressors better. These skills can be learned or strengthened.
- Continuity of personnel and having as few people as possible providing services leave the client with more energy to deal with the problem at hand.
- Timing is important. Individuals have personal time clocks that order their peak efficiency daily, monthly, and developmentally; use the best times to introduce change.
- Another aspect of timing to consider is the timing of stresses. More energy will be needed to integrate events that have occurred within the previous 6 weeks, 6 months, or 1 year than those occurring in the remote past.

- Older people often experience multiple, simultaneous stresses, and reduction of anxiety is necessary before options for intervention can be considered.
- Some older people are in a chronic state of grief because losses are never fully resolved before another one occurs; stress then becomes a constant state of being.
- The individual needs to understand that resolution may be slower then expected if he or she has recently been bombarded with change.
- Do not infantilize. Make yourself aware of the person's strengths. Analysis of past accomplishments and clear definition of the present problem contribute to crisis resolution and a higher level of functioning.
- Your interpersonal relationship is an important aspect of assisting individuals with crisis resolution. Therapeutic relationships encourage expression of feelings, support, education, and anticipatory guidance.
- Leave the person with a summary of coping mechanisms and accomplishments during crisis intervention. State clearly how assistance can be secured in further crisis.

- Provide information about available resources.
- Follow up after resolution of the crisis to determine level of adaptation.

Further guidelines for planning crisis intervention with older people are presented in Box 24-7.

EMOTIONS AND ILLNESS

Much remains unknown about the connection between emotions and health and illness, but it is known that the mind and body are integrated and cannot be approached as separate entities (Kelley, 2001). We know some emotions for some people result in physical illness, particularly negative emotions (Kiecolt-Glaser et al., 2002a). Data suggest that persons with low psychosocial resources are vulnerable to illness and mood disturbance when their stress levels increase, even if they generally have few current stressors in their lives. Sustained stress can lead to such physical consequences as heart disease, hypertension, bowel irritation, and skin disorders. These conditions, when identified with stress as a major factor, are called *stress-related diseases*.

Some researchers have found that early life events, such as parental loss, continue to exact an emotional price throughout life (Johnson and Barrer, 2002). Resurgence of traumatic memories is often triggered by current crises and losses. In addition, the weighting of events at any given time depends on concurrence of both positive and negative events; recency of exposure; timing, interval, and duration of the event; number of roles occupied by the individual; and the general affective state of the person.

Psychoneuroimmunology

From the seminal thoughts of Cannon, Meyer, and Selye decades ago, hundreds of studies and a whole science of psychoneuroimmunology have emerged, most within the past decade. It is generally accepted that emotions can wreak havoc with health and may be the source of many illnesses. Diseases thought to be triggered by psychological factors that influence the immune system include cardiovascular disease, osteoporosis, arthritis, type 2 diabetes, certain cancers, frailty, and functional decline (Kiecolt-Glaser et al., 2002b). In recent years, research has increased dramatically related to the psychobehavioral modulation of immune function and attempts to assay the actual stress-related impairment of the immune system.

Learned Helplessness

Helplessness may be the result of repeated ineffective attempts to deal with stressors or crises. Seligman (1975) introduced the concept of "learned helplessness" into the vernacular of gerontologists. It is based on studies of mice that show they will continue to seek food through a maze even when they receive a predictable electric shock. However, when the shocks become unpredictable, they cease trying. Extrapolated to humans, we believe that actions with unpredictable results over time eventually result in the individual's retreat into helplessness. In uncertain and inconsistently demanding situations, helplessness, powerlessness, and perceived lack of control erode the personality of the individual. The loss of health is often the precursor to loss of control. Uncertainty of illness outcome is seen as a particularly debilitating situation in which coping may be seriously

---

BOX 24-8 Sources of Feelings of Helplessness

- An unsuccessful illness-related regimen
- The implacable structure of the health care environment
- Interpersonal interactions
- A lifestyle of helplessness
- Repeated attempts to exert control that have failed
- Inability to predict a consistent outcome of certain actions

The pervasiveness of the powerless feeling can be categorized from the most to the least severe in the following manner:

- Verbalization of lack of influence over outcome
- Depression when condition deteriorates in spite of compliance with health regimen
- Apathy
- Nonparticipation in care or decisions when opportunities are provided
- Expressed frustration over limitations
- Expressed doubt regarding role performance
- Passivity
- Disinterest in information regarding care
- Dependency on others with the accompanying feelings of resentment, anger, and guilt
- Reluctance to express true feelings
- Agreeing readily to whatever may be suggested
- Expressed uncertainty about fluctuations in energy and functional ability

---

undermined (Mishel, 1988). Nurses, remembering this, must make special efforts to reinstitute personal control, particularly with the ill or institutionalized older person. Feelings of powerlessness and helplessness can arise from any of the sources identified in Box 24-8.

Establishing Control

The nursing function is to redirect any evidence of control toward preserving the integrity, personality, and self-esteem of the individual. Even when people are unable to make decisions regarding their own personal care, they may still be able to participate if given direction and assistance. For example, giving the patient a washcloth and standing by to help if requested, rather than doing for the patient, reinstates an element of control. Nurses must examine their capacity to tolerate untidiness, inefficiency, and delay in the interest of promoting some measure of independence. The most constructive role the nurse can assume is that of confidante, advocate, counselor, and encouraging supporter. These roles foster independence within the confines of the older person's capacity. In some cases, the older person may seek an ally to whom he or she can temporarily relinquish control. The nurse must be alert to this need for short-lived splinting support (Wolanin and Phillips, 1981). The individual, injured and limping psychologically, physically, or both, needs a support person to help him or her regain psychic stability. The immediate availability of such support in a crisis may be the most critical element in achieving higher levels of function.

COPING

Coping strategies are the stabilizing factors that help individuals maintain psychosocial balance during stressful periods. More broadly, coping strategies are any efforts toward stress management—things that people do to avoid being harmed by life strains or overt and covert behaviors to reduce or eliminate psychological distress (Ahmad et al., 2005). Two major categories of coping behaviors are those that actively and directly deal with the problem and those that are designed to avoid the problem.

Lazarus and Folkman (1984) distinguish between problem-focused strategies and those that are emotion focused. Problem-focused coping is aimed at managing or altering the problem, whereas emotion-focused coping focuses on regulating the emotional response to the problem (Ahmad et al., 2005). For example, if one's elderly parent makes excessive demands on an adult daughter, a problem-focused strategy to solve the problem would be to discuss with the elder the assistance that can realistically be given and what is needed. Emotion-focused strategies might include reducing emotional frustration by avoiding the problem, taking a tranquilizer and going to bed, hoping that the problem would eventually resolve itself. Some emotion-focused strategies may be healthy, such as centering oneself or meditating, but may still be avoidance of the actual issue (Box 24-9). Ahmad et al. (2005) suggest that nurses need to be aware of the importance of appraisal style when helping patients cope with illnesses or other losses.

Older people more frequently have a decreased ability to cope with daily hassles, cumulative life events, and other stressors because of their waning energy and adaptive capacity. The deficits in adaptability are most evident in neuroendocrine interactions and in the responsiveness of the nervous and endocrine systems. Regardless of whether stress is physical or emotional, older people require more time to recover or return to prestress levels than when they were younger.

Various means of stress reduction exist, such as meditation, biofeedback, tai chi, progressive relaxation, and visualization (see Chapter 3). Moderately vigorous exercise is one of the best ways to handle stress (Woods et al., 2002). Other methods include yoga, prayer, deep breathing, imagery, laughter, and massage. Elders respond positively to most of these interventions. Some individuals use one; others use a combination of holistic methods to achieve inner balance (Maes, 2001). Mind-body therapies that integrate cognitive, sensory, expressive, and physical aspects are most helpful (Bauer-Wu et al., 2002; Eliopoulos, 2000). These data are significant for nurses as they identify and reinforce successful coping mechanisms. Because nurses often focus exclusively on the problem-solving mode, they may forget that there are many ways to solve a problem besides resolving it.

BOX 24-9   Coping Strategy Items

ACTIVE-COGNITIVE STRATEGIES

Prayed for guidance and strength
Prepared for the worst
Tried to see the positive side of the situation
Considered several alternatives for handling the problem
Drew on my past experiences
Took things a day at a time
Tried to step back from the situation and be more objective
Went over the situation in my mind to try to understand it
Told myself things that helped me feel better
Made a promise to myself that things would be different next time
Accepted it; nothing could be done

ACTIVE-BEHAVIORAL STRATEGIES

Tried to find out more about the situation
Talked with spouse or other relative about the problem
Talked with friend about the problem
Talked with professional person (e.g., physician, lawyer, clergy)
Got busy with other things to keep my mind off the problem

Made a plan of action and followed it
Tried not to act too hastily or follow my first hunch
Got away from things for a while
Knew what had to be done and tried harder to make things work
Let my feelings out somehow
Sought help from persons or groups with similar experiences
Bargained or compromised to get something positive from the situation
Tried to reduce tension by exercising more

AVOIDANCE STRATEGIES

Took it out on other people when I felt angry or depressed
Kept my feelings to myself
Avoided being with people in general
Refused to believe that it happened
Tried to reduce tension by drinking more
Tried to reduce tension by eating more
Tried to reduce tension by smoking more
Tried to reduce tension by taking more tranquilizing drugs

From Holahan C, Moos R: Personal and contextual determinants of coping strategies, *J Pers Soc Psychol* 52(5):946-955, 1987.

As elders confront problems that cannot be reversed or logically resolved, they obviously resort to other mechanisms that help them successfully cope with the issue. Encouraging the sharing of early memories is often useful in comprehending the coping style of an elder and helping the elder remember how he or she coped successfully. Application of what one has learned from a previous situation can help dissipate the intensity of stress.

Occasionally getting lost in some creative pursuit is an excellent means of dealing with stress. For some, knitting is helpful, whereas others find that painting a pastoral scene or the side of the house may be satisfying. Stroking a pet, rocking on a porch, or watching fish swim in an aquarium can be a tranquilizer. Others enjoy fishing, a game of golf, reading a book, or listening to music. Still others find writing poetry a means of releasing frustration and stress. Physical activity is an appropriate means of handling stress for some individuals. These activities provide time to revitalize after a stressful incident, although if used continually as a means of avoiding resolutions, they may become less effective (Box 24-10).

Many older people, especially African-American elders, rely on spiritual and religious beliefs to help them cope with life's stresses and crises. A belief system and greater spiritual perspective have been identified to be associated with emotional well-being, decreased loneliness and depression, coping with chronic illness and pain, terminal or life-threatening illness, bereavement, and levels of hope (Ark et al., 2006; Dunn and Horgas, 2000; Koening and Brooks, 2002; Miller and Thoresen, 2003; Touhy 2001a, 2001b; Touhy and Zerwekh, 2006). In a study by Dunn and Horgas (2000), 96% of the participants reported the use of prayer as a coping strategy, with women and African-

BOX 24-10   Ways of Coping Checklist Responses

MOST FREQUENT RESPONSES

Pray
Remind self that things could be worse
Maintain pride
Look for the silver lining
Turn to work or activity
Keep feelings from interfering
Try to analyze the problem

LEAST FREQUENTLY USED COPING ACTIVITIES

Talk with someone who can help
Get professional help
Apologize
Take it out on others

Americans using prayer more often than men and white persons. When working with older adults, it is especially important to include assessment of their religiosity and spiritual perspectives and how they influence their health (Box 24-11). Spirituality is discussed in Chapter 27.

Personal and Contextual Determinants of Coping

Factors such as sociodemographics, personal disposition, and contextual issues all affect ability to cope with crises. Contextual issues include such things as education, marriage and economic status, personal flexibility, logical choice, and problem-focused coping strategies.

BOX 24-11   **Evidence-Based Practice: Religiosity, Religious Coping Styles, and Health Service Use**

PURPOSE

The purpose of the study was to examine racial differences in religiosity and religious coping styles and to explore possible racial differences in the effects of religiosity and religious coping styles on health service use among elderly women living in standardized high-rise complexes.

SAMPLE/SETTING

Secondary analysis of religiosity, religious coping styles, and health service use was conducted using data from the Nashville Elderly Depression study. Analyses were conducted on 274 female residents ages 55 through 95 (M 73.5) years living in publicly subsidized high-rise community apartments for older adults in the Nashville, Tennessee, area. 40.5% of the participants were African-American.

METHOD

Three dimensions of religiosity were measured: feelings related to religion and perceived closeness with God, organizational religious behavior, and non-organizational religious behavior (items from the General Social Survey). Instruments used have been validated in past as well as the current study. Religious coping styles were measured using Pargament's Scale of Religious Coping and measured three types of religious coping (self-directed, deferring, and collaborating). Health service use was measured by self-reports of physician visits in the past 6 months, emergency room visits within the past 12 months, and inpatient days within the past 12 months.

Bivariate analysis was tested for racial differences in religiosity, religious coping styles, and health service use. Multivariate analyses and regression models were used to examine the effects of religiosity and religious coping styles on each of the health service use outcome variables.

RESULTS

African-American women perceived themselves to be more religious than white women, and both organizational religious behavior and non-organizational religious behavior scores were also higher in African-Americans. Self-directing coping style was associated with higher levels of health care use for white women but lower levels of use for African-American women. The deferring coping style was associated with greater physician visits and inpatient days among white women but fewer inpatient days among African-American women. The collaborative coping style was associated with higher inpatient days among African-American women but had no significant effect on use patterns for white women. Study limitations include the self-report nature of the data and the non-random relatively small sample size.

IMPLICATIONS

Racial and ethnic differences in religiosity and religious coping styles may have an effect on the use and choice of health services as well as compliance with treatment plans. Determination of religiosity and coping styles of older people may be an important part of nursing assessment and have implications for health promotion and disease prevention.

Data from Ark P et al: Religiosity, religious coping styles, and health service use, *J Gerontol Nurs* 32(8):20-29, 2006.

Most elders during the aging process are confronted with loss, threats, and deprivation when their socioeconomic status is likely to be reduced and their health compromised. On the positive side, they have developed, over time, numerous survival strategies that have been effective to one degree or another and they are likely to have developed an internal locus of control. This should be the focus on an interaction with any elder: identify past patterns that have been productive. Ongoing demands of a situation, up to a point, engender an increase in coping efforts, but just as there are individual pain thresholds, there are also stress thresholds.

Hardiness and Buffers

Hardiness and "buffers" are concepts that attempt to explain the ability of some individuals to withstand enormous stress. *Hardiness* is a term that has captured the imagination of researchers interested in determining the differences in coping capacity of ostensibly similar elders. The cornerstones of hardiness are control, competence, and compassion (Kobasa, 1979). Hardiness, the combination of personality characteristics of vigor, resilience, commitment, and control, apparently buffers the illness-related effects of stress (Felton and Hall, 2001; Hagberg et al., 2002). Buffers against decompensation with stress come from social supports and are usually

seen as the most important coping resource. Life goals and a sense of purpose or meaning undergird hardiness.

The relevance of hardiness to nursing practice is in assisting individuals to regain a sense of control over their lives, to feel committed or deeply involved with some activity that gives meaning, and to anticipate change as exciting. These may seem lofty goals, but they have been observed under the most extenuating circumstances.

Central to hardiness is the viewpoint that stress is a decision-making challenge and that meaning comes from making decisions. Stressful situations are seen as opportunities for growth. Clients should be apprised of any evidence of hardiness in their actions. This can reinforce their strength and coping abilities. Individuals should be asked the meaning of certain events in their lives and what they are learning from these challenging situations.

Resilience

Resilience is a concept closely related to hardiness that is associated with coping with stress and crises. The process of resilience is characterized by successfully adapting to difficult and challenging life experiences, especially those that are highly stressful or traumatic (O'Leary and Ickovics, 1995). Beliefs, attitudes, behaviors, and even physiology may help some people do better in adverse situations and recover more

BOX 24-12   Coping Strategies of Older Adults

- Using more active strategies to avoid negative situations in the first place. When uncontrollable stress occurs, older adults do not add to this by getting involved in other stressful situations.
- Using good cognitive strategies to manage negative emotions. Keep things in perspective and avoid overreacting.

- Staying focused on positive things they can do or positive events happening at the same time.
- Actively compare current stressors to things they have experienced and coped with in the past.
- Maximize good emotional experiences by selecting activities with familiar positive impact—they turn to the really meaningful people and activities in their life during hard times.

From American Psychological Association: *Fostering resilience in response to terrorism: for psychologists working with older adults,* 2007 (website): *www.apa.org.*

Human Needs and Wellness Diagnoses

Self-Actualization and Transcendence
(Seeking, Expanding, Spirituality, Fulfillment)
Incorporates daily methods of relaxation/meditation
Recognizes situations that require new coping skills
Recognizes potential for personal growth through crises
Seeks ways to develop new adaptive strategies
Seeks transcendent meanings in trauma

Self-Esteem and Self-Efficacy
(Image, Identity, Control, Capability)
Maintains a personally satisfactory stress threshold
Recognizes own personality strengths and idiosyncrasies
Anticipates and plans for crises that are predictable
Regains maximum resolution of stress toward least discomfort
and high-level wellness

Belonging and Attachment
(Love, Empathy, Affiliation)
Allows others to provide assistance as necessary
Allows self brief periods of dependency
Develops a cadre of relationships that can be
relied on in emergencies

Safety and Security
(Caution, Planning, Protections, Sensory Acuity)
Seeks assistance when crises occur
Maintains as many comfortable routines as possible
Has only brief periods of anxiety, extra discomfort, and insecurity
Maintains comforting contacts until stability returns

Biological and Physiological Integrity
(Air, Fluids, Comfort, Activity, Nutrition, Elimination, Skin Integrity)
Recognizes and responds to increased requirements for
rest, fluids, and nutrition during crises and
stressful situations

These are not all the possible wellness diagnoses that may be identified. The above are examples of nursing diagnoses that should be considered when planning care for the older adult.

quickly from traumatic events. Resilient people "bend rather than break during stressful conditions" and are able to return to adequate (or sometimes better) functioning after stress. Resilient individuals have a more positive outlook and a greater sense of personal mastery, and they actively cope with stressors and find meaning in their lives. Older people may demonstrate greater resilience and ability to maintain a positive emotional state under stress than younger persons. Box 24-12 presents stress and coping behaviors that may be found in older people.

▲ PROMOTING HEALTHY AGING: IMPLICATIONS FOR GERONTOLOGICAL NURSING

This chapter presents situations that often confront people in the aging process. With some people, events become catastrophic, whereas others seem to handle similar events well. Some events present immediate crises, and others result in stress overload and breakdown of coping mechanisms. Many of these factors are discussed here. A half century after Selye's (1956) seminal observations of the relationship of stress and illness and the numerous studies of psychoneuroimmunology, we still have only a beginning understanding of the mechanisms that create positive adaptations. Stress is a constant in our lives and those of our clients.

During the later years, many situations and conditions erode confidence in one's self and stir negative feelings. Restoration of a sense of control is basic to moving beyond the helplessness experienced during crises, stress, and illness. No generation has faced so many changes or had its mettle so tested. This provides a beginning focus of discussion with elders feeling uncertain and incapable of making changes in their situation. It is sometimes necessary to remind elders of all the major events they have survived and help them call upon the coping strategies used that may be helpful in dealing with the current crisis. Our task is to restore faith in one's adaptive capacity. The gerontological nurse is in a position to assist an individual seek meaning from untoward events. The presence of the nurse and his or her sensitivity in attending to the individual's immediate situation in a way that moves an individual toward higher levels of wellness is truly the art and the joy of nursing.

KEY CONCEPTS

- Disturbing emotions experienced over extended periods may result in depletions of the immune system and resulting illnesses.
- Crises and stressors are experienced by older people less frequently than among younger adults but often have more devastating consequences.
- Crises have the potential for producing individual growth and higher levels of function as a result of successful mastery of the situation.
- If timely support and appropriate interventions are not activated during a crisis situation, the individual is likely to stabilize at a lower level of function than that before the crisis.
- Methods of assessing the impact of stressful events are inadequate if they do not consider chronic stressors that may exist over long periods, the particular population profile of the individuals being assessed, the individual's personality, the recency and frequency of events, and very early traumatic events that erode the individual's sense of security.
- Stress management strategies must be designed to meet individual needs because some methods may in fact be experienced as an additional stressor; for example, a shy, reticent elder would be unlikely to find body massage soothing and relaxing.

- Though helplessness and dependency are often seen as negative qualities, they may be temporarily adaptive and stress reducers in certain situations within the family or institutions.
- Reestablishing feelings of adequacy and control is the *sine qua non* of crisis resolution and stress management.
- Psychoneuroimmunology is attracting considerable attention as the relationship of emotions and disease and the particular physiological responses involved are becoming clearer.

RESEARCH QUESTIONS

What items would be important in the development of age-specific tools to determine the nature of anxiety in the old?

What are the events that are particularly problematic crises for elders?

In what areas of life do elders feel they have the least control?

What are the most common or frequent worries of elders?

What is the impact on stress management of various personality gender differences?

Develop a tool for measuring coping capacity of elders on a scale of 1 to 10 (similar to pain assessment tools).

RESOURCES

Registered Nurses Association of Ontario (RNAO): *Supporting and strengthening families through expected and unexpected life events supplement*, Toronto (ON), 2006. (website): *www.guidelines.gov.*

Registered Nurses Association of Ontario (RNAO): *Crisis intervention supplement*, Toronto (ON), 2006. (website): *www.guidelines.gov.*

REFERENCES

Ahmad M et al: Prostate cancer: appraisal, coping, and health status, *J Gerontol Nurs* 31(10):34-43, 2005.

American Psychological Association: Fostering resilience in response to terrorism: for psychologists working with older adults, 2004 (website): *www.apa.org.* Accessed August 8, 2006.

Ark P et al: Religiosity, religious coping styles, and health service use, *J Gerontol Nurs* 32(8):20-29, 2006.

Bauer-Wu SM: Psychoneuroimmunology: Part II: Mind-body interventions, *Clin J Oncol Nurs* 6(4): 243, 2002.

Butler RN: The crises of old age, *RN* 30:47, 1967.

Dunn KS, Horgas AL: The prevalence of prayer as a spiritual self-care modality in elders, *J Holist Nurs* 18:337-353, 2000.

Eliopoulos C: Using complementary and alternative techniques—boosting immunity, *Director* 8(4):142, 2000.

Fakouri C, Lyon B: Perceived health and life satisfaction among older adults: the effects of worry and personal variables, *J Gerontol Nurs* 31(10):17-24, 2005.

Felton BS, Hall JM: Conceptualizing resilience in women older than 85: overcoming adversity from illness and loss, *J Gerontol Nurs* 27(11):46, 2001.

Hagberg M et al: The significance of personality factors for various dimensions of life quality among older people, *Aging Ment Health* 6(2):178, 2002.

Iwasiw C et al: Resident and family perspectives on the first year in a long-term care facility, *J Gerontol Nurs* 29(12):45-54, 2003.

CASE STUDY: Stress and Crisis in Aging

Aaron and Anna had a comfortable existence as the managers of a small hotel in upstate New York. They had downgraded from a large and lovely home when they retired but had been able to move most of their treasured possessions to the manager's cottage they occupied adjacent to the hotel. At 75 years old, they felt fortunate to remain active, healthy, and generating an income. Their lives had provided much satisfaction, and this was a time to enjoy the rewards for long years of hard work and relative success. Their duties at the hotel were not strenuous because employees took care of the manual duties. They were in the control center—guiding, problem solving, and delegating—their dream retirement! One night while they were at a concert, their cottage caught fire and almost all their possessions were destroyed before the blaze was brought under control. Aaron repeatedly said, "I'm so glad we were not there and that we are safe." Anna wrung her hands constantly and chanted over and over, "My mother's photos are gone; my grandmother's quilts are gone; my Spode china is black." Clearly, for Aaron this was another hazard of living; for Anna it was the loss of the substance of her existence, definitions of her identity. Ordinarily one thinks of rape, traumatic injury, or cataclysmic events as precipitants of later post-traumatic stress disorder (PTSD). In Anna's case this was truly a cataclysmic event. Fortunately, the firemen recognized the magnitude of Anna's crisis reaction and called for assistance. An alert public servant called a crisis counselor to spend some time with Anna.

Based on these case studies, develop a nursing care plan using the following procedure*:

- List Aaron's and Anna's comments that provide subjective data.
- List information that provides objective data.
- From these data, identify and state, using accepted format, two nursing diagnoses you determine are most significant to Aaron and Anna at this time. List two of their strengths that you have identified from data.
- Determine and state outcome criteria for each diagnosis. These must reflect some alleviation of the problem identified in the nursing diagnosis and must be stated in concrete and measurable terms.

- Plan and state one or more interventions for each diagnosed problem. Provide specific documentation of the source used to determine the appropriate intervention. Plan at least one intervention that incorporates Aaron's and Anna's existing strengths.
- Evaluate the success of the intervention. Interventions must correlate directly with the stated outcome criteria to measure the outcome success.

Critical Thinking Questions

1. Discuss differences between crises and stress, and describe methods to discriminate between the two situations.
2. Ask elders in your neighborhood about their crises and stressors within the past 6 months or 1 year. How frequently did they experience the loss of a friend or relative? Interview an elder in a nursing home and ask about the events or situations that are most troubling to him or her. List the crises and stressors you have experienced in the past year, and compare the differences and similarities in the three lists.
3. Discuss your thoughts about the science of psychoneuroimmunology.
4. Explain methods of restoring a sense of control and averting excessive dependency.
5. Discuss the meanings and the thoughts triggered by the students' and elders' viewpoints expressed at the beginning of the chapter. How do these vary from your own experience?
6. As a group project, develop a life events rating scale for an elderly population that includes the following considerations:
   - Events and other possible sources of social stress
   - Significance of event in relation to age, gender, cohort, and culture
   - Desirable and undesirable events
   - Comprehensiveness of events listed
   - Roles occupied by the individual at the time of the survey
   - Affect of the individual at the time of the survey
   - Time frame, recency, and duration of event
7. Construct a life chart for yourself and consider events around times when you were greatly stressed.

* Students are advised to refer to their nursing diagnosis text and identify possible or potential problems.

Johnson CL, Barrer BM: Life course effects of early parental loss among very old African Americans, *J Gerontol B Psychol Sci Soc Sci* 57(2):S108, 2002.

Kelley KW: It's time for psychoneuroimmunology, *Brain Behav Immun* 15(1):1, 2001.

Kiecolt-Glaser JK et al: Psychoneuroimmunology: psychological influences on immune function and health, *J Consult Clin Psychol* 70(3):537, 2002a.

Kiecolt-Glaser JK et al: Psychoneuroimmunology and psychosomatic medicine: back to the future, *Psychosom Med* 64(1):15, 2002b.

Kobasa SC: Stressful life events, personality and health: an inquiry into hardiness, *J Pers Soc Psychol* 37(1):1, 1979.

Koening HG, Brooks RG: Religion, health and aging: implications for practice and public policy, *Public Policy Aging Rep* 12:13-19, 2002.

Lazarus R, Folkman S: *Stress appraisal and coping*, New York, 1984, Springer.

Lindemann E: Symptomatology and management of acute grief, *Am J Psychiatry* 101:141, 1944.

Maes S: Nurses explore relationships among mind, body, spirit, *ONS News* 16(9):1, 2001.

Meyer A: The life chart and the obligation for specifying positive data in psychopathological diagnosis. In Winters EE, editor: *The collected papers of Adolph Meyer*, vol 3, Baltimore, 1951, Johns Hopkins University Press.

Miller WR, Thoresen CE: Spirituality, religion and health: an emerging research field, *Am Psychol* 58:3-16, 2003.

Mishel M: Uncertainty in illness, *Image J Nurs Sch* 20(4):225, 1988.

O'Leary VE, Ickovics JR: Resilience and thriving in response to challenge: an opportunity for a paradigm shift in women's health, *Womens Health* 1(2):121-142, 1995.

Powers CB et al: Age differences and correlates of worrying in young and elderly adults, *Gerontologist* 32(1):82, 1992.

Seligman M: *Helplessness: on depression, development and death*, San Francisco, 1975, Freeman.

Selye H: *The stress of life*, New York, 1956, McGraw-Hill.

Stetson B: Holistic health stress management program: nursing student and client health outcomes, *J Holist Nurs* 15(2):143, 1997.

Touhy T: Touching the spirit of elders in nursing homes: ordinary yet extraordinary care, *Int J Human Caring* 6(1):12-17, 2001a.

Touhy T: Nurturing hope and spirituality in nursing homes, *Holist Nurs Pract* 15(4):45-56, 2001b.

Touhy T, Zerwekh J: Spiritual caring. In Zerwekh J: *Nursing care at the end of life*, Philadelphia, 2006, FA Davis.

Wolanin MO, Phillips L: *Confusion: prevention and care*, St Louis, 1981, Mosby.

Woods JA et al: Can exercise training improve immune function in the aged? *Ann N Y Acad Sci* 959:117, 2002.

CHAPTER 25

Emotional Health in Late Life

Theris A. Touhy

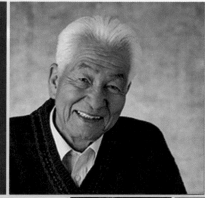

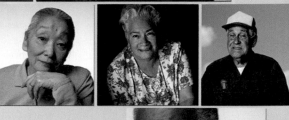

A STUDENT SPECULATES

The process of aging scares me. Aging brings up emotions such as low self-esteem, powerlessness, and hopelessness. An old person has to accept the existing gap between the young and the old. I still remember telling my grandmother she was old-fashioned and out of touch. Now, I realize how rude I was to her. By the time I am about 75 years old, I will be just as depressed as some of the elderly I work with.

Rossana, age 28

AN ELDER SPEAKS

I am very irritable and quick to anger, and this is increasing as I age. I think people's strengths increase as they age, and their weaknesses do also.

Madeline, age 78

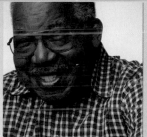

LEARNING OBJECTIVES

On completion of this chapter, the reader will be able to:

1. Discuss factors contributing to emotional health in late life.
2. List symptoms of late-life depression, and discuss assessment, treatment, and nursing responses.
3. Recognize elders who are at risk for suicide, and utilize appropriate techniques for suicide assessment.
4. Explain therapies that are useful in the care of elders with mental health concerns.
5. Evaluate interventions aimed at promoting emotional health in older adults.
6. Specify several indications of the possibility of substance abuse, and discuss appropriate nursing responses.
7. Develop an individualized nursing care plan for an older person with a depression and bipolar disorder.

This chapter presents concepts of mental and emotional health and disturbances common in late life and provides specific nursing responses to maintain and promote mental health wellness, self-esteem, and psychological health of older individuals to the optimum of their capacity. The chapter is divided into three major sections: considerations in emotional health of older adults, cognitive disturbances created by psychiatric problems, and therapeutic interventions. Developmental transitions, life events, and situations requiring psychic energy may interfere with the ability to concentrate in many older adults. These factors, though not unique to the old, often influence adaptation.

In previous chapters, we examined these challenges in Maslow's hierarchical fashion. Nurses caring for older people need to consider the person's basic human needs when attempting to assess emotional health and adaptation. Anyone who has survived 80 or so years has been exposed to many stressors and crises and has developed tremendous resistance. Most older people face life's challenges with grace, equanimity, good humor, and courage. It is our task to discover the strengths and adaptive mechanisms that will assist them to cope with the challenges and create relationships and systems of care that not only meet basic needs but also contribute to health, happiness, and meaning throughout life, even at the end of life.

Special thanks to Ann Schmidt Luggen, the previous edition contributor, for her content contributions to this chapter.

BOX 25-1 *Healthy People 2010:* Mental Health and Substance Abuse Goals and Objectives

- Increase the proportion of adults with recognized depression who receive treatments
- Reduce deaths and injury caused by alcohol- or drug-related motor vehicle crashes
- Reduce number of cirrhosis deaths
- Reduce alcohol-related hospital emergency department visits
- Reduce intentional injuries resulting from alcohol-related violence
- Reduce the proportion of adults using any illicit drug during the past 30 days
- Reduce the proportion of adults who engage in binge drinking of alcohol beverages during the past month
- Reduce average annual alcohol consumption
- Reduce the treatment gap for alcohol problems
- Increase the number of people referred for follow-up care for alcohol problems

From U.S. Department of Health and Human Services: *Healthy People 2010: national health promotion and disease prevention objectives,* Washington, DC, 2000, The Department.

HEALTHY PEOPLE 2000/2010

As discussed in *Healthy People 2010,* approximately 20% of the U.S. population of all ages are affected by mental illness during a given year. Depression is the most common disorder, with more than 19 million adults affected. Major depression is the leading cause of disability and the cause of more than two thirds of suicides each year. In addition, alcohol and illicit drug use are leading concerns in the United States and are associated with violence, injury, and human immunodeficiency virus (HIV) infection.

Healthy People 2010 has set goals and objectives for mental health and substance abuse that are discussed in this chapter. Box 25-1 presents some of those objectives.

EMOTIONAL HEALTH IN LATE LIFE

Mental health of the elderly is difficult to define because a lifetime of living results in many variations of personality, coping, and life patterns. One can say what 5-year-olds or 15-year-olds in general are like, but the same is not true for older people. Each individual becomes more uniquely himself or herself the older he or she becomes. Well-being in late life can be predicted by cognitive and affective functioning earlier in life (Qualls, 2002). The accumulation of life experiences, one's culture, and particular situations emphasize certain aspects of personality and appearance and diminish others. Some apparently negative personality characteristics, such as being crusty, disagreeable, grouchy, or grumpy, may be adaptive. Thus an old man coping with a severe illness and stoically protecting others from awareness of his pain might be mentally healthy although extremely cantankerous.

Emotional health can be simply defined as a satisfactory adjustment to one's life stage and situation. An emotionally healthy person is "one who accepts the aging self as an active being, engaging available strengths to compensate for weaknesses in order to create personal meaning, maintain maximum autonomy by mastering the environment, and sustain positive relationships with others" (Qualls, 2002, p. 12). Put quite simply, "We all try to do the best with what we have" (Kivnick, 1993, p. 24).

Emotional health is not different in late life, but the level of challenge may be greater. What it means to be emotionally healthy is subject to many interpretations and familial and cultural influences. Emotional health, as with general health, can be thought of as being on a fluctuating continuum from wellness to illness. The absence of emotional illness does not mean that one is emotionally healthy, nor does the presence of psychological symptoms mean one is emotionally or mentally ill. No one is entirely mentally unhealthy, and no one is fully healthy at all times. Individuals move back and forth on the continuum as stressors, supports, health, and resources are ample or scarce (Figure 25-1, A). Erikson thought autonomy, intimacy, integrity, and generativity were all aspects of mentally healthy adult adaptation. These concepts are culture-bound and to some extent dependent on semantics. We can help the elder seek to maximize the healthiest self-attributes. Using Maslow's hierarchical need model, we might assume that the higher one rises in terms of needs met, the more likely one is to be emotionally healthy (Figure 25-1, B).

Demographics and Services

Nearly 20% of people older than 55 years experience emotional disorders that are not part of normal aging, and these figures are expected to significantly increase in the next 25 years. The figures may be even higher because emotional disorders are underreported. The most prevalent disorders are anxiety, severe cognitive impairment, and mood disorders. The rate of suicide is higher in older adults than in any other age-group, with men 85 years and older having the highest suicide rate.

Stigma about having a mental or emotional disorder ("being crazy"), particularly for older people, discourages many from seeking treatment. Fewer than one half of elders who acknowledge mental health problems receive any treatment from any provider (APA Fact Sheet, 2004). The rate of utilization of mental health services for elders, even when available, is less than that of any other age-group. Lack of knowledge on the part of health care professionals about emotional health in late life presents another barrier to appropriate diagnosis and treatment.

Compounding the problem of inadequate services is the limited coverage for mental health care under Medicare and Medicaid. Medicare provides health insurance, but the coverage is not comprehensive. Only 50% of mental health services are covered, although recently, Medicare is providing more coverage for care of people with Alzheimer's disease and other dementias. A 190-day lifetime limit still re-

A.   1. Optimal psychological vitality   2. Satisfactory functioning with   3. Limited functioning or   4. Serious mental illness
                                                modest distress or limitation   meaningful distress

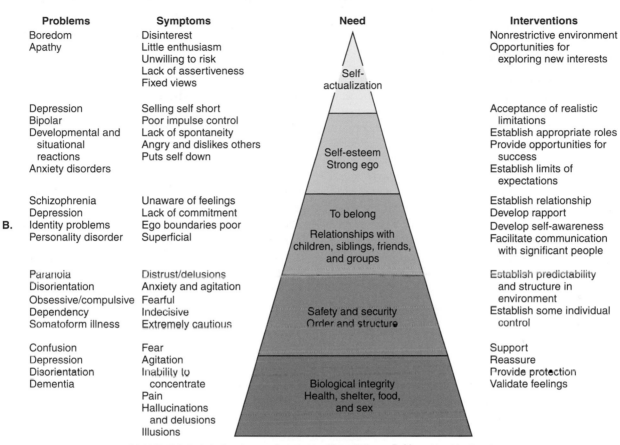

Problems	Symptoms	Need	Interventions
Boredom	Disinterest	Self-actualization	Nonrestrictive environment
Apathy	Little enthusiasm		Opportunities for
	Unwilling to risk		exploring new interests
	Lack of assertiveness		
	Fixed views		
Depression	Selling self short	Self-esteem Strong ego	Acceptance of realistic limitations
Bipolar	Poor impulse control		Establish appropriate roles
Developmental and situational reactions	Lack of spontaneity Angry and dislikes others		Provide opportunities for success
Anxiety disorders	Puts self down		Establish limits of expectations
Schizophrenia	Unaware of feelings	To belong	Establish relationship
Depression	Lack of commitment	Relationships with children, siblings, friends, and groups	Develop rapport
Identity problems	Ego boundaries poor		Develop self-awareness
Personality disorder	Superficial		Facilitate communication with significant people
Paranoia	Distrust/delusions	Safety and security Order and structure	Establish predictability and structure in environment
Disorientation	Anxiety and agitation		
Obsessive/compulsive	Fearful		
Dependency	Indecisive		Establish some individual control
Somatoform illness	Extremely cautious		
Confusion	Fear	Biological integrity Health, shelter, food, and sex	Support
Depression	Agitation		Reassure
Disorientation	Inability to concentrate		Provide protection
Dementia	Pain		Validate feelings
	Hallucinations and delusions		
	Illusions		

FIGURE 25-1 A, Continuum of mental health and illness. B, Mental health disorders.

mains on treatment in inpatient mental health facilities. Psychiatric services may be delivered by a psychiatrist, psychologist, nurse practitioner, geropsychiatric nurse, or licensed social worker. Many health maintenance organizations (HMOs) provide mental health counseling services, as well as programs for special problems such as addictions. This trend portends somewhat better and more available care.

Nursing homes and, increasingly, assisted living facilities (ALFs), although not licensed as psychiatric facilities and seldom staffed to provide continual mental health assessment or care, are providing the majority of care given to elders with psychiatric conditions (Becker et al., 2002). An estimated 65% to 70% of nursing home residents have significant mental disorders, and 30% to 40% with dementia have behavioral and psychiatric symptoms (Kaldy, 2005). An insufficient number of trained personnel affects the quality of mental health care in nursing homes and often causes great stress for staff. Some of the obstacles to mental health care in nursing homes are (1) shortage of trained personnel, (2) lack of in-service training in nursing homes related to mental health and illness, (3) inadequate Medicaid and Medicare reimbursement for mental health services, and (4) limited availability of psychiatric services. A survey of

900 nursing home directors of nursing revealed that 40% of the residents needed formal psychiatric services but only 50% of the facilities surveyed had adequate availability of these services. This was especially true of smaller nursing homes and those in rural areas (Lebowitz, 2002).

Recommendations of the U.S. Health Resources and Services Administration (USHRSA) report include additional funding for training, reimbursement, psychiatric and behavioral therapies, and consumer education. This financial support is unlikely, given the shift to state fiscal responsibility. However, some progress is being made in nursing homes and long-term care facilities. The various revisions of the Omnibus Budget Reconciliation Act (OBRA) and the implementation of the Minimum Data Set (MDS) have resulted in more resident-oriented and holistic care and the reduction of chemical and physical restraints, but more attention must be paid to the mental health of older people in these settings. A guide for screening for mental illness in nursing facility applicants (Linkins et al., 2001) offers screening guidelines and federal requirements.

Gerontological nurses must be advocates for better and more appropriate treatment of mental health needs for older people and should closely monitor proposals for federal and state revisions to services and budget cuts in this area. Geropsychiatric nursing is the specialty care that nurses provide to elders with mental health disorders across the continuum of care (Kaas, 2006). Few educational programs focus on this specialty and, unfortunately, few professional curricula include adequate content on mental health and aging.

Cultural and Ethnic Disparities

Lack of knowledge and awareness of cultural differences about the meaning of mental health, differences in the way concerns may present, the lack of culturally competent mental health treatment, and limited research in this area must be addressed in light of the rapidly increasing ethnic elderly population (Abramson et al., 2002; Zhan, 2004). Culturally and ethnically diverse older people have less access to mental health services and receive poorer quality mental health care (U.S. Department of Health and Human Services [USDHHS], 2001). Some identified barriers to use of services include a lack of bilingual and bicultural staff and a lack of awareness of the existence of services (Abramson et al., 2002).

It is important to include a cultural assessment and a discussion of what culturally and ethnically diverse older adults believe about their mental health problems in all assessment situations. Culturally appropriate education about mental health concerns is also important. Further, improving mental health for ethnic older adults, according to Zahn (2004, p. 3):

> …requires strong and collective commitments to overcome the multifaceted barriers of poverty, discrimination and prejudice, linguistic difficulty, cultural conflicts, social stigma, and a lack of coordinated and culturally competent health services, and build a care system that is equal, affordable, available, and acceptable.

Research on all aspects of culture and mental health care is critically needed. Chapter 21 discusses culture in depth.

Psychological Assessment of Elders

Moorhead and Brighton (2001) report several studies suggesting that a substantial number of elders are suffering anxiety, substance abuse, and somatoform disorders that are unrecognized and untreated. Medical patients present with psychiatric disorders in 25% to 33% of cases, although they are often unrecognized by primary health care providers. It is well-known that depression in the elderly is highly prevalent and treatable but is infrequently recognized or treated. These findings serve only to confirm the increasing prevalence and neglect of emotional concerns in elders.

General issues in the psychological assessment of older adults involve distinguishing among normal, idiosyncratic, and diverse characteristics of aging and pathological conditions. Baseline data are often lacking from the individual's earlier years. Using standardized tools and functional assessment is valuable, but the data will be meaningless if not placed in the context of the patient's early life and hopes and expectations for the future. Distinguishing normal from pathological aging in a particular individual depends on these factors. Although some age-appropriate assessment

instruments are available, many of the tools available were developed for younger people. Further research is needed in developing appropriate tools, especially for culturally and ethnically diverse elders and those with dementia.

Assessment of mental health includes examination for cognitive function or impairment and the specific conditions of anxiety and adjustment reactions, depression, paranoia, substance abuse, and suicidal risk. Assessment of mental health must also focus on social intactness and affectual responses appropriate to the situation. Attention span, concentration, intelligence, judgment, learning ability, memory, orientation, perception, problem solving, psychomotor ability, and reaction time are assessed in relation to cognitive intactness and must be considered when making a psychological assessment. Assessment includes specific processes that are intact, as well as those that are diminished or compromised. The Mental Health Toolkit (available from The National Conference of Gerontological Nurse Practitioners [2005] [*www.ncgnp.org*] is an excellent resource for assessment, evaluation, and treatment of mental health concerns in older people. Assessment for specific mental health concerns is discussed throughout this chapter and in Chapter 6. Assessment of cognitive function is discussed in Chapter 23.

Obtaining assessment data from elders is best done during short sessions after some rapport has been established. Performing repeated assessments at various times of the day and in different situations will give a more complete psychological profile. It is important to be sensitive to a patient's anxiety, special needs, and disabilities and vigilant in protecting the person's privacy. The interview should be focused so that attention is given to strengths and skills, as well as deficits. A global assessment of functioning is useful (Box 25-2) in assessing the older adult. Also useful is an inventory of the psychogeriatric client (Box 25-3). See Appendix 25-A for depression rating scales.

Defenses

"Defense mechanisms (or coping styles) are automatic psychological processes that protect the individual against anxiety and from the awareness of internal or external dangers or stressors" (American Psychiatric Association [APA], 2000, p. 751). In the *Diagnostic and Statistical Manual of Mental Disorders,* 4th edition (DSM-IV), the defenses have been grouped in the Defensive Functioning Scale. These hierarchical categories allow the practitioner to categorize coping styles and then indicate the predominant defensive level that the individual exhibits. A glossary of defense mechanisms, somewhat different and healthier than classic definitions, assists in evaluation. This Defensive Functioning Scale holds promise for evaluating an elder's adaptation. As with all evaluative efforts, micro and macro timing are important, as are fatigue, pain, and stress levels. Some defensive mechanisms of older people are healthy and effective in reducing anxiety, and some are inhibitory. Some of the most predominant are presented here, and others are found in Box 25-3.

	BOX 25-2 Global Assessment of Functioning (GAF) Scale

Consider psychological, social, and occupational functioning on a hypothetical continuum of mental health and mental illness. Do not include impairment in functioning caused by physical (or environmental) limitations.

Code	(NOTE: Use intermediate codes when appropriate [e.g., 45, 68, 72].)
100 91	Superior functioning in a wide range of activities (e.g., life's problems never seem to get out of hand) is sought out by others because of his or her many positive qualities. No symptoms are present.
90 81	Absent or minimal symptoms (e.g., mild anxiety before an examination), good functioning in all areas, interested and involved in a wide range of activities, socially effective, generally satisfied with life, no more than everyday problems or concerns (e.g., an occasional argument with family members).
80 71	If symptoms are present, they are transient and expectable reactions to psychosocial stressors (e.g., difficulty concentrating after family argument), no more than slight impairment in social, occupational, or school functioning (e.g., temporarily falling behind in schoolwork).
70 61	Some mild symptoms (e.g., depressed mood and mild insomnia) OR some difficulty in social, occupational, or school functioning (e.g., occasional truancy, theft within the household), but generally functioning well; has some meaningful interpersonal relationships.
60 51	Moderate symptoms (e.g., flat affect, circumstantial speech, occasional panic attacks) OR moderate difficulty in social, occupational, or school functioning (e.g., few friends, conflicts with peers or co-workers).
50 41	Serious symptoms (e.g., suicidal ideation, severe obsessional rituals, frequent shoplifting) OR any serious impairment in social, occupational, or school functioning (e.g., no friends, unable to keep a job).
40 31	Some impairment in reality testing or communication (e.g., speech is at times illogical, obscure, or irrelevant) OR major impairment in several areas, such as work or school, family relations, judgment, thinking, or mood (e.g., depressed man avoids friends, neglects family, is unable to work, child frequently beats up younger children, is defiant at home, is failing at school).
30 21	Behavior is considerably influenced by delusions or hallucinations OR serious impairment in communication or judgment (e.g., sometimes incoherent, acts grossly inappropriately, suicidal preoccupation) OR inability to function in almost all areas (e.g., stays in bed all day; no job, home, friends).
20 11	Some danger of hurting self or others (e.g., suicide attempts without clear expectation of death, frequently violent, manic excitement) OR occasionally fails to maintain minimal personal hygiene (e.g., smears feces) OR gross impairment in communication (e.g., largely incoherent or mute).
10 1	Persistent danger of severely hurting self or others (e.g., recurrent violence) OR persistent inability to maintain minimal personal hygiene OR serious suicidal act with clear expectation of death.
0	Inadequate information.

Reprinted with permission from American Psychiatric Association: *Diagnostic and statistical manual of mental disorders*, ed 4, Washington, DC, 2000, The Association.

Denial. Denial of illness, aging, loss, death, or incapacity helps ease one through some of the difficulties of late life. Denial may be difficult to assess because many older people avoid discussion of major concerns and losses, not because they are unaware but because they have a strong enculturation to stoic endurance or have great courage. If denial is present, it is necessary and should be addressed directly only when the elder shows signs that it is interfering with decision making and judgment and always within the context of a caring relationship.

Projection. Projection is when the individual attributes his or her own unacceptable feelings, impulses, or thoughts to another. Fear, anxiety, and anger accompanying uncer-

tainty about one's situation are often not perceived as part of one's repertoire of feelings but rather are projected onto others with whom one comes in contact. A common projection of elders is rejection of others who are old or disabled, for example, "You won't catch me at the senior center with all those old fogies. All they do is complain about their illnesses—an organ recital I call it."

Altruism. Altruism is a highly valuable defense against meaninglessness. Elders often become involved in helping others or dedicating their efforts to a good cause. The individual is gratified by the appreciation of others and by personal satisfaction. For example, Laura volunteers to take school children on nature walks. The clear observations and

BOX 25-3 Inventory of Psychogeriatric Client: Function and Care Plan

1. List client's strengths:
   - Ability to take initiative in caring for self, finances, work project
   - Ability to express feelings
   - Ability to stand up for his or her rights
   - Ability to make decisions
   - Ability to care for self; for example, dressing, going to meals
   - Ability to share with others or show concern for others
   - Enjoyment of music and arts
   - Active participation in organizations
   - Interest in sports
   - Enjoyment of reading
   - Imagination and creativity
   - Special aptitudes; for example, mechanical ability, gardening
2. Identify predominant defensive coping styles:
   - Denial
   - Projection
   - Displacement
   - Passive aggression
   - Positive identification
3. Identify highly adaptive coping styles:
   - Affiliation
   - Altruism
   - Humor
   - Self-assertion
   - Sublimation
4. Identify defensive breakdown patterns:
   - Delusional projection
   - Psychotic suspiciousness
   - Psychotic denial
   - Immobilizing fears
   - Psychotic distortions
   - Apathetic withdrawal
5. Determine client's needs and problems based on the following:
   - Reason for seeking assistance by client, family, and others

- Medical history and findings (physical, mental, neurological, and psychological examinations and tests)
- Drug use profile (use of prescribed and nonprescribed drugs)
- Laboratory and diagnostic tests
- Psychiatric history
- Social history
- Mental status
- Other background information provided by client, family, and each staff person who has interviewed the client
6. Develop a nursing care plan considering:
   - Client's problems, needs, and strengths
   - Mutually identified short-term goals
   - Mutually identified long-term goals
7. State expected outcome of care in terms that can be measured. The following are examples of goals stated in measurable terms:
   - Socializes more
   - Dresses appropriately—puts on coat or jacket when going outside in cold weather
   - Improves personal hygiene—brushes teeth daily without being reminded
   - Shows improvement in problem areas
   - Improves attitude—discusses problems or concerns instead of hitting or resisting
   - Increases functional independence
   - Reduces hostility—responds when spoken to in a friendly manner
   - Improves self-esteem—goes 1 day without self-criticism
   - Reduces depression—expresses interest in one outside activity
   - States increased enjoyment of activities
   - Reduces suspiciousness—eats a meal without expressing fear of poisoning
8. Review progress periodically, and revise goals as necessary and appropriate.

unique views of these children restore her youth as she teaches them and as they all commune with nature. We find this attribute one of the transcendent mechanisms and prefer to categorize it as quite beyond a defense mechanism.

Positive Identification. Positive identification is not listed among the defensive mechanisms in the DSM-IV, but it appears to be a healthy coping activity. Some older individuals in poor health identify with others who are more physically and psychologically intact, and because of this identification, these elders appraise themselves as more able. Positive identification seems to be a process embodying both hope and affiliation. If Bob Hope and George Burns could be clever, rich, and functional at their ages, then the elder can claim their success through cohort affiliation. These successful people were contemporaries and make the elder feel more effective because of affiliation with the respect they generated.

All of us use defensive strategies, some quite conscious and others that are far beyond our awareness. The more vulnerable we become, the more these defenses are needed. If the individual is maintaining sufficient supports and life satisfactions in the situation he or she is in, do not disturb the balance, no matter how precarious. Shore up the foundations of strength.

PSYCHIATRIC DISORDERS OF AGING

Adjustment Disorders

Adjustment disorders are diagnosed when one develops significant emotional or behavioral responses to an identifiable psychosocial stress or stressors (APA, 2000). Clinical significance is noted when the distress that the elder exhibits is in excess of that expected by the nature of the stressor (Box 25-4). The stressors may be single or multiple, recurrent or continuous, and some are more prominent than others in cer-

---

BOX 25-4   Diagnostic Criteria for Adjustment Disorders

A. The development of emotional or behavioral symptoms in response to an identifiable stressor(s) occurring within 3 months of the onset of the stressor(s).
B. These symptoms or behaviors are clinically significant as evidenced by either of the following:
   (1) Marked distress that is in excess of what would be expected from exposure to the stressor
   (2) Significant impairment in social or occupational (academic) functioning
C. The stress-related disturbance does not meet the criteria for another specific axis I disorder and is not merely an exacerbation of a preexisting axis I or axis II disorder.
D. The symptoms do not represent bereavement.
E. Once the stressor (or its consequences) has terminated, the symptoms do not persist for more than an additional 6 months.

Specify if:
Acute: if the disturbance lasts less than 6 months
Chronic: if the disturbance lasts for 6 months or longer

From American Psychiatric Association: *Diagnostic and statistical manual of mental disorders,* ed 4, Washington, DC, 1994, The Association.

BOX 25-5   Criteria for Generalized Anxiety Disorder

Excess worry and anxiety about many things more often than not for more than 6 months
Inability or difficulty controlling the worry and anxiety
Worry and anxiety associated with three or more of the following:
- Muscle tension
- Irritability
- Difficulty concentrating; mind going blank
- Sleep disturbances
- Easily fatigued
- Restless, on edge

Worry and anxiety focus on routine life situations, circumstances that may shift from one concern to another
Worry and anxiety not caused by physical effects of drug abuse or medication or by a medical condition and do not occur during a mood disorder or psychotic disorder

---

tain developmental periods, such as a move into a dependent situation, which many elders must confront (see Chapter 24).

Assessing excessive emotional reactions to certain adjustments required of older people may be difficult because personality, gender, and cultural factors must be considered, as well as the availability of supportive relationships. Adjustment disorders may be exhibited by profound depression, with or without anxiety, and behavioral disturbances.

Nursing interventions should include anticipatory rehearsal of the event and establishment of a reliable and ongoing support system available to the individual before and after the occurrence. In addition, options and alternatives related to the particular adjustment should be thoroughly discussed and considered, which will reduce the sense of helplessness and irreversibility. Consider the following scenario:

George had all of his teeth removed and both upper and lower dentures put in place in 1 day. The analgesics made him nauseated, pain kept him awake, and he lost interest in food. These not unusual occurrences continued to be a focus of attention and complaint for him for several months. Whenever anyone said, "How are you?" George would go into a litany about his teeth. Insomnia and weight loss became serious problems, and he became increasingly nonfunctional.

When the complaints persisted for several months, and after many visits to the dentist because the teeth "didn't fit properly," the prosthodontist recognized an extreme adjustment reaction and referred George for a psychiatric consult. The geriatric nurse practitioner (GNP) who saw George convinced him to accompany her to the senior center, which he had previously avoided because of "all the old folks there." The GNP introduced him to some of the elders in her caseload who attended the center's meals and activities.

Fortunately, the GNP was able to establish a tentative relationship between George and a lady who had experienced similar difficulties adjusting to dentures. Much later, George told the GNP that she had literally saved his life. He found others who had been as distressed as he was about adjusting to dentures, and he established a friendship with the lady to whom he had first been introduced. To avoid such an intense adjustment, there should have been much preparatory work and discussion of options by George and his dentist and sufficient time elapsed to incorporate the idea of this major change in appearance, self-perception, and sensual pleasure.

Anxiety Reactions

A general definition for anxiety is unpleasant and unwarranted feelings of apprehension, which may be accompanied by physical symptoms. Anxiety itself is a normal human reaction and part of a fear response; it is rational, within reason. Anxiety becomes problematic when it is prolonged and exaggerated and begins to interfere with function. Anxiety meeting the criteria for a diagnosable disorder affects from 3.5% to 10% of older people. In women older than 65 years, 10% to 15% find anxiety symptoms sufficiently distressing to visit a physician (Hegel et al., 2002). Risk factors for anxiety disorders include the following: female; urban living; history of worrying or rumination; poor physical health; low socioeconomic status; high stress events; and depression and alcoholism.

Generalized anxiety disorder (GAD) is the most common anxiety disorder in the elderly, although it is underdiagnosed and undertreated. GAD is commonly related to life events such as illness, bereavement, social and financial status changes, and cognitive impairment. Worry is the primary feature of GAD, and anxiety symptoms frequently co-exist with depression (Frampton, 2004). The criteria for GAD are listed in Box 25-5. Other anxiety disorders that occur in older people include phobic disorder, obsessive-compulsive disorder, and panic disorders. Very little research has been done on anxiety in older adults (Burke, 2004).

▲ *Promoting Healthy Aging: Implications for Gerontological Nursing*

Assessment. The general and pervasive nature of anxiety may make diagnosis difficult in older adults. In addition, older adults tend to deny psychological symptoms, attribute anxiety-related symptoms to physical illness, and have co-existent medical conditions that mimic symptoms of generalized anxiety. Some of the medical disorders that cause anxiety responses include cardiac arrhythmias, delirium, dementia (probably the most common cause of anxiety), chronic obstructive pulmonary disease (COPD), congestive heart failure, hyperthyroidism, hypoglycemia, postural hypotension, pulmonary edema, and pulmonary emboli. Anxiety is frequently the presenting symptom of depression in older people. Anxiety is also a common side effect of many drugs including anticholinergics, digitalis, theophylline, antihypertensives, beta-blockers, beta-adrenergic stimulators (albuterol), corticosteroids, and over-the-counter (OTC) medications such as appetite suppressants, nicotine, and cough and cold preparations. Caffeine, alcohol, and benzodiazepine misuse are often causes of anxiety. Withdrawal from alcohol, sedatives, and hypnotics will cause symptoms of anxiety.

It is important to assess the older adult for anxiety symptoms and to investigate other possible causes such as depression and medical conditions. Clinical signs that suggest an anxiety reaction include restlessness, edginess, fatigue, difficulty concentrating, irritability, tension, and sleep disturbances. When co-morbid conditions are present, they need to be treated. A review of medications is in order, eliminating those that cause anxiety.

Interventions. When dealing with anxiety reactions, look for daily disturbances such as staff or caregiver changes, room changes, and other events over which the individual feels a lack of control or influence. By themselves, these circumstances seldom provoke an anxiety reaction, but they may be the "straw that breaks the camel's back." Anxiety embodies an overwhelming sense of being out of control of one's life and destiny. Restoring the individual's sense of control as quickly as possible is critical. Discuss feelings and actions that can be taken. In a room change, for instance, how can the individual be alerted in sufficient time to incorporate the idea? How can the new room be personalized? Is there a choice of rooms? We can assist by focusing attention away from the body and onto feelings and problem solving.

Providing a structured environment may alleviate anxiety in older people experiencing dementia. Nurses need to be alert to signs of anxiety in frail older people or those with dementia, since they may be unable to tell us how they are feeling. Carefully observing behavior and searching for possible reasons for changes in behavior or patterns are important (see Chapter 23). Interventions such as cognitive-behavioral therapy, relaxation training, exercise, anxiety management, and interpersonal psychotherapy, often in combination with medication, have been shown to be beneficial.

Medications found to be especially useful are paroxetine and venlafaxine, particularly when depression is present (Reuben et al., 2003). Benzodiazepines (lorazepam, oxazepam) may be recommended for short-term therapy. These medications can have problematic side effects such as sedation, falls, altered mental status, and dependence (see Chapter 12). Although useful, they are often prescribed without adequate assessment of the multitude of factors contributing to anxiety symptoms. Non-benzodiazepine anxiolytic agents (e.g., buspirone) are preferred. Buspirone has fewer side effects but requires a longer dosing time for effectiveness.

Posttraumatic Stress Disorder

Posttraumatic stress disorder (PTSD) has become a part of our national vocabulary and reminds us of the deep and lasting toll that national disasters take. PTSD was early recognized as an outcome of overwhelmingly stressful experiences of individuals in the war in Vietnam. Only recently realized is that many World War II veterans have lived most of their lives under the shadow of PTSD without it being recognized. Seniors under our care now have also experienced the Great Depression, the Holocaust, racism, and the Korean conflict (Kennedy, 2001).

Now we know from community surveys that PTSD is fairly common, occurs increasingly in women, and has a lifetime prevalence of 7% to 12% (Culpepper, 2000). Rape is the most likely specific trauma that will result in long-lived PTSD in women, followed by child abuse, then being threatened with a weapon, molested, neglected as a child, and physical violence. For men, the greatest trauma is also rape, followed by abuse as a child, neglect as a child, combat, and being molested.

According to the DSM-IV, PTSD (recognized by the DSM over 20 years ago) is a syndrome characterized by the development of symptoms after an extremely traumatic event that involves experiencing, witnessing, or unexpectedly hearing about an actual or threatened death or serious injury to oneself or another closely affiliated person. Individuals often reexperience the traumatic event in episodes of fear and experience symptoms such as helplessness, flashbacks, intrusive thoughts, memories, images, emotional numbing, loss of interest, avoidance of any place that reminds of the traumatic event, startle reactions, poor concentration, irritability, jumpiness, and hypervigilance (Culpepper, 2000). These episodes may occur periodically for years, though they frequently remain submerged until activated by the losses of aging. These individuals may have ongoing sleep problems, somatic disturbances, anxiety, depression, and restlessness. Over the long term, these people are typically impaired in work, have maladaptive lifestyles, and do not develop close relationships. Consider the following example:

Ernie may have had PTSD, though it was only speculative after his suicide. On his eighteenth birthday, Ernie joined the U.S. Army Air Corps (precedent to our present U.S. Air Force) in 1941. He was quickly trained and sent to Burma to "fly the hump," the Himalayan mountains in Burma, China, and India. During his 3-year stint, Ernie survived two airplane crashes, saw several of his companions mutilated in crashes, watched the torture of captured Japanese, and witnessed the capture of some of his friends. When Ernie returned to the United States, his hair had turned from deep auburn to pure white. He retired from the service after 20 years but was never really able to work after his retirement. Ernie's life was filled with episodes of alcoholic binges, outbursts of anger, and episodes of abusing others, all seemingly quite out of his control. One friend remained from his "service" days and visited him periodically until his death in 1996. Other relationships seemed to have been superficial and to have had little meaning for Ernie. On his seventy-eighth birthday, which he spent alone, Ernie shot himself. One must wonder how many of the elderly veterans of World War II, the most highly suicidal group in the United States, are suffering from PTSD.

A person who becomes cognitively impaired may no longer be able to control thoughts, flashbacks, or images. This can be the cause of great distress that may be exhibited by aggressive or hostile behavior. An example of this occurred in a Veterans Administration (VA) nursing home with an 80-year-old WW II veteran resident with dementia who became very agitated and attempted to hit others around him when he was placed in the large day room with other residents. The staff recognized this as a PTSD reaction from his years as a prisoner of war. They always placed him in a smaller dayroom near the nursing station away from the other residents. The aggression stopped without the need for medication. Bludau (2002) described the concept of second institutionalization that occurs in nursing home residents who are Holocaust survivors.

▲ Promoting Healthy Aging: Implications for Gerontological Nursing

Assessment and Interventions. PTSD prevention and treatment are only now getting the research attention that other illnesses have received over the years (Culpepper, 2000). The care of the individual with PTSD involves awareness that certain events may trigger inappropriate reactions and the pattern of these reactions should be identified when possible. Cognitive-behavioral therapy with pharmacological therapy will be useful for supporting the patient with PTSD (Culpepper, 2000). Sertraline and paroxetine have U.S. Food and Drug Administration (FDA) approval to treat PTSD.

Nursing supports also include humor, distraction, teaching relaxation techniques, back massage, support groups with guided imagery, therapeutic touch, and information provided to family members (Moorhead and Brighton, 2001). Effective coping with extremely traumatic events that created intense fear and helplessness seems to be associated with secure and supportive relationships; the ability to freely express or fully suppress the experience; favorable circumstances immediately after the trauma; productive and active lifestyles; strong faith, religion, and hope; a sense of humor; and biological integrity. An instrument to assess PTSD can be found at *www.hartfordign.org*.

Obsessive-Compulsive Disorders

Obsessive-compulsive disorder (OCD) is characterized by recurrent and persistent thoughts, impulses, or images (obsessions) that are repetitive, purposeful, and intentional urges or ritualistic behaviors (compulsions) that improve comfort level but are recognized as excessive and unreasonable. OCD is an anxiety disorder that significantly impairs function and consumes more than 1 hour each day (APA, 2000). OCD is common among elderly people, seems to have a genetic component, and occurs mainly in women. These disorders are exaggerated manifestations of a need for control and order and a way of warding off anxiety. In elderly people, symptoms often are not sufficient to seriously disrupt function and thus may not be considered a true disorder but rather a coping strategy. If symptoms progress to a point at which they disrupt lifestyle, the elder will need clinical attention.

Interventions. As in other anxiety disorders, exercise and cognitive-behavioral therapy have been effective in managing OCD in combination with pharmacological therapy if indicated. Sertraline, paroxetine, fluoxetine, and fluvoxamine are recommended (Reuben et al., 2003).

Excessive Suspicion and Paranoia

Paranoia is characterized by suspiciousness and insecurity. Many older people without a history of mental disturbance develop a suspicious or paranoid viewpoint. Various estimates of the prevalence of paranoia range from 5% to 10% of the older adult population. These reactions are sometimes induced by alcoholism or medications, and hearing impairment may accentuate these feelings. Fear and a lack of trust originating from a reality base may become magnified, especially when one is isolated from others and does not receive reality feedback. The majority of reactions, however, originate in attempts to exert control in an unsatisfactory situation or to feel capable. Inability to correctly evaluate the social milieu because of isolation or cognitive impairment is a significant factor.

Paranoia is an early symptom of Alzheimer's disease, appearing approximately 20 months before diagnosis. In his description of a woman with a peculiar disease of the cerebral cortex, Dr. Alois Alzheimer described the first noticeable symptoms of the illness as suspiciousness of her husband and believing that people were out to murder her. Memory loss and forgetfulness may result in an elder being convinced that items are being stolen or that medications are not the correct ones. The dynamics seem to be loss of control, inability to evaluate the social milieu appropriately, and the feeling of external forces controlling one's life, which in many instances is true.

In addition to these dynamics, an unknown number of elders have a paranoid personality disorder that has simply grown old and more pronounced. These individuals have had a pervasive distrust and suspiciousness of others' motives all of their adult life, assuming that others will harm, exploit, or even deceive them though they have no basis to support these beliefs. It is sometimes difficult to determine the reality of an apparent paranoid reaction. Many cases have been encountered in which plots against an older person were real.

Delusions

Delusions are beliefs that guide one's interpretation of events and help make sense out of disorder. The delusions may be comforting or threatening, but they always form a structure for understanding situations that otherwise might seem unmanageable. A delusional disorder is one in which conceivable ideas, without foundation in fact, persist for more than 1 month. These beliefs are not always bizarre and do not originate in psychotic processes. Common delusions are of being poisoned, being followed, their children taking their assets, being held prisoner, or being deceived by a spouse or lover. Delusional disorders in the absence of psychoses usually begin earlier in life but may continue into old age. In older adults, delusions often incorporate significant persons rather than the global grandiose or persecutory delusions of younger persons. When an individual becomes incapable of obtaining life's satisfactions or of maintaining function or adequate supplies, the delusions may allow the individual to avoid depression and maintain self-esteem by projecting blame onto others or society.

One older woman persistently held onto the delusion that her son was coming to pick her up and take her home, although her son had been dead for 10 years. The events of her day, her hopes, and her status were all organized around this belief. Clearly, without her delusion, she would have felt forlorn, lost, and abandoned. Many delusions related to family members and their actions or intentions occur among institutionalized older people. Some may aid in coping, whereas others may be troubling to the person. One study found that 21% of 125 new nursing home residents had delusions (Grossberg, 2000).

▲ Promoting Healthy Aging: Implications for Gerontological Nursing

Assessment and Interventions. The assessment dilemma is often one of determining the truth of the delusional belief and avoiding assumptions. Concluding that someone is delusional is never safe unless you have thoroughly investigated his or her claims. In one case, an elderly man insisted that he must visit his mother. His thoughts seemed clear in other respects, which is often the case with people who are delusional. One of the authors (PE) suspected that he had

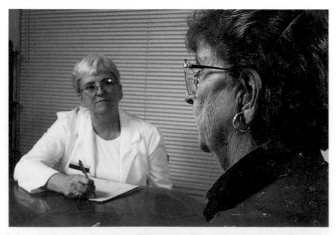

Demonstrating respect and a willingness to listen is the foundation for a caring nurse-patient relationship. (From Harkreader H, Hogan MA: *Fundamentals of nursing: caring and clinical judgment,* ed 2, St Louis, 2004, Saunders.)

some unresolved conflicts about his dead mother or needed comforting and caring. She did not argue with him about his dead mother because arguing is never a useful approach to people with delusions. Rather, she used the best techniques she was able to recall to assure him that she was interested in him as a person and recognized that he must feel very lonely sometimes. He continued to say he must leave and go to his mother. When she could no longer delay his leaving, she walked with him to the nurses' station and found that his 103-year-old mother did indeed live in another wing of the institution and he visited her every day.

Frightening delusions (e.g., the world is coming to an end; one is being poisoned) are usually in response to anxiety-provoking situations and are best handled by reducing situational stress, being available to the client, and attending to the fears more than the content of the delusion. Other suggestions are to avoid television, which can be confusing, especially if the patient awakens and finds it on. Also, reduce clutter in the patient's room, eliminate large mirrors, and eliminate shadows that can appear threatening. Provide glasses and hearing aids to maximize sensory input and decrease misinterpretations.

Direct confrontation is likely to increase anxiety and agitation, the sense of vulnerability, and the need for the delusion; it may also disrupt the relationship. A more useful approach is to establish a trusting relationship that is nondemanding and not too intense. It is important to identify the client's strengths and build upon them. This will reduce the alienation and feelings of insignificance that underlie paranoid ideation. Demonstrating respect and a willingness to listen to complaints and fears is important. It is important that the nurse be trustworthy, give clear information, and present clear choices. Do not pretend to agree with paranoid beliefs; instead, ask what is troubling the person and provide reassurance of safety.

Clear information should be given and clear choices should always be presented to the patient. When offering food, medication, treatments, or resources, relevant information should be given. When patients refuse necessary treatments, their decision must be respected. Focusing on decision-making power will probably be beneficial. For example, "Mrs. S., it seems you are reluctant to take these medications. I respect the fact that you are cautious about such things. I will get you more information about these drugs. Are there particular reactions you are concerned about? Let me know if you decide to take them"; or "Mrs. J., many people feel angry or afraid when they are ill. Is there anything I can do to make you more comfortable?" Other strategies include not arguing with the patient about disappearing items or trying to rationally explain them. Whispering in the presence of the patient will increase suspiciousness and should be avoided.

When encountering suspicious elderly, the nurse's primary concern is first directed at establishing the reality of the feeling, but if the suspicions are not substantiated, the elder should not be challenged. Other strategies include not arguing with the person or giving false reassurance. Paranoia may act as an effective shield against intrusion into one's

BOX 25-6 Guidelines for Nursing Care of Suspicious Patients

- Remember that anger is pervasive and is not meant for the nurse per se.
- Anger is a legitimate expression of feeling.
- Suspicious patients will look for flaws or indications of injustice.
- Attempt to accept criticism without resentment or defensiveness.
- Arguing only increases the struggle for control.
- The quality of nursing care may not be measurable by patient progress, particularly if the goals are unrealistic or not relevant to the patient. In other words, paranoia may lift slowly or not at all.
- Nursing care should provide for the following needs:
  1. Suspicious patients need to learn to trust themselves. Allow the patient to function independently in areas in which success can be achieved and identified.
  2. Suspicious patients need to be able to trust others. Nurses should state what they are willing and able to do. Vague promises, such as "I'll be around whenever you need me," only increase opportunities for distrust and disappointment.
  3. Suspicious patients need to test reality. When the larger reality is distorted, focus on smaller aspects of reality, for example:

     Mrs. J: The whole world is against me.

     Nurse: What in this room gives you that feeling? Are there certain times when you feel that most strongly?
  4. Contact with the nurse and his or her accepting responses reassure the person and decrease the need for a protective delusion.
  5. Suspicious persons need outlets for their anger.

vulnerable state and as such may be a useful defensive posture. The presence of paranoid ideation is a problem only if it disturbs the patient or others in his or her environment. If symptoms are interfering with function, antipsychotic drugs may be needed for effective management. The newer atypical antipsychotics (risperidone, olanzapine) are preferred. Careful monitoring for side effects is essential. Box 25-6 presents other guidelines for care.

Hallucinations

Hallucinations are best described as sensory perceptions of a nonexistent object stimulus and may be spurred by the internal stimulation of any of the five senses. Although not attributable to environmental stimuli, hallucinations may occur because of the total environmental impact. Hallucinations arising out of psychological conflicts tend to be less predominant in old age, and those that are generated as security measures tend to increase as the person ages. These hallucinations are thought to germinate in situations in which one is feeling alone, abandoned, isolated, or alienated. To compensate for insecurity, a hallucinatory experience, often a companion, is imagined. Imagined companions may fill the

intense void and provide some security, but they may become accusing and disturbing.

The character and stages of hallucinatory experiences have not been adequately defined in late life. Many hallucinations are in response to physical disorders, such as dementia, Parkinson's disease, physiological and sensory disorders, and medications. Hallucinations of older adults most often seem mixed with disorientation, illusions, intense grief, and immersion in retrospection, the origins being difficult to separate. Psychotic symptoms arising in late life may be associated with cognitive decline.

The onset of true psychotic disorders is low among older people, but psychotic manifestations may occur as a secondary syndrome in a variety of disorders, the most common being Alzheimer's disease. Psychotic symptoms in Alzheimer's disease require different assessment and treatment than do long-standing psychiatric disorders. Alzheimer's disease and other dementias are discussed in Chapter 23.

Older people with severe vision and hearing deficits may also hear voices or see people and objects that are not actually present (illusions). Some have explained this as the brain's attempt to create stimulation in the absence of adequate sensory input. If these illusions are not disturbing to the person, they do not need treatment. One older woman in the nursing home who had Alzheimer's disease and was experiencing agnosia would look in the mirror and talk to the "nice lady I see in there." "Do you want to eat or go for a walk with me?" she would ask. It was comforting to her and therefore she did not need medication for her "hallucinations," as some would have labeled her behavior.

Determining whether the hallucinations are the result of dementia, psychoses, deprivation, or overload is important for nurses because the treatment will vary. An isolated older person who is admitted to the hospital in a hallucinatory state must be carefully and thoroughly assessed physically and then gradually brought into socializing experiences. A subdued environment with staff continuity is important, and the person should be allowed peripheral participation and retreat when necessary. Individuals in the community who develop hallucinations must be assessed in terms of threats to security, severe physical or psychological disruptions, withdrawal symptoms, medications, and overload of stimuli. Antipsychotic medications are used for management of hallucinations that impair function but must be monitored closely for correct dosage and side effects.

Schizophrenia

The onset of schizophrenia usually occurs between adolescence and the mid-30s, and the occurrence of schizophrenia is rare in older people. Older adults with late-onset schizophrenia show less formal thought disorder than younger people (Palmer et al., 2002). Theories suggest that many elderly people who are homeless may have chronic schizophrenia; discharged from state hospitals years ago after spending their young adulthood institutionalized, they were simply unable to develop satisfactory living situations. An estimated 43% of elderly schizophrenics now reside in nursing homes (Frampton, 2004). Individuals with severe, persis-

TABLE 25-1

Factors in the Self-Management Process for Persons with Bipolar Disorder

	Self-Management Efforts		
Motivators	**Successful**	**Unsuccessful**	**Self-Assessment Parameters**
Wanting to live	Follow professional advice	Deny there is a problem	How you feel
Wanting mental wellness	Talk with people	Overextend self	Intervention frequency
Wanting to get along with others	Take medication	Expect too much from misinformed	Common sense
Wanting love	Set goals	Stay to oneself	How people treat you
To become productive	Follow schedule	Be open with family*	How you treat people
To feel better about self	Be prepared	Do street drugs	Positive results
To avoid problems in the family	Stay active	Rely on others for information	Decreased hospital stay
Self-love	Seek information	Self-start and stop medication	Behavior
Because of barriers	Read	Let problems overwhelm	Able to manage daily activities
Receiving help	Groups	Get angry	
Finally knew what was wrong	Therapy	Watch TV all the time	
Costs (e.g., relationships, jobs)	Selective disclosure	Not coping with stress	
Duration of illness	Do not let things get to you	Not seeking help	
Symptoms	Hospitalization		
Being hospitalized			
Self-management not an option			

From Pollack LE: Inpatient self-management of bipolar disorder, *Appl Nurs Res* 9(2):71, 1996.
*An unsuccessful intervention for one person may be helpful for another in differing circumstances.

tent mental illness such as schizophrenia form a disenfranchised group whose access to medical care has been limited, leading to greater functional declines and mortality; this is demonstrated by statistics that show that individuals with schizophrenia have a life expectancy 20% lower than the general population (Davis, 2004).

Assessment. Every patient presenting with psychosis should be evaluated for depression, dementia, suicidal and homicidal risk, extrapyramidal effects (if the patient has been taking antipsychotic drugs), and irreversible movement disorders such as tardive dyskinesia (TD) (Antai-Otong, 2000). The Abnormal Involuntary Movement Scale (AIMS) is useful for evaluating early symptoms of TD.

Support. Environmental intervention is the most successful, least expensive, and safest form of treatment (Beers and Berkow, 2000). Appropriate behaviors should be supported, maintaining safety of the person. Physical activity is important to avoid emotional or physical outbursts and to promote sleep. Getting to know patients well helps the nursing staff know what kinds of cues the patient gives before a burst of agitation; sometimes pacing the floor is a precipitant to an outburst. Medications are used when the environmental changes are not enough to maintain a safe and tolerable milieu. OBRA guidelines for the use of antipsychotic medications in the nursing home provide the indications for use of these medications in schizophrenia. The newer atypical antipsychotics (risperidone, olanzapine, quetiapine), given in low doses, are less likely to cause the irreversible side effects of TD and seem to be very effective in late-onset schizophrenia (Frampton, 2004).

Bipolar Disorders

Bipolar disorders, characterized by periods of mania and depression, often level out in late life, and individuals tend to have longer periods of depression (National Institutes of Mental Health [NIMH], 2002). However, frequent relapses may occur with aging and may be precipitated by medical problems. Mania does occur in older adults and is a distinct period lasting at least 1 week during which an abnormally and persistent elevated, expansive, or irritable mood is exhibited (Beers and Berkow, 2000). Mania may present as irritability or agitation and is often misdiagnosed as something other than bipolar disorder. As people with bipolar disorder get older, they become "rapid cyclers." They can cycle from mania to deep depression in days or weeks as opposed to month or years typical in the younger patient (Sattinger, 2006). An individual with a bipolar disorder is afflicted with a chemical imbalance and must be treated as such. A thorough history and physical examination are imperative in making a diagnosis. Thyroid dysfunction should always be part of the differential diagnosis. Lithium, the most commonly used substance for individuals with bipolar disorders, has neurological effects that make it difficult for older people to tolerate; it also has a long half-life (more than 36 hours). Careful monitoring of blood levels and patient response is important (Tabloski, 2006).

Treatment. Benzodiazepines, antipsychotics, antidepressants, and mood-stabilizing agents such as carbamazepine or valproic acid may be effective. Balancing the appropriate medication dosage and monitoring side effects is particularly precarious in elders and requires very careful and consistent attention. Use of selective serotonin reuptake in-

TABLE 25-2

Self-Management Information Needed
for Groups of Patients with Bipolar Disorder

Area of Concern	Information Needed
Understanding bipolar disorder	Education for self and others Importance of medication Importance of groups Importance of therapy How to deal with the disorder How to manage yourself Follow medical advice The need to get help
Managing daily life	Set goals Schedule self-seek support Manage stress Daily functioning Enjoy life Importance of exercise
Living in society	Stress management Money management Society reentry
Relating to others	Anger management Need for support Be self-aware and independent
Relating to self	Need for good self-esteem Avoid substances Think positively Take responsibility for your life Assess self Solve problems Help self Attend groups Seek spiritual strength Deal with situations Seek support Meditate Exercise mind and body

From Pollack LE: Inpatient self-management of bipolar disorder, *Appl Nurs Res* 9(2):71, 1996.

hibitors (SSRIs) in people with undiagnosed bipolar disorder can lead to manic behaviors shortly after the first administration and may be a significant diagnostic clue that the person has bipolar disorder (Sattinger, 2006). Patient and family education is essential. The family must understand that the individual is not able to control mania and irritating behaviors because of a chemical imbalance in the brain. Family members also need a great deal of support and information (Tables 25-1 and 25-2).

Depression

Depression is the most common mental health problem of late life, affecting up to 15% of individuals older than 65 years. Depression remains underdiagnosed and undertreated among this population, with only about 15% of older people with depression receiving appropriate treatment (Gum et al., 2006; Lawrence et al., 2006, Loughlin, 2004). Estimates of the prevalence of depression in homebound elderly adults is between 26% and 44% (Loughlin, 2004). Box 25-7 presents the results of a study of the prevalence of depression in homebound elders. An estimated 30% to 50% of older adults will experience a depressive episode that will seriously affect function at some time in their life (Tanner, 2005).

Race and culture may affect perceptions of the meaning of depression as well as the likelihood of seeking treatment. In addition, assessment of depression in racial and ethnic populations is affected by cultural beliefs of the patient and the provider, as well as linguistic differences and the lack of culturally appropriate assessment tools. Further study of cultural and racial differences is needed, but estimates are that minor depression may affect as many as 10% of older African-Americans, 15% of older Latinos, and 12% of older Asians, with even lower levels of service use than other cultures (Hegel et al., 2002; Lawrence et al., 2006). Native Americans also have very high rates of depression (Kennedy-Malone et al., 2000). Some studies have reported that African-Americans with depression may exhibit more hostility and irritability as well as a greater frequency of somatic complaints. African-Americans may also rely more on informal support from family, friends, and ministers than on the formal health care system (Kales and Mellow, 2006). However, this may also be a result of the lack of culturally competent health care services. A recent cross-cultural study (Lawrence et al., 2006) emphasized the importance of being sensitive to the way different ethnic and cultural groups describe depression (e.g., excessive thinking within the South Asian group; weighed down and low spirited within the Afro-Caribbean group) in recognition and assessment.

More than 15% of older adults with chronic physical conditions are depressed, and depression may be initiated or complicated by physical illness. Poststroke depression is very common, and administration of antidepressants within the first 3 months of stroke has been shown to prevent depression and improve performance in self-care activities (Frampton, 2004). The prevalence of depression in long-term care may be as high as 25% and has been attributed to stressors such as chronic illness and disability, dementia, chronic pain, preexisting depressive disorder, death of a spouse, and relocation to an institution (Frampton, 2004; Ugarriza, 2002). The prevalence of depression in nursing home residents increases with severe cognitive impairment and pain, making assessment of these variables important in this population (Kenefick, 2004).

Many drugs and medical conditions common to the elderly are associated with depression. In addition, the life situations of elders may result in depression. Depression may be considered a chronic illness in late life, with estimates that 30% of depressed older adults remain chronically depressed, take longer to recover from depression, and have shorter relapse times than do younger persons (Gallo and Coyne, 2000; Reynolds et al., 2002).

BOX 25-7 Evidence-Based Practice: Depression and Social Support: Effective Treatments for Homebound Older Adults

PURPOSE

The purposes of this pilot study were to identify the prevalence of depression in homebound elderly adults receiving home care services and to examine the relationship between depression and social support systems.

SAMPLE/SETTING

A convenience sample of 25 older people (75-98 years of age) receiving home health services in the Chicago area. 80% of the participants were white and 20% were African-American. 19 were female and 6 were male.

METHOD

Participants were screened for depression using the long form of the GDS. Social support was defined as the quantity and quality of social interaction. Participants indicated the number of formal social support services they received and completed the short form of the social support questionnaire, which measures perceived social support. The reliability of both instruments has been demonstrated with older adult populations. Chi square was used to determine statistical associations between depression severity and perceived quality and quantity of social support using the SPSS program.

RESULTS

55% of the white and 40% of the African-American participants reported depressive symptoms, with more men than women reporting mild depression. Formal measures of social support and living alone were not found to be related to depression. Using Pearson's correlation, depression was positively associated with being a man, being unmarried, and needing formal social supports in the home.

IMPLICATIONS

The non-random sample and small sample size limit the interpretation and generalizability of the findings. The prevalence of depression found in this study is similar to other studies of homebound older adults and indicates a need to address depression in this population. Findings that functional decline contributed more to depression than lack of social support have also been reported in other studies in this population. Further research is needed to examine the relationship between social support and depression in older adults. Identification and treatment of depression in homebound elders are important roles for home health nurses and nurse practitioners working in home settings. A team approach involving nurses, social workers, families, primary care providers, and the patient is recommended. Education in self-management skills to cope with chronic illness is suggested as an effective nursing intervention to prevent depression.

Data from Loughlin A: Depression and social support: effective treatment for homebound older adults, *J Gerontol Nurs* 30(5):11-15, 2004.
GDS, Geriatric depression scale; *SPSS,* statistical package for the social sciences.

Subsyndromal Depression. A new class of disorders called *subsyndromal* or *subthreshold mental disorders* (*minor depression* and *subthreshold generalized anxiety disorders*) is emerging as a significant concern. These disorders do not meet the full criteria for classification as specific mental disorders; however, they are associated with clinically significant distress and impairment and are associated with an increased risk of developing major depression (NIMH, 2007). Minor depression is defined as the presence of at least two but fewer than five depressive symptoms, including depressed mood or loss of interest in normal daily activities during the same 2-week period with no history of a major depressive episode or dysthymic disorder but with clinically significant impairment or distress. A sense of hopelessness, sleep problems, memory problems, lethargy, and decreased appetite may be presenting symptoms. An estimated 10% of older adults in the community experience minor depression (Hegel et al., 2002).

Differing Presentation of Depression in Elders. "Depression may be even more difficult to understand and diagnose than other illnesses and conditions because depression may take on different meanings when subjected to age and cultural variables" (Ugarriza, 2002, p. 22). To understand depression, the nurse must understand the influence of late-life stressors and changes, culture, and the

beliefs older people, society, and health professionals may have about depression and its treatment. Depressive symptoms may be seen as normal in older adults. Older people may not say they are depressed. The stigma associated with depression may be more prevalent in older people; and many, particularly those who have survived the depression, World Wars, the Holocaust, and other tragedies, may see depression as shameful, evidence of flawed character, self-centered, a spiritual weakness, and sin or retribution (Reynolds et al., 2002; Ugarriza, 2002; Whall and Hoes-Gurevich, 1999). Culturally and ethnically diverse older people (particularly South Asian and Black Caribbean elders) may see depression as a sign of weakness or deficiency of character, and fear of being ostracized by peers may make individuals less likely to seek help (Lawrence et al., 2006).

Older people who are depressed report more somatic complaints, such as physical symptoms, insomnia, fatigue, loss of appetite and weight loss, anxiety, memory problems (often called *pseudodementia*), or chronic pain. Depressed older adults may perform poorly on cognitive assessment examinations and are more likely to simply not answer or say they do not care rather than make up answers (confabulation) as seen in people with dementia. They are less likely to have feelings of guilt and worthlessness seen in younger depressed individuals. Hypochondriasis is also common, as are constant complaining and criticism, which may actually be

TABLE 25-3
Symptoms of Depression and Related Behavior in Older Adults

Symptoms of Depression	Behavior
Decrease of energy, motivation, interest, social engagement	Decreased self-care ability: (1) refuses to do tasks requiring physical exertion; (2) asks staff to do total care when not medically indicated; (3) change in socialization patterns and attendance at activities
Frequent somatic complaints, worry	Frequently uses signal light; numerous physical complaints that do not resolve with usual nursing-measures
Decreased or increased appetite	Takes inadequate nutrition, refuses food and fluids, overeats
Perceived cognitive deficits	Complains of being forgetful; loses familiar objects but performs well on mental status examination, poor on concentration; gives "I don't know" answers
Critical and envious of others	Complains about poor care, criticizes family and staff; may tell you others are getting better treatment
Decreased concentration and indecisiveness	Cannot keep his or her mind on what you are saying, especially patient teaching; has difficulty with decisions (e.g., "When would you like your bath?", "I don't know, I don't care, leave me alone.")
Loss of self-esteem, decreased sense of lifelong accomplishments	Ignores appearance; has no positive feelings about his or her life, hobbies, marriage, family, accomplishments; shares pessimism about future, little about self
Combative or resistive behavior	May strike out at staff or be verbally abusive when being cared for or may lash out verbally or physically at another patient who he or she may consider a "brother"
"Model patient" who never uses signal light	"Don't bother with me"; rarely complains or asks for anything, passive and apathetic

Adapted from Dreyfus JK: Depression assessment and intervention in medically frail elderly, *J Gerontol Nurs* 14(9):27-36, 1988; Tanner E: Recognizing late-life depression: why is this important for nurses in the home setting? *J Gerontol Nurs* 26(3):145-149, 2005.

expressions of depression. Decreased energy and motivation, lack of ability to experience pleasure, hopelessness, increased dependency, poor grooming and difficulty completing activities of daily living (ADLs), withdrawal from people or activities enjoyed in the past, decreased sexual interest, and a preoccupation with death or "giving up" are also signs of depression in older people (Meiner and Lueckenotte, 2006). Agitated behavior in persons with dementia may be a symptom of depression. A summary of symptoms of depression in late life and related behavior is presented in Table 25-3.

Etiological Factors of Depression. Depression in older adults differs in several ways from that in younger adults. One of the major differences is the insidious manner in which depression develops and the concurrency with other events, which results in depression frequently going unrecognized and untreated. In fact, the cause of depression in elders is biopsychosocial (Beers and Berkow, 2000). Some of the medical disorders that cause depression are cancers; cardiovascular disorders; endocrine disorders, such as thyroid problems; neurological disorders, such as Alzheimer's disease, stroke, and Parkinson's disease; metabolic and nutritional disorders, such as vitamin-B_{12} deficiency and malnutrition; viral infections, such as herpes zoster and hepatitis; and advanced macular degeneration. Elders with macular degeneration have twice the prevalence of depression compared with the general population of older adults (Brown, 2001).

Medications may result in depressive symptoms including antihypertensives (beta-blockers, calcium channel blockers, angiotensin-converting enzyme [ACE] inhibitors, methyldopa, reserpine, guanethidine, antiarrhythmics, anticholesterolemics, antibiotics, analgesics, corticosteroids, digoxin,

BOX 25-8 Common Risk Factors for Depression in Older Adults

- Chronic medical illnesses, disability, functional decline
- Alzheimer's disease and other dementias
- Bereavement
- Caregiving
- Female (2:1 risk)
- Lower SES
- Family history of depression
- Previous episode of depression
- Admission to long-term care or other change in environment
- Medications
- Alcohol or substance abuse
- Living alone
- Widowhood
- New stressful losses, including loss of autonomy; loss of privacy; loss of functional status; loss of independence; loss of body part; loss of family member, roommate, or pet

Adapted from Tanner E: Recognizing late-life depression: why is this important for nurses in the home setting? *J Gerontol Nurs* 26(3):145-148, 2005.
SES, Socioeconomic status.

progesterone, and L-dopa (Tanner, 2005). Other important factors influencing the development of depression are alcohol abuse, cognitive dysfunction, loss of a spouse or partner, loss of social supports, lower income level, and gender (depression occurs more often in women). Heredity is also a factor, especially in late-life onset of depression (Beers and Berkow, 2000). Some common risk factors for depression are presented in Box 25-8.

Diagnosis. Both physicians and patients have difficulty identifying the signs of depression (NIMH, 2007). The Geriatric Depression Scale (GDS), the Hamilton Depression Rating Scale, and the Beck Depression Inventory are often used to screen for depression. The Zung Self-Rating Depression Scale was developed specifically for use in elders with depression and is a self-report instrument. A five-item version of the GDS has been evaluated for reliability and validity and is as effective as the 15-item version, making it even more convenient to use in screening. The Cornell Scale for Depression is used to assess depression in elders with dementia. The Dementia Mood Picture Test (Tappen and Barry, 1995), a series of faces depicting moods, is another instrument being investigated for assessment of depression in older people with dementia.

We encourage staff nurses to use the simple and reliable tools provided in Appendix 25-A and to alert geriatric nurse practitioners and physicians when evidence of depression exists. A key to depression management is early identification, diagnosis, and management (Beers and Berkow, 2000). Family members and caregivers should be alert to subtle changes in personality, especially spontaneity, loss of sense of humor, new onset of forgetfulness, loss of appetite, agitation, and new sleep disturbance. Other signs may include wringing the hands, hypersomnia, recurrent thoughts of death, inattention to personal cleanliness or dress, persistent sadness, anxiety, and irritability (Kennedy-Malone et al., 2000).

Grief. Grief is a normal process that often occurs or begins before an anticipated death or loss. Dynamics include loss of control, preparation for loss, fear of separation, an uncertain future, and suffering (Beers and Berkow, 2000). Chronic grief and multiple losses may result in profound depression, apathy, and withdrawal from life. Grief is discussed fully in Chapter 26. Loss of a spouse or long-time partner is one of the most grievous losses in late life. Adjustment to bereavement is an ongoing life process with no precise point when grieving is over and mourning ends. The pain of loss may remain for a lifetime, felt in a different manner as time passes. Widowhood is discussed in Chapter 20.

▲ Promoting Healthy Aging: Implications for Gerontological Nursing

Assessment. Assessment involves a systematic and thorough evaluation using a depression screening instrument, interview, history and physical and laboratory tests, medication review, determination of iatrogenic or medical causes, family interview, and mutual decision making regarding treatment. It is most important that the nurse recognize suicidal potential in the depressed elder, inquire about suicidal thoughts, and provide necessary protection. For those suffering from iatrogenic or medical-induced depression, restoring basic function—sleep, nutrition, hydration, exercise, comfort, and pain control—often will help. Assessment of depression in elders is complicated by the fact that some somatic changes that occur normally in aging, such as tendencies toward constipation, early-morning awakening, and

slowed motor activity, which would indicate depression in a young adult, may be the normal consequence of aging. If depression is diagnosed, treatment should begin as soon as possible and appropriate follow-up should be provided. Depressed people are usually unable to follow through on their own and may be candidates for deeper depression or suicide without appropriate treatment and monitoring.

Goals of Treatment. The goals of treatment for depression include (1) decreasing symptoms, (2) reducing risk of relapse and recurrence, (3) increasing quality of life, (4) improving medical health status, and (5) decreasing health care costs and mortality. In treating depression in the older adult, consider the following:

- There are several types of depression. It is important that a comprehensive evaluation be made before a conclusion is reached.
- Biochemical and hormonal changes of aging may intensify depression in the older adult (e.g., neurotransmitters change with aging; most hormones, particularly thyroid hormones, are reduced).
- Drugs that are used for medical problems may intensify depression (e.g., hypotensives, psychotropics, cardiotonics, hypnotics).
- Antidepressant drugs may have idiosyncratic effects, toxic accumulation, and/or paradoxical effects. They should be used with expert knowledge, discrimination, and adequate observation (see Chapter 12).
- Knowledge of the presence of depression may be helpful when assisting the older person to understand and cope with some of the unexplained symptoms that he or she is experiencing. Clients should be involved in the assessment and discussion of depression, the available treatment, and the positive outcomes of treatment. Having the individual assess the level of depression immediately engages the person actively in examining his or her own feelings. To assist in overcoming the stigma of depression in older people, it is sometimes helpful to explain the neurochemical changes accompanying aging that may predispose to depression.
- The importance of restoring a sense of control, choice, and mastery needs to be recognized.
- Often, increased socialization and relief from physical discomfort and ailments will significantly lift depression.
- One must be alert to early signs of recurrent depression because this is common in major depressions.
- To decrease depression and raise self-esteem, defensive structures should be supported unless they are clearly detrimental to the client or family.

Interventions. Depression is often reversible with prompt and appropriate treatment; and 80% of older people will improve on appropriate medication, psychotherapy and psychosocial interventions, or a combination (NIMH, 2007). Interventions are individual and are based on history, what has previously been effective, concurrent illnesses, and se-

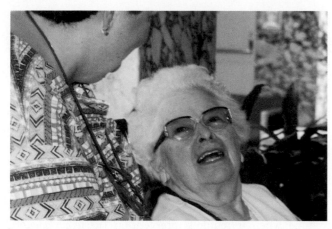

Creating hopeful environments in which meaningful activities and supportive relationships can be enjoyed is an important nursing role in the treatment of depression. (From Christensen B, Kockrow E: *Foundations of nursing*, ed 5, St Louis, 2006, Mosby.)

verity of illness (Reuben et al, 2003). Gum et al. (2006) stress the importance of a collaborative care model in treatment planning. Asking about prior treatment experiences in terms of tolerance and helpfulness is important, as well as providing education about treatment options. Family and social support, grief management, exercise, humor, spirituality, cognitive-behavioral therapy, interpersonal therapy, reminiscence, life review therapy, and problem-solving therapy have all been noted to be helpful in depression (Jones, 2003; Reuben et al., 2003).

In one of the largest studies examining treatment preferences of older, depressed primary care patients, most of the participants desired active treatment, particularly counseling, although it was rarely available. Electroconvulsive therapy (ECT) is being used more frequently for older people with psychotic depression or for those individuals who do not respond to antidepressant medications. People who received no treatment, treatment of short duration, or treatment with inadequate doses of medication may respond quite well to ECT. It is hypothesized that people who suffer depression for a long time may experience neuronal degeneration that impairs their ability to recover. ECT is much improved, but older people will need a careful explanation of the treatment since they may have many misconceptions. The relapse rate using ECT with antidepressant therapy is 10% to 20%. ECT is contraindicated in patients with increased intracranial pressure, severe heart disease, recent myocardial infarction, and aortic aneurysm, related to the risk of arrhythmia and death (Tabloski, 2006). Expert consensus guidelines for the management of depression in late life have been developed by Alexopoulos et al. (2001) (*www.psychguides.com*). The Nursing Standard of Practice Protocol: Depression in the Elderly (Kurlowicz, 2003, and the NICHE faculty [*www.guidelines.gov*]) is another nursing protocol. Other resources are in the Resource section at the end of this chapter.

Pharmacological Treatment. Drug therapies are very effective in managing depression. The addition of pharmaceuticals seems to have the most beneficial effect; 80% of elders will improve on appropriate medication, psychotherapy, or the combination (NIMH, 2007). The newer SSRIs are the drugs of choice for most elders with depression. Choice of medication depends on co-morbidities, drug side effects, and type of effect desired. People with agitated depression and sleep disturbances may benefit from medications with a more sedating effect, whereas those who are not eating may do better taking medications that have an appetite-stimulating effect such as mirtazapine (Remeron). If depression is immobilizing, psychostimulants may be used. Continuing treatment may be necessary, since depression is considered a relapsing and chronic illness.

If the person is in remission after a single lifetime episode of depression, 1 year of treatment may be necessary. If the person had two episodes of depression, treatment for 2 years or longer may need to be considered (Reynolds et al., 2002). More severe depression complicated by psychosis or suicide intent may require lifetime medication therapy. The side effects of antidepressants need to be monitored closely, and several different medications may be tried before improvement is noted. Most medications take about 6 weeks to completely resolve symptoms, and inadequate dosing or duration of treatment is common (Kennedy, 2001). The occurrence of hyponatremia within several weeks of starting therapy with SSRIs, particularly in patients known to be at risk, calls for careful observation of changes in mental status and electrolyte evaluation (Burke, 2004). See additional discussion of antidepressant medication in Chapter 12.

A strategy developed fully in Chapter 27 is the use of dreams for self-expression, understanding, and reestablishing control. One of the authors (PE) has found this strategy useful because many very depressed people seem to live more in their dream time than they do while awake. This finding has not been corroborated with studies. Reminiscing serves somewhat the same functions, though a very depressed elder may not reminisce spontaneously. Reminiscence and life review therapy are discussed on p. 624. In all interventions with depressed elders, the goal is to stimulate them to take control and make the decisions and to explain what they want and what they enjoy or appreciate.

Cognitive-Behavioral Therapy. Cognitive-behavioral therapy is designed to modify thought patterns, improve skills, and alter the environmental states that contribute to the onset or perpetuation of emotional disorders. Cognitive-behavioral group therapy, focused visual imagery group therapy, and education and discussion groups on cognition, depression, and hopelessness have been used with moderate improvement in cognitive function in people with mild depression. These approaches are more effective than analytic therapy or nondirective therapies (Beers and Berkow, 2000). Cognitive-behavioral therapy focuses on negating cognitive errors that are common to mildly depressed elderly: (1) overgeneralizing; (2) "awfulizing"; (3) exaggerating own importance; (4) demanding of others; (5) expecting mind reading; (6) self-blame; and (7) unrealistic expectations.

Nurses may help themselves and the client by being present, accepting the client's limited amount of interaction,

BOX 25-9   Interpersonal Support by Family and Professionals

- Provide structured, noncompetitive activities.
- Provide opportunities for decisions and to exercise control.
- Focus on spiritual renewal and rediscovery of meanings.
- Help the person write a guided autobiography.
- Engage the person in self-analysis through journals and dreams.
- Reactivate latent interests or develop new ones.
- Validate depressed feelings as aiding recovery; do not try to bolster the person's mood or deny his or her despair.
- Provide an accepting atmosphere and an empathic response.
- Share yourself.
- Demonstrate faith in the person's strengths; remind of past challenges and positive coping.
- Praise all efforts at recovery, no matter how small.
- Assist in expressing and dealing with anger.
- Do not stifle the grief process; grief cannot be hurried.
- Create a hopeful environment in which self-esteem is fostered and life is meaningful.
- Assist in dealing with guile, real or neurotic.
- Foster development of connections with others.
- Help the person become aware of the presence of depression, the nature of the symptoms, and the time limitation of depression. For example, do not try to talk the person out of being depressed; do not console with "life is worth living" or other clichés that only confirm the nurse's inability to comprehend the pain.
- Create your own support system and care for yourself, because working with elders who are depressed can be especially challenging.

and continually giving the client choices and clear feedback. When certain expectations of the client exist, state them in the form of options; for example, "It is important for you to get up and get dressed. Movement will increase your circulation and your energy levels. Do you want to get up before breakfast or after breakfast?" The client may respond that he does not want to get up. In that case, the nurse might reply, "You do have the right not to participate. I will return in 30 minutes, after you have given it more thought." On returning, the nurse may ask, "What is your decision?" Use humor: "Do I understand you intend to remain in bed? Remaining in bed ensures that you won't get up on the wrong side!"

Getting into a power struggle over involvement in activities only ensures that the nurse will lose. If this event occurs inadvertently, stop as soon as you recognize it and bring it to the attention of the client; for example, "You will win this game. You can choose to remain in bed, and there is little I can do about that." Suggestions for interpersonal support by family and professionals are presented in Box 25-9.

To be successful, treating depression must include considerations of the individual's premorbid personality, determination of reactive or endogenous origins, symptom relief, social

support manipulation, and the importance of a positive relationship with health care providers. The ability to tolerate depression enhances the person's coping capacity in later years. All older people will be depressed at some time and may better survive these episodes if they can develop a perspective that allows depression to be viewed as a valid and healing life process. Factors cited as protective against depression include hardiness, resilience, and the development of healthy attitudes toward death (Meiner and Lueckenotte, 2006).

Some experts express concern about the overdiagnosis of depression, particularly in long-term care settings, and caution that a certain amount of this entity called *depression* may be an expected reaction of sadness and grief and to determine when it requires intervention (*www.mhaging.org/info/improve_service.htm*). A depressive episode may be time needed for psychological wound repair, cleansing tears, protection of the wounded psyche by withdrawal, and the facilitation of repair and restoration of vitality, enthusiasm, and spontaneity. Nurses can facilitate this process by validation and ongoing support. An extensive nursing care plan based on Maslow's Hierarchy of Needs to be used in the care of a depressed patient is presented in Table 25-4.

Suicide

Although elders make up 13% of the population, they commit 20% of suicides (McAndrews, 2001). White men older than 85 years commit suicide at a rate approximately six times the national rate (NIMH, 2007). Older African-Americans have much lower suicide rates (men, 18 per 100,000; and women, less than 1 per 100,000); however, suicide rates of elderly black males is increasing. Results of a recent study (Joe et al., 2006) suggest that health care providers should enhance their skills in talking with black patients about risks for suicide, providing interventions, and referring for diagnosis and treatment. In most cases, depression and other mental health problems contribute significantly to suicide risk. Sixty percent of suicides are related to depression. Suicide may have some familial tendencies, with estimates that a suicide in the family of one parent is associated with a sixfold risk of suicide to the children (Kennedy, 2004). One of the significant differences in suicidal behavior in the old and young is lethality of method. Eight of ten suicides of men older than 65 years were with firearms. Elderly people rarely threaten to commit suicide; they just do it.

Up to 75% of older adults who die by suicide visited a physician within 1 month before death (NIMH, 2007). Twenty percent of the elders visited the physician on the same day of the suicide, 40% within 1 week, and 70% within 1 month. This statistic suggests that opportunities for intervening are present but the need for intervention is not seen as urgent or is not even recognized. As with depression, physical complaints are the primary reason for seeking medical treatment. Consequently, it is very important to recognize warning signs and risk factors as well as to assess for suicidal thoughts and ideas. The PROSPECT study to reduce suicidal ideation and risk in elders in primary care settings investigates the effect of a program to improve recognition and treatment of late-life depression on decreasing risk factors for suicide. Study findings support that treatment of depression in programs such as PROSPECT reduces suicidality (Bruce et al., 2004).

Common precipitants of suicide include physical or mental illness, death of spouse, substance abuse, and pathological relationships. Contrary to general opinion, the majority of elderly people who committed suicide were not physically ill. Most of these individuals were depressed (65%) or had other mental health problems. Other behavioral clues and risk factors are presented in Box 25-10. Elderly widowers are thought to be most vulnerable, because they have often depended on their wives to maintain the comforts of home and the social network of relatives and friends. Older white men may also suffer the most status loss, because the American white male society is almost totally devoted to occupational success, often to the neglect of other social roles. Women in all countries have much lower suicide rates, possibly because of greater flexibility in coping skills based on multiple roles that women fill throughout their lives. Suicide may also be less socially acceptable than for men. The more children a woman has, the lower her risk of suicide (Holkup, 2003).

▲ Promoting Healthy Aging: Implications for Gerontological Nursing

Assessment. Older people with suicidal intent are encountered in many settings. It is our professional obligation to prevent whenever possible an impulsive destruction of life that may be a response to a crisis or a disintegrative reaction. The lethality potential of an elder must always be assessed when elements of depression, disease, and spousal loss are evident. Any direct, indirect, or enigmatic references to the ending of life must be taken seriously and discussed with the elder. Elderly Suicide. Secondary Prevention (Holkup, 2003) is available at *www.guideline.gov*.

The most important consideration is for the nurse to establish a trusting and respectful relationship with the person. Because many older people have grown up in an era when suicide bore stigma and even criminal implications, they may not discuss their feelings in this respect. Also important to remember is that in older people, typical behavioral clues such as putting personal affairs in order, giving away possessions, and making wills and funeral plans are indications of maturity and good judgment in late life and cannot be considered indicative of suicidal intent. Even statements such as "I won't be around long" or "I'm ready to die" may be only a realistic appraisal of the situation in old age.

To increase communication and expression of feeling, depersonalizing the subject and discussing it on a more philosophical basis are often helpful, using questions such as the following:

- "Under what conditions do you think a person has a right to take his life?"
- "What are your opinions about the present interest in active euthanasia and assisted suicide?"
- "Do you think suicide is a sign of weakness or strength?"
- "Suicide is a taboo subject that many people are uncomfortable discussing, but as a health professional I think it is very important. Have you ever believed that you would be better off dead?"

Use open-ended questions such as "Could you tell me how it is for you to feel so alone right now?" when asking people to describe their emotions, and ask for clarification if needed.

In evaluating lethality potential, the informed nurse will recognize the high-risk patient: male, old, widowed or divorced, white, in poor health, retired, alcoholic, with a family history of unsatisfactory relationships and mental illness. A cluster of these factors should be a red flag of distress to all health professionals. Recent traumatic changes, mild dementia, depression, or cerebrovascular disease also increase the danger. Present relationships that are unsatisfactory, critical, or rejecting greatly enhance the potential for suicide.

If there is suspicion that the elder is suicidal, use direct and straightforward questions such as the following:

- Have you ever thought about killing yourself?
- How often have you had these thoughts?
- How would you kill yourself if you decided to do it?

The following must also be considered in assessing lethality potential:

- Internal resources (personality factors, coping strategies)
- External resources (money, family, friends, services)
- Communication skills (ability to ask for help and express feelings)

Interventions. Community health nurses, visiting nurses, and other professionals have a case-finding role in the community that extends beyond traditional boundaries; the role includes awareness and use of resources within the high-risk populations and providing depression screening clinics at nutrition sites, senior centers, industrial health sites, churches, and community clubs. Establishing lifesaving connections with individuals and groups that can be available on demand and that can provide ongoing, long-term counseling, emotional support, and reassurance is the approach to the suicidal elder. Improvement of the social network could reduce suicides by 25% (Beautrais, 2002).

If suicidal intent has been established, the following interventions, arranged in order of immediacy, are necessary:

- Reduce immediate danger by removing hazardous articles.
- Do not leave the person alone; evaluate the need for constant attendance; and arrange for family, friend, or professional to be present during the period of immediate danger.
- Provide an honest expression of concern, such as "I do not want you to take your life. I will help you with this troubling situation."

TABLE 25-4

Dealing with Depression: The Nursing Process and Maslow's Hierarchy of Needs

Needs	Assessment	Identifying Problems	Establishing Goals	Intervention	Evaluation
PHYSIOLOGICAL NEEDS					
Food and fluid Shelter and warmth Air Rest and sleep Avoidance of pain Sex	Usual and present nutritional, elimination, sleep, and sexuality patterns Physical activity—exercise pattern Emotional pain and discomfort Suicide potential Physical health Medications	Nutritional deficit Dehydration Constipation Sleep pattern disturbance Sexual dysfunction Self-destructive behavior Medication or physical illnesses that may cause depression	Establishing and maintaining adequate biologic functioning in areas of sleep, nutrition, and elimination Relief from emotional pain and discomfort Elimination of drug- or disease-induced depression	Assist with ADLs Support of self-care abilities Encouragement to start a physical activity regimen Teach side effects of antidepressants Treat medical problems under poor control Change medications that may cause depression	Feelings of physical satiation Homeostasis Optimal health
SAFETY AND SECURITY NEEDS					
Feel free from danger Need for a predictable, lawful, orderly world Need to feel in control	Home environment assessment Mental status examination Assessment of visual acuity and hearing Knowledge of disease process Physical mobility	Perceived inability to control feelings or behavior Perceived powerlessness Translocation syndrome Cognitive impairment Alteration in sensory perceptions Impaired physical mobility	Establish predictability and structure in environment Maintenance of a safe environment Realistic understanding of disease course and expected outcome Reversal of treatable confusion	ECT, hospitalization, antidepressive medications for the severely depressed Avoid relocations when possible Correct environmental hazards Encourage a structured daily routine Instruct about disease course and prognosis	Feeling in control of one's disease and optimistic about the future Confidence in the future Feelings of safety, peace, security, protection, lack of danger, and threat

Need	Assessment	Problems	Goals	Interventions	Outcomes
NEED FOR LOVE, BELONGING, AND AFFECTION					
Need for contact and intimacy Need for friends Need for a feeling of having a place, "belonging" Need for interactions with others	Family relationships and members Friends that are supportive Recent losses Present and past social interactions	Disruption in significant relationships Social isolation Lack of contact with or absence of significant others Alterations in socialization with reduced social interactions	Maintenance of significant relationships with family and friends Establish community support system Resumption of previous level of social activity	Encourage social interactions that have been enjoyed in the past Encourage interactions with family members, friends, and health caregivers Provide reassuring, supportive atmosphere	Feelings of loving and being loved, of being one of a group, of acceptance
NEED FOR ESTEEM AND SELF-RESPECT					
Need for achievement, mastery, and competence Need for reputation or prestige, appreciation, and dignity Need for love of self	Amount of pleasurable pursuits Emotional or mood assessment Role patterns Coping—stress tolerance pattern Attitude about self, the world, the future	Negative feelings or conception of self Loss of significant roles Unrealistic self-expectations Anxiety Lifestyle change Dependency on others	Acceptance of realistic limitations Establish appropriate roles Achieve self-acceptance Accept ownership of consequences of one's own behavior	Teach problem-solving skills Cognitive therapy Promote self-care Counseling Behavior therapy Relaxation techniques	Feelings of self-confidence, worth, strength, capability, adequacy, and of being useful and necessary in the world
NEED FOR SELF-ACTUALIZATION					
Need for beauty Need for self-expression Need for new situations and stimulation	Occupation, job history Value-belief patterns	Distress of human spirit Loss of zest for life	Expression of self through meaningful recreational activities Exploring new interests	Encourage a nonrestrictive environment Provide beauty in environment Read to the sick or hard of hearing Music	Autonomy Freshness of appreciation Creativeness Spontaneity Feelings of self-fulfillment

From Ronsman K. *J Gerontol Nurs* 13(12):21, 1987. Reprinted with permission from SLACK, Inc., Thorofare, NJ.
ADLs, Activities of daily living; *ECT,* electroconvulsive therapy.

BOX 25-10 Suicide Risk and Recovery Factors

RISK FACTORS

Depression

Paranoia or a paranoid attitude

Rejection of help; a suspicious and hostile attitude toward helpers and society

Major loss, such as the death of a spouse

History of major losses

Recent suicide attempt

History of suicide attempts

Major mental, physical, or neurologic illness

Major crises or transitions, such as retirement or imminent entry into a nursing home

Major crises or changes in others, especially among family members

Typical age-related blows to self-esteem, such as loss of income or loss of meaningful activities

Loss of independence, when dependency is unacceptable

Expressions of feeling unnecessary, useless, and devalued

Increased irritability and poor judgment, especially after a loss or some other crisis

Alcoholism or increased drinking

Social isolation: living alone; having few friends (The social isolation of the couple is also associated with suicide.)

Expression of the belief that one is in the way, a burden harmful to others

Expression of the belief that one is in an insoluble and hopeless situation

Communication of suicidal intent: direct or indirect expression of suicidal ideation or impulses and symptomatic acts, such as giving away valued possessions, storing up medications, or buying a gun

Intractable, unremitting pain—mental, or physical—that is not responding to treatment

Feelings of hopelessness and helplessness in the family and social network

Feelings of hopelessness in the therapist or other helpers; desire to be rid of the patient

Acceptance of suicide as a solution

RECOVERY FACTORS

A capacity for:

    Understanding

    Relating

    Benefiting from experience

    Benefiting from knowledge

    Accepting help

    Being loving

    Expressing wisdom

    Displaying a sense of humor

    Having a social interest

    Accepting a caring and available family

    Accepting a caring and available social network

    Accepting a caring, available, and knowledgeable professional and health network

From Richman J: A rational approach to rational suicide. In Leenaars AA et al, editors: *Suicide and the older adult,* New York, 1992, The Guilford Press.

- Evaluate the need for consultation with a mental health professional and possible hospitalization.
- Sometimes a no-suicide contract can be initiated. If the person demonstrates a high risk of suicide, a no-suicide contract cannot be relied on as a preventive measure.
- Evaluate the need for medication.
- Focus on the current hazard or crisis that gives the client the most present distress.
- Mobilize internal and external resources by getting the person reinvolved with external supports and reconnected with internal capabilities. The health professional or the family or caregiver may need to take the initiative to find activities, support systems, transportation, and other resources for the individual.
- Implement a specific plan of action with an ongoing structured program. Develop a lifeline of individuals who can be called on at any hour of distress, and plan regular calls and follow-up for the individual.

Suicide is a taboo topic for most of us, and there is a lingering fear that the introduction of the topic will be suggestive to the patient and may incite suicidal action. Precisely the opposite is true. By introducing the topic, we demonstrate interest in the individual and open the door to honest human interaction and connection on the deep levels of psychological need. Superficial interest and mechanical questioning will not, of course, be meaningful. It is the nature of our concern and ability to connect with the alienation and desperation of the individual that will make a difference. Working with isolated, depressed, and suicidal elders continually challenges the depths of nurses' ingenuity, patience, and self-knowledge.

Substance Abuse

Alcohol. Substance abuse often arises in old age as a coping mechanism to deal with loss, anxiety, depression, or boredom. Alcohol-related problems in the elderly often go unrecognized although the residual effects of alcohol abuse complicate the presentation and treatment of many chronic disorders of older people. The current DSM-IV (APA, 2000) criteria for abuse (failure to fulfill major role obligations at work, school, or home; physically hazardous situations; substance-related legal problems; or recurrent social or interpersonal problems) may not adequately describe consequences of alcohol use in older adults (Finfgeld-Connett, 2004). In the general population, alcohol abuse is readily recognized because of social or work problems; however, elders may live alone and not come under scrutiny at work. They may easily hide their drinking.

The misuse and abuse of alcohol is prevalent among older adults and are significant public health concerns. An estimated 2% to 17% of elders older than 60 years abuse alcohol or are alcohol-dependent (probably underreported) (Blow et al., 2002), but prevalence is likely to increase with the aging of the "baby boomers" who had more access to drugs, alcohol, and other substances (Goodman, 2003). An estimated 35% of older primary care patients consume alcohol at levels that place them at risk for harm, and up to 50% of nursing home patients have a history of alcohol abuse. Hospital admissions for alcohol-related problems may be equal to admission rates for myocardial infarction (Masters, 2003). The actual prevalence of alcohol-related hospitalizations is most likely greater than reported, and many studies have shown that older adults are less likely to receive a primary diagnosis of alcoholism that are younger adults (Culberson, 2006a).

Genetic predisposition, limited education, poverty, depression, and being male are risk factors for alcohol abuse (Tabloski, 2006). Men (particularly older widowers) are four times more likely to abuse alcohol than women, but prevalence in women may be underestimated (Finfgeld-Connett, 2004). Most severe alcohol abuse is seen in people ages 60 to 80 years, not in those older than 80 years. Two thirds of elderly alcoholics are early-onset drinkers (alcohol use began at 30 or 40 years of age), and one third are late-onset drinkers (after age 60 years). Late-onset drinking may be related to situational events such as illness, retirement, or death of a spouse and includes a higher number of women (Finfgeld-Connett, 2005).

Gender Issues. An estimated 7% of women older than 59 years abuse alcohol. Women of all ages are significantly more vulnerable to the effects of alcohol misuse, including cirrhosis of the liver and a higher death rate. Often, alcohol abuse in women is undetected until the consequences are severe (Finfgeld-Connett, 2004).

Drug Effects. Many drugs that elders use for chronic illnesses cause adverse effects when combined with alcohol. Some drugs can increase alcohol levels by 30% to 40%; cimetidine is one commonly used drug that produces this increase, as are sedatives (Kennedy-Malone et al., 2000). Medications that interact with alcohol include analgesics, antibiotics, antidepressants, benzodiazepines, H2 receptor blockers, nonsteroidal antiinflammatory drugs (NSAIDs), and herbal medications (Echinacea, valerian) (Masters, 2003). Also, some mouthwash and cough and cold preparations have up to 40% alcohol content (Letizia and Reinboltz, 2005). Acetaminophen taken on a regular basis, when combined with alcohol, may lead to liver failure. Alcohol diminishes the effects of oral hypoglycemics, anticoagulants, and anticonvulsants (Kennedy-Malone et al., 2000). All older people should be given precise instructions regarding the interaction of alcohol with their medications.

Other effects of alcohol in older people include urinary incontinence, which results from rapid bladder filling and diminished neuromuscular control of the bladder; gait disturbances from alcohol-caused cerebellar degeneration and peripheral neuropathy; depression and suicide; sleep distur-

bances and insomnia; and dementia or delirium. Elderly who drink to excess are susceptible to cognitive decline, physical decline, functional decline, and increased risk for injury.

Physiology. Older people develop higher blood alcohol levels because of age-related changes (increased body fat, decreased lean body mass and total body water content) that alter absorption and distribution of alcohol (Culberson, 2006a). Reduced liver and kidney function slow alcohol metabolism and elimination. A decrease in gastric alcohol dehydrogenase enzyme results in slower metabolism of alcohol and higher blood levels for a longer time (Finfgeld-Connett, 2004). Risks of gastrointestinal ulceration and bleeding may be higher in older people because of the decrease in gastric pH that occurs in aging (Letizia and Reinboltz, 2005).

▲ Promoting Healthy Aging: Implications for Gerontological Nursing

Assessment. Screening for alcohol abuse is not routinely conducted in primary or long-term care settings. Emergency room personnel fail to recognize 23% of acutely intoxicated patients; female gender and older age increase the likelihood that alcohol problems will be missed (Masters, 2003). Reasons for the low rates of alcohol detection among older adults by health care professionals include poor symptom recognition, inadequate knowledge about screening instruments, lack of age-appropriate diagnostic criteria for abuse in older people, and ageism. Finfgeld-Connett (2004) reported that 37% of primary care physicians overlooked alcohol abuse among older women because "It is one of the few pleasures they have left" (p. 32).

Alcoholism is a disease of denial and not easy to diagnose, particularly in older people with psychosocial and functional decline from other conditions that may mask decline caused by alcohol. Health care providers tend to overlook substance abuse disorders and misuse among older people, mistaking the symptoms for those of dementia, depression, or other problems common to older adults. Early signs such as weight loss, irritability, insomnia, and falls may not be recognized as indicators of possible alcohol problems and may be attributed to "just getting older." Box 25-11 presents signs and symptoms that may indicate potential alcohol problems in older adults.

The possible health benefits of alcohol in moderation have been reported in the literature (reduced risk of coronary artery disease, ischemic stroke, Alzheimer's disease, and vascular dementia). As a result, older people may not perceive alcohol use as potentially harmful, but clinically significant adverse effects can occur in some individuals consuming as little as two to three drinks per day over an extended period. Alcohol screening with older adults suggests that 15% of men regularly drink more than 14 drinks per week and that 12% of women regularly drink more than 7 drinks per week (National Institute on Alcohol Abuse and Alcoholism, 2005). Because of the increased risk of adverse effects from alcohol use, the National Institute on Alcohol Abuse and Alcohol-

BOX 25-11	Signs and Symptoms of Potential Alcohol Problems in Older Adults

Anxiety
Irritability (feeling worried or "crabby")
Blackouts
Dizziness
Indigestion
Heartburn
Sadness or depression
Chronic pain
Excessive mood swings
New problems making decisions
Lack of interest in usual activities
Falls
Bruises, burns, or other injuries
Family conflict, abuse
Headaches
Incontinence
Memory loss
Poor hygiene
Poor nutrition
Insomnia
Sleep apnea
Social isolation
Out of touch with family or friends
Unusual response to medications
Frequent physical complaints and physician visits

Adapted from National Institute on Alcohol Abuse and Alcoholism: Older adults and alcohol problems, Participant Handout, 2005 (website): *www.niaaa.nih.gov*, and Geriatric Mental Health Foundation: Substance Abuse and Misuse Among Older Adults: Prevention, Recognition and Help, 2006 (website): *www.gmhfonline.org*.

BOX 25-12	Standard Drink Equivalents

In assessing for alcohol use, a standard drink contains about 0.6 ounces of pure alcohol. Many drinks are sold in containers that hold multiple standard drinks (e.g., malt liquor in 16-, 22-, or 40-ounce containers holding 2-5 standard drinks and wine in 750-mL bottles holding 5 standard drinks). It is important to determine what types of containers are used by the person (e.g., 6-oz glass of beer or 22-oz bottle).

STANDARD DRINK EQUIVALENTS

- 12 oz beer or cooler
- 8-9 oz malt liquor
- 5 oz table wine
- 3-4 oz sherry or port
- 2-3 oz liqueur or aperitif
- 1.5 oz brandy (single jigger)
- 1.5 oz spirits (jigger of gin, vodka, whiskey, etc.)

From Letizia M, Reinboltz M: Identifying and managing acute alcohol withdrawal in the elderly, *Geriatr Nurs* 26(3):176-183, 2005.

BOX 25-13	Questions Regarding Abuse of Alcohol

- Are you upset when people criticize your drinking? How do you handle that?
- Do you believe that you sometimes drink too much? Are there particular occasions when that occurs?
- Do you feel disturbed about your alcohol consumption?
- Do you drink when you are feeling lonely?
- Have you identified a pattern regarding your drinking?
- Would you like to stop drinking?

ism (NIAAA) has recommended that individuals over the age of 65 limit alcohol consumption to no more than one standard drink per day. The Substance Abuse and Mental Health Services Administration (SAMSHA) recommends a maximum of two drinks on any drinking occasion (holidays or other celebrations) and somewhat lower limits for women. Health professionals need to share information with older people about safe drinking limits and the deleterious effects of alcohol intake. Box 25-12 presents standard drink amounts for use in assessment of alcohol intake.

Alcohol users often reject or deny the diagnosis, or they may take offense at the suggestion of it. Feelings of shame or disgrace may make elders reluctant to disclose a drinking problem. This may be especially true among ethnically or culturally diverse older women from a background in which alcohol use is highly discouraged (Finfgeld-Connett, 2004). Families of older people with substance abuse disorders, particularly their adult children, may be ashamed of the problem and choose not to address it. Health care providers may feel helpless over alcoholism, uncomfortable with direct questioning, or may approach the person in a judgmental manner. Many of the traditional ways of dealing with alcoholism have a punitive sound; for example, "Have you ever thought you were drinking too much?" A far more productive approach is to discuss the issue factually. For example, "Many elders find

that the stresses, loneliness, and losses of aging are very hard to bear. Some retreat into alcohol use as a way of coping. There are treatments and groups that assist individuals in these difficult adjustments. If this is a problem for you or if it becomes a problem, please let us know so we may provide resources or referrals for you." It is always important to search for the pain beneath the behavior. Box 25-13 presents some suggested questions to be used in assessment.

Culberson (2006b) suggests that the use of a simple question—"Have you had a drink containing alcohol within the past 3 months?"—be included in an assessment to identify clients in whom further screening is indicated. This may be followed by administration of a screening instrument such as The Michigan Alcoholism Screening Test—Geriatric Version (MAST-G) (available at *www.hartfordign. org*) or The Alcohol Use Disorders Identification Test (AUDIT) to identify problem drinking or dependence. AUDIT, a 10 minute questionnaire completed by patients or with family assistance, may also be used to identify hazardous or harmful drinking and may have better reliability for elders and for culturally or ethnically diverse clients. The focus of this instrument is on the relationship between alcohol consumption and declining health, medication use, and functional status (Culberson, 2006b; Finfgeld-Connett 2004, 2005; Masters, 2003). Assessment of depression is also

BOX 25-14 Summary of A-Frames Brief Intervention Model

Most frequent problems in late life caused by depression:
1. Social isolation, loss of important social support systems
2. Loss of autonomy (psychiatric and physical illness, physical disability)
3. Inactivity (retirement)
4. Loss of reputation, financial problems
5. Relocation of residence
6. Severe insomnia

Data from Finfgeld-Connett D: Treatment of substance misuse in older women: using a brief intervention model, *J Gerontol Nurs* 30(8):30-37, 2004. From Müller-Spahn F, Hock C: Clinical presentation of depression in the elderly, *Gerontology* 40(suppl 1):10, 1994.

important, as discussed on p. 612. Alcohol and depression screenings should be offered routinely at health fairs and other sites where older people may seek health information and should be included as part of the assessment of all older adults and a prerequisite to the prescription of new medications (Finfgeld-Connett, 2005; Masters, 2003). Diagnostic tests should include a complete blood count (CBC), liver function tests, chemistries, and an electrocardiogram.

Interventions. Abstinence from alcohol is seen as the desired goal, but a focus on alcohol reduction and reducing harm is also appropriate (Finfgeld-Connett, 2005). Unless the person is in immediate danger, a stepped-care approach beginning with brief interventions followed by more intensive therapies if necessary should be utilized in intervention. Brief interventions may range from one meeting to four or five short sessions (Finfgeld-Connett, 2005). Brief intervention is a time-limited, patient-centered strategy focused on changing behavior and assessing patient readiness to change. Sessions can range from one meeting of 10 to 30 minutes to 4 or 5 short sessions. The goals of brief intervention are to (1) reduce or stop alcohol consumption, and (2) facilitate entry into formalized treatment if needed. Research results indicate that this type of intervention has positive outcomes when used by primary care providers (Culberson, 2006b). Barry and colleagues (2001) have published a workbook for brief intervention therapy that professionals will find useful in guiding this intervention.

A very useful framework (A-Frames) for assessment and intervention of alcohol-related problems in older women has been developed by Finfgeld-Connett (2004, 2005) (Box 25-14). Elements included in intervention are appropriate feedback on the patient's risk or impairment and discussion of the effects of alcohol on function and physical health status; the provision of clearly written advice and instructions for appropriate use of alcohol; suggestions on how to limit alcohol use to recommended guidelines or quit drinking; measures to enhance self-efficacy such as demonstrating faith in the person's ability to change; an empathetic approach; and understanding of the challenges lifestyle changes present (Finfgeld-Connett, 2005). Models such as the Gerontology Alcohol

Project (GAP) have also been effective for individuals who were not successful with brief interventions. This program focuses on increasing behavioral coping skills and self-efficacy in high-risk situations (Finfgeld-Connett, 2005).

Other treatment and intervention strategies include cognitive-behavioral approaches, individual and group counseling, medical and psychiatric approaches, referral to Alcoholic Anonymous, family therapy, case management and community and home care services, and formalized substance abuse treatment. Long-term self-help treatment programs for elders show high rates of success, especially when social outlets are emphasized and cohort supports are available. A significant concern is the lack of programs designed specifically for older people whose concerns are very different from those of a younger population who abuse drugs or alcohol. Estimates are that fewer than one in five existing substance abuse programs offer services specifically designed for older adults (Schultz et al, 2002). The cost of care is another issue, since Medicare covers only hospital-based detoxification and limits coverage of outpatient counseling services to 50%. Health status, availability of transportation, and mobility impairments further may limit access to treatment (Finfgeld-Connett, 2004). Additional information on late-life addictions can be found in Substance Abuse Among Older Adults Treatment Improvement Protocol (TIP) available from *www.samhsa.gov*.

Other Substance Abuse Concerns. A more common concern seen among older people, particularly older women, is the inappropriate use of psychoactive prescription and OTC medications. Nicotine, more common than alcohol abuse, and caffeine may also be misused by the elderly person. The inappropriate use of psychoactive medications, particularly benzodiazepines, is especially problematic for older women, who are 37% more likely than men to receive prescriptions for these drugs (Finfgeld-Connett, 2004).

Some of the reasons for abuse of psychoactive prescription medications may be the inappropriate prescribing and ineffective monitoring of response and follow-up. In many instances, older people are given prescriptions for benzodiazepines because of complaints of insomnia or nervousness, without adequate assessment for depression or other conditions that may be causing the symptoms. Older people may not be informed of the side effects of these medications including interactions with alcohol, dependence, and withdrawal symptoms. More important, conditions such as depression may not be recognized and treated appropriately. Blow et al. (2002) note that increases in illness and mortality are associated with misusing prescription and nonprescription medications, although this is not considered a disorder by DSM-IV.

Acute Alcohol Withdrawal. Older people who drink are at risk of experiencing acute alcohol withdrawal if admitted to the hospital. All patients admitted to acute care settings should be screened for alcohol use and assessed for signs and symptoms of alcohol-related problems. Older people with a long history of consuming excess alcohol, previous episodes of acute withdrawal, and a history of prior detoxification are at increased risk of acute alcohol withdrawal (Letizia and Reinboltz, 2005). Symptoms of acute alcohol withdrawal vary but may be more severe and last longer in older people. Minor withdrawal (withdrawal tremulousness) begins 6 to 12 hours after a patient has consumed the last drink. Symptoms include tremor, anxiety, nausea, insomnia, tachycardia, and increased blood pressure and frequently may be mistaken as common problems in older adults. Major withdrawal is seen 10 to 72 hours after cessation of alcohol, and symptoms include vomiting, diaphoresis, hallucinations, tremors, and seizures (Letizia and Reinboltz, 2005).

Delirium tremens (DTs) is the term used to describe alcohol withdrawal delirium and usually occurs 24 to 72 hours after the last drink but may occur up to 10 days later. DTs occur in 5% of patients with acute alcohol withdrawal and is considered a medical emergency with a mortality rate from respiratory failure and cardiac arrhythmia as high as 15%. Other signs and symptoms include confusion, disorientation, hallucinations, hyperthermia, and hypertension. The Clinical Institute Withdrawal Assessment (CIWA) scale is recommended as a valid and reliable screening instrument (*www.pubs.niaa.nih.gov*) (Letizia and Reinboltz, 2005).

Recommended treatment is the use of benzodiazepines (Ativan, Serax) at one-half to one-third the normal dose around the clock or as needed during withdrawal. The CIWA aids in medication adjustments. The use of oral or intravenous alcohol to prevent or treat withdrawal is not established. Other interventions include assessing mental status, monitoring vital signs, and maintaining fluid balance without overhydrating. Calm and quiet surroundings, no unnecessary stimuli, consistent caregivers, frequent reorientation, prevention of injury, and support and caring are additional suggested interventions. Nutritional assessment is indicated, as well as addition of a multivitamin containing folic acid, pyridoxine, niacin, vitamin A, and thiamine (Letizia and Reinbolz, 2005).

Risk, prevention, assessment, and treatment of alcohol and substance abuse have not been sufficiently studied among older people. Diagnostic criteria to identify alcohol and prescription drug misuse among older adults, particularly older women and culturally and ethnically diverse elders, also need further investigation (Finfgeld-Connett, 2004). This is a particularly salient issue for gerontological nursing research in light of the growing numbers of older people, many of whom have a history of alcohol and drug use.

THERAPEUTIC STRATEGIES TO PROMOTE MENTAL HEALTH

Mental health promotion and treatment strategies for the elderly are based primarily in the community and nursing homes, though some geropsychiatric units and some mental health units provide excellent care for elders with emotional concerns. Community-based mental health centers, senior partial hospitalization programs or day treatment programs where people receive treatment and return home in the afternoon, home care services, and clinics or offices of psychiatrists, licensed social workers, or nurse practitioners are other sites of care. Models of primary care that integrate mental health services using nurses or social workers as case managers have been successful in some settings and may be preferred by older people (Oxman and Dietrich, 2002). Psychiatric care in the home is provided by nurses experienced in mental health nursing, often by master's level clinical nurse specialists. This type of care is particularly appropriate for patients with psychiatric diagnoses who reside in the community but have functional limitations affecting their ability to live independently or for medically ill patients who also have psychiatric illnesses. Home health care is an underutilized source of mental health care for older people and has many advantages (Bruce, 2002).

Extensive psychotherapy is rarely reported, and most treatment is somatic. Effective treatment modes include psychoanalysis, psychotherapeutic reminiscence therapy, brief psychotherapy and crisis intervention, somatotherapy, behavioral therapy, family and couples therapy, and life review therapy (Bartels et al., 2002). The choice of therapy depends on the needs of the client and method of reimbursement. Some of these modalities are discussed in the following section.

Community-Based Psychiatric Care

Elderly psychiatric patients have had "Band-Aid treatment" and are then dismissed and frequently forgotten. Now, with the trend of all health care to move the majority of care provision to the community, mental health providers are creating new comprehensive community psychogeriatric care systems. Canadians in Ontario have found this method most satisfactory. Case finding may be from several sources, and initial screening is often in response to a crisis call from a client, family member, or professional in the community or based in an institution.

When completed, an assessment provides the base for a holistic plan of care. The client and care planning team determine what is both desired and feasible. The range of options is thoroughly examined. Only then is the needed level of support determined and whether a move may be necessary. Wherever the site in which the care plan is activated, the client is still provided access to the community-based services identified in the care plan. Periodic assessment of progress toward goals involves all team members, the client, and the family. This community case-managed model can be effectively implemented in any community. As the program becomes more fully developed, an increasing number of caregivers and local resources can be involved. Overall, these programs have demonstrated economic and humanistic effectiveness. Institutions and community groups have worked together to maintain continuity of efforts and consistency of service. The programs appear to be more cost-effective than institutionalization.

Brief Psychotherapy and Crisis Intervention

These modalities are often surprisingly successful because the elderly are acutely aware that their time is limited and their problems are often clearly apparent. Crisis intervention is discussed in Chapter 24. Brief psychotherapy is often the treatment of choice for the elderly who need to resolve interpersonal problems and develop more effective coping strategies. Generally, brief psychotherapy is limited to less than 15 weeks. The emphasis is on important problems in the person's life; goals are limited. The therapist is active in providing direction, guidance, and environmental manipulation.

Psychodrama

Psychodrama has been infrequently used with older individuals because they have been considered poor candidates for developing insight and personality change. Nonetheless, the approach can be used effectively. Residents of nursing homes can participate in expressive groups for the purpose of dramatizing physical limitations, death of self and loved ones, and dependencies. These topics, frequently avoided when working with older people, are potent issues that need to be handled openly and in depth. The participants confront issues that cause conflict and develop insight into anxieties. Dramatic role-playing not only resolves past issues but also brings about reinvestment in the present relationships in a group.

Psychodrama and life review have been used successfully to enhance adaptation and life satisfaction. Psychodrama emphasizes the reenactment of troublesome memories that are consuming psychic energy and producing incongruence in an individual's self-concept. The life review and reminiscence activity can be effectively implemented using the techniques of psychodrama. Although used with adolescents, dreams have also been incorporated into psychodrama for further understanding. Imagery-based cognitive training techniques have also been used successfully with elders. The particular techniques used include visual imagery elaboration, verbal judgment, and relaxation. Elders who are intuitive seem to benefit most from psychodrama, life review, and imagery.

Institutionally Based Care

Typically, as mentioned earlier, nursing homes have, by default, been given the task of caring for older people with emotional health problems. Many facilities have done an excellent job of implementing programs and providing psychiatric consultation to improve care. Reminiscence therapy and other memory-stimulating groups can be successful interventions that can be implemented rather easily, benefitting both residents and staff. Some long-term care facilities use reminiscence boxes containing things familiar to older people that can be taken to individual patient units and used to encourage sharing memories. Having the residents and/or their families make memory boxes unique to important things in their lives is another way to encourage sharing and coming to know. Music and pictures are other props to memory sharing. Community learning circles and life story circles also are successful techniques (*www.culturechange.not.com/stories/storytelling.html*).

Monthly psychiatric consultation in nursing homes is another method to serve the mental health needs of residents. Geropsychiatric nursing consultation can be particularly beneficial on an ongoing basis to improve mental health care and enhance staff competencies. The consultations are useful primarily to increase staff understanding and acceptance of the emotional problems of residents. Beck et al. (2002) suggest that better education and support programs for nursing assistants, the front-line caregivers in nursing homes, will improve quality and consistency of mental health and behavioral interventions. Better understanding will also encourage staff members to increase the number of therapeutic programs offered. It is particularly important that consulting mental health professionals involved in the care of nursing home residents utilize a multidisciplinary approach, seeking input from staff and family members about patient needs, behavior, and response to therapy. Treatment based on inadequate knowing of the person can be problematic.

Animal-Assisted Therapy

Animal-assisted (pet) therapy in nursing homes is generally used to bridge the gap between the resident and the therapist. The dog or cat helps the resident break through apathy and depression, and the resident is then better able to respond to caregivers and interact with other residents. Positive effects of animal-assisted therapy and activity include relaxation, motivation, and improvement of communication. Animal-assisted therapy may have other positive health benefits. The effect of animal-assisted therapy on pain in cancer patients is also being studied. Hooker et al. (2002) provides an historical review of pet therapy research with a review of nursing research on this topic. For more information on guidelines for animal-assisted therapy, see the Resources section at the end of this chapter.

Typically, pet therapy consists of a brief session each month in which well-behaved cats and dogs are brought to nursing homes for residents to play with and hold. Animals are selected based on their good temperament and ability to withstand the confusion and the number of people who will hold and play with them; the animals must have appropriate health clearance and vaccinations. Volunteers from the animal shelter usually accompany pets to ensure the safety of both animals and residents. Nursing homes sometimes adopt an animal that becomes the mascot, and various residents take responsibility for caring for the animal. This has been a successful strategy in culture change efforts such as the Eden Alternative. The Humane Society of the United States offers the following points to consider before initiating pet therapy in a nursing home:

1. What does the staff think about the project?
2. Will the facilities lend themselves to such a program?
3. Is space available where the animal can retreat and also be kept out of the way of residents who have no interest in pets or are afraid of them?

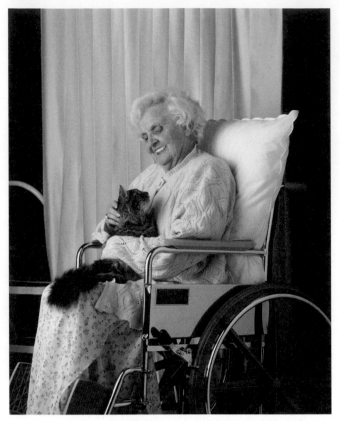

A nursing home resident enjoying pet therapy. (Courtesy Corbis.)

4. Can a program schedule be set up to include an animal on a routine basis?
5. Is the local humane society or animal shelter willing to become involved in such a project?
6. If adopting a resident mascot, are adequate food, shelter, and water available for the mascot at all times and will designated people be consistently responsible for the care of the animal?

A novel type of animal-assisted therapy being researched in Japan is the use of mental commit robots, which have the appearance of real animals. Paro, a seal-like robot, was developed with tactile, vision, audition, and posture sensors and a behavior-generation system that stimulates the behaviors of a real animal. A seal was chosen since it is a nonfamiliar animal and it is thought that people may accept it more easily without preconception. Early research has shown decreased stress levels, enhanced communication, and improvement of mood among nursing home elders who were exposed to Paro, which is amazingly lifelike, even able to respond and turn its head in response to voices and touch. This may well be an example of the unique kind of assistive technology we have to look forward to in the future. (See *http://paro.jp/english* for more information on Paro.)

Reminiscence and Life Review

Reminiscence and life review are therapeutic modalities for the treatment of depression. The life story as constructed through reminiscing, journaling, psychotherapy, or guided autobiography has fascinated gerontologists in the past quarter century. The universal appeal of the life story as a vehicle of culture, a demonstration of caring and generational continuity, and an easily stimulated activity has allured many professionals. Stories are a gift in that they image those life events most dear to the storyteller. Stories are an invaluable means of coming to know the beauty, wholeness, and uniqueness of the person (Boykin et al., 1998). Stories are important; as Robert Coles states (1989, p. 7):

> The people who come to see us bring us their stories. They hope that they tell them well enough so that we understand the truth of their lives. They hope we understand how to interpret their stories correctly.

The literature is vast, and some especially good sources for further study are cited in the Resources section at the end of this chapter. The work of Haight and Webster (1995, 2002) is among the most comprehensive emanating from the nursing profession. Cole (1992), Birren and Deutchman (1991), and Birren and Cochran (2001) have also been influential in describing the importance of seeking life stories. The International Institute for Reminiscence and Life Review, an interdisciplinary organization bringing together participants to study reminiscence and life review, is another valuable resource for nurses and members of other disciplines involved in research or practice in the field.

An older person is a living history book, but unlike written history, the story remains flexible and changeable, similar to a kaleidoscope. Each shift, however minor, in the person's self-esteem or interaction brings forth another pattern and colorful image. The most exciting aspect of working with older adults is being a part of the emergence of the life story—the shifting and blending patterns. When we are young, it is important for our emotional health and growth to look forward and plan for the future. As we age, it becomes more important to look back, talk over experiences, review and make sense of it all, and end with a feeling of satisfaction with the life lived. This is important work and the major developmental task of older adulthood that Erik Erikson called *ego integrity versus self despair*. Ego integrity is achieved when the person has accepted both the triumphs and disappointments of life and is at peace and satisfied with the life lived.

A memory is an incredible gift to the nurse, a sharing of a part of oneself when one may have little else to give. The more personal memories are saved for persons who will patiently wait for their unveiling and who will treasure them. Especially with older adults, listening to stories is a more complete way to know them. Older people bring us complex stories derived from long years of living. Through attentiveness to the stories of those cared for, the gerontological nurse can unfold many wraps of life that influence the present experiences and enhance person-focused care (Boykin et al., 1998). From Maloney (1995, p. 108):

> Storytelling can be thought of as a way of caring: caring for the individual who is telling the story by providing a vehicle for looking over his or her life, and caring for the listener who gains from the wisdom of the storyteller's experiences.

BOX 25-15	Suggested Applications of Memories

- Life story recording for family
- Legacy identification
- Products
- Contributions
- Qualities of character
- Talents
- Scrapbooks
- Photo albums
- Establishment of rituals of security and comfort
- Work history
- Life's turning points—can be mapped out as a road map
- Fantasy trips—follow the alternate road
- Grief resolution
- History of homes
- Mapping of life geographically
- Historical events—cohort identification
- Life history of significant persons and why significant
- Sensory stimulation
- Development of memory chains
- Inventory of significant items and why significant—to whom would he or she like to give them?
- Dietary history (significant foods of the past may stimulate appetite)
- Resolution of disappointment
- Entertainment

BOX 25-16	Reminiscence as a Developmental and Therapeutic Strategy

- Maintain continuity
- Extract meaning
- Define and develop personal philosophy
- Identify cycles and themes
- Recapitulate learning and growth
- Evolve identity
- Provide insight and growth
- Integrate and accept regrets and disappointments
- Perceive universality

Reminiscence. *Reminiscing* is an umbrella term that can include any recall of the past. Robert Butler (2002) pointed out that 50 years ago, reminiscing was thought to be a sign of senility or what we now call Alzheimer's disease. Older people who talked about the past and told the same stories again and again were said to be boring and living in the past. From Butler's seminal research (1963), we now know that reminiscence is the most important psychological task of older people. The work of several gerontological nursing leaders, including Irene Burnside, Priscilla Ebersole, and Barbara Haight, has contributed to the body of knowledge about reminiscence and its importance in nursing. Box 25-15 lists several ways that memories and reminiscences can be used effectively for the enrichment of the aging process.

Reminiscing occurs from childhood onward, particularly at life's junctures and transitions. Reminiscing cultivates a sense of security through recounting comforting memories, belonging through sharing, and self-esteem through confirmation of uniqueness. For the nurse, reminiscing is a therapeutic intervention important in assessment and understanding.

Reminiscence can have many goals. It not only provides a pleasurable experience that improves quality of life but also increases socialization and connectedness with others, provides cognitive stimulation, improves communication, and can be an effective therapy for depressive symptoms (Bohlmeijer et al., 2003; Haight and Burnside, 1993). Reminiscence is important to personal development and is also a very accessible activity with therapeutic implications, as can

be seen in Box 25-16. The process of reminiscence can be structured as in a nursing history, or it can occur in a group where each person shares memories and listens to others share memories (Haight and Burnside, 1993). The nurse can learn much about a resident's history, communication style, relationships, coping mechanisms, strengths, fears, affect, and adaptive capacity by listening thoughtfully as the life story is constructed. Box 25-17 provides some suggestions for encouraging reminiscence. The concept of reminiscence also fits well with mechanisms of crisis and grief resolution and is a fitting tool to use to accomplish some of the work in these situations.

Life Review. Butler (1963) first noted and brought to public attention the review process that normally occurs in the older person as the realization of one's approaching death creates a resurgence of unresolved conflicts. Butler called this process *life review.* Life review occurs quite naturally for many persons during periods of crisis and transition; however, Butler (2002) noted that in old age, putting one's life in order increases in intensity and emphasis. Life review occurs most frequently as an internal review of memories, an intensely private, soul-searching activity. It often occurs sporadically in a long-term trusted relationship.

The goals of life review include the following (Butler, 2002, p. 2):

> …resolution of past conflicts and issues, atonement for past acts or inaction, and reconciliation with family members or friends …The overall benefit of a life review is that it can engender hard-won serenity, a philosophical acceptance of what has occurred in the past, and wisdom. When people resolve their life conflicts, they have a lively capacity to live in the present.

Life review should occur not only when we are old or facing death but also frequently throughout our lives. This process can assist us examine where we are in life and change our course or set new goals. Butler commented that one might avoid the overwhelming feelings of despair that may surface when there is no time left to make changes.

Life review can be considered a psychotherapeutic process or technique and involves the review of remote memories (self-revelation), the expression of related feelings (catharsis), the recognition of conflicts (insight), and the relinquishment of viewpoints that are self-inhibiting

---

BOX 25-17   Suggestions for Encouraging Reminiscence

- Listen without correction or criticism. Older adults are presenting their version of their reality; our version belongs to another generation.
- Encourage older adults to cover various ages and stages. Use questions such as "What was it like growing up on that farm?" "What did teenagers do for fun when you were young?" "What was WW II like for you?" If reluctant to share because they don't feel their life was interesting, reassure them that everyone's life is valuable and interesting and that their memories are important to you and others.
- Be patient with repetition. Sometimes people need to tell the same story often to come to terms with the experience, especially if it was very meaningful to them. If they have a memory loss, it may be the only story they can remember and it is important for them to be a member of the group and contribute. If group members seem bothered by repetition, be sure to acknowledge the person's contribution and then direct conversation to include others.
- Be attuned to signs of depression in conversation (dwelling on sad topics) or changes in physical status or behavior, and provide appropriate assessment and intervention.
- If a topic arises that the person does not want to discuss, change to another topic.
- Keep in mind that reminiscing is not an orderly process. One memory triggers another in a way that may not seem related; it is not important to keep things in order or verify accuracy.
- Keep the conversation focused on the person reminiscing, but do not hesitate to share some of your own memories

that relate to the situation being discussed. Participate as equals, and enjoy each other's contributions.
- Listen actively, maintain eye contact; do not interrupt.
- Respond positively and give feedback by making caring, appropriate comments that encourage the person to continue.
- Use props and triggers such as photographs, memorabilia (e.g., a childhood toy or antique), short stories or poems about the past, favorite foods.
- Use open-ended questions to encourage reminiscing. You can prepare questions in advance, or you can ask the group to pick a topic that interests them. One question or topic may be enough for an entire group session. Consider using questions such as the following:

 How did your parents meet?
 What do you remember most about your mother? Father? Grandmother? Grandfather?
 What are some of your favorite memories from childhood?
 What was the first house you remember?
 What were your favorite foods as a child?
 Did you have a pet as a child?
 Tell me about your first job.
 How did you celebrate birthdays or other holidays?
 Tell me about your wedding day.
 What was your greatest accomplishment or joy in your life?
 What advice did your parents give you? What advice did you give your children? What advice would you give to young people today?

(decathexis). The process of life review is very directive and structured and occurs on a one-to-one basis. Gerontological nurses participate with older adults in both reminiscence and life review, and it is important to acquire the skills to be effective in achieving the purposes of both.

Life review therapy (Butler and Lewis, 1983), guided autobiography (Birren and Deutchman, 1991), and structured life review (Haight and Webster, 1995) are psychotherapeutic techniques based on the concept of life review. An important setting for life review therapy is in hospice and palliative care. The Hospice Foundation of America published *A Guide for Recalling and Telling Your Life Story* that nurses and families may find helpful (*www.hospicefoundation.org*). When working with the elderly in a life review process, it is important to have a clear understanding of goals:

1. Is the person reviewing the life course preparatory to letting go? If so, the main goal will be acceptance of what has been.
2. Is the individual facing a major crisis in self-esteem or need? The goal will be to identify past coping strategies and, from those, gather strategies that will be currently effective. Evaluating times when one was effective will sustain confidence in future effectiveness.
3. Is the individual bound in a morass of regret? The goal will be to reenergize the person for present and future

functioning by developing alternative views of past failures.
4. Is the individual suffering the effects of institutionalization? The goal will be to stimulate clear memories of what one has been and has accomplished to reaffirm uniqueness and individuality.
5. Has the person held long-standing grievances against significant others? The goal will be to explore the complexity of those relationships and provide opportunities for interpersonal resolution with the individuals involved.

These and many other exploratory statements will facilitate the life review. Do not ask if you are not prepared to listen carefully and without judgment or advice. It is usually helpful to begin with descriptions of events, since those are less threatening than sharing fears, failures, and feelings. During any interview, it is important to comment on increasing evidence of anxiety and tension and ask if the interviewee wishes to continue, to sit quietly, or to be left alone. When life review occurs during group reminiscing, it can produce anxiety or agitation in the individual. In that situation, the nurse would verbally validate the discomfort and move the focus to another group member by saying, "I can see that this was a very difficult experience for you. When the group is over, I would like to spend a few minutes alone with you."

BOX 25-18   Guidelines for Life Review Therapy

1. Share with older adults the characteristics and normalcy of the life review process.
2. Provide opportunities for older adults to recapitulate events in their lives (e.g., "What has most influenced the course of your life?" "Who has most influenced the course of your life?").
3. Assist older adults to view their life experiences in a broader or different context (e.g., "As you explain your regrets, can you think of other factors that contributed to those events?" "How would you have changed your life then?" "What factors influenced your course of action?" "What would you do differently now, and what difference might it have made?")
4. Facilitate connections among past hopes, present events, and future expectations.
5. Be aware that the process may be carried out sporadically over several months. It can be a painful examination of the past and is sometimes avoided. Be open and encourage sharing, but do not force it.
6. As difficult events are remembered, focus on affirming and acknowledging the strengths of the person. Coping strategies that got them through can be brought forward to deal with current difficulties.
7. Conflicts or regrets may emerge, and the process may assist the individual to come to terms with these feelings or events. This may involve reconciling with an estranged friend or family member, or it may mean forgiving oneself or another and letting go of the negative feelings associated with the memory. This may give new meaning to life and assist in preparation for death by decreasing anger, fear, and anxiety.
8. Life review can be thought of as a time of "sorting," a time of doing a "balance sheet" and ending up with the feeling that despite some rocky times, people did the best they could. The outcome of life review is to achieve resolution, celebrate a life well lived, provide hope, and encourage personal growth and integrity.
9. Goals of life review include integrity, resolution of conflicts, serenity and peace, and preparation for death.
10. Life review therapy requires a skilled listener with knowledge and experience in psychotherapeutic techniques.

Sometimes memories are painful and may produce tears or lead to anxiety, guilt, or depression. The nurse must be skilled in providing support and appropriate interventions and referrals if indicated. Box 25-18 provides guidelines for life review therapy.

Reminiscing and Storytelling with Individuals Experiencing Cognitive Impairment. Cognitive impairment does not necessarily preclude older adults from participating in reminiscence or storytelling groups. Opportunities for telling the life story, enjoying memories, and achieving ego integrity and self-actualization should not be denied to individuals based on their cognitive status. Modifications must be made based on the cognitive abilities of the person, and although individual life review from a psychotherapeutic approach is not an appropriate modality, individuals with mild to moderate memory impairment can enjoy and benefit from group work focused on reminiscence and storytelling, and the modality may improve mood and self-esteem (Moss et al., 2002; Bastings, 2003, 2006). Storytelling and group work with elders who have cognitive impairment is discussed in more detail in Chapter 23.

When the nurse is working with a group of cognitively impaired older adults, the emphasis in reminiscence groups is on sharing memories, however they may be expressed, rather than specific recall of events. The individual should not be pressured to answer questions such as "Where were you born?" or "What was your first job?" Rather, discussions may center on jobs people had and places they have lived. Additional props, such as music, pictures, and familiar objects (e.g., an American flag, an old coffee grinder) can prompt many recollections and sharing. The leader of a group with participants who have memory problems needs to be more active. Many resources are available to guide these groups, including books such as *I Remember When* (Thorsheim and Roberts, 2000), that offer numerous ways to adapt the reminiscing process for those with cognitive impairment. Other helpful resources are listed in the Resources section at the end of this chapter.

Group Psychotherapy

The group psychotherapy approach may be more practical and acceptable than individual psychotherapy for people with limited incomes and psychological distress resulting from the aging process. Cohort groups sharing common problems reduce feelings of alienation and ineffectiveness. Intergenerational groups are also successful in promoting understanding of common human needs and conflicts.

Goals of group therapy with older people are as follows:
1. Reduction in stress-related anxiety
2. Short-term treatment of specific disorders
3. Acceptance of the aging process
4. Resolution of conflicts

Special Considerations for Groups of Older Adults. Group work with older adults is different from that with younger age-groups, and some unique aspects require special skills, training, and an extraordinary commitment on the part of the leader. Although these unique aspects may not apply to all types of groups of older adults, some of the differences are presented in Box 25-19.

Grief Support Therapy

The most common problem of aging, grief resolution, is seldom addressed in the care of the institutionalized elderly. Worley (1996), an experienced grief therapist, has contracted

---

BOX 25-19   Suggestions for Group Work with Elders

1. The leader must pay special attention to sensory losses and compensate for vision and hearing loss.
2. Pacing is different, and group leaders must slow down in both physical and psychological actions.
3. Group members often need assistance or transportation to the group, and adequate time must be allowed for assembling the members and assisting them to return to their homes or rooms.
4. Time of day to schedule a group is important. Meeting time should not conflict with bathing and eating schedules, and evening groups may not be good for older people who may be tired by then. For community-based older people, transportation logistics may become complicated in the evening.
5. A warm and friendly climate of acceptance of each member and showing appreciation and enjoyment of the group and each member's contribution are important. As a result of ageist attitudes in society, older people's wisdom and contributions are not often valued, making them feel useless or a bother.
6. They may need more stimulation and be less self-motivating. (This is, of course, not true of self-help and senior activist groups such as the Gray Panthers.)
7. Groups generally should include people with similar levels of cognitive ability. Mixing very intact elders with those who have memory and communication impairments requires special skills. Burnside* suggested that in groups of people with varying abilities, alert persons tend to ask, "Will I become like them?," whereas the people with memory and communication impairments may become anxious when they are aware that they cannot perform as well as the other members.

8. Many older people likely to be in need of groups may be depressed or have experienced a number of losses (health, friends, spouse). Discussion of losses and sad feelings can be difficult for group leaders. A leader prone to depression would not be appropriate.
9. Leaders must be prepared for some members to become ill, deteriorate, and die. Plans regarding recognition of missing members will need to be clear. The following example that occurred during a reminiscence group conducted by one of the authors (TT) illustrates: "As I arrived at the nursing home one week for the group, I was told by the nursing home staff that one of our members had died. One of the members had been a priest so we asked him to say a prayer for our deceased group member. He did so beautifully, and the group was grateful. The next week, to our surprise, the supposedly deceased member showed up for the group (she had been in the hospital). We didn't know how to handle the situation, but the other members came to our rescue by saying, 'Father's prayers really worked this time.'" Older people's wisdom and humor can teach us a lot.
10. Leaders are continually confronted with their own aging and attitudes toward it. Group leaders need to plan to incorporate a consistent support person in the group if possible. Co-leaders are ideal. If this is not feasible, someone must be available for planning and recapitulation of group sessions. Students generally should work in pairs and will need supervision. Skills in developing and implementing groups for older adults improve with experience. Burnside* reminds us that "all new group leaders should have guidance from an experienced leader to help them weather the difficult times" (p. 43).

*Burnside I: Group work with older persons, *J Gerontol Nurs* 20(1):43, 1994.

---

with several long-term care facilities in California to provide grief counseling and has found the response encouraging. With continuation of these efforts and measurement of efficacy, it is hoped that greater interest will develop in implementing grief counseling in nursing homes for both residents and staff. In addition, similar group sessions are conducted on a weekly basis for community residents recovering from losses. Hospitals provide these opportunities as part of community outreach efforts. These "drop-in" groups are open to all community residents and are focused on warm acceptance; immediate support; sharing of feelings; provision of specific information, guidance, and resources in written form; and referral for individual therapy when needed. Although these groups are not limited to older people, the great majority of participants are older than 60 years. Some participants attend weekly for several years, and some attend a few times or drop in sporadically as they feel the need. The individual is not "expected" to follow any particular pattern.

Somatotherapies

Promoting health, nutrition, activity, and rest is crucial to the success of any psychotherapeutic venture. These activi-

ties are discussed in many ways throughout this text. A balance of sleep and activity is important in maintaining mental health. Sleep not only is essential to daily restoration of function but also is the domain of the psyche. Interference with sleep delays the integration and resolution of daily events. Psychological work is accomplished during dream or rapid-eye-movement (REM) sleep, and this work may not proceed efficiently during drugged sleep. The dilemma for nurses is to support the need for rest and dream sleep. Activity during the day and anxiety-reduction exercises before sleep may have beneficial results in promoting the natural healing tendencies of the psyche during sleep.

NONTRADITIONAL THERAPY AND COUNSELING

Nontraditional therapies are nonthreatening and designed to enhance coping, self-esteem, and respect for individuality. Developing an individualized nursing care plan is essential. Motivating the older person to use traditional counseling and psychotherapy has always been a factor in underuse of mental health facilities. Nontraditional therapeutic pro-

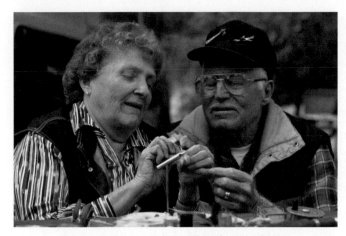

Elders enjoying an activity together. (Courtesy Corbis.)

grams and approaches may be more acceptable to older people than those that have the mental illness stigma.

Peer Counseling

In peer counseling, people without professional training but of similar age and experience help other people. The approach is appealing to both the helper and the one being helped and is nonthreatening. The peer concept can facilitate the development of a genuinely supportive relationship and a special rapport. The older person providing service enhances his or her own mental health through the opportunity to engage in productive, other-directed activities. Elders have been used to provide services for other elders in the following ways:

- Counseling people in retirement transition about benefits, income tax, insurance and investment, and retirement adjustment
- Counseling elders about legal issues and social and personal problems
- Providing for developmentally disabled adults
- Providing senior companions, visitation, and support to residents in nursing homes and to the homebound
- Providing older adult advocacy by indigenous elders for minorities

Volunteers in peer support programs need special training in the following:

- Empathic interviewing and listening skills
- Aspects of normal aging
- Special problems of the elderly
- Self-awareness
- Problem-solving methods
- Information and resources available to older people

Particular topics that may be introduced in peer counselor training sessions include the following:

- Assertiveness training
- Management of depression
- Death and dying, grief
- Evaluation of institutional care
- Working with the disabled
- Use of reminiscence
- Human sexuality

Self-Help Programs

Self-help programs have flourished in the past two decades, as has the use of peer counselors and volunteers. Self-help programs usually follow a "train the trainer" model and recruit from churches, community colleges, and universities in which vital and engaged older individuals can be found. Community and news announcements are also effective in recruiting trainees.

Screening of volunteers is a sensitive issue and must in no way erode the self-esteem of the individual volunteer. Throughout the process of selection and training, the emphasis must be on the strengths that the volunteer brings. If the qualities necessary for counseling are not present, the person must be routed early to an activity fitting his or her skills.

Providing scheduled supervision and support is necessary, as are providing tokens and awards of appreciation and planning activities in which the peer counselors have opportunities to share and learn from each other. Failure to plan for these needs of the peer counselor or volunteers is likely to result in unsatisfactory results from them as counselors. Volunteer activity is further discussed in Chapter 20.

Mobile Clinics

A psychogeriatric clinic may become a vital addition to the elder services. The clinic offers multidisciplinary assessment and treatment services. Home assessments, follow-up visits, and psychosocial, nursing, medication, and occupational therapy consultation are included in the comprehensive care plans. Referrals are accepted from anyone in the community. The clinic also provides consultation to nursing homes and ongoing support groups for elders at risk, including such foci as relaxation, memory strengthening, and peer counseling.

Within the home, providing such services is not only cost-effective but also more attendant to the holistic perspective of an individual's needs. Also, identifying high-risk individuals such as those who are living alone, homebound, recently bereaved, or suffering from repeated falls or hospitalizations and mental deterioration and providing preventive supports might best be accomplished by mobile mental health units. A similar model uses the services of a psychologist, nurse, geriatric NP, and psychiatrist to provide individuals with comprehensive physical and mental health assessments and problem management.

Multidisciplinary community mental health teams will continue to grow because of the multiple health and social needs of the older population and the limited availability of appropriate psychogeriatric institutional care. The geropsychiatric nurse's role is becoming a critical component of human services.

▲ PROMOTING HEALTHY AGING: IMPLICATIONS FOR GERONTOLOGICAL NURSING

The development of holistic and humanistic models of care for elders experiencing emotional health disturbances is critically important in gerontological nursing. Much of the

Human Needs and Wellness Diagnoses

Self-Actualization and Transcendence
(Seeking, Expanding, Spirituality, Fulfillment)
Participates in energizing activities: music, dance, laughter
Seeks meaning appropriately
Demonstrates consistent values
Appreciates beauty; can enjoy leisure time
Substances are sometimes used to achieve spiritual enlightenment

Self-Esteem and Self-Efficacy
(Image, Identity, Control, Capability)
Makes decisions and follows through
Respects other's rights
Recognizes impact of psychotropic substances on personality
Keeps physician informed of medication regimen
Recognizes transient nature of medication-induced affectual changes
Requests information when needed
Grooms self

Belonging and Attachment
(Love, Empathy, Affiliation)
Validates perceptions with trusted others
Develops reciprocal relationships

Safety and Security
(Caution, Planning, Protections, Sensory Acuity)
Seeks manageable level of stimulation
Accepts reorientation and/or protection when needed
Is able to follow rules and appropriate limits
Structures day

Biological and Physiological Integrity
(Air, Fluids, Comfort, Activity, Nutrition, Elimination, Skin Integrity)
Maintains nutrition
Is able to sleep
Seeks social services for basic needs when appropriate

These are not all the possible wellness diagnoses that may be identified. The above
are examples of nursing diagnoses that should be considered when planning care
for the older adult.

distress associated with emotional illness in late life can be relieved through competent, caring, and compassionate nursing care. Awareness of appropriate assessment and treatment of the distressing reactions that can occur in late life as presented in this chapter is an important component of best practice care. However, knowing and appreciating each elder's uniqueness, his or her past and present experiences, and how they color the present may contribute far more to healthy aging and emotional well-being than medications and therapy. Believing in and supporting the strength and wisdom of older people restores self-confidence and feelings of worth, an important component of emotional health. Appreciating the nature of grief in old age means that gerontological nurses listen, really listen, and offer support to

weather the storm. Nurses' work needs to focus on the development of environments of care that enhance both physical and emotional functioning, create conditions of hope, and support elders in the often difficult journey in late life.

KEY CONCEPTS

- Emotional health in late life is difficult to determine because the accrual of life experiences makes for great variations. Emotional health must be determined by the gratification or satisfaction that individuals feel within their particular situation.
- Mental health is a fluctuating situation for most individuals, with peaks and valleys of happiness and pain.

- Elders are not well served within the mental health system as it exists today. Neither practitioners nor reimbursement mechanisms are adapted to their needs.
- Psychological assessment of elders that is based on the common psychometric instruments will usually show deficits because these instruments, with few exceptions, have been designed to test the mental health of young adults.
- Classic defense mechanisms, such as denial, displacement, and identification, when used by the elderly, are often life enhancing and necessary to their function.
- The incidence of late-life onset of psychotic disorders is low among older people, but psychotic manifestations can occur as a secondary syndrome in a variety of disorders, the most common being Alzheimer's disease. Psychotic symptoms in Alzheimer's disease require different assessment and treatment than long-standing psychotic disorders.
- Anxiety disorders are common in late life and are best managed by restoring some sense of control to the situation that the individual perceives as out of control.
- PTSD is finally being recognized in older people who have been subjected to extremely traumatic events. Programs are now available to provide support and insight for these individuals.

- Depression is the most common emotional disorder of aging and similarly the most treatable. Unfortunately, depression is often neglected or assumed to be a condition one must "learn to live with." Nurses may be instrumental in ensuring that elders are assessed properly and treated for depression.
- Grief is a component of aging for most individuals as they confront various losses. Grief is not a mental illness, but it often requires grief counseling and support for resolution.
- Suicide is a significant problem among older men. Assessment for suicidal intent is important especially in light of loss, trauma, or catastrophe. Many present to the health care professional with physical complaints shortly before they commit suicide.
- Substance abuse and addictions are growing and often under-recognized and undertreated problems of older adults, particularly older women. Screening and appropriate assessment and intervention are important nursing interventions in all settings.
- Further research is needed to fully understand the cultural and ethnic differences in mental health concerns, as well as appropriate assessment and treatment in culturally and ethnically diverse older people.

CASE STUDY: Bipolar Disorder

Myra is a 71-year-old white woman who was admitted to the geropsychiatry inpatient unit for alcohol abuse and noncompliance with her lithium, which had been prescribed for a diagnosed bipolar disorder. Myra's primary mode of coping with her depression and mood swings has been to drink alcohol, meet abusive men, and play bingo. However, when she stops taking her dose of lithium, she begins to have flights of ideas, argues with her daughters, and tries to pick up men in her apartment complex. After seeing her at home, you discover that she has a long history of being physically abused by her husband, now deceased for 8 years, and has been living with one daughter who also has emotionally and physically abused her, causing her to be hospitalized. Myra's ability to test reality is compromised because of years of denial and low self-esteem. She says, "I used to have lots of times when I felt really good in between the depressions. Now I feel depressed most of the time." She tells you that her daughters harass her and interfere in her life. Your goals as a community-based nurse are to facilitate her independence (being able to live in her own apartment), to assist her with medication compliance, and to intervene with Myra to improve relationships with her daughters. Home visits are approved through Medicare for 2 months after hospital discharge.

Based on the case study, develop a nursing care plan using the following procedure*:
- List Myra's comments that provide subjective data.
- List information that provides objective data.
- From these data, identify and state, using accepted format, two nursing diagnoses you determine are most significant to Myra at this time. List two of Myra's strengths that you have identified from the data.
- Determine and state outcome criteria for each diagnosis.

These criteria must reflect some alleviation of the problem identified in the nursing diagnosis and must be stated in concrete and measurable terms.
- Plan and state one or more interventions for each diagnosed problem. Provide specific documentation of the sources used to determine the appropriate intervention. Plan at least one intervention that incorporates Myra's existing strengths.
- Evaluate the success of the intervention. Interventions must correlate directly with the stated outcome criteria to measure the outcome success.

Critical Thinking Questions

1. How will you evaluate Myra's ability to live independently?
2. What particular strategies are necessary to meet the goals of the nursing care plan?
3. Given that Myra's primary coping strategy is drinking alcohol, how will you facilitate her sobriety and help her deal with stress?
4. How much involvement with Myra's daughters do you believe is necessary to assist with her transition back into her own apartment?
5. Given the limited number of visits covered by Medicare, what information does Myra need to provide self-care? In other words, the nurse must be teaching Myra how to live independently after discharge from home health care. What does Myra need to know?
6. Discuss the meanings and the thoughts triggered by the student's and the elder's viewpoints expressed at the beginning of the chapter. How do these vary from your own experience?

* Students are advised to refer to their nursing diagnosis text and identify possible or potential problems.

CASE STUDY: Depressive Disorder with Suicidal Thoughts

Jake had cared for his wife Emma during a long and painful illness until she died 4 years ago. He found that alcohol provided a way to cope with the stress. Within a year after her death, Jake met a lady to whom he was very attracted, and a few months later, she moved in with him. Jake managed to move his things around until some space was made for her personal items, but neither of them was very comfortable with this. He really did not like to move his things from their usual place and, because her allotted space was so small, she felt like an intruder. He collected guns, and she shuddered when she saw them. He was an avid fan of John Wayne movies, and she preferred going to the symphony. He liked meat and potatoes, and she was a vegetarian. She also disapproved of his increasing reliance on alcohol. The blending of two such different lifestyles proved difficult. In a few months she moved out, and Jake blamed himself. He said over and over, "I should have done more for her. I'm not good for anything anymore." His friends began to pull away from him, just when he needed them most, because he seemed to talk of nothing but his various aches, pains, and pills and his general discouragement with life. Jake's consumption of alcohol increased markedly. He had some health problems: a mild heart failure, a lack of exercise, dairy products gave him diarrhea, he was somewhat obese, and his knees were painful most of the time. He routinely visited his allergist, his internist, his orthopedist, and his cardiologist. However, it seemed the more he went to these specialists, the worse he felt. He was taking several medications, and each time he saw one of his clinicians, he came away with another prescription. No one asked about his drinking, and he never mentioned it. He awoke one morning feeling very dizzy, so he went to his internist later in the day. He began to share the litany of his discomforts, and the physician reminded him that at 76 years of age he could not expect to always feel in top shape.

When he returned from seeing the physician, Jake called his daughter and surprised her by saying he had just decided he would take a week off and go to Hawaii to see if the sun and sand would revive him. Jake was not usually impulsive. His daughter, fortunately, was a psychiatric nurse and was concerned about the change in his behavior.

Based on the case study, develop a nursing care plan using the following procedure*:

- List Jake's comments that provide subjective data.
- List information that provides objective data.
- From these data, identify and state, using accepted format, two nursing diagnoses you determine are most significant to Jake at this time. List two of Jake's strengths that you have identified from the data.
- Determine and state outcome criteria for each diagnosis. These criteria must reflect some alleviation of the problem identified in the nursing diagnosis and must be stated in concrete and measurable terms.

- Plan and state one or more interventions for each diagnosed problem. Provide specific documentation of the source used to determine the appropriate intervention. Plan at least one intervention that incorporates Jake's existing strengths.
- Evaluate the success of the intervention. Interventions must correlate directly with the stated outcome criteria to measure the outcome success.

Critical Thinking Questions

1. Discuss the variations in symptoms of depression in the old and the young.
2. Describe some of the reasons that elders are more vulnerable to depression than younger people are.
3. Describe a time when you were depressed and the feelings you had. What did you do about it?
4. Given the situation in this case, discuss what your thoughts would be if you were Jake's daughter.
5. Given his daughter's background, what are her responsibilities in this case?
6. What is the responsibility of a student nurse in the case of suspected suicidal thoughts?
7. Would you address the possibility of suicidal thoughts if you were the nurse in the physician's office? When and how would you take on this task?
8. What action should be taken for Jake's protection?
9. Would you expect that Jake is still grieving over the death of his wife? What are your thoughts about this situation?
10. What are the clues or indications that an elder is thinking of committing suicide?
11. What are some of signs of suicidal intent in young adults? How are these signs different from those of elders?
12. Under what conditions do you think a person has a right to take his or her life?
13. What are your thoughts about Jake's use of alcohol?
14. Do you think suicide is a sign of weakness or strength?
15. Do you agree or disagree with the following statements based on the evidence about depression and suicide in older adults?
    - Normally older people feel depressed much of the time.
    - Older people are more likely than young people to admit to depression.
    - Most older people talk about suicide but rarely try to kill themselves.
    - Depression of the elderly is helped by medications.
    - Depression may be the cause of forgetfulness.
    - Depression in the elderly is often linked with illness and alcoholism.

* Students are advised to refer to their nursing diagnosis text and identify possible or potential problems.

RESEARCH QUESTIONS

What is the prevalence of emotional disorders in community-dwelling older adults? What mental health care is nursing able to provide in the home?

How common is alcohol abuse a strategy of self-care used by the older adult with emotional concerns?

What types of interventions are most appropriate for older adults with alcohol or drug abuse problems?

Is psychiatric home care a more cost-effective alternative than institutional care?

Determine in what circumstances antidepressants are useful in grief reactions.

What are the cardinal symptoms of depression in the oldest-old?

Although the general status of older white males is thought to be the best it has been from a socioeconomic perspective, inexplicably, suicide has begun to increase since 1981. What factors may be contributing to this increase?

How many physicians consider or evaluate for the presence of depression in elders who see them for physical complaints?

What are the most reliable tools for identifying depression in cognitively intact and cognitively impaired elderly?

In what present cultures are older adults most comfortable and honored?

What is the meaning of depression in older people of different cultures and ethnicity?

What type of assessment and interventions are culturally appropriate for diverse older people?

RESOURCES

Alternative Solutions in Long-Term Care
Animal-assisted therapy
www.activitytherapy.com/pet.htm

American Association for Geriatric Psychiatry
7910 Woodmont Ave., Suite 1050
Bethesda, MD, 20814-3004
(301) 654-7850
www.aagponline.org

AssessmentPsychology.com
Professional information and resources for mental health practitioners, educators, and consumers

Bi-Folkal Reminiscing Kits
Check with your local library to see if they have these kits
Bifolkal Productions, Inc.
809 Williamson St.
Madison, WI 53703
(800) 568-5357
www.bifolkal.org

Connecticut Association of Therapeutic Recreation Directors, Inc.
Several videos to use in reminiscence groups
www.catrd.com/resources/videos

Delta Society
Animal-assisted therapy
www.deltasociety.org/animalsaaaabout.htm

Helping Older Adults Overcome Alcohol or Medication Dependence
www.agingaddictions.net

Hyer L, Intrieri R: *Geropsychological interventions in long-term care*, New York, 2006, Springer.

International Psychogeriatric Association
5215 Old Orchard Rd., Suite 340
Skokie, IL 60077
(847) 663-0574
www.ipa-online.org

International Society for Reminiscence and Life Review
Center for Continuing Education/Extension
University of Wisconsin-Superior
PO Box 2000
Superior, WI 54880-4500
(800) 370-9882
www.reminiscenceandlifereview.org

In Times Past: Radio Days
An entertaining history of the golden days of radio bringing back many wonderful memories
Terra Nova Films
www.terranova.org

Mental Health and Aging Network
American Society on Aging
833 Market St., No. 511
San Francisco, CA 94103-1824
(800) 537-9728
www.asaging.org

National Institute of Mental Health
Office of Communications
6001 Executive Blvd., Room 8184, MSC 9663
Bethesda, MD 20982-9663
(866) 615-6464
www.nimh.gov

National Coalition on Mental Health and Aging
3003 W. Touhy
Chicago, IL 60645
(773) 508-4745
www.ncmha.org

National Institute on Alcohol Abuse and Alcoholism
5635 Fishers Lane, MSC 9304
Bethesda, MD 20892
www.niaaa.nih.gov

National Institute on Drug Abuse
Self-Administered Assessment of Drug and Alcohol Abuse
www.dapaonline.com

National Time Slips Project
Center on Age & Community
PO Box 413
Milwaukee, WI 43211
(414) 229-2740
www.timeslips.org

Substance Abuse and Mental Health Services Administration
Substance Abuse Among Older Adults Treatment Improvement Protocol (TIP)
www.samhsa.gov

Tell Me a Story
A simple reminiscence tool for visitors as well as family and professional caregivers of people with Alzheimer's disease.
Elder Books
Forest Knolls, CA

The Baby Boomer Memory Bank
www.boomerbaby.com

The Fifties Web Site
www.fiftiesweb.com

The San Francisco SPCA's Animal Assisted Therapy Program
www.sfspca.org/att/index.shtml

Well into Your Future: Mental Health and Aging
3-hour documentary series
www.wellme.stateart.com

REFERENCES

Abramson T et al: Culture and mental health: providing appropriate services for a diverse older population, *Generations* xxvi(1):21-27, 2002.

Alexopoulos GS et al: The Expert Consensus Guidelines Series: pharmacotherapy of depressive disorders in older patients, *Postgrad Med Spec Rep*, October 2001.

American Psychiatric Association (APA): *Diagnostic and statistical manual of mental disorders (DSM-IV)*, ed 4, Washington, DC, 2000, The Association.

Antai-Otong D: Schizophrenia in the elderly, *Adv Nurse Pract* 8(3):39, 2000.

APA: *Fact sheet on mental health and aging*, 2004. (website): *www.apa.org*. Accessed July 12, 2006.

Barry K et al: *Alcohol problems in older adults: prevention and management*, New York, Springer, 2001.

Bartels S et al: Implementing evidence-based practices in geriatric mental health, *Generations* xxvi(1):90-98, 2002.

Bastings A: Reading the story behind the story: context and content in stories by people with dementia, *Generations* xxv(3):25-29, 2003.

Bastings A: Arts in dementia care: "this is not the end...it's the end of this chapter," *Generations* xxx(1):16-20, 2006.

Beautrais AL: A case control of suicide and attempted suicide in older adults, *Suicide Life Threat Behav* 32(1):1-9, 2002.

Beck C et al: Nursing assistants as providers of mental health care in nursing homes, *Generations* xxvi(1):66-71, 2002.

Becker M et al: Assisted living: the new frontier for mental health care? *Generations* xxiv(1):72-77, 2002.

Beers MH, Berkow R: *Merck manual of geriatrics*, ed 3, Whitehouse Station, NJ, 2000, Merck Research Laboratories.

Birren JE, Cochran KN: *Telling the stories of life through guided autobiographical groups*, Baltimore, 2001, Johns Hopkins University Press.

Birren JE, Deutchman DE: *Guiding autobiography groups for older adults: exploring the fabric of life*, Baltimore, 1991, Johns Hopkins University Press.

Blow F et al: Misuse and abuse of alcohol, illicit drugs, and psychoactive medications among older people, *Generations* xxvi(1):50-54, 2002.

Bludau J: Second institutionalization: impact of personal history on patients with dementia, *Caring for the Ages* 3(5):3-4, 2002.

Bohlmeijer E et al: Effects of reminiscence and life review on late-life depression: a meta-analysis, *Int J Geriatr Psychiatry* 18(12):1088-1094, 2003.

Boykin A et al: Discovering the beauty of older adults—opening doors, *J Clin Psychol* 4(3):205-210, 1998.

Brown SI: Depression common among adults with advanced macular degeneration, *Ophthalmology* 108:1893, 2001.

Bruce M: Mental health services in home healthcare, *Generations* xxvi(1):78-82, 2002.

Bruce ML et al: Reducing suicide ideation and depressive symptoms in depressed older primary care patients: a randomized controlled trial, *JAMA* 291(9):1081-1091, 2004.

Burke W: Management of anxiety in late life, *Ann Long-Term Care* 12(8):28-33, 2004.

Burnside I: Group work with older persons, *J Gerontol Nurs* 20(1):43, 1994.

Butler R: *Age, death and life review*, 2002. (website): *www.hospicefoundation.org*. Accessed June 24, 2004.

Butler RN: The life review: an interpretation of reminiscence in the aged, *Psychiatry* 26:65-76, 1963.

Butler R, Lewis M: *Aging and mental health: positive psychosocial approaches*, ed 3, St Louis, 1983, Mosby.

Cole TR: *The journey of life: a cultural history of aging in America*, Cambridge, UK, 1992, Cambridge University Press.

Coles R: *The call of stories*, Boston, 1989, Houghton-Mifflin.

Culberson J: Alcohol use in the elderly: beyond the CAGE. Part 1 of 2: prevalence and patterns of problem drinking, *Geriatrics* 61(10): 23-27, 2006a.

Culberson J: Alcohol use in the elderly: beyond the CAGE. Part 2 of 2: screening instruments and treatment strategies, *Geriatrics* 61(11): 20-26, 2006b.

Culpepper L: Recognizing and treating post-traumatic stress disorder, *Hippocrates* 14(6):40-52, 2000.

Davis B: Assessing adults with mental disorders in primary care, *Am J Primary Health Care* 29(5):19-27, 2004.

Finfgeld-Connett DL: Treatment of substance misuse in older women: using a brief intervention model, *J Gerontol Nurs* 30(8):31-37, 2004.

Finfgeld-Connett D: Self-management of alcohol problems among older adults, *J Gerontol Nurs* 31(5):51-58, 2005.

Frampton K: The state of geriatric mental health services in LTC, *Caring for the Ages* 5(4):47-51, 2004.

Gallo JJ, Coyne JC: The challenge of depression in later life: bridging science and service in primary care, *JAMA* 284(12):1570-1772, 2000.

Geriatric Mental Health Foundation: Substance abuse and misuse among older adults: prevention, recognition, and help, 2006 (website): *www.gmhonline.org*. Accessed May 24, 2007.

Goodman A: Update: geriatric psychiatry, *Caring for the Ages* 4(8):16-17, 2003.

Grossberg GT: Diagnosis and treatment of late-life psychosis in the elderly, *Long-term Care Forum* 1(3):7, 2000.

Gum A et al: Depression treatment preferences in older primary care patients, *Gerontologist* 46(1):14-22, 2006.

Haight BK, Burnside IM: Reminiscence and life review: explaining the differences, *Arch Psychiatr Nurs* 7(2):91-98, 1993.

Haight BK, Webster J: *The art and science of reminiscing: theory, research, methods and applications*, Washington, DC, 1995, Taylor & Francis.

Haight B, Webster J: *Critical advances in reminiscence work: from theory to application*, New York, 2002, Springer.

Hegel M et al: Minor depression and subthreshold anxiety symptoms in older adults: psychosocial therapies and special considerations, *Generations* 26(3):44-49, 2002.

Holkup P: Evidence-based protocol: elderly suicide—secondary prevention, *J Gerontol Nurs* 29(6):4-17, 2003.

Hooker SD et al: Pet therapy research: a historical review, *Holist Nurs Pract* 16(5):17-23, 2002.

Joe S et al: Prevalence of and risk factors for lifetime suicide risks among blacks in the United States, *JAMA* 296(17): 2112-2123, 2006.

Jones ED: Reminiscence therapy for older women with depression: effects of nursing intervention classification in assisted-living long-term care, *J Gerontol Nurs* 29(7):26-33, 2003.

Kaas M: Geropyschiatric nursing practice in the United States: present trends and future directions. *J Am Psychiatr Nurs Assoc* 12(3): 142-155, 2006.

Kaldy J: Managing mental health, *Caring for the Ages*, 6: 17-18, 2005.

Kales H, Mellow A: Race and depression: does race affect the diagnosis and treatment of late-life depression? *Geriatrics* 61(5):18-21, 2006.

Kenefick A: Pain treatment and quality of life, *J Gerontol Nurs* 30(5):22-29, 2004.

Kennedy G: Prevention of suicide in older persons: lessons and limitations of evidence-based interventions, *Ann Long-Term Care* 12(8):43-48, 2004.

Kennedy GJ: Psychopharmacology of late-life depression, *Ann Long-Term Care* 9(3):35-40, 2001.

Kennedy-Malone L et al: *Management guidelines for gerontological nurse practitioners*, Philadelphia, 2000, FA Davis.

Kivnick HQ: Everyday mental health: a guide to assessing life's strengths. In Smyer MA, editor: *Mental health and aging*, New York, 1993, Springer.

Kurlowicz LH: Depression in older adults. In Mezey M et al, editors: *Geriatric nursing protocols for best practice*, ed 2, New York: Springer, 2003. (website): *www.guidelines.gov.*

Lawrence V et al: Concepts and causation of depression: a cross-cultural study of the beliefs of older adults, *Gerontologist* 46(1):25-32, 2006.

Lebowitz B: Trends in mental illness among nursing home patients, *Long-term Care Forum* 1(2), 2002 (website): *www.aagponline.org.* Accessed July 28, 2002.

Letizia M, Reinboltz M: Identifying and managing acute alcohol withdrawal in the elderly, *Geriatr Nurs* 26(3):176-183, 2005.

Linkins K et al: *Screening for mental illness in nursing facility applicants: understanding federal requirements*, SAMSHA Pub No (SMA) 01-3543, Rockville Md, Center for Mental Health Services, Substance Abuse and Mental Health Services Administration, July 2001.

Loughlin A: Depression and social support: effective treatments for homebound elderly adults, *J Gerontol Nurs* 30(5):11-15, 2004.

Maloney MF: A Heideggerian hermeuneutical analysis of older women's stories of being strong, *Image J Nurs Sch* 27(2):104-109, 1995.

Masters J: Moderate alcohol consumption and unappreciated risk for alcohol-related harm among ethnically diverse urban-dwelling elders, *Geriatr Nurs* 24(3):155-161, 2003.

McAndrews MM: Lighting the darkness, *Adv Providers Post-acute Care* 73(Sept/Oct):40, 2001.

Meiner S, Lueckenotte A: *Gerontological nursing*, ed 3, St Louis, 2006, Mosby.

Moorhead SA, Brighton VA: Anxiety and fear. In Maas ML et al, editors: *Nursing care of older adults: diagnoses, outcomes, and interventions*, St Louis, 2001, Mosby.

Moss S et al: Reminiscence group activities and discourse interaction in Alzheimer's disease, *J Gerontol Nurs* 28(8):36-44, 2002.

National Conference of Gerontological Nurse Practitioners: *Mental health toolkit: meeting the needs of your older patients*, 2005 (website): *www.ngna.org.*

National Institute on Alcohol Abuse and Alcoholism: older adults and alcohol problems, Participant Handout, 2005 (website): *www.niaaa.nih.gov.* Accessed May 24, 2007.

National Institutes of Mental Health (NIMH): *A story of bipolar disorder*, 2002. (website): *www.nimh.nih.gov/pub licat/bipol-story08.cfm.*

National Institutes of Mental Health (NIMH): *Older adults: depression and suicide facts*, 2007. (website): *www.nimh.nih.gov/publi-cat/elderlydepsuicide.cfm.* Accessed July 19, 2007.

Oxman T, Dietrich A: The key role of primary care physicians in mental health care for elders, *Generations* xxvi(1):59-65, 2002.

Palmer B et al: Psychotic disorders in late life: implications for treatment and future directions for clinical services, *Generations* 26(1):28-31, 2002.

Qualls S: Defining mental health in later life, *Generations* xxvi(1):9-13, 2002.

Reuben DB et al: *Geriatrics at your fingertips*, 2003 edition, Malden, Mass, 2003, American Geriatric Society Blackwell.

Reynolds C et al: Geriatric depression: diagnosis and treatment, *Generations* xxvi(1):28-31, 2002.

Sattinger A: 'Rapid cycles' are growing problem for older patients with bipolar disorder, *Caring for the Ages* 7(7):10, 2006.

Schultz S et al: Alcohol use among older persons in a rural state, *Am J Geriatr Psychiatr* 10:750-753, 2002.

Tabloski P: *Gerontological nursing*, Upper Saddle River, NJ, 2006, Pearson Prentice Hall.

Tanner E: Recognizing late-life depression: why is this important for nurses in the home setting? *Geriatr Nurs* 26(3):145, 2005.

Tappen R, Barry C: Assessment of affect in advanced Alzheimer's disease: the dementia mood picture test, *J Gerontol Nurs* 21(3):44-46, 1995.

Thorsheim H, Roberts B: *I remember when: activity ideas to help people reminiscence*, Forest Knolls, Calif, 2000, Elder Books.

Ugarriza DN: Elderly women's explanation of depression, *J Gerontol Nurs* 28(5):22-29, 2002.

U.S. Department of Health and Human Services (USDHHS), Office of the Surgeon General, SAMSHA: *Culture, race, and ethnicity: a supplement to the mental health report of the Surgeon General*, Washington DC, 2001, USDHHS.

Whall AL, Hoes-Gurevich ML: Missed depression in elderly individuals: why is this a problem? *J Gerontol Nurs* 25(6):44-46, 1999.

Worley A: *Grief group counseling in nursing homes and community "drop-in" grief support groups*, Unpublished manuscript, 1996.

Yesavage J et al: Development and validation of a geriatric depression screening scale: a preliminary report, *J Psychiatr Res* 12:63, 1983.

Zhan L: Improving mental health for ethnic older adults, *J Gerontol Nurs* 30(8):3, 2004.

Zung W: A self-rating depression scale, *Arch Gen Psychiatry* 12:63, 1965.

Depression Rating Scales

The Zung Self-Rating Depression Scale (SDS) is probably the most widely used test of depression in the elderly. The SDS is a self-administered questionnaire consisting of 20 items that measure areas associated with depression such as mood, well-being, optimism, and somatic symptoms (Zung, 1965). The scale incorporates both positive and negative responses. The items are scored on a 4-point scale, ranging from "a little of the time," "some of the time," "a good part of the time," to "most of the time." The responses are given a score of 1 to 4, arranged such that the higher the score, the greater the depression: the statements designated with (1) are given "1" for response "most of the time," and those with (2) are given "4" for "most of the time." The score is derived by dividing the sum of the 20 items (which are rated from 1 to 4) by the maximum score of 80 to arrive at a number expressed as a decimal. Scores above 0.38 (or a raw score of 50 and over) were associated with depression requiring hospital treatment (Zung, 1965).

The Center for Epidemiologic Studies Depression Scale (CES-D) was developed by the Center for Epidemiologic Studies at the National Institutes of Mental Health for use in studies of depression in community samples. The CES-D contains 20 items. Respondents are asked to report the amount of time they have experienced symptoms during the past week. Typically, a threshold of 17 and above is taken as defining "caseness," although higher cutoff points (e.g., 24 and above) have been suggested.

The General Health Questionnaire (GHQ) is a 60-item self-administered instrument, the purpose of which is to detect the presence of psychiatric distress. A scaled version has been devised and consists of 28 items that test four general categories (seven questions each): somatic symptoms, anxiety and insomnia, social dysfunction, and depression. The GHQ is unusual in that it was developed specifically for use in the primary care setting.

Using the GHQ, respondents rate the presence of anxious and depressive symptoms "over the past few weeks" into one of four categories: "not at all" (coded 1); "no more than usual" (coded 2); "more than usual" (coded 3); or "much more" (coded 4). Each question has four responses: score 1 for either of the two answers consistent with depression and 0 for the other two.

Zung Self-Rating Depression Scale

1. (−) I feel down-hearted and blue.
2. (+) Morning is when I feel the best.
3. (−) I have crying spells or feel like it.
4. (−) I have trouble sleeping at night.
5. (+) I eat as much as I used to.
6. (+) I still enjoy sex.
7. (−) I notice that I am losing weight.
8. (−) I have trouble with constipation.
9. (−) My heart beats faster than usual.
10. (−) I get tired for no reason.
11. (+) My mind is as clear as it used to be.
12. (+) I find it easy to do the things I used to.
13. (−) I am restless and can't keep still.
14. (+) I feel hopeful about the future.
15. (−) I am more irritable than usual.
16. (+) I find it easy to make decisions.
17. (+) I feel that I am useful and needed.
18. (+) My life is pretty full.
19. (−) I feel that others would be better off if I were dead.
20. (+) I still enjoy the things I used to do.

Adapted from Zung WK. *Arch Gen Psychiatry* 12:65, 1965, © 1965, American Medical Association, with permission.

All depression checklists in Gallo JJ et al: *Handbook of geriatric assessment*, ed 2, Gaithersburg, Md, 1995, Aspen Publishers.

Center for Epidemiologic Studies Depression Scale

INSTRUCTIONS FOR QUESTIONS: Below is a list of the ways you might have felt or behaved. Please tell me how often you have felt this way during the past week.

Rarely or none of the time (less than 1 day)
Some or a little of the time (1-2 days)
Occasionally or a moderate amount of time (3-4 days)
Most or all of the time (5-7 days)

During the past week:

1. I was bothered by things that usually don't bother me.
2. I did not feel like eating; my appetite was poor.
3. I felt that I could not shake off the blues even with help from my family or friends.
4. I felt that I was just as good as other people.
5. I had trouble keeping my mind on what I was doing.
6. I felt depressed.
7. I felt that everything I did was an effort.
8. I felt hopeful about the future.
9. I thought my life had been a failure.
10. I felt fearful.
11. My sleep was restless.
12. I was happy.
13. I talked less than usual.
14. I felt lonely.
15. People were unfriendly.
16. I enjoyed life.
17. I had crying spells.
18. I felt sad.
19. I felt that people dislike me.
20. I could not get "going."

From Center for Epidemiologic Studies, National Institutes of Mental Health.

Items from the Scaled U.S. Version of the General Health Questionnaire

A. Somatic symptoms
  A1. Been feeling in need of some medicine to pick you up?
  A2. Been feeling in need of a good tonic?
  A3. Been feeling run down and out of sorts?
  A4. Felt that you are ill?
  A5. Been getting any pains in your head?
  A6. Been getting a feeling of tightness or pressure in your head?
  A7. Been having hot or cold spells?

B. Anxiety and insomnia
  B1. Lost much sleep over worry?
  B2. Had difficulty staying asleep?
  B3. Felt constantly under strain?
  B4. Been getting edgy and bad-tempered?
  B5. Been getting scared or panicky for no reason?
  B6. Found everything getting on top of you?
  B7. Been feeling nervous and uptight all the time?

C. Social dysfunction
  C1. Been managing to keep yourself busy and occupied?
  C2. Been taking longer over the things you do?
  C3. Felt on the whole you were doing things well?
  C4. Been satisfied with the way you have carried out your tasks?
  C5. Felt that you are playing a useful part in things?
  C6. Felt capable of making decisions about things?
  C7. Been able to enjoy your normal day-to-day activities?

D. Depression
  D1. Been thinking of yourself as a worthless person?
  D2. Felt that life is entirely hopeless?
  D3. Felt that life isn't worth living?
  D4. Thought of the possibility that you might do away with yourself?
  D5. Found at times you couldn't do anything because your nerves were too bad?
  D6. Found yourself wishing you were dead and away from it all?
  D7. Found that the idea of taking your own life kept coming into your mind?

Adapted from Psychological Medicine. © 1979, Cambridge University Press.

In scoring the Social Dysfunction Rating Scale, the rater assigns a score based on the following six gradations: not present (score 1); very mild (score 2); mild (score 3); moderate (score 4); severe (score 5); and very severe (score 6). This instrument, although not designed to measure degrees of depression, is very useful when assessing the impact of depression on quality of life. The Geriatric Depression Scale (GDS) exists in both short and long forms (Yesavage et al., 1983). The original 30-item form of the GDS has been shown to be an effective screening test for depression in a variety of settings. The short, 15-item version of the GDS was developed primarily for brevity and, in particular, for use in populations such as the medically ill or those with dementia, in which the longer form might be burdensome. How well this short form works in these populations, however, is largely undetermined.

The short version of the GDS, similar to its longer predecessor, is an effective screening tool in the cognitively intact. However, in a population of subjects with mild dementias of the Alzheimer's type (DAT), the short form does not appear to retain its validity.

The Short Form of the Geriatric Depression Scale

1. Are you basically satisfied with your life?
2. Have you dropped many of your activities and interests?
3. Do you feel that your life is empty?
4. Do you often get bored?
5. Are you in good spirits most of the time?
6. Are you afraid that something bad is going to happen to you?
7. Do you feel happy most of the time?
8. Do you often feel helpless?
9. Do you prefer to stay at home, rather than going out and doing new things?
10. Do you feel you have more problems with memory than most?
11. Do you think it is wonderful to be alive?
12. Do you feel pretty worthless the way you are now?
13. Do you feel full of energy?
14. Do you feel that your situation is hopeless?
15. Do you think that most people are better off than you?

From Yesavage J et al: Development and validation of a geriatric depression screening scale: a preliminary report, *J Psychiatr Res* 17(1):37, 1982-1983.

Social Dysfunction Rating Scale

SELF-ESTEEM

1. Low self-concept (feelings of inadequacy, not measuring up to self-ideal)
2. Goallessness (lack of inner motivation and sense of future orientation)
3. Lack of a satisfying philosophy or meaning of life (a conceptual framework for integrating past and present experiences)
4. Self-health concern (preoccupation with physical health, somatic concerns)

INTERPERSONAL SYSTEM

5. Emotional withdrawal (degree of deficiency in relating to others)
6. Hostility (degree of aggression toward others)
7. Manipulation (exploiting of environment, controlling at other's expense)
8. Overdependency (degree of parasitic attachment to others)
9. Anxiety (degree of feeling of uneasiness, impending doom)
10. Suspiciousness (degree of distrust or paranoid ideation)

PERFORMANCE SYSTEM

11. Lack of satisfying relationships with significant persons (spouse, children, kin, significant persons serving in a family role)
12. Lack of friends, social contacts
13. Expressed need for more friends, social contacts
14. Lack of work (remunerative or nonremunerative, productive work activities that normally give a sense of usefulness, status, confidence)
15. Lack of satisfaction from work
16. Lack of leisure time activities
17. Expressed need for more leisure, self-enhancing, and satisfying activities
18. Lack of participation in community activities
19. Lack of interest in community affairs and activities that influence others
20. Financial insecurity
21. Adaptive rigidity (lack of complex coping patterns to stress)

From Linn MW et al: A social dysfunction rating scale, *J Psychiatr Res* 6:300, 1969. © 1969, Pergamon Journals Ltd.

CHAPTER 26

Loss, Death, and Dying in Late Life

Kathleen Jett

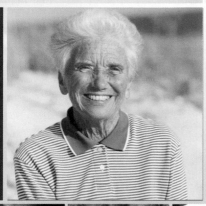
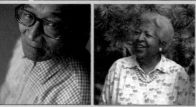
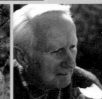
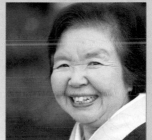

AN ELDER SPEAKS

When we were in our 60s, my friends and I met over cards, went on trips, and experienced all of the joys of retirement. We didn't have much time to worry about aches and pains. In our 70s we had less time to play because we were busy visiting one another in the hospital or in nursing homes. In our 80s we met frequently again, but it was usually at our friends' funerals, leaving little time for cards or travel. Now that I am in my 90s, hardly any of my friends are still alive; you know it gets kind of lonely, so you just have to make new younger friends!

Theresa, age 93

LEARNING OBJECTIVES

On completion of this chapter, the reader will be able to:

1. Differentiate between loss and grief.
2. Explain the different types of grief and the dynamics of the grieving process.
3. Explain the attributes that are required of the nurse to be able to intervene effectively in grief and mourning.
4. List interventions that are helpful to the newly bereaved and those whose grief is established.
5. Discuss the process of dying and the pros and cons of the various theories and frameworks for the dying process.
6. Identify and discuss the needs of the dying and appropriate interventions.
7. Differentiate among the types of advance directives, and explain the role and responsibilities of the nurse as they relate to each of them.
8. Develop an understanding of end-of-life issues.
9. Describe palliative nursing care and the competencies it requires.
10. Suggest the pros and cons of active and passive euthanasia.

LOSS, GRIEF, AND BEREAVEMENT

Loss, dying, and death are universal, incontestable events of the human experience that cannot be stopped or controlled. With age, the number of losses increases (Box 26-1). Some of these are associated with the normal changes with aging, such as the loss of flexibility in the joints, and some are related to the normal changes in everyday life and life transitions, such as moving and retirement. Other losses are those of loved ones through death. Some deaths are considered normative and expected, such as older parents and friends. Other deaths are considered nonnormative and unexpected, such as the death of adult children or grandchildren.

Regardless of the type of loss, each one has the potential to trigger grief and a process we call *bereavement* or *mourning*.

Grief and mourning are commonly used synonymously. However, grief is an individual's response to a loss. Mourning is an active and evolving process (also called the *grieving process* and *bereavement*). Mourning includes those behaviors used to incorporate the loss into one's life. Mourning behaviors are strongly influenced by social and cultural norms that proscribe the appropriate ways of both reacting to the loss and coping with it (Spector, 2003). It is important to realize that there is no single way to grieve or respond to loss. Responses will vary widely among individuals and across cultures.

Although certain behaviors are expected for grief related to loss through death, no guidelines exist for behavior when the loss is of another type (Shield, 1997). For example, an individual who is seriously ill, who moves to a nursing home (loses one's home), or who retires (willingly or unwillingly)

Special thanks to Patricia Hess, the previous edition contributor, for her content contributions to this chapter.

BOX 26-1   Examples of Losses in Late Life

LOSS OF RELATIONSHIPS	LIFE TRANSITIONS
Significant others	Significant roles
Social contacts through:	Financial security
• Illness	Independence
• Death	Physical health
• Distance	Mental stability
• Decreased mobility	Life-death

---

may be very sad, irritable, and forgetful. The person may be suspected of developing dementia when he or she is actually grieving (Hegge and Fischer, 2000). Too often the individual is labeled *depressed* rather than grieving.

Multiple loss experiences through acute and chronic illness may be superimposed on relocation, a shrinking support network, economic changes, or role change. This phenomenon can lead to a continual state of grieving, known as *bereavement overload*. No sooner has the individual begun to grieve for one loss than another occurs, and so forth. When the losses accumulate in quick succession, the griever may become incapacitated and require careful and skilled support and guidance.

The gerontological nurse needs to have basic knowledge of the grieving process and how to comfort and care for grievers, including one another. Additional knowledge and skills are needed of the dying process and care of the dying person and his or her survivors. The purpose of this chapter is to provide the basic information needed to promote effective grieving, peaceful dying, and good and appropriate deaths.

THEORETICAL MODELS FOR UNDERSTANDING GRIEF

Researchers have tried for years to understand the grieving process, resulting in a number of proposed models and theories to explain and predict the experience. The majority of these models evolved between the early 1900s and early 1980s and influence what caregivers and society in general have been taught about grief. Although intended to describe death-related grief, these same models can be applied to any of the losses in the lives of older adults that are considered significant or meaningful.

All early models proposed that grief work or mourning occurred in varying numbers of stages (Bowlby, 1961; Engel, 1967; Worden, 1991). Regardless of the theorist, each proposes that grief has a *beginning* with physical and psychological manifestations, a *middle* (considered the work of grieving or mourning) when the mourner's day-to-day functioning may be affected, and an *end* with the individual emerging refocused having adjusted to whom or what has been lost.

The implication of stages or phases has been that grievers go through grief or mourning in a linear pattern. This view suggests that each stage must be achieved sequentially if one is to grieve well. The individual is expected to progress toward an ending, completion, or resolution of the grief. If this goal is not accomplished, the individual is thought to have grieved poorly or has not adjusted to the loss. Recently, the linear stages or phases of grief have been questioned. Grief work is now seen as a process, more circular than linear, and is not considered as rigidly structured and predictable.

Contemporary studies show grief resolution to be more complex than simply letting go and moving on with life after a loss. Examples of ongoing attachments, which to some have been labeled as unhealthy or problematic, are pilgrimages to the Vietnam War Memorial, the Wailing Wall, and family gravesites. Each year, individuals visit the Vietnam War Memorial in Washington, D.C., to remember and leave items that connect them to those who have died. Similarly, individuals make pilgrimages to the Wailing Wall in Jerusalem, praying and placing prayer papers in the crevices of the wall. In Mexico, there is an annual holiday called "Day of the Dead" at which time people visit the graves of their family members, leave food, grieve anew, and feel a renewed sense of connection with their relatives who have died. These practices may instead be considered healthy and restorative for those who participate.

It is important to remember that theories are attempts to address the grieving process; they are helpful to our understanding of grief. Similarities and differences exist, behavior may be the same or different, and the process of grief has been approached differently by those who have developed models, but they should not be imposed on the survivor. Nurses need to know about grief work to be helpful to the older adult and to understand the dynamics of their own grief.

Loss-Restoration Model

Stroebe and Schut (1999) proposed a dual process model, that of a weaving of loss and restoration. It uses aspects of previous theories but suggests a dynamic and interactive process that goes back and forth (oscillation) between loss-oriented and restoration-oriented bereavement not unlike the cyclical expanding and contracting movement seen in the nursing theory of Martha Rogers. Stroebe and Schut do not focus on outcomes but, rather, on coping with primary and secondary losses and sources of stress. For example, loss-oriented coping involves not only dealing with the loss per se but also coping with ties or bonds to that which has been lost. Loss-oriented coping includes concentrated thinking about life before the loss or with the person and circumstances and events surrounding the death or loss. Restoration-oriented coping includes doing new things, distracting oneself from grief, avoiding or denying grief, assuming new roles, and transcendence. The changes can result in new perspectives in self-actualization. The person in grief alternates between loss-oriented and restoration-oriented coping, which is comparable to confrontation and avoidance

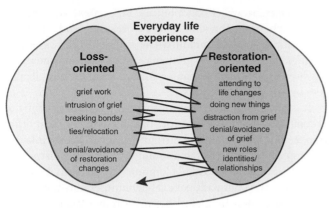

FIGURE 26-1 A dual process model of coping with bereavement. (From Stroebe M, Schut H: The dual process model of coping with bereavement: rationale and description, *Death Stud* 23:197-224, 1999. Reproduced by permission of Taylor & Francis Group, LLC, London, *http://www.taylorandfrancis.com*.)

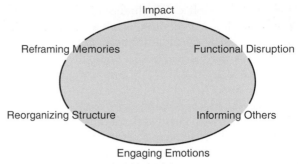

FIGURE 26-2 The loss response model. (From Jett KF: *The loss response model,* Unpublished manuscript, 2004. Adapted from Giacquinta B: Helping families face the crisis of cancer, *Am J Nurs* 77[10]:1585-1588, 1977.)

of the stressors associated with bereavement. The individual will avoid memories and seek relief by focusing on other things. As stated by Stroebe and Schut (1999, p. 216), "sometimes there may simply be no alternative but to attend to additional stressors (e.g., managing household chores or earning a living)."

Oscillation and mental and physical health are necessary for optimal adjustment over time: the person may take *time off*, be distracted, or need to attend to new things. Or confronting some aspect may be too painful at times, and thus it is voluntarily or involuntarily repressed. Over time, repeated exposure and confrontation may lead to the reaction response weakening and the individual no longer thinks about specific aspects of the loss. In other words, over time, the emotional experience of grief will lessen or fewer incidents of the intrusion of grief in one's emotional and physical life will occur. This model has the potential to be applicable to differences in culture, as well as gender differences, and emphasizes coping with bereavement rather than outcomes (Figure 26-1).

A Loss Response Model

Nurse Barbara Giacquinta proposed a model of families facing the crisis of cancer (1977). Through modification and incorporation of a systems approach, the Loss Response Model (Jett, 2004) lends itself to an understandable and usable model of the grieving process from which nursing interventions are easily developed. In the Loss Response Model, the family and the person are viewed as a system that strives to maintain equilibrium.

When loss occurs within the system, the *impact* is experienced as acute grief. The system's equilibrium is in chaos and is seen as a *functional disruption*; that is, the system cannot perform its usual activities; either the person or the members are in a state of disequilibrium. The loss seems unreal. The family or individual then *searches for meaning*: why did this happen to them? How will they survive the loss? If an elder is responding to the loss of a child or a grandchild, thoughts

of "why wasn't it me?" are common. The family then may become active in *informing others*. Each time the story is repeated, the loss becomes more real and the system moves toward a new steady state. Informing others involves *engaging emotions* that may have been previously withheld or subdued because of the shock of the impact. The expression of emotions can release energy that can be used to *reorganize* the family *structure*. As roles change, adaptation and accommodation are necessary. Someone else steps in to perform the roles of the person who is now absent or to complete the tasks no longer possible in the presence of the loss. For example, when the elder patriarch dies, the eldest son may step up and assume some of his father's roles and responsibilities. Finally, if the system is to survive, it will need to redefine itself. One of the ways that it does this is by *reframing its memories*; that is, families accept that portraits and reunions are still possible, just different from how they were before the loss, or they accept that a person can still be vital, active, and important even after the loss of the ability to drive a car, to walk unassisted, or to live alone (Figure 26-2).

GRIEF WORK

Grieving takes enormous amounts of physical and emotional energy. It is the hardest thing anyone can do and may be especially hard for older adults. The potential intensity of emotions may appear as confusion, depression, or preoccupation with thoughts of the deceased or loss; these emotions may be mistaken for another condition such as dementia, when it probably is a type of delirium, something that requires care. The gerontological nurse will probably work with elders who are experiencing anticipatory grief, acute grief, or chronic grief. A fourth type, disenfranchised grief, may be occurring and hidden but nonetheless significant.

Anticipatory Grief

Anticipatory grief is the response to a real or perceived loss before it occurs—a dress rehearsal, so to speak. One observes this grief in preparation for potential loss, such as loss of belongings (e.g., selling a home), moving (e.g., into a nursing home), or knowing that a body part or function is going to change (e.g., a mastectomy), or in anticipation of the loss of a spouse or oneself either through a progressive illness such as dementia or Parkinson's disease or through death. Behaviors that may signal anticipatory grief include preoccupation with the particular loss, unusually detailed planning, or a sudden change in attitude toward the thing or person to be lost.

The grieving process described by the models just mentioned will occur, with one significant difference: the loss has not yet occurred. If the loss is certain but no one can say when it will occur or if it does not occur when or as expected, those awaiting the actual loss or death may become irritable, hostile, or impatient, not because they want the loss to occur but in response to the emotional ups and downs of the waiting. Glaser and Strauss (1968) describe what they call an *interruption in the sentimental order of a nursing unit* when this occurs—no one quite knows how to behave. Professional grievers, such as nurses, as well as family and friends, usually deal much more easily with known losses at a known time or in a set manner (Glaser and Strauss, 1968). Some individuals feel more in control of the situation because anticipatory grief facilitates planning and preparation for death by saying goodbyes in special ways (Zilberfein, 1999).

Very similar to the Loss Response Model (Jett, 2004), Futterman and colleagues (1970) conceptualized anticipatory grief as having five functionally related aspects: (1) acknowledgment—convinced the inevitable will occur; (2) grieving—experiencing and expressing the emotional impact of the anticipated loss and the physical, psychological, and interpersonal turmoil associated with it; (3) reconciliation of the situation; (4) detachment—withdrawal of the emotional investment from the situation; and (5) memorialization—developing a relatively fixed conscious mental representation of that which will be lost. One frequently sees the struggle of anticipatory grief in families with elders who have been diagnosed with Alzheimer's disease.

Anticipatory grief can result in the phenomenon of premature detachment from an individual who is dying or detachment of the dying person from the environment. Pattison (1977) called the premature withdrawal of others *sociological death* and the premature withdrawal of the person *psychological death*. In either case, the person who is dying is no longer involved in day-to-day activities of living and essentially suffers a premature death.

Acute grief after anticipatory grief has not been found to be less painful but may help the griever develop some coping skills (Parks and Weiss, 1983). In contrast, Dessonville and colleagues (1983) found that anticipatory grief not only did not lessen the eventual acute grief but also in some cases may actually be associated with a poorer adjustment. Anticipatory grief, then, can be helpful or harmful to the griever but is recognized as a legitimate phenomenon.

Acute Grief

Acute grief is a crisis. It has a definite syndrome of somatic and psychological symptoms of distress that occur in waves lasting varying periods of time. These symptoms may occur every time the loss is acknowledged, others are informed, or another person offers condolences. Preoccupation with the loss is a phenomenon similar to daydreaming and is accompanied by a sense of unreality. Depending on the situation, feelings of self-blame or guilt may be present and manifest themselves as hostility or anger toward usual friends, depressive signs, or withdrawal.

It is often difficult for persons who are acutely grieving to accomplish their usual activities of daily living or meet other responsibilities (functional disruption). Even if the tasks are accomplished, the person may complain of feeling distracted, restless, and "at loose ends." Common, simple activities such as dressing that normally take a few minutes may take much longer; deciding which clothing to wear may seem too complex a task. Fortunately the signs and symptoms of acute grief do not last forever or none of us could survive. Acute grief will be the most intense in the months immediately after the loss, with the intensity of feelings lessening over time. Acute grief was experienced at a national level in the United States after the attack and collapse of the World Trade Centers in New York City in 2001 (Neimeyer et al., 2004).

Disenfranchised Grief

The person whose loss cannot be openly acknowledged or publicly mourned experiences what is called disenfranchised grief. The grief is socially disallowed or unsupported (Doka, 1989). The person does not have a socially recognized right to be perceived or function as a bereaved person. In other words, a relationship is not recognized; the loss is not sanctioned; or the griever is not recognized. Disenfranchised grief has frequently been associated with domestic partnerships in which the family of the deceased does not acknowledge the partner of the dead person or in secret relationships in which the involved party cannot tell others of the meaning or depth of the attachment. Disenfranchised grief can also occur in situations of family discord in which a member of the family is considered the "black sheep." The person in late life can experience this disenfranchisement when family or friends do not understand the full meaning, for example, of a retiree's retirement, the death of a pet, or gradual losses caused by chronic conditions. Families coping with a member who has Alzheimer's disease may also experience disenfranchised grief, particularly when others perceive death of the elder as a blessing and fail to support the griever or caregiver who has struggled for years with anticipatory grief and now must cope with the actual death.

Chronic Grief

Grief work or mourning takes time, sometimes much longer than anyone anticipates. Lund and colleagues (1986) and Arbuckle and de Vries (1995) found that it may take older widows and widowers much longer to reach the same level of adjustment than younger spouses. Horacek (1991) referred to this lingering grief as *shadow grief*. It may temporarily inhibit some activity but is considered a normal response. The intermittent pain of grief is often exacerbated on anniversary dates (birthdays, holidays, wedding anniversaries).

For the survivors of tragedies, such as war, the Oklahoma City bombing, and the 9/11 attack, the "shadows" may never completely go away.

However, some chronic grief is more than that of shadow grief and crosses over the boundary to what we call *impaired*, *pathological*, *abnormal*, *dysfunctional*, or *maladaptive grief*. It has been thought that pathological chronic grief begins with normal grief responses but obstacles interfere with its normal evolution toward adjustment, toward the reestablishment of equilibrium. The memories resist being reframed. Issues of guilt, anger, and ambivalence toward the individual who has died are factors that will impede the grieving process until these issues are resolved. Reactions are exaggerated, and memories are experienced as recurrent acute grief—repeatedly, months and years later. Signs of possible pathological grief include excessive and irrational anger, outbursts in social settings, and insomnia that lingers for an extended time or surfaces months or years later, or a grief episode may trigger a major depressive episode. This type of grief requires the professional intervention of a grief counselor, a psychiatric nurse practitioner, or a psychologist who is skilled in helping grieving elders. Guidelines for supporting the bereaved older adult are found in Box 26-2.

Factors Affecting Coping with Loss

Coping as it relates to loss and grief is the ability of the individual or family to find ways to deal with the stress. In the language of the Loss Response Model (Jett, 2004), it is the ability to move from a state of chaos and disequilibrium to one of reorder, equilibrium, and peace. Many factors affect the ability to cope with loss and grief (Box 26-3).

Those at special risk for significantly adverse effects of grief are spouses and life partners. Studies have consistently found that widowed persons have an usually high mortality rate after bereavement. The risky times have been found from the week after the death to up to 2 years; however, most

---

BOX 26-2 Guidelines for Supporting the Bereaved Person

- Permit and help the person put into words and nonverbal expression the pain, sorrow, and finality of bereavement.
- Review the relationship of the person with the deceased (i.e., a life history approach).
- Encourage the patient to discuss feelings of love, guilt, and hostility toward the deceased.
- Help the person recognize the alterations in cognition, affect, and behavior secondary to bereavement.
- Work with the patient to find an acceptable balance for the future incorporated memory of the deceased.
- Avoid interpretations of long-dormant, highly charged intrapsychic conflicts.
- Support existing coping mechanisms.
- Reassure the patient that the intense suffering and pain are transient.
- Facilitate the transfer of dependency from the deceased to other sources of gratification when necessary.
- Decrease sessions with the patient upon improvement, but avoid abrupt termination.
- Refer to grief counseling specialists as needed.

BOX 26-3 Factors Influencing the Grieving Process

PHYSICAL

Illness involves numerous losses.

Sedatives deprive experience of reality of loss that must be faced.

Nutritional state, if inadequate, leads to the inability to cope or meet demands of daily living and numerous symptoms that grief can cause.

Inadequate rest leads to mental and physical exhaustion, disease, and unresolved grief.

Exercise, if inadequate, limits emotional outlet; increases aggressive feelings, tension, and anxiety; and leads to depression.

PSYCHOLOGICAL

Unique nature and meaning of loss

Individual qualities of the relationship

Role body part, self-image, aspect of self was to the individual, family, or both

Individual coping behavior, personality, and mental health

Individual level of maturity and intelligence

Previous experience with loss or death

Social, cultural, ethnic, religious, or philosophic background

Sex-role conditioning

Immediate circumstances surrounding loss

Timeliness of the loss

Perception of preventability (sudden vs. expected)

Number, type, and quality of secondary losses

Presence of concurrent stresses or crises

SOCIAL

Individual support systems and the acceptance of assistance of its members

Individual sociocultural, ethnic, religious, or philosophic background

Educational, economic, and occupational status

Ritual

SPECIFIC TO DYING AND DEATH (IN ADDITION TO THE ABOVE)

Role that the deceased occupied in family or social system

Amount of unfinished business

Perception of deceased's fulfillment in life

Immediate circumstances surrounding death

Length of illness before death

Anticipatory grief and involvement with dying patient

From Beare PG, Myers JL: *Adult health nursing*, ed 3, St Louis, 1998, Mosby.

emphasize the 6- to 12-month–period after death (Erlangsen et al., 2004; Kaprio et al., 1987; Manor and Eisenbach, 2003; Schaefer et al., 1995).

Unfortunately, this increased risk for death includes the risk for suicide, especially among widowed men (Kaprio et al., 1987) . Mittleman (1996) found that heart attack risk was five times higher than normal 2 days after the death of a significant person and remained elevated for approximately 1 month after the death. Pietruszka (1992) noted that bereaved elders may present clinical symptoms that mimic the signs and symptoms of serious medical and psychological conditions of the deceased person, which presents a diagnostic challenge to primary care providers.

A risk factor profile for bereaved spouses was developed by Steele (1992) to identify individuals whose behaviors are suggestive of risk for physical or emotional disturbances. For example, a 70-year-old, middle-class widow exhibiting despair or pessimism, loss of vigor, depersonalization, physical and somatic symptoms, anger, and social isolation may be at risk.

Those who are more likely to effectively deal with loss Weisman calls the "good copers" (1979, p. 42). These are individuals or families who have experience with the successful management of crisis. They are resourceful, and they are able to draw on techniques that have worked in the past. Weisman (1979, pp. 42-43; 1984) found persons who cope effectively with cancer are those who do the following:

- Avoid avoidance
- Confront realities, and take appropriate action
- Focus on solutions
- Redefine problems
- Consider alternatives
- Have good communication with loved ones
- Seek and use constructive help
- Accept support when offered
- Can keep up their morale

In other words, the persons who will cope with loss most effectively are those who can acknowledge the loss and try to make sense of it. They can maintain composure, use generally good judgment, and can remain optimistic without denying the loss. These good copers seek guidance when they need it.

On the contrary, those who cope less effectively have few if any of these abilities. They tend to be more rigid and pessimistic, appear demanding, and experience emotional extremes. They are more likely to be dogmatic and expect perfection from themselves and others. Ineffective copers are also more likely to live alone, socialize little, and have few close friends or have an ineffective support network. They may have a history of mental illness, or they may have guilt, anger, and ambivalence toward the individual who has died or that which has been lost. Those at risk for pathological grief will more likely have unresolved past conflicts or be facing the loss at the same time as other secondary stressors. They will have fewer opportunities as a result of the loss. They are the elders who are most in need of the expert interventions of grief counselors and skilled gerontological nurses.

Grief and Gender Differences

Three of four women will be widowed at some time in their lives. Women live longer and frequently marry older men. Theories suggest that widowhood is less difficult for women than retirement is for men because other widows are available with whom to share leisure time and activities. In many instances, a woman's status increases with widowhood whereas a man's decreases with retirement (DeSpelder and Strickland, 1996). The abundance of literature on bereavement focuses on women. This emphasis has lead to the use of the feminine model of grief, which most health professionals use with both men and women, not realizing that perhaps differences in the grief response do exist. Loss and mourning models shed little light on how men bereave, particularly for spousal loss in which males are the survivors. The assumption is that men are less emotionally involved in the conjugal relationship than women and therefore are less likely to grieve or express their grief. This assumption was found not to be true (Brabant et al., 1992; Martin and Doka, 1996, 1998). Evidence shows that men hurt and knew they hurt but did not reach out to others for help.

Hopmeyer and Werk (1994) found that women placed *sharing feelings and emotions* first in coping with grief. Men, however, were reluctant to share or seek help. Most men wanted to learn how others solved problems that were similar to their own at first, wanted to be self-reliant next, and then immersed themselves in work. The identification of the feminine and masculine grief response does not mean that every man and every woman follows the pattern ascribed to him or her. What has been derived from these responses is that men and women often mix these gender-specific responses or reverse them, with women responding as men do, and vise versa. Gender and grief work remains an area for further research.

Grief as a Growth Opportunity

Survivor coping ability improves when the person is aware that death and bereavement can lead to growth. Changes in thinking from limits to potential, from coping to growth, and from problems to challenges are perceptual mindsets that help move one toward growth. Resolving loss and working through the grief process provide incentives, enabling possible important life changes. Transformation from intense focus on self-awareness evolves into a new sense of identity. The loss is placed within the context of growth and life cycles—the lost relationship is changed, not ended. By turning to the inner resources, creativity can arise from the experience of grief.

▲ Promoting Healthy Aging: Implications for Gerontological Nursing

Loss, grief, and death are parts of the lives of all and occur with increasing frequency as one ages. The goal of the gerontological nurse is not to prevent grief but to support those who are grieving. Although the acute emotions associated with loss will go away, the potential long-term detrimental effects can be ameliorated. While promoting healthy aging, the nurse works with grieving elders as part of the normal workday and this is a special privilege. It is one of the few areas in nursing in which small actions can make a large difference in the quality of life for the persons to whom we provide care.

Assessment.   The goal of the grief assessment is to differentiate those who are likely to cope effectively from those who are at risk for ineffective coping so that appropriate interventions can be planned. A grief assessment is based on knowledge of the grieving process. Data are obtained through observation of behavior of the individual, keeping gender and cultural context in mind (Goldstein et al., 2004). Behaviors may range from the stoic response of a person from a German or English heritage to the highly vocal expressions typical of persons from some Hispanic groups (Lipson et al., 1996).

A thorough grief assessment includes questions about recent significant life events, life or religious values, and relationship to that which has been lost and that which has been "gained." How many other stressful or demanding events or circumstances are going on in the griever's life? Information about these concurrent life stresses will help determine who may be at more risk for impaired grieving. The more concurrent stressors the person is dealing with, the more he or she will need the nurse or grief specialists. What stress management techniques are normally used, and are they potentially helpful (e.g., talking) or potentially harmful (e.g., substance use or abuse)? What are the individual's usual coping strategies and support systems? Was the griever's identity closely tied to that which is lost, such as a lifelong athlete who is faced with never walking again? If the loss is of a partner, how was the relationship? The loss of an abusive or controlling partner may liberate the survivor, who may feel guilty for not feeling the amount of grief that is expected. For many older women who depended on their spouses financially, death may leave them impoverished, significantly complicating their grief. A survivor may be suddenly homeless after the loss of a domestic partner in jurisdictions in which such relationships are unrecognized. Knowing more about the loss and the effect of the loss on the elder's life will enable the nurse to construct and implement appropriate and caring responses.

Interventions.   One of the goals of intervention is to help the individual (or family) attain a healthy adjustment to the loss experience. Actions that can meet this goal are basic and simple; however, the emotional overlay of providers may make the simple difficult. The nurse who is confronted with a person's grief for the first time may feel intense discomfort, fear, and insecurity. The tendency is to be sympathetic rather than empathetic. Confronting one's own mortality complicates the interactions. Questions arise in one's mind: What do I say? Should I be cheerful or serious? Should I talk about or even mention the dead person's name? What if this should happen to me or to someone I love?

Nurses commonly provide crisis intervention with the newly bereaved, largely because the majority of deaths occur

---

BOX 26-4   Nursing Actions Families Have Reported Helpful
• Kept me informed
• Asked how I was doing and offered support
• Put an arm around me when I cried
• Brought me food
• Knew my name
• Cried with me
• Brought a bed and encouraged me to stay in the room with my dying husband
• Told me to hold my husband's hand while he was dying
• Held my hand
• Got the chaplain for me
• Let me take care of my husband
• Stayed with me after their shift was over

From Richter J: Support: a resource during crisis of mate loss, *J Gerontol Nurs* 13(11):18-22, 1987. Reprinted with permission from Slack, Inc., Thorofare, NJ.

in the institutional setting and most of these deaths are of older adults. Up to 20% of all deaths in the United States occur in nursing homes (Weitzen et al., 2003). A study from the late 1980s has served as a guide for nurses' responses to families who are experiencing the loss of a loved one (Richter, 1987) (Box 26-4). These actions may assist nurses in gaining a clearer perspective of comfort interventions.

Nursing interventions, especially when elders are in crisis, begin with gently establishing rapport. Nurses introduce themselves and explain their roles (e.g., charge nurse, staff nurse, medication nurse) and the time they will be available to the elder or survivor. If it is the time of impact (e.g., just after a new serious diagnosis, at the death of a family member, or as a new but resistant resident of a long-term care facility), the most nurses can do is to provide support and a safe environment and ensure that basic needs, such as meals, are met. The nurse must also be ready to listen. Active listening is an important skill for the nurse who serves as a support person for the griever. Giving advice on how to solve a problem is far easier than allowing a grieving person time and space to express feelings. The nurse can soften the despair by fostering reasonable hope, such as, "You will survive this time, one moment at a time, and I will be here to help."

Nurses observe for *functional disruption* and offer support and direction. They may have to help the family figure out what needs to be done immediately and find ways to do it—the nurse either offers to complete the task or finds a friend or family member who can step in so the disruption does not have any deleterious effects.

As grievers *search for meaning,* they may need help finding what they are looking for and spend time *talking it out.* Sometimes what they are looking for is information about a disease, a situation, or a person, and the nurse can assist in obtaining the information whenever possible. Talking it out requires active listening when grievers are trying to make sense of the loss and find meaning in it, questioning their values, and constructing new ones to account for the change in their reality. The expressions of grief and feelings and sharing them with others and the momentary panics, hysteria, and other sensations accompanying the grief are less frightening when heard by a caring person who can validate their appropriateness.

At other times, the nurse can help the persons "feel it out." *Feeling it out* is a cathartic experience. In many instances, the nurse allows the griever to express hurt, anger, crying, and so forth. The nurse may have to say, "It's okay to [have whatever feelings the griever has]." Sometimes it is a spiritual search and help in finding a resource or a place of peace, such as the chapel. Often, needed most is someone to listen to the "whys" and "hows"—which cannot always be answered.

Sometime nurses offer to *inform others* for the grievers, thinking that this is something that will help. Because it usually is therapeutic for grievers to talk to others about the losses, nurses should refrain from helping in this way. Instead, the nurse can offer to find a phone number or hold the griever's hand during the conversation or just "be there" when the news is being shared. In this way the nurse can be available to provide support when the griever's emotions engage.

As the elder moves forward in adjusting to the loss, such as a move from home to a nursing home, the nurse can help the person *reorganize* this new life. The nurse talks with the elder about what was most valued about living at home and what habits were comforting and finds ways to incorporate these in a new way to the new environment. If the elder does not have access to a kitchen and always had a cup of tea before bed, this can become part of the individualized plan of care.

For the cycle of grieving to be completed, at least according to the Loss Reaction Model, *new memories* are needed. The grandmother who had always hosted her eldest daughter's birthday party can still do that even if she is now a resident in a long-term care facility. When the nurse has the information about this important ritual, he or she can help the person reserve a private space, send out invitations, and have the birthday party as always but now reframed as it is catered by the facility in the elder's new "home."

Often reminiscence is helpful in creating new memories. Listening to the same thing, endlessly repeated, is difficult for the nurse and others. However, reminiscing is important to the griever. Reminiscing helps work through the loss. Reminiscence is a means by which denial can fall by the wayside and allow reality of the loss to filter slowly into the conscious mind. Reminiscence helps the griever acknowledge that the loss is indeed real and that life can go on, even though the future will be difficult and experienced in a different way.

Kelly (1992) talks about re-forming one's life story. By incorporating the loss and putting the deceased into the life story in a new way (re-forming the story), energy can be invested in all other relationships that exist or may come to be. Drawing out anecdotes and vignettes of the relationship helps the griever keep control over the story of his or her life and reframe it into a new, updated memory. Encourage

TABLE 26-1
Caring Behaviors

Behavior	Caring Action
Advocacy	Extend oneself to find proper help
	Work to grant reasonable requests
Authenticity	Sharing feelings appropriately
	Honesty
	Use of healing touch
Responsiveness	Be available
	Interact verbally
	Provide comfort
	Provide privacy
	Be nonjudgmental
Commitment and presence	Provide the little extras
	Grooming
	Quiet for talking
	Time
	Presence
Competence	Perform tasks consistently
	Radiate self-assurance in care giving
	Teach simply and completely
Give positive meaning to another's life	Listen
	Touch*
	Point out reactions to family
	Praise when appropriate
	Help them gain a sense of control

From Krohn B: When death is near: helping families cope, *Geriatr Nurs* 19(5):276-278, 1998.
*The appropriateness of the use of touch varies greatly by culture (see Chapter 21).

the griever to talk and tell the story of the relationship as it had been. Keeping the continuity of the presence of the deceased alive permits the griever to feel the influence of the dead in life.

The nurse's role is also as an advocate who displays the behavioral qualities of responsiveness, authenticity, commitment, and competence (Krohn, 1998). Table 26-1 correlates caring behaviors with caring actions or interventions by the nurse.

Countercoping. Avery Weisman (1979) described the work of health care professionals related to grief as "countercoping." Although he was speaking of working with people with cancer, it is equally applicable to working with people who are grieving. "Countercoping is like counterpoint in music, which blends melodies together into a basic harmony. The patient copes; the therapist [nurse] countercopes; together they work out a better fit" (Weisman, 1979, p. 109). Weisman suggests four specific types of interventions or countercoping strategies: (1) clarification and control, (2) collaboration, (3) directed relief, and (4) cooling off.

Clarification and Control. The nurse helps elders cope with dying by helping them confront the loss by getting or receiving information, considering alternatives, and finding a way to make the grief manageable. The nurse helps per-

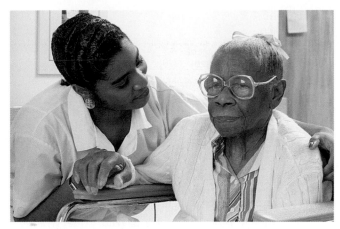

Use touch to calm the person (From Sorrentino SA, Gorek B: *Mosby's textbook for long-term care assistants,* ed 5, St Louis, 2007, Mosby.)

sons resume control by encouraging them to avoid acting on impulse.

Collaboration. The nurse collaborates by encouraging the griever to share stories with others and repeat the stories as often as is necessary as he or she "talks it out." The nurse as a collaborator is more directive than usual; it may be acceptable to say, "No, this is not a good time to make any major decisions."

Directed Relief. Some temporary directed relief may be necessary, especially during acute grief. Catharsis may be helpful. In many instances, the nurse encourages the griever to cry or otherwise express feelings such as hurt or anger. The nurse may have to say something like, "Expressing your feelings is important." Activity may also be recommended as a natural extension of feelings. Intense physical activity gives one some control over emotions. In some cultures, people may tear their clothes or cut their hair. There are numerous ways of acting out feelings—from throwing things, to taking a walk, to busying oneself with tasks, to expressing feelings through creative works.

Cooling Off. From time to time the griever might be encouraged to temporarily avoid processing the grief through diversions that worked in the past during times of stress, especially when things need to be done or decisions need to be made. The nurse may need to suggest new tactics that may prove helpful. Cooling off also means encouraging the person to modulate emotional extremes and to think about ways to make sense of the loss, to build a new sense of self-esteem after the loss and to reestablish life patterns.

In all interventions related to grief, the nurse must be skilled in therapeutic communication. Active listening is greatly preferable to giving advice. When listening, the nurse soon discovers that it is not the actual loss that is of utmost concern but, rather, the fear associated with the loss. If the nurse listens carefully to both the stated and the implied, expressions such as the following may be heard: "How will I go on?" "What will I do now?" "What will become of me?" "I don't know what to do." "How could he (she) do this to me?" Because the nurse knows there is resolution, such comments may seem exaggerated or melodramatic, but to the one who is grieving, there seems to be no end to the pain. The person who is actively grieving cannot yet look ahead and know that the despair and other feelings will resolve. Like good copers, good gerontological nurses must be flexible, practical, resourceful, and abundantly optimistic.

DYING AND DEATH

A major question arises when considering dying and death in late life. When is a person with multiple chronic or repeated acute or progressive health problems considered to be "dying"? Although sometimes confused with the onset of acute, treatable health problems, the consensus is that physical deterioration is the prime indicator of dying. However, other, more subtle cues may be present. An approaching death is also suspected when coded communication is used by the individual, such as saying good-bye instead of the usual good night, giving away cherished possessions as gifts, urgently contacting friends and relatives with whom the person has not communicated for a long time, and direct or symbolic premonitions that death is near. Anxiety, depression, restlessness, and agitation are behaviors that are frequently categorized as manifestations of confusion or dementia but, in reality, may be responses to the inability to express feelings of foreboding and a sense of life escaping one's grasp.

Many people have said that death is not the problem; it is the dying that takes the work. This is true for all involved: the person, the loved ones, the professional caregivers such as the nurses, and, especially in long-term care facilities, the nursing assistants.

Before the 1900s, most women and men died at home. Women died during childbirth, and men died of unknown causes. During times of war, most men died in battle or from battle-associated injuries. Now most women live well after menopause, and both men and women die most often from heart disease. Life expectancy went from about 49 years in the late 1800s to 74 years for men and 79 years for women by the end of the 1900s with variation by race and ethnicity (Federal Interagency Forum on Aging-Related Statistics, 2002). Today, persons usually die in acute and long-term care settings.

Dying is both a challenging life experience and a private one. How one deals with dying is often a reflection of the way the person has handled earlier losses and stressors. Most people probably die as they have lived. Although not all older adults have had fulfilling lives or have a sense of completion, transcendence, or self-actualization, their deaths at the age or after that of their parents are considered normative. If the dying process is particularly long or the death occurs after a painful illness, we may rationalize it or view it as relief, at least in part. Death at a younger age or as the result of trauma or catastrophe is viewed as tragic and sometimes incomprehensible. After 9/11 no one rationalized the

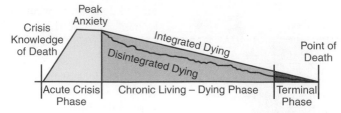

FIGURE 26-3 The living-dying interval. (From Pattison EM: *The experience of dying,* Englewood Cliffs, NJ, 1977, Prentice-Hall.)

deaths of the older victims as a relief; all deaths were considered an unacceptable loss of human potential.

Conceptual Model for Understanding the Dying Process

As models have been proposed to explain the grieving process, so have they been proposed for the process of dying. One of the most well-known has been that of Elisabeth Kübler-Ross, MD. In her book *On Death and Dying* (1969), she reported on observations of predominately middle-aged in-patients on the psychiatric ward where she did her psychiatry residency. She proposed the stages of dying as denial, anger, bargaining, depression, and acceptance. Nurses and many others have tried to help the dying work through denial to achieve acceptance before their deaths. However, we have come to realize that the "stages" are actually types of emotional reactions to dying that people experience and not a step-wise model at all. A discussion of a useful alternative model follows.

The Living-Dying Interval

Whereas physically we may begin dying early in life as proposed by the theories of aging (see Chapter 2), in personal terms, dying begins at a moment called the "crisis knowledge of death" (Pattison, 1977, p. 44) and ends at the moment of physiological death. Pattison (1977) calls the time between these two points the *living-dying interval*, made up of the acute, chronic, and terminal phases. The chronological time of the living-dying interval is accordion-like because of remissions and exacerbations in the terminal diagnosis; it may last days, weeks, months, or years. The manner in which one faces dying is an expression of personality, circumstances, illness, and culture.

The *crisis knowledge of death* occurs when someone receives the information that he or she will not live as long as previously anticipated. Certainly it would appear that the more the discrepancy between the previously believed length of life and the newly projected length of life, the more the adjustment and perhaps the intensity of the grief experienced.

The point of crisis is a moment in time that is followed by an *acute phase*. It is usually the peak time of stress and anxiety as the life and future of the individual and the family are thrown into disequilibrium. Crisis intervention is most effective here because the individual, family, and caregivers are struggling to come to terms with the knowledge. A significant amount of anticipatory grieving may be observed.

Because no one can live with a crisis indefinitely, most of the dying time is spent in the *chronic phase*. During this time, the dying and those about them are forced to resume some sense of normalcy. Bills still need to be paid, dishes still need to be washed, and life can still be lived. The challenge for persons with terminal diagnoses and their families is to work toward living while dying and not dying while dying. Entertainment, work, and relationships can be maintained as normally as the individual's condition permits. Life goes on despite the anticipation of its end.

The *terminal phase* is reached when the speed of the physical dying is accelerated and the dying person no longer has the energy to maintain the activities of everyday life. The terminal phase is ushered in by withdrawal or turning away from the outside world in response to internal body signals that tell the dying person to conserve energy. The focus then turns to preserving energy and completing life's journey. In some cultures this period is called the "death watch" and is associated with proscribed rituals. It is especially important for the nurse to understand and respect the cultural expectations of his or her patients at this time (Goldstein et al., 2004).

The living-dying interval can reflect an integrated or disintegrated experience (Pattison, 1977). The interval is integrated when each new crisis occurs, is dealt with effectively, and the quality of life while dying is preserved. The interval is disintegrated if one crisis tumbles onto the next one without any effective resolution; the quality of life while dying is compromised (Figure 26-3). Martocchio (1982) describes living-dying patterns as peaks and valleys, descending (stepwise) plateaus, and progressive downward slopes. The patterns may be singular or in combination and may or may not be related to the pathological parameters of the disease.

Theories suggest that any approach to coping with dying should consider a basic understanding of all dimensions and all the individuals involved and tasks associated with each phase of living-dying (Table 26-2). The approach should foster empowerment by emphasizing the options available while the person lives on, emphasizing participation or shared aspects of coping with dying (interpersonal network), and providing guidance for care providers and helpers.

The Family

Older adults of today are usually members of a multigenerational family. Although members may be geographically separated, some degree of filial tie exists. When an elder becomes seriously or terminally ill and cannot uphold his or

TABLE 26-2

Tasks Associated with Phases Along the Living-Dying Interval

General	Acute Phase	Chronic Phase	Terminal Phase
1. Responding to the physical fact of disease 2. Taking steps to cope with the reality of disease 3. Preserving self-concept and relationships with others in the face of disease 4. Dealing with effective and existential or spiritual issues created or reactivated by the disease	1. Understanding the disease 2. Maximizing health and lifestyle 3. Maximizing one's coping strengths and limiting weaknesses 4. Developing strategies to deal with the issues that the disease creates 5. Exploring the effect of the diagnosis on a sense of self and others 6. Ventilating feelings and fears 7. Incorporating the present reality of diagnosis into one's sense of past and future	1. Managing symptoms and side effects 2. Carrying out health regimens 3. Preventing and managing health crisis 4. Managing stress and examining coping 5. Maximizing social support and minimizing isolation 6. Normalizing life in the face of the disease 7. Dealing with financial concerns 8. Preserving self-concept 9. Redefining relationships with others throughout the course of the disease 10. Ventilating feelings and fears 11. Finding meaning in suffering chronicity, uncertainty, and decline	1. Dealing with symptoms, discomfort, pain, and incapacitation 2. Managing health procedures and institutional stress 3. Managing stress and examining coping 4. Dealing effectively with caregivers 5. Preparing for death and saying goodbye 6. Preserving self-concept 7. Preserving appropriate relationships with family and friends 8. Ventilating feelings and fears 9. Finding meaning in life and death

From Coolican MB et al: Education about death, dying, and bereavement in nursing programs, *Nurse Educ* 19(6):35-40, 1994.

her role or obligation, the family balance or dynamics are significantly altered. Even the elderly person who is single and relies on friends and neighbors finds a change in the relationships. Depending on the role the individual has in the family/friend constellation, problems often begin at the time of diagnosis or shortly thereafter. Roles and traits of the person who is now considered to be dying may create adjustment difficulties in the soon-to-be survivors, whether they are partners, spouse, adult children, or grandchildren. Adult children often begin to see their own mortality through the death of their parent with the re-forming and reframing of a new family order.

The idea that family members can remain involved with the dying person can be a constant struggle as they try to withdraw and try to readjust their lives without the dying member. This change requires enormous energy by family members who are already burdened with their own anticipatory grief, daily living, and, in many cases, raising their own children and possibly grandchildren. The conflict is grieving not only for the dying but also for a part of themselves that will be lost with the death of the parent or significant family member. A number of adaptive tasks may facilitate healthy resolution of the loss of a family member.

At times, family members have to separate their own identities from that of the patient and learn to tolerate the reality that the family member will die while they live on. The ability of the family members to truly support, love, and provide intimacy may lead to exhaustion, impatience, anger, and a sense of futility if the patient's dying is prolonged. Family members may be at different points in grief than the patient is, which can hinder communication between the patient and family members. As the illness worsens, physical disability increases and the patient's needs intensify family members' feelings of helplessness, and frustration.

Experiencing the effects of grief requires acknowledging current feelings that surface as anticipatory grief. Coming to terms with the reality of the impending loss means that family members must go through many emotional responses in achieving acceptance of the loved one's approaching death. Because people are "supposed to" die in old age according to social norms, the grief responses may not be exceptionally intense; on the other hand, many filial relationships that seem superficial can result in very deep and acute grief responses.

Family members may feel extremely pressured during the final days of a relative's life and need the support of the nurse. These individuals may be caught between experiencing the present and remembering the patient as he or she was, between pushing for more interventions or letting life take its course, and occasionally wanting to retreat because of a discordant relationship with the patient. Families frequently feel guilt-ridden if they believe they are thinking more about their needs than those of the dying patient.

Despite the family's grief and pain, the family must give the patient permission to die; let the patient know that it is all right to let go and leave. This gesture is the last act of love and dignity that the family can offer the dying patient. Occasionally, no family is available to say, "It's okay to let go." The task then falls to the nurse who has developed a meaningful relationship with the patient through care.

Religiosity and Death Anxiety

One of the most common ways researchers have used to attempt to understand the relationship between religiosity and death or dying is to consider the concept of death anxiety. The pioneer of this body of knowledge was Herman Feifel, who began his considerable volume of work in the late 1950s. He was probably the first person to study the attitudes toward death held by older adults (Neimeyer et al., 2004). For a long time there was a belief that persons who were more religious were able to accept death more easily. Later researchers found an increase in anxiety among elders with complex medical problems and less life satisfaction but again, weaker religious beliefs (Fortner and Neimeyer, 1999). Closer examination, however, found considerable variation by individual and by ethnicity.

As research became more sophisticated, the idea of religiosity was dissected. Extrinsic religiosity or that which reflects a "utilitarian view of religion" was associated with increased anxiety (Neimeyer et al., 2004, p. 324). On the other hand, those with lowered anxiety specifically had what was called *intrinsic religiosity*, or a deeper sense of faith and connection with a higher power. Others have found conflicting levels of anxiety related to beliefs in an afterlife. Although positive anticipation was associated with lower levels of anxiety and despair (McClain-Jacobson, et al., 2004), some who were only moderately religious had more anxiety related to fears of punishment in the afterlife (Neimeyer et al., 2004).

▲ Promoting a Good Death: Implications for Gerontological Nursing

The needs of the dying are like threads in a piece of cloth. Each thread is individual but necessary to the integrity and completeness of the fabric. If one thread is pulled, it touches the other threads, affecting the fabric's appearance, the thread placement, and the stability of the piece. When one need is unmet, it will affect all others because they are all interwoven. Separating the physical and psychological needs of the dying in late life to identify specific interventions and approaches is difficult because of their interconnection (Tables 26-3 and 26-4).

The responsibility of the nurse is to provide safe conduct as the dying and their families navigate through unknown waters to a good and appropriate death. A good and appropriate death is one that a person would choose if choosing were possible (Box 26-5). A good and appropriate death is one in which one's needs are met to the extent possible. There are several ways to approach an understanding of the needs of persons who are dying and the responsibilities of the

TABLE 26-3

Physical Signs and Symptoms Associated with the Terminal Phase of the Living-Dying Interval: Rationales and Nursing Interventions

Physical Signs and Symptoms	Rationale	Intervention (If Any)
Coolness, color, and temperature change in hands, arms, feet, and legs; perspiration may be present	Peripheral circulation diminished to facilitate increased circulation to vital organs	Place socks on feet; cover with light cotton blankets; keep warm blankets on person, but do not use electric blanket.
Increased sleeping	Conservation of energy	Spend time with the patient; hold the hand if appropriate; speak normally to the patient, even though response may be lacking.
Disorientation, confusion of time, place, person	Metabolic changes	Identify self by name before speaking to patient; speak softly, clearly, and truthfully.
Incontinence of urine, bowel, or both	Increased muscle relaxation and decreased consciousness	Maintain vigilance; change bedding as appropriate; use bed pads; try not to use an indwelling catheter.
Congestion	Poor circulation of body fluids, immobilization, and the inability to expectorate secretions causes gurgling, rattles, bubbling	Elevate the head with pillows, or raise the head of the bed, or both; gently turn the head to the side to drain secretions.
Restlessness	Metabolic changes and decrease in oxygen to the brain	Calm the patient by speech and action; reduce light; gently rub back, stroke arms, or read aloud; play soothing music; do not use restraints.
Decreased intake of food and fluids	Body conservation of energy for function	Do not force patient to eat or drink; give ice chips, soft drinks, juice, popsicles, as possible; apply petrolatum jelly to dry lips; if patient is a mouth breather, apply protective jelly more frequently as necessary.
Decreased urine output	Decreased fluid intake and decreased circulation to kidney	None
Altered breathing pattern	Metabolic and oxygen changes	Elevate the head of bed; speak gently to patient.

From Hess PA: Loss, grief, and dying. In Beare P, Myers J: *Adult health nursing,* ed 3, St Louis, 1998, Mosby.

nurse in the promotion of a healthy death (Figure 26-4). The approaches apply the care of the nurse to the needs identified by noted thanatologist Charles Corr and his colleagues and psychiatrist Avery Weisman.

Corr et al. (2000) suggest the tasks that dying persons need to address: (1) maintaining sense of self; (2) participating in decisions regarding their life; (3) being assured that their life has value; and (4) receiving appropriate and adequate health care. Within these tasks, the need for freedom from pain, freedom from loneliness, conservation of energy, and maintenance of self-esteem can be identified.

Similarly, Weisman (1979) identified six needs of the dying: care, control, composure, communication, continuity, and closure (the 6 Cs). The importance of each to the person is influenced by his or her background, culture, experiences, religious and philosophical orientation, the prior degree of life involvement, and perhaps gender. Weisman's and Corr's works are incorporated in the following discussion with the clear implications for the gerontological nurse.

The 6 Cs Approach

Care. The dying person should have the best care possible; this means freedom from pain, conservation of energy, expert management of symptoms, and support at all times. It means that needed expert medical care is received. Of primary importance is adequate pain relief. Uncontrolled pain can occupy the patient's whole attention, isolating him or her from the world. Pain can be relieved by administering analgesics given properly, by positioning, and by other adjuvant approaches (see Chapter 11). Persons with chronic pain do not respond to the usual methods used with acute pain. Unfortunately, many nurses make no distinction between the two types of pain and chronic pain is undertreated, especially in the nursing home setting (see Chapter 11).

Pain management for the person with a terminal illness requires the nurse to use a double standard. When a person is experiencing acute pain that is expected to dissipate, the nurse is often concerned about addiction and sometimes abuse. The stronger or longer-acting narcotics are used for as short a time as possible. The chronic pain associated with dying is not going to stop and usually requires a regimen of narcotic and adjuvant drug therapy administered around the clock and on time, not just as requested by the patient. Narcotic addiction is not the issue in care of the dying person; relief of pain is paramount (see Chapter 11 for a detailed discussion of pain management).

Care also goes beyond physical to psychological pain, induced by depression, anxiety, fear, and other unresolved emotional concerns that are just as strong and just as real. When emotional needs are not met, the total pain experience, physical and psychological, may be exacerbated or intensified. Medication alone cannot relieve this pain. Instead, empathetic listening and allowing the dying person to verbalize what is on his or her mind are important interventions that must be based on the energy level of the one who is dying. If tears and sadness are present, silence and touch are worth more than words can convey. Gentleness of touch, closeness, and sitting near the person may be appropriate if within the boundaries of culture (see Chapter 21).

Diversional activity can sometimes ease pain: a backrub to relieve tension, a foot massage, access to a radio or television set, or exposure to art and music. If hearing is impaired, an amplifier close to the patient's ear may help. If vision is impaired, talking books (with or without headphones) can be obtained, or a volunteer reader might help. In many instances, psychological pain can be relieved if the person feels safe and has someone close by to converse, to listen, and to be with.

Care also means helping the person conserve energy. Dying requires much energy to cope with the physical assault of illness on the body and the emotional unrest that dying initiates. How much can the individual do without becoming physically and emotionally taxed? What activities of

TABLE 26-4

Emotional or Spiritual Symptoms of Approaching Death, Rationale, and Interventions

Emotional or Spiritual Symptoms	Rationale	Intervention
Withdrawal	Prepares the patient for release and detachment and letting go of relationships and surroundings	Continue communicating in a normal manner using a normal voice tone; identify self by name.
Vision-like experiences (dead friends or family, religious vision)	Preparation for transition	Do not contradict or argue regarding whether this is or is not a real experience; if the patient is frightened, reassure them that the feeling is normal.
Restlessness	Tension, fear, unfinished business	Listen to patient express his or her fears, sadness, and anger associated with dying; give permission to die.
Decreased socialization	As energy diminishes, the patient begins making his or her transition	Express support; give permission to die.
Unusual communication: out of character statements, gestures, requests	Signals readiness to let go	Say what needs to be said to the dying patient; kiss, hug, cry with him or her as appropriate.

From Hess PA: Loss, grief, and dying. In Beare P, Myers J: *Adult health nursing*, ed 3, St Louis, 1998, Mosby.

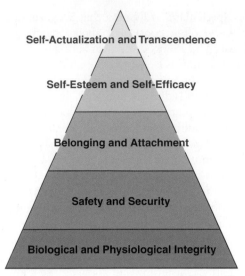

To share and come to terms with the unavoidable future
To perceive meaning in death

Self-Actualization and Transcendence

To maintain respect in the face of increasing weakness
To maintain independence
To feel like a normal person, a part of life right to the end
To preserve personal identity

Self-Esteem and Self-Efficacy

To talk
To be listened to with understanding
To be loved and to share love
To be with a caring person when dying

Belonging and Attachment

To be given the opportunity to voice hidden fears
To trust those who care for him or her
To feel that he or she is being told the truth
To be secure

Safety and Security

To obtain relief from physical symptoms
To conserve energy
To be free from pain

Biological and Physiological Integrity

FIGURE 26-4 Hierarchy of the dying person's needs.

BOX 26-5   Indicators of an Appropriate and Good Death

- Care needed is received, and it is timely and expert.
- One is able to control one's life and environment to the extent that is desired and possible and in a way that is culturally consistent with one's past life.
- One is able to maintain composure when necessary and to extent desired.
- One is able to initiate and maintain communication with significant others for as long as possible.
- Life continues as normal as possible while dying with the added tasks that may be needed to deal with and adjust to the inevitable death. One can maintain desirable hope at all times.
- One is able to reach a sense of closure in a way that is culturally consistent with one's practices and life patterns.

---

daily living are most important for the person to do independently? How much energy is needed for the patient to talk with visitors or staff without becoming exhausted? Only the person who is dying can answer these questions, and the nurse can advocate for the person to be given the opportunity to do so; in doing so, the patient is able to remain in better control and maintain composure. By meeting the needs for freedom from pain and conservation of energy, the nurse has already begun to intervene on behalf of maintaining self-esteem.

Control. While proceeding along the living-dying interval, one often feels that control over his or her life has been lost. This is a particular concern to the person who is dying. The person is in the process of losing everything he or she has ever known or would ever know. The potential loss of identity, independence, and control over body functions can lead to a sense of loss of control and self-esteem. The person may begin to feel ashamed, humiliated, and like a "burden." Control is the need to remain in a collaborative role relating to one's own living and dying and as active a participant in the care as desired. The nurse can help the person meet these needs by taking every opportunity to return the control to the person and, in doing so, bolster self-esteem. Essential to the facilitation of self-esteem is the premise that the values of the patient must figure significantly in the decisions that will affect the course of dying. Whenever possible, the nurse can have the person decide when to groom, eat, wake, sleep, and so on. The nurse never has the right to determine the activities of the individual, especially relating to visitors and how time is spent.

Composure. Dying is usually an emotional activity—for dying persons and for those around them. The need for composure is that which enables the person to modulate emotional extremes within cultural norms as is appropriate. This is not to avoid the sadness; this is to have moments of relief. The nurse may use many of the countercoping techniques previously discussed to help persons maintain composure as they desire.

Communication. The need for communication is broad, from the need for information to make decisions to the need to share information. Although the type and content of communication that is acceptable to the person vary by culture, the nurse has a responsibility to ensure that the dying person has an opportunity for the communication he or she desires.

Communication includes auditory, visual, and tactile stimulation to appropriately nurture and foster quality of life while dying. Verbal and nonverbal communication are necessary to convey positive messages; hand-holding, placing an arm around the shoulder, or sitting on the edge of the bed as culturally appropriate conveys to the dying person that the nurse or caregiver is available to listen.

In a classic study of communication about terminal illness and among the patient, family, and hospital staff, Glaser and Strauss (1963) identified four types: closed awareness, suspected awareness, mutual pretense, and open awareness. Each of these influenced the work on the hospital unit. *Closed awareness* is described as "keeping the secret." Hospital staff and the family and friends know that the patient is dying, but the patient does not know it or knows and keeps the secret as well. Generally, caregivers invent a fictitious future for the patient to believe in, in hopes that it will boost the patient's morale. Although this happens less today with the legislation related to patients' rights, it still occurs. In *suspected awareness*, the patient suspects that he or she is going to die. Hints are bandied back and forth, and a contest ensues for control of the information.

Mutual pretense is a situation of "let's pretend." Everyone knows the patient has a terminal illness and may be dying, but the patient, family, friends, nurses, and physicians do not talk about it—real feelings are kept hidden, and too often, so are questions. *Open awareness* acknowledges the reality of approaching death. The patient, family, friends, nurses, and physicians openly acknowledge the eventual death of the patient. The patient may ask, "Will I die?" and "How and when will I die?" The patient becomes resigned to dying, and the family grieves with the patient rather than for the patient. The nurse can encourage open awareness whenever possible while respecting the patient's cultural patterns and behaviors. In some cultures, talking about an anticipated death is deemed helpful. In others, one can be aware of the dying but talking about it openly may be taboo (Irish et al., 1993).

Continuity. The need for continuity is fulfilled by preserving as normal a life as possible while dying; by transcending the present, continuity helps to maintain self-esteem. Often a dying patient can feel shut off from the rest of the world at a time when he or she is still capable of being involved and active in some way. Providing stimuli such as photographs and mementos, enabling the individual to stay at home, or enabling individuality in the institutional setting engenders continuity and self-esteem. Self-esteem and dignity complement each other. Dignity involves the individual's ability to maintain a consistent self-concept.

Loneliness is the result of a loss of continuity with one's life and a diminution of one's concept of self. The nurse may ask about the person's life and those things most valued and work with the family and the patient or resident on a plan to remain engaged in as many of the activities and past roles as possible. A father who watches a certain ballgame with his son every Sunday can continue to do this regardless of the need to be in a hospital, a nursing home, or an in-patient hospice unit. If the person is at home and is bed-bound, it may be more practical to have the bed in a central area rather than in a distant room. Treating the dying elderly person as an intelligent adult, holding a hand, or putting an arm around a shoulder if culturally acceptable says, "I care" and "You're not alone" and "You are important."

Yet some prefer some time alone and have valued solitude (Box 26-6). This too can be respected as a way of enhancing the continuity of a long life. The nurse can find out the

---

BOX 26-6   Meditation Coping

Mrs. Jones was a spry 76-year-old white woman. She was the sole caregiver of her husband with mid-stage Alzheimer's disease. The hospital had arranged for her husband to share a room with her while her diagnostic tests were completed and her symptoms stabilized before she went home. She had just been diagnosed with metastatic breast cancer, with a terminal diagnosis. The nurses thought that she was becoming increasingly irritable and agitated after her initial calmness. As an advanced practice nurse on an oncology unit, I was called to assess Mrs. Jones and recommend a treatment plan. We talked for awhile—about her life, her plans for the future, and her usual coping. She explained that she had everything under control, had already made arrangements for homecare in the process of planning for the eventual long-term care needs of her husband. As she started to cry, she said, "It's just so hard with my life disrupted here. Every morning for years I have meditated for 30 minutes. My husband respects my need for quiet, and afterward I think I can do anything! I have not been able to meditate since I have been here; the nurses and staff are always coming in my room or calling on the room's intercom—I can't find any moments of peace!" The nurses and I worked out a plan with Mrs. Jones. Every morning between 6 and 6:30 AM she would not be disturbed. A "Do Not Disturb" sign would be placed on the intercom at the nurses' station and on her door. A noticeable change was seen in just a few days; Mrs. Jones was calmer and coping well again. She was most appreciative to "have my life back again."

Kathleen Jett

---

personal and cultural preferences and values of the person and work toward honoring these.

Legacies can take many different forms and may range from memories that will live on in the minds of others to bequeathed fortunes. A grandmother who is likely to die before a favorite grandchild's wedding can be asked to participate in anticipatory planning, regardless of the age of the grandchild, thereby leaving an enduring and special legacy. The nurse can assist older adults in meeting continuity needs by helping them think about a possible legacy, by doing the following:

- Find out lifestyle interests.
- Establish a method of recording.
- Identify recipients (either generally or specifically).
- Help record the legacy.

Legacies are also a part of Maslow's transcendence and are discussed in more detail in Chapter 27.

Closure. The need for closure is the need for the opportunity for reconciliation, transcendence, and self-actualization, the highest of Maslow's Hierarchy. Reminiscence is one way of putting one's life in order, to evaluate the pluses and minuses of life. It is a means of resolving conflicts, giving up possessions, and making final good-byes. Learning to say "good-bye" today leaves open the possibility of many more "hellos." Pain and other symptoms that are not well cared for may interfere with this reconciliation, making appropriate interventions by the nurse especially important.

For some, closure means coming to terms with their spiritual selves, with Jesus, God, Allah, or Buddha. If the expressions of the patient have spiritual overtones, arranging for pastoral care may be offered but should never be done without the person's permission. The nurse can foster transcendence by providing patients with the time and privacy for self-reflection and an opportunity to talk about whatever they need to talk about, especially about the meanings of their lives and the meanings of their deaths (see Chapter 27).

The fabric of needs of the dying person comprise the six Cs. The influence of communication and control is omnipresent in the other needs; without them, the cloth will fray and attempts to meet the needs will be limited.

Spirituality and Hope.
Spirituality is the basic human quality for hope. Without one's own spiritual nourishment, one cannot meet the same needs in others. The spiritual dimension of a person is that from which one draws meaning for both life and death and connection to some force outside of oneself. Spirituality is the manner in which one integrates one's knowledge or belief system, inner life experiences, and exterior life and institutional activities in support of these beliefs (Thibault et al., 1991). The spiritual dimension deals with the transcendental relationship between the dying person and another—between the person and his or her god or the person and significant others (see Chapter 27).

Nurses can tend to the spiritual needs of dying elders in the following ways:

- Ask the individual his or her source of strength and hope.
- Ask if the individual sees any connection between physical health and spiritual beliefs.
- Discuss his or her sources of spiritual strength throughout life.

Signs of spiritual distress while dying include doubt, despair, guilt, boredom, and anger at the supernatural force in their lives. Interventions may involve calling their choice of a religious leader; sharing spiritual readings that are consistent with their beliefs, meditative poems, and music of the person's choice; obtaining religious articles such as amulets, a Bible, or a rosary; or praying. The nurse is cautioned that these interventions must be consistent with the culture and wishes of the patient and not expressions of the nurse's belief system.

Hope is expectancy of fulfillment, an anticipation, or relief from something. Hope is based on the belief of the possible, support of meaningful others, a sense of well being, overall coping ability, and a purpose in life. Erickson equates hope with integrity; it is also comparable to Maslow's self-actualization. Hope empowers, generates courage, motivates action and achievement, and can strengthen physiological and psychological functioning.

Hope involves faith and trust. Hope can be classified as desirable or expectational (Pattison, 1977). Expectational hope sounds like "I hope to get better" or "I hope my children get here in time." If this hope is a reflection of expectations that are not realistic, they can increase stress for the person and caregiver. However, this hope can be modified without being lost. In desirable hope, the wishes are something that would be appreciated if it were to occur without the fixed expectation that it will or must occur. The nurse can respond to the comment "I hope I get better" from someone who is rapidly declining with "That would be really great; in the meantime, there is so much we can do for you such as keep you comfortable." Desirable hope may be related to a cure, a holiday, the birth of a grandchild, or reconciliation.

Nurses seldom recognize the small things they do, routinely and unconsciously, to impart hope. The act of helping with grooming conveys a quiet belief that the person matters. Pain relief and comfort measures reinforce the recognition of an individual's needs and reinforce the value of the person. Several approaches that may help the nurse more clearly foster and sustain hope in the physically failing elder are to (1) confirm the value of life, (2) establish a support system, (3) incorporate humor, (4) incorporate the person's religion, and (5) set realistic goals (Hickey, 1986).

Like Weisman's countercoping, Sister Rosemary Donley defines the nursing role in the spiritual search of suffering persons as compassionate accompaniment—entering into another's reality and quietly, attentively sharing the experience. "Nurses need to be with people who suffer, to give meaning to the reality of suffering, and insofar as possible, to remove suffering and its causes. Here lies the spiritual dimension of health care" (Donley, 1991, p. 180).

Assessment.
Few, if any, tools are available to assess dying patients. Caregivers, for the most part, have to depend on their understanding of the grieving and dying processes and draw carefully from the literature appropriate behavioral responses. A danger exists among health professionals of superimposing what they think the patient should feel and do in the dying process. The purpose of knowing about theories of grief and dying is to recognize emotions and behaviors and to plan interventions accordingly as they appear. An extensive list of items to assess for the dying patient and grieving family appears in Box 26-7.

As an individual nears the final days and hours of life, physical, psychological, and emotional events occur that provide clues to the impending death. Nurses, families, and patients are too often unaware and unprepared for these signs and responses. Tables 26-3 and 26-4 provide guidance for these responses.

The Family.
The nurse is often present and supporting the family at the moment of death and in the moments preceding it. Regardless of the age of the surviving family members, as spouse, partner, children, or friends, they too have needs

BOX 26-7 Assessment of the Dying Patient and Family

PATIENT

Age
Gender
Coping styles and abilities
Social, cultural, ethnic background
Previous experience with illness, pain, deterioration, loss, grief
Mental health
Lifestyle
Fulfillment of life goals
Amount of unfinished business
The nature of the illness (death trajectory, problems particular to the illness, treatment, amount of pain)
Time passed since diagnosis
Response to illness
Knowledge about the illness or disease
Acceptance or rejection of the diagnosis
Amount of striving for dependence or independence
Feelings and fears about illness
Comfort in expressing thoughts and feelings and how much is expressed
Location of the patient (home, hospital, nursing home)
Relationship with each member of the family and significant other since diagnosis
Family rules, norms, values, and past experiences that might inhibit grief or interfere with a therapeutic relationship

FAMILY

Family makeup (members of family)
Developmental stage of the family
Existing subsystems
Specific roles of each member

CHARACTERISTICS OF THE FAMILY SYSTEM

How flexible or rigid
Type of communication
Rules, norms, expectations
Values, beliefs
Quality of emotional relationships
Dependence, interdependence, freedom of each member
How close to or disengaged from the dying member
Established extrafamilial interactions
Strengths and vulnerabilities of the family
Style of leadership and decision-making
Unusual methods of problem solving, crisis resolution
Family resources (personal, financial, community)
Current problems identified by the family
Quality of communication with the caregivers
Immediate and long-range anticipated needs

From Hocc PA: Loss, grief, and dying. In Deare P, Myers J. *Adult health nursing*, ed 3, St Louis, 1998, Mosby.

and nurses have a responsibility to care for them. Newly bereaved persons were asked what they had found most helpful (Merlevede et al., 2004; Richter, 1987). They most appreciated nurses who did the following:

- Kept me informed
- Asked how I was doing and offered support
- Put an arm around me when I cried
- Brought me food
- Knew my name
- Cried with me
- Brought a bed and encouraged me to stay in the room with my dying husband
- Told me to hold my husband's hand while he was dying
- Held my hand
- Got the chaplain for me
- Let me take care of my husband
- Stayed with me after their shift was over

Although these will not provide comfort to all nor are all these behaviors always possible, they can be used as starting points. See Table 26-5 for sample care plans for survivors.

DYING AND THE NURSE

Nurses are professional grievers. We invest time and caring, and if working with older adults, especially those who are frail and in acute and long-term care settings, we repeatedly experience the death of patients and residents. Some consider the death of a patient as a failure—they have "lost" the person they cared for. However, when it is a good death, it can be viewed as a professional success because the nurse provided safe conduct for the dying elder and gently cared for the survivors. We can use the reminders of our own mortality as motivation to live the best we can with what we have. Nurses can seek support and support each other. As grievers, we too may need to tell the story of the dying person to those professionals around us, either in formal or informal support groups; and we need to listen to our colleagues' stories.

Caring for older adults requires knowledge of the grieving and dying processes as well as skills in providing relief of symptoms or palliative care. However, it is also acknowledged that working daily with the grieving or dying is an art. The development of the art necessitates inner strength. The nurse needs to have spiritual strength, strength from within. This does not mean that the nurse must have a specific religious orientation or affiliation but, rather, that he or she has a positive belief in self and a belief that life has meaning. The effective nurse has developed a personal philosophy of life and of death. Although this may change over time and cannot be assumed to be held by anyone else, one's beliefs about life and death will help the nurse through difficult times. Emotional maturity allows the nurse to deal with disappointment and postponement of immediate wants or

TABLE 26-5
Nursing Care Plan for Survivors

Nursing Diagnosis	Expected Outcomes	Interventions
LONELINESS, SOCIAL ISOLATION RELATED TO LOSS OF SPOUSE, SEXUAL PARTNER, FRIEND, COMPANION, OR CONFIDANT		
Manifestations: teariness, crying, sleep disturbance, weight gain, compulsive eating, weight loss, anorexia, fatigue, confusion, forgetfulness, withdrawal, disinterest, indecisiveness, inability to concentrate, guilt feelings; displays feelings of detachment, inferiority, rejection, alienation, emptiness, isolation; unable to initiate social contacts; seeks attention	*Short-term and intermediate goals:* The survivor will: Develop or use immediate support systems Express feelings of security Exhibit meaningful social relationships Show decreasing signs of depression *Long-term goal:* The survivor will: Demonstrate readiness to build a new life as a single person	Attempt to develop a therapeutic relationship through touch, empathy, and listening. Listen to perceived feelings. Help person realize that grief is a painful but normal transitional process. Encourage relationships with other persons as support systems. Encourage balance between *linking phenomena* (mementos, photographs, clothes, furniture) associated with the deceased and the *bridging phenomena* (new driving skills, evening classes, new job). Program for counseling if appropriate. Refer to appropriate agencies as needed.
ANXIETY RELATED TO INCREASED LEGAL, FINANCIAL, AND DECISION-MAKING RESPONSIBILITIES		
Manifestations: anger, nervousness, palpitations, increased perspiration, face flushing, dyspnea, urinary frequency, nausea, vomiting, restlessness, apprehension, panic, fear, headache	*Short-term and intermediate goals:* The survivor will demonstrate adequate decision-making skills in financial and legal matters as evidenced by: Seeking legal aid as needed Writing or calling appropriate agencies Formulating a realistic budget *Long-term goals:* The survivor will: Cope and deal with legal, financial, and decision-making responsibilities with only a moderate degree of anxiety Make rational decisions about single life	Assist in obtaining attorney if necessary. Encourage contact of Social Security and spouse's employer to ensure receipt of all benefits. Encourage contact of insurance agencies if applicable. Discourage immediate decision-making regarding assets (e.g., home, investments). Encourage seeking of advice from individuals who are trusted. Contact proper social agencies if indigent or in need. Assist in seeking employment if health permits and client so desires. Offer alternatives for decision-making. Refer to any other proper community agencies that offer needed assistance.

Adapted from Alexander J, Kiely J: Working with the bereaved, *Geriatr Nurs* 7(2):85-86, 1986.

desires. Maturity means that the nurse can reach out for help for self when needed. Finally, to provide comfort to grieving persons, nurses must be comfortable with their own lives or at least be able to set aside their own sadness and grief while working with the sadness and grief of others.

It is always important to remember that some nurses are unable to care for the dying because of their own unresolved conflicts and should not be expected to function in these situations. This may be a temporary situation associated with events in the nurse's life or something deeper, such as a traumatic experience in the death of a loved one. The nurse should recognize his or her limitations, and another nurse who is better able should instead provide care.

Palliative Care

Gerontological nurses routinely care for elders who have irreversible and progressive conditions, such as Alzheimer's disease or Parkinson's disease. Other elders have exhausted

all treatment options or have decided that they want no further treatment for conditions such as cancer or end-stage heart or renal disease. A nursing home resident may elect to remain at the facility rather than return to a hospital, even if faced with an acute event such as a myocardial infarction (MI) or stroke. These persons should receive *palliative care*—that which focuses on comfort rather than cure, on the treatment of symptoms rather than disease, and on quality of life left rather than quantity of life foreseen. Palliative care is much of what is given in gerontological nursing and may indeed be the heart of caring. Palliative care can be provided anywhere by anyone sharing these goals and skills. See Box 26-8 for core competencies for palliative/end-of-life care.

The scope and specialty of this knowledge base have grown considerably over the years; research has been conducted, professional organizations have been formed, and, most recently, standardized curricula have been developed. With the support of the American Association of Colleges

BOX 26-8   Core Competencies for Palliative/ End-of-Life Care

The nurse should be able to:
- Talk to patients and families about dying.
- Be knowledgeable about symptom control and pain-control techniques (opioid dosing and other pharmacological interventions).
- Provide comfort-oriented nursing interventions.
- Provide palliative treatments.
- Recognize physical changes that precede eminent death.
- Deal with own feelings.
- Deal with angry patients and families.
- Be knowledgeable and deal with the ethical issues in administering end-of-life palliative therapies.
- Be knowledgeable, and inform patients about ADs.
- Be knowledgeable of the legal issues in administering end-of-life palliative care.
- Be adaptable and sensitive to religious and cultural perspectives.
- Explain the meaning of hospice.

Modified from White KR et al: Are nurses adequately prepared for end-of-life care? *J Nur Scholarsh* 33(2):147, 2001, Sigma Theta Tau International.
ADs, Advance directives.

of Nursing and City of Hope Medical Center, a broad initiative was established to train nurses through the End-of-Life Nursing Education Consortium (ANA-ELNEC). It is hoped that by training nurses and faculty, nursing as a profession can provide the highest level of palliative care (Matzo and Sherman, 2004).

Whereas initially palliative care was the specialty of community-based hospices, specialized units and staff are now seen in long-term care and acute care facilities across the United States. Palliative care was once not a well-reimbursed service, but since a hospice benefit was added to Medicare Part A in the 1980s, the number of private insurance companies and health maintenance organizations (HMOs) offering a hospice option has increased and programs have grown considerably (Matzo and Sherman, 2004).

Hospice: An Alternative

Hospice is described as the link among the needs of the terminally ill, their families, and the staff; it employs the medieval concept of hospitality in which a community assists the traveler at dangerous points along his or her journey. It returns nursing to its roots—as humane, compassionate care, an ideal that has been the basis of nursing for centuries. The dying are indeed travelers—travelers along the continuum of life—and the community consists of friends, family, and specially prepared people to care—the hospice team. The philosophy of hospice care is that "the last stages of life should not be seen as defeat, but rather as life's fulfillment. It is not merely a time of negation, rather an opportunity for positive achievement..." (Ulrich, 1978, p. 20). A summary of the philosophy and principles that guide hospice is presented in Box 26-9. Hospice is a reorientation for the patient and family to palliative care.

The model for hospice and its concepts was based on way stations, which cared for the sick and tired during the crusades. More than 40 years ago under the direction of Dr. Cicely Saunders, Saint Christopher's Hospice in London implemented this concept for people who were dying of cancer. The hospice movement, which began in the United States in 1971, has made hospice a familiar word to many health care professionals and the lay public. However, the meaning attached to hospice is still subject to a variety of interpretations.

Today, hospice organizations, some nonprofit and others for-profit, are throughout the United States and some parts of Canada. The variations in origins and style reflect the particular needs of the community, the style of leadership, funding sources, political forces, and available resources for health and social services in each community in which hospices are established.

Hospice programs provide comprehensive and interdisciplinary care to persons in the last 6 months of life. Under the U.S. Medicare plan, hospice provides, at a minimum, medical, nursing, nursing assistant, chaplain, social work, and volunteer support available 24 hours per day. Potential services may also include music, art, and pet therapy and inpatient services in a homelike setting. Hospices provide care not only to the dying but also to their families and friends through support groups before and after the deaths. Hospice services are usually available to individuals and families regardless of ability to pay because of the generous support of donors and volunteers.

The majority of hospice care is provided in people's homes to support the informal caregiver. The home becomes the primary center of care, and care is provided by family members or friends, who are taught basic nursing care, including diet, exercise, and medication needed to care for the dying individual. Hospice is available 24 hours every day of the year for its clients, providing the services of the interdisciplinary team as needed.

Hospice facilitates a redefinition of relationships. The spouse may not always be the caregiver; it might be a friend or child. For individuals without family, hospice staff and, at times, friends become the patient's family. Some hospice programs are able to provide volunteer or staff relief to the caregivers. Whenever possible, neither the dying person nor the family is alone during the dying process or during the months of bereavement that follow. Much personal contact, interaction, and sharing take place between the family and hospice team. Hospice volunteers provide direct or indirect assistance. Chores are performed, and friendship and companionship are provided to the patient and family.

The unprecedented contribution of hospice continues to be the reestablishment of control for the dying person. Through polypharmaceutical means, control of distressful symptoms and pain has been accomplished without denying the patient full alertness and the ability to communicate to others. This gift, so to speak, allows addressing all of Weisman's Six Cs: care, control, composure, communication, continuity, and closure. The crux of accomplishing this end

BOX 26-9   Summary of Hospice Philosophy and Principles

- Hospice is a philosophy, not a facility, one in which the primary focus is on palliative care.
- Hospice affirms life, not death.
- Hospice strives to maximize present quality of living.
- Hospice offers palliative care to all people and their family members, regardless of age, gender, nationality, race, creed, or sexual orientation, who are coping with a life-threatening illness, dying, death, and bereavement.
- The hospice approach offers care to the patient and family as a unit.
- Hospice programs make service available on a 24-hour-a-day, 7-day-a-week basis without interruption, even if the patient care setting changes.
- Participants in hospice programs give special attention to supporting each other.
- Hospice is holistic care.
- A highly qualified, specially trained team of hospice professionals and volunteers work together to meet the physiological, psychological, social, spiritual, and economic needs of patient and family facing terminal illness and bereavement.

- Hospice offers a safe, coordinated program of palliative and supportive care, in a variety of settings, from the time of admission through bereavement, with the focus of keeping the terminally ill patient in his or her home as long as possible.
- Hospice offers continuing care and ongoing support to bereaved survivors after the death of someone they love.
- Hospice is accountable for the appropriate allocation and utilization of its resources to provide optimum, culturally competent care consistent with patient and family needs and desires.
- Hospice has an organized governing body that has complete and ultimate responsibility for the organization. The governing body entrusts the hospice administrator with overall management responsibility for operating hospice, including planning, organizing, staffing, and evaluating the organization and its services.
- Hospice is committed to continuous assessment and improvement of the quality and efficiency of its services.

Data from Hospice Standards of Practice, National Hospice and Palliative Care Organization, 2000.

is the anticipation of symptoms and intervention by the caregiver before problems occur. Pain and symptom control and the opportunity to die at home are the key ideas and activities that people associate with hospice. Actually, hospice represents much more. It supports and guides the family in patient care and ensures that the patient will not die alone and that the family will not be abandoned. Bereavement services for the family extend for a period of time on an emergency and regular basis after the death of the patient. Life is made as meaningful as possible.

Nursing practice and hospice incorporate the mind-body continuum. Nursing is considered the cornerstone of hospice care. The nurse provides much of the direct care and functions in a variety of roles: as staff nurse giving direct care, as coordinator implementing the plan of the interdisciplinary team, or as executive officer responsible for research and educational activities, and as advocate for the patient and hospice in the clinical and political arena. Nursing practice in hospice and palliative care is guided by two sets of standards as noted in the following sections.

Palliative/Hospice Care in the Long-Term Care Setting

Although it is not uncommon for residents of long-term care facilities to die, the use of formal hospice services is very limited (Stillman et al., 2005). As a result of this and the lack of emphasis on palliative care in facilities, research findings have supported the claims that advance care planning and terminal pain management are inadequate and support of the grieving family may be nonexistent (Stillman et al., 2005, p. 259). Yet studies have also found that the care of residents with hospice services and those who are identified

as dying in the general population may receive similar care, but a conclusion has not been reached (Munn et al., 2006).

Philosophically, most nurses believe that hospice services have the potential to increase the comfort for long-term care residents while they are dying. Hospice enrollees are able to receive services beyond those which are available to the general population of residents. Some facilities have special palliative care units or rooms that are staffed with specially trained nurses, but this is the exception (Kayser-Jones et al., 2005). In most cases those identified as terminally ill remain in their own rooms. In other cases the local hospice programs have nurses and staff dedicated to working with the residents of select nursing facilities. At all times the palliative care services are expected to meet the principles derived from the American Geriatrics Society or those established by the American Nurses Association and the National Hospice and Palliative Care Organization (NHPCO) (*www.hpna.org*; www.nho.org) (Box 26-10). The NHPCO is committed to developing education in the hospice concept and promoting appropriate legislation, regulation, and reimbursement.

Recently a variety of intervention studies have been conducted to increase the use of hospice in long-term care settings. For example, Stillman and colleagues (2005) used an educational intervention to teach palliative care approaches with some increase in the comfort level and knowledge of the staff. Another intervention study demonstrated that those facilities that identified and trained a "Palliative Care Leadership Team" increased the number of referrals to hospice, improved pain management, and increased the number of advance care planning discussions (Hanson et al., 2005).

BOX 26-10   Standards and Scope of Hospice and Palliative Nursing Practice

In recent years the number of available standards of practice and nursing in palliative and hospice care has multiplied significantly. The cornerstone for nurses has been standards of practice approved by the American Nurses Association (*www.nursingworld.org*), and these standards may have helped form the basis for many more. Other resources for information about standards of care and practice can be found at the websites listed below. The user may need to go into the website and search for "palliative care standards" for current access to specific location.

- The International Association for Hospice and Palliative Care includes links to standards in a number of countries worldwide (*www.hospicecare.com*).
- The Joint Commission provides those standards expected of all approved health care facilities in the United States (*www.jointcommission.org*).
- The National Institutes of Health provides several sets of standards of care specific to identified terminal conditions. These are available in the related Institute (*www.nih.gov*).
- Australia provides well-developed standards as well as links to sources from other countries (*www.pallcare.org.au*).

DECISION MAKING AT THE END OF LIFE

Who makes end-of-life decisions has been the subject of research, debate, and federal legislation. The individual adult is generally recognized as the decision maker; however, this assumption is based on a very Euro-American or Western perspective. Persons who are from non-Western traditions place less emphasis on the individual and more on the needs of the family or community (Blackhall et al., 1995; Mazanec and Tyler, 2003). The nurse is obligated to know legal expectations and then work with the elder and the family on how these will fit with their cultural patterns and needs related to end-of-life decisions.

Decision making on life-prolonging procedures when death is inevitable has become a legal, ethical, medical, and professional issue today. The blurring of the lines between living and dying results from technological advances, the ambivalence of whether death is to be fought or accepted, and the dilemma brought about by medical technologies. Decision making at the end of life has become increasingly complex because most people die in advanced age from chronic illnesses; that is, they die over a period of years, slowly declining from degenerative conditions such as Alzheimer's disease, Parkinson's disease, and heart failure.

Advance Directives

Although people have always had opinions about their wishes, their right to refuse medical treatment was legislated in the United States through the Patient Self-Determination Act (PSDA) enacted by Congress in October 1990 and was implemented in all states in December 1991. Under the PSDA, the adult was recognized as the ultimate authority in the decisions to forego life-sustaining treatment for himself or herself, rather than a physician or a health care agency. In other words, through the PSDA, adults were granted the legal authority to complete what are known as *advance directives (ADs)*—or statements about their wishes or directions to others determined before the need for decisions (in other words, in advance). These directives may be as detailed or as vague as desired, from "no treatment if I am terminally ill" to a breakdown of decisions about dialysis, antibiotics, tube feedings, cardiopulmonary resuscitation (CPR), and so on. Through the PSDA, any adult also may appoint any other adult (not necessarily next of kin or relative) to speak for him or her and make decisions if the patient is unable to do so.

An AD can be revoked only by the individual, either verbally or in writing. The person may also indicate revocation by tearing, burning, or destroying the document, preferably in front of witnesses. Directives may also be amended; formal language is not necessary, and one can add items in writing or cross out unwanted passages. If the person becomes incompetent, revocation is no longer possible, and the last statement stands.

Two common forms of ADs are known as *living will* and *durable power of attorney for health care (DPAHC)*, also called *advance health care directive (AHCD)*. A living will (Figure 26-5) is restricted to representing a person's wishes specific to the condition of a terminal illness and applies only in that situation. In most states, a proxy may be appointed in a living will to speak on behalf of the person if he or she is unable to do so. A living will (LW) is not the same as a do-not-resuscitate (DNR) order, which is a medical directive to health care professionals and is not a personal directive.

In contrast, a DPAHC appoints a person, called a *health care surrogate*, to speak for the other in all matters of health care (not to be confused with the power of attorney discussed in Chapter 17). However, in some cases the DPAHC cannot make decisions related to withdrawal of life support, at which time both the DPAHC and LW are needed. Both the proxy and the health care surrogate are expected to make the decisions for the person that he or she would make if able to do so, using what is known as *substituted judgment*. Although advance directives are considered morally binding, they are legally binding only when declared so in state statutes.

All agencies that receive Medicare and Medicaid funds are mandated to disseminate PSDA information to their clients and inquire as to the existence of living wills (Berrio and Levesque, 1996; Mezey, 1996; Mezey et al., 1994). Hospitals and long-term care facilities are responsible for providing written information at the time of admission about the individual's rights under law to refuse medical and surgical care and the right to initiate this in a written advance directive. HMOs are required to do the same at the time of membership enrollment, and home health agencies are required to do it before the patient comes under the care of the agency. Hospices are obliged to inform patients of their self-determination rights on the initial visit (Berrio and Levesque,

Florida Living Will

Declaration made this _____ day of _____ , 20_____.
I, _____ , willfully and voluntarily make known my desire that my dying not be artificially prolonged under the circumstances set forth below, and I do hereby declare:

If at any time I have a terminal condition and if my attending or treating physician and another consulting physician have determined that there is no medical probability of my recovery from such condition, I direct that life-prolonging procedures be witheld or withdrawn when the application of such procedures would serve only to prolong artificially the process of dying, and that I be permitted to die naturally with only the administration of medication or the performance of any medical procedure deemed necessary to provide me with comfort care or to alleviate pain.

It is my intention that this declaration be honored by my family and physician as the final expression of my legal right to refuse medical or surgical treatment and to accept the consequences for such refusal.

In the event that I have been determined to be unable to provide express and informed consent regarding the witholding, withdrawal, or continuation of life-prolonging procedures, I wish to designate, as my surrogate to carry out the provisions of this declaration:
Name: _____
Address: _____
Zip code: _____
Phone: _____

I wish to designate the following person as my alternate surrogate to carry out the provisions of this declaration should my surrogate be unwilling or unable to act on my behalf:
Name: _____
Address: _____
Zip code: _____
Phone: _____

Additional instructions (optional):
I understand the full import of this declaration and I am emotionally and mentally competent to make this declaration.
Signed: _____
Witness 1: _____
Signed: _____
Address: _____
Witness 2: _____
Signed: _____
Address: _____

FIGURE 26-5 Living will declaration. (Courtesy Choice in Dying, Inc.)

1996; Mezey, 1996). Providers (physicians and nurse practitioners) are encouraged but not obligated to provide this same information to their patients.

Although the exact format and signature (e.g., notary) requirements vary from state to state, the PSDA is a federal mandate and applies to persons in all jurisdictions. There are several clearinghouses of related information, including *www.fivewishes.com,* wherein persons can obtain information relevant to their state and forms can be ordered or downloaded.

Barriers to Completing Advance Directives. Studies have indicated inaccessible documents, level of education, income, younger age, and race as impediments to executing an AD (Douglas and Brown, 2002; Habel, 2001; Havens, 2000; Mezey et al., 2000). Individuals with high school or lower education, who are non-white, and who exist on a low income tend not to have completed an AD. This tendency is the result in part of the lack of information about ADs and lack of information about subsequent consequences of treatment choices or refusal of treatments. In some groups and cultures, the family is the decision maker of care issues, not the patient. Finding someone to serve as proxy and the fear of putting things in writing also influence the completion of a directive. Interpreters, used to assist the health care professional with explanations to their non–English-speaking patients, may not facilitate a clear translation of an AD because of cultural beliefs surrounding death or anticipation of poor health (Douglas and Brown, 2002; Havens, 2000; Mezey et al., 2000; Morrison, 1998). The nurse must consider all these factors when attempting to ensure that a patient has an AD.

Nurse's Role and Advance Directives. Although the nurse cannot provide legal information, he or she does serve as a resource person ready to answer many of the questions people have about end-of-life decision making and care. The nurse may be responsible to inquire about the presence of an existing advance directive, to offer and explain the option, and to ensure that any existing directive still reflects the person's wishes. The nurse also is responsible for ensuring that existing or newly created advance directives are available in the appropriate locations in the medical record.

The nurse can help the elder understand treatments that are available to sustain life and the implications of interventions such as resuscitation efforts (CPR), intubation, and artificial nutrition, as well as the technical terms associated with them. However, in providing this information, the nurse must avoid injecting personal bias into the discussion. The gerontological nurse is an advocate for the patient regardless of the setting but is particularly important in the long-term care setting (Kayser-Jones, 2002). There, the nurse advocates for the self-determination of all patients, even those with questionable cognitive functioning.

In a small study of older patients who were diagnosed as demented by standard tests, 30% were found to possess the mental ability to understand the nature of a health care proxy and designate a relative as their decision maker. Of the participants, 27% were able to express their preference for or against a DNR option; 21% were able to make a decision about both a DNR and a health care proxy (Schmitt, 1996). Although this study was limited, it suggests that decision-making capacity is not always accurately predicted by screening tests such as the Folstein Mini-Mental State Examination (MMSE) or the Global Deterioration Scale (GDS-2) (see Chapters 6 and 23). Further, the question is raised as to who is making the decision of mental capacity. The implication for elders in long-term care facilities is that these elders should not be automatically excluded from discussions or decision making related to ADs.

As a provider of information, the nurse needs to be aware of the types of directives that are legally recognized in the state in which the nurse practices and the terminology associated with directives; for example, *surrogate* is not always recognized as interchangeable with *proxy* or *agent* (Weenolsen, 1996). The nurse should also be familiar with the AD form or forms used by the organization in which he or she is employed. Forms vary from state to state and from institution to institution and may still be recognized as legal documents.

The nurse acts as a patient advocate by bringing family members and the elder together to discuss the difficult issues addressed in making a directive or to simply discuss the elder's wishes. The nurse may be the one who brings the patient and the physician together to ensure that both parties agree on the terms of the directive and that the physician can honor the patient's wishes. The nurse may also be the one who obtains the appropriate AD form for the elder who is well or ill. Several studies have concluded that counseling hospitalized patients by hospital representatives, nurses, and others is an effective and generalized way of improving recognition and execution of advance directives (Meier et al., 1996).

No one can think of all possible contingencies that might require decisions with serious illness or a current condition. The use of values assessment may help clarify what the elder holds important in his or her life and how this relates to his or her desires for health care and quality of life. Does the elder want measures to be taken to prolong life at all costs, or does he or she wish for a natural death if the alternative may mean being prolonged artificially with today's technology? Are there any persons the elder feels comfortable with who can act as a proxy to ensure that the elder's wishes will be carried out? Answers to these questions are helpful when discussing the elder's wishes. Before a directive is completed, the family and perhaps the clergy and friends should discuss whether those who are to be involved are comfortable with the decisions and will adhere to the directive. For elders without family, the nurse may become a sounding board.

Euthanasia

The recognition of a patient's right to refuse life-sustaining medical measures renewed age-old questions over the patient's right to make decisions about the continuation of life. Some people, especially those who were suffering at the end of life, have ended their lives, either passively in refusal of food or more actively in the refusal of treatments or other more dramatic ways. The number of successful suicides increases with age, particularly with older men. The incidence of suicide in men older than 65 years is second only to male teens, with the preferred mode a gun. Others, especially those who are extremely debilitated, have asked for assistance in accomplishing this in the most painless way possible.

In May 1992 the *Journal of the American Medical Association* reported that 73% of the general public in a large sample approved of some form of euthanasia. *Physician-assisted death, physician-assisted suicide, physician aid in dying,* and *passive* and *active euthanasia* are all terms that are heard. An example of physician-assisted suicide might be the physician providing the patient with sleeping pills and instructions about a lethal dose. This form is considered passive euthanasia because the physician has not administered the lethal dose. The person who injects poison or a lethal dose of a medication into a patient who voluntarily requested to be helped to die would be practicing active euthanasia.

In 1994 and again in 1997, voters in the state of Oregon passed the Death with Dignity Law, and Oregon became the only state in the United States to legalize physician-assisted suicide in the form of passive euthanasia. This law enables an Oregon resident who (1) is a terminally ill adult, (2) has less than 6 months to live, and (3) is judged to be mentally competent to obtain the assistance of a physician for the purpose of a dignified death at a time and manner of his or her choosing. The additional criteria required before the request can be granted are stringent and include one written and two oral requests at 15-day intervals followed by a 15-day waiting period to certify the person's desire to end his or her life. Two physicians must certify the diagnosis, prognosis, competency, and voluntary nature of the request. The individual must be counseled on alternatives and receive counseling from a pharmacist. If these criteria are met, the patient's request can be granted and he or she may receive a prescription of a lethal dose of a medication from the physician. The person then decides if and when the dose is taken, and it cannot be in the presence of the prescribing physician. Lethal injection or active euthanasia is not allowed. In 1998 the U.S. Attorney General tried various ways of preventing the enactment of this law; however, the voters' rights to make this decision have been upheld by the Supreme Court.

The impact of the Death with Dignity law has led to the establishment of universal hospice availability and an increase in providers' knowledge of pain and symptom man-

agement in Oregon. Between 1997 and 2003, only 57 per 100,000 persons were reported to have committed suicide. This number amounts to only ⅐ of 1% of all deaths. Eighty-nine percent of all persons who ingested a lethal dose of a medication were receiving hospice care. Although the majority of these persons had cancer, the actual percentage is greatest for persons with ALS (5%), compared with only 0.4% of all persons with cancer. It is interesting to note that 97% of those persons who elected to commit suicide were white (Lunge, et al., 2004).

Nurses have had strong opinions pro and con on the topic. The American Nurses Association position statement on assisted suicide was developed to provide nurses with a point of reference for discussion and understanding of the

Human Needs and Wellness Diagnoses

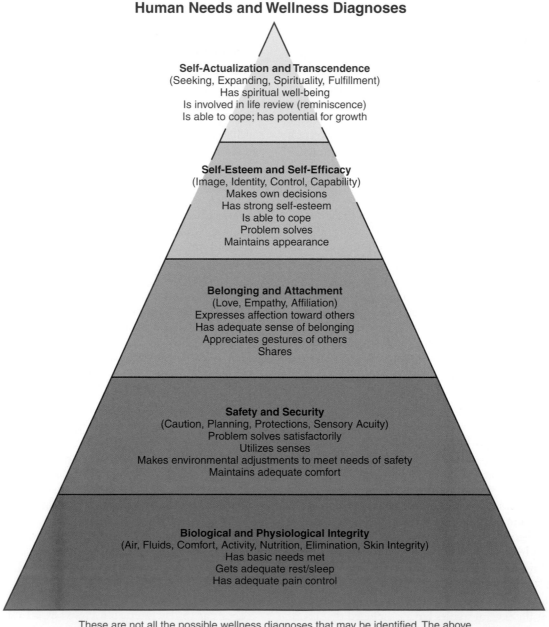

Self-Actualization and Transcendence
(Seeking, Expanding, Spirituality, Fulfillment)
Has spiritual well-being
Is involved in life review (reminiscence)
Is able to cope; has potential for growth

Self-Esteem and Self-Efficacy
(Image, Identity, Control, Capability)
Makes own decisions
Has strong self-esteem
Is able to cope
Problem solves
Maintains appearance

Belonging and Attachment
(Love, Empathy, Affiliation)
Expresses affection toward others
Has adequate sense of belonging
Appreciates gestures of others
Shares

Safety and Security
(Caution, Planning, Protections, Sensory Acuity)
Problem solves satisfactorily
Utilizes senses
Makes environmental adjustments to meet needs of safety
Maintains adequate comfort

Biological and Physiological Integrity
(Air, Fluids, Comfort, Activity, Nutrition, Elimination, Skin Integrity)
Has basic needs met
Gets adequate rest/sleep
Has adequate pain control

These are not all the possible wellness diagnoses that may be identified. The above are examples of nursing diagnoses that should be considered when planning care for the older adult.

many difficulties involved in the issue of a patient's request to terminate his or her life. The American Nurses Association advises nurses not to participate in assisted suicide, citing such action a "violation of the Code for Nurses with Interpretive Statements and the ethical traditions of the profession" (Canavan, 1996, p. 8). The nurse is involved in many end-of-life care situations because he or she is the primary care provider who implements decisions of others around end-of-life care. Such advice does not mean patients who want their life terminated should be abandoned.

Considerable confusion exists regarding terminology and interpretation of what effects the nurse's role may have. Many nurses believe that turning off the ventilator, turning off tube feedings, stopping intravenous fluids, or giving as much pain medication as needed when a possible side effect is death constitutes assisted suicide. Nurses must also consider the possibility that the withdrawal of devices such as feeding tubes and ventilators allows a natural, anticipated death to occur (Huang and Ahronheim, 2000; Kuebler and McKinnon, 2002).

The general trend in American law is toward greater freedom for the individual to choose when and how to die. Many people believe that patient-assisted suicide might soon be reality based on constitutional grounds of the right to privacy (Messinger, 1993) or the due process clause of the Fourteenth Amendment to the U.S. Constitution (Carter, 1996; Sedler, 1993; Wilkes, 1996). In the years ahead, nurses and nursing organizations will be challenged to rethink their approach to both terminal care and the choices individuals will make about their living and their dying.

KEY CONCEPTS

- Grief is an emotional and behavioral response to loss.
- Many theories or frameworks have been offered that outline grief responses. However, grief responses are individual.
- One never completely resolves grief. Instead, the individual incorporates the loss as a part of his or her life.
- Dying is a multifaceted active process. Everyone involved is affected: the one who is dying, the family, significant others, and the professional caregivers.
- The person with a terminal illness and the dying person attempts to complete tasks in the acute, chronic, and terminal phases of his or her illness.
- An individual is living until he or she has died.

CASE STUDY: Coping with Dying

Jesse was simply unable to believe that his wife was dying. The physician told Jesse that Jeannette was in the early stages of multiple myeloma, and she might die in less than a year or she might have remissions and live another decade. Jesse and his wife had worked hard all their lives and raised two sons. Now they were both retired and financially secure and thought the best years of their lives were ahead of them. However, both Jesse and Jeannette were the type who approached a problem head on. They gathered all the relevant material they could find about multiple myeloma and assiduously studied it. Jeannette said that she did not want to mention her problem to others because she thought that she was unable to deal with "their piteous cancer looks." She also stressed that she expected to have long remissions and to live to be 75 years of age, at least. So why trouble friends and family? As a result of her decision, Jesse was unable to share his fear and grief because he had promised to respect Jeannette's wishes in that regard. She began a series of chemotherapeutic drugs, and friends began to notice her lethargy. They began to worry about her, but she insisted, "I'm just fine." Six months passed with a steady downward course in Jeannette's condition. Her sons began to suspect she had a malignancy, and one son, Rob, asked outright, "Are you hiding a serious illness from us?" She denied it, but Rob also noticed that Jesse was withdrawing into himself and that he was drinking more than usual. Rob knew something was wrong but was at a loss. When Rob went to the family physician for his annual checkup, the office nurse said, "Oh, Rob, how is your mother doing?"

Discuss your rationale and feelings as the office nurse, and determine a plan of action that seems appropriate at this time. Develop a long-range plan of care for this family.

Based on the case study, develop a nursing care plan using the following procedure*:
- List Jeanette's comments that provide subjective data.
- List information that provides objective data.
- From these data, identify and state, using accepted format, two nursing diagnoses you determine are most significant to Jeanette at this time. List two of Jeanette's strengths that you have identified from the data.
- Determine and state outcome criteria for each diagnosis. These criteria must reflect some alleviation of the problem identified in the nursing diagnosis and must be stated in concrete and measurable terms.
- Plan and state one or more interventions for each diagnosed problem. Provide specific documentation of the sources used to determine the appropriate intervention. Plan at least one intervention that incorporates Jeanette's existing strengths.
- Evaluate the success of the intervention. Interventions must correlate directly with the stated outcome criteria to measure the outcome success.

Critical Thinking Questions

1. Considering the situation and the current regulations about the protection of patient privacy, how would you respond to the son's next question if you were the nurse?
2. As a nurse, how could you promote communication within this family to help them move toward open awareness?
3. What is your priority in attending to the needs of Jesse? Of Jeanette?

* Students are advised to refer to their nursing diagnosis text and identify possible or potential problems.

- The dying older adult is a living person, with all the same needs for good and natural relationships with people as others have.
- Hope is empowering; it generates courage and motivates action and achievement. The degree of hope that a dying individual possesses depends on a caring relationship with others.
- The health professional who cares for the dying must have outside interests, support systems, and emotional maturity before considering care of the dying.
- Hospice is a process or unique ideology that links the needs of the terminally ill, the family, and staff to fulfill the remainder of a dying individual's life by enabling or returning control to the dying person.
- Advance directives allow an individual control over life and death decisions by written communication and allow an appointed person to be his or her spokesperson when he or she is not able to communicate desires personally.
- Oregon is the first state in the United States to legalize assisted suicide in tightly controlled situations. As a result of the law, the care of the dying has improved.

RESEARCH QUESTIONS

Explore your responses to being given a terminal diagnosis. What coping mechanisms work for you?

With which level of awareness approach would you be most comfortable? As a nurse? As a patient?

If you believe that you are able, discuss your grief process when you dealt with the loss of someone special in your life.

Practice with a partner several methods that you will use to introduce the topic of dying with a client who is critically ill and is not expected to live.

Describe how you would deal with a dying person and his or her family when these family members are especially protective of each other.

Discuss and strategize how you would bring up the topic of advance directives.

What advance directive is legally recognized in your state?

Explore with family and friends their thoughts on completing an advance directive.

What nursing actions do you consider assisted suicide?

REFERENCES

Arbuckle NW, deVries B: The long-term effects of late life spousal and parental bereavement on personal functioning, *Gerontologist* 35(5):637, 1995.

Berrio MW, Levesque ME: Advance directives: most patients don't have one. Do yours? *Am J Nurs* 96(8):25, 1996.

Blackhall LJ et al: Ethnicity and attitude toward patient autonomy, *JAMA* 274(10):820-825, 1995.

Bowlby J: Process of mourning, *Int J Psychoanal* 42:317-340, 1961.

Brabant S et al: Grieving men: thoughts, feelings and behaviors following deaths of wives, *Hosp J* 8(4):33, 1992.

Canavan K: ANA advises nurses not to participate in assisted suicide, *Am Nurs* 28(4):8, 1996.

Carter SL: Rush to a lethal judgment, *Time Magazine*, July 2, 1996.

Corr CA et al: *Death and dying, life and living*, ed 3, Stamford City, Conn, 2000, Wadsworth.

DeSpelder LA, Strickland AL: *The last dance: encountering death and dying*, ed 4, Mountainview, Calif, 1996, Mayfield Publishing.

Dessonville CL et al: The role of anticipatory bereavement in the adjustment to widowhood in the elderly, *Gerontologist* 23(special issue):309, 1983.

Doka KJ: Disenfranchised grief. In Doka KJ, editor: *Disenfranchised grief: recognizing hidden sorrow*, Lexington, Mass, 1989, Lexington Books.

Donley R: Spiritual dimensions of health care: nursing's mission, *Nurs Health Care* 12(4):178-183, 1991.

Douglas R, Brown HN: Patients' attitudes toward advance directives, *J Nurs Scholarsh* 34(1):61, 2002, Sigma Theta Tau International.

Engel G: Grief and grieving, *Am J Nurs* 64:93, 1967.

Erlangsen A et al: Loss of partner and suicide risk among the oldest old: a population-based register study, *Age Ageing* 33(4):378-383, 2004.

Federal Interagency Forum on Aging-Related Statistics: *Older Americans 2000: key indicators of well-being*, Washington, DC, 2002. Administration on Aging. (website): *www.aoa.gov*.

Fortner BV, Neimeyer RA: Death anxiety in older adults: a quantitative review, *Death Stud* 23:387-411, 1999.

Futterman EH et al: Parental anticipatory mourning. In Schoenberg B et al, editors: *Psychosocial aspects of terminal care*, New York, 1970, Columbia University Press.

Giacquinta B: Helping families face the crisis of cancer, *Am J Nurs* 77(10):1585-1588, 1977.

Glaser B, Strauss A: *Awareness of dying*, Chicago, 1963, AVC.

Glaser BG, Strauss AL: *Time for dying*, Chicago, 1968, Aldine.

Goldstein C et al: Research guiding practice related to cultural issues at end-of-life care, *Geriatr Nurs* 25(1):58-59, 2004.

Habel M: Advance directives, a long way to go, *NurseWeek* 4(22):21, October 22, 2001.

Hanson LC et al: A quality improvement intervention to increase palliative care in nursing homes, *J Palliat Med* 8(3):576-584, 2005.

Havens GAD: Differences in execution/nonexecution of advance directives by community dwelling adults, *Res Nurs Health* 23(4):319, 2000.

Hegge M, Fischer C: Grief responses of senior and elderly widows: practice implications, *J Gerontol Nurs* 26(2):25-43, 2000.

Hickey SS: Enabling hope, *Cancer Nurs* 9(3):133-137, 1986.

Hopmeyer E, Werk A: A comparative study of family bereavement groups, *Death Stud* 18:243, 1994.

Horacek BJ: Toward a more viable model of grieving and consequences for older persons, *Death Stud* 15(5):459, 1991.

Huang ZB, Ahronheim JC: Nutrition and hydration in terminally ill patients: an update, *Clin Geriatr Med* 16(2):313, 2000.

Irish DP et al: *Ethnic variations in dying, death, and grief: diversity in universality*, Philadelphia, 1993, Taylor & Francis.

Jett KF: *The loss response model*, Unpublished manuscript, 2004.

Kaprio J et al: Mortality after bereavement: a prospective study of 95,647 widowed persons, *Am J Public Health* 77(3):283-287, 1987.

Kayser-Jones J: The experience of dying: an ethnographic nursing home study, *Gerontologist* 42(special no. 3):11-19, 2002.

Kayser-Jones J et al: A model long-term care hospice unit: care, community and compassion, *Geriatr Nurs* 26(10:16-20, 2005.

Kelly JD: Grief: re-forming life's story, *J Palliat Care* 8(2):33, 1992.

Krohn B: When death is near, helping families cope, *Geriatr Nurs* 19(5):276, 1998.

Kübler-Ross E: *On death and dying*, New York, 1969, MacMillan.

Kuebler S, McKinnon S: Dehydration. In Kuebler KK et al, editors: *End-of-life care: clinical practice guidelines*, Philadelphia, 2002, Saunders.

Lipson JG et al: *Culture and nursing care: a pocket guide*, San Francisco, 1996, UCSF Nursing Press.

Lund DA et al: Gender differences through two years of bereavement among the elderly, *Gerontologist* 26(3):314, 1986.

Lunge R et al: Oregon's Death with Dignity law and euthanasia in the Netherlands: factual disputes, 2004, Vermont Legislation Council (website): www.leg.state.vt.us/reports/04Death/Death_with_Dignity_Report.htm. Accessed July 17, 2007.

Manor O, Eisenbach Z: Mortality after spousal loss: are there sociodemographic differences? *Soc Sci Med* 56(2):405-413, 2003.

Martin TL, Doka KJ: Masculine grief. In Doka KJ, editor: *Living with grief after sudden loss: suicide, homicide, accident, heart attack, stroke*, Washington, DC, 1996, Hospice Foundation of America.

Martin TL, Doka KJ: Revisiting masculine grief. In Doka KJ, Davidson JD, editors: *Living with grief: who are we, how we grieve*, Washington, DC, 1998, Hospice Foundation of America.

Martocchio BC: *Living while dying*, Bowie, Md, 1982, RJ Brady.

Matzo ML, Sherman DW: *Gerontologic palliative care nursing*, St Louis, 2004, Mosby.

Mazanec P, Tyler MK: Cultural considerations in end-of-life care: how ethnicity, age & spirituality affect decisions when death is imminent, *Am J Nurs* 103(3):50-59, 2003.

McClain-Jacobson C et al: Belief in an afterlife, spiritual well-being and end-of-life despair in patients with advanced cancer, *Gen Hosp Psychiatry* 26(6):484-486, 2004.

Meier DE et al: Marked improvement in recognition and completion of health care proxies: a randomized controlled trial of counseling by hospital patient representatives, *Arch Intern Med* 156(11):1227, 1996.

Merlevede E et al: Perceptions, needs and mourning reactions of bereaved relatives confronted with a sudden unexplained death, *Resuscitation* 61(3):341-348, 2004.

Messinger TJ: A gentle and easy death: from ancient Greece to beyond Cruzan—toward a reasoned legal response to the societal dilemma of euthanasia, *Denver Univ Law Rev* 71(1):229, 1993.

Mezey M: Geriatric nursing standard of practice protocol: advance directives—nurses helping to protect patient rights, *Geriatr Nurs* 17(5):204, 1996.

Mezey M et al: Making the PSDA work for the elderly, *Generations* xviii(4):13, 1994.

Mezey MD et al: Why hospital patients do and do not execute an advance directive, *Nurs Outlook* 48:165, 2000.

Mittleman M: Taking grief to heart, *Harvard Health Letter* 21(8):8, 1996.

Morrison RS: Barriers to completion of health care proxies: an examination of ethnic differences, *Arch Intern Med* 158(12):2439, 1998.

Munn JC et al: Is hospice associated with improved end-of-life care in nursing homes and assisted living facilities, *J Am Geriatr Soc* 54(3):490-495, 2006.

Neimeyer RA et al: Psychological research on death attitudes: an overview and evaluation, *Death Stud* 28:309-340, 2004.

Parks CM, Weiss RS: *Recovery from bereavement*, New York, 1983, Basic Books.

Pattison EM: The experience of dying. In Pattison EM (Ed.), *The experience of dying*. Englewood Cliffs, NJ, 1977, Prentice-Hall.

Pietruszka FM: Management of bereavement in the elderly, *Phys Assist* 16(4):31, 1992.

Richter J: Support: a resource during crisis of mate loss, *J Gerontol Nurs* 13(11):18, 1987.

Schaefer C et al: Mortality following bereavement and the effects of a shared environment, *Am J Epidemiol* 141(12):1177-1178, 1995.

Schmitt L: *The right to choose: capacity study of demented residents in nursing homes* (Executive summary), Chicago, 1996, Franciscan Sisters of the Poor Hospital Systems.

Sedler RA: The constitution and hastening inevitable death, *Hasting Cent Rep* 23(5):20, 1993.

Shield RR: Liminality in an American nursing home: the endless transition. In Sokolovsky J, editor: *The cultural context of aging: worldwide perspectives*, Westport, Conn, 1997, Bergin & Garvey.

Spector R: *Cultural diversity in health and illness*, ed 6, Upper Saddle River, NJ, 2003, Prentice-Hall.

Steele L: Risk factor profile for bereaved spouses, *Death Stud* 16(5):387, 1992.

Stillman D et al: Staff perceptions concerning barriers and facilitators to end-of-life care in nursing homes, *Geriatr Nurs* 26(4):259-264, 2005.

Stroebe M, Schut H: The dual process model of coping with bereavement: rationale and description, *Death Stud* 23:197, 1999.

Thibault JM et al: Conceptual framework for assessing spiritual functioning and fulfillment of older adults in long-term care settings, *J Relig Gerontol* 7(4):29, 1991.

Ulrich LK: The challenge of hospice care, *Bull Am Protestant Hosp Assoc* 21:6, 1978.

Weenolsen P: *The art of dying*, New York, 1996, St Martin's Press.

Weisman A: *Coping with cancer*. New York, 1979, McGraw-Hill.

Weisman A: *The coping capacity: on the nature of being mortal*, New York, 1984, Human Sciences Press.

Weitzen S et al: Factors associated with site of death: a national study of where people die, *Med Care* 41(2):323-335, 2003.

Wilkes P: The next pro-lifers, *New York Times Magazine*, July 21, 1996.

Worden JW: *Grief counseling and grief therapy: a handbook for mental health practitioners*, ed 2, New York, 1991, Springer.

Zilberfein F: Coping with death: anticipatory grief and bereavement, *Generations* xxxiii(1):69, 1999.

CHAPTER 27

Self-Actualization, Spirituality, and Transcendence

Theris A. Touhy

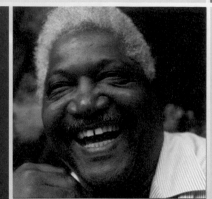
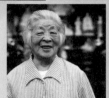
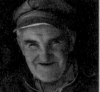

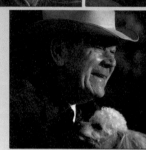

A STUDENT LEARNS

Well, I always went to church with my parents when I was a child, but it was really boring. Now, I sometimes go with my Grandmother to make her happy. I see how important it is to her, and I wonder if it will be important to me when I get really old. I'm just too busy right now.

Lori, age 22

AN ELDER SPEAKS

This is a real problem! I have three children and don't want them to squabble over my things when I'm gone. I would like it if they would each choose something special that would remind them of me, but every time I bring it up they cut me off and won't talk about it. I know there will be a big fight over the piano!

Mabel, age 74

LEARNING OBJECTIVES

On completion of this chapter, the reader will be able to:

1. Provide a comprehensive definition of self-actualization and identify several qualities to expect in self-actualized elders.
2. Describe several learning opportunities that are available to elders and the special characteristics and growth factors predominant in each.
3. Discuss the nursing role in relation to the self-actualization of elders.
4. Describe several evidences of transcendence as experienced by older people.
5. Specify several types of creative self-expression, including those that are less often visible to the public.
6. Understand the meaning of spirituality in the lives of older people and discuss nursing responses to facilitate spiritual well-being.
7. Define the concept of legacy and name several types of legacies and what the nurse can do to facilitate their expression.

Self-actualization, spirituality, and transcendence are vague, ambiguous terms that mean whatever the theorist thinks. These expressions also serve as umbrella terms for other conditions and situations that are addressed throughout this chapter. These terms overlap a great deal, but we have attempted to tease out the meanings for the reader, knowing that the perception of the reader will cast a particular interpretation that we may not have thought or intended. These conditions are ineffable, within the awareness of the individual but often inexpressible. We have used Maslow as our guide to comprehend self-actualization and Jung and many others to grasp transcendence. Spirituality embodies religion, faith, and beliefs that sustain individuals through the vicissitudes of life. Why, if these concepts are so obscure, do we include them as the final chapter in a text for nurses working with elders? Because these concepts are the life tasks of aging, seldom fully approached earlier. Concerns of the young are to become established as adults; middle-aged persons are overwhelmed with the requirements of success and survival. Ferreting out the reason for being and the meaning of life is the concern of elders.

Nurses will likely see numerous older people who are apparently not seeking any of these esoteric states of existence and have never tried to cultivate their deepest *inner*

Special thanks to Priscilla Ebersole, the previous edition contributor, for her content contributions to this chapter.

nature (Maslow, 1970). We live in a mechanistic, scientifically based culture in which cultivation of immeasurable states of being has not been necessarily highly regarded or regarded at all. The dramatic increase in the population of older people has been considered a problem to be solved in an era of *dwindling resources*. Attempting to sort, dissect, and classify everything is a hazard of our society. In all of human efforts for several millennia, we have not been able to grasp or dissect the soul. Therefore, with effrontery and apologies, we will devote this last chapter to just that! I have many times approached this subject incorrectly by asking individuals what it is like to be old. Now that I am old, *what it is like* seems too concrete. What is the meaning of this stage of life? Every nurse must ask this question of his or her older clients, friends, and parents. Do not ask on your way out the door. For many people, this notion will take some pondering; for some, it will open the door of their later lives just a crack; others will be enlightened and will teach you a great deal.

SELF-ACTUALIZATION

Self-actualization is the highest expression of one's individual potential and implies inner motivation that has been freed to express the most unique self or the "authentic person" (Maslow, 1959, p. 3). The crux of self-actualization is defining life in such a way as to allow room for continual discovery of self. Self-actualization is an evolution of maturity and emotions that many writers have identified in one way or another. We have chosen Maslow's model because it moves one forward in continual self-development toward the most unique possibilities. Maslow's model can be viewed as a development model, a need model, and an evolutionary humanistic model that within existential psychology is investigated through phenomenology. This idea, simply stated, means human potential is unknown and unknowable, but our present understanding is based on analysis of individual experiences, always unique to that person. A child's first need is to be given food, shelter, safety, security, and love. An adult, who has moved to sufficient levels of maturity to give to the child, fulfills this need. In adolescence, the focus on self reaches narcissistic proportions and development is powered by the need to be accepted. As one experiences love outside the family, goals enlarge. A pyramidal model of need appears to convey a narrowing, rising principle. True human development might be viewed as an inverted triangle. We might conceptualize energy that is focused in an intense, narrow manner on lower-level needs, becoming less focused and intense as one moves upward in maturity. The inverted pyramid concept shows development as a process of enlarging concerns (Figure 27-1). At the top level, universal and world concerns and ethics transcend self, family, community, and nation.

Anywhere along the developmental continuum, concerns may again become constricted. A self-actualized person may, under threat of illness, become self-centered and

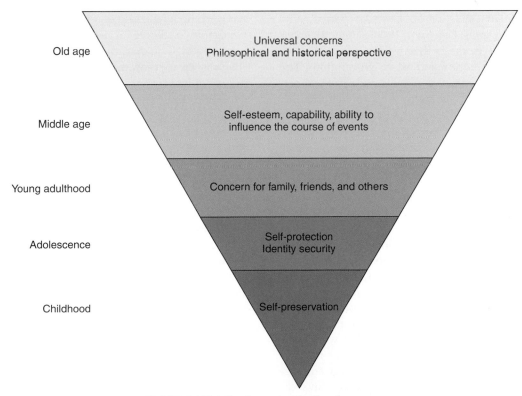

Old age — Universal concerns
Philosophical and historical perspective

Middle age — Self-esteem, capability, ability to influence the course of events

Young adulthood — Concern for family, friends, and others

Adolescence — Self-protection
Identity security

Childhood — Self-preservation

FIGURE 27-1 Development: expansion of concerns.

BOX 27-1   Traits of Self-Actualized People

- Time competent: The person uses past and future to live more fully in the present.
- Inner directed: The person's source of direction depends on internal forces more than on others.
- Flexible: The person can react situationally, without unreasonable restrictions.
- Sensitive to self: The person is responsive to his or her own feelings.
- Spontaneous: The person is able and willing to be self.
- Values self: The person accepts and demonstrates strengths as a person.
- Accepts self: The person approves of self, in spite of weaknesses or deficiencies.
- Positively views others: The person sees both the bad and the good in others as essentially good and constructive.
- Positively views life: The person sees the opposites of life as meaningfully related.
- Acceptance of aggressiveness: The person is able to accept own feelings of anger and aggressiveness.
- Capable of intimate contact: The person is able to develop warm interpersonal relationships with others.

narrow. The task of nursing is to assist these individuals in achieving their highest potential within their present situation, "maximizing the potential of which an individual is capable within the environment where functioning occurs" (Hemstrom, 2000, p. 42).

McLeod (2001) interviewed Sue Bender regarding her spiritual trilogy, *Plain and Simple, Everyday Sacred,* and, most recently, *The Daring That Starts From Within.* Bender's thesis in all of these works is that we are constrained by self-judgment, past memories, and future expectations. The need to be and look good to others may stifle the real person who can emerge with *daring* to face our self-imposed limits and be who we are. Bender's message is particularly relevant to aging individuals in that she challenges herself and others to accept our *limping* selves, with the assurance that the body is a healer and teacher if we remain in the present and approach ourselves with a caring spirit and body awareness. Bender challenges us to not become a smaller person with age but to grow new habits of accepting who we are.

A critical consideration in developing self-actualization is an underlying sense of mastery and a sense of coherence in the life situation. This effort depends to a large extent on individual attributes, as well as self-esteem. Informal social support is essential for most people, though some relatively isolated individuals have such a strong sense of self that they reach a satisfactory self-actualized state with few supports (Forbes, 2001). In this unit, we hope to expose the nurse to the myriad evidences of self-actualization in old age and suggest ways in which the nurse can assist older people in seeking their own unique way of living and growing. The focus is

on nursing actions that may encourage elders to seek new possibilities within themselves. Holistic health practices, examined in depth in Chapter 3, are somewhat relevant to self-actualization because they are the first step in acknowledging one's active participation in becoming truly whole. For additional thoughts on wellness and self-actualization, see the wellness paradigm in Chapter 3.

Characteristics of the Self-Actualized

In old age, threats to self-esteem are strong if value is measured only by attainment, containment, power, and influence. Ethics, values, humor, courage, altruism, and integrity flourish in people who continue to grow toward self-actualization. Numerous other attributions can be mentioned. We focus only on those qualities that seem most pertinent to the older people that health care professionals are serving (Box 27-1).

Courage. Courage is the quality of mind or spirit that enables a person to conquer fear and despair in the face of difficulty, danger, pain, or uncertainty. We believe that facing a long, painful, and restricted existence requires the highest level of courage. An older man with diabetes, amputations, and failing vision sits in his room at the retirement home, looking out the window for hours each day, for weeks, months, and years. This is courage. An older lady crippled with arthritis attends her ailing spouse, who no longer recognizes her. This is courage.

When asking older people how they keep going day by day, various answers are given. No one has ever said to me, "It is because I am courageous." Older people need to be told. A gold star can be given to people who have lived and survived the long battle of a mediocre existence. In current vernacular, mediocre means *ordinary.* These individuals are not ordinary. The origins of the word mediocre translate to "halfway up a stony mountain" (Merriam-Webster, 1974, p. 274). Many elders are enduring the climb up a stony mountain, and they are the epitome of courage. Memorials are made for people who die in battle, but few monuments are raised to those who courageously wake every morning with no great purpose or challenge to push them out of bed. Believing that older people are unable to be self-actualized unless they are energetic, healthy, and wealthy is a mistake. The capacity of the spirit to find meaning in existence is often remarkable. Nurses may ask, "What sustains you in your present situation?"

Altruism. A high degree of helping behaviors is present in many older people. The very old will remember the Great Depression and the altruism that kept people physically and spiritually alive. Neighbor helped neighbor long before the government came to the rescue. Apparently, a sense of meaning in life is strongly tied to survival and is derived from the conviction of, in some way, being needed by others. Many nurses are in the field because of altruistic motives and can understand the importance. This idea might be discussed with the elder.

Volunteering often involves new role development and endeavors that expand one's awareness. When volunteer services are considered as a means of personal enrichment and an expression of altruism, it is important for the elder to augment some latent interest areas and launch into pursuits perhaps unavailable earlier because of time constraints or other commitments. Nurses may question elders about latent interests and talents that they may want to cultivate. Volunteer activities are discussed in Chapter 20.

Humor. Metcalf (1993) explains humor: originating in the Latin root *humor,* meaning *fluid and flexible,* able to flow around and wear away obstacles. In the same way that water sustains our life and well-being, humor sustains our mental well-being. Cousins (1979) and many other researchers have recognized the importance of humor in recovery from illness. The physiological effects of humor stimulate production of catecholamines and hormones and increase pain tolerance by releasing endorphins.

Elders often initiate humor, and in our seriousness, we may overlook the dry wit or, worse, perceive it as confusion. Older people are not a humorless group and frequently laugh at themselves. Objections to jokes about old age seem to emanate from the young far more than the old. Perhaps the old, from the vantage point of a lifetime, can more clearly see human predicaments. Ego transcendence (Peck, 1955) allows one to step back and view the self and situation without the intensity and despair of the egocentric individual.

Continuous Moral Development. The moral development of mankind, on an individual and collective basis, has been of interest to philosophers and religious leaders throughout history. The driving forces of morality are love (Plato) and intellect (Aristotle).

Kohlberg's refinements of his original theories have focused on the evidence, derived from autobiographies, that in maturity, transformations of moral outlook take place. Kohlberg posited old age as a seventh stage of moral development that goes beyond reasoning and reaches awareness of one's relative participation in universal morality. This stage of moral development involves identification with a more enduring moral perspective than that of one's own life span (Kohlberg and Power, 1981). This effort involves moral expansion and the exemplary impact of the fully developing elder on the following generations, born and unborn. We have come to believe that these exemplary lives may be the most important function of elders as we decry the honor and recognition given to individuals who seem to have little integrity or reliability. Each individual carries a mass of motivations and desires. Some people are stunted, and some will flourish. Youngsters must have models of honorable, truthful, and honest elders if we hope to cultivate these qualities in society and human experience.

Self-Renewal

Self-renewal is an ongoing process that ideally continues through adult life as one becomes self-actualized (Hudson,

1999). According to Hudson, self-renewal involves the following:

- Commitment to beliefs
- Connecting to the world
- Times of solitude
- Episodic breaks from responsibility
- Contact with the natural world
- Creative self-expression
- Adaptation to changes
- Learning from down times

Travel

Travel is a route many elders take to achieve knowledge while increasing pleasure and renewal through new experiences. The self-actualization in travel often occurs as one becomes immersed in another culture and sees facets of the human experience through an unfamiliar lens.

The number of traveling elders is a reflection of the increased affluence and energy of older people today. Intergenerational travel seems to be increasing, with many elders traveling with grandchildren. The Grandtravel Agency and Elderhostel offer vacations specially designed for grandparents and grandchildren (*www.elderhostel.org*).

For people who have a strong desire to travel and to seek new lands and scenes, many opportunities are available if they are physically and economically able. For elderly who are less affluent and content to stay closer to home territory, many organized low-cost tours explore unusual sites near one's area. The American Bed and Breakfast Association (*www.abba.com*) can provide information regarding providers nationwide who belong to the organization and offer inexpensive lodging and breakfast.

The personal effects of travel are as variable as the individuals and the places they select to see. Nursing involvement will be most useful in addressing potential problems and assisting elders in planning ahead for contingencies. Pets must be placed appropriately, house-sitting services are sometimes necessary, and physical limitations must be considered (Box 27-2). People often find travel after retirement a vehicle for learning and growing. Careful planning will make travel safer and more enjoyable. Suggestions for travel are summarized in Box 27-3.

Elderhostel. The Elderhostel program, an adult education program originally based on the youth hostel concept, was originated by Marty Knowlton in 1974 at the University of New Hampshire and now offers a wide variety of programs around the world, in addition to those in the United States and Canada. Elderhostel offers opportunities for service, as well as learning. In addition, the program has recently added a discussion board to its well-established website (*www.elderhostel.org*) (Elderhostel, 2003).

Elderhostel is a nonprofit international program that provides low-cost room and board and specially designed classes for elders on college campuses, conference centers, state and national parks, museums, theaters, environmental outdoor education centers, and other sites. The program mails its

---

BOX 27-2 Considerations for Travel

- Whom will you contact in an emergency? Is this person's phone number in your billfold? Is your blood type also noted?
- What health care and travel insurance coverage do you have? Is the coverage adequate for unforeseen illness?
- Do you have sufficient medications, hearing aid batteries, and extra eyeglasses?
- What immunizations will you need, and where can you obtain them?
- Do you have a safe place on your body for money?
- From where are you obtaining prior information about the places you intend to go?
- Are the areas you wish to see accessible in terms of your mobility and energy?
- Do you desire accommodations similar to those provided by locals or Western-type hotels?
- What is the usual weather during the time you will be visiting?
- Have you considered changes in water, altitude, and climate and how this might affect you?

BOX 27-3 Travel Tips for Elders

- Many organizations offer special group rates and tours planned for elders.
- Travel agencies can give information about reduced rates for charter flights or about less-popular travel months. Choose the off-season to avoid crowds and to get best rates.
- Some air carriers have reduced rates for the elderly or handicapped.
- Many countries offer special rates to older travelers. Information should be obtained from the tourist bureau of the countries on the itinerary.
- Medicare coverage does not extend outside the United States and its territories; however, many European countries have national health services that are extended to travelers. Supplementary health insurance is a good idea.
- Passports should be applied for well in advance if birth certificates are not readily available. Visas are required for many countries.
- Immunizations are required to travel in certain countries. Check with the U.S. Public Health Service.
- Take a medical travel kit containing sufficient medication for any chronic condition; first aid equipment; medications for diarrhea, dyspepsia, and nausea; an extra pair of eyeglasses; and records of medical problems, medications, physician contact information, allergies, and blood type.
- Take extras of equipment needed, such as hearing aid batteries, eyeglasses, braces, and orthopedic shoes.

---

catalogs to over 500,000 people, and each year nearly 300,000 people older than 55 years or who have a spouse older than 55 years participate in this phenomenally successful educational program for older adults. About one half of people who participate in the Elderhostel program live in dormitories and eat in college dining halls while taking brief noncredit college courses taught by regular faculty members or specialists in a particular field.

The national Elderhostel concept is a response to the awareness that the elderly want to continue learning and contributing in their later years. Some scholarships are offered for programs within the United States. Some of the reasons for attending Elderhostel are (1) change—opportunity to go somewhere or do something different; (2) time—short time frame for learning; (3) cost—low fixed cost; (4) courses—suitable course content; (5) absence of evaluation—no tests or homework; and (6) learning—opportunities to develop new interests and re-explore old ones. Programs of special interest include hiking and biking trips, historic houses, folk colleges, and study cruises. The opportunities for study address almost every interest one can imagine. Classes, taught by academics, specialists, and local experts, cover a broad range of subjects, such as jazz, art, religion, astronomy, history, and mythology. Older citizens who may wish intellectual stimulation and personal enrichment should be encouraged to investigate these programs. We encourage nurses to become aware of programs offered for elders in their community.

Learning and Growing in Late Life

Opportunities for elders to learn are available in many formal and informal modes: self-teaching, college attendance, participation in seminars and conferences, public television programs, videotapes, courses via telecommunications, and countless other modes. The Internet has become one of the major vehicles of learning for older adults. Part of the nurse's function is to be informed and assist an elder in finding the learning mode and setting that is appropriate to his or her need or desire.

In most universities, older people are taking classes of all types. Fees are usually lower for individuals older than 60 years, and elders may choose to work toward a degree and complete all assignments or audit classes just for enrichment and enjoyment. Many opportunities are available also for distance learning and external degrees.

On-campus classrooms provide older persons the opportunity to share their perspective from a long-range view and for youth to interject theirs of immediacy and energy. The results are increased positive attitude toward older people among the youth and elevated self-esteem in the elders who compete and achieve academic success, as well as increased understanding of the concerns of young adults. (See Chapter 23 for further discussion of learning in late life.)

Education for Elders with Special Needs

Homebound Elderly. Education has become accessible to many homebound individuals through public television, teleconferencing, the Internet, and radio. Many methods are available for implementing educational outreach programs. With increasingly adaptable telecommunications

---

BOX 27-4   **Suggestions for Older People as Advocates of the Public Interest**

- Identify and document the social issue, problem, or need. Providers delivering services to individuals should record cases, instances of critical need, scope, extent of deprivation, alienation, and that which needs to be changed.
- Bring together the victims of discrimination, abuse, and oppression to discuss their problems, understand their situation, and examine the interaction between personal need and public response.
- Raise the consciousness of victims, and educate them about the societal aspects, roots, and causes of their dilemmas.
- Organize victims to develop support groups for mutual support and empowerment, to confront oppressors, and to find local support from established bodies and agencies (insiders!).
- Map strategies for action, including new models for dealing with particular issues, legislative initiatives, court action, and forming coalitions of groups with similar problems.
- Go public: organize a rally with posters, speeches, marches to public places where public officials, interested people,

- agency heads, and boards can become aware and be held accountable. Go before television cameras with street theater. Go to press with well-prepared press releases.
- Present testimony in public hearings: set up e-mail and telephone campaigns pressing for redress and change.
- Take stock of your advances or setbacks, evaluate results, and consider the next steps.
- Report back to groups for their information and encouragement. Keep communication open with members and coalitions.
- Draft legislation, or prepare for legal action in the courts. Marshal arguments; collect cases, including horror stories; and evoke interest.
- Celebrate victories, even the small ones. Coverage in the press and on television may be significant to successes. Even failures should be recognized and evaluated.
- Regroup to fight on with increased knowledge, broader impact, and enlarged constituencies!

Data from Kuhn M: Advocacy in this new age, *Aging* 3:297, Jul/Aug, 1979.

---

technology and cost reductions, these opportunities are becoming common.

Reading for Self-Development. Bond and Miller (1987) call *reading* an ageless activity and find that institutionalized elders often much prefer the individual, passive involvement in reading to the group activities that are planned for them. Group reading and discussion can also be enjoyable, as demonstrated in the Great Books discussion groups that meet routinely in many libraries. When an array of books is available, many older people find them sustaining. Books extend boundaries imposed by physical limitations, allow exploration into untouched arenas of thought, and enrich the individual. For many elders, reading has been a major pleasure throughout life and, common as it seems, should not be underestimated as a form of self-discovery and actualization.

Many libraries across the country have developed creative programs to serve elders. Some of these programs include talking books for the blind, large-print books and magazines, mail delivery to the homebound, low-vision reading aids, 24-hour audio reader service through a closed-circuit radio station, kits designed to provoke reminiscing, and one-to-one reading service in several languages.

COLLECTIVE ACTUALIZATION

The collective power of self-actualized older people has already brought about many changes in society. *Power* is a term describing the capacity of an individual or group to accomplish something, to take command, to exert authority, and to influence. The self-actualized older person is

powerful and confident. Power is the gateway to resources and recognition.

The age-equality movement, older citizens returning to school, and the revolution of older people in movements such as the Gray Panthers have produced major changes in the status and recognition of older people. Gray Panthers recognize that issues of aging are not narrow or exclusive but, rather, are representative of human rights for people of all ages.

Maggie Kuhn (1979), founder of the Gray Panthers, died in 1995 at the age of 89, but her beliefs and followers survive. Kuhn perceived that the issues confronting older people are not those of self-interest but, rather, as "elders of the tribe," the old should seek "survival of the tribe" (Kuhn, 1979, p. 3). Box 27-4 presents steps suggested by Kuhn by which older people can be advocates of the public interest.

Politics and Power

Older people are a powerful political group. Older voters generally recognize their power, as do politicians. Elders can be counted on to vote, but their voting behaviors demonstrate their diversity. Aside from issues of Medicare and Social Security, elders do not form strong voting blocks because they are individualistic. However, any politician who wishes to remain in office must gently manipulate sacrosanct programs such as Social Security and Medicare. Older voters are often more concerned about a candidate's character and experience than about party affiliation. Hooyman and Kiyak (2005) discuss the concept of generational investment and the politics of *new aging*, which seek to unite all age-groups in identifying how all generations contribute to a new society. In the new politics, advocacy and lobbying should be redirected from special interest issues toward policies and programs that benefit all age-groups and future generations.

Nurses attuned to the political concerns of elders will find that these concerns are numerous and include the following:

- Comprehensive health care in rural areas
- Available mental health services
- Supports for their caregivers
- Affordable medications
- Transportation adapted to their needs
- Better training and screening of service providers
- Concern about the shortage of nurses

CREATIVITY

Creativity is a bridge between the growing self and the transcending of self. Creativity may be the transit mechanism between self-actualization (the reaching of one's highest potential) and the step beyond, to transcend the limitations of ego. "Creativity has always been at the heart of our experience as human beings…this need for creativity never ends" (Perlstein, 2006, p. 5). American culture has neglected to recognize the innate creativity in elders who are too often viewed as debilitated, in need of medical attention, and the focus of societal problems. Recently, our understanding of aging has expanded to a view that older people possess unique strengths and wisdom. The American Society on Aging has included this focus in its new strategic plan, and the National Center for Creative Aging, established in 2001, is dedicated to fostering the relationship between creative expression and quality of life for older people. *Generations*, journal of the American Society on Aging, devoted an entire issue to aging and the arts (30[1]: entire issue, 2006).

Emphasis is renewed on the relationship between arts and creative expression and well-being and health in aging (Cohen, 2006; Perlstein, 2006). "The Creativity and Aging Study is the first formal experimental study investigating the influence of professionally conducted, participatory arts programs on the general health, mental health, and social activities of older people" (Cohen, 2006, p. 11). Preliminary results indicate that participation in the arts programs has positive effects on physical health, independence, and morale when compared with the control group (Cohen, 2006).

Products of creativity are less important than creative attitudes. Curiosity, inquisitiveness, wonderment, puzzlement, and craving for understanding are creative attitudes. Much of the natural creative imagination of childhood is subdued by enculturation. In old age, some people seem able to break free of excessive enculturation and again express their free spirit when practical matters no longer demand their sole attention.

Creativity is often considered in terms of the arts, literature, and music. A truly self-actualized person may express creativity in any activity. Breaking through the habitual or traditional mode into authentic expression of self is creativity, whether it is through cooking, cleaning, planting,

poetry, art, or teaching. Creative expression does not necessarily mean that the older person has to create a work of art. Subtler ways of expressing creativity are present even in the frailest of older people. Consider Priscilla Ebersole's description of Catherine at 100 years old and living in a nursing home:

> Catherine was self-actualized and creative to the extent possible. Her physical constraints were enormous: she had no material assets, her range of activity was limited to her small cubicle in a skilled nursing facility, and her body was frail. However, her spirit was strong, and she knew and used her potential. Catherine's creativity was expressed at each meal when she rearranged, mixed, and added to her food. She carefully chopped a pickle and sprinkled it on her cottage cheese and added a little honey to her applesauce. Each meal was a small adventure. Several friends would visit regularly and bring Catherine small items she enjoyed. They could always count on being entertained with creatively embroidered tales of the past. The gifts they brought were always used in extraordinary ways. A scarf might be tied around her head. Powder, perfume, books, and other things would be bartered for favors from staff members or given as gifts. Her radio brought news of the day interspersed with classical music. Catherine created a milieu in which she enjoyed life and maintained her self-esteem. That she was self-actualized was never in doubt. Her artistry overflowed in myriad small gestures.

Creative Arts for the Elderly

Maximizing the use of self in the later years in unique ways might be termed *creative self-actualization*. Many individuals will need the stimulus of an interested person to uncover latent interests and talents. Other people will need encouragement to try new avenues of self-expression—some will be fitting for them and others not. Several ideas are presented here for nurses working with older people who may need an introduction to creative use of leisure time.

Many aspects of the developmental needs of older people are met by artistic expressions. Among these achievements are (1) conflict resolution, (2) clarification of thoughts and feelings, (3) creation of balance and an inner order, (4) a sense of being in control of the external world, (5) creation of something positive from defeating experiences or in the face of paralyzing depression, (6) artistic communication as an integral part of human experience, and (7) the sustenance of human integrity. Wikstrom (2004, p. 30) suggests that art and aesthetics "help individuals know themselves, become more alive to human conditions, provide a new way of looking at themselves and the world, and offer opportunities for participation in new visual and auditory experiences." Each person has a private, symbolic, feeling world that can be brought out by certain expressive activities.

The creative process is any activity in which the unconscious can be expressed in an integrated unique manner. To accomplish this task, an atmosphere of trust is essential. Trust is attained through rules, structure, and acceptance of all efforts without approval or disapproval. When this atmosphere is provided, creative expressions begin to occur. At that time, the facilitator needs to relax rules and structure and cultivate individualistic expressions. Useful concepts and guidelines for people who wish to involve the elderly in creative artistic expressions are noted in Boxes 27-5 and 27-6.

Creative Arts and People with Dementia

Creative and expressive activities are not limited to the cognitively intact elder. Art, poetry, dance, music, drama, and storytelling activities are therapeutic interventions that offer great value to people with dementia. According to Bastings (2006, p. 17):

> To people with dementia, the arts bring tools that enable them to express themselves and their vision of the world. The arts operate on an emotional level, one needn't have

control of rational language to write a poem, create a dance, or take a photograph. Where rational language and factual memory have failed people with dementia, the arts offer an avenue for communication and connection with caregivers, loved ones, and the greater world.

The National TimeSlips Project (Bastings, 2006) is an example of a creative storytelling program designed for people with dementia (see Chapter 23). Arts for Alzheimer's, Arts for the Aged, and the Age Exchange Theater are other examples of creative arts programs for people with dementia. At the Louis and Anne Green Memory and Wellness Center in the Christine E. Lynn College of Nursing at Florida Atlantic University, the "Artful Memories" program provides opportunities for individuals with mild to moderate dementia to learn techniques of artistic creation and expression in artistic media in a supportive and nonjudgmental environment. Works created are on display at the Center and have been made into a calendar as well. Participants have derived a great deal of pleasure, pride, stimulation, and camaraderie from the time spent creating art (Figure 27-2). The arts offer people with dementia the opportunity for expression of feelings, connections, and joy and hold tremendous promise to improve the quality of life for people with dementia (Bastings, 2006). A list of suggested resources is in the Resources section at the end of this chapter.

Creative Arts and Theater

Endowment grants are available to ensure the continued contributions of elders as artists, teachers, mentors, students, volunteers, patrons, and consumers of the arts. Some of the programming grants have supported drama groups, storytelling, dance, and singing. These activities are designed for older people of all levels of ability; some are teachers and

---

BOX 27-5	How to Begin Involving Older Adults in the Arts

- Develop program ideas using older adults as advisors.
- Plan specific ways that older adults can participate.
- Survey Office of Aging, senior centers, nursing homes, adult day care centers, and community-dwelling elders regarding their needs, sources of talent, and possible contributions.
- Contact local resource people who may be of assistance.
- Consider access issues such as cost, transportation, and time of day.
- Seek local and national funding.
- Publicize.
- Orient elders who are interested in participating.
- Provide incentives for participating: awards, receptions, and refreshments.

BOX 27-6	Ideas for Developing Creative Abilities

ART

Using oil pastels, create a drawing that represents self, or select three colors you like and three colors you dislike, using all six colors to create a self-portrait.

Draw a representation of your world.

Create a collage or mobile out of an assortment of materials and pictures that can represent subjects such as the self, part of self you like or dislike, the family, etc.

In small groups, use clay to create an *art piece* or a statement.

MUSIC

Play a variety of music; focus discussion on imagery and any feelings that the music evokes.

Discuss or have clients bring in music that elicits feelings of sadness, happiness, etc.

Show a picture (can be cut from a magazine) and ask members to see if they can imagine the sounds that might go with the picture.

Express self or group through dance and movement to select music.

MOVEMENT

Create a movement to fit the way you are feeling while introducing self to group.

Have members stand and initiate a slow, swaying motion (good exercise with which to end the group session).

Have members mirror each other's movements, such as hands or the entire body, creating a duet.

IMAGERY

Use guided fantasies and imagery to facilitate stress reduction and relaxation, awareness, the power of one's own healing capability, and self-expression through symbols and symbolisms.

WRITING

Encourage journals or diaries; set a group time available to write and share ideas.

In small groups, create a group poem.

Read selected poems or stories as a group, and then share reactions and feelings from the readings.

Create a *book* to be distributed to group consisting of a collection of members' writings.

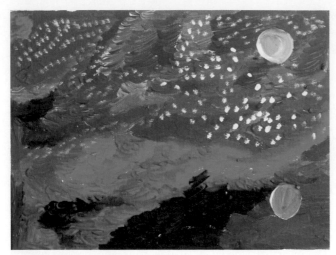

FIGURE 27-2 Artwork created by Frances Hope Goldstein in the Florida Atlantic University (FAU) Memory and Wellness Center "Artful Memories" program.

BOX 27-7   **Creative Use of Poetry with Older Adults**

- Translate poetry if an older person speaks or reads a second language.
- Recite poetry individually and in groups.
- Memorize poetry.
- React to a poem.
- Listen to poetry recorded or recited by poets in the community.
- Create a group poem.
- Copy favorite poems (to develop handwriting or calligraphy skills).
- Illustrate a poem.
- Sing a poem, setting it to familiar music.
- Investigate and discuss children's poetry.
- Discuss a contemporary poem.
- Make a poetry notebook.
- Compose nonsense or humorous poetry.
- Make a literary analysis of a poem.
- Rewrite a poem (start with a famous first line and then improvise).
- Write a poem about a favorite object.
- Create or read haiku.
- Find poetry from various cultures and identify themes and differences.
- Listen for the meter in a poem; illustrate it with hand movements.
- Find a favorite poem and discuss its appeal for you.
- Try choral reading of poetry in small groups.

mentors, some are entertainers, and some are participants, purely for the joy of living. According to Hillary Rodham Clinton (Sherman, 1996, p. 1):

> Some of our most powerful works of art have been produced by older Americans by hands that have engaged in years of hard work, eyes that have witnessed decades of change, and hearts that have felt a lifetime of emotions. Our whole society benefits when older Americans use their talents and experiences to become involved in the arts as creators, teachers, mentors, volunteers and audiences.

Creative Expression Through Music, Poetry, and Dance

Rhythms infiltrate life on every level from individual cellular functions to the constantly expanding and contracting universe. Unseen and unfelt oscillating waves surround us. Felt waves—pulsating, vibrating, and undulating—stimulate us. These waves are intrinsic to existence and may somewhat explain the healing power of music, poetry, and repetitive movement. Life itself is an ongoing dance. In many countries, song, dance, and poetic history flow as naturally as breath and are inextricably interwoven in daily existence.

Music. Music is a familiar and universal experience. Tonal or rhythmic music can be an inward experience or an outward expression. As such, music is adaptable to each individual. Deanna Edwards (1977) was one of the first nurses to use music to assist the ill and the dying in coping with and transcending their physical limitations. Many nurses have used music in myriad ways since that time.

Music therapy is an individual music program prescribed by a professional music therapist to bring about desirable changes in behavior. The self-determined use of music as a means of enjoyment and personal expression can be achieved by listening, meditating, improvising, relaxing, moving to music, creative dancing, composing, learning new songs, studying music history, rhythmic patterning, mastering an instrument, building an instrument, or in any other manner

an individual chooses to adapt music toward self-fulfillment. Music can be a comforting, structured expression, a therapeutic tool, or it can provide the opportunity for creative and imaginative self-expression. People with dementia often respond to music, moving to the rhythms and singing the words to old songs, even when their verbal communication skills are quite impaired.

Poetry. Music and poetic expression are similar in rhythmic beauty. Traditionally, poetry has been judged and categorized by its rhythmic meter; however, modern poetry may have style and quality without a categorical rhythm. Older people enjoy the traditional patterns, rhyming qualities, and free verse. Many people who never thought of themselves as poets have discovered a talent for poetic expression.

Killick (1997, 2000) has done beautiful work with poetry writing with persons with dementia. Killick (2005) has said that "people with dementia can often find a real solace and satisfaction and a creativity in speaking in this way and having it recognized as being of value because they're so used to being put down." (*www.bbc.co.uk/radio4/youandyours/transcript_2005_46_fri_02.shtml*).

Koch (1977) wrote a delightful book explaining the way he began poetry groups with elderly individuals who did not think of themselves as poets. Matsumoto (1978) modified Koch's techniques and applied them with older people in senior centers, day-care centers, and residential housing complexes. Box 27-7 provides suggestions on the creative use of poetry.

BOX 27-8   Resources That Can Enhance Recreational Activities and Programs

- Local florists may present a flower show or provide a flower-arranging activity.
- Police/fire departments may give safety presentations.
- Local ministers may lead Bible readings and discussions.
- Craft suppliers can give demonstrations.
- Local pharmacists may give talks on medication use.
- Clothing stores can sponsor fashion shows.
- Bakeries may give demonstrations of pastry decoration.
- Beauty supply houses may give makeup demonstrations.
- Travel agencies may present slide shows.
- Librarians may institute great book discussions or other activities.

- Students from community colleges may provide numerous educational events and activities.
- Garden clubs or horticultural groups may provide gardening classes.
- Collector's clubs may talk about collecting stamps, antiques, coins, memorabilia.
- Historical societies may give tours to historic places of interest.
- Whenever possible, events should be planned as field trips to the sites of the locals involved because trips add elements of additional interest, stimulation, and involvement in the community at large.

Modified from Leitner MJ, Leitner SF: *Leisure in later life,* ed 2, New York, 1996, Haworth Press.

RECREATION

Recreation is akin to creation. The wisdom of regularly scheduled periods of recreation and recuperation following creative acts can be traced to early Jewish writings and the creation story. If God needed time to rest and recuperate, we certainly do. Inherent in creative acts is time for renewal, time for re-creation. Burnout and boredom are companions of monotony and shorten the perceived life span by emptiness and vanished time. A change of scene or companions may be exhilarating. Retreats from routine to periods of recreation are important as are retreats following intensive efforts.

An important point is that the lower four levels of need must be met to some degree before one is ready for recreation and creative acts. The individual struggling with feelings of insecurity needs predictable routines. Nurses need to assess readiness (in terms of needs met) for challenge, change, and creative expression. Many intricate plans for recreation and creative expression fail because (1) the individual is focusing energy on meeting needs at a more basic level or (2) the individual has not been consulted about his or her particular interests or talents.

Mass activities often provide a sense of belonging, body integration, and better function, but they do not necessarily supply self-esteem or the opportunity for self-actualization. Self-esteem grows out of individual accomplishments and personal recognition. Self-actualization flows from confidence and a milieu in which self-expression is cultivated and valued.

To facilitate a milieu conducive to revitalizing recreation, the following suggestions may be helpful:

1. Assess individual level of needs met.
2. Provide activities structured to meet needs of people who are dealing with the first three levels.
3. Explore individual needs, talents, interests, vocations, and hobbies to promote self-esteem and self-actualization.
4. Encourage individual activities and projects. Group activities are most appropriate in meeting the need for belonging and gaining group esteem. Self-esteem may arise from group esteem but still depends on the group until one gains the capacity of self-validation.

5. Provide materials and a milieu in which one may try new means of self-expression.

Leitner and Leitner (1996) provide an extensive list of resources that may be helpful in generating activities and obtaining donated items and volunteer assistance to provide stimulation and opportunities for elders in institutional or community settings (Box 27-8).

BRINGING YOUNG AND OLD TOGETHER

Larson (2006, p. 39) suggests that intergenerational programs can "help older and younger people look beyond their generational stereotypes and know each other (body, mind, and spirit)" (p. 39). Intergenerational programs can be those in which older people assist younger people (tutoring, mentoring, childcare, foster grandparent programs); those in which younger people assist older people (social visits, meal assistance); and those in which younger and older people serve together. Benefits of intergenerational programs for younger people include increased self-esteem and self-worth, improved behavior, increased involvement and success in school work, and a sense of historical and personal continuity. For older people, contact with younger people can promote life satisfaction, decrease isolation, help develop new skills and insights, promote fulfillment, establish new and meaningful relationships, and provide a sense of meaning and purpose (Larson, 2006). Examples of such programs include Stagebridge Theater Company's program *Grandparent Tales* (*www.stagebridge.org*); Elders Share the Arts, Roots and Branches Theatre, and the Liz Lerman Dance Exchange (*www.danceexhange.org*).

Recognizing the developmental significance of contact between the generations, many plans and projects have flourished in attempts to bring them together. Some institutions have included children in their milieu in various ways:

- As residents (children with profound developmental disabilities or severe neurological disabilities): elders rock, stroke, and cuddle these children, providing stimulation for both.
- As a service to employees (day care centers for children of employees): elders sometimes assist in the

care and special programs for the children, such as reading stories or teaching basic skills (tying shoes, telling time).

- In adopt-a-grandparent programs: one child affiliates with one institutionalized person with periodic visits, cards, and inclusion of grandparent in some special family events.

Nurses in the community may want to explore potential intergenerational experiences that may be of interest to their older clients. Although we recommend intergenerational contact when desired by the older person, certain pitfalls must be considered. Contacts with the very young, energetic child must be brief or the elder is likely to be exhausted and the benefits will decrease. In intergenerational programs, young people need consistent supervision, support, and training in the developmental aspects of old age. Similarly, elders will also benefit from education and support in understanding developmental tasks of children, as well as effective methods of intergenerational communication.

▲ PROMOTING HEALTHY AGING: IMPLICATIONS FOR GERONTOLOGICAL NURSING

In this unit, we have considered what aging can be and that the last years can truly actualize the most unique capacities of older people. Our functions as nurses who value self-actualization are (1) to continually spur our clients to ask, "What is possible and suitable for me?" and (2) to assist them in finding appropriate resources and, when needed, assist in implementing activities toward self-actualization. The nature of self-actualization is self-determination and direction. Nurses are ancillary to the process but may be needed to stir the beginnings of the search. In doing so, we may move forward with our own search.

Self-actualization implies that one actualizes the potential of self through various mechanisms. We have mentioned only a few of these mechanisms in a somewhat cursory manner, knowing that these individually instituted actions have a force of their own and that once activated go far beyond the professionals' involvement. Activities such as yoga, focused meditation, the discipline of karate, and other forms of centered concentration are segued into spirituality and transcendence.

SPIRITUALITY

Spirituality is a rather indescribable need that drives individuals throughout life to seek meaning and purpose in their existence. We recognize that our readers will see great overlap and fuzzy boundaries between transcendence and spirituality. Spirituality is difficult to define, though many people have tried. We can observe the body and we can imagine the mind in operation and measure intelligence, but there is no computerized tomography (CT) scan of the spirit (Bell and Troxel, 2001). Understanding spirituality is far more elusive than learning about the pathology associated with disease and illness.

Moberg (1996), one of the major contributors to our understanding of spirituality and aging, defines spirituality as the (p. 2):

...totality of man's inner resources, the ultimate concerns around which all other values are focused, the central philosophy of life that guides conduct, and the meaning-giving center of human life which influences all individual and social behavior.

Spirituality can be defined in terms of personal views and behaviors that express a sense of relatedness to a transcendent dimension or to something greater than self. The sense of relatedness may be experienced intrapersonally (connectedness with oneself); interpersonally (in relation to others and the environment), and transpersonally (relatedness to God or a power greater than self). Spirituality is manifested through these observable human experiences of connectedness. Examples of these experiences include religious behaviors, mystical experiences, meaningful and reciprocal relationships with others, the discovery of meaning in suffering, and the experience of forgiveness (Reed, 1991a, 1992; Touhy, 2001a, 2001b).

Spiritual well-being can be considered the ability to experience and integrate meaning and purpose in life through connectedness with self, others, art, music, literature, nature, or a power greater than oneself (Gaskamp et al., 2006; NANDA International, 2004). Spiritual distress or spiritual pain is "an individual's perception of hurt or suffering associated with that part of his or her person that seeks to transcend the realm of the material. Spiritual distress is manifested by a deep sense of hurt stemming from feelings of loss or separation from one's God or deity, a sense of personal inadequacy or sinfulness before God and man, or a pervasive condition of loneliness" (Gaskamp et al., 2006, p. 9). The person experiencing spiritual distress is unable to experience meaning, hope, connectedness, and transcendence. Spiritual distress may be manifested by anger, guilt, blame, hatred, expressions of alienation and turning away from family and friends, inability to enjoy, and inability to participate in religious activities that have previously provided comfort (Doenges et al., 2004; Touhy and Zerwekh, 2006) (Box 27-9).

The spiritual path leads one into self-discovery, self-acceptance, affirmation of self-love, and a connection with all others that are brought about by loving the most unlovable aspects of self and of others. At the deepest level of spirituality, a profound connection exists with all living things, the universal awareness of which Jung was cognizant (Freke and Gandy, 2001). True spirituality endeavors to make the world a better place, often in small daily acts or in a larger sense. The enormity of the actions and where they occur are not as significant as the love that produces them.

Spirituality and Religion

Distinguishing between religion and spirituality is a concern for many health professionals. Religious beliefs and church participation are often the avenues of spiritual expression, but they are not necessarily interchangeable. "Religion can

BOX 27-9   Assessing and Intervening in Spiritual Distress

ASSESSMENT

Brief history:
- Losses
- Challenged belief, value system
- Separation from religious and cultural ties
- Death
- Personal and family disasters

Symptoms (defining characteristics) such as the following:
- Unmet needs
- Threats to self
- Change in environment, health status, self-concept, etc.
- Questioning meaning of own existence
- Depression
- Feeling of hopelessness, abandonment, fear

Assessment of the cause of spiritual distress
- Depletion anxiety
- Helplessness, hopelessness

- Perceived powerlessness
- Medication reaction
- Hormonal imbalances

INTERVENTIONS

Create a therapeutic environment.

Assess the support system.

Assess past methods of decreasing distress (e.g., prayer, imagery, healing, memories-reminiscence therapy, medication, relaxation).

Determine environmental changes needed to enhance function.

Assess and assist implementation of coping mechanisms.

Refer to clergy.

Evaluate effects of nursing interventions.

Activate and evaluate appropriate community referrals.

Use techniques to assist client and family in reducing spiritual distress.

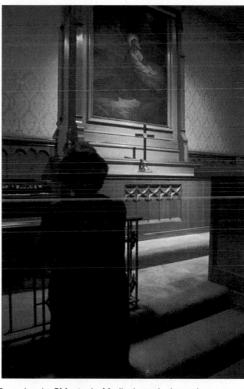

Prayer. (From Lewis SM et al: *Medical-surgical nursing: assessment and management of clinical problems*, ed 7, St Louis, 2007, Mosby.)

be described as a social institution that unites people in a faith in God a higher power, and in common rituals and worshipful acts. A god, divinity, and/or soul is always included in the concept" (Strang and Strang, 2002, p. 858). Each religion involves a particular set of beliefs. Spirituality is a broader concept than religion and encompasses a person's search for meaning, relationships with a higher power, with nature, and with other people.

For some people, particularly older people, formalized religion helps them feel fulfilled. According to Touhy and Zerwekh (2006, p. 215):

> Religion may be considered one path by which some people create a sense of the spiritual and support the personal sense of self. Everyone has a spirit or is spiritual whether or not they consider themselves religious or belong to an organized religion or faith community. Religious systems and needs are not universal and are different for each individual. Spiritual needs, on the other hand, are essentially the same for everyone. The way people meet those needs will be different and will change over the course of a person's life, but the core spiritual needs are universal. The concept of spirituality is found in all cultures and societies.

Spirituality and Aging

Life satisfaction, happiness, morale, and health have all been studied in relation to religion and spiritual expression. Although successful aging has been studied in numerous ways, Crowther and colleagues (2002) contend that spirituality must be considered a significant factor. Rowe and Kahn's (1998) prevalent model of successful aging includes active engagement in life, minimal risk and disability, and the maximum physical and mental abilities. Crowther and colleagues maintain that positive spirituality must be the fourth element of the model and is interrelated with all the others.

Gerontologists appreciate the significance of religion and spirituality to the well-being of elders. Aging as a biological process has been studied extensively. Less attention has been paid to the study of aging as a spiritual process. In the past few years, we have seen a revival of interest in philosophy, religion, and spirituality. Henderson (1996) calls the movement a spiritual renaissance that has captured the interest of professionals. This description has certainly been observed in the past 5 years given that the focus of conferences of the American Society on Aging and the Gerontology Society of America (previously the bastion of medical research) has had spiritual overtones in many of the symposia and presentations.

Some people see the essence of aging as a spiritual journey in which one connects with the transcendent self and the route of spiritual growth (Berggren-Thomas and Griggs, 1995). Hungelmann et al. (1985) interviewed 31 older adults to determine the defining characteristics of spiritual well-being. The model generated from the research describes spiritual well-being in old age as a (p. 21):

> ...sense of harmonious interconnectedness between self, others, and nature, and an Ultimate Other which exists throughout and beyond time and space. It is achieved through a dynamic and integrative growth process which leads to a realization of the ultimate purpose and meaning of life.

"Although aging changes can affect the body and the mind, there is no evidence that the spirit succumbs to the aging process, even in the presence of debilitating physical and emotional illness" (Heriot, 1992, p. 23). For some older people, particularly those who are frail or cognitively impaired, meeting spiritual needs may be a greater challenge than for healthier elders. Functional decline and dependence can threaten the sense of identity and connection with others and the world, thus causing a loss of spirit (Leetun, 1996; Touhy 2001b). The spiritual aspect transcends the physical and psychosocial to reach the deepest individual capacity for love, hope, and meaning. The spiritual person can rise above that which is humanly expected in a situation. For example, a dying elder in great pain to whom one of the authors (TT) was attending said, "This is so hard for you." That he was able to see beyond himself at that time was difficult to believe.

▲ Promoting Healthy Aging: Implications for Gerontological Nursing

As people age and move closer to death, spirituality may become more important. Declining physical health, loss of loved ones, and a realization that life's end may be near often challenge older people to reflect on the meaning of their lives (Touhy, 2001b). The older person may have a pressing need to talk about philosophy and spiritual development. Private time for prayer, meditation, and reflection may be needed. Nurses may neglect to explore this issue with elders because religion and spirituality may not seem the high priority. The client should be assured that religious longings and rituals are important and that opportunities will be made available as desired (Hermann, 2000). Nurses need to be knowledgeable and respectful about the rites and rituals of varying religions, cultural beliefs, and values (see Chapter 21). Religious and spiritual resources such as pastoral visits should be available in all settings where older people reside. It is important to avoid imposing one's own beliefs and respecting the person's privacy on matters of spirituality and religion (Touhy and Zerwekh, 2006).

Although religious needs are important for many older people, spiritual needs are much broader and more personal

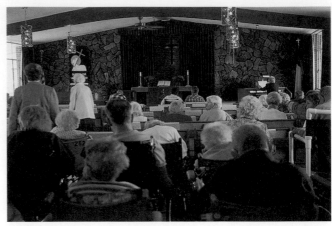

Residents attend a religious service at a nursing center. (From Sorrentino SA, Gorek B: *Mosby's textbook for long-term care assistants*, ed 5, St Louis, 2007, Mosby.)

than any particular religious persuasion. Spiritual care entails assisting patients to find a sense of meaning and reconciliation with others and with a transcendent reality, encouraging patients to strengthen their spiritual life as they choose (Touhy and Zerwekh, 2006). Nurses may not lead individuals to soul growth and acceptance when facing illness and disability but may have the privilege of accompanying them on the journey. Reflection, feedback, comfort, and affirmation are all a part of being with the elder, providing the supports that release energy for spiritual seeking.

An emphasis on spirituality in nursing is not new; nursing has encompassed the spiritual from its origin. The science of nursing was not seen as separate from the art and spirit of the discipline. Florence Nightingale's view of nursing was derived from her spiritual philosophy, and she considered nursing a spiritual experience, "intrinsic to human nature, our deepest and most potent resource for healing" (Macrae, 1995, p. 8). Many nursing theories address spirituality, including those of Neuman, Parse, and Watson (Martsolf and Mickley, 1998). Nursing and medicine are beginning to reclaim some of the essential healing values from their roots.

The essence of being spiritual is being whole or holistic, and attention to the spiritual needs of patients is a critical dimension of holistic nursing care. Yet surveys with practicing nurses suggest that most have had little, if any, education in spiritual care. Many nurses view spiritual nursing responses in religious terms and may feel that spirituality is a religious matter better left to clergy and religious leaders. Heriot (1992) suggested that nurses need to understand care of the human spirit both within and outside the context of religion. "Incorporating spirituality into the caring dimension of nursing requires a sensitivity to the many ways in which spirituality may be experienced and thus expressed" (Dyson et al., 1997, p. 1186).

Goldberg (1998) asserted that the connection in the nurse-patient relationship is central to spiritual care but that most nurses are "carrying out spiritual interventions at an unconscious level" (p. 840). She called for education and research to help nurses become more aware of the impor-

BOX 27-10	Identifying Elders at Risk for Spiritual Distress

- Individuals experiencing events or conditions that affect the ability to participate in spiritual rituals
- Diagnosis and treatment of a life-threatening, chronic, or terminal illness
- Expressions of interpersonal or emotional suffering, loss of hope, lack of meaning, need to find meaning in suffering
- Evidence of depression
- Cognitive impairment
- Verbalized questioning or loss of faith
- Loss of interpersonal support

Data from Gaskamp C et al: Evidence-based guideline: promoting spirituality in the older adult, *J Gerontol Nurs* 32(11): 8-11, 2006.

BOX 27-11	Brief Assessment of Spiritual Resources and Concerns

Instructions: Use the following questions as an interview guide with the older adult (or caregiver if the older adult is unable to communicate).

- Does your religion/spirituality provide comfort or serve as a cause of stress? (Ask to explain in what ways spirituality is a comfort or stressor).
- Do you have any religious or spiritual beliefs that might conflict with health care or affect health care decisions? (Ask to identify any conflicts.)
- Do you belong to a supportive church, congregation, or faith community? (Ask how the faith community is supportive.)
- Do you have any practices or rituals that help you express your spiritual or religious beliefs? (Ask to identify or describe practices.)
- Do you have any spiritual needs you would like someone to address? (Ask what those needs are and if referral to spiritual professional is desired.)
- How can we (health care providers) help you with your spiritual needs or concerns?

From Gaskamp C et al: Evidence-based guideline: promoting spirituality in the older adult, *J Gerontol Nurs* 32(11):8 11, 2006, p. 10. Adapted from Meyer CL. *Dissertation Abst Int* 55(6):2158B, UMI No 9428614, 2003; Koenig HG, Brooks RG: Religion, health, and aging: implications for practice and public policy, *Public Policy Aging Rep* 12(4):13, 2002.

tance of connection and use of self in relationships as ways of bringing the elements of spiritual care into conscious awareness. From Gaskamp et al. (2006, p. 8):

> Nursing studies of spirituality and aging indicate that spirituality increases in importance (Lowry and Conco, 2002), is a source of hope (Touhy, 2001a), aids in adaptation to illnesses such as arthritis (Potter and Zauszniewski, 2000), and has a positive influence on quality of life in chronically ill older adults (O'Brien, 2003). The ultimate goal for promoting spirituality is to support and enhance quality of life.

An evidence-based guideline for promoting spirituality in the older adult (Gaskamp et al., 2006) provides a framework for spiritual assessment and interventions. The guideline identifies older adults who may be at risk for alterations in spirituality and who might be most likely to benefit from use of the guideline (Box 27-10).

Spiritual Assessment. Patients welcome a discussion of spiritual matters and want health professionals to consider their spiritual needs (O'Brien, 1999; Post et al., 2000; Touhy and Zerwekh, 2006). A spiritual history opens the door to a conversation about the role of spirituality and religion in a person's life. People often need permission to talk about these issues. Without a signal from the nurse, patients may feel that such topics are not welcome or appropriate.

Obtaining a spiritual history involves simply listening to patients as they express their fears, hopes, and beliefs. A spiritual assessment is intended to elicit information about the core spiritual needs and how the nurse and other members of the health care team can respond to them (Touhy and Zerwekh, 2006). Several spiritual assessment instruments are available such as the Faith, Importance/Influence, Community and Address (FICA) Spiritual History (Puchalski and Romer, 2000) and the Brief Assessment of Spiritual Resources and Concerns (Koenig and Brooks, 2002; Meyer, 2003) (Box 27-11).

Hungelmann and colleagues (1996) have developed an assessment tool that emphasizes strengths, as well as possible spiritual distress (Figure 27-3). The scale is multidimensional and includes factors that affect psychological and physical

welfare. The authors identify the following areas of nursing interventions: affirmation through listening and discovering the gift and identifying the need; therapeutic communication as a vehicle for identifying strengths, as well as pain; and referral to clergy or another health professional when desire or need is indicated. Open-ended questions within the context of the nurse-patient relationship can also be used to begin dialogue about spiritual concerns (Blues and Zerwekh, 1984; Touhy and Zerwekh, 2006) (Box 27-12). For older people with cognitive impairment, information about the importance of spirituality and religious beliefs can be obtained from family members (Gaskamp et al., 2006). Nurses often see cognitive impairments as obstacles or excuses to providing spiritual care to people with dementia (Heriot, 1992). Nurturing mind, body, and spirit is part of holistic nursing, and nurses must provide opportunities to all elders, no matter how impaired, to live life with meaning, purpose, and hope (Touhy, 2001a).

Spiritual Responses. The caring relationship between nurses and persons nursed is the heart of nursing that touches and supports the spirit. Knowing persons in their complexity, responding to that which matters most to them, identifying and nurturing connections, listening with one's being, using presence and silence, and fostering connections to that which is held sacred by the person are spiritual nursing responses that arise from within the caring, connected relationship (Touhy, 2001b).

Interventions identified as particularly important in spiritual nursing care include the following (Emblem and Hal-

Jarel Spiritual Well-Being Scale

DIRECTIONS: Please circle the choice that **best** describes how much you agree with each statement. Circle <u>only</u> one answer for each statement. There is no right or wrong answer.

	Strongly Agree	Moderately Agree	Agree	Disagree	Moderately Disagree	Strongly Disagree
1. Prayer is an important part of my life.	SA	MA	A	D	MD	SD
2. I believe I have spiritual well-being.	SA	MA	A	D	MD	SD
3. As I grow older, I find myself more tolerant of others' beliefs.	SA	MA	A	D	MD	SD
4. I find meaning and purpose in my life.	SA	MA	A	D	MD	SD
5. I feel there is a close relationship between my spiritual beliefs and what I do.	SA	MA	A	D	MD	SD
6. I believe in an afterlife.	SA	MA	A	D	MD	SD
7. When I am sick I have less spiritual well-being.	SA	MA	A	D	MD	SD
8. I believe in a supreme power.	SA	MA	A	D	MD	SD
9. I am able to receive and give love to others.	SA	MA	A	D	MD	SD
10. I am satisfied with my life.	SA	MA	A	D	MD	SD
11. I set goals for myself.	SA	MA	A	D	MD	SD
12. God has little meaning in my life.	SA	MA	A	D	MD	SD
13. I am satisfied with the way I am using my abilities.	SA	MA	A	D	MD	SD
14. Prayer does not help me in making decisions.	SA	MA	A	D	MD	SD
15. I am able to appreciate differences in others.	SA	MA	A	D	MD	SD
16. I am pretty well put together.	SA	MA	A	D	MD	SD
17. I prefer that others make decisions for me.	SA	MA	A	D	MD	SD
18. I find it hard to forgive others.	SA	MA	A	D	MD	SD
19. I accept my life situations.	SA	MA	A	D	MD	SD
20. Belief in a supreme being has no part in my life.	SA	MA	A	D	MD	SD
21. I cannot accept change in my life.	SA	MA	A	D	MD	SD

FIGURE 27-3 Jarel Spiritual Well-Being Scale. (From Hungelmann J, Kenkel-Rossi E, Klassen L, Stollenwerk R: Marquette University College of Nursing, ©1987, Milwaukee, WI.)

Continued

BOX 27-12   Questions to Begin Dialogue about Spiritual Concerns

- Tell me more about your life.
- What has been most meaningful in your life?
- To whom do you turn when you need help?
- What brings you joy and comfort?
- What are you most proud of?
- How have you found strength throughout your life?
- What are you hopeful about?
- Is spiritual peace important to you? What would help you achieve it?

- Is your religion or God significant in your life? Can you describe how?
- Is prayer or meditation helpful?
- What spiritual or religious practices bring you comfort?
- Are there religious books or materials that you want nearby?
- What are you afraid of right now?
- What do you wish you could still do?
- What are your concerns at this time for the future?
- What matters most to you right now?

Adapted from Touhy T, Zerwekh J: Spiritual caring. In Zerwekh J: *Nursing care at the end of life: palliative care for patients and families,* Philadelphia, 2006, Davis; Hospice of the Florida Suncoast, 2001; Blues A, Zerwekh J: *Hospice and palliative care nursing,* Orlando, 1984, Grune & Stratton.

Jarel Spiritual Well-Being Scale

Factor I Faith/Belief Dimension

(Scoring: SA = 6   SD = 1)

Item 1 _____
Item 2 _____
Item 3 _____
Item 4 _____
Item 5 _____
Item 6 _____
Item 8 _____   Subscore _____

Factor II Life/Self Responsibility

(Reverse Scoring: SA = 1   SD = 6)

Item 7 _____
Item 12 _____
Item 14 _____
Item 17 _____
Item 18 _____
Item 20 _____
Item 21 _____   Subscore _____

Factor III Life Satisfaction/Self-Actualization

(Scoring: SA = 6   SD = 1)

Item 9 _____
Item 10 _____
Item 11 _____
Item 13 _____
Item 15 _____
Item 16 _____
Item 19 _____   Subscore _____   Total score _____

FIGURE 27-3, CONT'D

stead, 1993; Gaskamp et al., 2006; Goldberg, 1998; Nagai-Jacobson and Burkhardt, 1989; Stiles, 1990; Touhy, 2001a, 2001b; Touhy et al., 2005; Touhy and Zerwekh, 2006; Zerwekh, 1993):

- Relief of physical discomfort, which permits refocus on the spiritual
- Comforting touch, which fosters nurse-patient connecting
- Authentic presence and being there
- Attentive listening
- Knowing the patient as a person
- Listening to life stories
- Sharing caring words and love
- Fostering forgiveness and reconciliation
- Fostering connections with that which is held sacred by the person
- Respecting religious traditions and rituals
- Referring the person to a spiritual counselor

Specific suggestions for spiritual nursing interventions are presented in Box 27-13.

BOX 27-13   Spiritual Nursing Responses

- Promote physical comfort (bathing, positioning, pain and symptom relief, touch, peaceful environment).
- Provide psychosocial comfort (active listening, sharing fears, listen to self-doubts or guilt, provide guidance in the forgiveness of others and self, authentic presence, family support and presence).
- Provide spiritual comfort (share love and caring words, reminiscence, listen to life stories, validate their lives, assure them that they will be remembered, provide hopeful environments, praying with and for, read scripture and Bible, refer clergy, provide for religious objects and rituals).

From Gaskamp C et al: Evidence-based practice guideline: promoting spirituality in the older adult, *J Gerontol Nurs* 32(11):8-11, 2006; Touhy T et al: Spiritual caring: end of life in a nursing home, *J Gerontol Nurs* 31(9):27-35, 2004; Touhy T, Zerwekh H: Spiritual caring. In Zerwekh J: *Nursing care at the end of life: palliative care for patients and families,* Philadelphia, 2006, FA Davis.

Nurturing the Spirit of the Nurse. "Because spiritual care occurs over time and within the context of relationship, probably the most effective tool at the nurse's disposal is the use of self" (Soeken and Carson, 1987, p. 607). Thinking about what gives your own life meaning and value helps in developing your spiritual self and assists you in being able to offer spiritual support to patients. Examples of activities include finding quiet

---

BOX 27-14 Personal Spirituality Questions for Reflection for Nurses

- What do I believe in?
- How do I find purpose and meaning in my life?
- How do I take care of my physical, emotional, and spiritual needs?
- What are my hopes and dreams?
- Who do I love, and who loves me?
- How am I with others?
- What would I change about my relationships?
- Am I willing to heal relationships that trouble me?

Adapted from Newshan G: Transcending the physical: spiritual aspects of pain in patients with HIV and/or cancer, *J Adv Nurs* 28(6):1236-1241, 1998. In Touhy T, Zerwekh J: Spiritual caring. In Zerwekh J: *Nursing care at the end of life: palliative care for patients and families,* Philadelphia, 2006, Davis.

---

time for meditation and reflection; keeping your own faith traditions; being with nature; appreciating the arts; spending time with those you love; and journaling (Touhy and Zerwekh, 2006). Giving your patient the best spiritual care stems from taking care of your own spiritual needs first (Bell and Troxel, 2001). Find ways to nourish your own spirit. Nurses often do not take the time to do so and become dispirited. This is especially true for nurses who work with dying patients and experience grief and loss repeatedly. Having someone to talk to about feelings is important. Practicing compassion for oneself is essential to authentic practice of compassion for others (Touhy and Zerwekh, 2006) (Box 27-14).

Know that caring for an aging body is the least of the work with the elderly. "Limiting care to the physical needs denies elders the opportunity to live out their life with meaning, purpose, and hope" (Touhy, 2001a, p. 45). Recognizing the primacy of the spirit is essential. Some very spiritual individuals are unable to articulate their knowing; do not negate that aspect of an individual's experience because it is not expressed verbally. Realizing that biopsychosocial aspects of aging are all shards of the spirit will integrate every aspect of your work in gerontological nursing. The results of a nursing study on spirituality and health are presented in Box 27-15.

BOX 27-15 Evidence-Based Practice: Spirituality and Health

PURPOSE

This study examined health and spirituality in women living in a rural senior high-rise apartment setting.

SAMPLE/SETTING

A purposive sample of 10 women living in a rural senior high-rise apartment setting in West Virginia who spoke English, were 65 years of age and older, able to give informed consent, and willing and able to share their experiences participated in the study. Range of ages of the participants was from 69 to 85 years (M = 76.5 years). Four were widowed; 1 was separated; 3 were single; and 2 were divorced. Number of years living in the high-rise ranged from 3 to 16 years (M = 7.6 years). Six considered themselves Protestant, and 4 considered themselves Catholic.

METHOD

Qualitative research design using a phenomenological approach was utilized. A demographic questionnaire was administered, and semi-structured interviews were conducted. A broad opening question was asked: "What is the meaning of living?" This was followed by broad questions asking the participants to describe the experience of health and spirituality. If spirituality was included in responses, participants were asked: "What does spirituality mean to you?" and "What life experiences brought you to your conclusions about spirituality?" Interviews lasted an average of 45 minutes and were audiotaped and transcribed verbatim. Field notes were kept. Themes and theme clusters were derived by the researchers to uncover the essential essence of the women's experiences using Coliazzi's method. Peer debriefing was used, and a second interview was conducted with the

participants to share the data and confirm or correct the researchers' impressions.

RESULTS

Three themes were identified: (1) health is functional; (2) spirituality is a personal relationship with a Higher Power or God; and (3) death is a part of nature for which one is never prepared. All of the participants described spirituality as a personal relationship with a Higher Power operationalized by faith, prayer, keeping busy, and having family support. Theme clusters around spirituality included: (1) coping is keeping busy, using prayer, and having faith; (2) God has the Higher Power but individuals also have some control; and (3) beauty is in nature, colors, and inner beauty.

IMPLICATIONS

Participants' perceptions of spirituality were consistent with those found in the literature. While most did not regularly attend church services at this time in their life, praying and reading Bible scriptures were important to their spiritual life. Spirituality was described as a way of coping. It is important for nurses to assess an elder's views of spirituality and a personal relationship with a Higher Power or God. Opportunities for prayer, worship, scripture, or religious readings should be made available to those for whom this is important. Appreciation of the interconnectedness of health and spirituality and the use of spirituality as a coping mechanism with life events and the effects of chronic illness is important in the lives of many elders and should be included in assessment, care planning, and education of nurses. Further research is needed with larger samples and diverse populations, as well as elders of other religious or non-religious backgrounds.

Data from Knestrick J, Lohri-Posey B: Spirituality and health: perceptions of older women in a rural senior high rise, *J Gerontol Nurs* 31(10):44-50, 2005.

Parish Nursing. Parish nursing has found a niche in the care of elders and has begun to flourish in the past decade. From the handful practicing in 1990, today 7000 parish nurses are practicing in a variety of roles in every state (Deaconess Parish Nurse Ministries, 2002). Religious communities and hospitals working together might provide for the preventive and health maintenance needs of many frail elders, as well as their spiritual needs. *Parish nurses* are becoming visible nationwide as churches and hospitals join forces to provide health maintenance and monitoring activities for parishioners. Parish nursing is also called *faith-based nursing* and is found among many denominations.

Many models of parish nursing have been developed, but the underlying motivation is to address and blend the maintenance of physical and spiritual health to the satisfaction of the parishioners. Weis and Schank (2000) found among over 400 subjects that health-seeking behavior was the primary reason for seeing the parish nurse for services, but unidentified needs were equal motivators. A very small number of people expressed spiritual distress (7% younger than 80 years and 5% older than 80 years). The most frequent nursing interventions were active listening, emotional support, and spiritual support. Touching and nursing presence were also valued.

Nurses who are involved in religious organizations can be advocates for increasing the attention given to the health needs of older people. Nurses may even spearhead particular services to older people, such as peer counseling, health screening activities, day care, home visitation programs, and respite for families. Many religious organizations reach out to homebound elders in their community by offering visits from clergy or church members, involvement in prayer circles, and other activities to maintain connection with their faith community. Communities nationwide have organized interfaith volunteer services to provide in-home services for isolated frail elders. Many of these efforts have been organized and supported by the Robert Wood Johnson Foundation, and the national Faith Based Initiative also provides support for faith-based programs.

TRANSCENDENCE

Transcendence is the high-level emotional response to religious and spiritual life and finds expression in numerous rituals and modes of cosmic consciousness. Rituals provide a means of connecting with everyone through the ages who have observed like rituals. These modes of thinking and feeling are sometimes unfamiliar to individuals who are immersed in the necessary materialistic concerns of young adulthood, yet moments do occur throughout life when one is deeply aware of being part of a larger scheme. Although some of the material in this chapter may be obscure, it is the springboard for learning to appreciate the full life cycle. The privilege of briefly walking alongside an elder on the last great journey can be truly inspiring.

Transcending is roused by the desire to go beyond the self as delimited by the material and the concrete aspects of living, to expand self-boundaries and life perspectives. "Transcendence involves detachment and separation from life as it has been lived to experience a reality beyond oneself and beyond what can be seen or felt" (Touhy and Zerwekh, 2006, p 229). Transcending embodies aspects of belonging, connecting, giving life, holding commitments, struggling with and surrendering ego, turning inward, and becoming free (Forbes, 1994). Creative thought and actions are vehicles of both self-actualization and self-transcendence, the bridge to universal expression and existence. Self-transcendence is generally expressed in five modes: creative work, religious beliefs, children, identification with nature, and mystical experiences (Reed, 1991b). This section of the chapter deals with various mechanisms by which one transcends the purely physical limitations of existence.

Self-transcendence is thought to be a developmental process that forestalls depression in middle age and aging (Ellerman and Reed, 2001). Using Reed's Self-Transcendence Scale, Ellerman and Reed revealed significant gender differences and increasing levels of self-transcendence in the aging process. The way one perceives the passage of time, experiences extensions of the self, and copes with the sure knowledge that death is inevitable may be the ultimate victory or defeat.

Some people may use asceticism, self-denial, and rigorous rituals to reach the peaks of human experience; many others find more prosaic approaches just as effective. The thesis of Maslow's writings is that mystic, sacred, and transcendent experiences frequently arise from the ordinary elements of one's life (Maslow, 1970). Planting and harvesting, one of the most persistent interests of elders, is the "substance of things hoped for, the evidence of things not seen" (Hebrews 11:1). Gardening, reading, holding an infant, dealing with loss, and numerous other normal events have elements of mystery.

With each death of a loved one, throughout life, one is reborn to a slightly altered state. When deaths of significant others abound in the later years, elders must be given opportunity to express how they personally have been altered by the loss. We can speculate that with each personal loss, one moves slightly closer to the universal and away from the individual until, toward the end, one feels an affiliation with all living things, animal, plant, and mineral. Some of the old have achieved a state of existence that transcends the limits of the failing body.

Gerotranscendence

Tornstam (1994, 1996, 2005) theorizes that human aging brings about a general potential for what he terms *gerotranscendence*, a shift in perspective from the material world to the cosmic and, concurrent with that, an increasing life satisfaction. Tornstam found in a survey of 912 Danish elders that shifts in cosmic awareness and ego transcendence were accompanied by satisfaction and a lesser need for social activity. The higher the level of transcendence, the more internal were the sources of satisfaction.

This satisfaction is qualitatively different from disengagement (Cumming and Henry, 1961) or the achievement of ego integrity (Erikson, 1950). Disengagement or activity is

---

BOX 27-16 Characteristics of Individuals with a High Degree of Gerotranscendence

- Have high degrees of life satisfaction
- Engage in self-controlled social activity
- Experience satisfaction with self-selected social activities
- Social activities not essential to their well-being
- Midlife patterns and ideals no longer prime motivators
- Demonstrate complex and active coping patterns
- Have greater need for solitary philosophizing
- May appear withdrawn when engaged in inner development
- Have accelerated development of gerotranscendence fomented by life crises
- Feel shifts in perception of reality

Data from gerotranscendence theory development of Lars Tornstam.

---

of little significance in this transformation. There is not an either-or duality but a more profound, all-pervasive change in perspective. Gerotranscendence is conceptualized as a metamorphosis, an alteration in conception of time, space, life, death, and self. Tornstam says, "Simply put, gerotranscendence is a shift in metaperspective, from a mid-life materialistic and rational vision to a more cosmic and transcendent one, accompanied by an increase in life satisfaction" (Tornstam, 1996, p. 38). Indices of gerotranscendence are summarized in Box 27-16. Gerotranscendence is thought to be a gradual and ongoing shift that is generated by the normal processes of living, sometimes hastened by serious personal disruptions.

Wadensten and Carlsson (2001) wondered if nurses recognized signs of gerotranscendence and how they were interpreted. In their study, nurses did recognize these signs (declining interest in social activity; alterations in perspectives of time, space, life, and death; increased life satisfaction) occurring in many old people but saw them as evidence of aging or pathological conditions rather than a natural developmental process of transcendence. However, given that this study was conducted in a nursing home in Sweden, the conclusions are limited. The results of an additional study conducted by Raes and Marcoen (2001) in Belgium, using a gerotranscendence scale developed by Tornstam, showed that individuals who had experienced a recent crisis had higher scores on the Transcendent Connection subscale. Apparently, specific attributes of gerotranscendence need to be articulated more clearly if nurses and others are to identify the process.

Time Transcendence

Life as experienced ordinarily involves the chronological passage of time. Some types of conscious experience alter our time perception, but the unconscious destroys time. Therefore the release of the unconscious transcends the limitations of time that conscious life experience generally imposes on us. If we conquer time, we conquer annihilation and the dimensions of time that lie within the mind. Recognizing the importance of time perception, particularly in old age, is

a fertile field to explore more fully. Influences on time perception include age, imminent death, level of activity, emotional state, outlook on the future, and the value attached to time. Conclusions from studies of older people generally support the view that elders perceive time as passing quickly and favor the past over the present or the future.

Altered Mind States

In every society and every age, humans have sought spiritual enlightenment through altered mind states by using substances, rituals, and deprivations. An inherent need seems apparent in almost every culture to incorporate methods of seeking some enlightenment outside the common daily experience. Some of these exceptional experiences are treasured, and some are feared. The ritual use of peyote by the Southwest Indians, sake by the Japanese, isolation and deprivation by some of the Northwest Native tribes, withdrawal into nirvana by East Indians, and mind-altering drugs by the flower children are only a few of the most obvious of these methods. These examples simply exemplify some of the routes individuals take to move out of the common thought modes that may keep them trapped in the mundane levels of existence.

Mystical experiences seem to strengthen the immune system in that spontaneous remissions of illness sometimes seem to result from moods and altered perceptions, sometimes in a religious manner or with psychedelic drugs. Roberts advances the idea that mystical experiences boost the immune system (Roberts, 1999).

For some people, mind states are altered without using a particular substance or mechanism. These altered mind states may be frightening. Professionals may validate the experiences and assist the person in achieving a coping style that balances the internal reality with the demands of daily living. In the following discussion of some of these situations, examples and suggestions are given for facilitating acceptance and valuing these extraordinary occurrences.

Peak Experiences. A peak experience is when one momentarily transcends self through love, wisdom, insight, worship, commitment, or creativity. These experiences are the extraordinary events in one's life that clearly demonstrate self-actualization and personal authenticity. Peak experience is the time when restrictive boundaries seem to vanish and one feels more aware, more complete, more ecstatic, or more concerned for others. Peak experiences include many modes of transcending one's ordinary limitations. Spiritual and paranormal experiences, creative acts, courage, and humor may all produce peak experiences. Levin (1993) defines these mystical experiences as including déjà vu, clairvoyance, and other occurrences in which the self-perceptions reach beyond the ordinary limits. These mechanisms move humans beyond the boundaries of visible, concrete reality and toward a wholly integrated self. The self, as conceptualized by Jung, means the supreme oneness of being: integration of aspects of self that are generative and destructive, light and dark, conscious and unconscious, male

BOX 27-17 Near-Death Experiences

- Be receptive and nonjudgmental when listening to an account of the event.
- Reassure the individual that although these experiences are not common, they have been reported and they are not evidences of psychoses.
- Recognize the emotional impact this experience may have on the individual, and explore the meaning attached to it.
- Anticipate anger from some people who felt compelled to come back from the near-death experience.
- Realize that, as in any major crisis, the individual may become obsessed with the experience and repeat it over and over whenever a willing or unwilling listener is present.
- Explore your own biases and keep an open mind to the unknown aspects of our universe.

BOX 27-18 Benefits of Meditation

- Increased measured intelligence
- Increased short-term and long-term recall
- Decreased anxiety, depression, and irritability
- Greater perceived self-actualization (realization of potential)
- Better mind-body coordination
- Increased perceptual awareness
- Normalization of blood pressure
- Relief from insomnia
- Normalization of weight

and female. The ability to embrace the possibility of every potential behavior as native to self instills compassion and a sense of oneness with the world. Keeping oneself open to transcendence involves finding the places in which such experiences can break through: soul-stirring concerts, sunrises, sunsets, or raging storms on mountaintops (Kimble, 1993). Each individual seeks states of being in which he or she feels part of a larger whole.

Near-Death Experience. From antiquity to the present, near-death experiences (NDE) have been reported that have given insight into the experience of death itself. Individuals who have survived tell us what it is like to ostensibly return from the dead. Feelings of peace, tranquility, and unconditional love were described. Some people do not wish to return but believe they must. The urge to express these transcendental experiences is often strong but is mixed with fears of being considered crazy. The health care provider must realize that these experiences may have profound significance and lasting impact on the individual who has experienced them. We know so little of the human limits, the mystical, and the universal. Let us keep ourselves open to the unknown and the immeasurable.

To elicit a discussion of an NDE, you might ask, "Do you recall any unusual feelings or perceptions during any critical episode you have survived?" Suggestions for working with people who have experienced these remarkable events are presented in Box 27-17.

Hallucinations and Visions. Hallucinations and visions have great meaning for some people. These experiences differ from ordinary fantasies in that the individual believes the origin is external. History has given us many examples of such events: Saint Paul's confrontation with God, the voices heard by Joan of Arc, and the vision of the Virgin at Lourdes. These phenomena are sometimes collectively witnessed. Most of these experiences seem to have some religious or ethereal motif and are mentioned because they are poorly

understood and often judged a psychotic symptom or a miracle. Religious old people sometimes report visions of angels or other heavenly emissaries. Most often, these individuals see a person who has died and may feel comforted.

Meditation. Many types and rituals of meditation have flourished in Western societies in the past two decades. Some methods of meditation have been used for thousands of years in Eastern cultures. Whatever the method, the goal is to quiet the mind and center oneself. When the mind slows, the body relaxes and less oxygen and nutrients are needed. Other benefits of meditation are presented in Box 27-18. These benefits are all significant to older people; the fact that we see the polar opposites of these benefits so frequently attests to the stress level of many older citizens, which might be reduced through meditation.

Effective meditation requires approximately 20 minutes of focusing on a sound, a thought, or an image. Practicing two or more times daily will bring calmness, better health, and higher energy levels in its wake. Although meditation can be accomplished in any setting, a place with few distractions is helpful. People who meditate with consistency often begin to be aware of a transcendent state of being. Although meditation has unique meanings for each person, some common dynamics that tend toward transcendence exist:
- It is noncompetitive.
- It integrates body-mind function.
- It does not depend on others.
- It taps into beliefs about oneself.
- There is always room for improvement.
- You are in control.
- You cannot fail.

Nurses may introduce the values of meditation to the elderly and serve as guides in the beginnings of such activities. Chanting psalms, reciting poetry by rote, praying, saying the rosary, practicing yoga, and playing a musical instrument are all mechanisms of release and renewal that may bring one into higher states of awareness.

Dreams—Personal and Collective. Jung's view of the work of dreams is most appropriate in a gerontology text. Jung believed that dreams promote growth and individuation and that they are sources of informative and creative power. Jung saw the goal of the last half of life as reconciliation of one's various repressions to become a whole person by using dreams, myths, and symbols. To discover the hidden and embrace the unconscious is the process of individuation and transcendence, which may occupy one intensely after mid-life. To explore the hidden, one may analyze dreams. Dreams are the window of the unconscious.

Jung believed each person was able to best analyze and interpret his or her own dreams by meditating on them and examining them in great detail. To understand the meaning, several steps are employed. Establish the context of the present life situation, and then examine each image or symbol carefully for all the possible meanings. Jung suggests a series of dreams may be a most satisfactory basis for interpretation, because important images occur repeatedly in dreams.

Following is an example of a dream an old woman had after the death of her roommate:

> I have dreamed of her every night since she died. She sometimes sings to me, and she is waiting for me on an island and says she won't go on without me. She's holding a big bowl of soup.

We talked about the dream, about death, and about the fear of dying alone. She spoke of how her roommate knew she enjoyed soup and was never able to get a bowl of hot soup in the nursing home. She also mentioned that her roommate had been deaf. The dream seemed to give her assurance that she would not be alone in death (a compensatory aspect of the dream because so many do die alone) and that physical limitations were conquered through death (the singing of her deaf roommate). In a symbolic sense, the soup might mean nourishment, love, a blending, an offering, or it might be from the present context of her life in which she seldom got the soup she so enjoyed. The old woman died 2 weeks after her roommate. Jung might call this a prospective dream because it prepared her for a future place and time.

Ron had a vivid dream a few months before he died in which he was planting corn in sequential plots on neatly terraced hillsides to be sure they would always be ripening and ready for his family. He was a very providential man, and the dream was prophetic of his death in one sense and a summary of his life in another.

Dreams provide access to the unconscious of the individual or the collective unconscious. The individual may express desires, conflicts, fears, prophecies, hidden aspects of personality, compensation, or modifications of recent or distant experiences. To fully use dream material for self-transcendence, the concept of collective unconscious must be explored. Jung (1961) viewed the collective unconscious as composed of archetypal images or symbols, which include powerful, collectively carried, instinctual reactions:

- *Anima*: Feminine principle
- *Animus*: Masculine principle
- *Wise old man*: King, hero, medicine man, savior
- *Great mother*: Infinite love, understanding, help, protection, tyranny over the dependent

Dreams that connect one with the collective unconscious may be very vivid, seem highly significant, and include surprising or incomprehensible symbols that seem to have no relationship to the dreamer's life. Jung believed that these dreams are especially significant in transcending the personal and deepening one's experience by connection with remote people through symbols significant to many. We believe nurses should express interest in the dreams of their elderly clients and explore meanings with them. Sharing a dream is a revealing and intimate activity.

Dombeck (1995) reports a dream-sharing group in which *dream telling* is a mechanism for increasing spiritual awareness. The session has been found to be a healing experience for victims of abuse, disadvantaged youths, and prisoners. No efforts to interpret dreams were made but only to explore feelings, commonalties with others, and speculations about personal meanings.

We did not find reports of such activity with elders but believe it might be very illuminating. We would be particularly interested in recurring dreams and the meaning for the elder. Dream research seems a fruitful area of study with elders and has been studied by Moody (2003). Most studies indicate a decreasing importance and intensity of daydreams and fantasies in old age. However, we must remember cohort effects and realize that people born 75 years ago were culturally conditioned in a way that put little importance on dreams and fantasies. We might assist the elderly to value their self-exploratory activities by giving credence to them.

Memories might well be included with dreams and fantasies because they become so intertwined in the later years. The conscious and unconscious seem to merge in a more holistic manner when the very old move backward and forward in time with ease, weaving recurrent dreams, hopes, and fantasies into their memories. We often mistakenly label this fluidity as confusion or inaccuracy if we hold strict boundaries and a segmented personal reality. We might take lessons from the old who have learned to make peace with their multiple realities.

Hope as a Transcendent Mechanism

Hope is the belief in the future and the expectation of fulfillment. Hope is the anchor that sustains life in the most difficult times and in the face of doubts and ennui. Some level of hope must be maintained to survive and to die in peace. Hope embodies desires and expectations and the limitless possibilities of humans in all times and places—present, past, and future. For many elders, hope is a major means of coping and those who lose hope lose the capacity and desire for survival.

In a study of variables influencing hope among a group of institutionalized elders, differences were not significant in the level of hope based on age, gender, marital status, education, length of stay, self-report of physical and mental health, functional ability, and social support. Spirituality emerged as the only significant predictor of hope in the study. To be able to maintain hope in the face of losses, both physical and emotional, requires deep inner strength and faith in something greater than self. Tapping into and supporting these strengths are important nursing interventions (Touhy, 2001a).

Hope is a powerful force against despair and helps patients and families journey through difficult times. At the end of life, hope is not just associated with cure but extends beyond a physical nature to that of a social, psychological, and spiritual nature. "Because we have declared limits on treatment or cure does not mean that we have pronounced the limits of human potential. Patients are invited to open themselves to new targets of hope, to draw on strengths not yet experienced" (Jevne, 1993, p. 126).

O'Connor (1996) enumerates the critical aspects of hope: (1) the presence of an inner human energy, (2) positive expectations for the future, (3) motivation for action, and (4) formulations of meaningful, realistic goals. O'Connor further states that a person without hope has no goals or expectations for the future. All practicing nurses have observed how a small goal or hope for the future can sustain an elder. The grandson's graduation from college, the daughter's return from her travels, even a birthday may keep an elder alive until the event is safely fulfilled.

▲ *Promoting Healthy Aging: Implications for Gerontological Nursing.* Central to the instillation of hope is the caring relationship between nurses and patients. Nursing responses that instill hope foster harmony, healing, and wholeness (Watson, 1988). Caring relationships characterized by unconditional positive regard, encouragement, and competence help patients feel loved and cared about, thus inspiring hope. A patient's hope for cure may change to a hope for freedom from pain, day-to-day experiences to enjoy precious moments of life, time to accomplish life goals before life is over, sharing love with family and friends, relief of suffering, death with dignity, and eternal life (Matzo, 2001, Touhy and Zerwekh, 2006). Grooming conveys a quiet belief that it matters; pain relief and comfort measures reinforce the recognition of an individual's needs and confirm the value of the individual. Nurses may foster hope by the following:

1. Presenting honestly the limits of human knowledge
2. Controlling symptoms and providing comfort
3. Encourage patient and family to become involved in positive experiences that transcend the current situation
4. Determining significant aspects of the individual's life
5. Fostering spiritual processes and finding meaning
6. Exploring beliefs and values of elder
7. Promoting connection and reconciliation
8. Providing opportunities for prayer, meditation, scripture reading, clergy visits, religious rituals, if meaningful for the elder

Other hope-promoting experiences are presented in Box 27-19.

Transcendence in Illness

Serious illnesses influence how one perceives the meaning of life. A distinct shift in goals, relationships, and values often occurs among people who have survived life-threatening episodes. A heightened awareness may occur of beauty and

---

BOX 27-19 Hope-Promoting Activities

- Feel the warmth of the sun.
- Share experiences children are having.
- See the crystal blue of the sky.
- Enjoy a garden or fresh flowers.
- Savor the richness of black coffee at breakfast.
- Feel the tartness of grapefruit to wake up the taste buds.
- Watch the activities of an animal in a tree outside the window.
- Benefit from each encounter with another person.
- Write messages to grandchildren, nieces, or nephews.
- Study a favorite painting.
- Listen to a symphony.
- Build highlights into each day such as meals, visits, Bible reading.
- Keep a journal.
- Write letters.
- Make a tape recording of your life story.
- Have hope objects or symbols nearby.
- Share hope stories.
- Focus on abilities, strengths, past accomplishments.
- Encourage decision making about daily activities; foster a sense of control.
- Extend caring and love to others.
- Appreciate expressions of caring concern.
- Renew loving relationships.

Adapted from Jevne R: Enhancing hope in the chronically ill, *Humane Med* 9(2):121-130, 1993; Miller, J: *Coping with chronic illness: overcoming powerlessness*, Philadelphia, 1983, FA Davis; Touhy T, Zerwekh J: Spiritual Caring. In Zerwekh J: *Nursing care at the end of life: palliative care for patients and families*, Philadelphia, 2006, FA Davis.

---

of caring relationships, but a long period of emotional "splinting" may be necessary while recovering from the psychic wound of body betrayal. Newman (1994) contends that disease can be a manifestation of health as one confronts the crisis and as it reveals special meanings.

▲ *Promoting Healthy Aging: Implications for Gerontological Nursing.* Steeves and Kahn (1987) found from their work in hospice care that certain conditions facilitate the search for meaning in illness, noting the following:

- Suffering must be bearable and not all-consuming if one is to find meaning in the experience.
- A person must have access to and be capable of perceiving objects in the environment. Even a small window on the world may be sufficient to match the limited energy one has to attend.
- One must have time that is free of interruption and a place of solitude to experience meaning.
- Clean, comfortable surroundings and freedom from constant responsibility and decision making free the soul to search for meaning.
- An open, accepting atmosphere in which to discuss meanings with others is important.

Accompanying someone in his or her grief and quest for meaning in painful events is a privilege nurses are often given. This spiritual intimacy means being willing to suffer with another, and both the nurse and the client will reap the benefits. One of the great rewards of working with older clients is observing and participating as they turn suffering into a spiritual event.

Sister Rosemary Donley (1991) defines the nursing role in the spiritual search of suffering individuals as compassionate accompaniment, meaning entering into another's reality and quietly, attentively sharing the experience. "Nurses need to be with people who suffer, to give meaning to the reality of suffering, and, in so far as possible, to remove suffering and its causes. Here lies the spiritual dimensions of health care" (Donley, 1991, p. 180). The challenge is to find meaning and some purpose in the affliction that, unchallenged, entwines and chokes identity. Holstein and Cole (1996, p. 18) say, "Thus, part of the 'work' of chronic illness is to tell a new story about the self that integrates the illness into the ongoing story."

LEGACIES

A legacy is one's tangible and intangible assets that are transferred to another and may be treasured as a symbol of immortality. The purpose of legacies is to supersede death. Courage, wisdom, and insights that we perceive in our elders become part of their legacy (Wyatt-Brown, 1996). Not only the giver but also the receiver are essential to the concept of legacy; reciprocity is also essential (Kivnick, 1996). The desire for meaning and immortality seems to be the basic motivation for leaving a legacy. Extending one's authentic self to others can be an important activity in the last years. Throughout life, shared experiences provide satisfaction, but in the last years this exchange allows one to gain a clearer perspective on how his or her movement on earth has had impact.

Older people must be encouraged to identify that which they would like to leave and who they wish the recipients to be. This process has interpersonal significance and prepares one to leave the world with a sense of meaning. A legacy can provide a transcendent feeling of continuation and tangible or intangible ties with survivors. Although we have not studied bonding with elders, it seems the shared authenticity is the glue that binds us together. Legacies are the evidence of this process.

Legacies are manifold and may range from memories that will live on in the minds of others to bequeathed fortunes. Box 27-20 is a partial list of legacies. The list is as diverse as individual contributions to humanity. Erikson's seventh stage of man identifies the generative function as the main concern of the adult years and the last stage (eighth) as that of reviewing with integrity or despair that which one has accomplished. Legacies are generative and are identified and shared best as one approaches the end of life. This activity reinforces integrity.

Autobiographies and Life Histories

Oral histories are an approach to immortality. As long as one's story is told, one remains alive in the minds of others.

BOX 27-20   Examples of Legacies

- Oral histories
- Autobiographies
- Shared memories
- Taught skills
- Works of art and music
- Publications
- Human organ donations
- Endowments
- Objects of significance
- Written histories
- Tangible or intangible assets
- Personal characteristics such as courage or integrity
- Bestowed talents
- Traditions and myths perpetuated
- Philanthropical causes
- Progeny children and grandchildren
- Methods of coping
- Unique thought: Darwin, Einstein, Freud, and others

Doers leave their products and live through them. Powerful figures are remembered in fame and infamy. The quiet, unobtrusive person survives in the memory of intimates and in family anecdotes. Everyone has a life story. The quest for immortality grew out of words—the human ability to articulate meaning and personality to others. Without words, experience would contain no past or future. The short span of one's days would amount to only a series of sensory impressions, not even rising to the perceptual level, because perceptions are formed through internalized concepts and words spoken to the self.

Autobiographies and recorded memoirs can serve a transcendent purpose for people who are alone—and for many who are not. Nurses can encourage older people to write, talk, or express in other ways the meaning of their lives. The human experience and the poignant anecdotes bind people together and validate the uniqueness of each brief journey in this level of awareness and the assurance that one will not be forgotten. Dying patients can express and order their memories through audiotapes, CDs, videotapes, or DVDs, which are then bequeathed to families if the elderly person desires. Sharing one's personal story creates bonds of empathy, illustrates a point, conveys some of the deep wisdom that we all have, and connects us with our deepest human consciousness.

These stories are influenced by gender, culture, history, social class and context, race, and ethnicity (Harrienger, 1996; Schuster, 1996). All facets come together to form a unique, never-to-be-reproduced individual legend. In addition, stories from a grandparent will bring to life historic periods that have previously seemed sterile (Kivnick, 1996). Reaching across generations in this way decreases self-absorption and releases "grand-generativity" that incorporates care for the present and concern for the future (Kivnick, 1993, p. 13).

Creating a Life History. Birren (Kleyman, 2000) says "Guided autobiography is a nontherapy. It's life centered, not problem-centered like psychotherapy." In an interview by Paul Kleyman, he quoted Malcolm Cowley from *The View from Eighty:* "Our lives that seemed a random and monotonous series of incidents are something more than that. Each of them has a plot" (p. 11).

Becoming whole requires one to integrate all of life's remembered experience into the self-concept in a way that sustains or enhances self-esteem. Numerous gerontological nurses have used reminiscence, individually and in groups, as a therapeutic strategy to achieve these goals. Because it is such a natural function of many elders, reminiscence is one of the simplest and most enriching interventions for elder and nurse. Haight (1992) (a nurse) has been the foremost researcher in the measurable aspects of reminiscing and continues to work in that field to illuminate the process. Haight is also the organizer and driving force of the *International Reminiscence and Life Review Organization.*

Possibilities grow out of life history. One's life history is a product of multiple histories that shift and change with the passage of time and development of maturity. Examining the peaks and valleys in one's life facilitates understanding. When both inner and outer structures are changed, reorganization becomes possible. The period of disequilibrium is necessary for growth. Periods of stability, crisis, and joy are necessary. Some theorists believe that the spacing of these elements is critical to the possibility for continued growth.

Grudzen and Soltys (2000, p. 8) state:

> It is only when people who have loved and cared for us reach the end of life that we see the full gift we have received from them. By leaving us their reminiscences, their spirits can continue in our lives as a living memorial.

See Chapters 23 and 25 for additional discussions of storytelling, reminiscence, and life review.

Creation of Self Through Journaling. Through the personal journal, one can, in thoughtful reflection, discover meaning and patterns in daily events. The self becomes a coherent story with successive revisions as old events are reread and perceived in new contexts. Dellasega (2001) used reflective writing to assist troubled individuals in self-discovery, strengthening identity and self-esteem.

The journals of elders provide rich descriptions of the interior lives of the authors. May Sarton (1984) and Florida Scott-Maxwell (1968) are two of the best-known authors. The study of these journals and of the journals of less-known and less articulate elders assists nurses in understanding the inner experience of older people and, perhaps, their own.

Collective Legacies

Each person is a link in the chain of generations (Erikson, 1963) and as such may identify with generational accomplishments. An old man may think of himself as a significant part of a generation that survived the Great Depression. A middle-aged man may identify with the generation that walked on the moon. The years of youthful idealism are impressed in one's memory by the political or ideological climate of the time. This time is the stage when one searches for a fit in the larger society.

The importance of collective legacies to nurses lies in how they use this knowledge. For instance, the nurse may ask, "Who were the great men of your time?" "Which ones were important to you?" "What events of your generation changed the world?" "What were the most important events you experienced?" Mentioning certain historic events and asking about individual reactions are sometimes helpful.

Childless individuals are becoming more prevalent with each passing generation, and they must find a way to outlive the self through a legacy. Many people choose a *social* legacy (Rubinstein, 1996). Florence Nightingale would be one such person, with the grand legacy she left to nurses.

Legacies Expressed Through Other People

One's legacy can be expressed in many ways through the development of others in a teaching or learning situation or through mentorship, patronage, shared talents, organ donations, and genetic transmission. Some creative works and research are legacies left to successive generations for continued modification and growth (Philip, 1995). In other words, one's legacy may be a product of his or her own brought to fruition through someone else who may also become an intermediary to later developments. Thus people and generations are tied in sequential progress. Some examples may illustrate this type of legacy:

> An older man cried as he talked of his grandson's talent as a violinist. Both the man and his grandson shared their love for violin, and the grandfather believed that he had genetically and personally contributed to his grandson's development as an accomplished musician.
>
> A professor emeritus spoke of visiting his son in a distant state and hearing him expound ideas that had been partially developed by the professor and his father before him.
>
> Great-aunt Laura worried about preserving the environment for future generations, so she took young children on nature walks to stimulate their interest in birds, plants, and animals. She also donated land for a natural park. Years later, her grandnephew became a park ranger and passed on the knowledge he had learned from her.
>
> People who amass a fortune and allocate certain funds for endowment of artists, scientific projects, and intellectual exploration are counting on others to complete their legacy.

The following are suggestions for assisting elders to identify and develop their legacy:

1. Find out lifelong interests.
2. Establish a method of recording.
3. Identify recipients—either generally or specifically.
4. Record the legacy.
5. Distribute the legacy as planned.
6. Provide for systematic feedback of results to the older person.

A legacy that can be converted into some tangible form can be gratifying to the older person, ensuring that it will not be

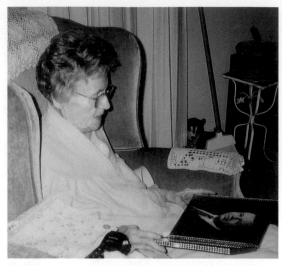

Widow reflecting on her deceased husband's legacy. (From Black JM, Hawks JH: *Medical-surgical nursing: clinical management for positive outcomes,* ed 7, St Louis, 2005, Saunders.)

readily dismissed or forgotten. The following vehicles can convey legacies:

- Summation of life work
- Photograph albums, scrapbooks
- Written memoir
- Taped memoirs (video or audio)
- Artistic representations
- Memory gardens
- Mementos
- Genealogies
- Recorded pilgrimages

Living Legacies

Many older people wish to donate their bodies to science or donate body parts for transplant. This mechanism is a means to transcend death. Parts of the body keep another person alive, or, in the case of certain diseases, the deceased body may provide important information leading to preventive or restorative techniques in the future. Donation of body parts in old age may not be encouraged because they are often less viable than those from younger people. Nonetheless, older bodies are welcome for use as cadavers. People who are interested in providing such a legacy should be encouraged to call the nearest university biomedical center and obtain more information. The nurse then has a postmortem obligation to the client to assist in carrying out his or her wishes.

Property and Assets

Wealth may be viewed as a means toward power more often than transcendence; therefore older people are often reluctant to disperse material goods before their death. Some elders use the future legacy as a means to exert power and control over offspring. One man said, "So long as I have that bankroll, they've got to treat me with re-

spect" (Lustbader, 1996). The power to exert influence, to punish, and to reward is often bound up in an anticipated estate distribution.

Estates can be planned in certain ways that are decidedly advantageous for the planner, as well as the recipient, in terms of control, avoidance of lengthy probate proceedings, and taxation. Because the laws are complex and ever-changing, using the services of an estate planner would be advisable. The nurse's responsibility regarding wills may be limited to advising older people to obtain legal counsel while they are healthy and competent and plan how they would like to distribute their worldly goods.

Knowledge

We carry thought legacies, without conscious awareness, of individuals, such as Lao-Tzu[1], Hippocrates[2], St. Augustine[3], James Madison[4], Nightingale[5], Darwin, Helen Hunt Jackson[6], Einstein, Freud, and others who underlie many of our thoughts and actions. Erik Homberg Erikson, one of the respected thinkers of our time, is just one of many formulators of human thought constructs who left numerous published works for future generations and has markedly influenced the understanding of life span development in our era. Erikson's legacy and that of many others continue with modifications and reinterpretations. As has been said in many ways before, we build on the thought and works of those who have preceded us. In a sense, all creative thinkers and teachers leave their legacy in their students and devotees.

Personal Possessions

Possessions carry more meaning as time passes; individuals change, but the possession remains much the same. A possession is a way of symbolically hanging on to individuals who are gone or times that are past. For some people, keeping personal possessions is a means of hanging on to the self that is changing with time. Cherished possessions passed on through several generations may have achieved meaning through the close family member to whom they belonged (Tobin, 1996). One's personally significant items become highly charged with memories and meaning, and transferring them to friends and kin can be a tender experience. Personal possessions should never be dispersed without the individual's knowledge. Because of the uncertainty of late life lucidity, these issues should be discussed early with older individuals.

---

[1] Lao-Tzu, Chinese founder of Taoism; circa 575 BC.
[2] Hippocrates, Greek "father of medicine"; circa 425 BC.
[3] St. Augustine, Christian theologian; circa 400 AD.
[4] James Madison, "father of the U.S. Constitution"; circa 1775 AD.
[5] Florence Nightingale, "mother of organized nursing"; circa 1860 AD.
[6] Helen Hunt Jackson, author defender of Native Americans, their rights, and intermarriage; circa 1884 AD.

People who are approaching death must be given the opportunity to distribute their important belongings appropriately to those who they believe will also cherish them. Nurses may encourage elders to plan the distribution of their significant items carefully. Deciding when and how best these possessions should be given is often difficult. Some people choose to distribute possessions before dying. In these cases, nurses often need to help family members accept these gifts, appreciating the meaning and recognizing the significance.

Certain questions allow the older person to consider a legacy if he or she is ready to do so; for example:

- What is the meaning to you of your life experience right now?
- Have you ever thought of writing an autobiography?
- If you were able to leave something to the younger generation, what would it be?
- Have you ever thought of the impact your generation has had on the world?
- What has been most meaningful in your life?
- What possessions have special meaning for you? Who else is interested in them?
- Do you see some of your genetic traits emerging in your grandchildren?

These suggestions should stimulate ideas for spontaneous statements, which are revealing in an interpersonal context.

Human Needs and Wellness Diagnoses

Self-Actualization and Transcendence
(Seeking, Expanding, Spirituality, Fulfillment)
Shares wisdom
Teaches others to live and die uniquely
Continues to develop curiosity
Seeks spiritual growth, transcends ego
Identifies a legacy and a plan of dispersal
Develops latent abilities that may be dormant

Self-Esteem and Self-Efficacy
(Image, Identity, Control, Capability)
Achieves inner peace and self-acceptance
Separates identity from work role
Cultivates the masculine and feminine principles
Develops flexible social roles
Accepts one's share of responsibility for the past

Belonging and Attachment
(Love, Empathy, Affiliation)
Accepts death of intimates
Serves as a historian for younger persons
Maintains significant relationships
Develops new relationships with old and young

Safety and Security
(Caution, Planning, Protections, Sensory Acuity)
Tolerates loss and depressive episodes
Accepts help when needed
Budgets income and energy to meet important needs
Finds the least restrictive suitable living situation

Biological and Physiological Integrity
(Air, Fluids, Comfort, Activity, Nutrition, Elimination, Skin Integrity)
Monitors body functions
Adapts to physical needs and limitations
Seeks health maintenance services as needed
May find transcendence from pain

These are not all the possible wellness diagnoses that may be identified. The above are examples of nursing diagnoses that should be considered when planning care for the older adult.

▲ PROMOTING HEALTHY AGING: IMPLICATIONS FOR GERONTOLOGICAL NURSING

"The responsibility of the nurse is not to make people well, or to prevent their getting sick, but to assist people to recognize the power that is within them to move to higher levels of consciousness" (Newman, 1994, p. xv). In this chapter, we have examined methods of expanding one's limited existence by developing the authentic self, transcendent self, spiritual self, and several mechanisms used to establish immortality through a legacy. These areas often become major issues in the latter part of life, and the nurse will find it a revealing, absorbing, and challenging task to be a part of this effort. An important point is that some people may avoid any such interest or concern, particularly when angry, in pain, or denying their own mortality. Nurses need not push the individual to accomplish this task but should be available to assist the person and family members.

The basic mysteries of life elude scientific researchers, yet they are the essence of existence with meaning. Remembering, feeling, dreaming, worshipping, and grasping one's connection to the universe are the realities of the human spirit. Being old is not the centrality of the self—spirit is. Spirit synthesizes the total personality and provides integration, energizing force, and immortality.

Nurses who care for older people have a great privilege in being able to accompany older persons on the final journey of their life. It calls for a nurse who is willing to enter into meaningful spirit-sharing relationships. Taking advantage of these opportunities will enrich our nursing, our inner selves, and the spiritual well-being of the elders whom we nurse. Such relationships have the potential to enhance inner harmony and healing. There may be no greater goal in caring for elders than helping a person see a life well lived and meaningful to themselves and others, thus providing hope that life's journey was not in vain. As we close this book, our hopes are that we have provided you with the knowledge to care for elders with competence and compassion and that you will find as much joy and fulfillment as we have in our nursing of older adults.

KEY CONCEPTS

- Self-actualization is a process of developing one's most authentic self. Maslow thought of self-actualization as the pinnacle of human development.
- Self-actualized individuals embody qualities of courage, humor, high moral development, and seeking to learn more about themselves and others.
- Opportunities for pursuing interests will assist individuals in developing latent talents, expressing their creativity, and rising beyond daily concerns.
- Groups working toward societal humanitarian advancement may accomplish collective actualization.
- Creativity emanates from people who are self-actualized and may be expressed in mundane activities, as well as the arts, music, theater, and literature.

- Transcending the material and physical limitations of existence through ritual and spiritual means is an especially important aspect of aging.
- Gerotranscendence is a theory proposed by Tornstam that implies a natural shift in concerns that occurs in the aging process. Elders are thought to spend more time in reflection, to spend less on materialistic concerns, and to find more satisfaction in life. This effort is an attempt to define aging not by the standards of young and middle adulthood but as having distinctive characteristics of its own.
- Illnesses that occur have the potential for altering one's fundamental beliefs and hopes. Nurses must give elders the opportunity to discuss the meanings of an illness. Some people find that these experiences bring new insights; others are angry. Empathic nurses will provide a sounding board while the elder makes sense of an illness within a satisfactory framework.
- Spiritual healing has ancient religious roots, but scientists are now recognizing and accepting the power of the mind in restoring health and, if not restoring health, enhancing one's ability to cope.
- Nurses need not neglect discussing spirituality with elders. Elders will respond only if it has significance for them.
- Spiritual nursing interventions emanate from the caring relationship between the older person and the nurse. The most important tool at the nurses' disposal is the use of self.
- Life satisfaction, happiness, morale, and health are related in some ways to beliefs, hope, and motivation that may be derived from a spiritual awareness.

RESEARCH QUESTIONS

Kane (1996) suggests the following aspects of legacies that need to be studied:

How do elders balance their own present needs against estate planning?

Who makes out wills and when?

How do bequests relate to gifts given during one's lifetime?

Is the perpetuation of one's name an important aspect of a legacy?

What are the motivating differences between gifts during life and those after one's death?

How do recipients view the adequacy of their legacy?

RESOURCES

American for the Arts
1000 Vermont Ave., N.W.
Washington, DC 20005
(202) 371-2830
www.artsusa.org

Bastings A, Killick J
The arts and dementia care: a resource guide.
Available from The National Center for Creative Aging
138 Oxford St.
Brooklyn, NY 11217
(718) 398-3870
www.creativeaging.org

CASE STUDY: Self-Actualization, Spirituality, and Transcendence

Melba had no children but numerous nieces and nephews, though she did not feel particularly close to any of them. She had been a nursing instructor at a community college and had enjoyed her students but had not developed a sustained relationship with any of them after they had completed her courses. At her level of nursing education, the opportunity for mentorship was lacking, though she had occasionally taken students under her wing and arranged special experiences that they particularly desired. Because she had taught several courses each year, Melba never really developed a strong affiliation to a specialty but considered herself a pediatric nurse. She had not made any major contributions to the field in terms of research or publications; a few reviews, continuing education workshops, and some nursing newsletters had really been the extent of her work outside of that which was required. Melba's husband died in 1988, and she had felt very much alone since that time, especially after her retirement 3 years ago. Before her husband's death, Melba had been too busy to think about the ultimate meaning of all her years of teaching and wifely activities. With time on her hands, she began to wonder what it all meant. Had she done anything meaningful? Had she really made a difference in anything or in anyone's life? Was anyone going to remember her in any special way? So many questions were making her morose. She had never been a religious person, though her husband had been a devout Catholic. He had believed that God had a purpose for him in life, and though he was not always able to understand what it might be, he seemed to have a sense of satisfaction. She began to wonder if she should go to church ... would that make her feel less depressed?

One Sunday morning, Melba had decided to attend her neighborhood Catholic church, but on her way out she slipped on the icy walkway and sustained bilateral Colles' fractures. After a brief emergency room visit for assessment, immobilization of the wrists, and medications, Melba was sent back home with an order for home health and social service assessment on the following day. Of course, she had extreme difficulty managing the most basic self-care while keeping her wrists immobilized and was very dejected. When the home health nurse arrived the next morning, to Melba's amazement, it was a former student who had graduated 4 years previously. Melba was more chagrined than pleased and greeted her with, "Oh, I hate to have you see me so helpless. I've been feeling so useless and, now with these wrists, I am totally useless." If you were the home health nurse, how would you begin working with Melba, knowing that your visits would be limited to just a few?

Based on the case study, develop a nursing care plan using the following procedure[*]:
- List Melba's comments that provide subjective data.
- List information that provides objective data.
- From these data, identify and state, using accepted format, two nursing diagnoses you determine are most significant to Melba at this time. List two of Melba's strengths that you have identified from the data.
- Determine and state the outcome criteria for each diagnosis. These must reflect some alleviation of the problem identified in the nursing diagnosis and must be stated in concrete and measurable terms.
- Plan and state one or more interventions for each diagnosed problem. Provide specific documentation of the sources used to determine the appropriate intervention. Plan at least one intervention that incorporates Melba's existing strengths.
- Evaluate the success of the intervention. Interventions must correlate directly with the stated outcome criteria to measure the outcome success.

Critical Thinking Questions

1. Discuss the meanings and the thoughts triggered by the student's and elder's viewpoints as expressed at the beginning of the chapter. How do they vary from your own experience?
2. How do nursing students learn about spirituality and spiritual nursing interventions?
3. What activities might be helpful in developing your own sense of spirituality?
4. How does culture affect one's concept of spirituality?
5. How can nurses enhance spiritual care, self-actualization, and transcendence of elders?

* Students are advised to refer to their nursing diagnosis text and identify possible or potential problems.

Center of Aging, Health & Humanities
George Washington University
10225 Montgomery Ave.
Kensington, MD 20895
(202) 895-1230
www.gwumc.edu/cahh

Center for Elders and Youth in the Arts
Institute on Aging
3330 Geary Blvd.
San Francisco, CA 94118
(415) 750-4111
www.ioaging.org/programs/art/ceya.html

Civic Ventures
139 Townsend St., Suite 505
San Francisco, CA 94107
(415) 430-0141
www.civicventures.org

Elders Share the Arts
138 Oxford St.
Brooklyn, NY 11217
(718) 398-3870
http://elderssharethearts.org

Generations United
1333 H St., N.W., Suite 500
Washington, DC 20005
(202) 289-3979
http://gu.org

International Society for Reminiscence and Life Review
Center for Continuing Education/Extension
University of Wisconsin-Superior
PO Box 2000
(800) 370-9882
www.reminiscenceandlifereview.org

National Center for Creative Aging
138 Oxford St.
Brooklyn, NY 11217
(718) 398-3870
www.creativeaging.org

National Time Slips Project
Center of Age & Community
PO Box 413
Milwaukee, WI 58211
(414) 229-2740
www.timeslips.org

North Carolina Center for Creative Retirement
Reuter Center, CPO #5000
The University of North Carolina at Asheville
One University Heights
Asheville, NC 28804
(828) 251-6140
www.unca.edu/nccr

Senior Corps
1201 New York Ave., N.W.
Washington, DC 20525
(800) 424-8867
www.seniorcorps.org

SeniorNET
1171 Homestead Rd., Suite 280
Santa Clara, CA 95050
(408) 615-0699
http://seniornet.org

Society for the Arts in Healthcare
1632 U St., N.W.
Washington, DC 20009
(202) 299-9770
http://theSAH.org

REFERENCES*

Bastings A: Arts in dementia care: "This is not the end…it's the end of the chapter," *Generations* 30(1):16-23, 2006.

Bell V, Troxel D: Spirituality and the person with dementia: a view from the field. *Alzheimer's Care Q* 2(2):31-45, 2001.

Berggren-Thomas P, Griggs MJ: Spirituality in aging: spiritual need or spiritual journey, *J Gerontol Nurs* 21(3):5, 1995.

Blues A, Zerwekh J: *Hospice and palliative care nursing*, Orlando, Fla, 1984, Grune & Stratton.

Bond C, Miller M: Reading: the ageless activity, *Geriatr Nurs* 8(4):910, 1987.

Cohen G: Research on creativity and aging: the positive impact of the arts on health and illness, *Generations* 30(1):7-15, 2006.

Cousins N: *Anatomy of an illness*, New York, 1979, WW Norton.

Crowther MR et al: Rowe and Kahn's model of successful aging revisited: positive spirituality—the forgotten factor, *Gerontologist* 42(5):613, 2002.

Cumming E, Henry WE: *Growing old: the process of disengagement*, New York, 1961, Basic Books.

Deaconess Parish Nurse Ministries: *Frequently asked questions*, July 1, 2002. (website): *www.parishnurses.org/faq.phtml*.

Dellasega CA: Using structured writing experiences to promote mental health, *J Psychosoc Nurs Ment Health Serv* 39(2):15, 2001.

Doenges M et al: *Nurses pocket guide: diagnoses, interventions, and rationales*, Philadelphia, 2004, FA Davis.

Dombeck M-TB: Dream telling: a means of spiritual awareness, *Holist Nurs Pract* 9(2):37, 1995.

Donley R: Spiritual dimensions of health care: nursing's mission, *Nurs Health Care* 12(4):178, 1991.

Dyson J et al: The meaning of spirituality: a literature review, *J Adv Nurs* 26:1183-1188, 1997.

Edwards D: *Presentation at American Nurses' Association Gerontological Nurses Conference*, St Paul, Minn, April 1977.

Elderhostel: *Elderhostel international catalog: 2003*, Boston, 2003, Elderhostel.

Ellerman CR, Reed PG: Self-transcendence and depression in middle-age adults, *West J Nurs Res* 23(7):698, 2001.

Emblem J, Halstead L: Spiritual needs and interventions: comparing the views of patients, nurses and chaplains, *Clin Nurs Spec* 7(4):176-182, 1993.

Erikson EH: *Childhood and society*, New York, 1950, WW Norton.

Erikson EH: *Childhood and society*, ed 2, New York, 1963, WW Norton.

Forbes DA: Enhancing mastery and sense of coherence: important determinants of health in older adults, *Geriatr Nurs* 22(1):29, 2001.

Forbes EJ: Spirituality, aging, and the community-dwelling caregiver and care recipient, *Geriatr Nurs* 16(6):297, 1994.

Freke T, Gandy P: *Jesus and the lost goddess: the secret teachings of the original Christians*, New York, 2001, Three Rivers Press.

Gaskamp C et al: Evidence-based guideline: promoting spirituality in the older adult, *J Gerontol Nurs* 32(11):8-11, 2006.

Goldberg B: Connection: an exploration of spirituality in nursing care, *J Adv Nurs* 27:836-842, 1998.

Grudzen M, Soltys FG: Reminiscence at end of life: celebrating a living legacy, *Dimensions* 7(3):4,5,8, 2000.

Haight B: Long term effects of a structured life review process, *J Gerontol* 47(5):P312, 1992.

Harrienger M: *Writing a life: the composing of grace*. Paper presented at the meeting of the Gerontological Society of America, Washington, DC, November 19, 1996.

Hebrews 11:1, *Holy Bible*, Chicago, 1964, John A Dickson.

Hemstrom MM: Wellness. In Fitzpatrick JJ et al, editors: *Geriatric nursing research digest*, New York, 2000, Springer.

Henderson R: The spirituality "renaissance": professional interest grows, *Aging Today* 17(2):11, 1996.

Heriot C: Spirituality and aging, *Holistic Nurs Pract* 7:22-31, 1992.

Hermann C: A guide to the spiritual needs of elderly cancer patients, *Geriatr Nurs* 21(6):324, 2000.

Holstein MB, Cole TR: Reflections on age, meaning, and chronic illness, *J Identity Health* 1(1):7, 1996.

---

* Many of the thoughts in this chapter cannot be attributed to a single or multiple sources because they are the conglomerate of numerous studies over the years. When possible, citations to specific theorist and researcher are given.

Hooyman N, Kiyak A: *Social gerontology: a multidisciplinary perspective*, Boston, 2005, Pearson.

Hudson F: *The adult years: mastering the art of self-renewal*, San Francisco, 1999, Jossey-Bass.

Hungelmann J et al: Spiritual well-being in older adults: harmonious interconnectedness, *J Relig Health* 24:147-153, 1985.

Hungelmann J et al: Focus on spiritual well-being: harmonious interconnectedness of mind-body-spirit—use of the Jarel Spiritual Well-Being Scale, *Geriatr Nurs* 17(6):262, 1996.

Jevne R: Enhancing hope in the chronically ill, *Humane Med* 9(2):121-130, 1993.

Jung C: *Memories, dreams, reflections*, translated by Jaffe A, editor, New York, 1961, Random House.

Kane RA: Toward understanding legacy: a wish list, *Generations* 20(3):92, 1996.

Killick J: *You are words*, London, 1997, Hawker Publications.

Killick J: *Openings*, London, 2000, Hawker Publications.

Killick J: *Dementia, You and yours transcript*, 2005. (website): *www.bbc.co.uk/radio4/youandyours/transcript_2005_46_fri_02.shtml*.

Kimble M: A personal journey of aging: the spiritual dimension, *Generations* 17(2):27, 1993.

Kivnick HQ: Everyday mental health: a guide to assessing life strengths, *Generations* 17(1):13, 1993.

Kivnick HQ: Remembering and being remembered: the reciprocity of psychosocial legacy, *Generations* 20(3):49, 1996.

Kleyman P: Life stories: a "nontherapy" for elders and their families, *Aging Today* 21(4):9,11, 2000.

Koch K: *I never told anybody*, New York, 1977, Random House.

Koenig HG, Brooks RG: Religion, health and aging: implications for practice and public policy, *Public Policy Aging Rep* 12(4):13, 2002.

Kohlberg L, Power C: Moral development, religious thinking and the question of a seventh stage. In Kohlberg L, editor: *The philosophy of moral development*, vol I, San Francisco, 1981, Harper & Row.

Kuhn M: Advocacy in this new age, *Aging* 3:297, Jul/Aug 1979.

Larson R: Building intergenerational bonds through the arts, *Generations* 30(1):38-42, 2006.

Leetun M: Wellness spirituality in the older adult, *Nurs Pract* 21:60-70, 1996.

Leitner MJ, Leitner SF: *Leisure in later life*, ed 2, New York, 1996, Haworth Press.

Levin JS: Age differences in mystical experience, *Gerontologist* 33(4):507, 1993.

Lowry LW, Conco D: Exploring the meaning of spirituality with aging adults in Appalachia, *J Holist Nurs* 20:388-402, 2002.

Lustbader W: Conflict, emotion and power surrounding legacy, *Generations* 20(3):54, 1996.

Macrae J: Nightingale's spiritual philosophy and its significance for modern nursing, *Image J Nurs Sch* 27(1):8-10, 1995.

Martsolf D, Mickely J: The concept of spirituality in nursing theories: differing world views and extent of focus, *J Adv Nurs* 27:294-303, 1998.

Maslow A: Creativity in self-actualizing people. In Anderson H, editor: *Creativity and its cultivator*, New York, 1959, Harper & Row.

Maslow A: *Religions, values and peak-experiences*, New York, 1970, Viking Press.

Matsumoto C: Class presentation in the Gerontological Certificate Program, Division of Continuing Education, San Francisco, 1978, San Francisco State University.

Matzo M: End-of-life care: nurses should help patients live fully, inspire hope, *Am Nurse*, September-October:1-4, 2001.

McLeod BW: The aging spirit: Sue Bender's stretching lessons extends spiritual reach, *Aging Today* 22(4):17, 2001.

Merriam-Webster: *Merriam-Webster dictionary*, New York, 1974, Simon & Schuster.

Metcalf CW: *Lighten up*, Niles, Ill, 1993, Nightingale Conant (audiotapes).

Meyer CL: How effectively are nurse educators preparing students to provide spiritual care? *Dissertation Abst Int* 55(6):2158B, UMI No 9428614, 2003.

Moberg DO: Religion in gerontology: from benign neglect to belated respect, *Gerontologist* 36(2):264, 1996.

Moody HR: *Oceans for the second half of life: human values in aging*, Newsletter April 1, 2003, UPDATE, 2002. Available at *hrmoody@yahoo.com*.

Morse JM, Doberneck B: Delineating the concept of hope, *Image J Nurs Sch* 27(4):277, 1995.

Nagai-Jacobsen M, Burkhardt M: Spirituality: cornerstone of holistic nursing practice, *Holist Nurs Pract* 3:18-26, 1989.

NANDA International: *Nursing diagnoses: definitions and classification 2003-2004*, Philadelphia, 2004, Author.

Newman MA: *Health as expanding consciousness*, ed 2, New York, 1994, National League for Nursing Press.

O'Brien ME: Sacred covenants: exploring spirituality in nursing, *AWHONN Lifelines* 3(2):69-72, 1999.

O'Brien ME: *Spirituality in nursing: standing on holy ground*, Boston, 2003, Jones & Bartlett.

O'Connor P: Hope: a concept for home care nursing, *Home Care Provider* 1(4):175, 1996.

Peck R: Psychological developments in the second half of life. In Anderson J, editor: *Psychological aspects of aging*, Washington, DC, 1955, American Psychological Association.

Perlstein S: Creative expression and quality of life: a vital relationship for elders, *Generations* 30(1):5-6, 2006.

Philip CE: Lifelines, *J Aging Stud* 9(4):265, 1995.

Post S et al: Physicians and spirituality: professional boundaries, competency, and ethics, *Ann Intern Med* 132(7):578-583, 2000.

Potter ML, Zauszniewski J: Spirituality, resourcefulness, and arthritis impact on health perception of elders with rheumatoid arthritis, *J Holist Nurs* 18:311-331, 2000.

Puchalski C, Romer A: Taking a spiritual history allows clinicians to understand patients more fully, *J Palliat Med* 3(4):129-137, 2000.

Raes F, Marcoen A: Gerotranscendence in the second half of life, *Tijdschr Gerontol Geriatr* 32(4):150, 2001.

Reed PG: Spirituality and mental health of older adults: extant knowledge for nursing, *Fam Community Health* 14:14-25, 1991a.

Reed PG: Toward a nursing theory of self-transcendence: deductive reformulation using developmental theories, *ANS Adv Nurs Sci* 13(4):64, 1991b.

Reed PG: An emerging paradigm for the investigation of spirituality in nursing, *Res Nurs Health* 15:349-357, 1992.

Roberts TB: Do entheogen-induced mystical experiences boost the immune system? Psychedelics, peak experiences, and wellness, *Adv Mind Body Med* 15(2):139, 1999.

Rowe JW, Kahn RL: *Successful aging*, New York, 1998, Pantheon–Random House.

Rubenstein RL: Childlessness, legacy, and generativity, *Generations* 20(3):58-61, 1996.

Sarton M: *At seventy: a journal*, New York, 1984, WW Norton.

Schuster E: *Transformative functions of life writing.* Paper presented at the meeting of the Gerontological Society of America, Washington, DC, November 19, 1996.

Scott-Maxwell F: *The measure of my days*, New York, 1968, Alfred A Knopf.

Sherman J: The arts and older Americans, monographs: National Assembly of Local Arts Agencies, *Americans for the Arts* 5(8):1, 1996.

Soeken K, Carson V: Responding to the spiritual needs of the chronically ill, *Nurs Clin North Am* 22:604-611, 1987.

Steeves R, Kahn D: Experience of meaning in suffering, *Image J Nurs Sch* 19(3):114, 1987.

Stiles M: The shining stranger, *Cancer Nurs* 13(4):235-245, 1990.

Strang S, Strang P: Questions posed to hospital chaplains by palliative care patients, *J Palliat Med* 5(6):857-864, 2002.

Tobin S: Cherished possessions: the meaning of things, *Generations* 20(3):46, 1996.

Tornstam L: Gerotranscendence: a theoretical and empirical exploration. In Thomas LE, Eisenhandler SA, editors: *Aging and the religious dimension*, Westport, Conn, 1994, Greenwood Publishing Group.

Tornstam L: Gerotranscendence: a theory about maturing into old age, *J Aging Identity* 1(1):37, 1996.

Tornstam L: *Gerontranscendence: a developmental theory of positive aging*, New York, 2005, Springer.

Touhy T: Nurturing hope and spirituality in the nursing home, *Holist Nurs Pract* 15(4):45-56, 2001a.

Touhy T: Touching the spirit of elders in nursing homes: ordinary yet extraordinary care, *Int J Human Caring* 6(1):12-17, 2001b.

Touhy T, Brown C, Smith C: Spiritual caring: end of life in a nursing home, *J Gerontol Nurs* 31(9):27-35, 2005.

Touhy T, Zerwekh J: Spiritual caring. In Zerwekh J: *Nursing care at the end of life: palliative care for patients and families*, Philadelphia, 2006, FA Davis.

Wadensten B, Carlsson M: A qualitative study of nursing staff members' interpretations of signs of gerotranscendence, *J Adv Nurs* 36(5):635, 2001.

Watson J: *Nursing: human science and human care*, New York, 1988, National League for Nursing.

Weis D, Schank MJ: Use of a taxonomy to describe parish nursing practice with older adults, *Geriatr Nurs* 21(3):125, 2000.

Wikstrom B: Older adults and the arts, *J Gerontol Nurs* 30(9):30-34, 2004.

Wyatt-Brown AM: The literary legacies: continuity and change, *Generations* 20(3):65, 1996.

Zerwekh J: Transcending life: the practice wisdom of nursing hospice experts, *Am J Hosp Palliat Care* 20(3):40-45, 1993.

Index

b indicates boxed material, *f* indicates illustrations, and *t* indicates tables.